D1573156

THE BIG KETO COOKBOOK FOR BEGINNERS 1500 RECIPES

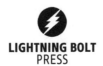

LIGHTNING BOLT
PRESS

For general information on our other products and services or to obtain technical support, please contact our Customer Care Department within the U.S. at (866) 744-2665, or outside the U.S. at (510) 253-0500.

Rockridge Press publishes its books in a variety of electronic and print formats. Some content that appears in print may not be available in electronic books, and vice versa.

TRADEMARKS: Rockridge Press and the Rockridge Press logo are trademarks or registered trademarks of Callisto Media Inc. and/or its affiliates, in the United States and other countries, and may not be used without written permission. All other trademarks are the property of their respective owners. Rockridge Press is not associated with any product or vendor mentioned in this book.

Cover and Interior Designer: Angie Chiu
Photo Art Director/Art Manager: Maya Melenchuk
Editor: Jacinta O'Halloran
Production Manager: Martin Worthington

Cover photography:
© Emulsion Studio, © Antonis Achilleos, © Biz Jones, © Annie Martin, © Darren Muir
Back cover photography:
© Annie Martin with food styling by Oscar Molinar, © Helene Dujardin, © Laura Flippen

ISBN: Print 978-1-63878-793-8
       eBook 978-1-68539-115-7
R0

CONTENTS

KETO 101   xvi

Smoothies 1

Kale Refresher Smoothie...................1
Spirulina Smoothie...........................1
Avocado-Matcha Smoothie...........1
Berry Green Smoothie......................1
Green Herb Smoothie.......................1
Creamy Kale Smoothie.....................1
Cucumber Green Smoothie.............1
Mean Green Smoothie......................2
Almond Kale Smoothie....................2
Cauliflower Smoothie.......................2
Green Goddess Smoothie...............2
Green Coconut Avocado Smoothie...2
Green Tea Smoothie.........................2
Lemon-Cashew Smoothie..............2
Avocado-Lime Smoothie...............2
Lemon Smoothie................................3
Spiced Orange-Pistachio
Smoothie..3
Spinach-Blueberry Smoothie........3
Blueberry Smoothie with Lemon
and Ginger..3
Strawberry Spinach Smoothie......3
Tropical Smoothie.............................3
Triple Berry Smoothie.....................3
Coconut Berry Smoothie................4
Avocado Blueberry Smoothie........4
Creamy Snickerdoodle Shake........4
Creamy Cinnamon Smoothie.........4
Nutty Chocolate Protein Shake....4
Peanut Butter Smoothie..................4
Peanut Butter Shake........................4
Peanut Butter Cup Protein
Smoothie..4
Chocolate, Peanut Butter, and
Banana Shake...................................4
Chocolate-Mint Smoothie.............5
Almond Butter and Cacao Nib
Smoothie..5

Double Chocolate Shake.................5
Chocolate Protein Shake................5
Vanilla Bean Smoothie....................5
Vanilla Shake.....................................5
Strawberries and Cream Shake....5
Cheesecake Smoothie......................5
Berry Cheesecake Smoothie..........6
Avocado Coconut Smoothie..........6
Pumpkin Pie Smoothie....................6
Buttered Coffee Shake....................6
Coffee Smoothie...............................6

Breakfast 6

Cherry-Coconut Pancakes.............6
Spiced Cream Cheese Pancakes....7
Winter Squash Pancakes................7
Almond Butter Pancakes................7
Almond and Vanilla Pancakes.......7
Cream Cheese Pancakes..................7
Lemon–Olive Oil Breakfast Cakes..7
Pumpkin Pancakes with Maple
Frosting...8
Chocolate, Chocolate Chip
Pancakes...8
Ricotta Pancakes..............................8
Banana Bread Blender Pancakes..8
Keto Blueberry Pancakes...............9
Chaffles...9
Spaghetti Squash Chaffles.............9
Belgian-Style Waffles....................9
Chaffle and Lox..............................10
Vanilla Belgian Waffles.................10
Coconut Flour-Based
Chocolate Chip Waffles...............10
Waffles with Whipped Cream....10
Coconut Flaxseed Waffles...........10
Ham and Swiss Waffles................11
Very Berry Waffles........................11
Meat Waffles...................................11

Quick and Easy Blueberry
Waffles...11
French Toast....................................12
Cinnamon French Toast Sticks....12
Sweet 'n' Savory Toast with
Burrata and Berries.......................12
Toast-less Blueberry French
Toast..12
Buttery Boiled Eggs......................13
Classic Bacon and Eggs...............13
Bacon-Wrapped Asparagus
and Eggs...13
Scotch Eggs.....................................13
Breakfast "Sandwich"....................13
Avocado and Eggs with
Shredded Chicken.........................13
Florentine Breakfast Sandwich....14
Avocado Toast................................14
Egg Baked in Avocado.................14
Eggs with Goat Cheese &
Asparagus..14
Creamed Spinach with Eggs.......14
Skillet-Baked Eggs with Yogurt
and Spinach....................................15
Italian Vegetable Egg Bake.........15
Mexican Egg Casserole................15
Egg & Cheese Biscuit Casserole....15
Denver Omelet Breakfast Bake....16
Loaded Denver Omelet.................16
Italian Omelet.................................16
Bacon-Artichoke Omelet.............16
Spanakopita Omelet......................16
Mushroom Cream Cheese
Omelet...17
Baked Omelet with Pancetta
and Swiss Cheese...........................17
Asparagus Gouda Frittata...........17
Asparagus, Mushroom & Fennel
Frittata..17

Mushroom and Bacon Frittata 17
Spinach, Mushroom, and
Cheddar Frittata 18
Mediterranean Frittata 18
Asparagus Frittata 18
Lemon-Herb Baked Frittata 18
Sausage and Cheese Frittata 19
Prosciutto Egg Cups 19
Baked Eggs in Ham Cups 19
Ham and Cheese Poached
Egg Cups 19
Bacon, Egg, and Cheese Cups 19
Bacon-Wrapped Egg Cups 19
Broccoli Bacon Egg Muffin Cups 20
Broccoli and Cheese
Quiche Cups 20
Bacon Eggs Benedict Cups 20
Egg Breakfast Muffins 20
Cheesy Sausage & Egg Muffins 20
French Toast Egg Muffins 21
Chorizo Egg Muffins 21
Simple Scrambled Eggs 21
Cheesy Scrambled Eggs 21
Ham and Cheese Egg Scramble 21
Chile Relleno Scrambled Eggs 21
Scrambled Eggs with Mackerel 22
Salmon and Egg Scramble 22
Tofu and Veggie Scramble 22
Brussels Sprouts & Ground
Beef Scrambled Eggs 22
Turkey Egg Scramble 22
Greek-Style Egg and Tomato
Scramble 22
Country Garden Scramble 23
Corned Beef Breakfast Hash 23
Roasted Vegetable Hash 23
Cabbage Sausage Hash Browns 23
Eggs Benedict with Bacon 23
Easy Eggs Benedict 24
Eggs Benedict with
Five-Minute Hollandaise 24
Eggs Benedict on Grilled
Portabella Mushroom Caps 24
Crustless Quiche Lorraine 24
Ham and Cheese Crustless
Quiche 25
Broccoli Quiche 25
Crustless Sausage and Green
Chile Quiche 25
Tuscan "Quiche" Bites 25

Crustless Cream Cheese and
Spinach Quiche 26
Breakfast Sausage 26
Bacon Broccoli Crustless
Quiche Cups 26
Sausage Verde Casserole 26
Breakfast Bowl with Cauliflower
Hash 26
Savory Sausage Balls 27
Sausage Egg Roll in a Bowl 27
Bagels with Smoked Salmon 27
Breakfast Pizza 27
Portabella Breakfast "Burger" 27
Biscuits and Sausage Gravy 28
Cheesy Sausage and Cabbage
Hash 28
Cheesy "Hash Brown"
Casserole 28
Chicken Brunch Pie with
Cheddar Pecan Crust 28
Breakfast Burrito Bowl 29
Classic Diner Hash Browns 29
Shakshuka 29
Crustless Greek Cheese Pie 29
Greek Yogurt Parfait 30
Simple Cheesy Yogurt 30
Chia Parfait 30
Yogurt Parfait with Chia Seeds 30
Coconut Yogurt Berry Parfait 30
Lemon Berry Yogurt Parfait 30
Peanut Butter Whipped
Greek Yogurt 30
Go Get 'Em Green
Smoothie Bowl 30
Pumpkin Pie Yogurt Bowl 31
Cinnamon-Nut Cottage Cheese 31
Overnight Chocolate Chia
Pudding 31
PB&J Overnight Hemp 31
Creamy Cinnamon Breakfast
Pudding 31
Nut Medley Granola 31
Keto Granola 32
Superfood Granola 32
Macadamia Nut Granola 32
Coconut Granola 32
Granola Cereal 32
Cacao Crunch Cereal 32
Toasty Granola Bars 33

Pumpkin-Pecan N'Oatmeal 33
Chocolate Coconut "Oatmeal" 33
Cinnamon Roll "Noatmeal" 33
Cauliflower N'Oatmeal 33
Nutty "Oatmeal" 33
Chia Almond "Oatmeal" 34
Almond Coconut Hot Cereal 34
Baklava Hot Porridge 34
Overnight Chia
Blueberry Pudding 34
Overnight Chia Pudding 34

Baked Goods 34

Biscuits with Sausage Gravy 34
Apricot Hot Cross Buns 35
Buttermilk Biscuits 35
Cheddar-Chive Biscuits 35
Easy Cheese Biscuits 36
Sesame Burger Buns 36
Cheesy Garlic Rolls 36
Everything Bagels 36
Chorizo Bagels 37
Classic Zucchini Bread 37
Slow Cooker Zucchini-Carrot
Bread 37
Onion Cheddar Bread 37
Basic Sandwich Bread 38
Onion-Garlic Pita Bread 38
Pizza Pull-Apart Bread 38
Garlic Cloud Bread 38
Jalapeño Cheese Bread 39
Rosemary Flatbread 39
Savory Naan 39
Herb and Olive Focaccia 40
Blackberry, Prosciutto, and
Goat Cheese Flatbread 40
Flax Meal Tortillas 40
Southern Sweet Corn Bread 41
Sour Cream Corn Bread 41
Tex-Mex Green Chile
Corn Bread 41
Bacon Cheddar Chive Scones 41
Raspberry Scones 41
Mixed Berry Scones with
Lemon Icing 42
Chocolate Chip Scones 42
Strawberry Rhubarb Scones 42
"Cornbread" Muffins 42
Cinnamon Muffins with Cream
Cheese Frosting 43
Applesauce Yogurt Muffins 43

Dairy-Free Churro Muffins............43
Cranberry Muffins............43
Glazed Dairy-Free Carrot
Cake Muffins............44
Glazed Cranberry-Orange
Muffins............44
Pancake Muffins............44
Banana Nut Muffins............44
Greens and Parmesan Muffins............45
Lemon Poppy Seed Muffins............45
Orange Olive Oil Poppy
Seed Muffins............45
Zucchini Muffins............45
Zucchini Chocolate Muffins............46
Cream Cheese Pumpkin
Muffins............46
Chocolate Cake Donuts............46
Jelly Donuts............46
Dairy-Free Chocolate Donuts............47
Baked Donut Bites with Jelly............47
Matcha Donuts............47
Cinnamon "Apple" Pecan
Coffee Cake............47
Cinnamon Coffee Cake............48
Lemonade Snack Cake............48
Old-Fashioned Lemon-Lime
Teacakes............48
Iced Cranberry-Gingerbread
Loaf............49
Pumpkin Spice Loaf with
Maple Icing............49
Cinnamon Swirl Bread............49
Chocolate Chip Banana Bread............50
Buttery Coconut Bread............50
Nut-Free Pumpkin Bread............50
Nut-Free Sunflower Bread............50
Cinnamon Rolls............51

Soups 51

Creamy Asparagus Soup............51
Creamed Cauliflower Soup............51
Cauliflower-Cheddar Soup............51
Spiced Pumpkin Soup............52
Broccoli Cheddar Soup............52
Creamy Broccoli, Bacon, and
Cheese Soup............52
Roasted Red Pepper Soup with Basil
and Goat Cheese............52
Cream of Mushroom Soup............53
Creamed Mushroom and

Fennel Soup............53
Tomato Basil Soup............53
Watercress-Spinach Soup............53
Loaded Miso Soup with Tofu
and Egg............53
Vegetarian French Onion Soup............54
French Onion Soup............54
Turnip and Thyme Soup............54
Creamy Tomato Soup............54
Easy Herbed Tomato Bisque............54
Hearty Cauliflower Soup............54
Egg Drop Soup............55
Spicy Serrano Gazpacho............55
Chilled Avocado-Cilantro Soup............55
Cream of Cauliflower Gazpacho............55
Loaded Baked "Fauxtato" Soup............56
Butternut Squash Soup with
Turmeric & Ginger............56
Cold Cucumber and
Avocado Soup............56
Avocado Gazpacho............56
Spring Pea Soup............56
Creamy Leek Soup............57
Miso Magic............57
Avocado-Lime Soup............57
Tuscan Kale Soup............57
Vegan Italian Wedding Soup............57
Easy Chicken Soup............58
Vegan Pho............58
Chicken Noodle Soup............58
Matzo Ball Chicken Soup............58
Chicken Tortilla Soup............59
Fiesta Lime Chicken Chowder............59
Tom Kha Gai............59
Chicken Marsala Soup............59
Peanut-Chicken Soup............59
Jalapeño-Chicken Soup............60
Greek Chicken and "Rice"
Soup with Artichokes............60
Spicy Creamy Chicken Soup............60
Chicken Ramen Soup............60
Southwest-Style Chicken Soup............60
Chicken and Baby Corn
Chowder............61
Chicken Taco Soup with
Cauliflower Rice............61
Italian Wedding Soup............61
Beef Pho............62

Zuppa Toscana (Sausage and
Kale Soup)............62
Country Pork and "Rice" Soup............62
Beef-Sausage Stew............62
Hearty Lamb Cabbage Soup............62
Creamy Seafood Stew with
Cauliflower Rice............63
Seafood Chowder with Lobster............63
Fennel and Cod Chowder with
Fried Mushrooms............63
New England Clam Chowder............64

Salads 64

Citrus Arugula Salad............64
Spinach Avocado Salad............64
Kale, Avocado & Tahini Salad............64
Vegan Niçoise Salad............64
Japanese Hibachi House Salad............64
Ranch Wedge Salad with
Coconut "Bacon"............64
Spinach Salad with Warm Bacon
Dressing............65
Strawberry Spinach Salad............65
Pistachio Pomegranate Salad............65
Bacon and Berry Harvest Salad............65
Classic Club Salad............66
Hemp Cobb Salad............66
Mediterranean Salad............66
Italian Garden Salad............66
Avocado and Asparagus Salad............66
Killer Kale Salad............66
Shaved Brussels Sprouts Salad
with Avocado Dressing............67
Tuscan Kale Salad with
Anchovies............67
Everyday Caesar Salad............67
Walnut-Fennel Salad with
Sherry Vinaigrette............67
Traditional Greek Salad............67
Weeknight Greek Salad............67
Powerhouse Arugula Salad............68
Tuna and Jicama Salad with
Mint Cucumber Dressing............68
Red Radish "Potato" Salad............68
Tuna Niçoise Salad............68
Creamy Dill and Radish
"Potato" Salad............68
Simple Egg Salad............69
Curried Egg Salad............69
Avocado Egg Salad............69

Turmeric and Avocado Egg Salad 69
Chicken, Avocado, and Egg Salad 69
Deviled Egg Salad with Bacon 69
Cool and Creamy Cucumber Tomato Salad 70
Greek Cottage Cheese Salad 70
Thai Noodle Salad 70
Smoked Salmon and Cucumber Noodles 70
Classic Chicken Salad 70
Buffalo Chicken Salad 70
Chicken Salad on Romaine Boats 71
Chicken Melon Salad 71
Lobster BLT Salad 71
Pecan Chicken Salad 71
Classic Tuna Salad 71
Lemony Chicken Salad with Blueberries and Fennel 72
Mayo-Less Tuna Salad 72
Italian Tuna Salad 72
Curried Tuna Salad with Pepitas 72
Caprese Stuffed Avocados 72
Crab Salad–Stuffed Avocado 72
Tuna-Stuffed Avocado 72
Turkey-Stuffed Avocados 73
Chicken Salad–Stuffed Avocados 73
Italian Green Bean Salad 73
Guacamole Salad 73
Avocado Caprese Lettuce Wraps 73
Broccoli Salad with Bacon 73
Creamy Broccoli Salad 74
Israeli Salad with Nuts and Seeds 74
Moroccan Cauliflower Salad 74
Cucumber and Tomato Feta Salad 74
Cucumber, Tomato, and Avocado Salad 74
Goat Cheese Caprese Salad 75
Sausage and Cauliflower Salad 75
Creamy Riced Cauliflower Salad 75
Apple Cabbage Cumin Coleslaw 75
Sesame Ginger Slaw 75
Crisp and Creamy Southern Coleslaw 75
Ranch Broccoli Slaw 76
Turkey and Kale Coleslaw 76
Roasted Chicken, Artichoke, and Hearts of Palm Salad 76

Chef Salad 76
Chopped Salad 76
Zesty Chicken Tender Salad 76
Grilled Chicken Cobb Salad 76
Chicken Caesar Salad 77
Essential Cobb Salad with Crumbled Bacon 77
Classic Steak Salad 77
Grilled Steak Salad with Cucumber and Mint 77
Sirloin Steak Salad with Goat Cheese and Pecans 77
Ground Beef Taco Salad with Peppers and Ranch 78
BLT Salad 78
Deluxe Sub Salad 78
Quick Fiesta Taco Salad 78
Spinach Salad with Bacon and Soft-Boiled Eggs 78
Asian Shrimp Salad 79
Shrimp & Avocado Salad 79
Crab Salad Lettuce Cups 79
Greek Salad with Shrimp 79
Smoked Trout Salad 79
Omega-3 Salad 80
Shrimp Ceviche Salad 80
Mint-Marinated Artichoke Hearts 80
Bacon-Wrapped Asparagus Bundles 80
Prosciutto-Wrapped Asparagus and Lemon Aioli 80
Sautéed Asparagus with Walnuts 81
Roasted Asparagus with Goat Cheese 81
Citrus Asparagus with Pistachios 81
Creamed Broccoli 81
Creamy Broccoli Casserole 81
Roasted Broccoli 81
Sesame-Roasted Broccoli 82
Broccoli Stir-Fry 82
Garlicky Broccoli Rabe with Artichokes 82
Brussels Sprouts Casserole 82
Crispy Brussels Sprouts 82
Roasted Brussels Sprouts & Poached Eggs 82
Brussels Sprouts with Bacon 83
Brussels Sprouts with Hazelnuts 83
Roasted Cabbage "Steaks" 83

Sweet-Braised Red Cabbage 83
Grilled Balsamic Cabbage 83
Asian Cabbage Stir-Fry 83
Thai-Inspired Peanut Roasted Cauliflower 84
Cauliflower Rice 84
Mexican Cauliflower Rice 84
Nutty Miso Cauliflower Rice 84
Green Goddess Buddha Bowl 84
Raw Tabouli 85
Mediterranean Cauliflower Tabbouleh 85
Mashed Cauliflower 85
Mashed Cauliflower with Yogurt 85
Cheesy Mashed Cauliflower 85
Cauliflower-Pecan Casserole 85
Cheesy Cauliflower Mac 'n' Cheese 86
Cauliflower Mac and Cheese 86
Cauliflower Pizza 86
Roasted Cauliflower Lettuce Cups 86
Celery Root Purée 86
Sautéed Swiss Chard 87
Braised Greens with Olives and Walnuts 87
Quick Pickled Cucumbers 87
Spiced Cucumbers 87
Eggplant Lasagna 87
Roasted Eggplant with Mint and Harissa 87
Stuffed Eggplant 88
Caramelized Fennel 88
Garlicky Green Beans 88
Southern Green Beans 88
Tofu Green Bean Casserole 88
Green Bean Casserole 88
Smoky Stewed Kale 89
Kale with Bacon 89
Garlicky Kale 89
Kale and Cashew Stir-Fry 89
Slow Cooker Mushrooms 89
Roasted Mushrooms 89
Pumpkin Seed and Swiss Chard-Stuffed Portabella Mushrooms 90
Mushrooms with Camembert 90
Stuffed Mushrooms 90
Herbed Ricotta–Stuffed Mushrooms 90

Portabella Mushroom Pizza 90
Portabella Mushroom Burger with Avocado 90
Wild Mushroom Stroganoff 91
Stuffed Portabella Mushrooms 91
Stuffed Cremini Mushrooms 91
Roasted Onions 91
Goat Cheese Stuffed Roasted Peppers 91
Creamy Stuffed Peppers 92
Chiles Rellenos 92
Carrot-Pumpkin Pudding 92
Herbed Pumpkin 92
Radishes with Olive Mayo 92
Creamed Spinach 93
Cheesy Spinach Bake 93
Spinach Soufflé 93
Golden Rosti 93
Twice-Baked Spaghetti Squash 93
Sautéed Summer Squash 93
Creamy Spaghetti Squash Bake 94
Fakeachini Alfredo 94
Ratatouille 94
Zucchini Noodles 94
Avocado Pesto Zoodles 94
Vegetarian Zucchini Noodle Carbonara 95
Greek Stewed Zucchini 95
Mediterranean Spiralized Zucchini 95
Sautéed Crispy Zucchini 95
Pesto Zucchini Noodles 95
Coconut-Zucchini Noodles 95
Zucchini Lasagna 95
Sautéed Zucchini with Mint and Pine Nuts 96
Stuffed Zucchini 96
Zucchini Fritters 96
Zucchini Mini Pizzas 96
Zucchini Pizza Boats 96
Mexican Zucchini Hash 97
Vegetable Hash 97
Cayenne Pepper Vegetable Bake 97
Creamed Vegetables 97
Crustless Spanakopita 97
Konjac Noodles with Spinach Hemp Pesto and Goat Cheese 98
North African Vegetable Stew 98
Mixed-Vegetable Lasagna 98
Mediterranean Spaghetti 98

Moroccan Vegetable Tagine 98
Pesto Sautéed Vegetables 99
Green Vegetable Stir-Fry with Tofu 99
Vegetable Vindaloo 99
Summer Vegetable Mélange 99

Fish & Seafood 99

Chili Fish Stew 99
Nut-Crusted Baked Fish 100
Easy Oven-Fried Catfish 100
Halibut Curry 100
Pecan-Crusted Catfish 100
Fish Tacos 101
Crispy Fried Cod 101
Mustard-Crusted Cod with Roasted Broccoli 101
Cod with Parsley Pistou 101
Roasted Cod with Garlic Butter and Bok Choy 101
Poached Cod over Brothy Veggie Noodles 101
Cod Cakes 102
Baked Halibut with Herb Sauce 102
Pesto Flounder with Bok Choy 102
Coconut Milk Baked Haddock 102
Cheesy Golden Fried Haddock 103
Crispy "Breaded" Haddock 103
Balsamic Teriyaki Halibut 103
Baked Nutty Halibut 103
Halibut in Tomato Basil Sauce 103
Blackened Redfish with Spicy Crawfish Cream Sauce 104
Macadamia-Crusted Halibut with Mango Coulis 104
Mackerel Escabeche 104
Turmeric Coconut Mahi-Mahi 104
Baked Mackerel with Kale and Asparagus 104
Garlic Parmesan Crusted Salmon 105
Salmon in Cream Sauce 105
Whole Roasted Sea Bass 105
Ginger Scallion Steamed Fish 105
Sesame Salmon 105
Teriyaki Salmon with Spicy Mayo and Asparagus 106
Salmon Poke 106
Charred Alaskan Salmon with Garlic Green Beans 106
Sushi 106

Smoked Salmon Avocado Sushi Roll 107
Moroccan Salmon with Cauliflower Rice Pilaf 107
Pepper-Crusted Salmon with Wilted Kale 107
Sheet Pan Salmon With Lemon Green Beans 107
Salmon with Spinach Hemp Pesto 108
Salmon in Lime Caper Brown Butter Sauce 108
Roasted Salmon with Black Olive Salsa 108
Lemon Salmon and Asparagus 108
Pan-Seared Dijon-Ginger Salmon 108
Glazed Salmon 108
Grilled Salmon Foil Packets 109
Salmon Gratin 109
Salmon with Tarragon-Dijon Sauce 109
Pecan-Crusted Salmon 109
Pan-Seared Lemon-Garlic Salmon 109
Salmon Oscar 110
Roasted Herb-Crusted Salmon with Asparagus and Tomatoes 110
Salmon Cakes 110
Curried Salmon Fish Cakes 110
Coconut Ginger Salmon Burgers 110
Salmon Cakes with Avocado 111
Snapper Veracruz 111
Rosemary-Lemon Snapper Baked in Parchment 111
Sole with Cucumber Radish Salsa 111
Sole Meunière 112
Swordfish in Tarragon-Citrus Butter 112
Parmesan-Crusted Tilapia with Sautéed Spinach 112
Brown Butter–Lime Tilapia 112
Pan-Fried Tilapia 112
Garlic Herb Marinated Tilapia 113
Parmesan Baked Tilapia 113
Cream-Poached Trout 113
Rainbow Trout with Cream Leek Sauce 113
Roasted Trout with Swiss Chard 113

Grandma Bev's Ahi Poke 114
Tuna Slow-Cooked in Olive Oil ...114
Sesame-Crusted Tuna with
Sweet Chili Vinaigrette 114
Seared Tuna with Steamed
Turnips, Broccoli, and
Green Beans 114
Tuna Casserole 114
Crab Cakes with Spicy
Tartar Sauce 115
"Spaghetti" with Clams 115
Crab Cakes with Cilantro
Crema 115
Classic Crab Cakes 115
Spicy Crab Cakes 116
Crab Cakes with Garlic Aioli ...116
Crab Cakes with Green
Goddess Dressing 116
Crab au Gratin 116
Crab-Stuffed Portabella
Mushrooms 117
Spicy Italian Sausage and
Mussels 117
Crab Fried Rice 117
Steamed Mussels with Garlic
and Thyme 117
Coconut Saffron Mussels 118
Pan-Fried Scallops 118
Sea Scallops with Curry Sauce ...118
Sea Scallops with Bacon
Cream Sauce 118
Pan-Seared Butter Scallops 118
Bacon-Wrapped Scallops and
Broccolini 118
Salt-and-Pepper Scallops and
Calamari 119
Seafood Coconut Stew 119
Sheet Pan Seafood Boil 119
Creamy Shrimp and Grits
Casserole 119
Seafood Fideo 120
Seafood Ceviche 120
Shrimp and "Grits" 120
Popcorn Shrimp 121
Shrimp Veracruz 121
Sheet-Pan Shrimp 121
Bacon-Wrapped Shrimp 121
Roasted Shrimp and Veggies 122
Shrimp Coconut Pad Thai 122
Chimichurri Shrimp 122

Oregano Shrimp with
Tomatoes and Feta 122
Cajun Shrimp and Cauliflower
Rice 122
Basil Butter Grilled Shrimp 122
Shrimp with Creamy Tomato-
and-Spinach Sauce 123
Shrimp and Sausage Jambalaya ...123
Shrimp Scampi with Zucchini
Noodles 123
Grilled Shrimp with Avocado
Salad 123
Vietnamese Shrimp Cakes 123
Bang Bang Shrimp 124
Shrimp and Vegetable Kebabs
with Chipotle Sour Cream Sauce ...124
Shrimp Fried Rice 124
Shrimp, Bamboo Shoot, and
Broccoli Stir-Fry 124
Shrimp in Creamy Pesto over
Zoodles 125
Coconut Shrimp 125
Garlicky Shrimp with
Mushrooms 125
Garlic and Herb Baked Shrimp
with Cauliflower Rice 125
Greek Stuffed Squid 125

Poultry 126
Chicken Vegetable Hash 126
Chicken Cutlets with Garlic
Cream Sauce 126
Loaded Chicken and
Cauliflower Nachos 126
Shredded Chicken 126
Roast Chicken with Cilantro
Mayonnaise 127
Buffalo Chicken Wings 127
Chicken Tenders 127
Almond Meal–Crusted
Chicken Fingers 127
Garlic Parmesan Wings 127
Chicken Paprikash 127
Paprika Chicken with Broccoli ...128
Chicken Parmesan 128
Stuffed Chicken Breasts 128
Coconut Chicken 128
Breaded Chicken Strip Lettuce
Wraps 129
Chopped Chicken-Avocado
Lettuce Wraps 129

BBQ Chicken Wraps 129
BBQ Chicken Skewers 129
Bacon-Wrapped Jalapeño
Chicken 129
Chicken Breast Tenders with
Riesling Cream Sauce 129
Curried Chicken Salad 130
Crispy Chicken Paillard 130
Chicken Kebabs with Spicy
Almond Sauce 130
Chicken Pot Pie 130
Chicken and Dumplings 131
Chicken Enchiladas 131
Chicken Fajitas 131
Chicken Cacciatore 131
Creamy Chicken and Spinach
Bake 132
Caprese Balsamic Chicken 132
Caprese-Stuffed Chicken
Breasts 132
Chicken Milanese 132
Bacon Ranch Cheesy Chicken
Breasts 133
Chicken Fajita Stuffed Bell
Peppers 133
Curried Chicken with Bamboo
Shoots 133
Basil Chicken Zucchini "Pasta" ...133
Lemon-Rosemary Spatchcock
Chicken 133
Moroccan Chicken and
Vegetable Tagine 134
Chicken Shawarma 134
Balsamic Chicken with
Asparagus and Tomatoes 134
Bacon Barbecued Chicken 134
Bacon-Wrapped Chicken 135
Cilantro Chili Chicken Skewers ...135
Carne Asada Chicken Bowls 135
Crispy Chicken Thighs with
Radishes and Mushrooms 135
Chicken Tenderloin Packets
with Broccoli, Radishes, and
Parmesan 135
Chicken Thigh Chili with
Avocado 136
Tomato Basil Chicken
Zoodle Bowls 136
Spaghetti Squash Chicken Bowls ...136
Chicken Teriyaki 136

Chicken Cordon Bleu 137
Thai Chicken Lettuce Cups 137
Chicken with Mushrooms, Port, and Cream 137
Chicken Cordon Bleu Casserole 137
Chicken Tikka Masala 137
Tandoori Vegetable Chicken Skewers 138
Kung Pao Chicken 138
Chicken Piccata 138
Baked Chicken Tenders 138
Chicken Nuggets 139
Harissa Chicken and Brussels Sprouts with Yogurt Sauce 139
Spinach and Bacon Stuffed Chicken Thighs 139
Chicken Piccata with Mushrooms 139
Greek Chicken Souvlaki 140
Feta and Olive Stuffed Chicken Thighs 140
Lemon Butter Chicken 140
Lemon Chicken and Asparagus Stir-Fry 140
Sesame Broiled Chicken Thighs 140
Roasted Chicken Thighs and Zucchini with Wine Reduction 141
Chicken Thighs with Lemon Cream Sauce 141
Chorizo, Chicken, and Salsa Verde 141
Herb-Infused Chicken 141
Mustard Shallot Chicken Drumsticks 142
Jamaican Jerk Chicken 142
Herb Roasted Whole Chicken with Jicama 142
Fried Chicken 142
Chicken Adobo 143
Southern Oven-Fried Chicken 143
Roasted Herb Chicken 143
Avocado Chicken Burger 143
Lettuce-Wrapped Chicken Burger 144
Chicken Bacon Burgers 144
White Chili 144
Spicy Kung Pao Chicken 144
Chicken Potstickers 144
Chicken Quesadillas 145
Smothered Sour Cream Chicken Thighs 145

Chicken and Cheese Quesadillas 145
Green-Chile Chicken Enchilada Casserole 145
Potluck Chicken Spaghetti Squash Casserole 146
Calabacitas Con Pollo 146
Cheesy Chicken and Rice Skillet Casserole 146
Jalapeño Popper Chicken Casserole 147
Golden Chicken Asiago 147
Chicken & Waffles 147
Tuscan Chicken 147
Chicken Salad–Stuffed Peppers 147
California Chicken Bake with Guacamole 148
Chicken Tamale Pie 148
Mezze Cake 148
Roast Turkey 149
Marinara Turkey Meatballs 149
Turkey Meatloaf 149
Turkey Meatloaf Muffins 149
Turkey and Cauliflower Rice–Stuffed Bell Peppers 149
Turkey Rissoles 149
Turkey Burgers 150
Avocado Turkey "Toast" 150
Turkey Enchilada Skillet 150
Turkey Thyme Burgers 150
Turkey Egg Roll in a Bowl 150
Turkey Pilaf 151
Turkey Florentine Bake 151
Turkey Bacon Ranch Casserole 151
Turkey Tetrazzini 151
Unstuffed Bell Pepper Skillet 152
Weeknight Texas Turkey Chili 152
Bacon-Wrapped Cajun Turkey Tenderloins with Roasted Brussels Sprouts 152

Meat 152

Breaded Pork Chops 152
Smothered Pork Chops with Onion Gravy 153
Pork Chops Smothered in Caramelized Onions & Leeks 153
Breaded Pork Chops with Creamy Mashed Cauliflower 153
Spiced Pork Chops 153
Cracked Pepper Fried Pork Chops 153

Pan-Fried Pork Chops with Peppers and Onions 154
Pork Chops with Mushroom Sauce 154
Nut-Stuffed Pork Chops 154
Ham-Stuffed Pork Chops 154
Cheese-Stuffed Pork Chops 155
Pork Pumpkin Ragout 155
Pork Fried Rice 155
Lemongrass Pork Noodle Bowls 155
Pork Pho with Shirataki Noodles 155
Rosemary Balsamic Pork Medallions 156
Pork Medallions with Blue Cheese Sauce 156
Glazed Pork Tenderloin 156
Balsamic–Thyme Pork Tenderloin 156
Stuffed Pork Loin with Sun-Dried Tomato and Goat Cheese 157
Bacon-Wrapped Pork Tenderloin 157
Jerk Pork Tenderloin 157
Spice-Rubbed Roasted Pork with Cilantro Pesto 157
Roasted Pork Loin with Grainy Mustard Sauce 158
BBQ Baby Back Ribs 158
Pork Ribs 158
Oven-Baked Country-Style Pork Ribs 158
Dry Rub Ribs 158
Barbecue Pork Ribs 159
Smoked Ribs 159
Pork and Sauerkraut 159
Spicy Barbecued Pork Wings 159
Roasted Pork Belly and Asparagus 160
Crispy Bourbon Pork Belly 160
Sriracha Pork Belly 160
Honey Glazed Ham 160
Spicy Sausage and Cabbage Casserole 160
Fried Ham "Rice" 161
Ham-Broccoli-Cauliflower Casserole 161
Cold Front Kielbasa and Cabbage Skillet 161

Keto Lasagna with Deli Meat "Noodles" ... 161

Creole Sausage and Rice ... 162

Sausage, Zucchini, and Green Bean Packets ... 162

Rich Sausage and Spaghetti Squash Casserole ... 162

Pork with Sesame Slaw ... 162

Pork Larb Lettuce Wraps ... 162

Baked Sausage and Shrimp with Turnips and Green Peppers ... 162

Spicy Pork and Eggplant Stir-Fry ... 163

Brussels Sprout Ground Pork Hash ... 163

Spaghetti Squash & Ground Pork Stir-Fry with Kale ... 163

Egg Roll in a Bowl ... 163

Pork Spring Rolls ... 164

Steak with Drunken Broccoli Noodles ... 164

Ginger Pork Meatballs ... 164

Beef Fajitas ... 164

Beef Stroganoff ... 165

Southwest-Style Fajita Bowls ... 165

Chicken-Fried Steak Fingers with Gravy ... 165

Garlic Steak Bites ... 166

Soy-Ginger Veggie Noodle Steak Roll-Ups ... 166

Flank Steak with Kale Chimichurri ... 166

Flank Steak with Orange-Herb Pistou ... 166

Tandoori Beef Fajitas ... 167

Pan-Seared Hanger Steak with Easy Herb Cream Sauce ... 167

Essential New York Strip Steak ... 167

Grilled Hanger Steak with Cilantro Crema ... 167

Grilled Sirloin Steak with Herbed Butter ... 168

Sirloin with Blue Cheese Compound Butter ... 168

Sheet Pan Sirloin Steak with Eggplant and Zucchini ... 168

Grilled Sirloin Steak, Roasted Red Pepper, and Mozzarella Lettuce Boats ... 168

Butter-Basted Rib Eye Steaks ... 169

Cast-Iron Blackened Rib Eye with Parmesan Roasted Radishes ... 169

Rib Eye Steaks with Garlic-Thyme Butter ... 169

Chipotle Coffee-Crusted Bone-In Rib Eye ... 169

Rib Eye Steak with Anchovy Compound Butter ... 169

Classic Prime Rib au Jus ... 170

Garlic Studded Prime Rib with Thyme au Jus ... 170

Bacon-Wrapped Beef Tenderloin ... 170

Rosemary Roasted Beef Tenderloin ... 170

Beef Stew ... 171

Beef Bourguignon Stew ... 171

Beef Taco Stew ... 171

Beef Pot Roast ... 171

Pot Roast with Turnips and Radishes ... 172

Spiced-Up Sunday Pot Roast and Sautéed Squash ... 172

Braised Beef Short Ribs ... 172

Slow-Cooked Shredded Beef ... 173

Garlic Braised Short Ribs ... 173

Brisket Nachos ... 173

Bacon and Egg Cheeseburgers ... 174

Beef Burgers with Bacon ... 174

Loaded Burgers ... 174

Grilled Burgers with Basil Aioli ... 174

Classic Meatloaf ... 175

Italian Beef Burgers ... 175

Mozzarella-Stuffed Burgers ... 175

Double Bacon Cheeseburger ... 175

Mini Burger Sliders ... 175

Oven Burgers ... 176

Cheeseburger Meatloaf ... 176

Zucchini Meatloaf ... 176

Southwest Meatloaf with Lime Guacamole ... 176

Herbed Meatloaf ... 176

Cheeseburger Casserole ... 177

Simple Reuben Casserole ... 177

Beefy Stuffed Cornbread Casserole ... 177

Cheesy Beef and Spinach Casserole ... 177

Southern-Style Shepherd's Pie ... 177

Cottage Pie ... 178

Broccoli and Beef Casserole ... 178

Cottage Pie Muffins ... 178

Moussaka ... 179

Cheesy Triple Meat Baked "Spaghetti" ... 179

Zucchini Lasagna ... 179

Beef Taco Lasagna ... 180

Philly Cheesesteak Stuffed Peppers ... 180

Beef-Stuffed Red Peppers ... 180

Moroccan Stuffed Peppers ... 180

Chili con Carne ... 181

Five-Alarm Beef Chili ... 181

Classic Beef Chili ... 181

Texas-Style Beef Chili ... 181

Zoodles Bolognese ... 182

Quick and Easy Dirty Rice Skillet ... 182

Ground Beef Cauli-Fried Rice ... 182

Salisbury Steak ... 182

Meatza ... 182

Texas Taco Hash ... 183

Ground Beef Taco Salad ... 183

Cilantro Lime Taco Bowls ... 183

Beef Tacos ... 183

Meatballs in Creamy Almond Sauce ... 184

Swedish Meatballs ... 184

Meatballs with Spaghetti Squash ... 184

Italian Meatballs ... 185

Baked Cheesy Meatballs ... 185

Beef Stroganoff Meatballs over Zoodles ... 185

Cheese-Stuffed Italian Meatballs ... 185

Bison Burgers in Lettuce Wraps ... 186

Rack of Lamb with Kalamata Tapenade ... 186

Herb-Crusted Lamb Chops ... 186

Broiled Lamb Chops with Mint Gremolata and Pan-Fried Zucchini ... 187

Grilled Moroccan Spiced Lamb Chops ... 187

Rosemary-Garlic Lamb Racks ... 187

Herb Mustard Lamb Racks ... 187

Leg of Lamb with Sun-dried Tomato Pesto ... 187

Lamb Meatball Salad with Yogurt Dressing ... 188

Lamb Chili 188
Simple Lamb Sausage 188
Savory Lamb Stew 188
Lamb Kofte with Yogurt Sauce ... 189
Greek Meatball Lettuce Wraps ... 189
Grilled Venison Loin with Dijon
Cream Sauce 189
Venison Pot Roast 189

Small Appliance Recipes 190

Pressure Cooker Sloppy Joes 190
Pressure Cooker Pot Roast
with Sour-Cream Gravy 190
Pressure Cooker Pork-and-Beef
Meatloaf 190
Lemon-Thyme Asparagus 190
Parmesan-Rosemary Radishes ... 190
Bacon-Wrapped Jalapeño
Poppers 191
Smoky Zucchini Chips 191
Lemon-Garlic Mushrooms 191
Spicy Roasted Broccoli 191
Buttery Green Beans 191
Sweet and Spicy Pecans 192
Veggie Frittata 192
Bacon and Spinach Egg Muffins ... 192
Pumpkin-Pie Breakfast Bars 192
Smoky Sausage Patties 193
Fried Chicken Breasts 193
Buffalo Chicken Wings 193
Buffalo Chicken Breakfast
Muffins 193
Broccoli-Stuffed Chicken 194
Chicken Parmesan 194
Lemon-Dijon Boneless Chicken ... 194
Spiced Chicken 194
Nashville Hot Chicken 195
Spice-Rubbed Turkey Breast 195
Buffalo Chicken Tenders 195
Barbecue Turkey Meatballs 195
Chicken Kiev 196
Maple-Glazed Salmon with
a Kick 196
Fish Fillets with Lemon-Dill
Sauce 196
Shrimp Caesar Salad 197
Crab Cakes 197
Scallops with Lemon-Butter
Sauce 197

Marinated Swordfish Skewers 197
Coconut Shrimp 198
Crispy Fish Sticks 198
Sweet and Spicy Salmon 198
Garlic Shrimp 198
Bacon Cheeseburger Meatloaf ... 198
Garlic-Marinated Flank Steak 199
Greek Beef Kebabs with
Tzatziki 199
Short Ribs with Chimichurri 199
Grilled Rib Eye Steaks with
Horseradish Cream 199
Goat Cheese–Stuffed
Flank Steak 200
Garlic Steak 200
Sausage-Stuffed Peppers 200
Pork Kebabs 200
Cream Cheese Sausage Balls 200
Parmesan-Breaded Boneless
Pork Chops 201
Sweet-and-Sour Pork Chops 201
Herb-Braised Pork Chops 201
Slow Cooker Pulled Pork 201
Pancetta-and-Brie–Stuffed
Pork Tenderloin 201
Dijon Pork Chops 202
Cranberry Pork Roast 202
Pork-and-Sauerkraut
Casserole 202
Carnitas 202
Asian Pork Spare Ribs 202
Bacon-Wrapped Pork Loin 203
Lemon Pork 203
Smoky Pork Tenderloin 203
Pork Taco Bowls 203
Tomato and Bacon Zoodles 203
Chocolate Chip–Pecan Biscotti ... 204
Pecan Squares 204
Air-Fried Vanilla and
Chocolate Layer Cake 204
Slow Cooker Breakfast
Sausage 204
Slow Cooker Huevos
Rancheros 205
Slow Cooker Mediterranean
Eggs 205
Greek Frittata with Olives,
Artichoke Hearts & Feta 205
Slow Cooker Layered Egg
Casserole 205

Slow Cooker Spanakopita
Frittata 205
Crustless Wild Mushroom–
Kale Quiche 206
Bacon-and-Eggs Breakfast
Casserole 206
Vegetable Omelet 206
Sausage-Stuffed Peppers 206
Dill-Asparagus Bake 206
Slow Cooker Grain-Free
Zucchini Bread 206
Cheddar Cheese Soup 207
Sausage-Sauerkraut Soup 207
Slow Cooker Grain-Free
Pumpkin Loaf 207
Spiced-Pumpkin Chicken Soup ... 207
Cheesy Bacon-Cauliflower
Soup 208
Turkey-Potpie Soup 208
Chicken-Nacho Soup 208
Faux Lasagna Soup 208
Chicken-Bacon Soup 208
Curried Broccoli, Cheddar &
Toasted Almond Soup 208
Chicken Chowder with Bacon ... 209
Mulligatawny Soup with
Cauliflower Rice 209
Homemade Sausage Soup 209
Cheeseburger Soup 209
Jambalaya Soup 209
Creamy Chicken Stew 210
Simple Chicken-Vegetable
Soup 210
Beef Stew 210
Curried Vegetable Stew 210
Turkey-Vegetable Stew 210
Simple Texas Chili 211
Simple Spaghetti Squash 211
Chipotle Chicken Chili 211
Slow Keto Chili 211
Vegetarian Mole Chili 211
Cheese-Stuffed Peppers 212
Deep-Dish Cauliflower Crust
Pizza with Olives 212
Vegan Pumpkin Curry 212
Thai Green Curry with Tofu &
Vegetables 212
Slow Cooker Eggplant
Parmesan 212
Enchilada Casserole 213

Mushroom No-Meatballs in Tomato Sauce 213
Squash Boats Filled with Spinach-Artichoke Gratin 213
White Chicken Chili 213
Coconut Chicken Curry 214
Mandarin Orange Chicken 214
Garlicky Braised Chicken Thighs 214
Chicken Mole 214
Chicken Cacciatore 214
Creamy Lemon Chicken 215
Hungarian Chicken 215
Bacon-Mushroom Chicken 215
Roasted Chicken Dinner 215
Herb-Infused Turkey Breast 215
Turkey-Pumpkin Ragout 216
Thyme Turkey Legs 216
Easy "Roasted" Duck 216
Duck Legs Braised in Olive Oil with Chive Cream 216
Duck with Turnips in Cream 216
Classic Sauerbraten 217
Pesto Roast Beef 217
Salisbury Steak 217
Tomato-Braised Beef 217
Beef and Bell Peppers 218
Ginger Beef 218
Carne Asada 218
Beef Goulash 218
Braised Beef Short Ribs 218
Stuffed Meatballs 218
Balsamic Roast Beef 219
Slow Cooker Barbacoa Pulled Beef with Cilantro Cauliflower Rice 219
Corned Beef & Cabbage with Horseradish Cream 219
Fiery Curry Beef 219
Slow Cooker Beef-Stuffed Cabbage in Creamy Tomato Sauce 220
Slow Cooker Brisket 220
Savory Stuffed Peppers 220
Mediterranean Meatloaf 220
Deconstructed Cabbage Rolls 220
Pork Chile Verde 221
Pork Loin with Creamy Gravy 221
Southeast Asian Lemongrass Pork 221

Slow Cooker Pork Chops with Creamy Bacon-and-Artichoke Sauce 221
Pork Loin with Ginger Cream Sauce 221
Mustard-Herb Pork Chops 222
Slow Cooker Pulled Pork with Cabbage Slaw 222
Slow Cooker Pork Carnitas 222
Slow Cooker Ranch Favorite Texas-Style Pulled Pork 223
Smoked Sausage with Cabbage & Onions 223
Slow Cooker Saucy Sausage-and-Beef Meatballs 223
Pork Belly with Brussels Sprouts & Turnips 223
Pork & Sausage Meatballs with Mushroom Ragout 223
Tunisian Lamb Ragout 224
Slow Cooker All-in-One Lamb-Vegetable Dinner 224
Wild Mushroom Lamb Shanks 224
Slow Cooker Braised Lamb with Fennel 224
Curried Lamb 225
Slow Cooker Lamb Stew with Turnips 225
Rosemary Lamb Chops 225
Tender Lamb Roast 225
Pumpkin-Nutmeg Pudding 225
Chocolate–Peanut Butter Fudge 226
Chocolate Walnut Fudge 226
Cinnamon-Cocoa Almonds 226
Chocolate Pot de Crème 226
Spicy Chai Custard 226
Coconut Custard 226
Tempting Lemon Custard 227
Vanilla Pudding 227
Pumpkin Spice Pudding 227
Pumpkin-Ginger Pudding 227
Spicy Chai Custard 227
Chocolate & Coconut Pudding 227
Berry-Pumpkin Compote 228
Blackberry Cobbler 228
Slow Cooker Sour-Cream Cheesecake 228
Peanut Butter Cheesecake 228

Blueberry Crisp 228
Tender Pound Cake 229
Almond Golden Cake 229
Delectable Peanut Butter Cup Cake 229
Coconut-Raspberry Cake 229
Warm Gingerbread 229
Carrot Cake 230
Lime-Raspberry Custard Cake 230
Slow Cooker Tangy Lemon Cake with Lemon Glaze 230
Brownie Chocolate Cake 230
Slow Cooker Moist Ginger Cake with Whipped Cream 231
Vanilla Cheesecake 231
Chocolate–Macadamia Nut Cheesecake 231
Toasted Almond Cheesecake 231
Slow Cooker Chocolate Chip Cookies 232
Chocolate Cake with Whipped Cream 232
Fudge Nut Brownies 232

Snacks & Apps 232

Bacon-Pepper Fat Bombs 232
Smoked Salmon Fat Bombs 233
Bacon Chive Fat Bombs 233
Sun-Dried Tomato and Feta Fat Bombs 233
Avocado Chili Fat Bomb 233
"Everything but the Bagel" Fat Bombs 233
Cheesy Dill Fat Bombs 233
Almond Crackers 234
Nut Crackers 234
Seedy Crackers 234
Crispy Parmesan Crackers 234
Flaxseed Chips and Guacamole 234
Spicy Cheddar Wafers 235
Triple Cheese Chips 235
Parmesan Zucchini Chips 235
Crispy Kale Chips 235
Margarita Pizza Chips 235
Garlic Pepperoni Chips 235
Savory Party Mix 236
Dips Herby Yogurt Dip 236
Bacon Guacamole 236
Coconut Tzatziki 236

Tzatziki Dip with Vegetables......236
Lemon-Turmeric Aioli......236
Guacamole......237
Olive and Artichoke Tapenade......237
Baba Ghanoush......237
Cauliflower Hummus......237
Zucchini Hummus......237
French Onion Dip......237
Pimento Cheese......238
Roasted Red Pepper Dip......238
Spinach-Artichoke Dip......238
Queso Dip......238
Queso Blanco Dip......238
Buffalo Chicken Dip......238
Taco Layer Dip......239
Crab and Artichoke Dip......239
Smoked Salmon and
Cucumber Bites......239
Black Forest Ham, Cheese,
and Chive Roll-Ups......239
Cheesy Shrimp Spread......239
Avocado and Smoked Salmon
Stack with Dill Caper Sauce......240
Salmon Salad Sushi Bites......240
BLTA Wraps......240
Party Deli Pinwheels......240
Turkey Spinach Roll-Ups......240
Smoked Salmon and Goat
Cheese Pinwheels......240
Dilled Tuna Salad Sandwich......241
Tuna Salad Wrap......241
Prosciutto-Wrapped
Mozzarella......241
Macadamia Nut Cream
Cheese Log......241
Mediterranean Cucumber Bites......241
Caprese Skewers......241
Turmeric Cauliflower "Pickles"......241
Anti-Inflammatory Power Bites......242
Marinated Antipasto Veggies......242
Grilled Avocados......242
Roasted Brussels Sprouts
with Tahini-Yogurt Sauce......242
Avocado Deviled Eggs......242
Bacon-Cheese Deviled Eggs......243
Bacon Deviled Eggs......243
Green Chile Deviled Eggs......243
Southern Fried Deviled Eggs......243
Antipasto Skewers......243

Rosemary Roasted Almonds......244
Smoked Almonds......244
Spicy Barbecue Pecans......244
Texas Trash......244
Marinated Artichokes......244
Fennel and Orange
Marinated Olives......244
Baked Olives and Feta......245
Baked Feta Blocks......245
Goat Cheese Nuggets......245
Almond Fried Goat Cheese......245
Feta Cheese Kebabs......245
Loaded Feta......246
Buffalo Roasted Cauliflower......246
Jalapeño Poppers......246
Cheesy Pork Rind Nachos......246
Jalapeño Firecrackers......246
Spicy Jalapeño Chips and
Ranch......247
Sriracha Artichoke Bites......247
Maple Bacon-Wrapped
Brussels Sprouts......247
Sausage and Spinach–Stuffed
Mushrooms......247
Pigs in a Blanket......248
Tofu Fries......248
Avocado "Fries"......248
Jicama Nachos......248
Cheesy Cauliflower
Breadsticks......249
Soft-Baked Pretzels with
Spicy Mustard Dip......249
Garlic Breadsticks......249
Classic Mozzarella Sticks......250
Bacon-Wrapped Mozzarella
Sticks......250
Prosciutto and Cream Cheese
Stuffed Mushrooms......250
Brown Sugar Bacon Smokies......250
Cheesy Baked Meatballs......250
Hot Dog Rolls......251
Empanadas......251
Beef Taquitos......251
Cheesy Chicken Taquitos......251
Thai Chicken Skewers with
Peanut Sauce......252
Sriracha Wings......252
Bacon-Wrapped Jalapeño
Chicken......252

Latkes with Sour Cream......252
Goat Cheese and Basil Pizza......253
Pesto Cauliflower Sheet-Pan
"Pizza"......253
Pepperoni Supreme Pizza......253
Meat Crust Pizza......254
Bacon and Egg Pizza......254

Sweets & Treats 254

Chocolate Sea Salt Almonds......254
Salted Caramels......254
Salted Caramel Cashew Brittle......255
White Chocolate Bark......255
Almond Chocolate Bark......255
Dairy-Free Chocolate Truffles......255
Candied Bacon Fudge......255
Pralines......256
Chocolate Peppermint Fudge......256
Cinnamon-Dusted Almonds......256
Cinnamon-Glazed Pecans......256
Coconut Truffles......256
Chocolate-Covered Bacon......256
Chocolate-Coconut Treats......257
Chocolate Peanut Butter Cups......257
Cookie Dough Balls......257
Almond Butter Fudge......257
Chocolate Fudge......257
Grilled Cantaloupe......257
Grilled Sweet Peaches......258
Chocolate-Covered
Strawberries......258
Mint Chocolate Fat Bombs......258
Salted Macadamia Fat Bomb......258
Roasted Strawberries with
Whipped Cream......258
Lime-Coconut Fat Bomb......258
Coconut Lemon Fat Bombs......259
Chocolate Peanut Butter
Fat Bombs......259
Nut Butter Cup Fat Bomb......259
Peanut Butter Cookie
Dough Fat Bombs......259
Marzipan Fat Bomb......259
Pumpkin Spice Fat Bombs......259
Creamy Banana Fat Bombs......260
Lime Almond Fat Bomb......260
Blueberry Fat Bombs......260
Spiced-Chocolate Fat Bombs......260
Key Lime Pie Fat Bombs......260

Salted Caramel Fudge Fat Bombs 260
Butter Pecan Cheesecake Truffle Fat Bombs 261
Cowboy Cookie Dough Fat Bombs 261
Cookie Dough Fat Bombs 261
Cheesecake Fat Bombs 261
Cinnamon Roll Fat Bomb 261
Strawberry Cheesecake Fat Bombs 262
Cinnamon Coconut Fat Bomb 262
Chocolate Almond Fat Bombs 262
Creamy Tiramisu Fat Bomb 262
Chai Tea Cookies 262
Peanut Butter–Chocolate Chip Cookies 262
Lemon Cookies 263
Chocolate Chunk Cookies 263
Double Chocolate Peppermint Cookies 263
Chocolate Sandwich Cookies 264
Sugar Cookie Balls 264
Chocolate Chip Brownies 264
Peanut Butter Cookies 265
Avocado Brownies 265
No-Bake Coconut Cookies 265
Lemon Snowball Cookies 265
Coconut Cookies 265
Nutty Shortbread Cookies 266
Almond Cookies 266
Chocolate Chip Cookies 266
Pecan Sandies 266
Chocolate Chip Cookie Dough Balls 266
Pistachio Cookies 267
Pumpkin Cookies 267
Salted Peanut Butter Cookies 267
Easy Peasy Peanut Butter Cookies 268
Lemon-Poppyseed Cookies 268
Iced Gingerbread Cookies 268
Snickerdoodle Cookies 268
Pecan Chocolate Chip Cookies 268
Carrot Cake Cookies 269
Fudgy Brownies 269
Coconut Macaroons 269
Coconut Lime Macaroons 270
Chewy "Noatmeal" Chocolate Chip Cookies 270

Almond Butter Oatmeal Cookies 270
Chocolate-Drizzled Pecan Shortbread 270
Classic Chocolate Brownies 270
Fluffy Lime-Meringue Clouds 271
French Meringues 271
No-Bake Brownie Bites 271
Pumpkin Cheesecake Brownies 271
Blondies 272
Blueberry Cheesecake Bars 272
Fudge Brownies 272
No-Bake Coconut Chocolate Squares 273
Raspberry Cheesecake Squares 273
Peanut Butter Cake Bars 273
Snickerdoodle Bars 273
Bourbon Pecan Pie Bars 274
Lemon Cheesecake Bars 274
Pecan Pie Bars 274
Coconut Cinnamon Bars 274
Cinnamon Popovers with Coconut Streusel 275
Ultra-Soft Pumpkin Chocolate Bars 275
Pistachio-Raspberry Chocolate Bark 275
Blackberry "Cheesecake" Bites 275
Salted Caramel Cupcakes 275
Coconut-Orange Cupcakes 276
Orange-Olive Oil Cupcakes 276
Almond Cake 276
Tiramisu 276
Strawberry Cheesecake 277
No-Bake Chocolate Raspberry Cheesecake 277
Quick Pressure Cooker Cheesecake 278
Pumpkin-Ricotta Cheesecake 278
Italian Cream Cheesecake 278
Butter Rum Pound Cake 279
Hazelnut-Chocolate Snack Cakes 279
Cream Cheese Pound Cake 279
Pumpkin Pound Cake 279
Raspberry-Lemon Pound Cake 280
Poppy Seed Pound Cake 280
Lemon Curd Layer Cake 280
Chocolate Marble Pound Cake 281
90-Second Lava Cake 281

Strawberry Shortcakes 281
Butter Cake with Cream Cheese Buttercream 282
Chocolate Mug Cake 282
Summer Squash Mock Apple Crumble 282
Jicama "Apple" Pie Filling 283
Strawberry Cream Pie 283
Apple Pie Bites 283
Keto-Friendly Key Lime Pie 284
"Buttermilk" Custard Pie Bars 284
Blackberry Cobbler 284
Fluffy Peanut Butter Pie 284
Fresh Berry Tart 285
Lemon Curd Tartlets 285
Chocolate Mousse Pie Cups 285
Pumpkin Pie 285
Pumpkin Pie 286
Raspberry Cream Cheese Tart Bars 286
Cinnamon Pecan "Apple" Crisp 286
Mixed Berry Crisp 287
Blueberry Crumble 287
Strawberry Rhubarb Cobbler 287
Chocolate Whoopie Pies 288
Maddie's Favorite Chocolate Malt 288
Chocolate Mousse 288
Peanut Butter Mousse 288
Pecan Pie Pudding 288
Bread Pudding 288
Banana Pudding 289
Mexican Chocolate Pudding 289
Almond Butter and Jelly Chia Pudding 289
Rice Pudding 289
Chocolate Avocado Pudding 289
Chocolate-Chia Pudding 290
Snickerdoodle Pudding 290
Whipped Cream-Chocolate Pudding Parfaits 290
Cookies and Cream Parfait 290
Creamy Panna Cotta 290
Double Coconut Panna Cotta 290
Vanilla Panna Cotta 291
Strawberry Panna Cotta 291
Crustless Cannoli 291
"Frosty" Chocolate Shake 291
Blueberry Cream Cheese Bites 291
Macadamia Lime Bites 291

Lemon-Blueberry Ice Cream . . . 292
Olive Oil Ice Cream . . . 292
Matcha Ice Cream . . . 292
Rich Vanilla Ice Cream . . . 292
Raspberry Maple Soft Serve . . . 292
Banana Pudding Ice Cream . . . 293
Mexican Chocolate Pudding . . . 293
Buttercream Pudding "Fluff" . . . 293
French Vanilla Ice Cream
with Hot Fudge . . . 293
Strawberry Avocado Ice Cream . . . 294
Raspberry Ice Cream . . . 294
Lavender Ice Cream . . . 294
Chocolate Coconut Milk
Ice Cream . . . 294
Mixed Berry Sherbet . . . 294
Strawberries and Cream
Ice Pops . . . 294
Sour Cream Ice Cream . . . 294
Strawberry Frozen Yogurt . . . 295
Chocolate-Dipped Peanut
Butter Ice Pops . . . 295
Sangria Granita . . . 295
Blueberry Mint Ice Pops . . . 295
Fudge Ice Pops . . . 295
Vanilla-Almond Ice Pops . . . 295
Orange Cream Ice Pops . . . 296
Churros and Chocolate Sauce . . . 296
Crème Brûlée . . . 296
Sweet Egg Salad . . . 296

Drinks 297

Buttered Coffee . . . 297
Pumpkin Spice Latte . . . 297
Bulletproof Coffee . . . 297
Matcha Coffee . . . 297
Earl Grey Rose Latte . . . 297
Coconut Iced Coffee . . . 297
Green Tea Latte . . . 297
Fat Chai . . . 297
Hot Cocoa . . . 298
Spicy Hot Chocolate . . . 298
Hot Almond Chocolate . . . 298
Bloody Mary . . . 298
Virgin (or Not) Eggnog . . . 298
Chocolate Martini . . . 298
Moscow Mule . . . 299

Virgin (or Not) Mojito . . . 299
Blueberry Mojito . . . 299
Hot Buttered Rum . . . 299
Spicy Margarita . . . 299
Lime Margarita . . . 299
Raspberry Mimosa . . . 300
Sangria . . . 300
Michelada . . . 300
Frosé Slushie . . . 300
Vesper Martini . . . 300
Negroni . . . 300
Tequila Sunrise . . . 300
Old-Fashioned . . . 300
Manhattan . . . 300
Gelatin Shooters . . . 301

Staples 301

Avocado-Herb Compound
Butter . . . 301
Cinnamon Butter . . . 301
Horseradish Compound
Butter . . . 301
Ghee . . . 301
Strawberry Butter . . . 301
Beef Bone Broth . . . 302
Rich Beef Stock . . . 302
Chicken Bone Broth . . . 302
Herbed Chicken Stock . . . 302
Herbed Vegetable Broth . . . 302
Fish Stock . . . 303
Italian Seasoning . . . 303
Ranch Seasoning . . . 303
Taco Seasoning . . . 303
Buttermilk Ranch Dressing . . . 303
Lemon-Garlic Dressing . . . 303
Green Basil Dressing . . . 303
Creamy Grapefruit-Tarragon
Dressing . . . 304
Harissa Oil . . . 304
Chimichurri . . . 304
Traditional Caesar Dressing . . . 304
Ranch Dressing . . . 304
Mustard Shallot Vinaigrette . . . 304
Herbed Balsamic Dressing . . . 305
Garlic-Rosemary Infused
Olive Oil . . . 305
Ginger-Lime Dressing . . . 305

Garlic Herb Marinade . . . 305
Lemon-Tahini Dressing . . . 305
Lemon Poppy Seed Dressing . . . 305
Bagna Cauda . . . 305
Pesto . . . 306
Hollandaise . . . 306
Herb-Kale Pesto . . . 306
Spinach Hemp Pesto . . . 306
Creamy Mayonnaise . . . 306
Zesty Orange Aioli . . . 306
Chimichurri Sauce . . . 307
Thai-Style Peanut Sauce . . . 307
Bleu Cheese Sauce . . . 307
Barbecue Sauce . . . 307
Garlicky Alfredo Sauce . . . 307
Sugar-Free Ketchup . . . 307
Alfredo Sauce . . . 307
Classic Bolognese Sauce . . . 308
Hot Crab Sauce . . . 308
Mustard Cream Sauce . . . 308
Enchilada Sauce . . . 308
Pico de Gallo . . . 308
Teriyaki Sauce . . . 308
Pasta Sauce . . . 309
Pizza Sauce . . . 309
Pesto Sauce . . . 309
Herbed Marinara Sauce . . . 309
Indonesian Peanut Sauce . . . 309
Herb Pesto . . . 309
Bacon Chutney . . . 310
Bacon Jam . . . 310
Cinnamon-Caramel Sauce . . . 310
Pastry Cream . . . 310
Cheesy-Crust Pizza . . . 310
Margherita Pizza . . . 310
Barbecue Onion and
Goat Cheese Flatbread . . . 311
Cauliflower Tortillas . . . 311
Versatile Sandwich Round . . . 311
Almond Butter Bread . . . 311
Coconut Almond Flour Bread . . . 311
Cheesy Taco Shells . . . 312
Cloud Bread . . . 312
Coconut Pie Crust . . . 312

KETO 101

Diets come and go: low-fat, low-calorie, gluten-free, Weight Watchers, South Beach, the list goes on. Most require you to go hungry, eat only boring food, count calories, or go through various entry phases. The major problem with these diets is that they aren't always nutritionally sound and they're not satisfying, so you're always feeling tired and hungry. They're simply not safe and definitely not sustainable.

What the more successful diets have in common is the reduction of foods high in carbohydrates. When you eat carbs, your body breaks them down into glucose, a simple sugar, which quickly and significantly raises your blood sugar levels. Then you produce insulin to reduce this spike in blood sugar. After years and years of this cycle, your body will need to produce more insulin at once to achieve the same results. You can quickly become insulin resistant, and very commonly this resistance turns into prediabetes, metabolic syndrome, and, eventually, type 2 diabetes.

When you reduce carbs, and eat lots of fat and high-protein foods instead, your body adapts and converts the fat and protein, as well as the fat you have stored, into ketone bodies, or ketones, for energy. This metabolic process is called ketosis. That's where the *ketogenic* in ketogenic diet originates from.

Studies consistently show that a keto diet helps people lose weight, improve energy levels throughout the day, and stay satiated longer. The increased satiety and improved energy levels are attributed to most of the calories coming from fat, which is very slow to digest and calorically dense, instead of fast-burning carbs and sugars. As a result, keto dieters commonly consume fewer calories because they don't feel the need to eat as much or as often. This decreased appetite, as well as maintaining a low-carb, high-fat diet is beneficial for weight loss. Most importantly, according to an increasing number of studies, it helps reduce risk factors for diabetes, heart diseases, stroke, Alzheimer's, epilepsy, and more.

The keto diet promotes fresh whole foods like meat, fish, veggies, and healthy fats and oils, and greatly reduces processed, chemically treated foods. It's a diet that you can sustain long-term and enjoy.

This book will provide you with everything you need to know to go keto, including 1,500 recipes that are macro-friendly. Whether your goal is sustainable weight loss, overall health, or a new way of cooking and eating, this book will help you achieve long-term success.

Go Keto

When you eat a ketogenic diet, your body becomes efficient at burning fat for fuel. This is great for a number of reasons, not the least of which is that fat contains more than double the calories of most carbs, so you don't need to eat as much to feel full and fuel your body. Your body also becomes more able to burn the fat it has stored (the fat you're trying to get rid of), resulting in weight loss. Using fat for fuel provides consistent energy levels, and it does not spike your blood glucose, so you don't experience the highs and lows—like a sugar rush—that can happen when eating large amounts of carbs. Consistent energy levels throughout your day means you can get more done and feel less tired doing so.

In addition to those benefits, eating a keto diet in the long term has been proven to:

- Result in more weight loss (specifically body fat)
- Reduce blood sugar and insulin resistance (often reversing prediabetes and controlling type 2 diabetes)
- Reduce triglyceride levels (having a high level of triglycerides in your blood can increase your risk of heart disease)
- Reduce blood pressure
- Improve levels of HDL (good) and LDL (bad) cholesterol
- Improve brain function

Ketosis

When eating a high-carb diet, your body is in a metabolic state of glycolysis, which simply means that most of the energy your body uses comes from blood glucose.

In contrast, a low-carb, high-fat diet puts your body into a metabolic state called ketosis. Your body breaks down fat into ketone bodies (ketones) to use as its primary source of energy. In ketosis, your body readily burns fat for energy, and fat reserves are constantly released and consumed. It's a normal state—whenever you're low on carbs for a few days (or even overnight), your body will do this naturally.

The main goal of the keto diet is to keep you in nutritional ketosis all the time. For those just starting the keto diet, to be fully keto-adapted usually takes anywhere from four to eight weeks.

Once you become keto-adapted, glycogen (the glucose stored in your muscles and liver) decreases, you carry less water weight, your muscle endurance increases, and your overall energy levels are higher than before. Also, if you fall out of ketosis by eating too many carbs, you can return to ketosis much sooner than when you were not keto-adapted. Additionally, once keto-adapted, many people can eat up to 50 grams of carbs per day and still maintain ketosis.

Macros

The keto diet is built on ratios of macronutrients. It's important to get the right balance of macronutrients so your body has the energy it needs and you're not missing any essential fat or protein in your diet. Macronutrients are what make up all food: fat, protein, and carbohydrates. Each type of macronutrient provides a certain amount of energy (calories) per gram consumed:

- Fat provides about 9 calories per gram
- Protein provides about 4 calories per gram
- Carbohydrates provide about 4 calories per gram

On the keto diet, 65 to 75 percent of the calories you consume should come from fat. About 20 to 25 percent should come from protein, and the remaining 5 percent or so from carbohydrates. The number of total calories you consume daily should be tailored to your body, activity levels, and goals. Total caloric intake depends on a few factors, including:

- Current lean body weight (total body weight minus body fat)
- Daily activity levels (do you work in an office, wait tables, compete as a professional athlete?)

- Workout regimen and type of workout
- Goals of those on a ketogenic diet might include:
- Lose weight
- Maintain a healthy weight
- Gain muscle
- Manage blood sugar

There are many ketogenic-based macro calculators available online. You'll be able to easily and quickly plug in your numbers and get an immediate estimation of your body's caloric needs. One of the great things about the keto diet is that it's not necessary to track each and every number—but if you want to track, it's a great way to speed up your progress.

Adjusting to Keto

You may have heard of the "keto flu" that some people experience when starting out the keto diet. This is primarily due to dehydration as your body flushes its sodium levels. It's crucial to drink plenty of water when beginning the keto diet. You may even notice that you're visiting the bathroom more often, and that's normal! This happens because you're cutting out a lot of processed foods and have started eating more whole, natural foods instead. Processed foods have a lot of added sodium, and the sudden change in diet causes a sudden drop in sodium intake.

Additionally, the reduction in carbs reduces insulin levels, which in turn tells your kidneys to release excess stored sodium. Between the reduction in sodium intake and flushing of excess stored sodium, the body begins to excrete much more water than usual, and you end up low on sodium and other electrolytes.

When this happens, you may experience symptoms such as fatigue, headaches, coughing, sniffles, irritability, and/or nausea. This state is generally known as the "keto flu." It's very important to know that this is not the actual influenza virus. It's called the keto flu only due to the similarity in symptoms, but it's neither contagious nor a real virus.

Many who experience these symptoms believe the keto diet made them sick and immediately go back to eating carbs. But the keto flu phase actually means your body is withdrawing from sugar, high carbs, and processed foods, and is readjusting so it can use fat as its fuel. The keto flu usually lasts just a few days while the body readjusts. You can abate its symptoms by temporarily adding more electrolytes to your diet.

5 Simple Steps to Go Keto

STEP 1: CLEAN OUT YOUR PANTRY

Out with the old, in with the new. Having tempting, unhealthy foods in your home is one of the biggest contributors to failure when starting any diet. Find a local food bank or homeless shelter to donate to, and look through your kitchen for any and all of the following:

Starches and Grains Cereal, pasta, rice, potatoes, corn, oats, quinoa, flour, bread, bagels, wraps, rolls, and croissants.

Sugary Foods and Drinks Refined sugar, fountain drinks, fruit juices, milk, desserts, pastries, milk chocolate, candy bars, etc.

Legumes Beans, peas, and lentils are dense with carbs.

Processed Polyunsaturated Fats and Oils Vegetable oils and most seed oils, including sunflower, safflower, canola, soybean, grapeseed, and corn oil, as well as trans fats like shortening and margarine—anything that says "hydrogenated" or "partially hydrogenated."

Fruits Many fruits are high in carbs, including bananas, dates, grapes, mangos, and apples. Dried fruit contains as much sugar as regular fruit but more concentrated, making it easy to eat a lot of sugar in a small serving. For comparison, a cup of raisins has over 100 grams of carbs while a cup of grapes has only 15 grams of carbs.

STEP 2: GO SHOPPING

It's time to restock your pantry, refrigerator, and freezer with delicious, keto-friendly foods that will help you lose weight, become healthy, and feel great!

The Basics
With these basics on hand, you'll always be ready to prepare healthy, delicious, and keto-friendly meals and snacks.

Water, coffee, and tea

All spices and herbs

Sweeteners such as stevia and erythritol

Lemon or lime juice

Low-carb condiments like mayonnaise, mustard, pesto, and sriracha

Broths (chicken, beef, bone)

Pickled and fermented foods like pickles, kimchi, and sauerkraut

Nuts and seeds, including macadamia nuts, pecans, almonds, walnuts, hazelnuts, pine nuts, flaxseed, chia seeds, and pumpkin seeds.

Meats
Any type of meat is fine for the keto diet, including chicken, beef, lamb, pork, turkey, game, etc. It's preferable to use grass-fed and/or organic meats if they're available and possible for your budget. You can and should eat the fat on the meat and skin on the chicken.

All wild-caught fish and seafood slide into the keto diet nicely. Try to avoid farmed fish.

Eat lots of eggs! Use organic eggs from free-range chickens, if possible.

Veggies
You can eat all nonstarchy veggies, including broccoli, asparagus, mushrooms, cucumbers, lettuce, onions, peppers, tomatoes, garlic (in small quantities—each clove contains about 1 gram of carbs), Brussels sprouts, eggplant, olives, zucchini, yellow squash, and cauliflower.

Avoid all types of potatoes, yams and sweet potatoes, corn, and legumes like beans, lentils, and peas.

Fruits
You can eat a small amount of berries every day, such as strawberries, raspberries, blackberries, and blueberries. Lemon and lime juices are great for adding flavor to your meals. Avocados are also low in carbs and full of healthy fat.

Avoid other fruits, as they're loaded with sugar. A single banana can contain around 25 grams of net carbs.

Dairy
Eat full-fat dairy like butter, sour cream, heavy (whipping) cream, cheese, cream cheese, and unsweetened yogurt. Although not technically dairy, unsweetened almond and coconut milks are great as well.

Avoid milk and skim milk, as well as sweetened yogurt, as it contains a lot of sugar. Avoid any flavored, low-fat, or fat-free dairy products.

Fats and Oils
Avocado oil, olive oil, extra-virgin olive oil, butter, lard, and bacon fat are the keto-friendly oils you want on hand. Avocado oil has a high smoke point (it does not burn or smoke until it reaches 520°F), which is ideal for searing meats and frying in a wok. Make sure to avoid oils labeled "blend"; they commonly contain small amounts of the healthy oil and large amounts of unhealthy oils.

STEP 3: SET UP YOUR KITCHEN

Preparing delicious recipes is one of the best parts of the keto diet, and it's easy if you have the right kitchen essentials. The following tools will make cooking simpler and faster. Each one is worth investing in, especially for the busy cook.

Food Processor

Food processors are critical to your arsenal. They are ideal for blending certain foods or processing foods together into sauces and shakes.

Spiralizer

Spiralizers make vegetables into noodles or ribbons within seconds. They make cooking a lot faster and easier—noodles have much more surface area and take a fraction of the time to cook. For example, a spiralizer turns a zucchini into zoodles which are delicious with some Alfredo or marinara sauce.

Electric Hand Mixer

If you've ever had to beat an egg white by hand until you get stiff peaks, then you know just how difficult it is. Electric hand mixers save your arm muscles and massive amounts of time, especially when mixing heavy ingredients.

Cast Iron Pans

Cast iron skillets don't wear out and are healthier to use (no chemical treatment of any kind), retain heat very well, and can be moved between the stove and oven. They are simple to clean up—just wash them out with a scrub sponge without soap, dry them off, and then rub them with cooking oil. This prevents rust and encourages the buildup of "seasoning," a natural nonstick surface. You can also purchase them pre-seasoned to save a step.

Sharpened Knives

Most of prep time is spent on cutting. You'll see your cutting speed skyrocket with a good, sharp knife set. Aim to sharpen your knives every week or so to keep them in good shape (professional chefs sharpen their knives before every use).

STEP 4: MEAL PLANNING & SHOPPING

Create a meal plan by strategizing what you want to cook (either ahead of time or day-of) for each meal in a given week (or two), and shopping for all the ingredients you need in one or two trips. With the 1,500 recipes in this cookbook, you'll have plenty of dishes to choose from! Using meal plans in the beginning of your diet greatly increases your chances of success by providing you with clear goals and day by day direction. If you know what you are planning to cook each day without thinking about it, you're less likely to give up, change your mind, and order food from your favorite takeout spot. Also, since you know what's coming next on your personal menu, you can look forward to it throughout the week.

When shopping for ingredients, especially when you're new to keto, be sure to look at the nutritional information provided for almost every packaged product. Some items may seem as though they'd be low on carbs, but many companies love to add sugar, so be on the lookout. Over your first few weeks, you'll get to know which products are reliable and which are not.

STEP 5: EXERCISE AND LIFESTYLE

As you start your diet and your energy levels rise and the pounds begin to fall off, think about how you can improve your health and feel even better. This is a great time to become more active through exercise.

Increase the amount you exercise relative to what you do now. If you don't exercise at all, start taking short walks or slow jogs, or a combination of both, for 15 minutes every other day. If you already go to the gym or lift weights, add a little cardio. If you have the time, try taking a class or practicing an activity that involves moving, like dancing or rec league basketball. It doesn't have to be competitive, and you don't need to have any previous experience. These activities can be a fun and easy way to get on your feet, and you can learn a new skill in the process.

Staying fit through regular physical activity has been proven to reduce blood pressure and cholesterol levels as well as reduce risk for various heart diseases and type 2 diabetes. In combination with the keto diet, your health will improve dramatically, and so will your energy levels. Remember that it doesn't matter what level you start at—all it takes to become healthier is to do a little more than you're doing now. Exercise is incremental, and every increment is a boost to your health.

With these changes in diet and exercise, you'll find that your body adapts to this new way of eating and moving, and the keto lifestyle will become second nature. Soon you won't need to count carbs or calculate macros, and your body will crave the kinds of foods and activities that keep you in ketosis and on your path to this healthier—and more delicious—lifestyle.

SMOOTHIES

Kale Refresher Smoothie

SERVES 1 | PREP TIME: 5 minutes

1 cup unsweetened almond, cashew, or coconut milk

½ medium cucumber, peeled and halved lengthwise

1 tablespoon vanilla protein powder (whey or vegan)

½ lime, peeled and deseeded

1 tablespoon hemp seeds

1 avocado, sliced

1 cup frozen kale, stems removed

1 tablespoon coconut oil, melted

5 to 6 stevia drops

1 cup ice cubes

In a high-powered blender, combine the milk, cucumber, protein powder, lime, hemp seeds, avocado, kale, and coconut oil. Blend for 30 seconds. Add the stevia and ice cubes, blend on high for 1 minute, and serve.

Per Serving: (1 smoothie): Calories: 634; Fat: 46g; Protein: 21g; Total Carbs: 32g; Fiber: 18g; Net Carbs: 14g; **Macros:** Fat: 65%; Protein: 15%; Carbs: 20%

Spirulina Smoothie

SERVES 1 | PREP TIME: 5 minutes

1 cup full-fat coconut milk

1 tablespoon coconut cream

1 teaspoon peeled and grated fresh ginger

½ teaspoon spirulina powder

¼ teaspoon ground cardamom

¼ teaspoon ground cinnamon

1 tablespoon vanilla protein powder (vegan or whey)

1 cup ice cubes

1 teaspoon flaxseed

In a high-powered blender, combine the coconut milk, coconut cream, ginger, spirulina, cardamom, and cinnamon. Blend for 30 seconds. Add the protein powder and ice cubes, and blend on high for 1 minute. Pour the smoothie into a glass, sprinkle with the flaxseed, and enjoy.

Per Serving: (1 smoothie) Calories: 708; Fat: 60g; Protein: 15g; Total Carbs: 27g; Fiber: 7g; Net Carbs: 20g; **Macros:** Fat: 77%; Protein: 8%; Carbs: 15%

Avocado-Matcha Smoothie

SERVES 1 | PREP TIME: 5 minutes

¼ cup full-fat canned coconut milk, divided

1½ teaspoons matcha green tea powder

1 small, very ripe avocado, peeled and pitted

1 cup unsweetened almond milk, plus more as needed

1 scoop unflavored collagen protein powder

½ teaspoon vanilla extract

1 to 2 teaspoons monk fruit extract or sugar-free sweetener

In a small microwave-safe bowl, heat 2 tablespoons of coconut milk in the microwave for 30 seconds. Whisk the matcha powder into the hot milk until smooth. In a blender, combine the avocado, matcha and cream mixture, remaining 2 tablespoons of coconut milk, almond milk, collagen powder, vanilla, and sweetener. Blend until smooth and creamy, adding more almond milk if needed.

Per Serving: Calories: 424; Fat: 34g; Protein: 17g; Total Carbs: 17g; Fiber: 11g; Net Carbs: 6g; **Macros:** Fat: 72%; Protein: 16%; Carbs: 12%

Berry Green Smoothie

SERVES 2 | PREP TIME: 10 minutes

1 cup water

½ cup raspberries

½ cup shredded kale

¾ cup cream cheese

1 tablespoon coconut oil

1 scoop vanilla protein powder

Put the water, raspberries, kale, cream cheese, coconut oil, and protein powder in a blender and blend until smooth.

Per Serving: Calories: 436; Fat: 36g; Protein: 28g; Total Carbs: 11g; Fiber: 5g; Net Carbs: 6g; **Macros:** Fat: 70%; Protein: 20%; Carbs: 10%

Green Herb Smoothie

SERVES 1 | PREP TIME: 5 minutes

1 cup unsweetened almond milk

1 cup ice

1 cup spinach

½ cup chopped fresh parsley

½ cup chopped fresh cilantro

½ avocado, pitted and peeled

1 tablespoon freshly squeezed lime juice

3 to 4 drops liquid stevia

In a blender, combine the milk, ice, spinach, parsley, cilantro, avocado, lime juice, and stevia. Blend until smooth, and serve immediately.

Per Serving: Calories: 208; Fat: 16g; Protein: 5g; Total Carbs: 13g; Fiber: 10g; Net Carbs: 3g; **Macros:** Fat: 70%; Protein: 10%; Carbs: 20%

Creamy Kale Smoothie

SERVES 2 | PREP TIME: 10 minutes

¾ cup unsweetened almond milk

¼ cup unsweetened apple juice

½ cup lightly steamed kale

¼ cup cream cheese

1 tablespoon hemp seeds

2 (7g) stevia packets

2 cups ice cubes

In a blender, blend the almond milk, apple juice, kale, cream cheese, hemp seeds, and stevia until combined. Add the ice, blend until smooth, and serve.

Per Serving: Calories: 152; Fat: 13g; Protein: 5g; Total Carbs: 4g; Fiber: 1g; Net Carbs: 3g; **Macros:** Fat: 76%; Protein: 13%; Carbs: 11%

Cucumber Green Smoothie

SERVES 2 | PREP TIME: 10 minutes

1 English cucumber

1 cup spinach

½ cup coconut milk

3 tablespoons egg white protein powder

1 tablespoon tahini

1 teaspoon coconut oil

2 cups ice cubes

In a blender, blend the cucumber, spinach, coconut milk, egg white protein powder, tahini, and coconut oil until combined. Add the ice cubes, blend until smooth, and serve.

Per Serving: Calories: 258; Fat: 21g; Protein: 10g; Total Carbs: 11g; Fiber: 3g; Net Carbs: 8g; **Macros:** Fat: 69%; Protein: 15%; Carbs: 16%

Mean Green Smoothie

SERVES 2 | PREP TIME: 10 minutes

1½ cups crushed ice, divided
1 cup kale, tightly packed, cleaned, stalks removed
½ cup spinach, cleaned, stalks removed

½ cup Swiss chard, cleaned, stalks removed
2 tablespoons coconut oil
2 tablespoons chia seeds
½ cup water

In a blender, combine ¾ cup of ice, kale, spinach, and Swiss chard and blend to combine. Add the coconut oil, chia seeds, remaining ¾ cup of ice, and water. Blend for 1 minute, or until smooth, and serve.

Per Serving: Calories: 293; Fat: 23g; Protein: 8g; Total Carbs: 15g; Fiber: 11g; Net Carbs: 3g; **Macros:** Fat: 70%; Protein: 11%; Carbs: 19%

Almond Kale Smoothie

SERVES 2 | TOTAL TIME: 10 minutes

1 cup crushed ice, divided
1 cup unsweetened almond milk
1 cup kale

1 tablespoon coconut oil
2 tablespoons almond flour
½ teaspoon almond extract

In a blender, blend ½ cup of ice, almond milk, kale, and coconut oil. Add the almond flour, almond extract, and remaining ½ cup of ice. Blend for 1 minute, or until smooth, and serve.

Per Serving: (½ of finished smoothie recipe): Calories: 396; Fat: 39g; Protein: 4g; Total Carbs: 11g; Fiber: 4g; Net Carbs: 7g; **Macros:** Fat: 85%; Protein: 4%; Carbs: 11%

Cauliflower Smoothie

SERVES 2 | PREP TIME: 5 minutes

1 scoop vanilla protein powder
1 cup unsweetened coconut milk or almond milk
1½ cups frozen cauliflower
½ cup puréed butternut squash (optional)

2 tablespoons erythritol
2 teaspoons vanilla extract
1 tablespoon sugar-free chocolate chips or 3 squares sugar-free chocolate bar

In a blender, combine the protein powder, coconut milk, frozen cauliflower, butternut squash (if using), erythritol, and vanilla extract and blend until the cauliflower is completely smooth. Add the chocolate chips, set the blender to the lowest setting possible, and blend for another 30 seconds. Pour the smoothie into glasses.

Per Serving: Calories: 392; Fat: 32g; Protein: 14g; Total Carbs: 12g; Fiber: 5g; Net Carbs: 6g; **Macros:** Fat: 73%; Protein: 14%; Carbs: 13%

Green Goddess Smoothie

SERVES 1 | PREP TIME: 5 minutes

1 ripe avocado, peeled and pitted
1 cup almond milk or water, plus more as needed

1 cup baby spinach leaves, stems removed
½ medium cucumber, peeled and seeded

1 tablespoon extra-virgin olive oil or avocado oil
8 to 10 fresh mint leaves, stems removed

Juice of 1 lime (about 1 to 2 tablespoons)

In a blender, combine the avocado, almond milk, spinach, cucumber, olive oil, mint, and lime juice and blend until smooth and creamy, adding more almond milk or water if necessary.

Per Serving: Calories: 330; Fat: 30g; Protein: 4g; Total Carbs: 19g; Fiber: 9g; Net Carbs: 10g; **Macros:** Fat: 77%; Protein: 4%; Carbs: 19%

Green Coconut Avocado Smoothie

1 SERVING | PREP TIME: 5 minutes

½ avocado, pitted and peeled
½ cup unsweetened full-fat coconut milk
½ cup cold water
1 teaspoon vanilla extract

1 tablespoon MCT oil
½ teaspoon stevia or 4 drops liquid stevia extract
1 cup fresh spinach
A few ice cubes (optional)

In a blender, combine the avocado, coconut milk, water, vanilla, MCT oil, stevia, spinach, and ice and blend until smooth.

Per Serving: Calories: 504; Fat: 48g; Protein: 5g; Total Carbs: 13g; Fiber: 9g; Net Carbs: 4g; **Macros:** Fat: 86%; Protein: 4%; Carbs: 10%

Green Tea Smoothie

SERVES 2 | TOTAL TIME: 10 minutes

1 cup crushed ice, divided
1 cup unsweetened almond milk
¼ cup heavy (whipping) cream
1 tablespoon coconut oil

3 tablespoons unsweetened vanilla protein powder
1½ teaspoons green tea powder

In a blender, blend ½ cup of ice, almond milk, heavy cream, and coconut oil. Add the vanilla protein powder, green tea powder, and remaining ½ cup of ice. Blend for 1 minute, or until smooth, and serve.

Per Serving: Calories: 442; Fat: 41g; Protein: 17g; Total Carbs: 7g; Fiber: 3g; Net Carbs: 4g; **Macros:** Fat: 79%; Protein: 15%; Carbs: 6%

Lemon-Cashew Smoothie

SERVES 1 | PREP TIME: 5 minutes

1 cup unsweetened cashew milk
¼ cup heavy (whipping) cream
¼ cup freshly squeezed lemon juice

1 scoop plain protein powder
1 tablespoon coconut oil
1 teaspoon sweetener

Put the cashew milk, heavy cream, lemon juice, protein powder, coconut oil, and sweetener in a blender and blend until smooth. Pour into a glass and serve immediately.

Per Serving: Calories: 503; Fat: 45g; Protein: 29g; Total Carbs: 15g; Fiber: 4g; Net Carbs: 11g; **Macros:** Fat: 80%; Protein: 13%; Carbs: 7%

Avocado-Lime Smoothie

SERVES 2 | PREP TIME: 10 minutes

1 cup unsweetened almond milk
Juice and zest of 1 lime

¼ avocado
2 tablespoons hemp seeds

1 teaspoon pure
   vanilla extract

2 (7g) stevia packets

2 cups ice cubes

In a blender, blend the almond milk, lime juice, lime zest, avocado, hemp seeds, vanilla, and stevia until combined. Add the ice cubes, blend until smooth and thick, and serve.

Per Serving: Calories: 114; Fat: 10g; Protein: 4g; Total Carbs: 5g; Fiber: 3g; Net Carbs: 2g; **Macros:** Fat: 71%; Protein: 13%; Carbs: 16%

Lemon Smoothie

SERVES 2 | PREP TIME: 10 minutes

1 cup unsweetened
   almond milk

½ cup coconut milk

2 tablespoons egg white
   protein powder

1 teaspoon pure
   vanilla extract

1 teaspoon lemon extract

2 (7g) stevia packets

2 cups ice cubes

In a blender, blend the almond milk, coconut milk, egg white powder, vanilla, lemon extract, and stevia until combined. Add the ice, blend until smooth and thick, and serve.

Per Serving: Calories: 172; Fat: 14g; Protein: 6g; Total Carbs: 4g; Fiber: 1g; Net Carbs: 3g; **Macros:** Fat: 76%; Protein: 15%; Carbs: 9%

Spiced Orange-Pistachio Smoothie

SERVES 1 | PREP TIME: 5 minutes

½ cup plain Greek yogurt

½ cup unsweetened almond
   milk, plus more as needed

Zest and juice of 1 clementine
   or ½ orange

1 tablespoon extra-virgin olive
   oil or MCT oil

1 tablespoon shelled pistachios, coarsely chopped

1 to 2 teaspoons monk fruit
   extract or stevia (optional)

¼ to ½ teaspoon ground
   allspice or unsweetened
   pumpkin pie spice

¼ teaspoon ground
   cinnamon

¼ teaspoon vanilla extract

In a blender, combine the yogurt, almond milk, clementine zest and juice, olive oil, pistachios, monk fruit extract (if using), allspice, cinnamon, and vanilla and blend until smooth and creamy, adding more almond milk if necessary.

Per Serving: Calories: 264; Fat: 22g; Protein: 6g; Total Carbs: 12g; Fiber: 2g; Net Carbs: 10g; **Macros:** Fat: 73%; Protein: 10%; Carbs: 17%

Spinach-Blueberry Smoothie

SERVES 2 | PREP TIME: 5 minutes

1 cup coconut milk

1 cup spinach

½ English cucumber, chopped

½ cup blueberries

1 scoop plain protein powder

2 tablespoons coconut oil

4 ice cubes

Mint sprigs, for garnish

Put the coconut milk, spinach, cucumber, blueberries, protein powder, coconut oil, and ice in a blender and blend until smooth. Garnish with the mint, and serve.

Per Serving: Calories: 353; Fat: 32g; Protein: 15g; Total Carbs: 9g; Fiber: 3g; Net Carbs: 6g; **Macros:** Fat: 76%; Protein: 16%; Carbs: 8%

Blueberry Smoothie with Lemon and Ginger

SERVES 1 | PREP TIME: 5 minutes

1 cup unsweetened almond
   milk, plus more as needed

¼ cup frozen blueberries

2 tablespoons coconut oil

1 to 2 teaspoons monk fruit
   extract or sugar-free
   sweetener (optional)

½ teaspoon vanilla extract

½ teaspoon ground ginger
   or 1 tablespoon minced
   fresh ginger

Zest of 1 lemon

In a blender, combine the almond milk, blueberries, coconut oil, sweetener (if using), vanilla, ginger, and lemon zest. Blend until smooth and creamy, adding more almond milk if necessary.

Per Serving: Calories: 319; Fat: 30g; Protein: 2g; Total Carbs: 10g; Fiber: 2g; Net Carbs: 8g; **Macros:** Fat: 85%; Protein: 3%; Carbs: 12%

Strawberry Spinach Smoothie

SERVES 2 | TOTAL TIME: 10 minutes

1 cup crushed ice, divided

½ cup unsweetened
   almond milk

2 cups fresh spinach

½ cup strawberries

1 tablespoon coconut oil

In a blender, blend ½ cup of ice, almond milk, spinach, strawberries, and coconut oil. Add the remaining ½ cup of ice. Blend for 1 minute, or until smooth, and serve.

Per Serving: Calories: 215; Fat: 21g; Protein: 2.5g; Total Carbs: 7g; Fiber: 3g; Net Carbs: 4g; **Macros:** Fat: 85%; Protein: 5%; Carbs: 10%

Tropical Smoothie

SERVES 2 | PREP TIME: 10 minutes

½ cup coconut milk

¼ cup plain Greek yogurt

2 tablespoons hemp seeds

2 (7g) stevia

1 teaspoon banana extract

2 strawberries

2 cups ice cubes

In a blender, blend the coconut milk, yogurt, hemp seeds, stevia, banana extract, and strawberries until combined. Add the ice, blend until smooth, and serve.

Per Serving: Calories: 201; Fat: 18g; Protein: 7g; Total Carbs: 5g; Fiber: 2g; Net Carbs: 3g; **Macros:** Fat: 77%; Protein: 13%; Carbs: 10%

Triple Berry Smoothie

SERVES 2 | PREP TIME: 10 minutes

1 cup crushed ice, divided

½ cup unsweetened
   almond milk

1 tablespoon coconut oil

½ cup blueberries

½ cup raspberries

½ cup blackberries

½ teaspoon pure
   vanilla extract

In a blender, blend ½ cup ice, almond milk and coconut oil. Add the blueberries, raspberries, blackberries, vanilla, and remaining ½ cup of ice. Blend for 1 minute, or until smooth, and serve.

Per Serving: Calories: 252; Fat: 22g; Protein: 3g; Total Carbs: 16g; Fiber: 6g; Net Carbs: 10g; **Macros:** Fat: 72%; Protein: 4%; Carbs: 24%

Coconut Berry Smoothie

SERVES 2 | PREP TIME: 10 minutes

1 cup crushed ice, divided
1 cup unsweetened, full-fat coconut milk
1 tablespoon coconut oil

½ cup raspberries
½ cup blackberries
2 tablespoons unsweetened coconut flakes

In a blender, blend ½ cup of the ice, coconut milk and coconut oil. Add the raspberries, blackberries, coconut flakes, and remaining ½ cup of ice. Blend for 1 minute, or until smooth, and serve.

Per Serving: Calories: 384; Fat: 38g; Protein: 4g; Total Carbs: 15g; Fiber: 7g; Net Carbs: 8g; **Macros:** Fat: 82%; Protein: 4%; Carbs: 14%

Avocado Blueberry Smoothie

SERVES 2 | PREP TIME: 10 minutes

1 cup crushed ice, divided
½ cup blueberries
¾ cup unsweetened almond milk

2 tablespoons heavy (whipping) cream
1 tablespoon coconut oil
1 avocado, peeled and pitted

In a blender, blend ½ cup of ice, blueberries, almond milk, heavy cream, and coconut oil. Add the avocado and remaining ½ cup of ice. Blend for 1 minute, or until smooth, and serve.

Per Serving: Calories: 543; Fat: 54g; Protein: 1g; Total Carbs: 1g; Fiber: 0g; Net Carbs: 1g; **Macros:** Fat: 98%; Protein: 1%; Carbs: 1%

Creamy Snickerdoodle Shake

SERVES 2 | PREP TIME: 5 minutes

1 cup full-fat coconut milk
1 cup water
1 teaspoon ground cinnamon

2 tablespoons chia seeds
2 tablespoons coconut oil
1 scoop vanilla protein powder

In a high-powered blender, combine the coconut milk, water, cinnamon, chia seeds, coconut oil, and protein powder and blend on high for 60 seconds. Divide the shake between two glasses and enjoy.

Per Serving: Calories: 535; Fat: 47g; Protein: 13g; Total Carbs: 15g; Fiber: 9g; Net Carbs: 6g; **Macros:** Fat: 79%; Protein: 10%; Carbs: 11%

Creamy Cinnamon Smoothie

SERVES 2 | PREP TIME: 5 minutes

2 cups coconut milk
1 scoop vanilla protein powder
5 drops liquid stevia

1 teaspoon ground cinnamon
½ teaspoon alcohol-free vanilla extract

Put the coconut milk, protein powder, stevia, cinnamon, and vanilla in a blender and blend until smooth. Pour into 2 glasses and serve immediately.

Per Serving: Calories: 492; Fat: 47g; Protein: 18g; Total Carbs: 8g; Fiber: 2g; Net Carbs: 6g; **Macros:** Fat: 80%; Protein: 14%; Carbs: 6%

Nutty Chocolate Protein Shake

SERVES 1 | PREP TIME: 5 minutes

1 cup unsweetened almond milk

1 cup ice

1 tablespoon peanut butter or almond butter

1 scoop chocolate protein powder

In a blender, blend the almond milk, ice, peanut butter, and protein powder until smooth. Serve immediately.

Per Serving: Calories: 368; Fat: 22g; Protein: 39g; Total Carbs: 12g; Fiber: 6g; Net Carbs: 6g; **Macros:** Fat: 54%; Protein: 41%; Carbs: 5%

Peanut Butter Smoothie

SERVES 2 | PREP TIME: 10 minutes

1 cup unsweetened almond milk
½ cup coconut milk
3 tablespoons natural peanut butter

1 teaspoon pure vanilla extract
2 (7g) stevia packets
2 cups ice cubes

In a blender, blend the almond milk, coconut milk, peanut butter, vanilla, and stevia until combined. Add the ice, and blend until smooth and thick.

Per Serving: Calories: 309; Fat: 27g; Protein: 9g; Total Carbs: 8g; Fiber: 4g; Net Carbs: 4g; **Macros:** Fat: 78%; Protein: 12%; Carbs: 10%

Peanut Butter Shake

SERVES 2 | PREP TIME: 10 minutes

1 cup crushed ice, divided
¼ cup powdered peanut butter (such as PB2)
¼ cup heavy (whipping) cream

2 tablespoons coconut oil
1 cup unsweetened almond milk

In a blender, blend ½ cup of ice, powdered peanut butter and heavy cream. Add the coconut oil, almond milk, and remaining ½ cup of ice. Blend for 1 minute, or until smooth, and serve.

Per Serving: (½ of finished smoothie recipe): Calories: 535; Fat: 51g; Protein: 13g; Total Carbs: 17g; Fiber: 7g; Net Carbs: 10g; **Macros:** Fat: 79%; Protein: 9%; Carbs: 12%

Peanut Butter Cup Protein Smoothie

SERVES 2 | PREP TIME: 5 minutes

1 cup water
¾ cup coconut cream
1 scoop chocolate protein powder

2 tablespoons natural peanut butter
3 ice cubes

Put the water, coconut cream, protein powder, peanut butter, and ice in a blender and blend until smooth.

Per Serving: Calories: 486; Fat: 40g; Protein: 30g; Total Carbs: 11g; Fiber: 5g; Net Carbs: 6g; **Macros:** Fat: 70%; Protein: 20%; Carbs: 10%

Chocolate, Peanut Butter, and Banana Shake

SERVES 2 | TOTAL TIME: 10 minutes

1 cup crushed ice, divided
3 tablespoons unsweetened chocolate protein powder
1 tablespoon unsweetened peanut butter
1 tablespoon coconut oil
1½ teaspoons cocoa powder

1 cup unsweetened almond milk
¼ cup heavy (whipping) cream
1 teaspoon banana extract
½ teaspoon pure vanilla extract

In a blender, blend ½ cup of ice, protein powder, peanut butter, and coconut oil. Add the cocoa powder, almond milk, heavy cream, banana extract, vanilla, and remaining ½ cup of ice. Blend for 1 minute, or until smooth, and serve.

Per Serving: Calories: 473; Fat: 46g; Protein: 10g; Total Carbs: 11g; Fiber: 4g; Net Carbs: 7g; **Macros:** Fat: 84%; Protein: 8%; Carbs: 8%

Chocolate-Mint Smoothie

SERVES 2 | PREP TIME: 10 minutes

1 cup unsweetened almond milk	1 teaspoon chopped fresh mint
2 tablespoons almond butter	2 (7g) stevia packets
2 tablespoons cocoa powder	1 cup ice cubes

In a blender, blend the almond milk, almond butter, cocoa powder, mint, and stevia until combined. Add the ice, and blend until smooth.

Per Serving: Calories: 129; Fat: 11g; Protein: 5g; Total Carbs: 6g; Fiber: 3g; Net Carbs: 3g

Almond Butter and Cacao Nib Smoothie

SERVES 1 | PREP TIME: 5 minutes

1 cup unsweetened almond milk	1 to 2 teaspoons monk fruit extract or sugar-free sweetener (optional)
¼ cup heavy (whipping) cream	½ teaspoon almond extract (optional)
2 tablespoons unsweetened almond butter	½ teaspoon ground cinnamon
1 tablespoon unsweetened cocoa powder	
1 tablespoon cacao nibs	

In a blender combine the almond milk, cream, almond butter, cocoa powder, cacao nibs, sweetener (if using), almond extract (if using), and cinnamon. Blend until smooth and creamy, adding more almond milk if needed. Serve garnished with additional cacao nibs if desired.

Per Serving: Calories: 506; Fat: 47g; Protein: 11g; Total Carbs: 16g; Fiber: 9g; Net Carbs: 7g; **Macros:** Fat: 84%; Protein: 9%; Carbs: 7%

Double Chocolate Shake

SERVES 2 | TOTAL TIME: 10 minutes

1 cup crushed ice, divided	1 tablespoon unsweetened cocoa powder
¾ cup unsweetened almond milk	1 tablespoon chopped 90 percent dark chocolate
¼ cup heavy (whipping) cream	1 tablespoon sugar-free chocolate syrup
1 tablespoon coconut oil	
3 tablespoons unsweetened chocolate protein powder	

In a blender, blend ½ cup of ice, almond milk, heavy cream, and coconut oil. Add the protein powder, cocoa powder, dark chocolate, chocolate syrup, and remaining ½ cup of ice. Blend for 1 minute, or until smooth, and serve.

Per Serving: Calories: 451; Fat: 41g; Protein: 10g; Total Carbs: 19g; Fiber: 6g; Net Carbs: 13g; **Macros:** Fat: 76%; Protein: 8%; Carbs: 16%

Chocolate Protein Shake

1 SERVING | PREP TIME: 5 minutes

1 cup unsweetened full-fat coconut milk	1 cup fresh spinach
1 scoop collagen powder	½ teaspoon stevia or 4 drops liquid stevia extract
1 teaspoon cacao powder	A few ice cubes (optional)
1 tablespoon MCT oil	

Place the coconut milk, collagen, cacao powder, MCT oil, spinach, stevia, ice (if using), and blend until smooth.

Per Serving: Calories: 631; Fat: 55g; Protein: 19g; Total Carbs: 15g; Fiber: 8g; Net Carbs: 7g; **Macros:** Fat: 78%; Protein: 12%; Carbs: 10%

Vanilla Bean Smoothie

SERVES 2 | PREP TIME: 10 minutes

1 cup almond milk	1 teaspoon coconut oil
½ avocado	Seeds of 1 vanilla bean
2 tablespoons egg white protein powder	¼ teaspoon ground cinnamon
	2 cups ice cubes

In a blender, blend the almond milk, avocado, egg white powder, coconut oil, vanilla bean seeds, and cinnamon until combined. Add the ice, and blend until smooth and thick.

Per Serving: Calories: 158; Fat: 13g; Protein: 6g; Total Carbs: 5g; Fiber: 4g; Net Carbs: 1g; **Macros:** Fat: 73%; Protein: 15%; Carbs: 12%

Vanilla Shake

SERVES 2 | TOTAL TIME: 10 minutes

1 cup crushed ice, divided	3 tablespoons unsweetened vanilla whey protein powder
1 cup unsweetened almond milk	1 teaspoon pure vanilla extract
¼ cup heavy (whipping) cream	
1 tablespoon coconut oil	

In a blender, blend ½ cup of ice, almond milk, heavy cream, and coconut oil. Add the protein powder, vanilla, and remaining ½ cup of ice. Blend for 1 minute, or until smooth, and serve.

Per Serving: Calories: 448; Fat: 41g; Protein: 17g; Total Carbs: 8g; Fiber: 2g; Net Carbs: 6g; **Macros:** Fat: 78%; Protein: 15%; Carbs: 7%

Strawberries and Cream Shake

SERVES 2 | PREP TIME: 10 minutes

1 cup crushed ice, divided	1 tablespoon coconut oil
¼ cup unsweetened almond milk	½ cup strawberries
½ cup heavy (whipping) cream	1 teaspoon pure vanilla extract

In a blender, blend ½ cup of ice, almond milk, heavy cream, and coconut oil. Add the strawberries, vanilla, and remaining ½ cup of ice. Blend for 1 minute, or until smooth, and serve.

Per Serving: Calories: 249; Fat: 25g; Protein: 2g; Total Carbs: 6g; Fiber: 1g; Net Carbs: 5g; **Macros:** Fat: 88%; Protein: 9%; Carbs: 3%

Cheesecake Smoothie

SERVES 2 | PREP TIME: 10 minutes

¾ cup unsweetened almond milk	¼ cup Greek yogurt
	2 tablespoons cream cheese

1 tablespoon heavy
(whipping) cream

2 (7g) stevia packets
2 cups ice cubes

1½ cups iced coffee

¼ cup heavy
(whipping) cream

In a blender, blend the almond milk, yogurt, cream cheese, cream, and stevia until combined. Add the ice, and blend until smooth and blend until smooth, and serve.

Per Serving: Calories: 113; Fat: 9g; Protein: 5g; Total Carbs: 2g; Fiber: 0g; Net Carbs: 2g; **Macros:** Fat: 74%; Protein: 19%; Carbs: 7%

In a blender, blend ½ cup of ice, butter, MCT oil, and coffee. Add the heavy cream and remaining ½ cup of ice. Blend for 1 minute, or until smooth, and serve.

Per Serving: Calories: 486; Fat: 55g; Protein: 1g; Total Carbs: 1g; Fiber: 0g; Net Carbs: 1g; **Macros:** Fat: 98%; Protein: 1%; Carbs: 1%

Berry Cheesecake Smoothie

1 SERVING | PREP TIME: 5 minutes

½ cup unsweetened full-fat
coconut milk
½ cup cold water
1 tablespoon MCT oil
¼ cup full-fat
cream cheese

½ teaspoon stevia or
4 drops liquid stevia
extract
¼ cup blueberries
A few ice cubes (optional)

Place the milk, water, MCT oil, cream cheese, stevia, blueberries, ice (if using), and blend until smooth.

Per Serving: Calories: 575; Fat: 55g; Protein: 7g; Total Carbs: 13g; Fiber: 4g; Net Carbs: 9g; **Macros:** Fat: 86%; Protein: 5%; Carbs: 9%

Avocado Coconut Smoothie

SERVES 2 | TOTAL TIME: 10 minutes

1 cup crushed ice, divided
1 avocado, peeled and pitted
1 cup unsweetened, full-fat
coconut milk

1 tablespoon coconut oil
1 tablespoon unsweetened
coconut flakes

In a blender, blend ½ cup of ice, avocado, coconut milk, and coconut oil. Add the remaining ½ cup of ice and coconut flakes. Blend for 1 minute, or until smooth, and serve.

Per Serving: Calories: 512; Fat: 51g; Protein: 4g; Total Carbs: 13g; Fiber: 7g; Net Carbs: 6g; **Macros:** Fat: 87%; Protein: 3%; Carbs: 10%

Pumpkin Pie Smoothie

SERVES 2 | PREP TIME: 5 minutes

1 cup canned pumpkin purée
¾ cup unsweetened
coconut milk
2 tablespoons vanilla
hemp protein
2 tablespoons erythritol

1 tablespoon coconut cream
or coconut yogurt
1 teaspoon vanilla extract
1 teaspoon pumpkin pie spice,
plus more for serving
Sugar-free maple syrup, for
serving (optional)

In a blender, combine the pumpkin purée, hemp milk, hemp protein, erythritol, coconut cream, vanilla extract, and pumpkin pie spice and blend until smooth. Pour into a glass and serve with an extra sprinkle of pumpkin pie spice, or you can drizzle some syrup on top.

Per Serving: Calories: 438; Fat: 30g; Protein: 14g; Total Carbs: 28g; Fiber: 13g; Net Carbs: 13g; **Macros:** Fat: 62%; Protein: 13%; Carbs: 25%

Buttered Coffee Shake

SERVES 1 | PREP TIME: 10 minutes

1 cup crushed ice, divided
2 tablespoons unsalted, butter

1½ tablespoons MCT oil, or
coconut oil

Coffee Smoothie

SERVES 2 | PREP TIME: 5 minutes

1 cup unsweetened hemp milk
½ cup ice
⅓ cup cold-brew coffee
½ avocado
2 tablespoons cacao powder

1 scoop plant-based, low-carb
protein powder (such as
Truvani or Sunwarrior
brands) (optional)
2 or 3 drops liquid stevia

Combine all the ingredients in a blender and blend on high until creamy and smooth.

Per Serving: Calories: 130; Fat: 9g; Protein: 3g; Total Carbs: 8g; Fiber: 4g; Net Carbs: 4g; **Macros:** Fat: 65%; Protein: 10%; Carbs: 25%

BREAKFAST

Cherry-Coconut Pancakes

SERVES 3 | PREP TIME: 5 minutes | COOK TIME: 25 minutes

1 cup fresh or frozen dark
cherries, thawed and
coarsely chopped
1 tablespoon water or lemon
juice, plus more if needed
1 teaspoon vanilla
extract, divided
2 to 4 teaspoons monk
fruit extract or powdered
sugar-free sweetener
(optional)

¼ cup almond meal
¼ cup coconut flour
¼ cup ground flaxseed
1 teaspoon baking powder
½ teaspoon ground cinnamon
½ cup heavy (whipping)
cream or full-fat canned
coconut milk
1 large egg
2 tablespoons coconut
oil, divided

In a small saucepan, heat the cherries, water, and ½ teaspoon of vanilla over medium-high heat for 5 to 6 minutes, until bubbly, add more water if it is too thick. Stir in the sweetener (if using). Mash the cherries and whisk until the mixture is smooth. Remove from the heat. In a large bowl, whisk the almond meal, coconut flour, flaxseed, baking powder, and cinnamon. Whisk in the cream, egg, 1 tablespoon of coconut oil, the remaining ½ teaspoon of vanilla, and a quarter of the cherry syrup mixture. In large nonstick skillet, heat the remaining 1 tablespoon of coconut oil over medium-low heat. Using about 2 tablespoons of batter for each, form three pancakes. Cook for 4 to 5 minutes, until bubbles begin to form, then flip. Cook for 2 to 3 minutes on the second side, until the pancakes are golden brown. Repeat this process with the remaining batter.

Per Serving: Calories: 511; Fat: 41g; Protein: 12g; Total Carbs: 27g; Fiber: 13g; Net Carbs: 14g; **Macros:** Fat: 72%; Protein: 9%; Carbs: 19%

Spiced Cream Cheese Pancakes

SERVES 4 | PREP TIME: 15 minutes | COOK TIME: 10 minutes

8 ounces cream cheese, at
   room temperature
6 large eggs
3 (7g) stevia packets
¾ cup almond flour

1 teaspoon ground cinnamon
¼ teaspoon ground nutmeg
Pinch ground allspice
¼ cup butter

In a blender, pulse the cream cheese, eggs, stevia, almond flour, cinnamon, nutmeg, and allspice until the mixture is very smooth. In a large skillet on medium-high heat, melt 1 tablespoon of butter. When the butter is sizzling, pour batter for 4 pancakes, about ¼ cup each, into the skillet. Cook until the underside is golden, and flip the pancakes over, about 2 minutes. Cook until the second side is golden, about 2 minutes. Transfer the pancakes to plates, and repeat the process with 1 tablespoon of butter and the remaining batter. Serve topped with butter.

Per Serving: (2 pancakes): Calories: 410; Fat: 33g; Protein: 17g; Total Carbs: 9g; Fiber: 3g; Net Carbs: 6g; **Macros:** Fat: 74%; Protein: 17%; Carbs: 9%

Winter Squash Pancakes

SERVES 1 | PREP TIME: 5 minutes | COOK TIME: 8 to 10 minutes

1 large egg
½ cup puréed
   butternut squash
3 tablespoons coconut flour
2 tablespoons erythritol

¼ teaspoon vanilla extract
1 tablespoon coconut oil
   or butter
Powdered coffee creamer or
   maple syrup (optional)

In a mixing bowl, combine the egg, butternut squash, flour, erythritol, and vanilla and stir together. In a small sauté pan over medium heat, melt the coconut oil or butter. Pour your batter in. Cook one side of the pancake until you can easily stick your spatula underneath all sides, 5 to 8 minutes. Carefully flip the pancake over and cook for another 3 to 4 minutes. Plate and top with creamer or syrup, if desired.

Per Serving: Calories: 331; Fat: 22g; Protein: 11g; Total Carbs: 25g; Fiber: 8g; Net Carbs: 17g; **Macros:** Fat: 58%; Protein: 13%; Carbs: 28%

Almond Butter Pancakes

SERVES 1 | PREP TIME: 5 minutes | COOK TIME: 10 minutes

Nonstick cooking spray
2 tablespoons almond butter
¼ cup unsweetened
   cashew milk
5 or 6 drops liquid stevia

1 tablespoon ground flaxseed
1 tablespoon coconut flour
½ teaspoon baking powder
½ teaspoon ground cinnamon
2 tablespoons butter

Spray a skillet with nonstick cooking spray. In a small bowl, combine the almond butter, cashew milk, and stevia. In a separate small bowl, combine the flaxseed, coconut flour, baking powder, and cinnamon. Mix well. Stir the wet ingredients into the dry and stir until smooth. Allow the batter to sit for 3 to 4 minutes to thicken. Heat the skillet over medium-high heat. When hot, pour the batter into 3- to 4-inch circles and

cook for about 4 minutes. Flip the pancakes and cook for an additional 2 minutes. Top with the butter and enjoy.

Per Serving: (3 pancakes) Calories: 573; Fat: 55g; Protein: 9g; Total Carbs: 11g; Fiber: 7g; Net Carbs: 4g; **Macros:** Fat: 86%; Protein: 6%; Carbs: 8%

Almond and Vanilla Pancakes

SERVES 4 | PREP TIME: 10 minutes | COOK TIME: 15 minutes

⅔ cup unsweetened
   almond milk
1 tablespoon apple
   cider vinegar
¼ cup coconut oil or
   vegan butter
1 teaspoon vanilla extract
1 cup coconut flour
1 cup almond flour

2 tablespoons ground
   flaxseed
½ teaspoon baking powder
Coconut oil cooking spray
Almond slivers, for serving
Vegan butter or coconut oil,
   for serving
Sugar-free maple syrup
   for topping

Preheat the oven to a warming setting. Blend the almond milk, vinegar, coconut oil, and vanilla in a high-powered blender until smooth. Add the coconut flour, almond flour, flaxseed, and baking powder. Blend for 3 minutes until the batter is full and fluffy. If the batter seems too thick, add a few tablespoons of water to thin it out. Heat a medium skillet over medium-low heat and coat it with coconut oil spray to prevent sticking. Once the skillet is hot, pour a small portion of batter into the pan, and cook for about 3 minutes (or until the top of the batter stops bubbling). Flip the pancake and cook until toasted on the opposite side. Place the finished pancake on a warming rack in the oven. Repeat steps 5 to 7 until all of the batter has been cooked. Top the pancakes with almond slivers, vegan butter, and maple syrup.

Per Serving: Calories: 426; Fat: 33g; Protein: 11g; Total Carbs: 28g; Fiber: 16g; Net Carbs: 12g; **Macros:** Fat: 66%; Protein: 9%; Carbs: 25%

Cream Cheese Pancakes

SERVES 1 | PREP TIME: 5 minutes | COOK TIME: 10 minutes

¼ cup cream cheese, at room
   temperature
2 large eggs

½ teaspoon stevia
¼ teaspoon nutmeg

Heat a griddle over medium-low heat. Place the cream cheese in a blender. Add the eggs, stevia, and nutmeg in a blender. Pulse until the batter is smooth. Slowly pour ⅛ cup of batter onto the griddle per pancake. The batter will be very thin and spread easily. Cook the pancake for just over 1 minute before gently flipping. Cook for another minute before removing from the pan. Repeat with the remaining batter.

Per Serving: (6 to 8 pancakes): Calories: 327; Fat: 29g; Protein: 15g; Total Carbs: 3g; Fiber: 0g; Net Carbs: 3g; **Macros:** Fat: 78%; Protein: 18%; Carbs: 4%

Lemon–Olive Oil Breakfast Cakes

SERVES 4 | PREP TIME: 5 minutes | COOK TIME: 10 minutes

For the pancakes

1 cup almond flour
1 teaspoon baking powder

¼ teaspoon salt

6 tablespoon extra-virgin
olive oil, divided

2 large eggs

For the berry sauce

1 cup frozen mixed berries

½ teaspoon vanilla extract

Zest and juice of 1 lemon

½ teaspoon almond or
vanilla extract

1 tablespoon water or
lemon juice, plus more
if needed

Combine the almond flour, baking powder, and salt in a large bowl
and whisk to break up any clumps. Add the ¼ cup olive oil, eggs,
lemon zest and juice, and almond extract and whisk to combine
well. In a large skillet, heat 1 tablespoon of olive oil and spoon about
2 tablespoons of batter for each of 4 pancakes. Cook until bubbles begin to form, 4 to 5 minutes, and flip. Cook for another 2 to
3 minutes on the second side. Repeat with remaining 1 tablespoon
olive oil and batter. In a small saucepan, heat the frozen berries,
water, and vanilla extract over medium-high for 3 to 4 minutes,
until bubbly, adding more water if mixture is too thick. Using the
back of a spoon or fork, mash the berries and whisk until smooth.

Per Serving: (2 pancakes with ¼ cup berry syrup): Calories: 275;
Fat: 26g; Protein: 4g; Total Carbs: 8g; Fiber: 2g; Net Carbs: 6g;
Macros: Fat: 83%; Protein: 6%; Carbs: 11%

Pumpkin Pancakes with Maple Frosting

PREP TIME: 10 minutes | COOK TIME: 20 minutes

For the maple cream cheese frosting

4 ounces (about ½ cup) cream
cheese, at room temperature

½ cup confectioners' erythritol–monk fruit blend

¼ cup sugar-free maple syrup

2 tablespoons heavy
(whipping) cream

½ teaspoon pure vanilla extract

¼ teaspoon ground cinnamon

⅛ teaspoon sea salt

For the pancakes

7 large eggs, at room
temperature

8 ounces (about 1 cup) cream
cheese, at room temperature

½ cup canned pumpkin purée

¼ cup heavy (whipping) cream

1 teaspoon pure
vanilla extract

½ cup coconut flour

½ cup granulated erythritol–
monk fruit blend

2 teaspoons baking powder

2 teaspoons ground cinnamon

½ teaspoon ground ginger

¼ teaspoon ground nutmeg

Pinch ground cloves

¼ teaspoon sea salt

2 to 3 tablespoons
butter, divided

In a medium bowl using an electric mixer, beat the cream cheese,
erythritol–monk fruit blend, maple syrup, cream, vanilla, cinnamon, and salt until it is a creamy consistency. Set aside. Using
a high-powered blender (or an electric mixer and a large mixing
bowl), blend the eggs, cream cheese, pumpkin purée, cream, and
vanilla, until fully combined. Add the coconut flour, sweetener,
baking powder, cinnamon, ginger, nutmeg, cloves, and salt. Mix
the pancake batter. In a nonstick skillet over medium heat, melt
1 teaspoon of butter. Using a ladle, add about 3 tablespoons of
batter to the hot skillet. Cook for about 2 minutes, or until bubbles
start to form. Flip, and cook for another 1½ to 2 minutes, or until
fully cooked. Repeat the process with the rest of the batter, adding
butter to the pan each time. Serve spread with the frosting.

Per Serving: Calories: 252; Fat: 21g; Protein: 8g; Total Carbs: 9g;
Fiber: 3g; Net Carbs: 6g; Macros: Fat: 75%; Protein: 13%; Carbs: 12%

Chocolate, Chocolate Chip Pancakes

MAKES 10 PANCAKES | PREP TIME: 10 minutes |
COOK TIME: 20 minutes

7 large eggs, at room
temperature

8 ounces (about 1 cup) cream
cheese, at room temperature

½ cup heavy (whipping) cream

1 teaspoon pure vanilla extract

½ cup granulated erythritol–
monk fruit blend

½ cup coconut flour

¼ cup unsweetened
cocoa powder

2 teaspoons baking powder

¼ teaspoon sea salt

2 to 3 tablespoons
butter, divided

¼ cup sugar-free
chocolate chips

Using a high-powered blender (or an electric mixer and a large
mixing bowl), blend the eggs, cream cheese, cream, and vanilla until
fully combined. Add the sweetener, coconut flour, cocoa powder,
baking powder, and salt. Blend the pancake batter, scraping down
the sides of the blender with a spatula a few times. In a nonstick
skillet over medium heat, melt 1 teaspoon of butter. Using a ladle,
add about 3 tablespoons of batter to the hot skillet, and sprinkle a
few chocolate chips over the top of the pancakes. Cook for about
2 minutes, or until bubbles start to form. Flip, and cook for another
1½ to 2 minutes or until fully cooked. Repeat with the rest of the
batter, adding butter before each new ladle of batter.

Per Serving: Calories: 249; Fat: 21g; Protein: 8g; Total Carbs: 11g;
Fiber: 4g; Net Carbs: 7g; Macros: Fat: 76%; Protein: 13%; Carbs: 11%

Ricotta Pancakes

SERVES 4 | PREP TIME: 5 minutes | COOK TIME: 20 minutes

5 ounces ricotta
cheese, drained

⅓ cup granular erythritol

2 teaspoons vanilla extract

2 tablespoons unsweetened
vanilla almond milk

1 cup almond flour

1 teaspoon baking powder

⅛ teaspoon cream of tartar

4 large eggs

¼ cup butter, divided

Preheat the oven to its lowest setting. Place a baking sheet in
the oven. In a large bowl, whisk the ricotta, erythritol, vanilla,
almond milk, almond flour, baking powder, cream of tartar, and
eggs until smooth. Thin the batter with almond milk if necessary. In a small nonstick skillet over medium-low heat, melt
1 tablespoon of butter. Pour ¼ cup of batter into the pan and
cook until golden, about 4 minutes per side. Transfer the pancake to the baking sheet in the oven. Repeat until the batter has
been used. Serve with your favorite toppings.

Per Serving: (1 pancake): Calories: 401; Fat: 35g; Protein: 15g;
Total Carbs: 25g; Fiber: 3g; Net Carbs: 6g; Macros: Fat: 75%;
Protein: 15%; Carbs: 10%

Banana Bread Blender Pancakes

SERVES 2 | PREP TIME: 10 minutes | COOK TIME: 10 minutes

2 large eggs

½ cup diced zucchini

¼ cup creamy almond butter,
well stirred

1 tablespoon coconut flour

2 teaspoons monk fruit/erythritol blend sweetener

¾ teaspoon ground cinnamon

¾ teaspoon banana extract

½ teaspoon vanilla extract

½ teaspoon baking powder

¼ teaspoon kosher salt

Coconut oil spray, or your favorite nonstick spray

1½ tablespoons finely chopped toasted pecans, divided, plus more for serving

Sugar-free syrup, for serving

In a blender, combine the eggs, zucchini, almond butter, coconut flour, sweetener, cinnamon, banana extract, vanilla, baking powder, and salt. Blend until smooth and silky. Coat a griddle pan with coconut spray and preheat it over medium heat. Pour about ¼ cup of batter onto the griddle for each pancake. Turn the heat to medium-low and cook the pancakes for 2 to 3 minutes until bubbles form on the surface and begin to burst around the edges. Sprinkle about 1 teaspoon pecans over each pancake. Using a spatula, carefully flip the pancakes and cook for about 1 minute on the second side. Repeat until all the batter is used. Serve warm with sugar-free syrup and more chopped pecans.

Per Serving: Calories: 350; Fat: 26g; Protein: 15g; Total Carbs: 14g; Fiber: 8g; Net Carbs: 6g; **Macros:** Fat: 67%; Protein: 17%; Carbs: 16%

Keto Blueberry Pancakes

MAKES 12 | PREP TIME: 10 minutes | COOK TIME: 20 minutes

2½ cups almond flour, sifted

2 teaspoons baking powder

4 large eggs, lightly beaten

⅔ cup almond milk

½ cup butter, melted, plus more for serving

1 teaspoon vanilla extract

½ cup fresh blueberries

Nonstick cooking spray

Sugar-free pancake syrup (optional)

In a large bowl, whisk the flour and baking powder until combined. Add the eggs, almond milk, butter, and vanilla and whisk until smooth. Carefully fold in the blueberries. Preheat a nonstick skillet or griddle over medium-high heat, and coat with cooking spray or brush lightly with oil. Working in batches, pour ¼ cup of batter into the skillet for each pancake. When bubbles start to appear on the surface of the pancakes, carefully flip. Cook for 2 to 3 minutes more, then transfer to a plate. Repeat with the remaining batter. Serve topped with melted butter.

Per Serving: Calories: 387; Fat: 35g; Protein: 11g; Total Carbs: 12g; Fiber: 4g; Net Carbs: 8g; **Macros:** Fat: 77%; Protein: 12%; Carbs: 11%

Chaffles

SERVES 1 | PREP TIME: 5 minutes | COOK TIME: 10 to 15 minutes

Nonstick cooking spray, butter, or oil for greasing the waffle maker

1 large egg

⅓ cup grated Cheddar cheese, divided

Grease and preheat a waffle maker. In a small bowl, whisk the egg and a third of the cheese. Sprinkle some grated cheese right onto the waffle maker and add half the egg and cheese mixture. Sprinkle a little more cheese on the mixture and close the lid on the waffle maker. Let the waffle cook for 4 to 5 minutes. If it's not as crispy as you'd like, flip and cook for 1 to 2 minutes more. Repeat the process with the remaining egg mixture and cheese.

Per Serving: Calories: 222; Fat: 17g; Protein: 16g; Total Carbs: 1g; Fiber: 0g; Net Carbs: 1g; **Macros:** Fat: 69%; Protein: 29%; Carbs: 2%

Spaghetti Squash Chaffles

SERVES 6 | PREP TIME: 10 minutes | COOK TIME: 1 hour 45 minutes

1 small spaghetti squash (about 1 pound)

1 tablespoon olive oil

½ teaspoon salt, divided

Oil or nonstick cooking spray, for greasing

3 large eggs

½ cup grated mozzarella cheese

1 cup grated Parmesan cheese, divided

½ teaspoon garlic powder

½ teaspoon minced garlic

Preheat the oven to 425°F, and line a baking sheet with parchment paper. Cut the squash in half horizontally, and scoop out the seeds and strings. Drizzle each half with the olive oil, and season with ¼ teaspoon of salt. Bake cut-side down for 30 minutes, flip, and cook 10 minutes. Remove from the oven. When, use a fork to rake the squash strands into a small colander or cheesecloth. Mash or squeeze out the excess water; then place the squash in a medium bowl, and use a fork to pull apart the strands. Grease and preheat a waffle maker. Add the eggs, mozzarella, ½ cup of Parmesan, the remaining salt, garlic powder, and minced garlic to the spaghetti squash and mix. Drop two spoonfuls of the squash mixture onto the waffle maker, just enough to cover and fill the waffle plate. Sprinkle with a little Parmesan cheese, and shut the lid for 4 minutes. Open the lid, flip the chaffle over, sprinkle a little Parmesan across the top, close, and cook another 4 minutes. Repeat with the remaining squash mixture.

Per Serving: (1 chaffle): Calories: 196; Fat: 15g; Protein: 9g; Total Carbs: 6g; Fiber: 1g; Net Carbs: 5g; **Macros:** Fat: 69%; Protein: 19%; Carbs: 12%

Belgian-Style Waffles

MAKES 4 | PREP TIME: 5 minutes | COOK TIME: 10 minutes

4 large eggs

4 ounces full-fat cream cheese, at room temperature

1 tablespoon melted butter

1 teaspoon vanilla extract

½ teaspoon maple extract (optional)

¼ cup fine almond flour

1 tablespoon coconut flour

½ tablespoon baking powder

2 tablespoons granular erythritol

Pinch sea salt

1 tablespoon unsweetened almond milk (optional)

Coconut cooking spray or butter, for greasing

Heat a waffle iron. Put the eggs, cream cheese, butter, vanilla, maple extract (if using), almond and coconut flours, baking powder, erythritol, and salt in a blender and blend on high speed until completely combined. Add the almond milk if you desire a thinner consistency and blend again until combined. Spray the waffle iron with cooking spray. Pour ¼ cup of batter onto the waffle iron and cook for 2 to 3 minutes or until browned and slightly crisped on both sides. Remove the waffle. Repeat to make 3 more waffles. Serve with your favorite toppings.

Per Serving: (1 waffle): Calories: 237; Fat: 20g; Protein: 10g; Total Carbs: 11g; Fiber: 1g; Net Carbs: 4g; **Macros:** Fat: 74%; Protein: 17%; Carbs: 9%

Chaffle and Lox

SERVES 4 | PREP TIME: 5 minutes | COOK TIME: 5 minutes

2 large eggs

1 cup shredded mozzarella cheese

¼ cup almond flour

1 teaspoon everything bagel seasoning, plus more for garnish

½ teaspoon baking powder

5 tablespoons extra-virgin olive oil, divided

4 ounces goat cheese

4 ounces smoked salmon

4 thin slices red onion

8 thin slices cucumber

1 tablespoon chopped capers

Heat a waffle maker over medium heat. In a medium bowl, whisk the eggs, cheese, almond flour, everything seasoning, baking powder, and 1 tablespoon of olive oil until smooth. When the waffle maker is hot, pour in half the batter and cook until done. Repeat with the remaining batter. Spread 1 ounce of goat cheese over each waffle and top with 1 ounce of smoked salmon, 1 slice of red onion, 2 slices of cucumber and chopped capers. Drizzle with olive oil and serve.

Per Serving: Calories: 466; Fat: 40g; Protein: 22g; Total Carbs: 4g; Fiber: 1g; Net Carbs: 3g; **Macros:** Fat: 77%; Protein: 19%; Carbs: 4%

Vanilla Belgian Waffles

SERVES 4 | PREP TIME: 10 minutes | COOK TIME: 20 minutes

8 large eggs, at room temperature

½ cup canned coconut milk

¼ cup butter, melted

½ teaspoon pure vanilla extract

½ cup coconut flour

¼ teaspoon baking soda

¼ teaspoon sea salt

In a large bowl, whisk the eggs until they are very frothy, about 3 minutes. Whisk in the coconut milk, butter, and vanilla until blended. Whisk the coconut flour, baking soda, and salt into the egg mixture until the batter is smooth and thick, about 1 minute. Let the batter rest for 15 minutes so the coconut flour can thicken it. Heat up the waffle maker, and make the waffles according to the manufacturer's directions. Serve.

Per Serving: Calories: 384; Fat: 31g; Protein: 16g; Total Carbs: 11g; Fiber: 7g; Net Carbs: 4g; **Macros:** Fat: 72%; Protein: 17%; Carbs: 11%

Coconut Flour–Based Chocolate Chip Waffles

SERVES 2 | PREP TIME: 10 minutes | COOK TIME: 8 to 10 minutes

½ cup coconut flour

3 tablespoons baking stevia

1 large egg

½ cup unsweetened coconut yogurt

1 teaspoon vanilla extract

2 tablespoons sugar-free dark chocolate chips

1 tablespoon coconut oil, for greasing

1 scoop So Delicious no-sugar-added coconut milk ice cream

1 to 2 tablespoons ChocoZero, or syrup of choice

½ cup whipped cream or coconut whipped cream

Preheat a waffle iron. In a bowl, mix the flour, stevia, egg, yogurt, vanilla, and chocolate chips until well combined. Grease the waffle iron well with coconut oil, butter, or nonstick spray. Pour in half the batter. Close and let cook for 8 to 10 minutes. Remove the waffle and transfer to a plate. Repeat with the remaining batter to make one more waffle. Scoop ½ cup of ice cream on top of each and drizzle the syrup over everything. Top each waffle with whipped cream.

Per Serving: Calories: 582; Fat: 44g; Protein: 12g; Total Carbs: 39g; Fiber: 19g; Net Carbs: 20g; **Macros:** Fat: 68%; Protein: 6%; Carbs: 26%

Waffles with Whipped Cream

MAKES 4 TO 5 WAFFLES | PREP TIME: 5 minutes | COOK TIME: 10 minutes

Cooking spray for waffle iron

¼ cup coconut flour

¼ cup almond flour

¼ cup flax meal

1 teaspoon baking powder

1 teaspoon stevia, or other sugar substitute

¼ teaspoon cinnamon

¾ cup egg whites (about 3 large whites)

4 large eggs

1 teaspoon pure vanilla extract

½ cup heavy (whipping) cream

1 teaspoon stevia, or other sugar substitute

Heat the waffle iron to medium-high heat. Coat with cooking spray. In a large bowl, whisk the coconut flour, almond flour, flax meal, baking powder, stevia, and cinnamon. In another medium bowl, beat the egg whites until stiff peaks form. Add the whole eggs and vanilla to the dry ingredients. Mix well to combine. Gently fold the beaten egg whites into the dry ingredients until fully incorporated. Pour the batter onto the preheated waffle iron. Cook according to waffle iron directions. In a medium bowl, whip the heavy cream for 3 to 4 minutes, until thick. Add the stevia. Continue to whisk until stiff peaks form, about 1 minute more. Top the waffles with whipped cream and serve.

Per Serving: (2 waffles; ½ of the whipped cream): Calories: 420; Fat: 27g; Protein: 27g; Total Carbs: 16g; Fiber: 9g; Net Carbs: 7g; **Macros:** Fat: 58%; Protein: 27%; Carbs: 15%

Coconut Flaxseed Waffles

SERVES 4 | PREP TIME: 15 minutes | COOK TIME: 5 minutes

Nonstick cooking spray

5 large eggs

½ cup water

⅓ cup coconut oil, melted

2 cups ground flaxseed

1 tablespoon baking powder

1 teaspoon salt

2 tablespoons unsweetened coconut flakes

5 to 6 drops liquid stevia

¼ cup butter

Spray a waffle iron with cooking spray and heat it to a medium-high temperature. Combine the eggs, water, and coconut oil in a blender. Blend on high speed for 30 to 40 seconds. In a medium bowl, mix the flaxseed, baking powder, and salt until combined. Pour the blender mixture into the flaxseed blend and stir. Allow to sit for 4 to 5 minutes to thicken. Add the coconut flakes and stevia, and mix well. Pour ¼ cup of batter onto the waffle iron and cook. Repeat until all the batter has been used. Top each waffle with 1 tablespoon of butter.

Ham and Swiss Waffles

SERVES 4 | PREP TIME: 10 minutes |
COOK TIME: 25 to 35 minutes

1 cup almond flour, measured and sifted	1 teaspoon pure vanilla extract
¼ cup coconut flour	5 large eggs, at room temperature
2 tablespoons granulated erythritol–monk fruit blend	¼ cup finely chopped ham
1 tablespoon psyllium husk powder	¼ cup finely chopped Swiss cheese
2 teaspoons baking powder	½ to ¾ cup water
½ teaspoon sea salt	2 tablespoons unsalted butter, melted
¼ teaspoon black pepper	
8 ounces (about 1 cup) cream cheese, at room temperature	

Preheat the waffle iron. In a large bowl, whisk the almond flour, coconut flour, sweetener, psyllium husk powder, baking powder, salt, and pepper, and set aside. In a medium bowl, using an electric mixer, combine the cream cheese and vanilla. Add the eggs one at a time, mixing after each. Add the egg mixture to the dry ingredients using a rubber spatula. Fold in the ham and Swiss cheese. Add ½ cup water, and stir to combine. Add up to another ¼ cup water as needed—the batter thickens as it sits. Grease a waffle iron well with the melted butter. Add spoonfuls of batter evenly. Close the waffle iron, and cook according to the manufacturer's instructions.

Per Serving: Calories: 583; Fat: 49g; Protein: 23g; Total Carbs: 17g; Fiber: 8g; Net Carbs: 9g; **Macros:** Fat: 76%; Protein: 16%; Carbs: 8%

Very Berry Waffles

SERVES 4 | PREP TIME: 10 minutes | COOK TIME: 25 to 35 minutes

For the mixed berry topping

½ cup water	¼ cup chopped strawberries
¼ cup blueberries, fresh or frozen	¼ cup granulated erythritol–monk fruit blend
¼ cup raspberries, fresh or frozen	

For the waffles

1 cup almond flour, measured and sifted	8 ounces (about 1 cup) cream cheese, at room temperature
¼ cup coconut flour	1 teaspoon pure vanilla extract
¼ cup granulated erythritol–monk fruit blend	5 large eggs, at room temperature
1 tablespoon psyllium husk powder	½ to ¾ cup water
2 teaspoons baking powder	2 tablespoons unsalted butter, melted
¼ teaspoon sea salt	

In a small saucepan over medium-low heat, gently simmer the water, blueberries, raspberries, strawberries, and sweetener for

7 to 10 minutes, or until the sauce reduces and thickens. Preheat the waffle iron. In a large bowl, whisk the almond flour, coconut flour, sweetener, psyllium husk powder, baking powder, and salt. Set aside. In a medium bowl, combine the cream cheese and vanilla. Add the eggs one at a time, mixing after each. Add the egg mixture to the dry ingredients, and combine using a rubber spatula. Add ½ cup water, and stir to combine. Add up to another ¼ cup water as needed—the batter thickens as it sits. Grease a waffle iron well with the melted butter. Add spoonfuls of batter evenly. Close the waffle iron, and cook according to the manufacturer's instructions. Serve the waffles topped with mixed berry topping.

Per Serving: Calories: 551; Fat: 46g; Protein: 19g; Total Carbs: 20g; Fiber: 9g; Net Carbs: 11g; **Macros:** Fat: 75%; Protein: 14%; Carbs: 11%

Meat Waffles

SERVES 4 | PREP TIME: 5 minutes | COOK TIME: 5 to 20 minutes

Avocado oil, coconut oil, or butter, for greasing	Salt
	Freshly ground black pepper
1 pound ground beef, turkey, pork, or bison	4 large eggs, sunny-side-up or over-easy, for serving (optional)
½ tablespoon garlic powder	
½ tablespoon dried oregano	Sliced cheese, for serving (optional)
½ tablespoon paprika	

Grease a waffle maker with oil or butter. In a bowl, mix your meat of choice with the garlic, oregano, paprika, salt, and pepper. Separate the meat mixture into 4 equal portions and press into the waffle maker. Cook for 3 to 5 minutes or until cooked through. Let cool slightly and serve warm, with a slice of cheese and an egg on top of each waffle, if desired.

Per Serving: Calories: 294; Fat: 19g; Protein: 29g; Total Carbs: 2g; Fiber: 0g; Net Carbs: 2g; **Macros:** Fat: 60%; Protein: 39%; Carbs: 1%

Quick and Easy Blueberry Waffles

SERVES 6 | PREP TIME: 5 minutes | COOK TIME: 30 minutes

1 cup almond flour	5 tablespoons plus 1 teaspoon butter, melted
¼ cup coconut flour	
¼ cup monk fruit/erythritol blend sweetener	2 tablespoons sour cream
	1 teaspoon vanilla extract
2½ teaspoons baking powder	½ cup frozen blueberries, thawed
¼ teaspoon kosher salt	
4 large eggs, slightly beaten	

Preheat a traditional waffle iron to high heat according to the manufacturer's instructions. In a medium bowl, stir the almond and coconut flours, sweetener, baking powder, and salt. In a small bowl, whisk the eggs, melted butter, sour cream, and vanilla until combined. Add the wet ingredients to the dry ingredients and whisk until thoroughly combined. Gently stir in the blueberries, breaking them up into the batter. Add about ½ cup of batter to the waffle iron and close the iron. Cook for 3 to 5 minutes, or until golden brown. Remove. Repeat with the remaining batter.

Per Serving: Calories: 240; Fat: 20g; Protein: 7g; Total Carbs: 8g; Fiber: 4g; Net Carbs: 4g; Macros: Fat: 75%; Protein: 12%; Carbs: 13%

French Toast

SERVES 3 | PREP TIME: 10 to 15 minutes | COOK TIME: 12 to 30 minutes

For the bread

1 tablespoon coconut oil or butter, for greasing

2 large eggs

1 (7-ounce) package cauliflower rice

6 tablespoons coconut flour

For the French toast

¼ cup coconut or almond milk

1 teaspoon ground cinnamon

1 teaspoon nutmeg

2 tablespoons erythritol

1 large egg

½ scoop protein powder

½ teaspoon vanilla extract

2 tablespoons butter-flavored coconut oil or butter

½ cup sugar-free syrup (optional, but highly recommended)

Preheat the oven to 400°F. Grease a bread loaf pan with oil or butter. In a bowl, combine the cauliflower rice, eggs, and flour and mix. Pour the mixture into the prepared loaf pan and bake for 15 to 20 minutes. Remove the bread from the oven. Let cool in the pan for 20 to 30 minutes, then carefully remove from the pan and cut into three equal pieces. To make the French toast: In a mixing bowl, combine the milk, cinnamon, nutmeg, erythritol, egg, protein powder, and vanilla and stir. Heat the coconut oil or butter in a shallow sauté pan over medium heat. Carefully dredge a bread slice it in the milk mixture, and place it in the warm sauté pan. Repeat with the remaining 2 bread slices. Cook on one side for about 6 minutes and then carefully flip and cook on the other side for another 6 minutes or so. Remove from the pan, transfer to plates, and drizzle sugar-free syrup over the top, if desired.

Per Serving: Calories: 506; Fat: 34g; Protein: 24g; Total Carbs: 26g; Fiber: 9g; Net Carbs: 17g; Macros: Fat: 61%; Protein: 19%; Carbs: 20%

Cinnamon French Toast Sticks

SERVES 16 | PREP TIME: 15 minutes | COOK TIME: 35 to 45 minutes, plus 15 to 20 minutes to cool

3 tablespoons golden flax meal

1½ cups almond flour

5 tablespoons granulated erythritol–monk fruit blend, divided

1 tablespoon psyllium husk powder

2 teaspoons baking powder

¼ teaspoon sea salt

⅛ teaspoon xanthan gum

1 cup warm water

4 large eggs, at room temperature, divided

1 tablespoon coconut oil, melted

½ cup heavy (whipping) cream

1 teaspoon ground cinnamon

1 teaspoon pure vanilla extract

3 tablespoons butter, divided

Sugar-free maple syrup (optional)

Preheat the oven to 375°F. Line a large baking sheet with parchment paper. Grind the flax meal in a coffee grinder until it's a fine powder. In a large bowl, combine the almond flour, flax meal powder, 3 tablespoons of sweetener, psyllium husk powder, baking powder, salt, and xanthan gum. Add the warm water,

2 eggs, and the coconut oil, and combine well using a rubber spatula to make a dough. Spread the dough onto the prepared baking sheet using a wet spatula. Bake for 25 to 30 minutes, or until lightly browned. Allow to cool on a wire rack for 15 to 20 minutes before slicing. Using a pizza cutter or sharp knife, cut the baked dough in half widthwise and then into 1½-inch wide strips. You should have 2 rows of 6 sticks. In a small bowl, prepare the egg wash by whisking the remaining 2 eggs, cream, cinnamon, remaining 2 tablespoons of sweetener, and vanilla. In a large skillet over medium heat, melt 1 tablespoon of butter. Dip 4 French toast sticks in the egg batter, and cook until lightly golden brown on both sides, or for 4 to 5 minutes total. Repeat with the remaining butter, French toast sticks, and batter.

Per Serving: Calories: 139; Fat: 13g; Protein: 4g; Total Carbs: 4g; Fiber: 2g; Net Carbs: 2g; Macros: Fat: 84%; Protein: 12%; Carbs: 4%

Sweet 'n' Savory Toast with Burrata and Berries

SERVES 2 | PREP TIME: 5 minutes

½ cup mixed frozen berries

Juice of 1 clementine or ½ orange (about ¼ cup)

½ teaspoon vanilla extract

1 slice of keto bread

2 ounces burrata cheese

In a small saucepan, heat the frozen berries, clementine juice, and vanilla over medium-high heat until simmering. Reduce the heat to low and simmer, stirring occasionally, until the liquid reduces and the mixture becomes syrupy. Cut the sandwich round in half horizontally and toast each half in a toaster or under a broiler. On a rimmed dish, slice the burrata into two slices, reserving the cream. Top each sandwich round half with 1 ounce sliced burrata cheese, the reserved cream, and ¼ cup berry sauce.

Per Serving: (1 toast): Calories: 221; Fat: 17g; Protein: 11g; Total Carbs: 6g; Fiber: 1g; Net Carbs: 5g; Macros: Fat: 69%; Protein: 20%; Carbs: 11%

Toast-less Blueberry French Toast

SERVES 6 | PREP TIME: 5 minutes | COOK TIME: 10 minutes

1 tablespoon butter

6 large eggs

¼ cup almond flour

3 ounces (6 tablespoons) mascarpone cheese

7 tablespoons sugar-free maple-flavored syrup, divided

½ teaspoon cinnamon

½ teaspoon vanilla extract

½ cup blueberries, divided

¼ cup chopped pecans, divided

1 teaspoon confectioners' erythritol blend, for dusting

Preheat the oven to broil. In a medium oven-safe skillet over medium heat, melt the butter. In a medium bowl, whisk the eggs for 30 seconds, and then add the flour, mascarpone, 1 tablespoon of syrup, cinnamon, and vanilla. Mash and stir with a spoon until the bigger chunks of mascarpone are broken up. The mixture will be lumpy. Pour into the skillet, and cook, undisturbed, for 5 minutes. After the first 3 minutes, scatter half the blueberries and half the pecans over the egg mixture. Transfer the skillet to the oven for 5 minutes. Remove from the oven, and scatter the remaining blueberries and pecans over top. Dust with the confectioners' sweetener. Cut into 6 wedges. Serve with syrup.

Per Serving: Calories: 210; Fat: 17g; Protein: 9g; Total Carbs: 7g; Fiber: 2g; Net Carbs: 5g; **Macros:** Fat: 73%; Protein: 17%; Carbs: 4%

Buttery Boiled Eggs

SERVES 1 | PREP TIME: 5 minutes | COOK TIME: 25 minutes

3 large eggs, at room
  temperature

2 teaspoons butter

⅛ teaspoon sea salt

⅛ teaspoon freshly ground
  black pepper

Place the eggs in a large pot. Add enough cold water to cover the eggs by a couple of inches. Slowly bring to a boil over medium-high heat. Once the water begins to boil, remove the pot from the stove and cover. After 15 minutes, transfer the eggs to a bowl of ice-cold water to cool. Peel eggs, place them in a bowl, and slice them up. Place the butter on top and sprinkle with the salt and pepper. Microwave for 30 to 40 seconds, mix, and enjoy.

Per Serving: (3 eggs) Calories: 265; Fat: 21g; Protein: 19g; Total Carbs: 1g; Fiber: 0g; Net Carbs: 1g; **Macros:** Fat: 70%; Protein: 29%; Carbs: 1%

Classic Bacon and Eggs

SERVES 2 | PREP TIME: 5 minutes | COOK TIME: 15 minutes

6 slices bacon

2 tablespoons butter

4 large eggs

Freshly ground black pepper
  (optional)

Preheat the oven to 350°F. Line a rimmed baking sheet with parchment paper. Line a plate with paper towels. Place the bacon slices in a single layer, not overlapping, on the prepared baking sheet. Bake for 13 to 17 minutes. Transfer to the prepared plate. While the bacon is baking, in a medium skillet over medium heat, melt the butter, swirling to coat the pan completely. Crack each egg into a measuring cup or bowl and pour each into the skillet. Allow the eggs to cook undisturbed for about 2 minutes, just until the whites are set. Slide a spatula under each egg and gently flip. Cook for another 1 to 2 minutes (shorter for a runny yolk, longer for a harder one). Season with pepper (if using) and serve with the bacon.

Per Serving: (3 bacon slices and 2 eggs): Calories: 328; Fat: 27g; Protein: 20g; Total Carbs: 1g; Fiber: 0g; Net Carbs: 1g; **Macros:** Fat: 73%; Protein: 26%; Carbs: 1%

Bacon-Wrapped Asparagus and Eggs

SERVES 2 | PREP TIME: 10 minutes | COOK TIME: 20 minutes

4 bacon slices

12 asparagus spears, divided

1 teaspoon minced garlic

½ teaspoon onion powder

½ teaspoon salt, divided

¼ teaspoon freshly ground
  black pepper, divided

1 tablespoon butter

4 large eggs

Preheat the oven to 400°F. Wrap one bacon slice around three asparagus spears and place them on a parchment-lined baking sheet. Sprinkle them with garlic, onion powder, ¼ teaspoon of salt, and a pinch of pepper. Bake for 12 minutes, or until the bacon crisps. In a large skillet over medium-high heat, melt the butter. Crack the eggs into the skillet and cook them to your desired doneness, about 5 minutes for a runny egg. Season with

the remaining ¼ teaspoon of salt and the remaining pepper. Serve two eggs atop two bundles of asparagus per serving.

Per Serving: (2 eggs with 2 bacon-wrapped asparagus bundles): Calories: 479; Fat: 36g; Protein: 33g; Total Carbs: 8g; Fiber: 3g; Net Carbs: 5g; **Macros:** Fat: 66%; Protein: 27%; Carbs: 7%

Scotch Eggs

SERVES 2 | PREP TIME: 15 minutes | COOK TIME: 25 minutes

½ cup breakfast sausage

½ teaspoon garlic powder

¼ teaspoon salt

⅛ teaspoon freshly ground
  black pepper

2 hard-boiled eggs, peeled

Preheat the oven to 400°F. In a medium bowl, mix the sausage, garlic powder, salt, and pepper. Shape the sausage into two ¼-inch-thick patty. Place them on a piece of parchment paper. Place one hard-boiled egg in the center of each patty and gently shape the sausage around the egg. Place the sausage-covered eggs on an ungreased baking sheet and bake for 25 minutes. Allow 5 minutes to cool, and then serve.

Per Serving: (1 sausage-wrapped egg): Calories: 258; Fat: 21g; Protein: 17g; Total Carbs: 1g; Fiber: 0g; Net Carbs: 1g; **Macros:** Fat: 72%; Protein: 26%; Carbs: 2%

Breakfast "Sandwich"

SERVES 4 | PREP TIME: 15 minutes | COOK TIME: 15 minutes

1 tablespoon extra-virgin
  olive oil

2 jalapeño peppers, seeded
  and chopped

1 red bell pepper, chopped

½ leek, white and green parts
  julienned

3 tablespoons butter, divided

4 (3½ ounce) peameal
  bacon slices

¼ cup cream cheese

4 large eggs

Sea salt

Freshly ground black pepper

1 teaspoon chopped fresh
  thyme, for garnish

In a large skillet over medium-high heat, heat the olive oil. Sauté the jalapeño peppers, bell peppers, and leeks until tender, about 4 minutes. Transfer the pepper-leek mixture to a small bowl, and set aside. Wipe out the skillet, and place it back over medium-high heat. Add 1½ tablespoons of butter. Cook the peameal bacon, turning once, until it is browned and cooked through, about 5 minutes total. Remove the bacon from the skillet, and place 1 piece on each plate. Place 1 tablespoon of cream cheese in the middle of each piece of bacon. Wipe the skillet out, and place it back over medium-high heat. Add the remaining 1½ tablespoons of butter, and fry the eggs until the whites are firm and the edges are lacy and brown, about 4 minutes. Top the cream cheese and bacon with 1 egg per plate, and season with salt and pepper. Divide the pepper-leek mixture evenly among the eggs, top each dish with a sprinkle of thyme, and serve.

Per Serving: Calories: 338; Fat: 26g; Protein: 22g; Total Carbs: 7g; Fiber: 2g; Net Carbs: 5g; **Macros:** Fat: 67%; Protein: 25%; Carbs: 8%

Avocado and Eggs with Shredded Chicken

SERVES 4 | PREP TIME: 10 minutes | COOK TIME: 20 minutes

2 avocados, peeled, halved
  lengthwise, and pitted

4 large eggs

1 (4-ounce) chicken breast,
  cooked and shredded

| ¼ cup shredded | Sea salt |
| Cheddar cheese | Freshly ground black pepper |

Preheat the oven to 425°F. Take a spoon and hollow out each side of the avocado halves until the hole is about twice the original size. Place the avocado halves in an 8-inch-square baking dish, hollow-side up. Crack an egg into each hollow and divide the shredded chicken between each half. Sprinkle with cheese and season lightly with the salt and pepper. Bake the avocados until the eggs are cooked through, about 15 to 20 minutes. Serve immediately.

Per serving: Calories: 324; Fat: 25g; Protein: 19g; Total Carbs: 8g; Fiber: 5g; Net Carbs: 3g; **Macros:** Fat: 70%; Protein: 20%; Carbs: 10%

Florentine Breakfast Sandwich

SERVES 1 | PREP TIME: 10 minutes | COOK TIME: 5 minutes

1 teaspoon extra-virgin	1 Versatile Sandwich Round
olive oil	(page 311)
1 large egg	1 tablespoon jarred pesto
¼ teaspoon salt	¼ ripe avocado, mashed
¼ teaspoon freshly ground	1 (¼-inch) thick tomato slice
black pepper	1 (1-ounce) slice fresh
	mozzarella

In a small skillet, heat the olive oil over high heat. When the oil is very hot, crack the egg into the skillet and reduce the heat to medium. Sprinkle the top of the egg with salt and pepper and let it cook for 2 minutes, or until set on bottom. Using a spatula, flip the egg to cook on the other side to desired level of doneness (1 to 2 minutes for a runnier yolk, 2 to 3 minutes for a more set yolk). Remove the egg from the pan. Cut the sandwich round in half horizontally and toast, if desired. Spread the pesto on a toasted bread half. Top with mashed avocado, the tomato slice, mozzarella, and the cooked egg. Top with the other bread half and eat warm.

Per Serving: Calories: 548; Fat: 48g; Protein: 21g; Total Carbs: 8g; Fiber: 3g; Net Carbs: 5g; **Macros:** Fat: 79%; Protein: 15%; Carbs: 6%

Avocado Toast

SERVES 2 | PREP TIME: 5 minutes | COOK TIME: 5 minutes

2 tablespoons ground	½ teaspoon garlic powder,
flaxseed	sesame seed, caraway
½ teaspoon baking powder	seed or other dried herbs
2 large eggs	(optional)
1 teaspoon salt, plus more	3 tablespoons extra-virgin
for serving	olive oil, divided
½ teaspoon freshly ground	1 medium ripe avocado,
black pepper, plus more	peeled, pitted, and sliced
for serving	2 tablespoons chopped ripe
	tomato or salsa

In a small bowl, combine the flaxseed and baking powder. Add the eggs, salt, pepper, and garlic powder (if using) and whisk well. Let sit for 2 minutes. In a small nonstick skillet, heat 1 tablespoon olive oil over medium heat. Pour the egg mixture into the skillet and let cook undisturbed until the egg begins to set on the bottom, 2 to 3 minutes. Using a rubber spatula, scrape

down the sides to allow uncooked egg to reach the bottom. Cook another 2 to 3 minutes. Once almost set, flip like a pancake and cook the other side, 1 to 2 minutes. Remove from the skillet and allow to cool slightly. Slice into 2 pieces. Top each "toast" with avocado slices, salt and pepper, chopped tomato, and drizzle with the remaining 2 tablespoons olive oil.

Per Serving: (1 toast): Calories: 287; Fat: 25g; Protein: 9g; Total Carbs: 10g; Fiber: 7g; Net Carbs: 3g; **Macros:** Fat: 76%; Protein: 12%; Carbs: 12%

Egg Baked in Avocado

SERVES 2 | PREP TIME: 5 minutes | COOK TIME: 15 minutes

1 ripe large avocado	2 tablespoons chopped
2 large eggs	tomato, for serving
Salt	2 tablespoons crumbled feta,
Freshly ground black pepper	for serving (optional)
¼ cup jarred pesto, for serving	

Preheat the oven to 425°F. Slice the avocado in half and remove the pit. Scoop out about 1 to 2 tablespoons from each half to create a hole large enough to fit an egg. Place the avocado halves on a baking sheet, cut-side up. Crack 1 egg in each avocado half and season with salt and pepper. Bake until the eggs are set and cooked to desired level of doneness, 10 to 15 minutes. Remove from the oven and top each avocado with 2 tablespoons pesto, 1 tablespoon chopped tomato, and 1 tablespoon crumbled feta (if using).

Per Serving: Calories: 302; Fat: 26g; Protein: 8g; Total Carbs: 10g; Fiber: 5g; Net Carbs: 5g; **Macros:** Fat: 75%; Protein: 10%; Carbs: 15%

Eggs with Goat Cheese & Asparagus

SERVES 1 | PREP TIME: 5 minutes | COOK TIME: 15 minutes

3 asparagus spears, woody	1 teaspoon extra-virgin olive
ends removed	oil, for drizzling
2 large eggs	A few leaves of cilantro or
1 tablespoon avocado oil	other fresh herbs (optional)
1 tablespoon goat cheese	

In a small skillet, heat 2 tablespoons of water over medium-high heat. Add the asparagus, cover, and steam until the asparagus is tender. Place the asparagus on a plate, slice them in half lengthwise, and set aside. In a small bowl, beat the eggs. Pour out any water left in the skillet. Add the avocado oil, and heat over medium heat. Add the eggs and goat cheese to the skillet, and season with salt and pepper. Cook until the eggs are set and the goat cheese is melted. Serve alongside the asparagus with the olive oil drizzled over top. Garnish with cilantro or fresh herbs of your choice.

Per Serving: Calories: 334; Fat: 29g; Protein: 14g; Total Carbs: 4g; Fiber: 2g; Net Carbs: 2g; **Macros:** Fat: 78%; Protein: 17%; Carbs: 5%

Creamed Spinach with Eggs

SERVES 4 | PREP TIME: 10 minutes | COOK TIME: 15 minutes

2 tablespoons butter	½ cup finely diced white onion
8 large eggs	2 garlic cloves, minced
Nonstick cooking spray	1½ tablespoons almond flour

1½ cups unsweetened almond milk

2 tablespoons grated Parmesan cheese

4 ounces Greek yogurt cream cheese

¾ teaspoon salt

½ teaspoon freshly ground black pepper

¼ teaspoon ground nutmeg

16 ounces frozen spinach, thawed, drained, and squeezed dry

Heat a large skillet over medium-high heat. Melt the butter, and then crack in the eggs. Reduce the heat to low and cook until the egg whites begin to thicken. Slide a spatula under each egg and carefully flip it over. Cook for another 3 to 4 minutes. Remove from the heat and set aside. Spray a large skillet with cooking spray. Over medium heat, sauté the onion and garlic for about 4 minutes. Whisk in the almond flour and cook for an additional minute. Reduce the heat to low and whisk in the milk, Parmesan cheese, Greek yogurt, cream cheese, salt, pepper, and nutmeg. Mix until completely smooth. Add the spinach and combine well. Cook for 1 more minute, or until the spinach is heated through. Place the over-easy eggs on top of the creamed spinach and divide into 4 equal servings.

Per Serving: Calories: 345; Fat: 25g; Protein: 20g; Total Carbs: 11g; Fiber: 4g; Net Carbs: 7g; **Macros:** Fat: 65%; Protein: 23%; Carbs: 12%

Skillet-Baked Eggs with Yogurt and Spinach
SERVES 4 | PREP TIME: 10 minutes | COOK TIME: 25 minutes

½ cup plain Greek-style yogurt

1 teaspoon freshly squeezed lemon juice

¼ teaspoon chili powder

2 tablespoons butter

2 tablespoons extra-virgin olive oil

½ white onion, diced

8 cups spinach

4 large eggs

1 teaspoon chopped fresh cilantro, for topping

In a small bowl, stir the yogurt, lemon juice, and chili powder, and set aside. Preheat the oven to 350°F. In a large, oven-proof skillet over medium heat, heat the butter and olive oil. Add the onion, and sauté until soft, about 5 minutes. Stir in the spinach, and sauté, tossing frequently, until wilted, about 5 minutes. Push the spinach to the side of the skillet, and spoon out any extra liquid. Arrange the spinach so it covers the entire bottom of the skillet, and use a spoon to make 4 wells in the greens. Break the eggs into the wells, and place the skillet in the oven. Bake until the whites are set, about 10 minutes. Spoon the yogurt mixture over the eggs, top with the cilantro, and serve.

Per Serving: Calories: 241; Fat: 23g; Protein: 9g; Total Carbs: 5g; Fiber: 2g; Net Carbs: 3g; **Macros:** Fat: 79%; Protein: 14%; Carbs: 7%

Italian Vegetable Egg Bake
SERVES 4 | PREP TIME: 10 minutes | COOK TIME: 30 minutes

Nonstick cooking spray

1 (10-ounce) package frozen spinach, thawed, drained, and squeezed dry

⅓ cup diced red bell pepper

1 garlic clove, minced

1 tablespoon minced fresh parsley

¾ cup diced and drained canned artichokes

1 cup black olives, sliced

½ cup diced scallions

¼ teaspoon cayenne pepper

12 large eggs

¼ cup heavy (whipping) cream

1¼ teaspoons salt

½ teaspoon freshly ground black pepper

Preheat the oven to 375°F. Spray a 9-by-13-inch baking dish with cooking spray and set aside. In a small bowl, combine the spinach, bell pepper, garlic, parsley, artichokes, olives, and scallions. Stir well. Add the cayenne pepper and mix until the vegetables are well coated. Spread the vegetables in the bottom of the baking dish. In a separate bowl, whisk the eggs, cream, salt, and pepper. Pour the egg mixture over the vegetables. Bake for 30 minutes, or until the eggs are set. Remove the dish from the oven and let stand for about 7 minutes before serving.

Per Serving: Calories: 337; Fat: 23g; Protein: 20g; Total Carbs: 10g; Fiber: 4g; Net Carbs: 6g; **Macros:** Fat: 61%; Protein: 24%; Carbs: 15%

Mexican Egg Casserole
SERVES 8 | PREP TIME: 15 minutes | COOK TIME: 45 minutes

Nonstick cooking spray

2 tablespoons olive oil

1 cup chopped green bell pepper

½ cup minced onion

2 garlic cloves, minced

3 cups raw spinach

Salt

Freshly ground black pepper

½ cup unsweetened almond milk

12 large eggs

1½ cups grated Cheddar cheese, divided

1 avocado, sliced

1 cup salsa

Preheat the oven to 375°F. Spray a nonstick 9-by-13-inch casserole dish with cooking spray and set aside. In a skillet over medium-high heat, warm the olive oil. Add the bell pepper, onion, and garlic, and sauté for about 3 minutes. Then add the spinach and allow to wilt. Season with a pinch of salt and pepper. Spread the veggies out in the casserole dish. In a medium bowl, whisk the milk, eggs, and 1 cup of Cheddar cheese and pour the egg mixture over the veggies. Top with the remaining ½ cup of Cheddar cheese. Bake for 40 minutes, or until the edges of the casserole are brown and the eggs are set. Divide the casserole between eight plates. Top with the avocado slices and salsa, and serve warm or cold.

Per Serving: Calories: 271; Fat: 21g; Protein: 15g; Total Carbs: 7g; Fiber: 3g; Net Carbs: 4g; **Macros:** Fat: 70%; Protein: 22%; Carbs: 8%

Egg & Cheese Biscuit Casserole
SERVES 9 | PREP TIME: 15 minutes | COOK TIME: 20 minutes

¼ cup butter, at room temperature, plus more for greasing the pan

½ cup coconut flour

2 teaspoons baking powder

¼ teaspoon salt

7 large eggs, divided

¼ cup sour cream

2 tablespoons heavy (whipping) cream

1 teaspoon salt

1 teaspoon freshly ground black pepper

1 cup grated Cheddar cheese

Preheat the oven to 400°F. Grease a 9-inch-square casserole dish and set aside. In a small bowl, whisk the coconut flour, baking powder, and salt. In a medium bowl, whisk 3 eggs, the sour cream, and butter. Pour the dry mixture into the egg mixture, and mix well until just a few lumps remain. Transfer the dough mixture to the casserole dish and spread it evenly across the bottom. In a small bowl, whisk the remaining 4 eggs and the heavy cream, salt, and pepper, and pour over the dough mixture. Bake for 15 minutes. Pull the casserole out and sprinkle the cheese across the top. Return to the oven for another 3 to 5 minutes or until the cheese is melted. Allow to rest for 5 to 10 minutes before serving.

Per Serving: (⅑ of casserole) Calories 280; Fat: 22g; Protein: 14g; Total Carbs: 9g; Fiber: 5g; Net Carbs: 4g; **Macros:** Fat: 68%; Protein: 19%; Carbs: 13%

Denver Omelet Breakfast Bake

SERVES 6 | PREP TIME: 15 minutes | COOK TIME: 40 minutes

Cooking spray	10 large eggs
1 tablespoon olive oil	½ cup heavy (whipping) cream
¼ cup diced white onion	Pinch nutmeg (optional)
½ large green bell pepper, diced	1½ cups cooked cubed ham
Sea salt	1 cup shredded Cheddar cheese, divided
Freshly ground black pepper	

Preheat the oven to 400°F. Spray a casserole dish with cooking spray. In a small saucepan over medium heat, heat the olive oil. Add the onion and sauté for 3 minutes or until soft and translucent. Add the bell pepper and season with salt and pepper to taste. Cook for another 2 minutes, stirring, and then set aside. In a large bowl, whisk the eggs, cream, and nutmeg (if using) until well combined. Stir in the onion, pepper, ham, and ¾ cup of cheese. Pour the omelet mixture into the prepared casserole dish. Top with remaining ¼ cup of cheese. Bake for 30 to 35 minutes or until a toothpick inserted in the center comes out clean. Serve.

Per Serving: Calories: 343; Fat: 26g; Protein: 23g; Total Carbs: 5g; Fiber: 0g; Net Carbs: 5g; **Macros:** Fat: 68%; Protein: 27%; Carbs: 5%

Loaded Denver Omelet

SERVES 1 | PREP TIME: 5 minutes | COOK TIME: 5 minutes

1 tablespoon butter	1 scallion, white and green parts thinly sliced
3 large eggs	¼ bell pepper, seeds and ribs removed, thinly sliced
Sea salt	
Freshly ground black pepper	2 tablespoons shredded Cheddar cheese
2 tablespoons diced ham	

Melt the butter in a small nonstick skillet over medium heat. Whisk the eggs in a small bowl and season with salt and pepper. Pour the eggs into the skillet and cook for 1 to 2 minutes, or until barely set around the edges. Lift up the edges with a spatula and tilt the pan so the liquid eggs slide underneath. Sprinkle the ham, scallion, bell pepper, and shredded cheese over the eggs and continue cooking for another minute. Fold the omelet in half and cook for 1 minute. Flip carefully and cook for 1 more minute or until the center of the omelet is no longer watery.

Per Serving: Calories: 415; Fat: 33g; Protein: 26g; Total Carbs: 4g; Fiber: 0g; Net Carbs: 4g; **Macros:** Fat: 72%; Protein: 25%; Carbs: 3%

Italian Omelet

SERVES 1 | PREP TIME: 5 minutes | COOK TIME: 10 minutes

1 tablespoon butter or ghee	1 prosciutto slice, chopped
4 cherry tomatoes, halved	1 teaspoon Italian Seasoning
¼ cup fresh spinach	1 tablespoon basil pesto
2 large eggs	

In a large skillet, melt the butter over medium heat. Add the prosciutto, tomatoes, and spinach, and cook for 2 minutes. In a small bowl, beat the eggs and the Italian seasoning. Pour the eggs into the skillet over the prosciutto, tomatoes, and spinach, and move the skillet around to spread them out evenly. When the omelet begins to firm up but has a little raw egg on top, ease around the edges with a spatula and then fold it in half. Let it cook for a few more minutes, checking to see when the bottom of the omelet looks golden brown. When golden brown, turn off the heat and slide the omelet onto a plate. Drizzle with the basil pesto.

Per Serving: Calories: 365; Fat: 29g; Protein: 21g; Total Carbs: 5g; Fiber: 1g; Net Carbs: 4g; **Macros:** Fat: 72%; Protein: 23%; Carbs: 5%

Bacon-Artichoke Omelet

SERVES 4 | PREP TIME: 10 minutes | COOK TIME: 10 minutes

6 large eggs, beaten	¼ cup chopped onion
2 tablespoons heavy (whipping) cream	½ cup chopped artichoke hearts (canned, packed in water)
8 bacon slices, cooked and chopped	Sea salt
1 tablespoon olive oil	Freshly ground black pepper

In a small bowl, whisk the eggs, heavy cream, and bacon until well blended, and set aside. Place a large skillet over medium-high heat and add the olive oil. Sauté the onion until tender, about 3 minutes. Pour the egg mixture into the skillet, swirling it for 1 minute. Cook the omelet, lifting the edges with a spatula to let the uncooked egg flow underneath, for 2 minutes. Sprinkle the artichoke hearts on top and flip the omelet. Cook for 4 minutes more, until the egg is firm. Flip the omelet over again so the artichoke hearts are on top. Remove from the heat, cut the omelet into quarters, and season with salt and black pepper.

Per serving: Calories: 435; Fat: 39g; Protein: 17g; Total Carbs: 5g; Fiber: 2g; Net Carbs: 3g; **Macros:** Fat: 80%; Protein: 15%; Carbs: 5%

Spanakopita Omelet

SERVES 4 | PREP TIME: 15 minutes | COOK TIME: 30 minutes

5 tablespoons butter, divided	12 large eggs, divided
2 teaspoons minced garlic	1 cup feta cheese
3 cups white mushrooms	Sea salt
10 cups spinach	Freshly ground black pepper

In a large skillet over medium heat, melt 2 tablespoons of butter. Sauté the garlic until it is softened, about 3 minutes. Add the mushrooms and sauté until they are light golden, about 5 minutes. Melt 2 tablespoons of butter in the skillet, and stir in the spinach. Sauté until the greens are wilted, about 3 minutes. Remove the skillet from the heat, and transfer the spinach, mushrooms, and garlic to a large bowl, leaving any excess liquid in the skillet. Wipe out the skillet, and place it back on the heat. Melt 1 tablespoon of butter in the skillet. Crack 3 eggs into a small bowl, and whisk to blend. Pour the eggs into the skillet, and swirl the pan so that the eggs keep moving for about 30 seconds to set on the bottom. Lift the edges of the cooked egg to allow the raw egg to flow underneath until the omelet is cooked through, about 3 minutes. Spoon ¼ of the spinach mixture onto the cooked egg, and sprinkle with ¼ cup of the feta. Flip one side over, slide the omelet onto a serving plate, and season with salt and pepper. Repeat to create 3 more omelets, and serve.

Per Serving: Calories: 548; Fat: 45g; Protein: 26g; Total Carbs: 8g; Fiber: 2g; Net Carbs: 6g; **Macros:** Fat: 75%; Protein: 19%; Carbs: 6%

Mushroom Cream Cheese Omelet

SERVES 2 | PREP TIME: 10 minutes | COOK TIME: 10 minutes

2 tablespoons butter, divided
2 cups sliced mushrooms
1 teaspoon minced garlic
4 large eggs
⅛ teaspoon salt
Freshly ground black pepper
½ cup cream cheese, cubed
1 scallion, white and green parts, thinly sliced

Melt 1 tablespoon of butter in a large skillet over medium-high heat. Sauté the mushrooms and garlic until lightly caramelized, about 5 minutes, and transfer to a plate. Place the skillet back on the heat and melt the remaining butter. In a medium bowl, whisk the eggs, salt, and pepper. Pour the egg mixture into the skillet. As the eggs set, lift the edges of the omelet to allow the uncooked eggs to flow underneath. When the eggs are just set, with no liquid left on top, arrange the mushrooms on one side and top with chunks of cream cheese. Fold the omelet in half and let stand for 1 minute to melt the cream cheese. Cut in half and serve topped with scallion.

Per Serving: Calories: 464; Fat: 41g; Protein: 19g; Total Carbs: 6g; Fiber: 1g; Net Carbs: 5g; **Macros:** Fat: 79%; Protein: 16%; Carbs: 5%

Baked Omelet with Pancetta and Swiss Cheese

SERVES 4 | PREP TIME: 10 minutes | COOK TIME: 40 minutes

1 tablespoon butter, plus more for greasing
1 cup diced pancetta
10 large eggs
1 cup canned coconut milk
1 cup shredded Swiss cheese
2 teaspoons chopped chives
Pinch sea salt
Freshly ground black pepper

Preheat the oven to 350°F. Lightly grease a 9-inch-square baking dish with butter, and set aside. In a large skillet over medium-high heat, melt the butter. Cook the pancetta, stirring, until it is crispy, about 4 minutes. Remove the skillet from the heat, and transfer the pancetta to a medium bowl. Add the eggs, coconut milk, cheese, and chives to the bowl, and whisk to blend. Season the egg mixture with salt and pepper. Pour the egg mixture into the baking dish, and bake the omelet until it is set, puffy, and golden, about 30 minutes, and serve.

Per Serving: Calories: 496; Fat: 41g; Protein: 27g; Total Carbs: 6g; Fiber: 1g; Net Carbs: 5g; **Macros:** Fat: 74%; Protein: 22%; Carbs: 4%

Asparagus Gouda Frittata

SERVES 4 | PREP TIME: 10 minutes | COOK TIME: 12 minutes

3 tablespoons butter, divided
½ onion, chopped
1 teaspoon minced garlic
2 cups asparagus, cut into 1-inch pieces
4 large eggs
¼ teaspoon sea salt
⅛ teaspoon freshly ground black pepper
1 cup shredded mild Gouda cheese
2 tablespoons chopped fresh parsley

Preheat the oven to broil. Melt half the butter in a medium oven-proof skillet over medium-high heat. Sauté the onion and garlic until softened, about 3 minutes. Add the asparagus and sauté until tender, about 4 minutes. Use a spoon to transfer the vegetables to a plate and wipe the skillet. In a medium bowl, whisk the eggs, salt, and pepper. Melt the remaining butter. Add the egg mixture to the skillet and cook until set, about 4 minutes, lifting the edges of cooked egg to allow the liquid to run underneath. When the eggs are just set, arrange the asparagus mixture evenly on top and top with cheese. Transfer to the broiler and broil until the cheese is melted, about 1 minute. Serve topped with parsley.

Per Serving: Calories: 271; Fat: 22g; Protein: 15g; Total Carbs: 6g; Fiber: 2g; Net Carbs: 4g; **Macros:** Fat: 73%; Protein: 20%; Carbs: 7%

Asparagus, Mushroom & Fennel Frittata

SERVES 4 | PREP TIME: 5 to 10 minutes | COOK TIME: 30 minutes

1 teaspoon coconut or regular butter, plus more for greasing
8 asparagus spears, diced
½ cup diced fennel
½ cup mushrooms, sliced (optional)
8 large eggs
½ cup full-fat regular milk or coconut milk
1 tomato, sliced
1 teaspoon salt
½ teaspoon freshly ground black pepper
Grated cheese (optional)

Preheat the oven to 350°F. Grease a pie dish with butter. Melt 1 teaspoon of butter in a medium skillet over medium-high heat and sauté the asparagus, fennel, and mushrooms (if using) for about 5 minutes, or until fork-tender. Transfer the vegetables to the prepared pie dish. Whisk the eggs and milk in a medium bowl until combined. Pour the egg mixture over the vegetables in the pie dish, season with salt and pepper, and lightly mix. Arrange the tomato slices on top and bake for about 30 minutes. Remove from the oven and let cool for 5 to 10 minutes. Slice into wedges and sprinkle with grated cheese, if desired.

Per Serving: Calories: 188; Fat: 12g; Protein: 14g; Total Carbs: 6g; Fiber: 2g; Net Carbs: 4g; **Macros:** Fat: 57%; Protein: 30%; Carbs: 13%

Mushroom and Bacon Frittata

SERVES 6 | PREP TIME: 10 minutes | COOK TIME: 15 minutes

2 tablespoons olive oil
1 cup sliced fresh mushrooms
1 cup shredded spinach
6 bacon slices, cooked and chopped
10 large eggs, beaten
½ cup crumbled goat cheese
Sea salt
Freshly ground black pepper

Preheat the oven to 350°F. Place a large ovenproof skillet over medium-high heat and add the olive oil. Sauté the mushrooms until lightly browned, about 3 minutes. Add the spinach and bacon and sauté until the greens are wilted, about 1 minute. Add the eggs and cook, lifting the edges of the frittata with a spatula so uncooked egg flows underneath, for 3 to 4 minutes. Sprinkle the top with the crumbled goat cheese and season lightly with salt and pepper. Bake until set and lightly browned, about 15 minutes. Remove the frittata from the oven, and let it stand for 5 minutes. Cut into 6 wedges and serve immediately.

Per serving: Calories: 316; Fat: 27g; Protein: 16g; Total Carbs: 1g; Fiber: 0g; Net Carbs: 1g; Macros: Fat: 80%; Protein: 16%; Carbs: 4%

Spinach, Mushroom, and Cheddar Frittata

SERVES 4 | PREP TIME: 5 minutes |
COOK TIME: 25 minutes, plus 5 minutes to rest

- 3 tablespoons olive oil or unsalted butter
- 1 (8-ounce) package white mushrooms, sliced
- 10 ounces fresh baby spinach
- 6 large eggs
- ¾ cup shredded Cheddar cheese, divided
- Salt
- Freshly ground black pepper
- Chopped fresh parsley, for garnish (optional)

Preheat the oven to 400°F. In a 12-inch oven-safe skillet, heat the oil over medium heat. Add the mushrooms and sauté for 5 minutes. Add the spinach in batches, letting it wilt down before stirring and adding more. Meanwhile, in a large bowl, beat the eggs with ¼ cup of Cheddar and season well with salt and pepper. Drain any excess liquid from the skillet, then add the egg mixture. Let cook without touching for 5 minutes, or until the edges start to set. Sprinkle the remaining ½ cup of Cheddar over the frittata, then bake for 10 minutes, or until set in the center. Remove from the oven and let rest for 5 minutes before serving. Garnish with the parsley, if using.

Per Serving: Calories: 298; Fat: 23g; Protein: 18g; Total Carbs: 5g; Fiber: 2g; Net Carbs: 3g; Macros: Fat: 70%; Protein: 24%; Carbs: 6%

Mediterranean Frittata

SERVES 2 | PREP TIME: 10 minutes | COOK TIME: 15 minutes

- 4 large eggs
- 2 tablespoons fresh chopped herbs, such as rosemary, thyme, oregano, basil or 1 teaspoon dried herbs
- ¼ teaspoon salt
- Freshly ground black pepper
- ¼ cup extra-virgin olive oil, divided
- 1 cup fresh spinach, arugula, kale, or other leafy greens
- 4 ounces quartered artichoke hearts, rinsed, drained, and thoroughly dried
- 8 cherry tomatoes, halved
- ½ cup crumbled soft goat cheese

Preheat the oven to broil on low. In a small bowl, whisk the eggs, herbs, salt, and pepper. Set aside. In a 4- to 5-inch oven-safe skillet heat 2 tablespoons of olive oil over medium heat. Add the spinach, artichoke hearts, and cherry tomatoes and sauté until just wilted, 1 to 2 minutes. Pour in the egg mixture and let it cook undisturbed over medium heat for 3 to 4 minutes, until the eggs begin to set on the bottom. Sprinkle the goat cheese across the top of the egg mixture and transfer the skillet to the oven. Broil for 4 to 5 minutes, or until the frittata is firm in the center and golden brown on top. Remove from the oven and run a rubber spatula around the edge. Invert onto a large plate or cutting board and slice in half. Serve warm and drizzled with the remaining 2 tablespoons olive oil.

Per Serving: Calories: 527; Fat: 47g; Protein: 21g; Total Carbs: 10g; Fiber: 3g; Net Carbs: 7g; Macros: Fat: 79%; Protein: 16%; Carbs: 5%

Asparagus Frittata

SERVES 4 | PREP TIME: 10 minutes | COOK TIME: 20 minutes

- ½ cup extra-virgin olive oil, divided
- ¼ cup finely chopped white onion (about ½ small onion)
- 1 pound medium-thin asparagus, rough stalks trimmed, cut into 1-inch pieces
- 2 medium garlic cloves, minced
- 6 large eggs
- 2 tablespoons vegetable broth
- 1 teaspoon salt
- ½ teaspoon freshly ground black pepper
- ¼ cup Zesty Orange for serving
- ½ cup chopped herbs (basil, parsley, or mint), for garnish (optional)

In a large skillet, heat ¼ cup of olive oil over medium heat. Add the onion and sauté for 3 to 4 minutes, until the onion begins to soften. Add the asparagus and garlic and cook until the asparagus is tender, 5 to 6 minutes. Transfer the cooked vegetables to a bowl and let cool. In a medium bowl, whisk the eggs, vegetable broth, salt, and pepper. Add the cooled asparagus and mix until well combined. In the same skillet, heat 2 tablespoons of olive oil over medium-high heat. Pour the egg mixture into the skillet and reduce the heat to medium-low. Let the eggs cook undisturbed for 2 to 3 minutes, or until the bottom begins to set. Cook, continuously moving the uncooked egg mixture until the top is a little wet but not liquid, 3 to 5 minutes. Place a large flat plate or cutting board on top of the skillet and quickly invert the tortilla. Add the remaining 2 tablespoons of olive oil to the skillet and carefully slide the tortilla back into the pan, uncooked-side down. Cook over low heat until cooked through, another 2 to 3 minutes. Transfer back to the plate or cutting board. Rest for 5 minutes before slicing. Serve warm.

Per Serving: Calories: 444; Fat: 40g; Protein: 12g; Total Carbs: 9g; Fiber: 3g; Net Carbs: 6g; Macros: Fat: 80%; Protein: 11%; Carbs: 9%

Lemon-Herb Baked Frittata

SERVES 4 | PREP TIME: 5 minutes | COOK TIME: 40 minutes, plus 10 minutes cooling time

- 6 tablespoons extra-virgin olive oil, divided
- 8 ounces feta cheese
- 2 tablespoons chopped fresh rosemary
- 1 tablespoon chopped fresh oregano
- 1 teaspoon garlic powder
- 1 teaspoon grated lemon zest
- ½ teaspoon freshly ground black pepper
- 4 large eggs
- ½ teaspoon baking powder

Preheat the oven to 350°F. Coat the bottom of an 8-inch square glass baking dish with 2 tablespoons of oil. In a medium bowl, crumble the feta and add the rosemary, oregano, garlic powder, lemon zest, and pepper and mix well. In a small bowl, whisk the eggs and baking powder. Add the egg mixture and remaining ¼ cup of olive oil to the feta mixture and whisk to combine well. Pour into the prepared baking dish and bake for 35 to 40 minutes, until lightly browned and set. Cool for 10 minutes before slicing.

Per Serving: Calories: 412; Fat: 38g; Protein: 15g; Total Carbs: 4g; Fiber: 0g; Net Carbs: 4g; **Macros:** Fat: 83%; Protein: 15%; Carbs: 2%

Per Serving: (2 eggs with 2 slices ham): Calories: 221; Fat: 14g; Protein: 21g; Total Carbs: 3g; Fiber: 1g; Net Carbs: 2g

Sausage and Cheese Frittata

SERVES 8 | PREP TIME: 10 minutes | COOK TIME: 35 minutes

¼ cup butter, melted, plus more for greasing pan
10 large eggs
¾ cup heavy (whipping) cream
½ teaspoon garlic powder
½ teaspoon onion powder
½ teaspoon paprika
½ teaspoon salt

½ teaspoon freshly ground black pepper
1 or 2 dashes favorite hot sauce (optional)
½ cup shredded Cheddar cheese
1 cup cooked ground breakfast sausage
½ cup diced scallion
½ cup diced red bell pepper

Preheat the oven to 350°F. Grease a 9-by-13-inch glass casserole dish with butter or cooking spray. In a large bowl, whisk the eggs, cream, butter, garlic powder, onion powder, paprika, salt, pepper, hot sauce (if using), and Cheddar until well combined. Pour into the prepared casserole dish. Evenly distribute the sausage, scallion, and bell pepper into the egg mixture. Place on the center rack of the oven and bake for 35 minutes or until the frittata is cooked through and the top is very lightly browned. Allow to rest for 5 minutes and serve.

Per Serving: Calories: 284; Fat: 25g; Protein: 12g; Total Carbs: 2g; Fiber: 0g; Net Carbs: 2g; **Macros:** Fat: 78%; Protein: 19%; Carbs: 3%

Prosciutto Egg Cups

SERVES 1 (2 CUPS PER PERSON) | PREP TIME: 5 minutes | COOK TIME: 30 minutes

2 large eggs
½ cup chopped fresh spinach
1 scallion, white and green parts finely sliced

1 tablespoon unsweetened full-fat coconut milk
1 teaspoon coconut oil
2 prosciutto slices, folded in half

Preheat the oven to 350°F. In a small bowl, beat the eggs, add the spinach and scallion, and mix. Mix in the coconut milk, and season with a little salt and freshly ground black pepper. Grease two cups of a muffin tin with the coconut oil, and line each cup with a folded slice of prosciutto. Fill each cup about two-thirds full with the egg mixture. Bake for 30 minutes, until the eggs are fully cooked.

Per Serving: Calories: 302; Fat: 22g; Protein: 23g; Total Carbs: 3g; Fiber: 1g; Net Carbs: 2g; **Macros:** Fat: 66%; Protein: 30%; Carbs: 4%

Baked Eggs in Ham Cups

SERVES 2 | PREP TIME: 5 minutes | COOK TIME: 15 minutes

Cooking spray for cupcake pan
4 slices Black Forest ham

4 large eggs
1 teaspoon dried parsley

Preheat the oven to 400°F. Spray the cupcake pan. Tuck one slice of ham into each cup. The ham will hang over the sides. Crack one egg into each cup and garnish with the parsley. Place the cupcake pan in the preheated oven. Cook for about 15 minutes, until the egg whites are cooked but the yolk is still runny.

Ham and Cheese Poached Egg Cups

MAKES 12 | PREP TIME: 5 minutes | COOK TIME: 20 minutes

Nonstick cooking spray
12 slices deli ham (about 1 pound)
1 cup shredded Cheddar cheese
12 large eggs

Salt
Freshly ground black pepper
Paprika (optional)
2 or 3 scallions (green parts only), sliced

Preheat the oven to 400°F. Lightly spray a muffin tin with cooking spray. Place a slice of ham over each muffin cup and press down to form a cup shape. Evenly divide the cheese among the 12 cups. Carefully crack 1 egg into each cup, keeping the yolk intact. Lightly season with salt, pepper, and a pinch of paprika (if using). Bake for 18 minutes or until the yolks are done to your liking. While still hot, garnish with the scallions, then allow to cool slightly before serving.

Per Serving: Calories: 172; Fat: 11g; Protein: 15g; Total Carbs: 2g; Fiber: 1g; Net Carbs: 1g; **Macros:** Fat: 59%; Protein: 37%; Carbs: 4%

Bacon, Egg, and Cheese Cups

SERVES 4 | PREP TIME: 5 minutes | COOK TIME: 35 minutes

6 bacon slices, divided
4 large eggs, beaten
½ cup heavy (whipping) cream
¼ teaspoon salt

⅛ teaspoon freshly ground black pepper
½ cup shredded Monterey Jack cheese, divided

Preheat the oven to 350°F. Wrap one bacon slice inside a cupcake tin around the edges, so it covers the sides of the tin. Repeat with three more slices in three more tins. Cut the remaining two bacon slices into 2-inch pieces. Place 2 to 3 bacon pieces at the bottom of each bacon-wrapped cupcake tin so each is fully covered. In a medium bowl, whisk the eggs, heavy cream, salt, and pepper. Pour the egg mixture evenly into the bacon-wrapped tins. Cover each with 2 tablespoons of cheese. Carefully place the cupcake pan in the oven to avoid spillage. Bake for 35 minutes or until golden brown.

Per Serving: (1 egg cup): Calories: 359; Fat: 29g; Protein: 23g; Total Carbs: 0g; Fiber: 0g; Net Carbs: 0g; **Macros:** Fat: 72%; Protein: 25%; Carbs: 3%

Bacon-Wrapped Egg Cups

SERVES 3 (MAKES 6 EGG CUPS) | PREP TIME: 10 minutes | COOK TIME: 20 minutes

6 bacon slices
1 teaspoon avocado oil
6 large eggs

2 tablespoons chopped scallions
¼ teaspoon salt
⅛ teaspoon black pepper

Preheat the oven to 375°F. Line a baking sheet with parchment paper. Add the bacon slides to the baking sheet and cook for 6 minutes in the oven. Remove the bacon slices from the oven and let cool slightly. Grease a six cup muffin pan with avocado oil. Carefully place each bacon slice inside the muffin cup creating a circle around the edge of each well. Crack one egg into each muffin cup; top with the scallions, salt, and pepper. Bake for 12 to 14 minutes, until the egg white is cooked but the yolk is still runny. Let cool for 1 to 2 minutes then remove each egg cup carefully with a spoon and serve.

Per Serving: Calories: 244; Fat: 18g; Protein: 19g; Total Carbs: 1g; Fiber: 0g; Net Carbs: 1g; **Macros:** Fat: 67%; Protein: 31%; Carbs: 2%

Broccoli Bacon Egg Muffin Cups

SERVES 4 | PREP TIME: 10 minutes | COOK TIME: 15 minutes

12 large eggs
Sea salt
Freshly ground black pepper

1 cup cooked broccoli florets
8 ounces bacon, cooked and crumbled

Preheat the oven to 350°F. Line a muffin tin with liners. In a large glass measuring cup or pitcher, whisk the eggs. Season with salt and pepper. Divide the broccoli and cooked bacon among the muffin cups. Pour the egg mixture into each of the muffin cups. Bake for 15 minutes, or until the eggs are set.

Per Serving: Calories: 338; Fat: 22g; Protein: 29g; Total Carbs: 4g; Fiber: 1g; Net Carbs: 3g; **Macros:** Fat: 62%; Protein: 34%; Carbs: 4%

Broccoli and Cheese Quiche Cups

SERVES 4 | PREP TIME: 10 minutes | COOK TIME: 35 minutes

Cooking spray for ramekins
½ teaspoon salt, plus additional for salting the cooking water
1½ cups broccoli florets
5 large eggs

¾ cup heavy (whipping) cream
¼ teaspoon freshly ground black pepper
½ teaspoon minced garlic
¾ cup shredded Cheddar cheese

Preheat the oven to 350°F. Spray four ramekins with cooking spray and place them on a baking sheet. Bring a medium pot of salted water to a boil. Add the broccoli. Cook for 1 minute. Drain the broccoli from the pot, pat dry with paper towels, and chop. In a large bowl, whisk the eggs, heavy cream, salt, and pepper. Fold in the broccoli, garlic, and cheese. Divide the egg mixture evenly among the ramekins. Place the baking sheet with the ramekins into the preheated oven. Bake until the egg and broccoli mixture has risen and is slightly browned, about 35 minutes.

Per Serving: (1 quiche cup): Calories: 255; Fat: 21g; Protein: 14g; Total Carbs: 4g; Fiber: 1g; Net Carbs: 3g; **Macros:** Fat: 72%; Protein: 21%; Carbs: 7%

Bacon Eggs Benedict Cups

SERVES 2 | PREP TIME: 10 minutes | COOK TIME: 20 minutes

Nonstick cooking spray
4 slices vegan bacon
4 large eggs, plus 3 egg yolks
½ cup butter (1 stick)
Juice of ½ lemon

⅛ teaspoon cayenne pepper
Chopped fresh parsley, for serving
1 avocado, pitted and sliced, for serving

Preheat the oven to 350°F. Spray 4 cups of a muffin tin generously with cooking spray. Line each muffin cup with a strip of

bacon, covering the sides as much as possible. Break 1 egg into each bacon nest. Bake the egg cups for 15 to 20 minutes, until the eggs are set in the center. While the eggs are cooking, melt the butter in a cup in the microwave for 30 to 40 seconds. In a blender, combine the egg yolks, lemon juice, and cayenne. With the blender on the lowest speed, slowly drizzle the melted butter into the blender until it is emulsified. Remove the egg cups from the oven and carefully remove each egg basket from the muffin tin. Drizzle the hollandaise sauce over the eggs. Sprinkle each cup with parsley and top with a few avocado slices.

Per Serving: (2 egg cups) Calories: 822; Fat: 78g; Protein: 19g; Total Carbs: 11g; Fiber: 7g; Net Carbs: 4g; **Macros:** Fat: 85%; Protein: 9%; Carbs: 6%

Egg Breakfast Muffins

SERVES 4 | PREP TIME: 5 minutes | COOK TIME: 16 minutes

1 tablespoon butter, for greasing
6 large eggs
1 cup heavy (whipping) cream
½ cup plus 2 tablespoons Cheddar cheese, divided

5 slices cooked bacon, chopped
½ teaspoon chopped cilantro
Pinch salt
Pinch freshly ground black pepper

Preheat the oven to 350°F. Lightly grease 8 muffin cups with the butter. In a medium bowl, whisk the eggs, cream, ½ cup of Cheddar, bacon, and cilantro. Season with salt and pepper. Evenly pour the egg mixture into the muffin cups. Bake the muffins until they are cooked through and lightly browned, about 15 minutes. Remove the muffin pan from the oven, and change the oven to broil. Sprinkle the remaining 2 tablespoons of Cheddar onto the muffins, broil until the cheese is melted and bubbly, about 1 minute, and serve.

Per Serving: (2 muffins): Calories: 346; Fat: 31g; Protein: 15g; Total Carbs: 2g; Fiber: 0g; Net Carbs: 2g; **Macros:** Fat: 80%; Protein: 17%; Carbs: 3%

Cheesy Sausage & Egg Muffins

SERVES 12 | PREP TIME: 10 minutes | COOK TIME: 30 minutes

Nonstick cooking spray (optional)
8 large eggs
6 ounces cream cheese
2 tablespoons butter

½ teaspoon freshly ground black pepper
½ teaspoon garlic powder
4 ounces cooked breakfast sausage
½ cup grated Cheddar cheese

Preheat the oven to 350°F. Prepare a 12-cup muffin pan with cooking spray or cupcake liners. In a blender, mix the eggs, cream cheese, butter, pepper, and garlic powder until fluffy. Divide the mixture evenly between the prepared muffin cups. Sprinkle each cup evenly with the sausage and cheese. Bake for 30 minutes. Serve warm.

Per Serving: (1 muffin) Calories: 168; Fat: 15g; Protein: 7g; Total Carbs: 1g; Fiber: 0g; Net Carbs: 1g; **Macros:** Fat: 81%; Protein: 17%; Carbs: 2%

French Toast Egg Muffins

SERVES 12 | PREP TIME: 10 minutes | COOK TIME: 20 to 25 minutes

Nonstick cooking spray (optional)

8 large eggs

1 (8-ounce) brick cream cheese

½ teaspoon cinnamon

2 tablespoons sugar-free maple syrup, plus ¾ cup for topping

1 tablespoon butter

1 teaspoon vanilla extract

1 teaspoon baking soda

Preheat the oven to 350°F. Prepare a 12-cup muffin pan with nonstick cooking spray or cupcake liners. In a blender, combine the eggs, cream cheese, 2 tablespoons of syrup, butter, vanilla, baking soda, and cinnamon and pulse until well blended. Divide the mixture evenly between the prepared muffin cups. Fill the cups all the way to the top. Bake for 20 to 25 minutes. Cool then drizzle with syrup and serve.

Per Serving: (1 muffin) Calories 122; Fat: 11g; Protein: 5g; Total Carbs: 1g; Fiber: 0g; Net Carbs: 1g; **Macros:** Fat: 80%; Protein: 16%; Carbs: 4%.

Chorizo Egg Muffins

SERVES 12 | PREP TIME: 10 minutes | COOK TIME: 32 minutes

Nonstick cooking spray

12 ounces Mexican chorizo, casing removed

1½ cups shredded Monterey Jack cheese, divided

6 large eggs

2 ounces cream cheese, at room temperature

2 tablespoons sour cream

1½ tablespoons salsa

½ teaspoon kosher salt

¼ teaspoon freshly ground black pepper

Preheat the oven to 325°F. Grease a muffin tin with cooking spray. In a large skillet over medium-high heat, cook the chorizo for 7 to 10 minutes, breaking it up into crumbles, until thoroughly cooked. Evenly divide the cooked chorizo and Monterey Jack cheese among the prepared muffin cups. In a blender, blend the eggs, cream cheese, sour cream, salsa, salt, and pepper. Evenly divide the egg mixture among the muffin cups, and bake for 20 to 25 minutes, or until set. Let the muffins cool in the pan for at least 20 minutes before removing them. Serve warm or at room temperature.

Per Serving: Calories: 240; Fat: 20g; Protein: 14g; Total Carbs: 1g; Fiber: 0g; Net Carbs: 1g; **Macros:** Fat: 75%; Protein: 23%; Carbs: 2%

Simple Scrambled Eggs

SERVES 4 | PREP TIME: 5 minutes | COOK TIME: 5 minutes

10 large eggs

½ cup heavy (whipping) cream

2 tablespoons butter

1 teaspoon chopped tarragon

Sea salt

Freshly ground black pepper

In a large bowl, whisk the eggs and heavy cream. Set aside. Place a large skillet over medium heat and melt the butter. Pour the egg mixture into the skillet and use a plastic spatula to pull the eggs into the center of the skillet as it cooks. Continue to scrape the skillet, creating moist, fluffy egg curds, until the eggs are just cooked, about 4 minutes. Stir in the tarragon, season the eggs with salt and pepper, and serve.

Per Serving: Calories: 282; Fat: 24g; Protein: 15g; Total Carbs: 2g; Fiber: 0g; Net Carbs: 2g; **Macros:** Fat: 76%; Protein: 21%; Carbs: 3%

Cheesy Scrambled Eggs

1 SERVING | PREP TIME: 5 minutes | COOK TIME: 8 minutes

1 tablespoon butter

1 tablespoon cream cheese

1 ounce cooked breakfast sausage

2 large eggs

½ teaspoon pepper

½ teaspoon garlic salt

¼ cup grated Cheddar cheese

½ avocado, sliced

In a small skillet over medium heat, melt the butter, then add the cream cheese, using a spatula to mix it with the butter. Add the breakfast sausage and mix well. Add the eggs and scramble until cooked. Season with the pepper and garlic salt. Top with the Cheddar cheese and avocado slices and enjoy.

Per Serving: Calories: 614; Fat: 54g; Protein: 27g; Total Carbs: 8g; Fiber: 5g; Net Carbs: 3g; **Macros:** Fat: 78%; Protein: 17%; Carbs: 5%

Ham and Cheese Egg Scramble

SERVES 1 | PREP TIME: 5 minutes | COOK TIME: 5 minutes

1 tablespoon butter

2 large eggs, whisked

Sea salt

Freshly ground black pepper

2 tablespoons diced ham

2 tablespoons shredded pepper Jack cheese

½ avocado, pitted, peeled, and thinly sliced

¼ cup diced tomatoes

Melt the butter in a small skillet over medium heat. Add the eggs to the skillet and season with salt and pepper. Stir in a circular pattern with a spatula for 3 to 4 minutes, or until nearly set. Stir in the ham and cheese, and stir just until the eggs are set and the cheese begins to melt, about 1 minute. Top with sliced avocado and tomatoes.

Per Serving: Calories: 546; Fat: 47g; Protein: 25g; Total Carbs: 11g; Fiber: 6g; Net Carbs: 5g; **Macros:** Fat: 77%; Protein: 18%; Carbs: 5%

Chile Relleno Scrambled Eggs

SERVES 1 | PREP TIME: 5 minutes | COOK TIME: 5 minutes

1 tablespoon butter

2 large eggs, whisked

Pinch sea salt

1 tablespoon chopped green chiles

1 ounce cream cheese, cut into ½-inch pieces

1 tablespoon minced fresh cilantro

Melt the butter in a small skillet over medium heat. Add the eggs, salt, and chiles to the pan and stir in a circular pattern with a spatula for 3 to 4 minutes, or until nearly set. Stir in the cream cheese, and stir just until the eggs are set and the cream cheese begins to melt, about 1 minute. Top with cilantro.

Per Serving: Calories: 346; Fat: 31g; Protein: 15g; Total Carbs: 3g; Fiber: 0g; Net Carbs: 3g; **Macros:** Fat: 81%; Protein: 16%; Carbs: 3%

Scrambled Eggs with Mackerel

SERVES 4 | PREP TIME: 5 minutes | COOK TIME: 10 minutes

6 large eggs

2 ounces goat cheese, at room temperature

7 tablespoons extra-virgin olive oil, divided

1 teaspoon garlic powder

½ teaspoon freshly ground black pepper

2 Roma tomatoes, finely chopped

2 tablespoons minced onion

1 (4-ounce) can olive oil-packed mackerel fillets, oil reserved and chopped

¼ cup chopped olives

2 tablespoons chopped fresh parsley, oregano, rosemary, or cilantro or 1 teaspoon dried herbs

In a small bowl, whisk the eggs, goat cheese, 2 tablespoons of olive oil, garlic powder, and pepper. In a medium nonstick skillet, heat 1 tablespoon of olive oil over medium-low heat. Sauté the tomato and onion for 2 to 3 minutes, until soft and the water from the tomato has evaporated. Add the egg mixture to the skillet and scramble for 3 to 4 minutes, until set and creamy. Remove the skillet from the heat and stir in the mackerel with the reserved oil, olives, and parsley. Serve warm with each serving drizzled with an additional 1 tablespoon of olive oil.

Per Serving: Calories: 479; Fat: 45g; Protein: 17g; Total Carbs: 4g; Fiber: 1g; Net Carbs: 3g; **Macros:** Fat: 85%; Protein: 14%; Carbs: 1%

Salmon and Egg Scramble

SERVES 6 | PREP TIME: 5 minutes | COOK TIME: 10 minutes

8 large eggs

2 tablespoons heavy (whipping) cream

¼ teaspoon salt

¼ teaspoon freshly ground black pepper

¼ cup butter

1 (6-ounce) salmon fillet, skinned and diced into small slivers

In a bowl, thoroughly whisk the eggs, cream, salt, and pepper. In a large nonstick skillet over medium heat, melt the butter. Add the eggs and salmon to the pan and cook over medium heat for 6 to 8 minutes or until the eggs are softly scrambled and the salmon pieces are cooked. Stir constantly to create creamy scrambled eggs.

Per Serving: Calories: 226; Fat: 18g; Protein: 15g; Total Carbs: 1g; Fiber: 0g; Net Carbs: 1g; **Macros:** Fat: 71%; Protein: 28%; Carbs: 1%

Tofu and Veggie Scramble

SERVES 2 | PREP TIME: 10 minutes | COOK TIME: 10 minutes

8 ounces firm tofu

¼ cup coconut oil, divided

2 tablespoons minced red onion

¼ red bell pepper, seeded and finely chopped

½ teaspoon ground turmeric

½ teaspoon salt

¼ teaspoon freshly ground black pepper

¼ teaspoon garlic powder

¼ cup chopped fresh cilantro or mint leaves

Cut the block of tofu lengthwise into 4 pieces. Lay them flat on a stack of paper towels and drain for 5 minutes, pressing down with additional dry paper towels to release water. Crumble the tofu into a in a large bowl. In a medium skillet, heat 2 tablespoons of coconut oil over medium heat. Add the onion and bell pepper

and sauté for 2 to 3 minutes, or until soft. Add the turmeric, salt, pepper, and garlic powder and sauté for 1 minute, or until fragrant. Add the remaining 2 tablespoons of coconut oil and stir to form a paste. Add the crumbled tofu to the skillet, increase the heat to medium high, and sauté for 3 to 4 minutes, until slightly crispy. Remove from the heat and stir in the cilantro. Serve warm.

Per Serving: Calories: 418; Fat: 37g; Protein: 20g; Total Carbs: 6g; Fiber: 3g; Net Carbs: 3g; **Macros:** Fat: 80%; Protein: 19%; Carbs: 1%

Brussels Sprouts & Ground Beef Scrambled Eggs

1 SERVING | PREP TIME: 10 minutes | COOK TIME: 10 to 15 minutes

1 tablespoon butter-flavored coconut oil

10 Brussels sprouts, halved

¼ pound ground beef (80 percent lean)

2 large eggs, beaten

Salt

Freshly ground black pepper

Sugar-free hot sauce (optional)

In a sauté pan over medium-high heat, melt the coconut oil and then add the Brussels sprouts. Stir, then cover and cook for 3 to 5 minutes. Add the ground beef and cook for another 3 to 5 minutes, stirring continuously. Add the eggs, season with salt and pepper, and scramble everything together for 2 to 3 minutes. Pour the mixture onto a plate and top with hot sauce.

Per Serving: Calories: 626; Fat: 46g; Protein: 38g; Total Carbs: 18g; Fiber: 7g; Net Carbs: 11g; **Macros:** Fat: 66%; Protein: 24%; Carbs: 10%

Turkey Egg Scramble

SERVES 1 | PREP TIME: 5 minutes | COOK TIME: 15 minutes

1 teaspoon avocado oil

¼ medium red onion, diced

¼ red bell pepper, diced

2 garlic cloves, minced

4 ounces ground turkey

¼ teaspoon chili powder

2 large eggs

¼ cup fresh spinach

In a skillet, heat the oil over medium heat. Add the onion, bell pepper, and garlic and sauté for 5 to 7 minutes until soft. Add the turkey, then season with the chili powder and salt and freshly ground black pepper to taste. Continue to cook until the turkey begins to brown. In a small bowl, beat the eggs, and pour them into the skillet over the turkey and vegetables. Layer the spinach on top of the eggs, stir to combine, and continue to cook until the eggs are set.

Per Serving: Calories: 367; Fat: 23g; Protein: 32g; Total Carbs: 8g; Fiber: 2g; Net Carbs: 6g; **Macros:** Fat: 56%; Protein: 35%; Carbs: 9%

Greek-Style Egg and Tomato Scramble

SERVES 4 | PREP TIME: 10 minutes | COOK TIME: 25 minutes

¼ cup extra-virgin olive oil, divided

1½ cups chopped fresh tomatoes

¼ cup finely minced red onion

2 garlic cloves, minced

½ teaspoon dried oregano or 1 to 2 teaspoons chopped fresh oregano

½ teaspoon dried thyme or 1 to 2 teaspoons chopped fresh thyme

8 large eggs

½ teaspoon salt

¼ teaspoon freshly ground black pepper

¾ cup crumbled   ¼ cup chopped fresh
    feta cheese   mint leaves

In a large skillet, heat the olive oil over medium heat. Add the chopped tomatoes and red onion and sauté until tomatoes are cooked through and soft, 10 to 12 minutes. Add the garlic, oregano, and thyme and sauté another 2 to 4 minutes, until fragrant and liquid has reduced. In a medium bowl, whisk the eggs, salt, and pepper. Add the eggs to the skillet, reduce the heat to low, and scramble until set and creamy, 3 to 4 minutes. Remove the skillet from the heat, stir in the feta and mint, and serve warm.

Per Serving: Calories: 338; Fat: 28g; Protein: 16g; Total Carbs: 6g; Fiber: 1g; Net Carbs: 5g; **Macros:** Fat: 74%; Protein: 19%; Carbs: 7%

Country Garden Scramble

SERVES 4 | PREP TIME: 20 minutes | COOK TIME: 10 minutes

8 large eggs   ¼ cup butter, divided
¼ cup sour cream   1 cup diced zucchini
1 tablespoon chopped   ½ cup chopped asparagus
    fresh parsley   ¼ cup diced red bell pepper
½ teaspoon kosher   2 tablespoons sliced scallion
    salt, divided   1 cup fresh baby spinach
¼ teaspoon freshly ground ½ cup shredded
    black pepper   Fontina cheese

In a large bowl, whisk the eggs, sour cream, parsley, ¼ teaspoon of salt, and pepper. Set aside. In a large skillet over medium heat, melt 2 tablespoons of butter. Add the zucchini, asparagus, red bell pepper, and remaining ¼ teaspoon of salt. Sauté for about 5 minutes until tender. Add the spinach and scallion. Cook for 1 minute just until the spinach wilts. Turn the heat to medium-low and add the remaining 2 tablespoons of butter to the skillet. Pour the egg mixture into the skillet. Scramble the eggs while mixing the veggies into the eggs. Cook for about 2 minutes more until the eggs are cooked and firm. Remove from the heat and sprinkle the Fontina cheese over the top. Serve immediately.

Per Serving: Calories: 332; Fat: 28g; Protein: 16g; Total Carbs: 4g; Fiber: 1g; Net Carbs: 3g; **Macros:** Fat: 76%; Protein: 19%; Carbs: 5%

Corned Beef Breakfast Hash

SERVES 4 | PREP TIME: 20 minutes | COOK TIME: 20 minutes

3 tablespoons butter, divided   Sea salt
8 ounces corned   Freshly ground black pepper
    beef, chopped   4 large eggs
2 cups chopped cauliflower   2 tablespoons parsley,
2 scallions, both white and   for garnish
    green parts chopped

In a large skillet over medium-high heat, melt 1½ tablespoons of butter. Sauté the corned beef for 5 minutes, until it is heated through and the fat renders. Stir in the cauliflower, and sauté until the cauliflower is tender and lightly caramelized, about 10 minutes. Add the scallions, and sauté 1 minute. Season the hash with salt and pepper. Remove the skillet from the heat, and set aside. In another large skillet over medium-high heat, melt the remaining 1½ tablespoons of butter. Fry the eggs sunny-side up in the butter until the whites are cooked through, about

4 minutes. Serve the hash topped with 1 egg per person and garnished with fresh parsley.

Per Serving: Calories: 251; Fat: 21g; Protein: 13g; Total Carbs: 4g; Fiber: 2g; Net Carbs: 2g; **Macros:** Fat: 74%; Protein: 20%; Carbs: 6%

Roasted Vegetable Hash

SERVES 1 | PREP TIME: 10 minutes | COOK TIME: 15 minutes

2 tablespoons coconut   Sea salt
    oil, divided   Freshly ground black pepper
1 cup diced zucchini   1 tablespoon minced
½ cup diced green bell pepper   fresh parsley
¼ cup diced red onion   2 large eggs

Heat 1 tablespoon of the coconut oil in a large skillet over medium-high heat. Season the zucchini, bell pepper, and onion with salt and pepper, and sauté until the vegetables are crisp-tender, about 5 minutes. Transfer them to a serving plate and sprinkle with the parsley. In the same skillet, heat the remaining tablespoon of coconut oil. When hot, crack in the eggs, season with salt and pepper, and cook for 3 to 4 minutes, or until the whites are set and the yolks are still runny or reach the desired level of doneness. Set them on top of the vegetable hash.

Per Serving: Calories: 443; Fat: 37g; Protein: 15g; Total Carbs: 16g; Fiber: 4g; Net Carbs: 12g; **Macros:** Fat: 75%; Protein: 12%; Carbs: 13%

Cabbage Sausage Hash Browns

SERVES 4 | PREP TIME: 10 minutes | COOK TIME: 10 minutes

2 cups shredded cabbage   1 teaspoon minced garlic
2 (4-ounce) cooked sau-   ½ teaspoon chopped
    sages patties, chopped   fresh thyme
    (8 ounces total)   2 tablespoons olive oil
2 large eggs, beaten   Freshly ground black pepper
½ onion, thinly sliced

In a large bowl, stir the cabbage, sausage, eggs, onion, garlic, and thyme and toss to combine. Heat the olive oil in a large skillet over medium-high heat. Divide the cabbage mixture into 4 equal patties and press them down with the flat of a spatula. Cook until golden on the bottom, flip, and repeat with the other side, about 10 minutes total. Season with pepper before serving.

Per Serving: Calories: 321; Fat: 27g; Protein: 15g; Total Carbs: 4g; Fiber: 1g; Net Carbs: 3g; **Macros:** Fat: 75%; Protein: 20%; Carbs: 5%

Eggs Benedict with Bacon

SERVES 2 | PREP TIME: 10 minutes | COOK TIME: 10 minutes

2 large eggs   ¼ cup butter, melted
1½ teaspoons freshly   ¼ teaspoon salt
    squeezed lemon juice

For the eggs
4 bacon slices   4 large eggs
1 teaspoon vinegar

In a large heat-safe bowl, whisk two eggs and the lemon juice vigorously until thick and almost double in volume. Fill a large skillet with 1 inch of water and heat to simmering. Reduce the heat to medium. Place the bowl with the eggs over the skillet, making sure it does not touch the water. Whisk the mixture for about 3 minutes, being careful not to scramble the eggs. Slowly add the butter to the egg mixture and continue to whisk until it thickens, about 2 minutes. Whisk in the salt. Refrigerate the sauce until cool. Pour the water out of the skillet and place it over medium-high heat. Place the bacon in the skillet. Cook for 3 minutes per side. Transfer the bacon to paper towels to drain. In a medium saucepan half full of water, add the vinegar and bring to a low boil. Gently crack the eggs into the water, being careful not to break the yolks. Reduce the heat to medium-low. Cook for 3 to 4 minutes. Remove the eggs. Allow them to drain and set aside. Break each bacon slice in half. Place two halves on each plate and top with one egg. Cover with hollandaise sauce.

Per Serving: (2 eggs; 2 bacon slices; ½ of the hollandaise sauce): Calories: 624; Fat: 54g; Protein: 33g; Total Carbs: 2g; Fiber: 0g; Net Carbs: 2g; **Macros:** Fat: 78%; Protein: 21%; Carbs: 1%

Easy Eggs Benedict

SERVES 4 | PREP TIME: 15 minutes | COOK TIME: 25 minutes

8 slices Canadian bacon
4 slices low-carb bread toasted
1 tablespoon white vinegar
8 large eggs, plus 3 large egg yolks, divided

1 tablespoon freshly squeezed lemon juice
⅛ teaspoon paprika
10 tablespoons melted salted butter

Preheat the oven to 325°F. Line a baking sheet with parchment paper. Place the bacon in an even layer on the baking sheet. Bake for 10 minutes, flip, and bake for another 10 minutes. Remove from the oven and set aside. Bring a large pot of water to a boil over high heat and then reduce the heat to low. Stir in the vinegar. Working with one egg at a time, crack it onto a small plate, allowing the runny white to separate from the solid white surrounding the yolk. Gently pour the egg into the water. Multiple eggs can cook together, but you want to pour them in individually. Set a timer for 3 minutes. When the eggs are done, remove them from the water with a slotted spoon. While the eggs cook, combine the egg yolks, lemon juice, and paprika in a blender and blend on high speed for about 30 seconds. Reduce the blender speed to its lowest setting. Drizzle in the melted butter and continue to blend for another 30 seconds or until completely incorporated. To serve, top each toast slice with 2 bacon slices, 2 eggs, and one-fourth of the hollandaise.

Per Serving: Calories: 852; Fat: 75g; Protein: 40g; Total Carbs: 8g; Fiber: 2g; Net Carbs: 6g; **Macros:** Fat: 77%; Protein: 19%; Carbs: 4%

Eggs Benedict with Five-Minute Hollandaise

SERVES 2 | PREP TIME: 10 minutes | COOK TIME: 20 minutes

Nonstick cooking spray
4 slices bacon
4 large eggs, plus 3 egg yolks
½ cup butter (1 stick)
Juice of ½ lemon

⅛ teaspoon cayenne pepper
Chopped fresh parsley, for serving
1 avocado, pitted and sliced, for serving

Preheat the oven to 350°F. Spray 4 cups of a muffin tin generously with cooking spray. Line each muffin cup with a strip of bacon, covering the sides as much as possible. Break 1 egg into each bacon nest. Bake the egg cups for 15 to 20 minutes, until

the eggs are set in the center. While the eggs are cooking, melt the butter in a cup in the microwave for 30 to 40 seconds. In a blender, combine the egg yolks, lemon juice, and cayenne. With the blender on the lowest speed, slowly drizzle in the melted butter until emulsified. Remove the egg cups from the oven and carefully remove each egg basket from the muffin tin. Drizzle the hollandaise sauce over the eggs. Sprinkle each cup with parsley and top with a few avocado slices.

Per Serving: (2 egg cups) Calories: 822; Fat: 78g; Protein: 19g; Total Carbs: 11g; Fiber: 7g; Net Carbs: 4g; **Macros:** Fat: 85%; Protein: 9%; Carbs: 6%

Eggs Benedict on Grilled Portabella Mushroom Caps

SERVES 1 | PREP TIME: 5 minutes | COOK TIME: 10 to 15 minutes

2 portabella mushroom caps stemmed
1 tablespoon avocado oil
2 large spinach leaves
2 bacon slices
2 large eggs
1 large egg yolk
¼ teaspoon freshly squeezed lemon juice

1½ tablespoons olive oil
Pinch salt
1 teaspoon paprika
Chopped fresh parsley, for serving
Sugar-free hot sauce, for serving (optional)

Preheat the oven to broil or to 400°F, or heat a grill. Rub the mushrooms all over with the avocado oil, place on a baking sheet, and broil or roast in the oven for 10 minutes, flipping them halfway through. In a large skillet while the mushrooms are baking, fry the bacon to your desired doneness. Remove from skillet and set aside. Remove the mushrooms from the oven or grill, transfer to a plate, and place the spinach leaves and bacon on top. To poach the eggs, fill a saucepan with water and bring to a boil, then lower the heat to a simmer. Crack the eggs into a small bowl and carefully pour them into the simmering water. Turn off the heat, cover the pan, and let the eggs cook for about 5 minutes. Carefully remove the eggs from the pan with a slotted spoon, and place on top of the crispy bacon, spinach, and mushroom caps. In a blender, combine the egg yolk, lemon juice, olive oil, and salt. Turn on the blender to its lowest setting and let the mixture whip. Pour the sauce over the mushrooms and sprinkle with the paprika and chopped parsley.

Per Serving: Calories: 841; Fat: 76g; Protein: 32g; Total Carbs: 14g; Fiber: 5g; Net Carbs: 9g; **Macros:** Fat: 80%; Protein: 14%; Carbs: 6%

Crustless Quiche Lorraine

SERVES 8 | PREP TIME: 20 minutes | COOK TIME: 25 minutes

Nonstick cooking spray
1 pound thick-cut bacon, grease reserved
1 tablespoon minced garlic
¼ cup minced onion
4 large eggs, beaten
1½ cups heavy (whipping) cream

1 cup shredded Swiss cheese
½ cup shredded Gruyère cheese
¾ teaspoon salt
¼ teaspoon freshly ground black pepper

Preheat the oven to 350°F. Lightly spray a 9-inch pie plate. In a large skillet over medium-high heat, cook the bacon until crispy, 6 to 8 minutes depending on thickness. Remove the bacon to drain on paper towels, reserving the bacon grease in the skillet. Once cooled, chop the bacon into small pieces. Lower the heat to medium, add the minced garlic and onions. Cook for 3 to 4 minutes, browning slightly. Remove the skillet from the heat. Spoon the onion and garlic mixture into a small bowl. Set aside to cool. In a large bowl, whisk the eggs and heavy cream for 2 minutes to combine. Whisk in the Swiss and Gruyère cheeses, reserved bacon, onions and garlic, salt, and pepper. Slowly pour the egg mixture into the prepared pie pan. Bake for 20 to 25 minutes, until the center has solidified. Remove the pan from the oven. Cool the quiche for 5 minutes before slicing and serving.

Per Serving: (⅛ of quiche): Calories: 498; Fat: 43g; Protein: 22g; Total Carbs: 2g; Fiber: 0g; Net Carbs: 2g; **Macros:** Fat: 80%; Protein: 18%; Carbs: 2%

Ham and Cheese Crustless Quiche

SERVES 6 | PREP TIME: 15 minutes | COOK TIME: 40 minutes

1 tablespoon butter or nonstick cooking spray, for greasing	½ cup grated Cheddar cheese
	1 cup heavy (whipping) cream
1 cup broccoli florets, steamed and chopped	6 large eggs
	2 ounces (¼ cup) cream cheese
6 ounces ham, cut into ¼-inch cubes	1 teaspoon garlic salt
½ cup grated mozzarella cheese	1 teaspoon freshly ground black pepper
	1 teaspoon paprika

Preheat the oven to 375°F. Grease a 9-inch pie plate with butter or cooking spray. Sprinkle the chopped broccoli, ham, mozzarella, and Cheddar cheese evenly in the pie pan. Using a hand mixer or blender, mix the cream, eggs, cream cheese, garlic salt, pepper, and paprika until well blended, about 15 seconds. Pour the egg mixture over the ham and broccoli mixture. Bake for 40 to 45 minutes, or until a knife inserted in the center comes out clean. Remove from the oven and allow to sit for 5 to 10 minutes before slicing and serving.

Per Serving: Calories: 357; Fat: 30g; Protein: 17g; Total Carbs: 4g; Fiber: 0g; Net Carbs: 4g; **Macros:** Fat: 76%; Protein: 19%; Carbs: 4%

Broccoli Quiche

SERVES 2 | PREP TIME: 10 minutes | COOK TIME: 30 minutes

Nonstick cooking spray	¼ teaspoon freshly ground black pepper
1 large egg, plus 5 egg whites	
½ cup plain nonfat Greek yogurt	1 tablespoon minced garlic
	1 cup broccoli florets
1 teaspoon salt	1 cup shredded Cheddar cheese

Preheat the oven to 400°F. Spray a 9-inch pie plate with cooking spray. In a medium bowl, mix the egg, egg whites, Greek yogurt, salt, pepper, and garlic. Fold in the broccoli and Cheddar cheese.

Pour the mixture into the pie plate and bake for 30 minutes, or until the eggs are set. Remove the quiche from the oven and allow it to cool for a few minutes before serving.

Per Serving: Calories: 352; Fat: 21g; Protein: 33g; Total Carbs: 8g; Fiber: 1g; Net Carbs: 7g; **Macros:** Fat: 54%; Protein: 38%; Carbs: 8%

Crustless Sausage and Green Chile Quiche

SERVES 8 | PREP TIME: 15 minutes | COOK TIME: 35 minutes

Nonstick cooking spray	3 ounces cream cheese, at room temperature
1 pound cooked pork breakfast sausage	
	½ cup sour cream
1 (7-ounce) can mild chopped green chilies	¼ cup heavy (whipping) cream
	½ teaspoon kosher salt
1 cup shredded Monterey Jack cheese, divided	¼ teaspoon freshly ground black pepper
6 large eggs	

Preheat the oven to 350°F. Lightly coat a 9-inch pie plate with cooking spray. In a medium bowl, stir the cooked sausage, green chilies, and ½ cup Monterey Jack cheese. Evenly spread the sausage mixture into the bottom of the pie plate. In a blender, combine the eggs, cream cheese, sour cream, heavy cream, salt, and pepper. Blend on low speed until well combined. Pour the egg mixture over the sausage and sprinkle the remaining Monterey Jack cheese evenly over the top. Bake for 35 to 45 minutes, or until set. Cover lightly with foil to prevent over-browning. Let cool for at least 20 minutes before serving.

Per Serving: Calories: 417; Fat: 37g; Protein: 17g; Total Carbs: 4g; Fiber: 1g; Net Carbs: 3g; **Macros:** Fat: 80%; Protein: 16%; Carbs: 4%

Tuscan "Quiche" Bites

SERVES 4 | PREP TIME: 15 minutes | COOK TIME: 45 minutes

2 tablespoons cold-pressed olive oil	¼ cup water
	2 tablespoons tahini
½ cup sliced cremini mushrooms	2 tablespoons nutritional yeast
⅓ cup chopped onion	1 teaspoon dried basil
¼ cup sliced cherry tomatoes	1 teaspoon dried oregano
1 teaspoon garlic powder	¼ teaspoon ground cumin
1 cup coarsely chopped fresh spinach	⅛ teaspoon turmeric powder
	½ teaspoon kala namak salt (optional)
¼ cup sliced black olives	
1 (14-ounce) block organic firm sprouted tofu, drained	Nonstick cooking spray

Preheat the oven to 350°F. Heat the olive oil in a large skillet over medium heat. Add the mushrooms, onion, tomatoes, and garlic powder, and sauté for about 5 minutes. Stir in the spinach and olives and set aside. In a blender, combine the tofu with the water, tahini, nutritional yeast, basil, oregano, cumin, turmeric, and salt (if using). Blend until it is a fluffy, consistency. Transfer the mixture to a large mixing bowl and fold in the sautéed vegetables. Coat a six-cup muffin pan with cooking spray. Divide the batter equally among the muffin cups. Bake in the preheated oven for 45 minutes until a toothpick inserted into the center of a quiche comes out clean. Allow the quiches to cool for 10 minutes before serving.

Per Serving: Calories: 241; Fat: 18g; Protein: 14g; Total Carbs: 7g; Fiber: 3g; Net Carbs: 4g; **Macros:** Fat: 66%; Protein: 23%; Carbs: 11%

Crustless Cream Cheese and Spinach Quiche

SERVES 8 | PREP TIME: 15 minutes | COOK TIME: 35 minutes

3 tablespoons butter, plus more for preparing the pie pan

¼ cup chopped onion

2 garlic cloves, finely chopped

4 large eggs, lightly beaten

4 ounces cream cheese, at room temperature

⅓ cup ricotta

¾ teaspoon kosher salt

¼ teaspoon freshly ground black pepper

10 ounces frozen chopped spinach, thawed and squeezed dry

3 tablespoons diced roasted red pepper

¼ cup shredded Parmesan cheese

Preheat the oven to 350°F. Coat a 9-inch pie plate with butter. In a small skillet over medium heat, melt the butter. Add the onion and garlic, and sauté for about 5 minutes until tender. Set aside. In a large bowl, whisk the eggs, cream cheese, ricotta, salt, and pepper. Stir in the onions and garlic, spinach, and roasted red pepper and mix well to combine. Pour the mixture into the pie plate and top with the Parmesan cheese. Bake for about 30 minutes, or until set. Let cool for 15 to 20 minutes before slicing.

Per Serving: Calories: 166; Fat: 14g; Protein: 7g; Total Carbs: 3g; Fiber: 1g; Net Carbs: 2g; **Macros:** Fat: 76%; Protein: 17%; Carbs: 7%

Breakfast Sausage

SERVES 4 | PREP TIME: 5 minutes | COOK TIME: 10 to 15 minutes

1 pound ground meat (pork, beef, turkey, chicken, or bison)

2 teaspoons erythritol "brown sugar" or sugar-free maple syrup

1 tablespoon dried sage

1 tablespoon dried thyme

1 teaspoon fennel seeds

1 teaspoon salt

1 teaspoon red pepper flakes

1 teaspoon garlic powder

½ teaspoon paprika

½ teaspoon onion powder

1 tablespoon chopped fresh parsley (optional)

1 tablespoon butter, coconut oil, or avocado oil

1 fried egg, for serving (optional)

Spinach, sautéed, for serving (optional)

In a bowl, mix the ground meat, erythritol, sage, thyme, fennel seeds, salt, red pepper flakes, garlic, paprika, onion powder, and parsley (if using) until well combined. Shape into 4 patties. Heat the butter or oil in a large skillet over medium-high heat. Place the meat patties in the skillet and cook about 5 minutes per side. Transfer to plates, and serve with a fried egg and some sautéed spinach, if desired.

Per Serving: Calories: 259; Fat: 19g; Protein: 20g; Total Carbs: 2g; Fiber: 1g; Net Carbs: 1g; **Macros:** Fat: 66%; Protein: 31%; Carbs: 3%

Bacon Broccoli Crustless Quiche Cups

MAKES 12 | PREP TIME: 10 minutes | COOK TIME: 20 minutes

Nonstick cooking spray

1 cup chopped fresh broccoli

1 cup shredded Cheddar or pepper Jack cheese

½ cup chopped cooked bacon

8 large eggs

½ cup heavy (whipping) cream

½ teaspoon onion powder

½ teaspoon salt

½ teaspoon freshly ground black pepper

Preheat the oven to 350°F. Thoroughly coat the cups of a 12-cup muffin tin with cooking spray. Evenly divide the broccoli, cheese, and bacon between the muffin cups. In a large bowl, whisk the eggs, cream, onion powder, salt, and pepper until well combined. Pour the egg mixture into the muffin cups, distributing it evenly. Bake for 18 minutes or until set.

Per Serving: Calories: 143; Fat: 12g; Protein: 8g; Total Carbs: 1g; Fiber: 0g; Net Carbs: 1g; **Macros:** Fat: 74%; Protein: 24%; Carbs: 2%

Sausage Verde Casserole

PREP TIME: 20 minutes | COOK TIME: 35 minutes | SERVINGS: 10

Oil or nonstick cooking spray (optional)

2 pounds hot breakfast sausage, cooked and drained

18 large eggs

1 (11-ounce) jar green pepper sauce

½ cup heavy (whipping) cream

2 cups shredded Cheddar cheese

¼ teaspoon salt

¼ teaspoon freshly ground black pepper

Preheat the oven to 350°F, and lightly grease a 9-by-13-inch baking dish or line with parchment paper. In a medium bowl, mix the cooked sausage, eggs, green sauce, heavy cream, cheese, salt, and pepper, and pour into the prepared baking dish. Bake for 35 minutes, or until the center is cooked through. Serve warm.

Per Serving: Calories: 566; Fat: 45g; Protein: 34g; Total Carbs: 5g; Fiber: 1g; Net Carbs: 4g; **Macros:** Fat: 72%; Protein: 25%; Carbs: 3%

Breakfast Bowl with Cauliflower Hash

SERVES 1 | PREP TIME: 10 minutes | COOK TIME: 15 to 20 minutes

2 tablespoons avocado oil or butter, divided

3 tablespoons finely diced onion

½ cup riced or diced cauliflower

¼ tablespoon garlic powder, plus ½ teaspoon

Salt

Freshly ground black pepper

1 large egg

½ cup peppers and onions

¼ cup shredded cheese, plus more for serving (optional)

½ cup raw spinach

¼ cup minced tomatoes

Melted ghee or MCT oil, for serving (optional)

In a large skillet, heat 1 tablespoon of avocado oil over medium heat. Add the onion and let cook for 1 minute. Add the cauliflower and cook for 3 minutes. Add ¼ tablespoon garlic powder, salt, and pepper and cook for 5 minutes more. While the cauliflower hash is cooking, in another skillet, cook a sunny-side-up or over-easy egg and heat up the peppers and onions with the remaining 1 tablespoon of avocado oil, salt, pepper, and the remaining ½ teaspoon of garlic powder. Turn off the heat for the cauliflower and add the cheese (if using). Place the raw spinach at the bottom of the bowl, then add your cauliflower hash. Top with the peppers and onions and egg. Then sprinkle with the tomatoes and top with cheese and drizzle with melted ghee or MCT oil.

Per Serving: Calories: 603; Fat: 47g; Protein: 29g; Total Carbs: 16g; Fiber: 5g; Net Carbs: 11g; Macros: Fat: 70%; Protein: 20%; Carbs: 10%

Savory Sausage Balls

MAKES 30 SAUSAGE BALLS | PREP TIME: 10 minutes | COOK TIME: 25 minutes

1 pound breakfast sausage
1 cup coconut flour
1½ cups shredded mozzarella cheese (or any other white cheese)
1 (5-ounce) package Boursin cheese, Garlic & Fine Herbs or any other flavor

2 large eggs
2 tablespoons butter, at room temperature
2 teaspoons baking powder
1 teaspoon garlic salt

Preheat the oven to 350°F. Line a baking sheet with parchment paper. In a large bowl, combine all the ingredients and mix well with your hands. Using a cookie scoop, drop scoopfuls into your hand, roll into balls, and place on the baking sheet. Bake for about 25 minutes or until golden brown.

Per Serving: (2 sausage balls) Calories: 254; Fat: 19g; Protein: 12g; Total Carbs: 9g; Fiber: 6g; Net Carbs: 3g; Macros: Fat: 67%; Protein: 19%; Carbs: 14%

Sausage Egg Roll in a Bowl

SERVES 4 | PREP TIME: 5 minutes | COOK TIME: 20 minutes

1 pound pork breakfast sausage
1 (1-pound) bag shredded cabbage or coleslaw mix

3 tablespoons soy sauce
3 garlic cloves, minced
1 tablespoon sesame oil
2 scallions, thinly sliced

In a skillet over medium heat, cook the breakfast sausage. Drain the grease. Add the cabbage mix, soy sauce, garlic cloves, and sesame oil to the skillet with the sausage and mix well. Cook for 5 to 10 minutes, until the cabbage is tender. Sprinkle with the scallions and serve warm.

Per Serving: (¼ skillet) Calories: 412; Fat: 33g; Protein: 20g; Total Carbs: 9g; Fiber: 3g; Net Carbs: 6g; Macros: Fat: 72%; Protein: 19%; Carbs: 11%

Bagels with Smoked Salmon

PREP TIME: 15 minutes, plus 30 minutes to rest | COOK TIME: 20 minutes | SERVINGS: 8

2½ cups grated mozzarella cheese
½ cup grated Parmesan cheese
2 ounces (¼ cup) cream cheese

1 cup almond flour
2 tablespoons coconut flour
2 teaspoons baking powder
1 teaspoon garlic powder

¼ teaspoon salt
2 large eggs, plus 1 egg for brushing on bagels
3 tablespoons everything bagel seasoning

4 ounces (½ brick) cream cheese
8 ounces smoked salmon, thinly sliced

Preheat the oven to 400°F, and line a baking sheet with parchment paper. In a medium microwave-safe bowl, combine the mozzarella, Parmesan, and cream cheese. Heat in 30-second increments until the cheeses are completely melted and smooth. In a small bowl, stir the almond flour, coconut flour, baking powder, garlic powder, and salt. Add half the flour mixture to the cheese mixture. Stir to blend. Add the eggs and remaining flour mixture, and mix until incorporated. Let the dough rest for 30 minutes. Spread a sheet of parchment paper on the counter. With damp hands, make a ball out of the dough, and split it in half. Place half onto the parchment paper on the counter, and split the dough into 4 equal parts. Using your palms, roll each part into a 6- to 8-inch snake on the paper. Shape each dough snake into a circle on the baking sheet, pinching the ends to connect. Repeat with the other half of the dough until you have 8 bagels. Whisk the remaining egg, and brush on top of each bagel. Sprinkle with the bagel seasoning and bake for 13 to 15 minutes, until golden brown. Slice the bagels horizontally and top each with 1 tablespoon of cream cheese, 1 ounce of salmon, and serve.

Per Serving: (1 bagel with cream cheese and salmon): Calories: 338; Fat: 26g; Protein: 21g; Total Carbs: 6g; Fiber: 2g; Net Carbs: 4g; Macros: Fat: 69%; Protein: 25%; Carbs: 6%

Breakfast Pizza

SERVES 4 | PREP TIME: 10 minutes | COOK TIME: 20 minutes

4 ounces Italian sausage
8 large eggs
½ cup half-and-half
½ cup almond flour
¼ teaspoon sea salt
Freshly ground black pepper

1 cup sliced roasted red bell peppers
1 cup shredded mozzarella cheese
1 tablespoon minced fresh oregano (optional)

Preheat the oven to 400°F. In a large ovenproof skillet, cook the sausage over medium heat until barely cooked through. Transfer to a small dish. In a blender, combine the eggs, half-and-half, almond flour, salt, and pepper. Blend until smooth. Pour the egg mixture into the skillet and cook over medium heat for 5 minutes. Top with the cooked sausage, red bell peppers, mozzarella cheese, and oregano (if using). Transfer the skillet to the oven and bake for 12 to 15 minutes, or until the eggs are completely set.

Per Serving: Calories: 431; Fat: 32g; Protein: 27g; Total Carbs: 8g; Fiber: 2g; Net Carbs: 6g; Macros: Fat: 67%; Protein: 25%; Carbs: 8%

Portabella Breakfast "Burger"

SERVES 1 | PREP TIME: 5 minutes | COOK TIME: 20 minutes

1 tablespoon olive oil
2 portabella mushroom caps, stemmed, gills removed

¼ cup ground breakfast sausage
2 (2-ounce) slices American cheese

In a medium nonstick skillet over medium heat, heat the olive oil for 1 minute. Add the mushrooms cap side up. Cook for about

5 minutes per side, or until browned. Heat medium skillet over medium-high heat. Form the breakfast sausage into a ½-inch-thick patty. Cook for 4 to 5 minutes. Flip and cook 2 to 3 minutes more. When the sausage is almost done, reduce the heat to low. Top the patty with the American cheese. Cook until the cheese melts. Transfer the mushroom caps from the skillet to a plate. Place the cheese-topped patty on one mushroom cap. Top with the remaining mushroom cap and serve.

Per Serving: (1 "burger"): Calories: 504; Fat: 41g; Protein: 24g; Total Carbs: 10g; Fiber: 3g; Net Carbs: 7g; **Macros:** Fat: 73%; Protein: 19%; Carbs: 8%

Biscuits and Sausage Gravy

SERVES 6 | PREP TIME: 20 minutes | COOK TIME: 30 minutes

For the biscuits

½ cup coconut flour
½ cup almond flour
2 teaspoons baking powder
1 teaspoon garlic powder
½ teaspoon onion powder
½ teaspoon salt

½ cup shredded
  Cheddar cheese
¼ cup butter, melted
4 large eggs
¾ cup sour cream

For the sausage gravy

1 pound ground break-
  fast sausage
1 teaspoon minced garlic
1 tablespoon almond flour
1½ cups unsweetened
  almond milk

½ cup heavy (whipping) cream
1½ teaspoons freshly ground
  black pepper
½ teaspoon salt

Preheat the oven to 350°F. Line a baking sheet with parchment paper. In a large bowl, combine the coconut flour, almond flour, baking powder, garlic powder, onion powder, and salt. Toss in the Cheddar cheese. In the center of the dry ingredients, create a well and add the melted butter, eggs, and sour cream. Fold together until a dough forms. Use a spoon to drop biscuits onto the baking sheet, about 1 inch apart. Bake the biscuits for 20 minutes, or until firm and lightly browned. Heat a large saucepan over medium-high heat. Add the ground sausage, breaking it up with a spoon and browning it on all sides. Once the sausage browns, add the minced garlic. Cook for 1 minute. Sprinkle in the almond flour. Reduce the heat to medium-low. Whisk into a light roux, stirring constantly, about 5 minutes. Slowly add the almond milk to the roux, stirring constantly. Add the heavy cream. Increase the temperature to medium-high, stirring and reducing the mixture for 3 minutes. Reduce the heat to medium-low. Add the pepper and salt. Cool the biscuits for 5 minutes. Reduce the heat again under the sausage gravy to low. Simmer while the biscuits cool. Plate 1 biscuit per person and top with ⅓ cup of gravy.

Per Serving: (1 biscuit; ⅓ cup sausage gravy): Calories: 559; Fat: 49g; Protein: 15g; Total Carbs: 14g; Fiber: 6g; Net Carbs: 8g; **Macros:** Fat: 79%; Protein: 11%; Carbs: 10%

Cheesy Sausage and Cabbage Hash

SERVES 6 | PREP TIME: 10 minutes | COOK TIME: 25 minutes

2 tablespoons olive oil or
  bacon fat

½ cup diced onion
1 garlic clove, minced

1½ pounds kielbasa sausage,
  cut into 1-inch rounds
4 cups chopped red or
  green cabbage
½ teaspoon salt

½ teaspoon freshly ground
  black pepper
1½ cups shredded
  Cheddar cheese

Preheat the oven to 400°F. Warm the oil in a large ovenproof skillet over medium heat, then add the onion and garlic. Sauté for 1 to 2 minutes until fragrant. Add the kielbasa and brown for 5 minutes, stirring regularly. Add the cabbage, salt, and pepper and sauté for 8 to 10 minutes. Top the cabbage and sausage mixture with the cheese. Bake for 10 minutes. Turn the broiler to high for the last minute to ensure the cheese is melted. Remove from the oven and serve.

Per Serving: Calories: 547; Fat: 48g; Protein: 20g; Total Carbs: 10g; Fiber: 2g; Net Carbs: 8g; **Macros:** Fat: 78%; Protein: 14%; Carbs: 8%

Cheesy "Hash Brown" Casserole

SERVES 8 | PREP TIME: 15 minutes | COOK TIME: 50 minutes

Nonstick cooking spray
2 pounds turnips, peeled and
  shredded
1¾ teaspoons kosher
  salt, divided
¼ cup butter
⅓ cup diced onion
¼ cup chicken stock
1 cup heavy (whipping) cream

¾ cup sour cream
¼ teaspoon freshly ground
  black pepper
¼ teaspoon garlic powder
2 cups shredded Cheddar
  cheese, divided
2 scallions, both white and
  green parts sliced

Preheat the oven to 350°F. Coat an 8-inch-square baking dish with cooking spray. Set aside. In a medium bowl, toss the turnips and 1 teaspoon of salt. Let sit for 10 minutes. Meanwhile, in a large skillet over medium heat, melt the butter. Add the onion and sauté for 5 to 7 minutes, or until the onion is translucent. Add the chicken stock and simmer for 1 to 2 minutes. Add the heavy cream and simmer for 5 to 7 minutes until the mixture is reduced and thick. Remove from the heat. Place the turnips between two paper towels, and squeeze to remove any excess liquid. Place the turnips in a large bowl. Add the sour cream, the remaining ¾ teaspoon of salt, the pepper, garlic powder, onion mixture, and 1½ cups of Cheddar cheese. Mix until thoroughly combined. Pour the mixture into the prepared baking dish and cover with aluminum foil. Bake for 35 minutes. Remove from the oven, top with the remaining ½ cup of Cheddar cheese, and bake for 10 more minutes. Garnish with scallions and serve warm.

Per Serving: Calories: 359; Fat: 31g; Protein: 10g; Total Carbs: 10g; Fiber: 3g; Net Carbs: 7g; **Macros:** Fat: 78%; Protein: 11%; Carbs: 11%

Chicken Brunch Pie with Cheddar Pecan Crust

SERVES 8 | PREP TIME: 20 minutes | COOK TIME: 1 hour

For the crust

1½ cups almond flour
¼ cup pecans, finely chopped
⅓ cup shredded
  cheddar cheese

¼ teaspoon freshly ground
  black pepper
Pinch kosher salt
3 tablespoons butter, melted

For the filling

1 cup sour cream

¼ cup mayonnaise

4 large eggs

¾ teaspoon kosher salt

¼ teaspoon freshly ground
black pepper

¼ teaspoon paprika

2 cups chopped
cooked chicken

½ cup shredded
Cheddar cheese

3 scallions, sliced

Preheat the oven to 350°F. In a small bowl, stir the almond flour, pecans, Cheddar cheese, pepper, and salt. Pour in the melted butter and stir until thoroughly incorporated. Firmly press the crust mixture evenly into the bottom and up the sides of a 9-inch pie plate. Bake for 12 to 15 minutes, or until the edges are golden brown. In a medium bowl, whisk the sour cream, mayonnaise, eggs, salt, pepper, and paprika until blended. Stir in the chicken, Cheddar cheese, and scallions, until thoroughly combined. Pour the mixture into the baked pie crust. Bake for 40 to 45 minutes, or until set. Let cool for at least 20 minutes before slicing.

Per Serving: Calories: 369; Fat: 29g; Protein: 20g; Total Carbs: 7g; Fiber: 2g; Net Carbs: 5g; Macros: Fat: 71%; Protein: 22%; Carbs: 7%

Breakfast Burrito Bowl

SERVES 6 | PREP TIME: 5 minutes | COOK TIME: 15 minutes

1 pound breakfast sausage

8 large eggs, beaten

Salt

Freshly ground black pepper

1 cup shredded Cheddar cheese

1 avocado, diced

½ cup salsa

½ cup sour cream

2 or 3 scallions, sliced

In a large skillet over medium heat, cook the breakfast sausage, breaking it up into small pieces, until browned. Remove from the skillet and divide among 6 bowls. In a medium bowl, beat the eggs and season with salt and pepper. Pour off all but about 1 tablespoon of fat from the skillet. Add the eggs to the skillet and cook over medium heat, stirring regularly to scramble. Divide the eggs among the 6 bowls. Top each bowl with the cheese, avocado, salsa, sour cream, and scallions.

Per Serving: Calories: 455; Fat: 35g; Protein: 26g; Total Carbs: 8g; Fiber: 3g; Net Carbs: 5g; Macros: Fat: 70%; Protein: 23%; Carbs: 7%

Classic Diner Hash Browns

SERVES 6 | PREP TIME: 10 minutes | COOK TIME: 30 minutes

3 cups radishes

2 large eggs

½ cup finely shredded
Parmesan cheese

½ teaspoon salt

½ teaspoon freshly ground
black pepper

Nonstick cooking spray or oil

Preheat the oven to its lowest setting. Using a box grater, grate the radishes. Place the radishes in a microwave-safe bowl with a plate on top, and microwave at full power for 3 minutes. Allow to cool. Turn out the radishes onto a clean tea towel or cheesecloth and squeeze well to remove as much liquid as possible. Return the radishes to the bowl. Add the eggs, cheese, salt, and pepper, and mix well with a fork. Preheat a large nonstick skillet over medium-high heat and coat with cooking spray. Form the radish mixture into 6 patties and flatten as thin as possible. Cook 3 patties at a time over medium heat for 4 to 5 minutes per side or until the patties are browned and crisp.

Per Serving: Calories: 68; Fat: 4g; Protein: 5g; Total Carbs: 3g; Fiber: 1g; Net Carbs: 2g; Macros: Fat: 52%; Protein: 30%; Carbs: 18%

Shakshuka

SERVES 4 | PREP TIME: 10 minutes | COOK TIME: 30 minutes

½ cup plus 2 tablespoons
extra-virgin olive oil, divided

½ small yellow onion,
finely diced

1 red bell pepper, finely diced

1 (14-ounce) can crushed
tomatoes, with juices

6 ounces frozen spinach,
thawed and drained
of excess liquid (about
1½ cups)

2 garlic cloves, finely minced

1 teaspoon smoked paprika

1 to 2 teaspoons red pepper
flakes (optional)

1 tablespoon roughly
chopped capers

6 large eggs

¼ teaspoon freshly ground
black pepper

¾ cup crumbled feta or
goat cheese

¼ cup chopped fresh flat-leaf
parsley or cilantro

Heat the broiler to low. In a medium, deep oven-safe skillet, heat 2 tablespoons of olive oil over medium-high heat. Add the onion and bell pepper and sauté until softened, 5 to 8 minutes. Add the crushed tomatoes and their juices, ½ cup olive oil, spinach, garlic, paprika, red pepper flakes (if using), and capers, stirring to combine. Bring to a boil, then reduce the heat to low, cover, and simmer for 5 minutes. Uncover the skillet and gently crack the eggs into the sauce, so they don't touch. Season with pepper, cover and cook, poaching the eggs until the yolks are just set, 8 to 10 minutes. Uncover the pan and spread the crumbled cheese over top of the eggs and sauce. Transfer to the oven and broil under low heat until the cheese is just slightly browned and bubbly, 3 to 5 minutes. Drizzle with the remaining 2 tablespoons olive oil, top with chopped parsley, and serve warm.

Per Serving: Calories: 476; Fat: 40g; Protein: 17g; Total Carbs: 12g; Fiber: 5g; Net Carbs: 7g; Macros: Fat: 76%; Protein: 14%; Carbs: 10%

Crustless Greek Cheese Pie

SERVES 6 | PREP TIME: 10 minutes | COOK TIME: 40 minutes

¼ cup extra-virgin olive
oil, divided

1¼ cups crumbled Greek feta

½ cup ricotta

2 tablespoons chopped
fresh mint

1 tablespoon chopped
fresh dill

½ teaspoon lemon zest

¼ teaspoon freshly ground
black pepper

2 large eggs

½ teaspoon baking powder

Preheat the oven to 350°F. Grease an 8-inch-square baking dish with 2 tablespoons of olive oil. In a medium bowl, combine the feta and ricotta. Stir in the mint, dill, lemon zest, and pepper and mix well. In a small bowl, beat the eggs and baking powder. Add to the cheese mixture and blend well. Pour into the prepared baking dish and drizzle the remaining 2 tablespoons of olive oil over top. Bake until lightly browned and set, 35 to 40 minutes.

Per Serving: Calories: 182; Fat: 17g; Protein: 7g; Total Carbs: 2g; Fiber: 0g; Net Carbs: 2g; Macros: Fat: 82%; Protein: 15%; Carbs: 3%

Greek Yogurt Parfait

SERVES 1 | PREP TIME: 5 minutes

½ cup plain Greek yogurt
2 tablespoons heavy (whipping) cream
¼ cup frozen berries, thawed with juices
½ teaspoon vanilla or almond extract (optional)

¼ teaspoon ground cinnamon (optional)
1 tablespoon ground flaxseed
2 tablespoons chopped nuts (walnuts or pecans)

In a small bowl or glass, combine the yogurt, heavy whipping cream, thawed berries in their juice, vanilla or almond extract (if using), cinnamon (if using), and flaxseed and stir well until smooth. Top with chopped nuts and enjoy.

Per Serving: Calories: 267; Fat: 19g; Protein: 12g; Total Carbs: 12g; Fiber: 4g; Net Carbs: 8g; **Macros:** Fat: 65%; Protein: 18%; Carbs: 17%

Simple Cheesy Yogurt

SERVES 4 | PREP TIME: 10 minutes

¾ cup coconut milk
¾ cup plain Greek yogurt

½ cup cream cheese, softened
¼ teaspoon stevia

In a medium bowl, whisk the coconut milk, Greek yogurt, cream cheese, and stevia until very smooth. Serve.

Per Serving: Calories: 242; Fat: 22g; Protein: 5g; Total Carbs: 6g; Fiber: 2g; Net Carbs: 4g; **Macros:** Fat: 82%; Protein: 8%; Carbs: 10%

Chia Parfait

SERVES 4 | PREP TIME: 5 minutes, plus at least 20 minutes to chill

2½ cups unsweetened almond milk
½ cup coconut cream
1 teaspoon ground cinnamon

¼ teaspoon ground cardamom
⅛ teaspoon ground nutmeg
1 teaspoon vanilla extract
¼ cup chia seeds

Pour the almond milk and coconut cream into a 32-ounce mason jar. Add the cinnamon, cardamom, nutmeg, vanilla, and chia seeds. Close the lid tightly and shake the jar vigorously. Place the jar in the refrigerator to set for at least 20 minutes or overnight.

Per Serving: Calories: 150; Fat: 11g; Protein: 4g; Total Carbs: 8g; Fiber: 6g; Net Carbs: 2g; **Macros:** Fat: 67%; Protein: 11%; Carbs: 22%

Yogurt Parfait with Chia Seeds

SERVES 1 | TOTAL TIME: 20 minutes

1 cup full-fat yogurt
¼ cup unsweetened almond milk
2 tablespoons chia seeds

6 teaspoons sliced almonds, divided
¼ teaspoon cinnamon, divided

In a medium bowl, mix the yogurt, almond milk, and chia seeds. Pour one-third of the yogurt mixture into a tall glass. Sprinkle 2 teaspoons of almonds and a dash of cinnamon on top. Repeat two more times with the remaining yogurt, 4 teaspoons of almonds, and cinnamon, forming three layers. Refrigerate to thicken for 5 to 10 minutes.

Per Serving: Calories: 434; Fat: 33g; Protein: 14g; Total Carbs: 19g; Fiber: 12g; Net Carbs: 7g; **Macros:** Fat: 69%; Protein: 18%; Carbs: 13%

Coconut Yogurt Berry Parfait

SERVES 1 | PREP TIME: 5 minutes | COOK TIME: 5 minutes

For the coconut topping (makes 4 servings)

1 teaspoon cinnamon
1 teaspoon raw honey

1 teaspoon filtered water
1 cup dried coconut flakes

For the parfait (makes 1 serving)

1 cup plain unsweetened coconut yogurt
1 teaspoon MCT oil

¼ cup Coconut Topping
¼ cup fresh raspberries

Preheat the oven to 300°F. Line a baking sheet with parchment paper. In a medium bowl, combine the cinnamon, honey, and water. Stir in the dried coconut flakes until they are fully coated. Spread the coconut flakes in an even layer on the baking sheet and bake for 15 to 20 minutes or until golden, stirring halfway. Let the coconut flakes cool completely before transferring to a sealed container. Refrigerate in a sealed container for up to a week. Scoop the coconut yogurt into a bowl and stir in the MCT oil. Top the yogurt with the coconut topping and raspberries.

Per Serving: Calories: 665; Fat: 65g; Protein: 8g; Total Carbs: 12g; Fiber: 3g; Net Carbs: 9g; **Macros:** Fat: 88%; Protein: 5%; Carbs: 7%

Lemon Berry Yogurt Parfait

SERVES 1 | PREP TIME: 5 minutes

5 ounces plain Greek yogurt
½ teaspoon lemon zest
1 to 2 drops liquid stevia (optional)

¼ cup roughly chopped pecans
¼ cup raspberries

In a small bowl, mix the yogurt, lemon zest, and stevia (if using). Place half of the yogurt into a small glass. Top with half of the raspberries followed by half of the pecans. Repeat with another layer each of yogurt, berries, and pecans. Serve immediately or cover and chill until ready to serve.

Per Serving: Calories: 331; Fat: 28g; Protein: 13g; Total Carbs: 12g; Fiber: 5g; Net Carbs: 7g; **Macros:** Fat: 76%; Protein: 16%; Carbs: 8%

Peanut Butter Whipped Greek Yogurt

SERVES 1 | PREP TIME: 5 minutes

5 ounces plain Greek yogurt
2 tablespoons creamy natural peanut butter

1 to 2 drops liquid stevia (optional)
15 no-sugar-added chocolate chips, such as Lily's brand

In a bowl, whisk the yogurt, peanut butter, and stevia (if using) until light and fluffy. Stir in the chocolate chips.

Per Serving: Calories: 322; Fat: 22g; Protein: 23g; Total Carbs: 11g; Fiber: 2g; Net Carbs: 9g; **Macros:** Fat: 61%; Protein: 28%; Carbs: 11%

Go Get 'Em Green Smoothie Bowl

SERVES 2 | PREP TIME: 5 minutes

2 cups fresh spinach
1 cup unsweetened almond milk

½ cup ice cubes
½ avocado
1 tablespoon MCT oil

1 tablespoon almond butter
1 handful fresh mint leaves
4 drops liquid stevia
½-inch fresh ginger, peeled

Optional toppings: hemp or chia seeds; coconut flakes; cacao nibs; fresh mint; sliced strawberries

Combine the spinach, almond milk, ice, avocado, MCT oil, almond butter, mint, stevia, and ginger in a high-powered blender. Blend on high until smooth and thick, adding a little extra liquid if needed. Scoop the smoothie mixture into a bowl and sprinkle with your choice of toppings.

Per Serving: Calories: 214; Fat: 20g; Protein: 3g; Total Carbs: 8g; Fiber: 5g; Net Carbs: 3g; **Macros:** Fat: 80%; Protein: 6%; Carbs: 14%

Pumpkin Pie Yogurt Bowl
SERVES 1 | PREP TIME: 10 minutes

1 tablespoon heavy (whipping) cream
½ cup plain whole milk Greek yogurt
1 tablespoon unsweetened pumpkin puree
1 teaspoon pumpkin pie spice

1 to 2 teaspoons monk fruit extract or sugar-free sweetener (optional)
½ teaspoon vanilla extract
2 tablespoons roughly chopped pecans

In a small bowl, whisk the cream for 2 to 3 minutes, until thick and doubled in volume. In a medium bowl, mix the yogurt, pumpkin, pumpkin pie spice, sweetener (if using), and vanilla. Place yogurt mixture in a medium bowl and top with the pecans and whipped cream.

Per Serving: Calories: 266; Fat: 20g; Protein: 13g; Total Carbs: 9g; Fiber: 2g; Net Carbs: 7g; **Macros:** Fat: 68%; Protein: 20%; Carbs: 12%

Cinnamon-Nut Cottage Cheese
1 SERVING | PREP TIME: 5 minutes

½ cup cottage cheese
1 stevia packet or a few squirts liquid stevia or substitute

2 teaspoons to 1 tablespoon cinnamon
¼ cup chopped pecans

In a bowl, combine the cottage cheese and stevia, mixing well. Add the cinnamon and mix just to incorporate. Add more cinnamon or stevia to taste. Sprinkle the pecans on top and enjoy!

Per Serving: Calories: 324; Fat: 27g; Protein: 15g; Total Carbs: 10g; Fiber: 4g; Net Carbs: 6g; **Macros:** Fat: 71%; Protein: 17%; Carbs: 12%

Overnight Chocolate Chia Pudding
MAKES 6 | PREP TIME: 5 minutes, plus overnight to chill

4½ cups unsweetened almond milk
9 tablespoons chia seeds
6 tablespoons unsweetened cocoa powder
1 sweetener of choice:

3 packets Splenda, or
10 to 12 drops liquid stevia, or
3 tablespoons sugar-free Torani syrup, or
3 tablespoons powdered erythritol blend

In a bowl, mix all the ingredients until well combined. Divide the mixture evenly among 6 (8-ounce or larger) glasses or canning jars. Cover and refrigerate overnight. The next morning, stir and serve.

Per Serving: Calories: 169; Fat: 9g; Protein: 4g; Total Carbs: 18g; Fiber: 9g; Net Carbs: 9g; **Macros:** Fat: 48%; Protein: 10%; Carbs: 42%

PB&J Overnight Hemp
SERVES 6 | PREP TIME: 5 minutes, plus overnight to set

3 cups unsweetened almond milk, plus more for serving
1 tablespoon sugar-free peanut butter
4 drops liquid stevia or sugar-free sweetener of choice

1½ cups hemp hearts
2 tablespoons chia seeds
¼ cup cacao nibs
⅛ cup unsweetened coconut flakes
¼ cup freeze-dried raspberries

In a large mixing bowl, whisk the almond milk, peanut butter, and stevia. Once well combined, add the hemp hearts, chia seeds, cacao nibs, coconut, and raspberries, and stir. Refrigerate in a sealed container for at least 8 hours. Divide the mixture among 6 small serving bowls and top with a splash of almond milk.

Per Serving: Calories: 324; Fat: 24g; Protein: 16g; Total Carbs: 10g; Fiber: 8g; Net Carbs: 2g; **Macros:** Fat: 68%; Protein: 20%; Carbs: 12%

Creamy Cinnamon Breakfast Pudding
SERVES 4 | PREP TIME: 2 minutes | COOK TIME: 11 minutes

2 cups cottage cheese
1 cup heavy (whipping) cream
4 large eggs
2 tablespoons flaxseed meal

4 (7g) stevia packets
½ teaspoon ground cinnamon
¼ teaspoon ground nutmeg
¼ cup butter, for topping

In a medium saucepan over medium-high heat, whisk the cottage cheese, heavy cream, and eggs to combine. Cook the cheese mixture, stirring occasionally, until the mixture starts to boil, about 5 minutes. Reduce the heat and simmer until the eggs are cooked through, about 4 minutes. Remove the saucepan from the heat, and stir in the flaxseed meal, stevia, cinnamon, and nutmeg. Top each serving with 1 tablespoon of butter and serve.

Per Serving: Calories: 401; Fat: 35g; Protein: 18g; Total Carbs: 7g; Fiber: 1g; Net Carbs: 6g; **Macros:** Fat: 76%; Protein: 17%; Carbs: 7%

Nut Medley Granola
SERVES 8 | PREP TIME: 10 minutes | COOK TIME: 1 hour

2 cups shredded unsweetened coconut
1 cup sliced almonds
1 cup raw sunflower seeds
½ cup raw pumpkin seeds

½ cup walnuts
½ cup melted coconut oil
10 drops liquid stevia
1 teaspoon ground cinnamon
½ teaspoon ground nutmeg

Preheat the oven to 250°F. Line a baking sheet with parchment paper. Toss the shredded coconut, almonds, sunflower seeds, pumpkin seeds, and walnuts in a large bowl until mixed. In a small bowl, stir the coconut oil, stevia, cinnamon, and nutmeg until blended. Pour the coconut oil mixture into the nut mixture and use your hands to blend until the nuts are very well coated. Spread the granola mixture on the baking sheet and bake, stirring every 10 to 15 minutes, until the mixture is golden brown and crunchy, about 1 hour. Let the granola cool, tossing it frequently to break up the large pieces.

Per Serving: Calories: 391; Fat: 38g; Protein: 10g; Total Carbs: 10g; Fiber: 6g; Net Carbs: 4g; **Macros:** Fat: 80%; Protein: 10%; Carbs: 10%

Keto Granola

SERVES 16 | PREP TIME: 10 minutes | COOK TIME: 3 to 4 hours on low

½ cup coconut oil, melted
2 teaspoons pure vanilla extract
1 teaspoon maple extract
1 cup chopped pecans
1 cup sunflower seeds
1 cup unsweetened shredded coconut

½ cup hazelnuts
½ cup slivered almonds
¼ cup granulated erythritol
½ teaspoon cinnamon
¼ teaspoon ground nutmeg
¼ teaspoon salt

Lightly grease the insert of the slow cooker with 1 tablespoon of the coconut oil. In a large bowl, whisk the remaining coconut oil, vanilla, and maple extract. Add the pecans, sunflower seeds, coconut, hazelnuts, almonds, erythritol, cinnamon, nutmeg, and salt. Toss to coat the nuts and seeds. Transfer the mixture to the slow cooker insert. Cover and cook on low for 3 to 4 hours, until the granola is crispy. Transfer the granola to a baking sheet covered in parchment to cool.

Per Serving: (⅓ cup) Calories: 236; Fat: 23g; Protein: 6g; Total Carbs: 5g; Fiber: 3g; Net Carbs: 2g; **Macros:** Fat: 82%; Protein: 10%; Carbs: 8%

Superfood Granola

SERVES 2 | PREP TIME: 5 minutes | COOK TIME: 20 minutes

½ cup unsweetened coconut flakes
2 tablespoons ground flaxseed
2 tablespoons pepitas
2 tablespoons sunflower seeds

3 tablespoons chopped pecans
2 tablespoons coconut oil, melted
1 teaspoon ground cinnamon
½ teaspoon ground ginger
1 teaspoon salt

Preheat the oven to 350°F. In a medium bowl, combine the coconut flakes, flaxseed, pepitas, sunflower seeds, and pecans, and mix well. Pour the coconut oil over the mixture and stir to coat well. Toss in the cinnamon, ginger, and salt. Spread the granola on a rimmed baking sheet and bake for 20 minutes, tossing the granola every 3 to 4 minutes. Remove from the oven once the mixture is light golden brown, and set aside to cool thoroughly.

Per Serving: Calories: 377; Fat: 35g; Protein: 6g; Total Carbs: 10g; Fiber: 7g; Net Carbs: 3g; **Macros:** Fat: 84%; Protein: 6%; Carbs: 10%

Macadamia Nut Granola

SERVES 6 | PREP TIME: 10 minutes | COOK TIME: 15 minutes

1 cup macadamia nuts
1 cup almonds
1 cup shredded unsweetened coconut
1 egg white, whisked

¼ cup coconut oil, melted
1 teaspoon vanilla extract
½ teaspoon liquid stevia
½ teaspoon sea salt

Preheat the oven to 325°F. In a food processor, pulse the macadamia nuts and almonds until the mixture is the texture of rolled oats. Add the coconut and pulse once or twice to mix. In a separate bowl, mix the egg white, coconut oil, vanilla, stevia, and sea salt. Pour this over the nut mixture and stir to mix. Spread

the granola into an 8-inch-square baking dish. Bake for 7 to 8 minutes. Stir and bake for another 7 to 8 minutes until the granola is golden brown. Allow to cool at room temperature.

Per Serving: (½ cup) Calories: 466; Fat: 43g; Protein: 8g; Total Carbs: 12g; Fiber: 7g; Net Carbs: 5g; **Macros:** Fat: 84%; Protein: 6%; Carbs: 10%

Coconut Granola

3 SERVINGS (½ CUP PER SERVING) |
PREP TIME: 5 minutes | COOK TIME: 20 minutes

½ cup chopped raw macadamia nuts
½ cup sliced raw almonds
¼ cup cacao nibs
2 tablespoons unsweetened coconut flakes

1 teaspoon vanilla extract
1 teaspoon ground cinnamon
¼ teaspoon salt
2 tablespoons melted coconut oil

Preheat the oven to 325°F. Line a baking sheet with parchment paper. Place the macadamia nuts, almonds, cacao nibs, coconut, vanilla, cinnamon, and salt in a medium bowl, add the coconut oil, and mix well. Spread the granola on the baking sheet in an even layer. Bake for 15 to 20 minutes or just until it is fragrant and toasted on the bottom.

Per Serving: Calories: 433; Fat: 43g; Protein: 8g; Total Carbs: 12g; Fiber: 8g; Net Carbs: 4g; **Macros:** Fat: 85%; Protein: 7%; Carbs: 8%

Granola Cereal

SERVES 8 | PREP TIME: 5 minutes | COOK TIME: 25 minutes

¼ cup creamy almond butter
2 tablespoons melted coconut oil
2 tablespoons sugar-free maple syrup
1 egg white
½ teaspoon vanilla extract
¼ teaspoon ground cinnamon

¾ cup unsweetened coconut flakes
¾ cup almond slivers
⅓ cup chopped pecans
2 tablespoons sugar-free chocolate chips
¼ teaspoon sea salt
Unsweetened nut milk, for serving

Preheat the oven to 300°F. Line a rimmed baking sheet with parchment paper. In a large bowl, whisk the almond butter, coconut oil, maple syrup, egg white vanilla, and cinnamon. Stir in the coconut flakes, almonds, pecans, and chocolate chips. Spread the mixture in an even layer on the prepared baking sheet. Sprinkle with the salt. Bake for 10 to 12 minutes, rotate the baking sheet without stirring the granola, and bake for another 10 to 12 minutes. It is done when the top browns. Remove the baking sheet from the oven and allow the granola to cool completely.

Per Serving: (¼ cup): Calories: 241; Fat: 22g; Protein: 5g; Total Carbs: 9g; Fiber: 5g; Net Carbs: 4g; **Macros:** Fat: 77%; Protein: 8%; Carbs: 15%

Cacao Crunch Cereal

SERVES 2 | PREP TIME: 5 minutes

½ cup slivered almonds
2 tablespoons unsweetened shredded or flaked coconut

2 tablespoons chia seeds
2 tablespoons cacao nibs

| 2 tablespoons | Unsweetened nondairy milk |
| sunflower seeds | of choice, for serving |

In a small bowl, combine the almonds, coconut, chia seeds, cacao nibs, and sunflower seeds. Divide into two bowls. Pour in the nondairy milk and serve.

Per serving: Calories: 325; Fat: 27; Protein: 10g; Total Carbs: 17g; Fiber: 12g; Net Carbs: 5g; **Macros:** Fat: 70%; Protein: 11%; Carbs: 19%

Toasty Granola Bars

MAKES 20 BARS | PREP TIME: 10 minutes | COOK TIME: 15 minutes

1 cup walnuts	1 large egg
1 cup unsweetened	½ cup natural peanut butter
shredded coconut	¼ cup coconut butter
1 cup slivered almonds	1 tablespoon pure
1 cup roasted sunflower seeds	vanilla extract
¼ cup egg white pro-	1 teaspoon ground cinnamon
tein powder	¼ teaspoon ground nutmeg

Preheat the oven to 350°F. In a food processor, pulse the walnuts, coconut, almonds, sunflower seeds, and egg protein powder to coarsely chop the ingredients. Transfer the nut mixture to a large bowl, and stir in the egg, peanut butter, coconut butter, vanilla, cinnamon, and nutmeg until well mixed. Press the granola bar mixture into a 9-by-13-inch baking dish. Using a paring knife, cut the mixture into 24 bars. Bake until the bars are firm and golden, about 15 minutes.

Per Serving: Calories: 148; Fat: 12g; Protein: 6g; Total Carbs: 4g; Fiber: 2g; Net Carbs: 2g; **Macros:** Fat: 73%; Protein: 16%; Carbs: 11%

Pumpkin-Pecan N'Oatmeal

SERVES 4 | PREP TIME: 10 minutes | COOK TIME: 8 hours on low

1 tablespoon coconut oil	2 tablespoons granulated
3 cups cubed pumpkin, cut	erythritol
into 1-inch chunks	1 teaspoon maple extract
2 cups coconut milk	½ teaspoon ground nutmeg
½ cup ground pecans	¼ teaspoon ground cinnamon
1 ounce plain protein powder	Pinch ground allspice

Lightly grease the insert of a slower cooker with the coconut oil. Place the pumpkin, coconut milk, pecans, protein powder, erythritol, maple extract, nutmeg, cinnamon, and allspice in the insert. Cover and cook on low for 8 hours. Stir the mixture or use a potato masher to create your preferred texture, and serve.

Per Serving: Calories: 292; Fat: 26g; Protein: 10g; Total Carbs: 9g; Fiber: 2g; Net Carbs: 7g; **Macros:** Fat: 75%; Protein: 13%; Carbs: 12%

Chocolate Coconut "Oatmeal"

SERVES 2 | PREP TIME: 5 minutes | COOK TIME: 5 minutes

½ cup unsweetened coco-	1 teaspoon vanilla extract
nut flakes	2 teaspoons cacao powder
¼ cup hemp hearts	1 tablespoon almond butter
1 tablespoon coconut flour	1 teaspoon low-carb dark
½ cup water	chocolate chips
⅓ cup canned full-fat	
coconut milk	

In a medium saucepan over medium-high heat, combine the coconut flakes, hemp hearts, coconut flour, water, and coconut milk. Bring the mixture to a boil and allow to cook for 2 minutes while stirring. Remove the pan from the heat and stir in the vanilla, cacao powder, and almond butter. Divide the "oatmeal" between two dishes and sprinkle with the chocolate chips.

Per Serving: Calories: 473; Fat: 37g; Protein: 16g; Total Carbs: 19g; Fiber: 12g; Net Carbs: 7g; **Macros:** Fat: 70%; Protein: 14%; Carbs: 16%

Cinnamon Roll "Noatmeal"

SERVES 2 | PREP TIME: 15 minutes | COOK TIME: 10 minutes

2 tablespoons butter	1 tablespoon desiccated
2 tablespoons chopped pecans	unsweetened coconut
¼ cup almond flour	1 tablespoon monk fruit/
1½ teaspoons coconut flour	erythritol blend sweetener
¼ cup unsweetened almond	1½ teaspoons golden flax meal
milk, plus more as needed	¼ teaspoon ground cinnamon
Pinch kosher salt	1 tablespoon heavy (whipping)
2 tablespoons hemp seeds	cream (optional)

In a small saucepan over medium-low heat, combine the butter and pecans. Cook for 3 to 4 minutes until the butter is golden brown and the pecans are toasted. Stir in the almond and coconut flours, almond milk, and salt. Cook for 3 to 4 minutes until thickened. Stir in the hemp seeds, coconut, sweetener, flax meal, and cinnamon. Cook for 1 to 2 minutes more. Remove from the heat and stir in the heavy cream (if using). Add additional almond milk, as needed, to reach your desired consistency.

Per Serving: Calories: 334; Fat: 29g; Protein: 10g; Total Carbs: 8g; Fiber: 5g; Net Carbs: 3g; **Macros:** Fat: 78%; Protein: 12%; Carbs: 10%

Cauliflower N'Oatmeal

1 SERVING | PREP TIME: 5 minutes | COOK TIME: 5 minutes

1 cup frozen cauliflower	1 tablespoon coconut oil
¼ cup unsweetened flax milk	Erythritol "brown sugar" or
1 scoop protein powder	sugar-free syrup (optional)
½ tablespoon ground	
cinnamon	

In a blender, combine the cauliflower, flax milk, protein powder, cinnamon, and coconut oil and purée. Transfer to a saucepan and warm over medium heat for about 5 minutes. Remove from the heat, pour into a bowl, and sprinkle sweetener or sugar-free syrup on top, if desired.

Per Serving: Calories: 242; Fat: 18g; Protein: 12g; Total Carbs: 8g; Fiber: 3g; Net Carbs: 5g; **Macros:** Fat: 67%; Protein: 20%; Carbs: 13%

Nutty "Oatmeal"

SERVES 6 | PREP TIME: 10 minutes | COOK TIME: 8 hours on low

1 tablespoon coconut oil	1 avocado, diced
1 cup coconut milk	2 ounces protein powder
1 cup unsweetened shred-	1 teaspoon ground cinnamon
ded coconut	¼ teaspoon ground nutmeg
½ cup chopped pecans	½ cup blueberries, for garnish
½ cup sliced almonds	
¼ cup granulated erythritol	

Lightly grease the insert of a slower cooker with the coconut oil. Place the coconut milk, shredded coconut, pecans, almonds, erythritol, avocado, protein powder, cinnamon, and nutmeg in the slow cooker. Cover and cook on low for 8 hours. Serve topped with the blueberries.

Per Serving: Calories: 365; Fat: 33g; Protein: 14g; Total Carbs: 10g; Fiber: 6g; Net Carbs: 4g; **Macros:** Fat: 76%; Protein: 14%; Carbs: 10%

Chia Almond "Oatmeal"

SERVES 4 | PREP TIME: 10 minutes, plus overnight to soak | COOK TIME: 5 minutes

2 cups water	¼ cup shredded unsweetened coconut
¾ cup coconut milk	¼ cup slivered almonds
1 vanilla bean, halved	3 (7g) stevia packets
½ cup chia seeds	¼ cup mixed berries

Pour the water and coconut milk into a medium saucepan, and use a paring knife to scrape the vanilla seeds out of the pod into the liquid. Add the bean pod as well. Place the saucepan over medium heat, and bring the liquid to a simmer, about 5 minutes. Remove the pan from the heat, and set aside to cool for 30 minutes. Remove and discard the vanilla bean. In a medium bowl, mix the chia seeds, coconut, and almonds. Pour the cooled coconut milk liquid over the chia seed mixture, and stir. Place the "oatmeal" in the refrigerator overnight, covered, to allow the chia seeds to soak up all the liquid. Stir in the stevia, divide the "oatmeal" evenly among 4 bowls, and serve topped with berries.

Per Serving: Calories: 281; Fat: 23g; Protein: 7g; Total Carbs: 16g; Fiber: 11g; Net Carbs: 5g; **Macros:** Fat: 68%; Protein: 9%; Carbs: 23%

Almond Coconut Hot Cereal

SERVES 1 | PREP TIME: 5 minutes | COOK TIME: 1 minute

¼ cup almond flour	3 tablespoons unsweetened shredded coconut
Pinch sea salt	½ cup coconut milk
¼ teaspoon ground cinnamon	

In a microwave-safe bowl, mix the almond flour, sea salt, cinnamon, and shredded coconut. Stir in the coconut milk, adding water if necessary to thin to the desired consistency. Microwave on high for 30 seconds. Stir and microwave for another 30 seconds or until heated through.

Per Serving: Calories: 395; Fat: 36g; Protein: 7g; Total Carbs: 13g; Fiber: 5g; Net Carbs: 8g; **Macros:** Fat: 82%; Protein: 7%; Carbs: 11%

Baklava Hot Porridge

SERVES 2 | PREP TIME: 5 minutes | COOK TIME: 5 minutes

2 cups cauliflower rice	2 teaspoons grated fresh orange peel (from ½ orange)
¾ cup unsweetened almond, flax, or hemp milk	½ teaspoon ground cinnamon
¼ cup extra-virgin olive oil, divided	½ teaspoon almond extract or vanilla extract
	⅛ teaspoon salt
¼ cup chopped walnuts, divided	1 to 2 teaspoons liquid stevia, monk fruit, or other sweetener of choice (optional)

In a medium saucepan, combine the cauliflower, almond milk, 2 tablespoons olive oil, grated orange peel, cinnamon, almond extract, and salt. Stir to combine and bring just to a boil over medium-high heat, stirring constantly. Remove from heat and stir in 2 tablespoons chopped walnuts and sweetener (if using). Stir to combine. Divide into bowls, topping each with 1 tablespoon of chopped walnuts and 1 tablespoon of the remaining olive oil.

Per Serving: Calories: 382; Fat: 38g; Protein: 5g; Total Carbs: 11g; Fiber: 4g; Net Carbs: 7g; **Macros:** Fat: 86%; Protein: 4%; Carbs: 10%

Overnight Chia Blueberry Pudding

1 SERVING | PREP TIME: 5 minutes, plus 2 hours to chill | COOK TIME: 2 hours

2 tablespoons chia seeds	¼ cup blueberries
1 cup unsweetened full-fat coconut milk	½ teaspoon stevia or 4 drops liquid stevia extract

In a mason jar, mix the chia seeds, coconut milk, blueberries, and stevia. Put the lid on the jar and shake to combine everything. Once the chia pudding mixture is well combined, put the jar in the refrigerator for at least 2 hours.

Per Serving: Calories: 599; Fat: 57g; Protein: 9g; Total Carbs: 17g; Fiber: 10g; Net Carbs: 7g; **Macros:** Fat: 85%; Protein: 5%; Carbs: 10%

Overnight Chia Pudding

1 SERVING | PREP TIME: 5 minutes, plus 2 hours to chill | COOK TIME: 2 hours

2 tablespoons chia seeds	½ teaspoon vanilla extract
1 cup unsweetened full-fat coconut milk	½ teaspoon stevia or 4 drops liquid stevia extract

In a mason jar, mix the chia seeds, milk, vanilla, and stevia. Put the lid on the jar and shake to combine everything. Once the chia pudding mixture is well combined, put the jar in the refrigerator for at least 2 hours.

Per Serving: Calories: 588; Fat: 57g; Protein: 9g; Total Carbs: 14g; Fiber: 10g; Net Carbs: 4g; **Macros:** Fat: 86%; Protein: 5%; Carbs: 9%

BAKED GOODS

Biscuits with Sausage Gravy

SERVES 4 | PREP TIME: 10 minutes | COOK TIME: 25 minutes

For the biscuits

½ cup, plus 2 tablespoons coconut flour	2 teaspoons apple cider vinegar
6 tablespoons plain unsweetened coconut yogurt	1 tablespoon plus 1 teaspoon baking powder

½ teaspoon salt

½ teaspoon onion powder

¼ cup frozen coconut oil chopped

1 tablespoon melted coconut oil

½ teaspoon garlic powder

For the sausage gravy

1 pound ground pork

1 teaspoon salt

2 teaspoons of fresh sage

1 teaspoon of fresh thyme

½ teaspoon of garlic powder

¼ teaspoon of onion powder

1 tablespoon coconut flour

1 cup coconut milk

Preheat the oven to 450°F. Line a baking sheet with parchment paper. In a medium bowl, mix the coconut flour, coconut yogurt, apple cider vinegar, baking powder, salt, garlic powder, and onion powder. Add the cold coconut oil to the flour mixture. Work the dough with your hands and break apart any solid coconut oil pieces. Form the dough into six biscuits. Arrange on the baking sheet and brush with melted coconut oil. Bake for 10 minutes or until golden brown. Combine the ground pork and spices in a medium bowl. Heat a large skillet over medium heat and brown the sausage. Once the sausage is cooked through, add the coconut flour and cook for 2 more minutes. Stir in the coconut milk and let the gravy cook for 5 to 10 minutes. Serve over the biscuits

Per Serving: Calories: 722; Fat: 62g; Protein: 24g; Total Carbs: 17g; Fiber: 8g; Net Carbs: 9g; **Macros:** Fat: 77%; Protein: 14%; Carbs: 9%

Apricot Hot Cross Buns

PREP TIME: 15 minutes | COOK TIME: 15 minutes | ROLLS: 12

¼ cup (½ stick) melted butter, plus more for greasing

1 cup whey protein isolate, unflavored

½ cup flaxseed meal

½ cup coconut flour

¼ cup granulated erythritol blend

2 teaspoons baking powder

3 large eggs separated

1 teaspoon xanthan gum

1 tablespoon olive oil

½ cup heavy (whipping) cream

1 teaspoon cream of tartar

¼ cup sugar-free apricot preserves

2 ounces (¼ cup) cream cheese, melted slightly in microwave

¼ cup confectioners' erythritol blend

Preheat the oven to 350°F, and heavily grease a muffin pan with melted butter. In a medium bowl, combine the whey protein, flaxseed, flour, sweetener, and baking powder. Add the egg yolks to the flour mixture, and put the whites in a medium bowl. Add the melted butter, olive oil, and cream to the flour mixture, and mix just until incorporated. Add the cream of tartar to the whites in the metal bowl. Using a mixer, beat the whites until they form small peaks. Gently fold the whites into the flour mixture until just incorporated. Evenly spoon the mixture into the 12 muffin holes, and bake for 10 minutes. Mix the melted cream cheese and confectioners' blend. Add the icing to a piping bag or resealable bag with the corner cut off. When the buns are baked, brush apricot preserves across the top of each bun. Pipe an icing cross on each one, and bake for another 3 to 5 minutes. Remove from the oven, and let them sit for about 5 minutes before removing from the pan.

Per Serving: (1 roll): Calories: 233; Fat: 14g; Protein: 21g; Total Carbs: 14g; Fiber: 4g; Net Carbs: 4g; **Macros:** Fat: 54%; Protein: 36%; Carbs: 6%

Buttermilk Biscuits

MAKES 8 BISCUITS | PREP TIME: 15 minutes | COOK TIME: 15 minutes

Oil or nonstick cooking spray, for greasing

½ cup almond flour

½ cup coconut flour

2 teaspoons granulated erythritol blend

1 teaspoon baking powder

½ teaspoon baking soda

¼ teaspoon salt

5 large eggs separated

½ teaspoons cream of tartar

¼ cup buttermilk

2 tablespoons cold butter, cubed, plus melted butter for brushing

1 tablespoon olive oil

Preheat the oven to 400°F, and grease a standard muffin pan. In a medium bowl, combine the almond flour, coconut flour, sweetener, baking powder, baking soda, and salt. Put the yolks in the flour mixture and the whites in another medium bowl. To the bowl with the egg whites, add the cream of tartar, and with an electric mixer, whip on high until stiff peaks form, about 1 minute. To the flour mixture, add the buttermilk, cold butter, and olive oil, and use your hands to mix until fully incorporated. Add the egg whites to the flour mixture, and gently fold over and over, until the whites are worked into the dough. It will be a little lumpy. Drop spoonfuls of dough evenly into 8 muffin holes, and bake for 10 minutes. Remove from the oven, brush with melted butter, and cook for 5 additional minutes, or until golden brown.

Per Serving: (1 biscuit): Calories: 164; Fat: 13g; Protein: 7g; Total Carbs: 7g; Fiber: 4g; Net Carbs: 3g; **Macros:** Fat: 71%; Protein: 17%; Carbs: 5%

Cheddar-Chive Biscuits

MAKES 10 BISCUITS | PREP TIME: 10 minutes | COOK TIME: 20 minutes

1¾ cup almond flour

2 tablespoons coconut flour

1 tablespoon baking powder

¼ teaspoon sea salt

½ cup sour cream

½ cup shredded Cheddar cheese

¼ cup (¼ stick) unsalted butter, melted, plus more for serving

2 large eggs, at room temperature

2 tablespoons finely chopped chives

2 tablespoons grated Parmesan cheese

Preheat the oven to 375°F. Line a large baking sheet with parchment paper. In a large bowl, sift the almond flour, coconut flour, baking powder, and salt. Add the sour cream, Cheddar cheese, melted butter, eggs, and chives. Use a fork to combine until fully incorporated. Drop the dough by large spoonfuls onto the baking sheet, and sprinkle the top of each biscuit with Parmesan cheese. Bake the biscuits for 20 minutes, or until lightly golden brown on top.

Per Serving: Calories: 229; Fat: 20g; Protein: 8g; Total Carbs: 7g; Fiber: 3g; Net Carbs: 4g; **Macros:** Fat: 79%; Protein: 14%; Carbs: 7%

Easy Cheese Biscuits

MAKES 8 BISCUITS | PREP TIME: 5 minutes |
COOK TIME: 15 minutes

4 large eggs, beaten
2 cups shredded
   Cheddar cheese
1 cup almond flour
2 teaspoons baking powder
1 teaspoon garlic powder

Freshly ground black pepper
2 tablespoons (1 ounce)
   unsalted butter, melted
1 tablespoon finely chopped
   fresh parsley, for garnish

Preheat the oven to 400°F. Line a large baking sheet with parchment paper. In a large bowl, mix the eggs, cheddar, almond flour, baking powder, garlic powder, and pepper. Use a large spoon or cookie dough scoop to portion out 8 biscuits, spacing them evenly on the baking sheet. Bake for 12 to 15 minutes, until they are brown at the edges. Transfer to a serving bowl and pour the melted butter over the top. Serve garnished with the parsley.

Per Serving (1-biscuit): Calories: 227; Fat: 19g; Protein: 12g; Total Carbs: 3g; Fiber: 1g; Net Carbs: 2g; **Macros:** Fat: 74%; Protein: 21%; Carbs: 5%

Sesame Burger Buns

MAKES 9 BUNS | PREP TIME: 10 minutes |
COOK TIME: 50 minutes to 1 hour, plus 20 minutes to cool

¼ cup (½ stick) unsalted
   butter, at room tem-
   perature, plus more for
   greasing the pan
¾ cup coconut flour
1 tablespoon psyllium
   husk powder
2 teaspoons baking powder
1 teaspoon granulated erythritol–monk fruit blend

½ teaspoon sea salt
4 ounces (about ½ cup)
   cream cheese, at room
   temperature
4 large eggs, at room
   temperature
¼ cup sour cream
2 tablespoons salted
   butter, melted
1 tablespoon sesame seeds

Preheat the oven to 350°F. Generously grease a 12-cup muffin top pan with butter. In a medium bowl, combine the coconut flour, psyllium husk powder, baking powder, erythritol–monk fruit blend, and salt. In a large bowl, using an electric mixer, beat the butter and cream cheese until light and fluffy. Add the eggs one at a time, mixing after each addition. Add the dry ingredients to the wet ingredients while mixing on low speed, scraping down the bowl a couple of times. Fold in the sour cream until fully incorporated into the batter, but not overmixed. Overfill the cups of the muffin top pan just slightly with batter. Brush the top of each muffin top with the melted butter and sprinkle the sesame seeds on top of 9 of the buns. Bake the buns for 25 to 30 minutes, or until lightly browned on the top and a toothpick inserted into the center comes out clean. Allow the buns to cool for 10 minutes in the pan before removing. Once the pan has cooled, regrease 6 openings, and bake the additional 6 buns. This will yield a total of 9 top and 9 bottom burger buns. Refrigerate for up to 5 days, or freeze for up to 3 weeks.

Per Serving: Calories: 209; Fat: 17g; Protein: 6g; Total Carbs: 9g; Fiber: 5g; Net Carbs: 4g; **Macros:** Fat: 73%; Protein: 11%; Carbs: 16%

Cheesy Garlic Rolls

MAKES 12 ROLLS | PREP TIME: 10 minutes | COOK TIME: 25 to 30 minutes

1½ cups shredded mozza-
   rella cheese
¼ cup cream cheese, at room
   temperature
2 large eggs, at room
   temperature
¾ cup almond flour, sifted
3 tablespoons salted butter

1 teaspoon extra-virgin
   olive oil
2 garlic cloves, minced
¼ teaspoon garlic salt
¼ cup grated Parme-
   san cheese
¼ cup chopped fresh
   flat-leaf parsley

Preheat the oven to 350°F. Line a baking sheet with parchment paper. Put the mozzarella cheese in a medium microwave-safe bowl. Microwave in 30-second increments, stirring each time, until fully melted. Add the cream cheese, and combine well. Allow the mixture to cool slightly and then stir in the eggs and almond flour. Using wet hands, separate the dough into 12 equal parts and shape into rounds. Place them on the baking sheet. In a small bowl, combine the butter, olive oil, garlic, and garlic salt. With a pastry brush, spread the garlic butter on top of each roll, and sprinkle with the Parmesan cheese. Bake for 25 to 30 minutes, or until lightly golden. Top with the parsley right out of the oven.

Per Serving: Calories: 148; Fat: 12g; Protein: 7g; Total Carbs: 3g; Fiber: 1g; Net Carbs: 2g; **Macros:** Fat: 73%; Protein: 19%; Carbs: 8%

Everything Bagels

MAKES 8 BAGELS | PREP TIME: 20 minutes, plus rising time | COOK TIME: 15 to 20 minutes

1 tablespoon yeast
1 teaspoon sugar
3 tablespoons warm water
2 cups shredded part-skim
   mozzarella cheese
2 tablespoons cream cheese,
   at room temperature
¾ cup coconut flour
2 teaspoons baking powder

¼ teaspoon xanthan gum
2 large eggs, at room
   temperature
2 tablespoons unsalted
   butter, melted
1 tablespoon everything
   bagel seasoning or coarse
   sea salt

Line a large baking sheet with parchment paper. Put the yeast and sugar in a small bowl. Add the warm water, and stir. Cover the bowl with a kitchen towel and rest for 10 minutes, until bubbly and expanded. Put the mozzarella cheese in a large microwave-safe bowl. Microwave in 30-second increments, stirring each time, until fully melted. Add the cream cheese to the melted mozzarella, and mix until combined. Add the coconut flour, baking powder, and xanthan gum, and mix well using a rubber spatula. Add the eggs and the proofed yeast, and mix. Once the dough comes together, with wet hands, lightly knead the dough. Divide the dough into 8 equal balls. On the baking sheet, using wet hands, form the bagels and smooth any cracks on the surface or sides. Brush the tops and sides of bagels with the melted butter. Allow the bagels to rise in a warm, draft-free place for 30 to 45 minutes. Preheat the oven to 375°F. After rising, sprinkle the bagels with the everything bagel seasoning. Bake for 18 to 20 minutes, or until the bagels are golden brown.

Chorizo Bagels

MAKES 8 BAGELS | PREP TIME: 20 minutes, plus rising time | COOK TIME: 15 to 20 minutes

1 tablespoon yeast	¼ teaspoon xanthan gum
1 teaspoon sugar	2 large eggs, at room
3 tablespoons warm water	temperature
2 cups shredded part-skim	¼ cup finely chopped fully
mozzarella cheese	cured Spanish chorizo,
2 tablespoons cream cheese,	casing removed
at room temperature	2 tablespoons unsalted
¾ cup coconut flour	butter, melted
2 teaspoons baking powder	Coarse sea salt

Line a large baking sheet with parchment paper. Put the yeast and sugar in a small bowl. Add the warm water and stir. Cover the bowl with a kitchen towel, and rest for 10 minutes, until bubbly and expanded. Put the mozzarella cheese in a large microwave-safe bowl. Microwave in 30-second increments, stirring each time, until fully melted. Add the cream cheese to the melted mozzarella, and mix until combined. Add the coconut flour, baking powder, and xanthan gum, and mix well using a rubber spatula. Add the eggs, chorizo, and proofed yeast, and combine well. With wet hands, lightly knead the dough and divide it into 8 equal balls. On the baking sheet, using wet hands, form the bagels, and smooth any cracks on the surface or sides. Brush the tops and sides of the bagels with the melted butter. Allow the bagels to rise in a warm, draft-free place for 30 to 45 minutes. Preheat the oven to 375°F. After rising, sprinkle the bagels with coarse sea salt. Bake for 18 to 20 minutes, or until the bagels are golden brown.

Per Serving: Calories: 204; Fat: 13g; Protein: 13g; Total Carbs: 10g; Fiber: 5g; Net Carbs: 5g; Macros: Fat: 57%; Protein: 25%; Carbs: 18%

Classic Zucchini Bread

SERVES 12 | PREP TIME: 20 minutes | COOK TIME: 1 hour

Nonstick cooking spray	1 teaspoon baking soda
8 large eggs	1 teaspoon ground cinnamon
1 cup almond flour	1 teaspoon vanilla extract
¾ cup coconut flour	½ teaspoon kosher salt
⅔ cup grated zucchini	5 tablespoons plus 1 teaspoon
½ cup monk fruit/erythritol	butter, melted
blend sweetener	3 tablespoons sour cream
1½ teaspoons baking powder	¼ cup chopped pecans

Preheat the oven to 350°F. Coat an 8-inch loaf pan with cooking spray and line it with parchment overhanging two sides. In a large bowl and using an electric hand mixer, whip the eggs for about 2 minutes until light and foamy. Add the almond and coconut flours, zucchini, sweetener, baking powder, baking soda, cinnamon, vanilla, and salt. Mix on medium speed until combined, stopping to scrape down sides at least once. Stir in the melted butter and sour cream until combined. Spoon the batter evenly into the loaf pan and smooth the top. Sprinkle

the pecans over the batter. Bake for 45 minutes to 1 hour, or until a toothpick inserted in the center comes out clean. If needed, cover the pan loosely with aluminum foil to prevent over-browning. Let cool in the pan for 30 minutes. Using the parchment, transfer the loaf to a wire rack to cool completely.

Per Serving: Calories: 186; Fat: 14g; Protein: 7g; Total Carbs: 8g; Fiber: 4g; Net Carbs: 4g; Macros: Fat: 68%; Protein: 15%; Carbs: 17%

Slow Cooker Zucchini-Carrot Bread

MAKES 8 SLICES | PREP TIME: 15 minutes | COOK TIME: 3 hours on high or 5 hours on low

2 teaspoons butter, for	½ teaspoon baking soda
greasing pan	¼ teaspoon salt
1 cup almond flour	4 large eggs
1 cup granulated erythritol	½ cup butter, melted
½ cup coconut flour	1 tablespoon pure
1½ teaspoons baking powder	vanilla extract
1 teaspoon ground cinnamon	1½ cups finely grated zucchini
½ teaspoon ground nutmeg	½ cup finely grated carrot

Lightly grease a 9-by-5-inch loaf pan with the butter and set aside. Place a small rack in the bottom of your slow cooker. In a large bowl, stir the almond flour, erythritol, coconut flour, baking powder, cinnamon, nutmeg, baking soda, and salt until well mixed. In a medium bowl, whisk the eggs, melted butter, and vanilla until well blended. Add the wet ingredients to dry ingredients and stir to combine. Stir in the zucchini and carrot. Spoon the batter into the prepared loaf pan. Place the loaf pan on the rack in the bottom of the slow cooker, cover, and cook on high for 3 hours. Remove the loaf pan, let the bread cool completely, and serve.

Per Serving: (1 slice): Calories: 217; Fat: 19g; Protein: 8g; Total Carbs: 5g; Fiber: 3g; Net Carbs: 2g; Macros: Fat: 77%; Protein: 14%; Carbs: 9%

Onion Cheddar Bread

SERVES 12 | PREP TIME: 15 minutes | COOK TIME: 42 minutes

2 tablespoons butter, plus	¼ teaspoon onion powder
more for preparing the pan	¼ teaspoon garlic powder
½ cup chopped Vidalia onion	¼ teaspoon freshly ground
8 large eggs	black pepper
1 cup almond flour	⅛ teaspoon cayenne pepper
½ cup coconut flour	5 tablespoons butter, melted
2 teaspoons baking powder	2 tablespoons sour cream
1 teaspoon baking soda	1 cup shredded
½ teaspoon kosher salt	Cheddar cheese

Preheat the oven to 350°F. Coat an 8-inch loaf pan with butter and line it with parchment paper overhanging two sides. Set aside. In a small skillet over medium heat, melt the butter. Add the onion and saute for 7 to 10 minutes until translucent and lightly caramelized. In a large bowl and using an electric hand mixer, whip the eggs for about 2 minutes until light and foamy. Add the almond and coconut flours, baking powder, baking soda, salt, onion powder, garlic powder, pepper, and cayenne. Mix on medium speed until combined, scraping down the sides at least once. Add the melted butter and sour cream and mix well to combine. Stir in the Cheddar cheese and cooked onion. Spoon the batter evenly into the prepared loaf pan and smooth the top. Bake for 45 to 55 minutes, or until a tester inserted into the center comes out clean. Let cool in the pan for 30 minutes. Using the parchment as an aid, transfer the loaf to a wire rack to cool completely.

Per Serving: Calories: 218; Fat: 18g; Protein: 8g; Total Carbs: 6g; Fiber: 3g; Net Carbs: 3g; **Macros:** Fat: 74%; Protein: 15%; Carbs: 11%

Basic Sandwich Bread

MAKES 12 SLICES | PREP TIME: 10 minutes |
COOK TIME: 30 to 40 minutes, plus 30 to 40 minutes to cool

1¼ cups almond flour, sifted

1 tablespoon psyllium husk powder

2 teaspoons baking powder

½ teaspoon sea salt

¼ cup (½ stick) unsalted butter, at room temperature, plus more to grease the pan

1 tablespoon granulated erythritol–monk fruit blend

3½ ounces (about 7 tablespoons) cream cheese, at room temperature

4 large eggs, at room temperature

2 tablespoons sesame seeds

Preheat the oven to 350°F. Grease a 9-by-5-inch loaf pan with butter. In a medium bowl, combine the almond flour, psyllium husk powder, baking powder, and salt. In a large bowl, using an electric mixer on medium-high speed, blend the butter and sweetener. Add the cream cheese, and combine well. Add the eggs one at a time, mixing well after each addition. Add the dry ingredients to the wet ingredients, and mix well until the batter is combined. Spread the batter in the prepared loaf pan, and sprinkle the sesame seeds on top. Bake the bread for 30 to 40 minutes, or until golden brown on top and a toothpick inserted into the center comes out clean. Allow to cool for about 10 minutes before removing from the pan. Place on a wire rack to cool for another 20 to 30 minutes to cool fully before slicing.

Per Serving: Calories: 165; Fat: 15g; Protein: 6g; Total Carbs: 4g; Fiber: 2g; Net Carbs: 2g; **Macros:** Fat: 82%; Protein: 15%; Carbs: 3%

Onion-Garlic Pita Bread

MAKES 6 PITAS | PREP TIME: 10 minutes | COOK TIME: 25 to 35 minutes, plus cooling time

3 tablespoons golden flax meal

3 cups almond flour, sifted

1 tablespoon psyllium husk powder

2 teaspoons sesame seeds

2 teaspoons baking powder

½ teaspoon xanthan gum

½ teaspoon sea salt

½ teaspoon onion powder

½ teaspoon garlic powder

1 cup hot water

1 tablespoon extra-virgin olive oil or melted coconut oil

2 large eggs, at room temperature

1 tablespoon salted butter, melted

¼ chopped parsley

Sea salt flakes

Preheat the oven to 400°F. Line a large baking sheet with parchment paper. In a coffee grinder, grind the flax meal until it's a fine powder. In a large bowl, combine the flax meal powder, almond flour, psyllium husk powder, sesame seeds, baking powder, xanthan gum, salt, onion powder, and garlic powder. Add the hot water, olive oil, and eggs and mix well. Scoop 6 equal portions of the dough onto the prepared baking sheet. With wet hands, form them into circles. Using a pastry brush, brush each pita with the melted butter. Sprinkle the tops of the breads evenly with the fresh parsley and sea salt flakes. Bake for 25 to 35 minutes, or until lightly browned. Allow to cool fully on the baking sheet before serving.

Per Serving: Calories: 409; Fat: 36g; Protein: 15g; Total Carbs: 15g; Fiber: 8g; Net Carbs: 7g; **Macros:** Fat: 79%; Protein: 15%; Carbs: 6%

Pizza Pull-Apart Bread

PREP TIME: 15 minutes, plus 30 minutes to chill |
COOK TIME: 30 minutes | SERVINGS: 8

Oil or nonstick cooking spray, for greasing

2½ cups grated mozzarella cheese

2 ounces (¼ cup) cream cheese

1¼ cups almond flour

2 tablespoons flaxseed meal

2 tablespoons coconut flour

2 large eggs

2 tablespoons whey protein isolate, unflavored

2 tablespoons finely grated Parmesan cheese

1 tablespoon baking powder

¼ teaspoon garlic salt

1 pound pork breakfast sausage, cooked and drained

30 pepperoni slices

Preheat the oven to 350°F, and grease a Bundt pan with butter. In a microwave-safe dish, combine the mozzarella and cream cheese, and heat in 20-second increments until the mozzarella is melted and smooth. Add the almond flour, flaxseed, coconut flour, and eggs. Using your hands, mix it and then into a ball, and refrigerate the ball for at least 30 minutes. In a small bowl, mix the whey protein, Parmesan, baking powder, and garlic salt. Spread a piece of parchment paper on the counter. Remove the dough from the refrigerator, and divide in half. Over the parchment, Divide the dough into 32 equal portions, and roll each into a ball. Roll each ball in the baking powder mixture, and set aside. Arrange a quarter of the sausage and pepperoni in the bottom of the Bundt pan, and then add 8 of the balls. Sprinkle in half the cheese, and then repeat, evenly adding more sausage, pepperoni, balls, and cheese, until it's all in the pan. Bake for 30 minutes. Remove from the oven, run a knife around the inside of the pan and place a plate on the top and flip it over.

Per Serving: Calories: 456; Fat: 36g; Protein: 26g; Total Carbs: 6g; Fiber: 3g; Net Carbs: 3g; **Macros:** Fat: 71%; Protein: 23%; Carbs: 3%

Garlic Cloud Bread

MAKES 12 SLICES | PREP TIME: 10 minutes |
COOK TIME: 25 minutes

Nonstick cooking spray

6 large eggs, separated

6 ounces cream cheese, at room temperature

Pinch cream of tartar

¼ cup (2 ounces) unsalted butter

1 teaspoon minced garlic

Freshly ground black pepper
½ cup shredded mozza-
  rella cheese

2 tablespoons finely chopped
fresh parsley, for garnish
(optional)

Preheat the oven to 300°F. Line two baking sheets with parchment paper and coat with cooking spray. In a large bowl with an electric hand mixer on medium speed, mix the egg yolks and cream cheese for 3 minutes, or until smooth. In another large bowl, with the mixer and clean beaters, beat the egg whites with the cream of tartar on high speed until stiff peaks form, 5 to 7 minutes. Add a spoonful of the egg yolk mixture to the egg whites and stir to combine. Add the remaining egg yolk mixture and fold everything together. Spoon out the mixture into 12 rounds (about 2 tablespoons for each) on the baking sheets. Bake for 20 minutes, or until golden on top. Meanwhile, prepare the garlic butter by melting the butter in a covered dish in the microwave, then stirring in the garlic and black pepper to taste. When the bread has cooked, remove it from the oven. Set the oven to broil. Brush the bread with the garlic butter, then sprinkle with the mozzarella. Broil for 2 minutes, or until the cheese has melted. Garnish with the parsley (if using) and serve.

Per Serving: (2-slice): Calories: 265; Fat: 24g; Protein: 10g; Total Carbs: 2g; Fiber: 0g; Net Carbs: 2g; Macros: Fat: 81%; Protein: 17%; Carbs: 2%

Jalapeño Cheese Bread

MAKES 12 SLICES | PREP TIME: 10 minutes |
COOK TIME: 50 minutes to 1 hour, plus 45 minutes to cool

¼ cup (¼ stick) unsalted
  butter, melted plus more to
  grease the pan
1 cup golden flax meal
¾ cup coconut flour
2 tablespoons granulated
  erythritol–monk fruit blend
3 tablespoons grated
  Parmesan cheese
1 tablespoon psyllium
  husk powder
2 teaspoons baking powder

1 teaspoon sea salt
¼ teaspoon black pepper
8 ounces (about 1 cup) cream
  cheese, softened
4 large eggs, at room
  temperature
3 cups shredded Cheddar
  cheese, divided
⅓ cup pickled jalapeño
  peppers, diced
1¼ cups coconut milk or
  almond milk

Preheat the oven to 375°F. Grease a 9-by-5-inch loaf pan with butter, and line the bottom of the pan with parchment paper. Grind the flax meal in a coffee grinder until it's a fine powder. In a large bowl, combine the flax meal powder, coconut flour, erythritol–monk fruit blend, Parmesan cheese, psyllium husk powder, baking powder, salt, and pepper. In another large bowl, using an electric mixer on high speed, combine the cream cheese and eggs. Add 2 cups of Cheddar cheese and the pickled jalapeño peppers, and stir until well incorporated. Add the dry ingredients to the wet ingredients, and combine well. Fold in the melted butter. Add the coconut milk, and mix until just combined. Spread the batter in the loaf pan. Top with the remaining 1 cup of Cheddar cheese. Bake for 50 minutes to 1 hour or until the top is lightly browned and a toothpick inserted into the center comes out clean. Check the bread after 45 minutes, cover with foil if it is too brown. Remove from the oven, and place on a wire rack. Allow to cool for at least 15 minutes before removing

from the loaf pan. Allow to cool for another 30 minutes on a wire rack before slicing.

Per Serving: Calories: 322; Fat: 26g; Protein: 13g; Total Carbs: 12g; Fiber: 6g; Net Carbs: 6g; Macros: Fat: 73%; Protein: 16%; Carbs: 11%

Rosemary Flatbread

MAKES 6 FLATBREADS | PREP TIME: 10 minutes |
COOK TIME: 25 to 35 minutes

1½ tablespoons golden
  flax meal
1½ cups almond flour,
  measured and sifted
2 teaspoons psyllium
  husk powder
1 teaspoon baking powder
¼ teaspoon xanthan gum
¼ teaspoon sea salt
¼ teaspoon onion powder

¼ teaspoon garlic powder
½ cup hot water
1 tablespoon extra-virgin olive
  oil, plus more for brushing
1 large egg, at room
  temperature
1½ tablespoons chopped
  fresh rosemary
Sea salt flakes

Preheat the oven to 400°F. Line a large baking sheet with parchment paper. In a coffee grinder, grind the flax meal until it's a fine powder. In a large bowl, combine the flax meal powder, almond flour, psyllium husk powder, baking powder, xanthan gum, salt, onion powder, and garlic powder. Mix in the hot water, olive oil, and egg. Scoop 6 equal portions of the dough onto the baking sheet. With wet hands, form the dough into circles. Use a pastry brush to brush each flatbread with olive oil. Sprinkle the tops evenly with the rosemary and sea salt flakes. Bake for 25 to 35 minutes, or until lightly browned. Serve this flatbread straight from the oven.

Per Serving: Calories: 225; Fat: 20g; Protein: 8g; Total Carbs: 8g; Fiber: 4g; Net Carbs: 4g; Macros: Fat: 80%; Protein: 14%; Carbs: 6%

Savory Naan

MAKES 6 NAAN | PREP TIME: 10 minutes | COOK TIME: 15 to
20 minutes, plus cooling time

1½ tablespoons golden
  flax meal
1½ cups almond flour, sifted
2 teaspoons psyllium
  husk powder
2 teaspoons sesame seeds
2 teaspoons baking powder
½ teaspoon onion powder
½ teaspoon garlic powder
¼ teaspoon xanthan gum
¼ teaspoon sea salt

1 cup hot water
1 teaspoon extra-virgin
  olive oil
2 large eggs, at room
  temperature
1 tablespoon salted
  butter, melted
2 tablespoons fresh flat-leaf
  parsley, chopped
2 teaspoons sea salt flakes

Preheat the oven to 375°F. Line a large baking sheet with parchment paper. In a coffee grinder, grind the flax meal until it's a fine powder. In a large bowl, combine the flax meal powder, almond flour, psyllium husk powder, sesame seeds, baking powder, onion powder, garlic powder, xanthan gum, and salt. Mix in the hot water, olive oil, and eggs. Scoop 6 equal portions of the dough onto the prepared baking sheet. With wet hands, form them into circles. Using a pastry brush, brush each naan with the melted butter. Sprinkle the tops of the naans evenly with the parsley and sea salt flakes. Bake for 15 to 20 minutes, or until lightly browned. Allow to cool slightly on the baking sheet before serving.

Per Serving: Calories: 227; Fat: 19g; Protein: 9g; Total Carbs: 9g; Fiber: 5g; Net Carbs: 4g; **Macros:** Fat: 75%; Protein: 16%; Carbs: 9%

Herb and Olive Focaccia

MAKES 10 SQUARES | PREP TIME: 10 minutes | COOK TIME: 25 to 35 minutes

For the bread

3 tablespoons golden flax meal

3 cups almond flour, sifted

1 tablespoon psyllium husk powder

2 teaspoons baking powder

½ teaspoon xanthan gum

½ teaspoon sea salt

½ teaspoon onion powder

½ teaspoon garlic powder

1 cup hot water

3 tablespoons extra-virgin olive oil, divided

2 large eggs, at room temperature

20 Kalamata olives, pitted

2 teaspoons sea salt flakes

¼ teaspoon red pepper flakes

For the bread dipping oil

½ cup extra-virgin olive oil

1 tablespoon sea salt

1 tablespoon dried oregano

1 tablespoon dried rosemary

2 teaspoons freshly ground pepper

2 teaspoons red pepper flakes

Preheat the oven to 400°F. Line a large baking sheet with parchment paper. In a coffee grinder, grind the flax meal until it's a fine powder. In a large bowl, combine the flax meal powder, almond flour, psyllium husk powder, baking powder, xanthan gum, salt, onion powder, and garlic powder. Mix in the hot water, 1 tablespoon of extra-virgin olive oil, and eggs. With wet hands, spread the dough evenly over the baking sheet. Using a pastry brush, spread the remaining 2 tablespoons of olive oil over the entire surface of the dough. Sprinkle the olives, sea salt flakes, and red pepper flakes over the top. Lightly press the olives into the dough. Bake for 25 to 35 minutes, or until lightly browned. While the bread is baking, combine the olive oil, salt, oregano, rosemary, pepper, and red pepper flakes in a small bowl. Remove the bread from the oven, and cut into 10 squares. Enjoy while still warm with the dipping oil.

Per Serving: Calories: 375; Fat: 36g; Protein: 9g; Total Carbs: 10g; Fiber: 5g; Net Carbs: 5g; **Macros:** Fat: 86%; Protein: 10%; Carbs: 4%

Blackberry, Prosciutto, and Goat Cheese Flatbread

MAKES 6 FLATBREADS | PREP TIME: 15 minutes | COOK TIME: 40 to 50 minutes, plus cooling time

For the flatbread

3 tablespoons golden flax meal

3 cups almond flour, measured and sifted

1 tablespoon psyllium husk powder

2 teaspoons baking powder

½ teaspoon xanthan gum

½ teaspoon sea salt

¼ teaspoon onion powder

¼ teaspoon garlic powder

1 cup hot water

1 tablespoon extra-virgin olive oil

2 large eggs, at room temperature

For the toppings

1 cup crumbled goat cheese, at room temperature, divided

¼ cup heavy (whipping) cream

2 tablespoons cream cheese, at room temperature

2 tablespoons unsalted butter, melted

½ pint fresh blackberries, quartered

½ cup fresh basil, chiffonade

6 slices prosciutto, torn into small pieces

1 tablespoon balsamic vinegar

Preheat the oven to 400°F. Line a large baking sheet with parchment paper. In a coffee grinder, grind the flax meal until it's a fine powder. In a large bowl, combine the flax meal powder, almond flour, psyllium husk powder, baking powder, xanthan gum, salt, onion powder, and garlic powder. Mix in the hot water, olive oil, and eggs. Scoop 6 equal portions of the dough onto the baking sheet. With wet hands, form the dough into circles. Bake for 25 to 35 minutes, or until lightly browned. Allow to cool completely on the baking sheet before topping. In a small bowl, combine ¾ cup of goat cheese, the heavy whipping cream, and cream cheese. Once the flatbreads have fully cooled, use a pastry brush to baste each flatbread with the melted butter. Spread the goat cheese mixture evenly on top, and top with the blackberries, basil, prosciutto, and remaining ¼ cup of goat cheese. Bake for another 15 minutes, or until the goat cheese has melted and slightly browned. Drizzle with the balsamic vinegar right before serving.

Per Serving: Calories: 574; Fat: 49g; Protein: 22g; Total Carbs: 20g; Fiber: 10g; Net Carbs: 10g; **Macros:** Fat: 77%; Protein: 15%; Carbs: 8%

Flax Meal Tortillas

MAKES 8 TORTILLAS | PREP TIME: 10 minutes, plus resting time | COOK TIME: 10 minutes

¾ cup golden flax meal

¼ cup coconut flour

1 tablespoon psyllium husk powder

½ teaspoon xanthan gum

½ teaspoon sea salt

1 cup hot water

1 tablespoon coconut or olive oil

In a coffee grinder, grind the flax meal until it's a fine powder. In a large bowl, combine the flax meal powder, coconut flour, psyllium husk powder, xanthan gum, and salt. Mix in the hot water and olive oil. Cover the dough with a kitchen towel, and rest for about 10 minutes. Use your hands to form the dough into 8 equal balls. Flatten each ball between 2 sheets of parchment paper or a tortilla press to form 8 (5-inch) tortillas. In a large nonstick skillet over medium heat, cook each tortilla for about 10 to 15 seconds per side until golden. Keep your tortillas warm by wrapping them in a kitchen towel. Serve immediately.

Per Serving: Calories: 79; Fat: 6g; Protein: 3g; Total Carbs: 7g; Fiber: 5g; Net Carbs: 2g; **Macros:** Fat: 68%; Protein: 15%; Carbs: 17%

Southern Sweet Corn Bread

MAKES 10 PIECES | PREP TIME: 10 minutes |
COOK TIME: 30 to 35 minutes, plus 10 minutes to cool

2 cups almond meal

½ cup granulated erythritol–
monk fruit blend

2 teaspoons baking powder

1 teaspoon sea salt

1 cup sour cream

¼ cup heavy (whipping) cream

6 drops OOOFlavors corn
bread extract

4 large eggs, beaten, at room
temperature

½ cup (1 stick) unsalted butter,
melted, plus 1 tablespoon

Preheat the oven to 375°F. Place the empty cast iron skillet in the preheated oven for 10 minutes. In a medium bowl, combine the almond meal, sweetener, baking powder, salt, and pepper, and set aside. In a large bowl, combine the sour cream, heavy whipping cream, corn bread extract, and eggs. Mix until fully combined. Add the dry ingredients to the wet ingredients, and stir until fully incorporated. Fold in ½ cup of melted butter, and stir gently until combined. Carefully remove the hot cast iron skillet, and add the remaining 1 tablespoon of butter to it. Swirl to cover the bottom and sides. Add the corn bread batter to the hot, greased skillet. Bake for 30 to 35 minutes. Allow to cool in the pan for 10 minutes before slicing into wedges.

Per Serving: Calories: 327; Fat: 31g; Protein: 9g; Total Carbs: 7g; Fiber: 2g; Net Carbs: 5g; **Macros:** Fat: 85%; Protein: 11%; Carbs: 4%

Sour Cream Corn Bread

SERVES 9 | PREP TIME: 10 minutes | COOK TIME: 30 minutes

5 tablespoons butter, melted,
plus more for prepar-
ing the pan

1 cup almond flour

2½ tablespoons coconut flour

2½ teaspoons baking powder

1 teaspoon monk fruit/
erythritol blend sweetener

½ teaspoon sea salt

¼ teaspoon baking soda

5 large eggs

2 tablespoons sour cream

Preheat the oven to 350°F. Thoroughly coat an 8-inch square baking pan with butter. In a medium bowl, stir the almond and coconut flours, baking powder, sweetener, salt, and baking soda. Using an electric hand mixer, mix in the eggs and sour cream, beating at medium speed until well combined. Stir in the melted butter. Pour the batter into the prepared pan. Bake for 25 to 30 minutes until golden brown and a toothpick inserted into the center comes out clean. Cut into squares and serve warm.

Per Serving: Calories: 157; Fat: 13g; Protein: 5g; Total Carbs: 5g; Fiber: 3g; Net Carbs: 2g; **Macros:** Fat: 76%; Protein: 12%; Carbs: 12%

Tex-Mex Green Chile Corn Bread

MAKES 10 PIECES | PREP TIME: 10 minutes | COOK TIME: 30 to 35 minutes

2 cups almond meal

2 tablespoons granulated
erythritol–monk fruit blend

2 teaspoons baking powder

1 teaspoon sea salt

¼ cup heavy (whipping) cream

1 cup sour cream

2 (7-ounce) cans green chiles,
drained and chopped

6 drops OOOFlavors corn
bread extract

4 large eggs, beaten, at room
temperature, at room
temperature

½ cup (1 stick) unsalted butter,
melted, plus 1 tablespoon

1 cup shredded Cheddar
cheese, divided

Preheat the oven to 375°F. Place the empty cast iron skillet in the preheated oven for 10 minutes. In a medium bowl, combine the almond meal, sweetener, baking powder, and salt, and set aside. In a large bowl, combine the heavy whipping cream, sour cream, green chiles, corn bread extract, and eggs. Mix until fully combined. Add the dry ingredients to the wet ingredients, and stir until fully incorporated. Fold in ½ cup of melted butter, and stir until combined. Then fold in ½ cup of Cheddar cheese. Carefully remove the hot cast iron skillet, and add the remaining 1 tablespoon of butter to the skillet. Swirl to cover the bottom and sides. Add the corn bread batter to the hot, greased skillet. Top with the remaining ½ cup of Cheddar cheese. Bake for 30 to 35 minutes. Allow to cool in the pan for 10 minutes before slicing into wedges.

Per Serving: Calories: 335; Fat: 31g; Protein: 9g; Total Carbs: 9g; Fiber: 3g; Net Carbs: 6g; **Macros:** Fat: 83%; Protein: 11%; Carbs: 6%

Bacon Cheddar Chive Scones

MAKES 10 SCONES | PREP TIME: 10 minutes | COOK TIME: 25 to 30 minutes, plus cooling time

¼ cup (¼ stick) unsalted
butter, melted and cooled,
plus 1 tablespoon to
grease the pan

½ cup full-fat sour cream

3 large eggs, at room
temperature

1½ cups almond flour, sifted

½ cup coconut flour

1½ teaspoons baking powder

½ teaspoon sea salt

¼ cup shredded Cheddar
cheese, divided

4 slices cooked bacon,
crumbled, divided

2 tablespoons chopped chives

Preheat the oven to 375°F. Grease a 9-inch cast iron skillet with butter. In a large bowl, using an electric mixer, combine the butter, sour cream, and eggs. Fold in the almond flour, coconut flour, baking powder, and salt with a rubber spatula until fully combined. Then fold in 2 tablespoons of Cheddar cheese and 2 slices of cooked crumbled bacon. Spread the batter in the skillet. Sprinkle the remaining 2 tablespoons of Cheddar cheese, remaining 2 slices of bacon, and the chives on top. Bake for 25 to 30 minutes, or until a toothpick inserted into the center comes out clean. Allow to cool completely in the skillet, then cut into wedges to serve.

Per Serving: Calories: 250; Fat: 21g; Protein: 9g; Total Carbs: 9g; Fiber: 4g; Net Carbs: 5g; **Macros:** Fat: 76%; Protein: 14%; Carbs: 10%

Raspberry Scones

SERVES 8 | PREP TIME: 10 minutes | COOK TIME: 15 minutes

1 cup almond flour

2 large eggs, beaten

⅓ cup Splenda, stevia, or other
sugar substitute

1½ teaspoons pure
vanilla extract

1½ teaspoons baking powder

½ cup raspberries

Preheat the oven to 375°F. Line a baking sheet with parchment paper. In a large bowl, combine the almond flour, eggs, Splenda, vanilla, and baking powder. Add the raspberries to the bowl and gently fold in. After the raspberries are incorporated, spoon 2 to 3 tablespoons of the batter, per scone, onto the parchment-lined baking sheet. Bake for 15 minutes, or until lightly browned. Remove the baking sheet from the oven. Place the scones on a rack to cool for 10 minutes.

Per Serving: (1 scone): Calories: 133; Fat: 9g; Protein: 2g; Total Carbs: 4g; Fiber: 2g; Net Carbs: 2g; **Macros:** Fat: 77%; Protein: 15%; Carbs: 8%

Mixed Berry Scones with Lemon Icing

MAKES 10 SCONES | PREP TIME: 10 minutes | COOK TIME: 25 to 30 minutes, plus cooling time

For the scones

¼ cup (½ stick) unsalted butter, melted and cooled, plus 1 tablespoon to grease the pan

½ cup granulated erythritol–monk fruit blend

½ teaspoon liquid lemon extract

3 large eggs, at room temperature

½ cup full-fat sour cream

1½ cups almond flour, sifted

½ cup coconut flour

1½ teaspoons baking powder

¼ teaspoon sea salt

¼ cup blueberries, fresh or frozen

¼ cup raspberries, fresh or frozen

¼ cup chopped strawberries, fresh or frozen

For the lemon icing

½ cup confectioners' erythritol–monk fruit blend

2 tablespoons freshly squeezed lemon juice

½ teaspoon liquid lemon extract

1 to 2 tablespoons heavy (whipping) cream

½ tablespoon grated lemon zest

Preheat the oven to 375°F. Grease a 9-inch cast iron skillet with butter. In a large bowl, using an electric mixer, combine the butter, sweetener, lemon extract, and eggs. Add the sour cream, and mix well. Add the almond flour, coconut flour, baking powder, and salt, and stir until fully combined. Fold the blueberries, raspberries, and strawberries into the batter. Spread the batter evenly in the skillet. Bake for 25 to 30 minutes, or until a toothpick inserted into the center comes out clean. Allow to cool completely in the skillet, then cut into wedges. In a medium bowl, combine the sweetener, lemon juice, and lemon extract. Add the heavy whipping cream, starting with 1 tablespoon. Add another tablespoon if the icing is too thick. Once the scones have fully cooled, drizzle with the icing, then sprinkle the lemon zest on top.

Per Serving: Calories: 232; Fat: 19g; Protein: 7g; Total Carbs: 10g; Fiber: 5g; Net Carbs: 5g; **Macros:** Fat: 74%; Protein: 12%; Carbs: 14%

Chocolate Chip Scones

MAKES 10 | PREP TIME: 10 minutes | COOK TIME: 30 minutes

¼ cup (½ stick) unsalted butter, melted, plus more for greasing

½ cup granulated erythritol–monk fruit blend

3 large eggs

½ cup full-fat sour cream

1½ cups almond flour, sifted

½ cup coconut flour

1½ teaspoons baking powder

¼ teaspoon sea salt

4 ounces sugar-free chocolate chips

2 tablespoons confectioners' erythritol–monk fruit blend, for dusting (optional)

Preheat the oven to 375°F. Grease the cast-iron skillet with butter and set aside. In the large bowl, using an electric mixer on medium high, mix the sweetener, melted butter, and eggs until well combined, scraping the bowl once or twice, as needed. Add the sour cream and mix well. Add the almond flour, coconut flour, baking powder, and salt, then stir until fully combined. Fold the chocolate chips into the batter. Spread the batter evenly into the cast-iron skillet. Bake for 25 to 30 minutes, or until a toothpick inserted into the center comes out clean. Allow the scones to cool completely. Dust with confectioners' sweetener (if using) and cut into 10 wedges before serving.

Per Serving: (1 scone): Calories: 268; Fat: 24g; Protein: 7g; Total Carbs: 8g; Fiber: 4g; Net Carbs: 4g; **Macros:** Fat: 78%; Protein: 10%; Carbs: 12%

Strawberry Rhubarb Scones

MAKES 10 | PREP TIME: 10 minutes | COOK TIME: 30 minutes, plus 20 minutes to cool

For the scones

¼ cup (½ stick) unsalted butter, melted, plus more for greasing

½ cup granulated erythritol–monk fruit blend

3 large eggs

½ cup full-fat sour cream

1½ cups almond flour, sifted

½ cup coconut flour

1½ teaspoons baking powder

¼ teaspoon sea salt

¾ cup fresh or frozen strawberries, thinly sliced

¾ cup fresh or frozen rhubarb, thinly sliced

For the icing

½ cup confectioners' erythritol–monk fruit blend

½ teaspoon vanilla extract

3 to 4 tablespoons heavy (whipping) cream

Preheat the oven to 375°F. Grease the cast-iron skillet with butter and set aside. In the large bowl, using an electric mixer on medium high, blend the sweetener, melted butter, and eggs, scraping the bowl once or twice, as needed. Add the sour cream and mix well. Add the almond flour, coconut flour, baking powder, and salt, then stir until fully combined. Fold the strawberries and rhubarb into the batter. Spread the batter evenly into the cast-iron skillet. Bake for 25 to 30 minutes, or until an inserted toothpick comes out clean. Cool completely, about 20 minutes. In a small bowl, combine the confectioners' sweetener and vanilla. Add the heavy cream, starting with 1 tablespoon. Drizzle the icing onto the cooled scones and cut into 10 wedges before serving.

Per Serving: (1 scone): Calories: 222; Fat: 20g; Protein: 6g; Total Carbs: 6g; Fiber: 3g; Net Carbs: 3g; **Macros:** Fat: 79%; Protein: 10%; Carbs: 11%

"Cornbread" Muffins

MAKES 12 MUFFINS | PREP TIME: 10 minutes | COOK TIME: 20 minutes

2 cups almond flour

2 tablespoons flaxseed meal

2 teaspoons baking powder

6 large eggs, beaten

½ cup plain Greek yogurt

½ teaspoon stevia

Preheat the oven to 350°F. Line a 12-cup muffin pan with paper liners, and set aside. In a large bowl, stir the almond flour, flaxseed meal, and baking powder. Stir in the eggs, yogurt, and stevia until the batter is smooth. Spoon the batter evenly among the muffin cups. Bake until the muffins are lightly browned and firm, about 15 minutes. Cool the muffins on wire racks, and serve.

Per Serving: Calories: 163; Fat: 13g; Protein: 4g; Total Carbs: 5g; Fiber: 2g; Net Carbs: 3g; **Macros:** Fat: 76%; Protein: 10%; Carbs: 14%

Cinnamon Muffins with Cream Cheese Frosting

SERVES 12 | PREP TIME: 15 minutes | COOK TIME: 25 minutes

1 cup almond flour
½ cup coconut flour
2 teaspoons baking powder
¼ cup erythritol, or other sugar substitute, like stevia
6 large eggs
½ cup butter, melted
½ cup sparkling water

1 teaspoon pure vanilla extract
1½ tablespoons cinnamon
8 ounces (1 package) cream cheese, at room temperature
1 tablespoon sour cream
½ teaspoon pure vanilla extract

Preheat the oven to 350°F. In a medium bowl, whisk the almond flour, coconut flour, baking powder, and erythritol. In a large bowl, whisk the eggs, melted butter, sparkling water, and vanilla. Whisk to combine. Add the dry ingredients to the wet ingredients. Mix well to combine. Spoon the batter evenly into a muffin pan. Top each muffin with an equal amount of cinnamon. Using a toothpick, swirl the cinnamon into the batter. Bake for 20 to 25 minutes, or until golden brown. Remove the pan from the oven and cool the muffins in the pan for 5 to 10 minutes. In a medium bowl, blend the cream cheese, sour cream, and vanilla. Distribute the frosting evenly on the muffins before serving.

Per Serving: (1 muffin with cream cheese frosting): Calories: 225; Fat: 19g; Protein: 5g; Total Carbs: 6g; Fiber: 3g; Net Carbs: 3g; **Macros:** Fat: 79%; Protein: 9%; Carbs: 12%

Applesauce Yogurt Muffins

MAKES 12 MUFFINS | PREP TIME: 10 minutes | COOK TIME: 18 minutes

½ cup almond flour
2 tablespoons flaxseed meal
½ teaspoon baking powder
½ teaspoon stevia
½ teaspoon ground cinnamon
½ teaspoon ground nutmeg
¼ teaspoon ground ginger
¼ teaspoon sea salt

3 large eggs
½ cup plain Greek yogurt
½ cup unsweetened applesauce
3 tablespoons butter, melted
1 teaspoon pure vanilla extract

Preheat the oven to 350°F. Line a 12-cup muffin pan with paper liners. In a large bowl, stir the almond flour, flaxseed meal, baking powder, stevia, cinnamon, nutmeg, ginger, and salt. In a medium bowl, whisk the eggs, yogurt, applesauce, butter, and vanilla. Add the wet ingredients to the dry ingredients, and stir to blend. Spoon the muffin batter into the muffin cups evenly. Bake until the muffins are golden and a knife inserted in the center of one comes out clean, about 18 minutes. Cool the muffins on wire racks, and serve.

Per Serving: Calories: 94; Fat: 8g; Protein: 3g; Total Carbs: 3g; Fiber: 1g; Net Carbs: 2g; **Macros:** Fat: 76%; Protein: 12%; Carbs: 12%

Dairy-Free Churro Muffins

MAKES 12 MUFFINS | PREP TIME: 5 to 10 minutes | COOK TIME: 20 to 25 minutes, plus 10 minutes to cool

For the churro topping

⅓ cup granulated erythritol–monk fruit blend

2 teaspoons ground cinnamon

For the muffins

¾ cup granulated erythritol–monk fruit blend
½ cup coconut oil, solid
2 large eggs, at room temperature
¼ cup coconut or almond milk

½ teaspoon pure vanilla extract
1½ cups almond flour, sifted
1¼ teaspoons baking powder
1 teaspoon ground cinnamon
¼ teaspoon ground nutmeg
¼ teaspoon sea salt

In a small bowl, combine the sweetener and cinnamon. Preheat the oven to 350°F. Line a 12-cup muffin pan with cupcake liners, or grease. In a large bowl, using an electric mixer, cream the sweetener and coconut oil until light and fluffy. Beat in the eggs one at a time. Add the coconut milk and vanilla, and combine well. In a medium bowl, combine the almond flour, baking powder, cinnamon, nutmeg, and salt. Add the dry ingredients to the wet ingredients, and mix well. Scoop or pour the batter into the muffin cups until they are mostly full. Sprinkle the churro topping evenly on top of the muffins before baking. Bake for 20 to 25 minutes, or until a toothpick inserted into the center comes out clean. Allow the muffins to cool in the pan for 10 minutes and then transfer to a wire rack to cool thoroughly.

Per Serving: Calories: 176; Fat: 17g; Protein: 4g; Total Carbs: 4g; Fiber: 2g; Net Carbs: 2g; **Macros:** Fat: 87%; Protein: 9%; Carbs: 4%

Dairy-Free Cranberry Muffins

MAKES 12 | PREP TIME: 10 minutes | COOK TIME: 25 minutes, plus 20 minutes to cool

½ cup coconut oil, solid, plus more for greasing
¾ cup granulated erythritol–monk fruit blend
2 large eggs, at room temperature
¼ cup coconut or almond milk
½ teaspoon orange extract

1½ cups almond flour, sifted
1¼ teaspoons baking powder
1 teaspoon ground cinnamon
¼ teaspoon ground nutmeg
¼ teaspoon sea salt
1 cup fresh or frozen cranberries

Preheat the oven 350°F. Grease the muffin pan generously with coconut oil and set aside. In a large bowl, using an electric mixer on medium high, cream the coconut oil and sweetener for 1 to 2 minutes, scraping the bowl once or twice, as needed, until light and fluffy. Beat in the eggs, one at a time. Add the coconut milk and orange extract and combine well. In another large bowl, combine the almond flour, baking powder, cinnamon, nutmeg, and salt. Add the dry ingredients to the wet ingredients and mix well. Fold in the cranberries. Pour the batter evenly into the muffin cups. Bake for 20 to 25 minutes, or until a toothpick inserted in a muffin comes out clean. Allow to cool for 15 to 20 minutes before serving.

Per Serving: Calories: 173; Fat: 17g; Protein: 4g; Total Carbs: 4g; Fiber: 2g; Net Carbs: 2g; **Macros:** Fat: 83%; Protein: 8%; Carbs: 9%

Glazed Dairy-Free Carrot Cake Muffins

MAKES 12 MUFFINS | PREP TIME: 5 to 10 minutes | COOK TIME: 20 to 25 minutes, plus 10 minutes to cool

For the churro topping

⅓ cup granulated erythritol–monk fruit blend

2 teaspoons ground cinnamon

For the muffins

¾ cup granulated erythritol–monk fruit blend

½ cup coconut oil, solid

2 large eggs, at room temperature

¼ cup coconut or almond milk

½ teaspoon pure vanilla extract

1½ cups almond flour, measured and sifted

1¼ teaspoons baking powder

1 teaspoon ground cinnamon

¼ teaspoon ground nutmeg

¼ teaspoon sea salt

In a small bowl, combine the sweetener and cinnamon. Set aside. Preheat the oven to 350°F. Line a 12-cup muffin pan with cupcake liners, or grease each opening. In a large bowl, using an electric mixer, cream the sweetener and coconut oil until light and fluffy. Beat in the eggs one at a time. Add the coconut milk and vanilla, and combine well. In a medium bowl, combine the almond flour, baking powder, cinnamon, nutmeg, and salt. Add the dry ingredients to the wet ingredients, and mix well. Scoop or pour the batter into the muffin cups until they are mostly full. Sprinkle the churro topping evenly on top of the muffins before baking. Bake for 20 to 25 minutes, or until a toothpick inserted into the center comes out clean. Allow the muffins to cool in the pan for 10 minutes and then transfer to a wire rack to cool thoroughly.

Per Serving: Calories: 176; Fat: 17g; Protein: 4g; Total Carbs: 4g; Fiber: 2g; Net Carbs: 2g; **Macros:** Fat: 87%; Protein: 9%; Carbs: 4%

Glazed Cranberry-Orange Muffins

MAKES 18 MUFFINS | PREP TIME: 10 minutes | COOK TIME: 20 to 30 minutes, plus 15 minutes to cool

For the muffins

1¼ cups almond flour, sifted

1½ teaspoons baking powder

¼ teaspoon sea salt

4 ounces (about ½ cup) cream cheese, at room temperature

¼ cup (½ stick) unsalted butter, at room temperature

¾ cup granulated erythritol–monk fruit blend

1 tablespoon grated orange zest

½ teaspoon liquid orange extract

4 large eggs, at room temperature

1 cup cranberries, fresh or frozen

For the orange glaze

½ cup confectioners' erythritol–monk fruit blend

1½ tablespoons freshly squeezed lemon juice

1 tablespoon heavy (whipping) cream

1 teaspoon freshly grated orange zest

½ teaspoon liquid orange extract

To make the muffins: Preheat the oven to 350°F. Add 18 cupcake liners to the 2 (12-cup) muffin pans (some cups will be empty), or grease 18 muffin openings. In a medium bowl, whisk the almond flour, baking powder, and salt. In a large bowl, using an electric mixer, beat the cream cheese and butter on high speed until light and fluffy. Add the sweetener orange zest, and orange extract, and whisk until combined. Add the eggs one at a time to the wet ingredients, mixing after each addition. Mix until they are well incorporated. Add the dry ingredients to the wet batter, and blend until fully combined. Fold in the cranberries. Scoop or pour the batter into the muffin cups until they are a little more than three-quarters full. Bake for 20 to 28 minutes, or until a toothpick inserted into the center comes out clean. Allow to cool completely on a wire rack for about 15 minutes before glazing. In a medium bowl, whisk the sweetener, lemon juice, heavy cream, orange zest, and orange extract until fully combined. Once the muffins have completely cooled, drizzle the glaze on top. If you are going to freeze them, leave off the glaze.

Per Serving: Calories: 111; Fat: 10g; Protein: 4g; Total Carbs: 3g; Fiber: 1g; Net Carbs: 2g; **Macros:** Fat: 81%; Protein: 14%; Carbs: 5%

Pancake Muffins

MAKES 6 MUFFINS | PREP TIME: 10 minutes | COOK TIME: 15 minutes

Nonstick cooking spray (optional)

¼ cup coconut flour

½ teaspoon cinnamon

⅛ teaspoon baking soda

Pinch sea salt

3 large eggs

¼ cup coconut milk

2 tablespoons sugar-free maple syrup

¼ teaspoon vanilla extract

6 tablespoons (¾ stick) butter, for serving

Preheat the oven to 350°F. Prepare a 6-cup muffin pan with cooking spray or cupcake liners and set aside. In a small bowl, mix the coconut flour, cinnamon, baking soda, and salt. In a medium bowl, whip the eggs, coconut milk, syrup, and vanilla until fluffy. Pour the flour mixture into the egg mixture and mix until just incorporated. The batter will be lumpy. Divide the mixture evenly between the prepared muffin cups. Bake for 15 minutes. Let rest a few minutes and then top each muffin with ½ tablespoon of butter.

Per Serving: (1 muffin) Calories: 208; Fat: 17g; Protein: 5g; Total Carbs: 9g; Fiber: 6g; Net Carbs: 3g; **Macros:** Fat: 73%; Protein: 10%; Carbs: 17%

Banana Nut Muffins

MAKES 12 | PREP TIME: 10 minutes | COOK TIME: 25 minutes

2½ cups fine almond flour

½ teaspoon baking soda

¼ teaspoon sea salt

1 teaspoon ground cinnamon

1½ teaspoons banana extract

2 large eggs, at room temperature

4 ounces full-fat sour cream

½ cup sugar-free maple syrup, plus 2 tablespoons, divided

⅓ cup chopped walnuts, plus 2 tablespoons, divided

1 tablespoon melted butter

Preheat the oven to 325°F. Line a 12-cup muffin tin with cupcake liners. In a large bowl, whisk the almond flour, baking soda, salt, and cinnamon. In another large bowl, combine the banana extract, eggs, sour cream, and ½ cup of syrup. Slowly pour the wet mixture into the dry mixture and thoroughly combine. Fold in ⅓ cup of walnuts. Divide the muffin mixture evenly among the muffin cups. Bake for 20 to 25 minutes, until a toothpick inserted into a muffin center comes out clean. Transfer to a wire rack to cool. In a small bowl, whisk the remaining 2 tablespoons of syrup, 2 tablespoons of walnuts, and the melted butter. When the muffins are cool enough to handle, spoon the walnut mixture evenly on top of each muffin and serve immediately.

Per Serving: (1 muffin): Calories: 224; Fat: 18g; Protein: 7g; Total Carbs: 12g; Fiber: 8g; Net Carbs: 4g; Macros: Fat: 69%; Protein: 11%; Carbs: 20%

Greens and Parmesan Muffins

SERVES 8 | PREP TIME: 15 minutes | COOK TIME: 20 minutes

For the collards

1½ tablespoons butter

1 garlic clove, finely minced

1½ cup frozen chopped collard greens

For the muffins

4 large eggs

½ cup almond flour

¼ cup coconut flour

¼ teaspoon onion powder

¼ teaspoon garlic powder

⅛ teaspoon cayenne pepper

2½ tablespoons butter, melted

2 tablespoons sour cream

2 tablespoons shredded Parmesan cheese, plus more for topping (optional)

3 crispy cooked bacon slices, finely chopped

In a medium skillet over medium heat, melt the butter. Add the collards and garlic. Sauté for 7 to 10 minutes until tender. Set aside to cool. Preheat the oven to 350°F. Prepare a standard muffin tin with eight liners. In a large bowl and using an electric hand mixer, whip the eggs for about 2 minutes until light and foamy. Add the almond and coconut flours, onion powder, garlic powder, cayenne, melted butter, and sour cream. Mix on medium speed until combined, scraping down the sides at least once. Stir in the Parmesan cheese, bacon, and cooled collard greens. Using a cookie scoop or spoon, evenly divide the batter among the prepared muffin cups. Top the muffins with additional Parmesan, if desired. Bake for 15 to 20 minutes, or until the tops are golden brown. Let the muffins cool in the pan for 10 minutes, then transfer to a wire rack to cool completely.

Per Serving: Calories: 190; Fat: 14g; Protein: 8g; Total Carbs: 8g; Fiber: 4g; Net Carbs: 4g; Macros: Fat: 66%; Protein: 17%; Carbs: 17%

Lemon Poppy Seed Muffins

MAKES 12 | PREP TIME: 5 minutes | COOK TIME: 25 minutes

¾ cup almond flour

⅓ cup coconut flour

½ cup erythritol sweetener

1 teaspoon baking powder

⅓ cup unsweetened almond milk

¼ cup melted butter

4 large eggs

Juice of 1 lemon (2 tablespoons)

Zest of 1 lemon (1 heaping tablespoon)

2 tablespoons poppy seeds

Preheat the oven to 350°F and place paper liners in the cups of a 12-cup muffin pan. In a large bowl, sift the almond flour, coconut flour, sweetener, and baking powder. In a medium bowl, whisk the almond milk, butter, eggs, lemon juice, and lemon zest. Combine the wet and dry ingredients and whisk. Fold in the poppy seeds. Fill the muffin cups evenly. Bake for 20 to 22 minutes until the muffins spring back when touched or a toothpick inserted into a center comes out clean. Allow to cool before serving.

Per Serving: Calories: 104; Fat: 8g; Protein: 4g; Total Carbs: 4g; Fiber: 1g; Net Carbs: 3g; Macros: Fat: 70%; Protein: 15%; Carbs: 15%

Orange Olive Oil Poppy Seed Muffins

MAKES 9 MUFFINS | PREP TIME: 15 minutes | COOK TIME: 20 minutes

4 large eggs

1 large egg yolk

1 cup almond flour

⅓ cup olive oil

6 tablespoons monk fruit/ erythritol blend sweetener

¼ cup coconut flour

2½ teaspoons baking powder

2 teaspoons grated orange zest

2 teaspoons poppy seeds

¼ teaspoon kosher salt

1 teaspoon vanilla extract

Preheat the oven to 350°F. Prepare a standard muffin tin with 9 liners. In a large bowl and using an electric hand mixer, whip the eggs and egg yolk for about 2 minutes until light and foamy. Add the almond flour, olive oil, sweetener, coconut flour, baking powder, orange zest, poppy seeds, salt, and vanilla. Mix on medium speed until well combined, scraping down the sides of the bowl at least once. Using a cookie scoop or spoon, evenly divide the batter among the prepared muffin cups. Bake for 15 to 20 minutes, or until golden brown on top. Let the muffins cool in the pan for 10 minutes, then transfer to a wire rack to cool completely.

Per Serving: Calories: 170; Fat: 14g; Protein: 5g; Total Carbs: 6g; Fiber: 4g; Net Carbs: 2g; Macros: Fat: 74%; Protein: 12%; Carbs: 14%

Zucchini Muffins

MAKES 16 MUFFINS | PREP TIME: 5 minutes | COOK TIME: 20 minutes

1 cup grated, drained zucchini

1 cup almond flour

¾ cup almond butter

3 large eggs

1 tablespoon honey

1 teaspoon pure vanilla extract

1 teaspoon baking powder

1 teaspoon cinnamon

Preheat the oven to 350°F. In a large bowl, combine the zucchini, almond flour, almond butter, eggs, honey, vanilla, baking powder, and cinnamon. Mix well. Line a cupcake pan with paper liners. Divide the batter evenly among the paper liners. Bake for 18 to 20 minutes, or until golden brown. Cool the muffins for 5 minutes before serving.

Per Serving: (1 muffin): Calories: 184; Fat: 15g; Protein: 5g; Total Carbs: 7g; Fiber: 2g; Net Carbs: 5g; Macros: Fat: 74%; Protein: 11%; Carbs: 15%

Zucchini Chocolate Muffins

MAKES 12 MUFFINS | PREP TIME: 5 minutes |
COOK TIME: 15 minutes

3 large eggs, beaten
2 cups shredded zucchini
½ cup cacao powder
½ cup coconut oil,
    slightly melted

1 teaspoon vanilla extract
⅓ cup granulated erythritol
2 tablespoons low-carb dark
    chocolate chips

Preheat the oven to 250°F. Grease the cups of a muffin tin (or use liners). In a medium bowl, mix the eggs, zucchini, cacao powder, coconut oil, vanilla, and erythritol. Pour the batter evenly into the 12 muffin cups. Sprinkle the chocolate chips on the tops of the muffins. Bake for about 15 minutes, or until a knife inserted into the middle of a muffin comes out clean. Transfer the muffins to a cooling rack.

Per Serving: Calories: 379; Fat: 35g; Protein: 7g; Total Carbs: 9g; Fiber: 4g; Net Carbs: 5g; **Macros:** Fat: 83%; Protein: 7%; Carbs: 10%

Cream Cheese Pumpkin Muffins

MAKES 12 MUFFINS | PREP TIME: 15 minutes |
COOK TIME: 20 minutes

Nonstick cooking spray
½ cup butter, at room
    temperature
⅔ cup erythritol, granulated
4 large eggs
¾ cup pumpkin purée
1 teaspoon vanilla extract
1½ cups almond flour
½ cup coconut flour

4 teaspoons baking powder
2 teaspoons pumpkin
    pie spice
½ teaspoon salt
8 ounces Greek yogurt
    cream cheese
Stevia
Ground cinnamon

Preheat the oven to 350°F. Line the cups of a muffin tin with liners or grease well with cooking spray. In a large bowl with a hand mixer, mix the butter and erythritol until creamy. Add the eggs one at a time, mixing thoroughly after each addition. Stir in the pumpkin and vanilla and mix well. In a small bowl, mix the almond flour, coconut flour, baking powder, pumpkin pie spice, and salt. Pour the flour mixture into the butter mixture and mix to combine. Divide the batter evenly between the muffin cups. In a small bowl, stir the cream cheese until softened. Add stevia to taste. Top each muffin with about 1 tablespoon of cream cheese. Sprinkle with cinnamon. Bake for about 20 minutes, or until the muffin tops are slightly brown.

Per Serving: (2 muffins): Calories: 447; Fat: 35g; Protein: 14g; Total Carbs: 19g; Fiber: 7g; Net Carbs: 12g; **Macros:** Fat: 70%; Protein: 13%; Carbs: 17%

Chocolate Cake Donuts

12 DONUTS | PREP TIME: 15 minutes |
COOK TIME: 20 minutes

Nonstick cooking spray
    (optional)
½ cup sugar substitute
¼ cup coconut flour

¼ cup unsweetened
    cocoa powder
½ teaspoon salt
¼ teaspoon baking powder

4 large eggs
½ cup (1 stick) butter, at room
    temperature
¼ cup buttermilk

Preheat the oven to 350°F. Prepare a donut pan or muffin pan with nonstick cooking spray or line a baking sheet with parchment paper. In a small bowl, mix the sugar substitute, coconut flour, cocoa powder, salt, and baking powder. In a medium bowl, whisk the eggs, butter, and buttermilk. Add the dry mixture to the egg mixture and mix until incorporated. Scoop the batter into the donut pan, or fill a piping bag and pipe circles onto the prepared baking sheet. Bake for 15 to 20 minutes, turning the pan halfway through the cooking time.

Per Serving: (1 donut) Calories: 114; Fat: 10g; Protein: 3g; Total Carbs: 3g; Fiber: 2g; Net Carbs: 1g; **Macros:** Fat: 78%; Protein: 11%; Carbs: 11%

Jelly Donuts

MAKES 6 | PREP TIME: 15 minutes | COOK TIME: 15 minutes

Cooking spray
1 cup chopped ripe
    strawberries
⅓ cup water
1 envelope (¼ ounce) unfla-
    vored gelatin
½ cup erythritol, divided, plus
    1 tablespoon

1 cup plus 2 tablespoons
    almond flour
½ teaspoon baking powder
2 large eggs
½ teaspoon apple
    cider vinegar
2 tablespoons unsweetened
    vanilla almond milk
2 tablespoons melted butter

Preheat the oven to 350°F. Spray 6 cups of a muffin tin with cooking spray. Puree the strawberries in a blender. Pour the water into a medium saucepan over medium heat. Sprinkle the gelatin on top and then add ¼ cup of erythritol. Whisk for 2 to 3 minutes until completely combined. Slowly whisk in the strawberries and allow the mixture to bubble. Turn the heat to low and cook, stirring occasionally, for 5 to 7 minutes until thickened. Remove from the heat and refrigerate to cool. In a large bowl, mix the almond flour, ¼ cup of erythritol, and the baking powder. Add the eggs, vinegar, and almond milk and mix into a thick dough. Divide the dough into 6 equal pieces and drop into the prepared muffin cups. Bake in the center of the oven for 12 to 15 minutes or until lightly golden on top. While the donuts bake, pour the strawberry jelly into a resealable plastic bag and cut off one of the corners. Pour the remaining 2 tablespoons of erythritol onto a small plate. Once the donuts are cooked, remove them from the muffin tin, pour the butter all over them, and roll each donut in the erythritol. Cut a deep slit into the side of each donut (not all the way through). Pipe strawberry jelly into each one. Serve immediately.

Per Serving: (1 donut): Calories: 193; Fat: 16g; Protein: 8g; Total Carbs: 24g; Fiber: 3g; Net Carbs: 3g; **Macros:** Fat: 72%; Protein: 15%; Carbs: 13%

Dairy-Free Chocolate Donuts

MAKES 12 | PREP TIME: 10 minutes | COOK TIME: 30 minutes, plus 20 minutes to cool

For the donuts

¼ cup coconut oil, melted, plus more for greasing

2 cups granulated erythritol–monk fruit blend

2 cups almond flour, sifted

¾ cup coconut flour

¾ cup unsweetened cocoa powder

1½ teaspoons baking powder

1½ teaspoons baking soda

½ teaspoon sea salt

1 cup full-fat coconut milk or almond milk

1 cup boiling water

1 teaspoon vanilla extract

3 large eggs

For the icing

4 ounces unsweetened baking chocolate, coarsely chopped

½ cup confectioners' erythritol–monk fruit blend

2 tablespoons coconut oil

¼ teaspoon sea salt

To make the donuts: Preheat the oven to 350°F. Grease the silicone molds well with coconut oil. In the large bowl, combine the sweetener, almond flour, coconut flour, cocoa powder, baking powder, baking soda, and salt. Add the coconut milk, boiling water, coconut oil, and vanilla. Add the eggs, one at a time, mixing well after each addition. Using an electric mixer on medium, mix the batter until fully incorporated, scraping the bowl once or twice, as needed. Pour the batter into the prepared molds and bake for 25 to 30 minutes, until a toothpick inserted in a donut comes out clean. Cool completely, 15 to 20 minutes, before taking the donuts out of the molds. Line the baking sheet with parchment paper and set aside. In the small microwave-safe bowl, melt the baking chocolate in the microwave in 30-second intervals. Add the confectioners' sweetener, coconut oil, and salt and combine until silky smooth. Once the donuts are fully cooled, dip each into the chocolate icing, taking care to evenly coat the tops. Place them on the prepared baking sheet and refrigerate until ready to serve.

Per Serving: Calories: 309; Fat: 28g; Protein: 8g; Total Carbs: 11g; Fiber: 6g; Net Carbs: 5g; Macros: Fat: 79%; Protein: 9%; Carbs: 12%

Baked Donut Bites with Jelly

15 DONUTS | PREP TIME: 5 minutes | COOK TIME: 10 minutes

Oil or nonstick cooking spray, for greasing

2 cups almond flour

3 tablespoons whey protein isolate, unflavored

½ cup confectioners' erythritol blend, plus 2 tablespoons for dusting

½ teaspoon baking powder

¼ teaspoon salt

4 large eggs

½ cup (1 stick) butter, room temperature or softened

¼ cup buttermilk

½ teaspoon vanilla extract

½ cup sugar-free strawberry jelly

Preheat the oven to 350°F, and lightly grease a mini muffin pan. In a large bowl, sift the almond flour, whey protein, ½ cup of confectioners' sweetener, baking powder, and salt. Add the eggs, butter, buttermilk, and vanilla, and mix well. Fill the muffin tins ⅔ full, and bake for 10 to 12 minutes, or until slightly golden brown. Remove from the oven, and allow to cool. Spoon the jelly into a small microwave-safe bowl. Microwave for 10 seconds,

and stir so it has a more liquid consistency. Transfer the donuts to a plate, and sift the remaining 2 tablespoons of sweetener over top. Serve with the warmed jelly on the side for dipping.

Per Serving: (2 donut bites with jelly): Calories: 185; Fat: 14g; Protein: 7g; Total Carbs: 14.5g; Fiber: 1.5g; Net Carbs: 1.5g; Macros: Fat: 58%; Protein: 13%; Carbs: 29%

Matcha Donuts

SERVES 6 | PREP TIME: 10 minutes | COOK TIME: 13 minutes

For the donuts

Nonstick coconut oil cooking spray

2 cups almond flour

⅓ cup powdered stevia

1½ tablespoons matcha powder

1 tablespoon baking powder

¼ teaspoon salt

¾ cup unsweetened hemp or almond milk

2 tablespoons freshly squeezed lemon juice

1 teaspoon vanilla extract

1 flax "egg"

6 tablespoons tahini

For the icing

¼ cup coconut oil

¼ cup powdered stevia

1 teaspoon vanilla extract

½ teaspoon matcha powder

Preheat the oven to 350°F. Grease a donut pan with cooking spray and set aside. In a large bowl, whisk the almond flour, stevia, matcha powder, baking powder, and salt. In a medium bowl, whisk the hemp milk, lemon juice, vanilla, flax "egg," and tahini. Pour the wet mixture into the dry mixture and stir to combine. Fill the prepared donut pan with the batter, and bake for 13 minutes or until a toothpick inserted in the center comes out clean Cool the donuts, in the pan, on a rack for about 15 minutes. In a small mixing bowl, whisk the coconut oil, stevia, vanilla, and matcha. Dip the top of the donuts into the icing and sprinkle with Matcha powder, if desired, and serve while still slightly warm.

Per Serving: Calories: 296; Fat: 28g; Protein: 8g; Total Carbs: 9g; Fiber: 5g; Net Carbs: 4g; Macros: Fat: 79%; Protein: 10%; Carbs: 11%

Cinnamon "Apple" Pecan Coffee Cake

SERVES 12 | PREP TIME: 15 minutes | COOK TIME: 35 minutes

For the "apple" topping

3 tablespoons butter

1 chayote squash, peeled and diced

¼ cup allulose blend sweetener

½ teaspoon ground cinnamon

⅛ teaspoon ground cloves

⅛ teaspoon ground nutmeg

⅓ cup chopped pecans

For the coffee cake

Nonstick cooking spray

1½ cups almond flour

¼ cup plus 2 tablespoons coconut flour

¼ cup monk fruit/erythritol blend sweetener

1 tablespoon baking powder

½ teaspoon ground cinnamon

½ teaspoon kosher salt

3 large eggs

½ cup unsweetened almond milk

2 teaspoons vanilla extract

¼ cup sour cream

6 tablespoons butter, melted

In a medium skillet over medium heat, melt the butter. Add the squash and sauté for about 7 minutes, or until the squash is tender.

Stir in the sweetener, cinnamon, cloves, nutmeg, and pecans. Cook for 2 to 3 minutes until the sweetener is dissolved and syrupy. Remove from the heat. Preheat the oven to 350°F. Lightly coat a 9-inch square pan with cooking spray and set aside. In a large bowl and using an electric hand mixer, mix the almond and coconut flours, sweetener, baking powder, cinnamon, and salt until combined. One at a time, add the eggs and mix well after each addition. Add the almond milk and vanilla, and mix until combined. Stir in the sour cream and melted butter. Pour the batter into the prepared pan and spread it evenly. Evenly distribute the squash mixture over the top of the batter and drizzle with the syrup from the pan. Bake for 20 to 25 minutes, or until a toothpick inserted into the center comes out clean. Let cool completely before slicing and serving.

Per Serving: Calories: 210; Fat: 18g; Protein: 5g; Total Carbs: 7g; Fiber: 3g; Net Carbs: 4g; **Macros:** Fat: 77%; Protein: 10%; Carbs: 13%

Cinnamon Coffee Cake

SERVES 16 | PREP TIME: 10 minutes | COOK TIME: 40 minutes

For the cake

2 cups almond flour

½ cup powdered erythritol

2 teaspoons baking powder

1 teaspoon ground cinnamon

¼ teaspoon ground nutmeg

Pinch salt

3 large eggs

5 tablespoons butter, at room temperature

½ cup sour cream

¼ cup unsweetened almond milk

1 teaspoon vanilla extract

For the cinnamon crumble

2 cups almond flour

¼ cup powdered erythritol

2 teaspoons ground cinnamon

¼ teaspoon ground nutmeg

¼ teaspoon salt

½ cup chopped walnuts

½ cup butter, melted

Preheat the oven to 350°F. Butter a 9-inch square baking dish or line it with parchment paper. Sift the almond flour, erythritol, baking powder, cinnamon, nutmeg, and salt into a large bowl and whisk to combine. In a mixing bowl, use a hand mixer to cream the eggs and butter until fluffy. Add the sour cream, almond milk, and vanilla. Mix to combine. Slowly add the dry ingredients and mix to combine. In a large bowl, combine the almond flour, erythritol, cinnamon, nutmeg, salt, and walnuts. Add the butter and mix. Pour half of the cake batter into the prepared baking dish. Sprinkle half of the crumble on top of the batter. Add the rest of the cake batter, then sprinkle the remaining crumble on top. Very gently press the crumble into the batter. Bake for 35 to 40 minutes or until a toothpick inserted comes out clean. Halfway through cooking, loosely cover the dish with aluminum foil to prevent the crumble burning. Allow to cool and serve.

Per Serving: Calories: 234; Fat: 22g; Protein: 5g; Total Carbs: 5g; Fiber: 3g; Net Carbs: 2g; **Macros:** Fat: 82%; Protein: 9%; Carbs: 9%

Lemonade Snack Cake

SERVES 12 | PREP TIME: 15 minutes | COOK TIME: 40 minutes

¼ cup butter, at room temperature, plus more for preparing the pan

1½ cups almond flour

2 tablespoons coconut flour

2 teaspoons baking powder

½ teaspoon kosher salt

4 ounces cream cheese, at room temperature

½ cup monk fruit/erythritol blend sweetener

4 large eggs, at room temperature

1 teaspoon vanilla extract

1½ tablespoons grated lemon zest

Preheat the oven to 350°F. Coat a 9-by-5-inch loaf pan with butter. In a medium bowl, stir the almond and coconut flours, baking powder, and salt. Set aside. In medium bowl and using an electric hand mixer, cream the butter, cream cheese, and sweetener until fluffy. One at a time, add the eggs, mixing well after each addition. Add the vanilla and lemon zest, and mix to combine. Add the flour mixture and mix until well combined. Pour the batter into the prepared pan. Bake for 35 to 40 minutes, or until a toothpick inserted into the center comes out clean. Let cool in pan for at least 20 minutes before transferring to a wire rack to cool completely before slicing.

Per Serving: Calories: 152; Fat: 13g; Protein: 5g; Total Carbs: 4g; Fiber: 2g; Net Carbs: 2g; **Macros:** Fat: 77%; Protein: 13%; Carbs: 10%

Old-Fashioned Lemon-Lime Teacakes

MAKES 20 | PREP TIME: 20 minutes | COOK TIME: 15 minutes

For the teacakes

½ cup unsalted butter, at room temperature

⅓ cup powdered erythritol

2 large eggs

3 tablespoons lemon juice

½ teaspoon vanilla extract

2¼ cup almond flour, sifted

½ cup oat fiber

1½ teaspoons baking powder

For the glaze

⅓ cup plus 1 tablespoon powdered erythritol

2 tablespoons lime juice

Zest of 1 lime

Preheat the oven to 350°F. Line a baking sheet with parchment paper. In a large bowl, cream the butter and erythritol for 3 to 4 minutes with a hand mixer until light and fluffy. Add the eggs one at a time and mix thoroughly after each addition. Add the lemon juice and vanilla. Mix well. In a medium bowl, whisk the almond flour, oat fiber, and baking powder until combined. Slowly add the dry ingredients to the wet ingredients and mix on medium speed for a minute. Using a 1-ounce scoop, place scoops of batter on the prepared baking sheet about 3-inches apart. Cover with more parchment paper and use a second baking sheet to press down on the cakes until they are ½-inch thick. Place the baking sheet of tea cakes in the refrigerator for 15 minutes. Bake for 15 minutes. The tea cakes should not be browned on top. Remove from the oven, and using a spatula, carefully move each cake to a cooling rack. In a small bowl, whisk the erythritol and lime juice. Transfer the glaze to a small zip-top bag and cut off a small portion of the corner plastic, and gently squeeze the glaze out across all the cookies. Sprinkle with the lime zest and allow the cookies and glaze to completely cool before storing.

Per Serving: Calories: 96; Fat: 9g; Protein: 3g; Total Carbs: 4g; Fiber: 1g; Net Carbs: 3g; **Macros:** Fat: 79%; Protein: 9%; Carbs: 12%

Iced Cranberry-Gingerbread Loaf

MAKES 10 SLICES | PREP TIME: 10 minutes |
COOK TIME: 45 minutes to 1 hour, plus cooling time

For the loaf

1¼ cups almond flour, sifted

1½ teaspoons baking powder

¼ teaspoon sea salt

1 tablespoon ground ginger

2 teaspoons ground cinnamon

½ teaspoon ground nutmeg

¼ teaspoon ground cloves

¼ teaspoon ground allspice

⅛ teaspoon pepper

4 ounces (about ½ cup) cream cheese, at room temperature

½ cup brown or golden granulated erythritol–monk fruit blend

¼ cup (½ stick) unsalted butter, at room temperature

1 teaspoon pure vanilla extract

4 large eggs, at room temperature

1 cup whole cranberries, fresh or frozen

¼ cup chopped walnuts

For the cream cheese icing

4 ounces (about ½ cup) cream cheese, at room temperature

2 tablespoons unsalted butter, at room temperature

½ confectioners' erythritol–monk fruit blend

¼ teaspoon pure vanilla extract

Pinch salt

½ cup heavy (whipping) cream

Preheat the oven to 350°F. Line a 9-by-5-inch loaf pan with parchment paper. In a medium bowl, combine the almond flour, baking powder, salt, ginger, cinnamon, nutmeg, cloves, allspice, and pepper. In a large bowl, using an electric mixer, mix the cream cheese, sweetener, butter, and vanilla until the mixture is light and fluffy. Add the eggs one at a time, mixing after each addition. Add the dry ingredients to the wet ingredients, and combine until well incorporated. Fold in the cranberries. Spread the batter into the prepared loaf pan, and sprinkle the top with the walnuts. Bake for 45 minutes to 1 hour, or until a toothpick inserted into the center comes out clean. Allow the loaf to cool for about 10 minutes before taking it out of the pan. Allow to cool completely before icing. In a large bowl, using an electric mixer, beat the cream cheese, butter, and vanilla until light and fluffy. Add the confectioners' sweetener and salt, and mix gently until just combined. Add the heavy cream a couple of tablespoons at a time, and beat until fully combined. Once the loaf has fully cooled, spread the icing on top, and serve.

Per Serving: Calories: 317; Fat: 30g; Protein: 8g; Total Carbs: 7g; Fiber: 2g; Net Carbs: 5g; **Macros:** Fat: 85%; Protein: 10%; Carbs: 5%

Pumpkin Spice Loaf with Maple Icing

MAKES 10 SLICES | PREP TIME: 10 minutes | COOK TIME: 45 to 50 minutes, plus cooling time

For the loaf

½ cup (1 stick) unsalted butter, at room temperature, plus more to grease the pan

1½ cups almond flour, measured and sifted

1½ tablespoons ground cinnamon

1½ tablespoons ground ginger

1½ teaspoons pumpkin pie spice

1½ teaspoons baking powder

¼ teaspoon ground nutmeg

¼ teaspoon sea salt

⅛ teaspoon ground cloves

¾ cup granulated erythritol–monk fruit blend

4 ounces (about ½ cup) cream cheese, at room temperature

½ cup canned pumpkin purée

For the maple icing

½ cup confectioners' erythritol–monk fruit blend

1 teaspoon ground cinnamon

¼ cup brown or golden granulated erythritol–monk fruit blend

1 teaspoon pure vanilla extract

3 large eggs, at room temperature

¼ cup heavy (whipping) cream

1 tablespoon sugar-free maple syrup

Preheat the oven to 350°F. Generously grease a 9-by-5-inch loaf pan with butter. In a medium bowl, sift the almond flour, cinnamon, ginger, pumpkin pie spice, baking powder, nutmeg, salt, and cloves. In a large bowl, using an electric mixer on high speed, beat the sweetener, butter, cream cheese, brown sweetener, and vanilla. Beat for 2 to 3 minutes, or until light and creamy. Add the pumpkin purée, and mix until just incorporated. Alternate adding the eggs one at a time with the dry ingredients. Be sure to mix thoroughly after each addition. Pour the batter into the prepared pan, and bake for 45 to 50 minutes, or until a toothpick inserted into the center comes out clean. Allow to cool in the pan for 10 minutes before removing. Allow to cool completely before icing. In a medium bowl, combine the confectioners' sweetener and cinnamon. Whisk in the heavy cream, fully incorporate the mixture. Add the maple syrup, and mix well. Once the loaf has fully cooled, spread the icing on top, and serve.

Per Serving: Calories: 270; Fat: 25g; Protein: 7g; Total Carbs: 7g; Fiber: 3g; Net Carbs: 4g; **Macros:** Fat: 83%; Protein: 10%; Carbs: 7%

Cinnamon Swirl Bread

MAKES 12 SLICES | PREP TIME: 10 minutes | COOK TIME: 45 minutes to 1 hour, plus 30 to 40 minutes to cool

½ cup (1 stick) unsalted butter, melted and cooled, plus more to grease the pan

1 cup coconut milk

6 large eggs, at room temperature

1 cup almond flour, sifted

¾ cup granulated erythritol–monk fruit blend, divided

½ cup coconut flour

½ cup psyllium husk powder

1½ teaspoons baking powder

½ teaspoon sea salt

2 tablespoons ground cinnamon

Preheat the oven to 350°F. Grease a 9-by-5-inch loaf pan with butter. In a large bowl, using an electric mixer, combine the coconut milk and butter, then add the eggs one at a time. Add the almond flour, ½ cup of sweetener, coconut flour, psyllium husk powder, baking powder, and salt. Mix the batter on medium speed for about 2 minutes, or until fully incorporated. In a small bowl, combine the remaining ¼ cup of sweetener and the cinnamon. Place half the batter into the loaf pan. Sprinkle the cinnamon mixture on top, reserving 2 teaspoons. Add the other half of the batter. Sprinkle the top of the bread with the reserved cinnamon mixture. Bake for 45 minutes to 1 hour, or until a toothpick inserted into the center comes out clean. Allow to cool for about 10 minutes before removing from the pan. Place on a wire rack for another 20 to 30 minutes to fully cool before slicing.

Per Serving: Calories: 210; Fat: 16g; Protein: 6g; Total Carbs: 13g; Fiber: 8g; Net Carbs: 5g; **Macros:** Fat: 69%; Protein: 11%; Carbs: 20%

Chocolate Chip Banana Bread

MAKES 12 SLICES | PREP TIME: 5 to 10 minutes |
COOK TIME: 35 to 40 minutes, plus cooling time

½ cup golden flax meal

1 cup almond flour, measured and sifted

½ cup coconut flour

1 tablespoon baking powder

1 tablespoon psyllium husk powder

2 teaspoons ground cinnamon

¼ teaspoon ground nutmeg

¼ teaspoon sea salt

¾ cup brown or golden granulated erythritol–monk fruit blend

½ cup coconut oil, melted

2 tablespoons sugar-free maple syrup

5 or 6 drops liquid banana extract

1 teaspoon pure vanilla extract

4 large eggs, at room temperature

½ cup coconut or almond milk

½ cup sugar-free chocolate chips, divided

Preheat the oven to 350°F. Line a 9-by-5-inch loaf pan with parchment paper. In a coffee grinder, grind the flax meal until it's a fine powder. In a medium bowl, combine the flax meal powder, almond flour, coconut flour, baking powder, psyllium husk powder, cinnamon, nutmeg, and salt. Set aside. In a large bowl, combine the sweetener, coconut oil, maple syrup, banana extract, and vanilla. Using an electric mixer, beat in the eggs one at a time until fully combined. Add the dry ingredients to the wet ingredients, and beat on medium-low speed until well incorporated. Add the coconut milk, and continue to mix. Reserve 1 tablespoon of the chocolate chips, then stir in the rest. Put the batter in the prepared loaf pan, and sprinkle the reserved chocolate chips on top. Bake for 35 to 40 minutes, or until a toothpick inserted into the center comes out clean. Allow to fully cool on a wire rack before slicing.

Per Serving: Calories: 254; Fat: 21g; Protein: 6g; Total Carbs: 16g; Fiber: 6g; Net Carbs: 10g; **Macros:** Fat: 74%; Protein: 9%; Carbs: 17%

Buttery Coconut Bread

MAKES 16 SLICES | PREP TIME: 10 minutes |
COOK TIME: 35 minutes

½ cup butter, melted, plus more for greasing

6 large eggs

½ teaspoon stevia

1 cup almond flour

½ cup coconut flour

1 teaspoon baking powder

1 teaspoon pure vanilla extract

Preheat the oven to 350°F. Lightly grease an 8-by-4-inch loaf pan with butter, and set aside. In a medium bowl, whisk the melted butter, eggs, and stevia until well blended. In a small bowl, stir the almond flour, coconut flour, and baking powder until mixed. Add the coconut flour mixture to the egg mixture, and stir to combine. Stir in the vanilla. Spoon the batter into the loaf pan, and bake the bread until it is golden brown, about 35 minutes. Cool the bread in the loaf pan for 15 minutes, and then turn the bread out onto a wire rack to cool completely.

Per Serving: (1 slice): Calories: 107; Fat: 9g; Protein: 4g; Total Carbs: 4g; Fiber: 2g; Net Carbs: 2g; **Macros:** Fat: 72%; Protein: 14%; Carbs: 14%

Nut-Free Pumpkin Bread

SERVES 12 | PREP TIME: 15 minutes | COOK TIME: 55 minutes, plus 30 minutes to cool

¼ cup (½ stick) unsalted butter, melted, plus more for greasing

1 cup granulated erythritol–monk fruit blend; less sweet: ½ cup

¾ cup canned pumpkin puree

1 teaspoon vanilla extract

4 large eggs, at room temperature

1½ cups sunflower seed flour

½ cup golden flaxseed meal, reground in a clean coffee grinder

1½ teaspoons baking powder

1 tablespoon psyllium husk powder

2 teaspoons ground cinnamon

1½ teaspoons ground ginger

½ teaspoon ground nutmeg

¼ teaspoon ground cloves

¼ teaspoon sea salt

Preheat the oven to 350°F. Grease 9-by-5-inch loaf pan with butter and set aside. In the large bowl, using an electric mixer on medium high, beat the butter, sweetener, pumpkin puree, and vanilla until well blended, scraping the bowl once or twice, as needed. Add the eggs, one at time, mixing well after each addition. Add the sunflower seed flour, flaxseed meal, baking powder, psyllium husk powder, cinnamon, ginger, nutmeg, cloves, and salt. Spread the batter into the prepared loaf pan. Bake for 40 to 55 minutes, or until a toothpick inserted into the center comes out clean. Let cool for 10 minutes in the pan. Remove the pumpkin bread from the pan and allow to cool 15 to 20 minutes. Refrigerate for up to 5 days or freeze for 3 weeks.

Per Serving: Calories: 195; Fat: 17g; Protein: 6g; Total Carbs: 7g; Fiber: 4g; Net Carbs: 3g; **Macros:** Fat: 75%; Protein: 12%; Carbs: 13%

Nut-Free Sunflower Bread

MAKES 12 SLICES | PREP TIME: 10 minutes |
COOK TIME: 45 minutes to 1 hour, plus 30 to 40 minutes to cool

Unsalted butter or coconut oil (to make the recipe dairy-free), for greasing the pan

1 cup coconut milk

½ cup coconut oil, melted and cooled

6 large eggs, at room temperature

1 cup sunflower seed flour

½ cup coconut flour

½ cup psyllium husk powder

½ cup granulated erythritol–monk fruit blend

1½ teaspoons baking powder

½ teaspoon sea salt

2 tablespoons sesame seeds

Preheat the oven to 350°F. Grease a 9-by-5-inch loaf pan with butter. In a large bowl, using an electric mixer, combine the coconut milk and coconut oil. Add the eggs one at a time, mixing after each addition. Add the sunflower seed flour, coconut flour, psyllium husk powder, sweetener, baking powder, and salt. Mix the batter well on medium speed for about 2 minutes, or until fully incorporated. Put the batter in the loaf pan. Sprinkle the sesame seeds on top. Bake for 45 minutes to 1 hour, or until a toothpick inserted into the center comes out clean. Allow to cool for about 10 minutes before removing from the pan. Place on a wire rack for another 20 to 30 minutes to cool fully before slicing.

Per Serving: Calories: 233; Fat: 18g; Protein: 7g; Total Carbs: 12g; Fiber: 8g; Net Carbs: 4g; **Macros:** Fat: 70%; Protein: 12%; Carbs: 18%

Cinnamon Rolls

MAKES 12 ROLLS | PREP TIME: 30 minutes |
COOK TIME: 15 minutes, plus 30 minutes to chill

For the dough
Butter or nonstick cooking spray, for greasing
½ cup coconut flour
2 tablespoons granulated erythritol blend
1 teaspoon baking powder
1 teaspoon cinnamon
Pinch salt
2 cups grated mozzarella cheese

5 tablespoons cream cheese
1 large egg

For the filling
5 tablespoons cold butter, cubed
¼ cup brown erythritol blend
1 tablespoon cinnamon
1½ teaspoons coconut flour

For the icing
¼ cup cream cheese
2 tablespoons butter
2 tablespoons sugar-free almond milk or milk of your choice

½ cup confectioners' erythritol blend
½ teaspoon vanilla extract

Preheat the oven to 400°F, and lightly grease a pie pan with butter. In a small bowl, combine the flour, sweetener, baking powder, cinnamon, and salt. In a large microwave-safe bowl, slowly melt the mozzarella and cream cheese, 30 seconds at a time, until the mozzarella is completely melted and smooth. Add the flour mixture, stir, and then stir in the egg. Using your hands, work the dough to form a ball. Lay the ball on a piece of parchment paper and, mash it down to begin making a rectangle. Lay another piece of parchment paper on top, and roll the dough ¼ inch thick. Take the top parchment paper off, and with your fingers, straighten the edges. Put a clean parchment paper on top and flip the dough over. Peel the top piece of parchment paper off. In a small bowl, mix the cubed butter, brown sweetener, cinnamon, and flour into a paste. Using a knife, spread it evenly over the dough. With a long end of the dough in front of you, roll the dough away from you into a tight log. Wrap the dough in a fresh piece of parchment paper, and freeze for 30 minutes to an hour. Remove the log from the freezer, and using a serrated knife, cut the log into 12 slices. Arrange the slices side by side in the greased pie pan, and cook for 12 to 15 minutes, or until golden brown. Using an electric mixer, mix the cream cheese, butter, milk, confectioners' blend, and vanilla until creamy in a medium bowl. Allow the cinnamon rolls to cool for about 5 minutes, and then spread or pipe the icing over the rolls. Cut and serve.

Per Serving: (1 roll): Calories: 189; Fat: 16g; Protein: 6g; Total Carbs: 15.5g; Fiber: 2.5g; Net Carbs: 2g; **Macros:** Fat: 62%; Protein: 11%; Carbs: 27%

Creamy Asparagus Soup

SERVES 4 | PREP TIME: 5 minutes | COOK TIME: 20 minutes

6 tablespoons extra-virgin olive oil, divided
1 pound asparagus, trimmed and cut into 2-inch pieces
½ cup chopped scallions, green parts only
4 garlic cloves, minced
1 teaspoon salt
½ teaspoon red pepper flakes

2 cups vegetable or chicken stock
1 cup water
¼ cup tahini (ground sesame seed paste)
Juice and zest of 1 lemon
2 tablespoons toasted pumpkin seeds, for garnish

In a medium saucepan, heat 2 tablespoons of olive oil over medium heat. Sauté the asparagus for 2 to 3 minutes, until just tender. Add the scallions, garlic, salt, and red pepper flakes and sauté for another 2 to 3 minutes, until fragrant. Add the stock and water, increase the heat to high, and bring to a boil. Reduce the heat to low, cover, and simmer for 8 to 10 minutes, or until the vegetables are tender. Remove from the heat and allow to cool slightly. Add the tahini, remaining ¼ cup of olive oil, and lemon juice and zest. Using an immersion blender, puree the soup until smooth and creamy. Serve warm garnished with toasted seeds.

Per Serving: Calories: 329; Fat: 30g; Protein: 7g; Total Carbs: 12g; Fiber: 4g; Net Carbs: 8g; **Macros:** Fat: 82%; Protein: 9%; Carbs: 9%

Creamed Cauliflower Soup

SERVES 4 | PREP TIME: 10 minutes | COOK TIME: 30 minutes

2 tablespoons butter
1 white onion, chopped
1 tablespoon minced fresh garlic
1 medium cauliflower, chopped into small florets
2 cups vegetable broth

1 bay leaf
1 cup grated Cheddar cheese
½ cup heavy (whipping) cream
1 teaspoon salt
½ teaspoon freshly ground black pepper

In a stockpot over medium-high heat, melt the butter. Add the onion and garlic and sauté for about 3 minutes. Add the cauliflower florets and cook, stirring, for another 2 to 3 minutes. Pour in the vegetable broth and add the bay leaf. Bring to a simmer and cook for about 20 minutes, or until the cauliflower is tender. Remove from the heat remove the bay leaf and stir in the cheddar cheese, cream, salt, and pepper. Stir until the cheese is totally melted. Divide into 4 portions and serve.

Per Serving: Calories: 351; Fat: 27g; Protein: 14g; Total Carbs: 13g; Fiber: 4g; Net Carbs: 9g; **Macros:** Fat: 69%; Protein: 16%; Carbs: 15%

Cauliflower-Cheddar Soup

SERVES 8 | PREP TIME: 10 minutes | COOK TIME: 30 minutes

¼ cup butter
½ sweet onion, chopped
1 head cauliflower, chopped
4 cups chicken stock
½ teaspoon ground nutmeg
1 cup heavy (whipping) cream

Sea salt
Freshly ground black pepper
1 cup shredded Cheddar cheese

Put a large stockpot over medium heat and add the butter. Sauté the onion and cauliflower until tender and lightly browned, about 10 minutes. Add the chicken stock and nutmeg to the pot and bring the liquid to a boil. Reduce the heat to low and simmer until the vegetables are very tender, about 15 minutes. Remove the pot from the heat, stir in the heavy cream, and purée the soup with an immersion blender or food processor until smooth. Season the soup with salt and pepper and serve topped with the Cheddar cheese.

Per serving: Calories: 227; Fat: 21g; Protein: 8g; Total Carbs: 4g; Fiber: 2g; Net Carbs: 2g; **Macros:** Fat: 80%; Protein: 14%; Carbs: 6%

Spiced Pumpkin Soup

SERVES 4 | PREP TIME: 5 minutes | COOK TIME: 1 hour on high or 2 hours on low

1 (15-ounce) can pump-kin puree	1 teaspoon ground cumin
1 (13.6-ounce) can unsweet-ened full-fat coconut milk	¼ teaspoon ground turmeric
	Salt
1 cup vegetable broth	Freshly ground black pepper
1 tablespoon onion powder	Fresh cilantro leaves, for garnish

In a slow cooker bowl, combine the pumpkin, coconut milk, broth, onion powder, cumin, and turmeric. Cover and cook for 1 hour on high or 2 hours on low. Season with salt and pepper to taste. Ladle the soup into serving bowls and garnish with cilantro.

Per Serving: Calories: 256; Fat: 22g; Protein: 5g; Total Carbs: 15g; Fiber: 3g; Net Carbs: 12g; **Macros:** Fat: 71%; Protein: 7%; Carbs: 22%

Broccoli Cheddar Soup

SERVES 6 | PREP TIME: 10 minutes | COOK TIME: 20 minutes

½ cup butter	4 ounces full-fat cream cheese, cubed, at room temperature
½ medium white onion, diced	
2 celery stalks, diced	
2 garlic cloves, minced	16 ounces Cheddar cheese, freshly grated, plus more for garnish
4 cups diced broccoli florets	
5 cups low-sodium chicken broth	
	Salt
1 cup heavy (whipping) cream	Freshly ground black pepper

In a large stockpot over medium heat, melt the butter. Add the onion, celery, and garlic, and sauté until the onion is soft and translucent, 8 to 10 minutes. Add the broccoli and cook for 5 minutes until the broccoli is vibrantly green and soft. Remove about ½ cup of broccoli and set aside for garnish. Add the broth and cream. Bring to a gentle boil then immediately lower the heat to low. Add the cream cheese and stir. Add the cheddar, stirring constantly to incorporate. Continue until all the cheese and stir until incorporated. Add salt and pepper to taste. Divide among bowls and garnish with the reserved broccoli and additional shredded cheddar.

Per Serving: Calories: 703; Fat: 63g; Protein: 26g; Total Carbs: 11g; Fiber: 2g; Net Carbs: 9g; **Macros:** Fat: 80%; Protein: 14%; Carbs: 6%

Creamy Broccoli, Bacon, and Cheese Soup

SERVES 6 | PREP TIME: 15 minutes | COOK TIME: 30 minutes

2 heads broccoli	1 cup heavy (whipping) cream
2 tablespoons olive oil	Sea salt
1 onion, chopped	Freshly ground black pepper
2 teaspoons minced garlic	1 cup shredded Cheddar cheese
4 cups low-sodium vegeta-ble stock	
½ teaspoon ground nutmeg	4 slices uncured bacon, cooked and chopped

Chop one head of broccoli, including the stem, and cut the remaining head into small florets and chop the stem. Set the florets aside. Heat the olive oil in a large saucepan over medium-high heat. Sauté the onion and garlic until tender, about 3 minutes. Add the chopped broccoli, stock, and nutmeg. Bring the soup to a boil, then reduce the heat to low and simmer until the vegetables are tender, about 25 minutes. While the soup is simmering, place a medium pot of water over high heat and bring to a boil. Blanch the florets until tender-crisp, about 3 minutes, and drain. Transfer the soup to a food processor or use an immersion blender and blend until smooth, then transfer back to the saucepan. Whisk in the cream and blanched florets. Season with salt and pepper. Serve topped with cheese and bacon.

Per Serving: Calories: 320; Fat: 29g; Protein: 10g; Total Carbs: 7g; Fiber: 2g; Net Carbs: 5g; **Macros:** Fat: 82%; Protein: 13%; Carbs: 5%

Roasted Red Pepper Soup with Basil and Goat Cheese

SERVES 4 | PREP TIME: 5 minutes | COOK TIME: 15 minutes

6 tablespoons extra-virgin olive oil, divided	½ teaspoon freshly ground black pepper
½ small onion, roughly chopped	3 cups vegetable or chicken stock
1 (16-ounce) jar roasted red peppers, drained and roughly chopped	1 cup water
	4 ounces goat cheese
2 garlic cloves, minced	½ cup chopped fresh basil leaves, plus more for garnish
1 teaspoon salt	2 tablespoons red wine vinegar

In a medium saucepan, heat 2 tablespoons of olive oil over medium heat. Sauté the onions for 3 to 4 minutes, until soft. Add the red peppers, garlic, salt, and pepper and sauté for 2 to 3 minutes more, until fragrant. Add the stock and water, increase the heat to high, and bring to a boil. Reduce the heat to low, cover, and simmer for 4 to 5 minutes. Remove from the heat and mix in the goat cheese, basil, remaining ¼ cup of olive oil, and vinegar. Using an immersion blender, puree the mixture until smooth and creamy. Serve warm garnished with additional basil leaves.

Per Serving: Calories: 331; Fat: 29g; Protein: 7g; Total Carbs: 10g; Fiber: 2g; Net Carbs: 8g; **Macros:** Fat: 79%; Protein: 8%; Carbs: 13%

Cream of Mushroom Soup

SERVES 4 | PREP TIME: 10 minutes | COOK TIME: 20 minutes

6 tablespoons butter, divided	2 tablespoons sherry
2 cups sliced mush-rooms, divided	(optional)
½ cup minced onions	Sea salt
1 teaspoon minced garlic	Freshly ground black pepper
1 teaspoon minced thyme	1 quart hot beef bone broth
	1 cup heavy (whipping) cream

Heat 2 tablespoons of the butter in a large pot over medium-high heat. Add ⅓ of the mushrooms to the pot and brown the mushrooms, about 1 minute on each side. Push the cooked mushrooms to the sides of the pot. Add another 2 tablespoons of butter and another third of mushrooms. Brown and repeat with the remaining butter and mushrooms. Reduce the heat to medium and add the onions, garlic, and thyme to the pan. Cook for 2 to 3 minutes, until the onions are beginning to soften. Add the sherry (if using), and deglaze the pan with it by scraping up all of the browned bits from the bottom of the pan. Season with salt and pepper. Pour in the beef broth and simmer gently until the mushrooms are tender, about 8 minutes. Stir in the heavy cream and cook over low heat until the soup is thick and velvety, about 2 minutes.

Per Serving: Calories: 335; Fat: 34g; Protein: 3g; Total Carbs: 6g; Fiber: 1g; Net Carbs: 5g; **Macros:** Fat: 91%; Protein: 4%; Carbs: 5%

Creamed Mushroom and Fennel Soup

SERVES 4 | PREP TIME: 10 minutes | COOK TIME: 25 minutes

2 tablespoons butter	1 teaspoon salt
1 cup sliced fennel bulb	½ teaspoon freshly ground
8 ounces mushrooms, preferably shiitake, sliced and divided	black pepper
	2 cups beef or vegetable stock
2 garlic cloves, minced	½ cup heavy (whipping) cream
2 tablespoons chopped fresh thyme or rosemary or 2 teaspoons dried thyme	2 tablespoons extra-virgin olive oil

In a medium saucepan, heat the butter over medium heat. Sauté the fennel for 5 to 6 minutes, until tender and slightly browned. Add 6 ounces of mushrooms, garlic, thyme, salt, and pepper and sauté for 3 to 4 minutes, until the mushrooms are soft. Add the stock, increase the heat to high, and bring to a boil. Reduce the heat to low, cover and simmer for about 5 minutes, until the vegetables are very tender. Remove from the heat and allow to cool slightly. Add the cream and olive oil and using an immersion blender, puree the mixture until smooth and creamy. Roughly chop the remaining 2 ounces of mushrooms. If using a blender, return the creamed soup to saucepan and heat over low. Add the mushrooms and cook, stirring constantly, until tender, 3 to 4 minutes. Serve warm.

Per Serving: Calories: 247; Fat: 24g; Protein: 4g; Total Carbs: 7g; Fiber: 2g; Net Carbs: 5g; **Macros:** Fat: 87%; Protein: 6%; Carbs: 7%

Tomato Basil Soup

SERVES 4 | PREP TIME: 5 minutes | COOK TIME: 20 minutes

¼ cup extra-virgin olive oil	2 cups vegetable broth or
1 cup diced onion	chicken bone broth
1 teaspoon minced garlic	¼ cup thinly sliced fresh basil
1 (28-ounce) can whole plum tomatoes with basil	

Heat the olive oil in a large pot over medium heat. Add the onion and garlic, and cook until soft and fragrant, about 10 minutes. Pour the tomatoes and broth into the pot and simmer uncovered for 10 minutes. Remove the soup from the heat. Use an immersion blender to purée the soup until very smooth. Stir in the fresh basil, and ladle the portions into soup bowls.

Per Serving: Calories: 167; Fat: 14g; Protein: 2g; Total Carbs: 11g; Fiber: 2g; Net Carbs: 9g; **Macros:** Fat: 75%; Protein: 5%; Carbs: 20%

Watercress-Spinach Soup

SERVES 4 | PREP TIME: 20 minutes | COOK TIME: 10 minutes

2 tablespoons coconut oil	4 cups spinach
½ sweet onion, chopped	1 cup coconut milk
2 teaspoons minced garlic	Sea salt
1 tablespoon arrowroot	Freshly ground black pepper
4 cups chicken stock	8 cooked turkey bacon slices,
4 cups watercress	chopped, for garnish

In a large saucepan over medium-high heat, heat the coconut oil. Sauté the onion and garlic in the oil until softened, about 3 minutes. Whisk in the arrowroot to form a paste. Whisk in the chicken stock until the mixture is smooth. Add the watercress, spinach, and coconut milk. Cook the soup until it is just heated through and the greens are still vibrant, about 3 minutes. Transfer the soup to a food processor, and purée. Transfer the soup back to the saucepan, and season with salt and pepper. Top with the bacon, and serve.

Per Serving: Calories: 280; Fat: 23g; Protein: 13g; Total Carbs: 7g; Fiber: 4g; Net Carbs: 3g; **Macros:** Fat: 72%; Protein: 18%; Carbs: 10%

Loaded Miso Soup with Tofu and Egg

SERVES 4 | PREP TIME: 10 minutes | COOK TIME: 20 minutes

3 cups water	1 (14-ounce) package firm
3 cups vegetable broth	tofu, drained and cut into
3 tablespoons white miso paste	bite-sized cubes
	2 cups spiralized zucchini (or
2-inch piece fresh ginger, peeled and minced	thinly sliced if preferred)
	2 hard-boiled eggs, peeled
4 baby bok choy, trimmed and quartered	and quartered
	2 nori seaweed sheets, cut into
2 cups thinly sliced shiitake mushrooms	2-inch very thin strips
	¼ cup avocado or olive oil
2 garlic cloves, very thinly sliced	2 tablespoons toasted sesame oil

In a large saucepan, bring the water and vegetable broth to a boil over high heat. Reduce the heat to low, whisk in the miso paste and ginger, cover, and simmer for 2 minutes. Add the bok choy, mushrooms, and garlic. Simmer, covered, another 5 minutes or until vegetables are tender. Remove from heat and stir in cubed tofu and zucchini. Divide the mixture between bowls. Add 2 egg quarters and seaweed strips to each bowl. Drizzle 1 tablespoon of avocado oil and ½ teaspoon of sesame oil over each bowl. Serve warm.

Per Serving: Calories: 378; Fat: 29g; Protein: 17g; Total Carbs: 14g; Fiber: 6g; Net Carbs: 8g; **Macros:** Fat: 69%; Protein: 18%; Carbs: 13%

Vegetarian French Onion Soup

SERVES 6 | **PREP TIME:** 10 minutes | **COOK TIME:** 30 minutes

1 tablespoon butter
2 large white onions, sliced
6 cups vegetable broth
1 tablespoon minced garlic
½ teaspoon salt
1 bay leaf
2 cups shredded
 Gruyère cheese

In a large stockpot on medium heat, melt the butter and sauté the onions until translucent, 4 to 5 minutes. Mix in the broth, garlic, salt, and bay leaf. Bring the soup to a simmer and cook for 20 to 25 minutes, or until the onions are very soft. Sprinkle with the cheese.

Per Serving: (1 cup) Calories: 222; Fat: 14g; Protein: 16g; Total Carbs: 8g; Fiber: 1g; Net Carbs: 7g; **Macros:** Fat: 57%; Protein: 29%; Carbs: 14%

French Onion Soup

SERVES 4 | **PREP TIME:** 10 minutes | **COOK TIME:** 80 minutes

2 tablespoons butter
2 tablespoons olive oil
3 yellow onions, halved and
 thinly sliced
Pinch sea salt
¼ cup dry red wine
1 quart beef bone broth
1 sprig fresh thyme
1 sprig fresh rosemary

Heat a large pot over medium heat and melt the butter and olive oil. Add the onions and season with the salt. Cover and cook for 30 minutes. Remove the lid and continue to cook until the onions are golden brown, about 30 more minutes. Pour in the red wine, broth, thyme, and rosemary. Bring to a simmer and cook for 20 minutes. Remove the herbs. Allow to cool for 10 minutes before serving.

Per Serving: Calories: 185; Fat: 13g; Protein: 7g; Total Carbs: 9g; Fiber: 2g; Net Carbs: 7g; **Macros:** Fat: 63%; Protein: 12%; Carbs: 15%

Turnip and Thyme Soup

SERVES 4 | **PREP TIME:** 10 minutes | **COOK TIME:** 20 minutes

2 tablespoons olive oil
1¼ pounds turnips (about
 4 medium), peeled
 and cubed
1 teaspoon dried thyme
½ teaspoon onion powder
3 cups chicken broth
Salt
Freshly ground black pepper
2 scallions, green and white
 parts, finely sliced
Fresh thyme leaves, for garnish

In a large stockpot, heat the oil over medium heat. Add the turnips, thyme, and onion powder. Cover and cook for about 10 minutes, or until the turnips are tender. Add the broth and bring to a boil. Reduce the heat to a simmer, cover, and cook for 10 minutes. Use an immersion blender to blend everything until smooth. Season

with salt and pepper to taste. Transfer to serving bowls, sprinkle with the scallions, and garnish with thyme.

Per Serving: Calories: 111; Fat: 7g; Protein: 2g; Total Carbs: 10g; Fiber: 3g; Net Carbs: 7g; **Macros:** Fat: 57%; Protein: 7%; Carbs: 36%

Creamy Tomato Soup

SERVES 3 | **PREP TIME:** 5 minutes | **COOK TIME:** 15 minutes

1 (14.5-ounce) can diced
 unsalted tomatoes
1 cup chicken bone broth
½ teaspoon salt
¼ teaspoon dried thyme
¼ teaspoon garlic powder
Pinch ground nutmeg
¼ cup heavy (whipping) cream
Freshly ground black pepper
 (optional)

In a medium saucepan over medium-high heat, combine the tomatoes, broth, salt, thyme, garlic powder, and nutmeg. Bring to a boil and then reduce the heat to low and simmer for 5 minutes. Either with an immersion blender or in a regular blender, puree the soup. Pour the soup back into the saucepan and turn the heat to medium low. Slowly whisk in the cream and continue whisking until well combined. Simmer for 5 more minutes. Portion into bowls and serve. Season with pepper (if using).

Per Serving: Calories: 119; Fat: 8g; Protein: 5g; Total Carbs: 8g; Fiber: 2g; Net Carbs: 6g; **Macros:** Fat: 55%; Protein: 18%; Carbs: 27%

Easy Herbed Tomato Bisque

SERVES 8 | **PREP TIME:** 15 minutes | **COOK TIME:** 25 minutes

3 tablespoons olive oil
½ cup diced onion
2 garlic cloves,
 roughly chopped
1 (28-ounce) can whole tomatoes (San Marzano style
 are best)
1 cup chicken stock or
 bone broth
1 tablespoon tomato paste
½ teaspoon dried basil
½ teaspoon dried thyme
1 tablespoon freshly squeezed
 lemon juice
½ cup heavy (whipping) cream

In a Dutch oven over medium heat, combine the olive oil and onion. Sauté for 5 minutes until the onion is translucent, but not brown. Add the garlic and cook for 1 minute more. Stir in the tomatoes, chicken stock, tomato paste, basil, and thyme, stirring to break up the chunks of tomato. Reduce the heat to low and simmer for 15 to 20 minutes. Transfer the soup to a blender and blend until smooth. Use caution while blending hot liquids and cover the lid with a towel. Pour the soup back into the pan and stir in the lemon juice and heavy cream.

Per Serving: (½ cup): Calories: 358; Fat: 30g; Protein: 10g; Total Carbs: 12g; Fiber: 6g; Net Carbs: 6g; **Macros:** Fat: 75%; Protein: 12%; Carbs: 13%

Hearty Cauliflower Soup

MAKES 4 CUPS | **PREP TIME:** 10 minutes |
COOK TIME: 50 minutes

4 cups cauliflower florets
¼ cup melted butter
¼ teaspoon sea salt
1 tablespoon olive oil
1 garlic clove, minced
¼ cup diced onion
Pinch ground nutmeg
⅛ teaspoon thyme
2 cups chicken bone broth

2 tablespoons mascarpone, at room temperature, divided

¼ cup heavy (whipping) cream

Sea salt

Freshly ground black pepper

Preheat the oven to 375°F. Line a baking sheet with parchment paper. In a large bowl, toss the cauliflower, butter, and salt until well combined. Pour the cauliflower onto the prepared baking sheet in a single layer. Bake for 30 minutes, until the cauliflower is fork-tender and begins to brown. In a large saucepan over medium-low heat, heat the olive oil. Add the garlic, stirring frequently, and cook for about 45 seconds. Stir in the onion, sprinkle in the nutmeg and thyme, and cook for another 5 to 7 minutes, until the onions are translucent. Transfer the roasted cauliflower to the saucepan. Add the chicken broth and bring the soup to a boil. Reduce the heat to medium-low and simmer for 15 to 20 minutes, until the vegetables are soft. Stir in the mascarpone ½ tablespoon at a time until melted. Slowly add the heavy cream, stirring constantly, until it is thoroughly incorporated. Season with salt and pepper. Transfer three-quarters of the soup to a blender and blend until smooth. Pour the blended soup back into the saucepan and stir to combine. Portion into bowls and serve.

Per Serving: (1 cup): Calories: 271; Fat: 24g; Protein: 8g; Total Carbs: 7g; Fiber: 2g; Net Carbs: 5g; **Macros:** Fat: 79%; Protein: 11%; Carbs: 10%

Egg Drop Soup

SERVES 6 | PREP TIME: 5 minutes | COOK TIME: 15 minutes

4 cups chicken broth or bone broth

4 cups vegetable broth

1 chicken bouillon cube

5 shiitake mushrooms, trimmed and thinly sliced

1 tablespoon soy sauce

1 tablespoon sesame oil

4 large eggs, beaten

2 scallions, green parts only thinly sliced, for garnish

In a medium pot over medium-high heat, combine the chicken broth, vegetable broth, bouillon cube, mushrooms, soy sauce, and sesame oil, and bring to a full boil. Reduce heat to a simmer. Use one hand to hold a fork on the edge of the egg bowl, and as you gently stir the pot with the other hand, slowly pour the eggs through the tines of the fork into the hot water. Pour into 6 bowls, top with the scallions, and serve.

Per Serving: (1½ cups): Calories: 112; Fat: 6g; Protein: 11g; Total Carbs: 4g; Fiber: 1g; Net Carbs: 3g; **Macros:** Fat: 44%; Protein: 39%; Carbs: 9%

Spicy Serrano Gazpacho

SERVES 4 | PREP TIME: 10 minutes

3 cups cored and diced vine-ripened tomatoes, divided

1 cucumber, peeled and diced, divided

1 serrano pepper, stem, seeds, and membranes removed, sliced in half

2 tablespoons red wine vinegar

¼ cup olive oil

Sea salt

Freshly ground black pepper

1 shallot, minced

2 tablespoons thinly sliced basil

In a blender, combine 1½ cups of the tomatoes, half of the cucumber, half of the pepper, the red wine vinegar, and the olive oil. Blend until smooth, and season with salt and pepper. Taste the soup for spiciness level. If desired, add the remaining half of the pepper and blend again until smooth. Stir in the remaining tomatoes, cucumber, shallot, and basil. Chill for 30 minutes before serving.

Per Serving: Calories: 156; Fat: 14g; Protein: 2g; Total Carbs: 8g; Fiber: 2g; Net Carbs: 6g; **Macros:** Fat: 81%; Protein: 5%; Carbs: 14%

Chilled Avocado-Cilantro Soup

SERVES 4 | PREP TIME: 10 minutes

2 very ripe avocados, peeled and pitted

½ cup plain Greek yogurt

½ cup chopped fresh cilantro leaves

¼ cup extra-virgin olive oil

¼ cup freshly squeezed lime juice (about 4 limes)

1 teaspoon salt

1 teaspoon onion powder

½ teaspoon freshly ground black pepper

½ teaspoon garlic powder

½ teaspoon ground turmeric

¼ cup roasted pumpkin seeds, to garnish (optional)

Add the avocados, yogurt, cilantro, olive oil, lime juice, salt, onion powder, pepper, garlic powder, and turmeric to a blender or a wide cylindrical container, if using an immersion blender. Blend until smooth and creamy. Serve chilled topped with pumpkin seeds (if using).

Per Serving: Calories: 268; Fat: 25g; Protein: 4g; Total Carbs: 9g; Fiber: 5g; Net Carbs: 4g; **Macros:** Fat: 84%; Protein: 6%; Carbs: 10%

Cream of Cauliflower Gazpacho

SERVES 4 TO 6 | PREP TIME: 15 minutes | COOK TIME: 25 minutes

1 cup raw almonds

½ teaspoon salt

½ cup extra-virgin olive oil, plus 1 tablespoon, divided

1 small onion, minced

1 small head cauliflower, stalk removed and broken into florets (about 3 cups)

2 garlic cloves, finely minced

2 cups chicken or vegetable stock or broth, plus more if needed

1 tablespoon red wine vinegar

¼ teaspoon freshly ground black pepper

Bring a small pot of water to a boil. Add the almonds to the water and boil for 1 minute. Drain in a colander and run under cold water. Pat dry and squeeze the meat of each almond out of its skin. Discard the skins. In a food processor or blender, blend the almonds and salt. With the processor running, drizzle in ½ cup extra-virgin olive oil, scraping down the sides as needed. Set the almond paste aside. In a large stockpot, heat the remaining 1 tablespoon olive oil over medium-high heat. Add the onion and sauté until golden, 3 to 4 minutes. Add the cauliflower florets and sauté for another 3 to 4 minutes. Add the garlic and sauté for 1 minute more. Add 2 cups of stock and bring to a boil. Cover, reduce the heat to medium-low, and simmer the vegetables until tender, 8 to 10 minutes. Remove from the heat and allow to cool slightly. Add the vinegar and pepper. Using an immersion blender, blend until smooth. With the blender running, add the almond paste and blend until smooth, adding extra stock if the soup is too thick. Serve warm, or chill in refrigerator at least 4 to 6 hours to serve a cold gazpacho.

Per Serving: Calories: 505; Fat: 45g; Protein: 10g; Total Carbs: 15g; Fiber: 5g; Net Carbs: 10g; **Macros:** Fat: 80%; Protein: 8%; Carbs: 12%

Loaded Baked "Fauxtato" Soup

SERVES 6 | PREP TIME: 15 minutes | COOK TIME: 20 minutes

3 tablespoons butter

1¼ pounds turnips, peeled and diced into 1-inch cubes

¼ cup chopped onion

1 teaspoon kosher salt, plus more as needed

½ teaspoon garlic powder

12 ounces cauliflower florets, fresh or frozen, steamed until just tender

2½ to 3 cups chicken stock, plus more as needed

⅓ cup heavy (whipping) cream

2 tablespoons sour cream

Freshly ground black pepper

Crispy, chopped cooked bacon, for garnish

Shredded Cheddar cheese, for garnish

Sliced scallion, for garnish

In a medium saucepan over medium heat, melt the butter. Add the turnips, onion, salt, and garlic powder. Sauté for 8 to 10 minutes until the onion is tender and add the cauliflower and cook for 1 to 2 minutes more. Add the chicken stock and bring the mixture to a boil. Lower the heat to maintain a simmer and cook for 7 to 8 minutes, or until the turnips are fork-tender. Remove from the heat and let cool a few minutes. Transfer the soup to a blender. Add the heavy cream and sour cream. Blend on high speed until smooth and creamy. Adjust the consistency with additional broth, and adjust the seasoning, as needed. Serve topped with bacon, cheese, and scallion.

Per Serving: Calories: 324; Fat: 24g; Protein: 14g; Total Carbs: 13g; Fiber: 4g; Net Carbs: 9g; **Macros:** Fat: 67%; Protein: 17%; Carbs: 16%

Butternut Squash Soup with Turmeric & Ginger

SERVES 8 | PREP TIME: 5 minutes | COOK TIME: 35 minutes

1 small butternut squash

3 tablespoons coconut oil

3 shallots, coarsely chopped

1-inch knob fresh ginger, peeled and coarsely chopped

1-inch knob fresh turmeric root, peeled and coarsely chopped

1 fresh lemongrass stalk, coarsely chopped

½ cup dry Marsala wine (optional)

8 cups miso broth

1 cup coconut cream

Cold-pressed olive oil, for drizzling

Handful toasted pumpkin seeds, for garnish (optional)

Preheat the oven to 365°F. Puncture the squash skin with a fork several times, put in a baking dish and bake for 30 minutes or until extremely tender. While the squash is baking, heat the oil in a large stockpot over medium heat. Add the shallots, ginger, turmeric, and lemongrass to the pan and sauté until the spices become fragrant and the shallots are tender. Deglaze the pot by pouring in the Marsala wine (if using), and stirring, scraping the bottom of the pot to loosen any stuck bits. Once the alcohol starts to reduce, add the miso broth and turn the heat to low. Remove the squash from oven when tender. Carefully cut the squash in half lengthwise, allowing any liquid to drain out. Once the squash is cool enough to handle, scoop out the seeds. With a paring knife, remove the skin. Roughly chop the squash and add it to the stockpot. Pour the coconut cream into the pot, bring to a simmer, and remove from the heat. Using an immersion blender, blend the soup thoroughly until smooth and velvety. Drizzle with olive oil, and top with toasted pumpkin seeds, if desired. Serve warm.

Per Serving: Calories: 149; Fat: 13g; Protein: 2g; Total Carbs: 10g; Fiber: 1g; Net Carbs: 9g; **Macros:** Fat: 71%; Protein: 5%; Carbs: 24%

Cold Cucumber and Avocado Soup

SERVES 4 | PREP TIME: 15 minutes

2 English cucumbers, cut into chunks

2 avocados, cubed

1 cup plain Greek yogurt

6 ounces firm tofu, diced

1 scallion, white and green parts, cut into chunks

Juice of 1 lemon

¼ jalapeño pepper

1 cup low-sodium chicken stock

2 tablespoons spinach hemp pesto

Sea salt

Freshly ground black pepper

½ cup mascarpone cheese

In a blender, purée the cucumber, avocados, yogurt, tofu, scallion, lemon juice, and jalapeño until very smooth. Add the chicken stock and pesto and blend until you have the desired texture and thickness. Season with salt and pepper and serve topped with mascarpone cheese.

Per Serving: Calories: 398; Fat: 33g; Protein: 10g; Total Carbs: 18g; Fiber: 7g; Net Carbs: 11g; **Macros:** Fat: 75%; Protein: 10%; Carbs: 15%

Avocado Gazpacho

SERVES 4 | PREP TIME: 15 minutes

2 cups chopped tomatoes

2 large ripe avocados, halved and pitted

1 large cucumber, peeled and seeded

1 medium bell pepper (red, orange or yellow), chopped

1 cup plain Greek yogurt

¼ cup extra-virgin olive oil

¼ cup chopped fresh cilantro

¼ cup chopped scallions, green part only

2 tablespoons red wine vinegar

Juice of 2 limes or 1 lemon

½ to 1 teaspoon salt

¼ teaspoon freshly ground black pepper

In a blender or in a large bowl, if using an immersion blender, combine the tomatoes, avocados, cucumber, bell pepper, yogurt, olive oil, cilantro, scallions, vinegar, and lime juice. Blend until smooth. Season with salt and pepper and blend to combine the flavors. Chill in the refrigerator for 1 to 2 hours before serving. Serve cold.

Per Serving: Calories: 392; Fat: 32g; Protein: 6g; Total Carbs: 20g; Fiber: 9g; Net Carbs: 11g; **Macros:** Fat: 73%; Protein: 7%; Carbs: 20%

Spring Pea Soup

SERVES 8 | PREP TIME: 5 minutes | COOK TIME: 15 minutes

3 tablespoons coconut oil

2 shallots, chopped

2 thyme sprigs

Sea salt

Freshly ground black pepper

4 cups fresh peas (frozen, if out of season)

8 cups vegetable broth

¼ cup chopped fresh mint

Juice of 1 lemon

Fresh pea shoots, for garnish

Heat the coconut oil in a large stockpot over medium heat. Toss in the shallots and the thyme. Season with salt and pepper. Sauté until the shallots becomes tender, about 3 minutes. Add the peas to the pan; stir to coat them with the oil, and allow them to toast. Add the vegetable broth and bring to a simmer. Remove the pot from the heat and stir in the mint and lemon juice. Using an immersion blender, blend the soup until silky smooth. Garnish with fresh pea shoots and serve hot.

Per Serving: Calories: 124; Fat: 5g; Protein: 4g; Total Carbs: 15g; Fiber: 5g; Net Carbs: 10g; **Macros:** Fat: 37%; Protein: 13%; Carbs: 50%

Creamy Leek Soup

SERVES 8 | PREP TIME: 10 minutes | COOK TIME: 30 minutes

¼ cup olive oil

1 yellow onion, coarsely chopped

Sea salt

3 cups coarsely chopped cauliflower

1 leek, white and pale green parts only, coarsely chopped

8 cups vegetable broth

1 cup coconut cream

2 rosemary sprigs

2 thyme sprigs

1 bay leaf

Juice of 1 lemon

Freshly ground black pepper

In a large stockpot over medium heat, warm the olive oil and add the onion. Season with salt. Sauté until the onion becomes translucent, about 3 minutes. Add the cauliflower and leek and stir for 5 minutes. Add the vegetable broth, coconut cream, rosemary, thyme, and bay leaf, and bring to a low simmer. Simmer for 20 minutes until the vegetables are extremely tender, then remove the pot from the heat and add the lemon juice. Fish out the rosemary and thyme sprigs and the bay leaf, then, using an immersion blender, blend the soup until silky smooth, adding a little water if needed. Garnish with fresh black pepper.

Per Serving: Calories: 158; Fat: 13g; Protein: 1g; Total Carbs: 9g; Fiber: 3g; Net Carbs: 6g; **Macros:** Fat: 75%; Protein: 2%; Carbs: 23%

Miso Magic

SERVES 8 | PREP TIME: 5 minutes | COOK TIME: 10 minutes

8 cups water

6 to 7 tablespoons miso paste

3 sheets dried seaweed

2 cups thinly sliced shiitake mushrooms

1 cup drained and cubed sprouted tofu

1 cup chopped scallions

1 teaspoon sesame oil

In a large stockpot over medium heat, add the miso paste and seaweed to the water and bring to a low boil. Toss in the mushrooms, tofu, scallions, and sesame oil. Allow to simmer for about 5 minutes and serve.

Per Serving: Calories: 80; Fat: 2g; Protein: 4g; Total Carbs: 12g; Fiber: 2g; Net Carbs: 10g; **Macros:** Fat: 22%; Protein: 20%; Carbs: 58%

Avocado-Lime Soup

SERVES 8 | PREP TIME: 5 minutes | COOK TIME: 20 minutes

2 tablespoons olive oil

½ yellow onion, chopped

1 teaspoon ground cumin

1 teaspoon ground coriander

1 teaspoon chili powder

¼ cup hemp hearts

1 medium tomato, chopped

1 cup chopped cabbage (set some aside for garnish)

½ cup chopped fresh cilantro

½ cup chopped celery

½ jalapeño pepper, chopped

8 cups vegetable broth

Juice of 2 limes

1 avocado, peeled, pitted, and cut into cubes

3 flax crackers

Heat the olive oil in a large stockpot over medium heat and add the onion, cumin, coriander, and chili powder. Sauté, stirring occasionally, until the onion becomes tender, about 5 minutes. Add the hemp hearts, tomato, cabbage, cilantro, celery, and jalapeño to the pot. Stir to coat the spices and allow to cook for 4 minutes. Pour the broth into the pot and simmer on low for 20 minutes. Remove the pot from the heat and stir in the lime juice. Divide the avocado equally among 4 serving bowls. Pour the soup over the avocado in the bowls and garnish with additional cabbage and cilantro. Break the flax crackers over the top of the soup to create a "tortilla soup" vibe.

Per Serving: Calories: 130; Fat: 9g; Protein: 3g; Total Carbs: 9g; Fiber: 4g; Net Carbs: 5g; **Macros:** Fat: 63%; Protein: 9%; Carbs: 28%

Tuscan Kale Soup

SERVES 8 | PREP TIME: 10 minutes | COOK TIME: 25 minutes

¼ cup cold-pressed olive oil

½ cup finely diced yellow onion

2 garlic cloves, chopped

2 tablespoons dried oregano

8 cups vegetable broth

¼ cup hemp hearts

3 cups kale, stems removed, and leaves cut into thin ribbons

1 cup chopped fresh parsley, plus a few sprigs for garnish

½ cup diced rutabaga

⅓ cup diced sun-dried tomatoes

⅓ cup diced carrot

Juice of 1 lemon

Sea salt

In a large stockpot over medium heat, heat the olive oil. Add the onion, garlic, and oregano and cook, stirring frequently to prevent sticking, until the onion is tender and the garlic is fragrant, about 5 minutes. Pour the broth into the pot and turn the heat to low. After the broth simmers for about 5 minutes, toss in the hemp hearts and simmer for another 15 minutes. Add the kale, parsley, rutabaga, sun-dried tomatoes, and carrot and simmer for another 5 minutes until the carrots are tender. Remove the pot from the heat and squeeze in the lemon juice, then throw in the entire lemon peel to allow the oils from the skin to get into the broth. Season with salt. Garnish the soup with parsley sprigs and serve hot.

Per Serving: Calories: 139; Fat: 9g; Protein: 3g; Total Carbs: 11g; Fiber: 3g; Net Carbs: 8g; **Macros:** Fat: 59%; Protein: 9%; Carbs: 32%

Vegan Italian Wedding Soup

SERVES 8 | PREP TIME: 10 minutes | COOK TIME: 15 minutes

1 tablespoon coconut oil

½ cup coarsely chopped yellow onion

1 teaspoon freshly ground black pepper

1 teaspoon dried oregano

1 bay leaf

⅓ cup coarsely chopped daikon radish

⅓ cup cauliflower rice

3 cups coarsely chopped fresh Italian parsley

3 cups coarsely chopped spinach

Juice of 1 lemon

½ cup coarsely chopped celery

8 cups vegetable broth

Warm the coconut oil in a large soup pot over medium heat. Add the onion, pepper, oregano, and bay leaf to the pot and sauté until the onion is translucent, about 3 minutes. Add the daikon, cauliflower rice, and celery to the pot and cook, stirring occasionally, for 5 minutes. Pour the vegetable broth over the sautéed vegetables and bring to a simmer. Remove the pot from the heat remove the bay leaf and stir in the parsley, spinach, and lemon juice. Serve hot.

Per Serving: Calories: 51; Fat: 2g; Protein: 1g; Total Carbs: 7g; Fiber: 3g; Net Carbs: 4g; Macros: Fat: 36%; Protein: 8%; Carbs: 56%

Easy Chicken Soup

SERVES 4 | PREP TIME: 15 minutes | COOK TIME: 1 hour 55 minutes

1 chicken carcass, including bones, skin, meat, and gelatin	2 bay leaves
8 cups water	½ teaspoon dried or fresh thyme
1 large carrot, roughly chopped	1 cup baby spinach
4 celery stalks, roughly chopped, divided	2 cups cooked chicken, diced
¼ cup chopped onion	¼ teaspoon red pepper flakes
2 medium turnips, peeled and diced	Salt
	Freshly ground black pepper
	Freshly grated Parmesan cheese, for serving

Place the chicken bones, skin, scraps of meat, and gelatin in a large stockpot. Add the water, carrot, half of the celery, and the onion. Bring to a boil, then cover and reduce to a simmer. Cook for 1 hour 30 minutes. Carefully remove any chicken pieces from the stock with a slotted spoon, or strain everything through a fine-mesh sieve. Add the turnips, remaining celery, bay leaves, and thyme and bring to a boil. Reduce to a simmer and cook for 10 minutes, or until the turnip is tender. Add the spinach and cook for 2 minutes to wilt, then add the chicken and warm through. Remove the bay leaf, season with the red pepper flakes, salt, and black pepper. Serve with a sprinkle of Parmesan.

Per Serving (2 cup): Calories: 206; Fat: 7g; Protein: 26g; Total Carbs: 7g; Fiber: 2g; Net Carbs: 5g; Macros: Fat: 56%; Protein: 31%; Carbs: 13%

Vegan Pho

SERVES 8 | PREP TIME: 10 minutes | COOK TIME: 20 minutes

8 cups vegetable broth	1 (8-ounce) package shirataki noodles
1-inch knob fresh ginger, peeled and chopped	2 cups shredded cabbage
2 tablespoons tamari	2 cups mung bean sprouts
3 cups shredded fresh spinach	Fresh Thai basil leaves, for garnish
2 cups chopped broccoli	Fresh cilantro leaves, for garnish
1 cup sliced mushrooms	Fresh mint leaves, for garnish
½ cup chopped carrots	1 lime, cut into 8 wedges, for garnish
⅓ cup chopped scallions	

In a large stockpot over medium-high heat, bring the vegetable broth to a simmer with the ginger and tamari. Once the broth is hot, add the spinach, broccoli, mushrooms, carrots, and scallions, and simmer for a few minutes, just until the vegetables start to become tender. Stir in the shirataki noodles, then remove the pot from the heat and divide the soup among serving bowls. Top each bowl with cabbage, sprouts, basil, cilantro, mint, and a lime wedge.

Per Serving: Calories: 47; Fat: 0g; Protein: 3g; Total Carbs: 10g; Fiber: 3g; Net Carbs: 7g; Macros: Fat: 0%; Protein: 23%; Carbs: 77%

Chicken Noodle Soup

SERVES 4 | PREP TIME: 20 minutes | COOK TIME: 15 minutes

2 tablespoons olive oil	2 cups shredded rotisserie chicken
2 baby carrots, diced	½ teaspoon dried thyme
1 garlic clove, minced	½ teaspoon dried oregano
¼ cup diced white onion	2 cups zucchini noodles
2 celery stalks, diced	Sea salt
4 cups chicken bone broth	Freshly ground black pepper

In a large saucepan over medium heat, heat the olive oil. Add the carrots and cook for 2 minutes. Stir in the garlic, onion, and celery and cook until softened, about 5 minutes. Stir in the broth, chicken, thyme, and oregano until well combined. Add the zoodles and stir again. Bring the soup to a boil; then reduce the heat to low and simmer for about 7 minutes or until the zucchini noodles are cooked but still have a little crunch. Season with salt and pepper to taste. Divide the soup into bowls and serve immediately.

Per Serving: (1¼ cups): Calories: 266; Fat: 11g; Protein: 26g; Total Carbs: 8g; Fiber: 2g; Net Carbs: 6g; Macros: Fat: 41%; Protein: 49%; Carbs: 10%

Matzo Ball Chicken Soup

SERVES 6 | PREP TIME: 10 minutes, plus 2 hours to chill | COOK TIME: 30 minutes

3 large eggs	2 tablespoons coconut flour
½ teaspoon salt	1 teaspoon baking powder
1 teaspoon freshly ground black pepper	1 tablespoon olive oil
2 cups almond flour	6 cups chicken bone broth
	1 carrot, shredded, for garnish

In a small bowl, whisk the eggs, salt, and pepper for 1 minute. In a large bowl, mix the almond flour, coconut flour, and baking powder. Add the egg mixture and oil to the flour mixture, and stir just until incorporated. Refrigerate covered for 2 hours or up to overnight. After chilling the dough, place a medium stockpot on the stove over medium heat, and pour the bone broth into the pot. Remove the mixture from the refrigerator, and using a cookie scoop, roll a ball the size of a Ping-Pong ball in the palm of your hand. Repeat for a total of 18 matzo balls. When the broth comes to a boil, carefully lower each ball into the pot using a slotted spoon, reduce heat to a simmer, and cook for 30 minutes. Ladle 1 cup of broth and 3 matzo balls into each bowl, and garnish with shredded carrots.

Per Serving: Calories: 297; Fat: 21g; Protein: 19g; Total Carbs: 8g; Fiber: 6g; Net Carbs: 2g; Macros: Fat: 64%; Protein: 26%; Carbs: 3%

Chicken Tortilla Soup

SERVES 2 | PREP TIME: 10 minutes | COOK TIME: 30 minutes

2 tablespoons avocado oil
¼ medium onion, diced
¼ red bell pepper, diced
1 garlic clove, minced
½ cup diced tomatoes, fresh or canned
1 tablespoon taco seasoning
4 cups chicken broth

1 tablespoon minced fresh cilantro
3 cooked boneless chicken thighs, shredded with a fork
Juice of ½ lime
½ avocado, pitted, peeled, and diced

In a medium pot, heat the oil over medium heat. Add the onion, bell pepper, and garlic, and sauté 5 to 7 minutes until soft. Add the tomatoes and taco seasoning; stir well. Let cook for 2 to 3 minutes. Add the chicken broth and cilantro, and stir everything together. Bring the soup up to a boil, then reduce the heat to low and let it simmer for 20 minutes. Add the cooked chicken and lime juice to the pot, and stir until everything is combined. Garnish with the diced avocado, more lime juice, or extra cilantro.

Per Serving: (2 cups): Calories: 529; Fat: 41g; Protein: 31g; Total Carbs: 9g; Fiber: 4g; Net Carbs: 5g; **Macros:** Fat: 70%; Protein: 23%; Carbs: 7%

Fiesta Lime Chicken Chowder

SERVES 4 | PREP TIME: 25 minutes | COOK TIME: 50 minutes

2 tablespoons extra-virgin olive oil
½ pound boneless, skinless chicken thighs, diced
1 sweet onion, chopped
1 jalapeño pepper, diced
2 teaspoons minced garlic
2 cups chicken stock

1 (14-ounce) can diced tomatoes
6 ounces cream cheese
½ cup coconut milk
Juice of 1 lime
2 tablespoons chopped fresh cilantro
½ cup shredded Cheddar cheese, for garnish

In a large saucepan over medium-high heat, heat the olive oil. Cook the chicken thigh until just cooked through, about 10 minutes, and use a slotted spoon to remove the poultry to a plate. Sauté the onion, jalapeño pepper, and garlic until the vegetables are softened, about 4 minutes. Add the chicken stock, diced tomatoes, and reserved chicken to the pot, and bring the liquid to a boil. Reduce the heat to low, and simmer for 30 minutes. Whisk in the cream cheese, coconut milk, lime juice, and cilantro. Cook until the soup is creamy, about 5 minutes. Top with the cheese, and serve.

Per Serving: Calories: 462; Fat: 36g; Protein: 28g; Total Carbs: 11g; Fiber: 3g; Net Carbs: 8g; **Macros:** Fat: 68%; Protein: 23%; Carbs: 9%

Tom Kha Gai

SERVES 2 | PREP TIME: 5 minutes | COOK TIME: 40 minutes

1 stalk fresh lemongrass, outer layers removed
1½-inch piece ginger, peeled
4 cups chicken broth
½ tablespoon lime zest
2 tablespoons lime juice

4 boneless and skinless chicken thighs, cut into 1-inch pieces
1 cup shiitake mushrooms, cut into pieces
1 cup full-fat coconut milk

1 tablespoon fish sauce
1 teaspoon raw honey

2 tablespoons fresh cilantro, chopped (optional)
1 lime, cut into 6 wedges

With the back of a knife, lightly smash the lemongrass and ginger. Cut the lemongrass into separate 4-inch pieces. In a large pot, bring the lemongrass, ginger, lime, and bone broth to a boil, then reduce the heat to low and let it simmer for 10 minutes. Strain the broth into a separate pot and discard the solids. Add the chicken and bring the soup to a boil, then reduce the heat to low and add in the mushrooms. Cook for 25 minutes then stir in the coconut milk, fish sauce, and honey. Garnish with cilantro and serve with lime wedges.

Per Serving: Calories: 556; Fat: 36g; Protein: 49g; Total Carbs: 9g; Fiber: 3g; Net Carbs: 6g; **Macros:** Fat: 60%; Protein: 35%; Carbs: 5%

Chicken Marsala Soup

SERVES 4 | PREP TIME: 10 minutes | COOK TIME: 30 minutes

2 tablespoons extra-virgin olive oil
1 pound chicken thighs, cut into 2-inch pieces
Sea salt
Freshly ground black pepper
1 onion, halved and thinly sliced

2 garlic cloves, smashed
¼ cup butter
2 cups cremini mushrooms, thinly sliced
½ cup Marsala wine
1½ quarts beef bone broth
1 sprig fresh rosemary

Place a large pot over medium-high heat and heat the olive oil. Season the chicken thighs with salt and pepper. Sear the chicken thighs until browned on both sides but not yet cooked through. Transfer the chicken to a separate dish. In the same pot, cook the onion and garlic until they begin to soften, about 5 minutes. Push them to the sides of the pot and melt the butter in the center. Brown the mushrooms in two or three batches, pushing them to the side as you go. Season with salt and pepper. Pour in the wine and beef stock, and add the rosemary. Return the chicken to the pot. Season with salt and pepper, cover, and simmer for 20 minutes.

Per Serving: Calories: 429; Fat: 26g; Protein: 38g; Total Carbs: 8g; Fiber: 1g; Net Carbs: 7g; **Macros:** Fat: 55%; Protein: 35%; Carbs: 10%

Peanut-Chicken Soup

SERVES 4 | PREP TIME: 10 minutes | COOK TIME: 15 minutes

2 cups chicken broth
1 cup coconut milk
½ cup natural peanut butter
2 tablespoons curry paste, or more if desired
1 cup diced tomatoes

1 cup shredded cooked chicken breast
1 teaspoon garlic powder
1 cup shredded spinach
1 tablespoon chopped fresh cilantro

In a large saucepan over medium-high heat, whisk the chicken broth, coconut milk, peanut butter, and curry paste. Bring the mixture to a boil, and reduce the heat to simmer for 4 minutes. Stir in the tomatoes, chicken, and garlic powder, and simmer until the mixture is completely heated through, about 5 minutes. Stir in the spinach and cilantro, and simmer until the greens are wilted, about 2 minutes. Remove from the heat, and serve immediately.

Jalapeño-Chicken Soup

SERVES 4 | PREP TIME: 20 minutes | COOK TIME: 45 minutes

1 tablespoon extra-virgin olive oil

½ pound boneless, skinless chicken thighs, cut into ½-inch pieces

1 sweet onion, diced

2 teaspoons minced garlic

1 carrot, peeled and diced

1 celery stalk, diced

4 jalapeño peppers, diced

1 cup diced tomatoes

2 cups chicken stock

2 teaspoons chili powder

1 teaspoon ground cumin

Pinch ground cayenne pepper

1 cup cream cheese

½ cup heavy (whipping) cream

¼ cup chopped fresh cilantro, for garnish

In a large saucepan over medium-high, heat the olive oil. Brown the chicken thighs until just cooked through, about 10 minutes. Using a slotted spoon, remove the chicken and set aside on a plate. Sauté the onion and garlic until softened, about 3 minutes. Stir in the carrot, celery, jalapeños, tomatoes, chicken stock, chili powder, cumin, cayenne, and the reserved chicken. Bring the soup to a boil, and then reduce the heat to low and simmer the soup until the vegetables are tender, about 30 minutes. Stir in the cream cheese and heavy cream until the cheese is melted. Garnish with the fresh cilantro, and serve.

Per Serving: Calories: 452; Fat: 35g; Protein: 25g; Total Carbs: 11g; Fiber: 3g; Net Carbs: 8g; Macros: Fat: 69%; Protein: 22%; Carbs: 9%

Greek Chicken and "Rice" Soup with Artichokes

SERVES 4 | PREP TIME: 10 minutes | COOK TIME: 15 minutes

4 cups chicken stock

2 cups cauliflower rice, divided

2 large egg yolks

¼ cup freshly squeezed lemon juice (about 2 lemons)

¾ cup extra-virgin olive oil, divided

8 ounces cooked chicken, coarsely chopped

1 (14-ounce) can artichoke hearts, drained and quartered

¼ cup chopped fresh dill

In a large saucepan, bring the stock to a low boil over medium-high heat. Reduce the heat to low and simmer, covered. Transfer 1 cup of the hot stock to a blender or food processor. Add ½ cup raw cauliflower rice, the egg yolks, and lemon juice and purée. While the processor or blender is running, stream in ½ cup olive oil and blend until smooth. Whisking constantly, pour the purée into the simmering stock until well blended and smooth. Add the chicken and artichokes and simmer until thickened slightly, 8 to 10 minutes. Stir in the dill and remaining 1½ cups of cauliflower rice. Serve warm, drizzled with the remaining ¼ cup olive oil.

Per Serving: Calories: 566; Fat: 46g; Protein: 24g; Total Carbs: 14g; Fiber: 7g; Net Carbs: 7g; Macros: Fat: 73%; Protein: 17%; Carbs: 10%

Spicy Creamy Chicken Soup

SERVES 15 | PREP TIME: 10 minutes | COOK TIME: 30 minutes

2 (32-ounce) cartons chicken broth or bone broth

1 (8-ounce) brick cream cheese, cubed

4 (13-ounce) cans chicken or 1¾ pounds chopped cooked boneless skinless chicken breasts or rotisserie chicken

2 (10-ounce) cans diced tomatoes and green chilies, undrained

½ cup ranch dressing

½ cup heavy (whipping) cream

1 teaspoon garlic powder

1 teaspoon sea salt

1 teaspoon freshly ground black pepper

15 ounces grated Cheddar cheese

In a stockpot over medium heat, combine the broth, cream cheese, chicken, tomatoes and green chilies, ranch dressing, heavy cream, garlic powder, salt, and pepper. Simmer for 30 minutes, stirring occasionally. Sprinkle each serving with ¼ cup of Cheddar cheese.

Per Serving: (8-ounce cup) Calories: 383; Fat: 27g; Protein: 27g; Total Carbs: 7g; Fiber: 0g; Net Carbs: 7g; Macros: Fat: 64%; Protein: 28%; Carbs: 8%

Chicken Ramen Soup

SERVES 4 | PREP TIME: 25 minutes | COOK TIME: 30 minutes

2 packages shirataki noodles

4 ounces shiitake mushrooms

1 teaspoon avocado oil

½ teaspoon sea salt

4 chicken bouillon cubes

4 cups water

1 tablespoon olive oil

2 garlic cloves, minced

¼ teaspoon ground ginger

3½ tablespoons shredded carrots

2½ tablespoons coconut aminos

2 cups shredded rotisserie chicken

4 soft boiled eggs, halved

1 scallion, white part only, diced (optional)

Hot sauce (optional)

Preheat the oven to 400°F. Line a baking sheet with paper towels. Line a baking sheet with parchment paper. Rinse and drain the noodles thoroughly. Place them on the towel-lined baking sheet and cover with more paper towels. Gently press to soak up the water. Discard the top layer of paper towels and let the noodles air-dry for 20 minutes. Place the mushrooms (stems and caps) on the parchment paper–lined baking sheet and drizzle with the avocado oil. Sprinkle with the salt. Bake for 20 minutes. In a medium saucepan over medium-high heat, warm the bouillon cubes and water until the bouillon dissolves. Turn off the heat. Pour the olive oil into a large saucepan over medium heat. Add the garlic, ginger, and carrots, and sauté until fragrant, 1 to 2 minutes. Add the noodles and stir-fry for another 2 to 3 minutes. Add the bouillon, coconut aminos, and chicken. Bring the mixture to a boil and then reduce the heat to low and simmer for 5 minutes. Divide the soup equally into four bowls. Top each bowl of ramen with a halved egg, equal portions of mushrooms, and equal portions of scallions (if using). Drizzle with hot sauce (if using).

Per Serving: (1 cup): Calories: 275; Fat: 12g; Protein: 21g; Total Carbs: 13g; Fiber: 7g; Net Carbs: 6g; Macros: Fat: 43%; Protein: 40%; Carbs: 17%

Southwest-Style Chicken Soup

SERVES 6 | PREP TIME: 10 minutes | COOK TIME: 55 minutes

2 tablespoons olive oil

1 medium white onion, diced

1 bell pepper, diced

1 jalapeño pepper, seeded and diced

3 garlic cloves, minced

1 tablespoon chili powder

1 teaspoon ground cumin

1 teaspoon dried oregano

1 teaspoon salt

1 teaspoon freshly ground black pepper

6 cups low-sodium chicken broth, divided

2 pounds boneless skinless chicken thighs

1 (10-ounce) can tomatoes and green chiles (such as Rotel brand)

4 ounces full-fat cream cheese, cubed, at room temperature

1 (15-ounce) can baby corn, drained and chopped

1 cup shredded Cheddar cheese

1 avocado, pitted and sliced

In a large soup pot, heat the oil over medium-high heat. Add the onion, bell pepper, jalapeño, and garlic. Sauté for 6 to 8 minutes or until the onion becomes translucent. Add the chili powder, cumin, oregano, salt, and pepper, and stir until fragrant, 1 to 2 minutes. Add 1 cup of broth to the pot and scrape the bottom with a wooden spoon to deglaze. Add the chicken thighs, pour in the remaining 5 cups of broth, and add the tomatoes and green chiles. Raise the heat to high. When the soup just comes to a boil, lower the heat to medium-low, cover, and cook for 45 minutes. Transfer the chicken to a cutting board. Using two forks, shred the meat and return it to the pot. Remove the pot from the heat and stir in the cream cheese and baby corn. Allow to sit for 10 minutes to combine. Serve in large bowls, garnished with the shredded cheese and avocado.

Per Serving: Calories: 524; Fat: 31g; Protein: 44g; Total Carbs: 23g; Fiber: 7g; Net Carbs: 16g; Macros: Fat: 52%; Protein: 33%; Carbs: 15%

Chicken and Baby Corn Chowder

SERVES 6 TO 8 | PREP TIME: 10 minutes | COOK TIME: 1 hour

½ pound bacon, cut into 1-inch slices

2 pounds boneless skinless chicken thighs, diced

3 tablespoons butter

1 medium white onion, diced

3 garlic cloves, minced

1 red bell pepper, diced

1 cup diced cauliflower florets

5 cups low-sodium chicken broth, divided

2 (15-ounce) cans baby corn, drained and chopped

1 teaspoon salt

1 teaspoon freshly ground black pepper

1½ cups heavy (whipping) cream

8 ounces full-fat cream cheese, cubed, at room temperature

2 or 3 scallions, both white and green parts sliced

In a large stockpot over medium heat, brown the bacon for 5 to 7 minutes or until crispy. Using a slotted spoon, transfer the bacon to a paper towel. In the bacon fat, cook the chicken until cooked through. Remove from the pan and set aside. Add the butter to the remaining fat, along with the onion, garlic, bell pepper, and cauliflower. Cook for about 8 minutes or until the onion starts to become translucent. Add 1 cup of broth and use a wooden spoon to scrape the bottom of the pot to deglaze. Return the chicken to the pot and add the remaining 4 cups of broth, baby corn, salt, and pepper. Turn up the heat to high, bring to a boil, turn the heat down to low, cover, and simmer for 35 to 40 minutes. Remove the pot from the heat and add the cream

and cream cheese. Stir well to melt. Taste for seasoning. Serve in large bowls, garnished with the bacon and scallions.

Per Serving: Calories: 846; Fat: 64g; Protein: 45g; Total Carbs: 24g; Fiber: 4g; Net Carbs: 20g; Macros: Fat: 67%; Protein: 22%; Carbs: 11%

Chicken Taco Soup with Cauliflower Rice

SERVES 6 TO 8 | PREP TIME: 30 minutes | COOK TIME: 30 minutes

¼ cup avocado oil

¾ cup diced celery with leaves

½ cup diced onion

1½ teaspoons kosher salt, divided

3 garlic cloves, minced

1 cup diced zucchini

2 tablespoons chili powder

1 tablespoon dried parsley

1¼ teaspoons granulated garlic

1¼ teaspoons ground cumin

1¼ teaspoons paprika

½ teaspoon freshly ground black pepper

½ teaspoon dried Mexican oregano

6 cups chicken stock or bone broth

3 cups shredded cooked chicken thighs

2 (12-ounce) packages frozen cauliflower rice

Chopped fresh cilantro, for garnish

Diced avocado, for garnish

In a large stockpot over medium heat, heat the avocado oil. Add the celery, onion, and ½ teaspoon of salt. Sauté for about 5 minutes, or until tender. Add the garlic cloves, zucchini, chili powder, parsley, granulated garlic, cumin, paprika, remaining 1 teaspoon of salt, the pepper, and oregano. Cook for 1 to 2 minutes more, stirring constantly. Stir in the chicken stock. Bring the mixture to boil and reduce the heat to maintain a simmer. Simmer, uncovered, for 10 to 15 minutes. Add the chicken and cauliflower rice. Simmer the soup for 10 minutes more, or until the veggies are tender. Serve warm topped with cilantro and avocado.

Per Serving: Calories: 262; Fat: 14g; Protein: 24g; Total Carbs: 10g; Fiber: 5g; Net Carbs: 5g; Macros: Fat: 48%; Protein: 37%; Carbs: 15%

Italian Wedding Soup

SERVES 4 | PREP TIME: 15 minutes | COOK TIME: 20 minutes

8 ounces ground beef

8 ounces ground pork

¼ cup chopped fresh parsley

¼ cup, plus 2 tablespoons freshly grated Parmesan cheese, divided

2 tablespoons finely minced onion

2 garlic cloves, minced

1 teaspoon salt

½ teaspoon freshly ground black pepper

8 cups chicken stock

½ cup extra-virgin olive oil

4 cups kale, thick stems removed and torn into bite-sized pieces

2 large eggs

In a large bowl, combine the beef, pork, parsley, ¼ cup of Parmesan, onion, garlic, salt, and pepper. Using your hands, form the mixture into 1-inch meatballs. In a large stock pot, combine the chicken stock and olive oil and bring to a boil over high heat. When the liquid is boiling, add the kale and carefully drop the meatballs into the pot. Reduce the heat to low, cover, and simmer for 8 to 10 minutes, until the meatballs are cooked through. In a small bowl, whisk the eggs and remaining 2 tablespoons of Parmesan. Using a large spoon, stir the soup in a circular direction and slowly stream in the egg and cheese mixture. Continue to cook, stirring over low heat for 1 minute, or until the egg is cooked through. Serve warm, garnished with additional cheese and parsley, if desired.

Per Serving: Calories: 597; Fat: 49g; Protein: 37g; Total Carbs: 3g; Fiber: 1g; Net Carbs: 2g; **Macros:** Fat: 74%; Protein: 25%; Carbs: 1%

Beef Pho

SERVES 6 | **PREP TIME:** 10 minutes | **COOK TIME:** 30 minutes

10 cups beef broth	1 pound flank steak, finely
1 (6-inch) piece of ginger,	sliced against the grain
peeled and cut in half	1 (7 ounce) package shirataki
lengthwise	noodles, prepared according
1 cinnamon stick	to the package instructions
4 garlic cloves	¼ cup whole Thai basil leaves,
¼ cup fish sauce	torn into pieces
2 teaspoons raw honey	¼ cup fresh cilantro, chopped
1 teaspoon salt	2 scallions, chopped
	1 lime, cut into 6 wedges

In a large pot, combine the bone broth, ginger, cinnamon, garlic, fish sauce, honey, and salt. Bring the broth to a boil, cover and reduce the heat to low, and let it simmer for at least 30 minutes. Strain the broth into a separate pot and discard the solids. Divide the steak, shirataki noodles, basil, cilantro, and scallions into 6 bowls and pour the hot broth into each one. Serve with lime wedges.

Per Serving: Calories: 190; Fat: 7g; Protein: 23g; Total Carbs: 7g; Fiber: 1g; Net Carbs: 6g; **Macros:** Fat: 34%; Protein: 51%; Carbs: 15%

Zuppa Toscana (Sausage and Kale Soup)

SERVES 6 | **PREP TIME:** 10 minutes | **COOK TIME:** 45 minutes

½ pound bacon, cut into	1 head cauliflower, stemmed
1-inch slices	and chopped
1 pound hot Italian sausage,	3 cups stemmed and chopped
casings removed	kale or baby spinach
1 medium onion, diced	½ cup heavy (whipping) cream
3 garlic cloves, minced	½ cup shredded
5 cups low-sodium	Parmesan cheese
chicken broth	

In a large soup pot over medium-high heat, brown the bacon for 5 to 7 minutes or until crispy. Using a slotted spoon or fork, transfer the bacon to a paper towel. Pour off all but 2 tablespoons of the fat. Lower the heat to medium. Add the sausage to the pot and cook until browned, about 5 minutes. Break up the sausage with the spoon. Add the onion and garlic and sauté until the onions are translucent, about 7 minutes. Add the broth. Use a wooden spoon to scrape the bottom of the pot to deglaze. Cover and simmer for 10 minutes. Add the cauliflower. Cover and simmer for 10 minutes or until the cauliflower is soft. Add the kale, cream, and reserved bacon, and simmer for 5 minutes to allow the kale to wilt. Serve in large bowls, garnished with the Parmesan.

Per Serving: Calories: 493; Fat: 40g; Protein: 24g; Total Carbs: 10g; Fiber: 2g; Net Carbs: 8g; **Macros:** Fat: 72%; Protein: 20%; Carbs: 8%

Country Pork and "Rice" Soup

SERVES 4 | **PREP TIME:** 25 minutes | **COOK TIME:** 1 hour, 20 minutes

2 tablespoons extra-virgin	1 cup coconut milk
olive oil	1 large tomato, chopped
1 pound boneless coun-	1 tablespoon chopped
try pork ribs, cut into	fresh thyme
1-inch pieces	2 cups finely chopped
½ sweet onion, chopped	cauliflower
2 teaspoons minced garlic	Sea salt
1 cup chicken stock	Freshly ground black pepper

In a large saucepan over medium-high heat, heat the olive oil. Brown the pork until it is almost cooked through, about 10 minutes. Using a slotted spoon, remove the pork, and set aside. Sauté the onion and garlic until softened, about 3 minutes. Add the pork back to the saucepan, and stir in the chicken stock, coconut milk, tomato, and thyme. Bring the soup to a boil, and then reduce the heat to simmer until the meat is very tender, about 1 hour. Stir in the cauliflower, and simmer the soup until the cauliflower is tender but not overcooked, about 3 minutes. Season the soup with salt and pepper, and serve.

Per Serving: Calories: 410; Fat: 32g; Protein: 25g; Total Carbs: 9g; Fiber: 4g; Net Carbs: 5g; **Macros:** Fat: 68%; Protein: 24%; Carbs: 8%

Beef-Sausage Stew

SERVES 4 | **PREP TIME:** 30 minutes | **COOK TIME:** 1 hour, 30 minutes

2 tablespoons extra-virgin	3 cups shredded cabbage
olive oil	½ cup sliced carrots
¼ pound chuck roast, cut into	½ cup peas
1-inch pieces	1 teaspoon chopped
1 sweet onion, chopped	fresh thyme
1 teaspoon minced garlic	2 tablespoons arrowroot
1½ cups beef broth, divided	Sea salt
½ pound cooked sausage, cut	Freshly ground black pepper
into ¼-inch rounds	

In a large saucepan over medium-high heat, heat the olive oil. Brown the beef on all sides, about 5 minutes. Using a slotted spoon, remove the beef to a plate and set aside. Sauté the onion and garlic until the vegetables are softened, about 3 minutes. Return the beef to the saucepan, and add 1¼ cups of beef broth and the sausage. Bring the liquid to a boil, and then reduce the heat to low and simmer, covered, until the beef is very tender, about 1 hour. Stir in the cabbage, carrots, peas, and thyme, and simmer for 15 minutes. In a small bowl, stir the remaining ¼ cup of beef broth and the arrowroot. Stir the arrowroot mixture into the stew, and stir until the sauce is thickened, about 4 minutes. Season the stew with salt and pepper, and serve.

Per Serving: Calories: 370; Fat: 27g; Protein: 24g; Total Carbs: 11g; Fiber: 4g; Net Carbs: 7g; **Macros:** Fat: 63%; Protein: 25%; Carbs: 12%

Hearty Lamb Cabbage Soup

SERVES 6 | **PREP TIME:** 15 minutes | **COOK TIME:** 35 minutes

3 tablespoons olive oil, divided	1 onion, chopped
1 pound ground lamb	2 celery stalks, chopped

2 teaspoons minced garlic

2 cups shredded
green cabbage

6 cups low-sodium
chicken stock

2 bay leaves

2 teaspoons chopped
fresh thyme

Sea salt

Freshly ground black pepper

Heat 1 tablespoon of olive oil in a large saucepan over medium-high heat. Sauté the lamb until cooked through, about 10 minutes, and transfer to a plate using a slotted spoon. Add the remaining olive oil and sauté the onion, celery, and garlic until the vegetables are tender, about 3 minutes. Add the cabbage, chicken stock, and bay leaves and bring the soup to a boil. Reduce the heat to low and simmer until the cabbage is tender, about 15 minutes. Add the cooked lamb and thyme and simmer until the lamb is heated through, about 5 minutes. Remove the bay leaves and season the soup with salt and pepper to serve.

Per Serving: Calories: 300; Fat: 25g; Protein: 15g; Total Carbs: 4g; Fiber: 1g; Net Carbs: 3g; **Macros:** Fat: 75%; Protein: 20%; Carbs: 5%

Creamy Seafood Stew with Cauliflower Rice

SERVES 6 | PREP TIME: 10 minutes | COOK TIME: 30 minutes

½ pound bacon, cut into
1-inch slices

½ medium white onion, diced

2 celery stalks, diced

3 garlic cloves, minced

2 cups frozen cauliflower rice

1 teaspoon salt

2 teaspoons freshly ground
black pepper

3 cups low-sodium
chicken broth

1 (8-ounce) jar clam juice

1 (6-ounce) can medium
shrimp, drained

1 (6-ounce) can crabmeat,
with juices

1 (10-ounce) can chopped
clams, with juices

1½ cups heavy
(whipping) cream

8 ounces full-fat cream cheese,
cubed, at room temperature

½ cup shredded
Cheddar cheese

In a large stockpot over medium heat, brown the bacon for 5 to 7 minutes or until crispy. Using a slotted spoon, transfer the bacon to a paper towel. Pour off all but 2 tablespoons of the fat. Raise the heat to medium high. Add the onion, celery, garlic, cauliflower rice, salt, and pepper. Sauté until the vegetables are soft, about 10 minutes. Add the chicken broth and use a wooden spoon to scrape the bottom of the pot to deglaze. Lower the heat to medium and allow to simmer for 15 minutes to continue to soften the vegetables. Turn the heat to low and add the clam juice and shrimp along with the crab and clams with their canning liquid. Stir to combine. Add the cream and cream cheese. Stir to melt the cream cheese and allow to sit, covered, on low heat for a few minutes to meld. Stir well and taste for seasoning. Serve in bowls, garnished with the bacon and cheddar.

Per Serving: Calories: 662; Fat: 55g; Protein: 32g; Total Carbs: 11g; Fiber: 1g; Net Carbs: 10g; **Macros:** Fat: 74%; Protein: 20%; Carbs: 6%

Seafood Chowder with Lobster

SERVES 4 | PREP TIME: 20 minutes | COOK TIME: 20 minutes

¼ cup coconut oil

1 sweet onion, finely chopped

2 celery stalks, finely chopped

2 garlic cloves, minced

2 tablespoons arrowroot

3 cups chicken broth

2 cups cooked, chopped lobster meat

¼ pound cooked
shrimp, chopped

1½ cups heavy
(whipping) cream

1 teaspoon chopped
fresh thyme

Sea salt

Freshly ground black pepper

2 tablespoons chopped
fresh chives

In a large saucepan over medium-high heat, melt the coconut oil. Sauté the onion, celery, and garlic until softened, about 5 minutes. Stir in the arrowroot, and cook for 2 minutes. Stir in the chicken broth, and cook, stirring constantly, until the soup thickens, about 5 minutes. Stir in the lobster meat, shrimp, cream, and thyme. Cook, stirring occasionally, until the soup is heated through, about 10 minutes. Season the soup with salt and pepper. Top with the chives, and serve.

Per Serving: Calories: 417; Fat: 32g; Protein: 26g; Total Carbs: 6g; Fiber: 1g; Net Carbs: 5g; **Macros:** Fat: 69%; Protein: 25%; Carbs: 6%

Fennel and Cod Chowder with Fried Mushrooms

SERVES 4 | PREP TIME: 20 minutes | COOK TIME: 35 minutes

1 cup extra-virgin olive
oil, divided

1 small head cauliflower, core
removed and broken into
florets (about 2 cups)

1 small white onion,
thinly sliced

1 fennel bulb, white part only,
trimmed and thinly sliced

½ cup dry white wine
(optional)

2 garlic cloves, minced

1 teaspoon salt

¼ teaspoon freshly ground
black pepper

4 cups fish stock, plus more
if needed

1 pound thick cod fillet, cut
into ¾-inch cubes

4 ounces shiitake mushrooms,
stems trimmed and thinly
sliced (⅛-inch slices)

¼ cup chopped Italian parsley,
for garnish (optional)

¼ cup plain Greek yogurt, for
garnish (optional)

In a large stockpot, heat ¼ cup olive oil over medium-high heat. Add the cauliflower florets, onion, and fennel and sauté for 10 to 12 minutes, or until almost tender. Add the white wine (if using), garlic, salt, and pepper and sauté for another 1 to 2 minutes. Add 4 cups of fish stock and bring to a boil. Cover, reduce the heat to medium-low, and simmer until vegetables are very tender, another 8 to 10 minutes. Remove from the heat and allow to cool slightly. Using an immersion blender, purée the vegetable mixture, slowly drizzling in ½ cup olive oil, until very smooth and silky, adding additional fish stock if the mixture is too thick. Turn the heat back to medium-high and bring the soup to a low simmer. Add the cod pieces and cook, covered, until the fish is cooked through, about 5 minutes. Remove from the heat and keep covered. In a medium skillet, heat the remaining ¼ cup olive oil over medium-high heat. When very hot, add the mushrooms and fry until crispy. Remove with a slotted spoon and transfer to a plate, reserving the frying oil. Toss the mushrooms with a sprinkle of salt. Serve the chowder hot, topped with fried mushrooms and drizzled with 1 tablespoon reserved frying oil. Garnish with chopped fresh parsley and 1 tablespoon of Greek yogurt (if using).

Per Serving: Calories: 658; Fat: 54g; Protein: 28g; Total Carbs: 15g; Fiber: 5g; Net Carbs: 10g; **Macros:** Fat: 74%; Protein: 18%; Carbs: 8%

New England Clam Chowder

SERVES 4 | PREP TIME: 10 minutes | COOK TIME: 20 minutes

8 ounces cauliflower florets (about 1 small head), roughly chopped

1½ cups chicken broth

¾ cup unsweetened almond milk

1 (6½-ounce) can chopped clams with liquid

1 celery stalk, finely chopped

½ cup heavy (whipping) cream

Salt

Freshly ground black pepper

Chopped fresh parsley, for garnish

Combine the cauliflower, broth, and almond milk in a stockpot. Bring to a boil, then reduce to a simmer. Cover and cook for about 10 minutes, or until the cauliflower is tender. Use an immersion blender to blend the cauliflower mixture until smooth. (You can also very carefully transfer the liquid to a blender. Work in batches, if necessary, to avoid spattering.) Add the clams, celery, and heavy cream. Warm through, then season with salt and pepper to taste. Pour into serving bowls and garnish with parsley.

Per Serving: Calories: 197; Fat: 13g; Protein: 14g; Total Carbs: 6g; Fiber: 2g; Net Carbs: 4g; Macros: Fat: 59%; Protein: 28%; Carbs: 13%

SALADS

Citrus Arugula Salad

SERVES 4 | PREP TIME: 5 minutes

1 pound arugula, washed

⅓ cup olive oil

Juice of 1 lemon

Sea salt

Freshly ground black pepper

1 avocado, cubed

½ grapefruit, peeled and sliced

¼ cup pine nuts

Dress the arugula lightly with the olive oil and lemon juice, and season with salt and pepper. Add the avocado and grapefruit to the dressed arugula. Top with the pine nuts and serve.

Per Serving: Calories: 328; Fat: 31g; Protein: 5g; Total Carbs: 12g; Fiber: 5g; Net Carbs: 7g; Macros: Fat: 80%; Protein: 6%; Carbs: 14%

Spinach Avocado Salad

SERVES 2 | PREP TIME: 10 minutes

1½ cups fresh spinach leaves

4 hard-boiled eggs, chopped

¼ cup chopped carrots

¼ cup chopped cucumbers

½ avocado, sliced

¼ cup diced tomatoes

1 tablespoon olive oil

1 tablespoon balsamic vinegar

Salt

Freshly ground black pepper

Place the spinach in a serving dish. Top with the eggs, carrots, cucumbers, avocado, and tomatoes. In a small bowl, mix the oil and vinegar. Pour the dressing on the salad and season with salt and pepper as needed.

Per Serving: Calories: 291; Fat: 23g; Protein: 13g; Total Carbs: 8g; Fiber: 4g; Net Carbs: 4g; Macros: Fat: 71%; Protein: 18%; Carbs: 11%

Kale, Avocado & Tahini Salad

SERVES 4 | PREP TIME: 5 minutes

1 bunch kale, stems removed, leaves cut into ribbons

¼ cup cold-pressed olive oil

4 to 5 tablespoons vegan dressing

1 avocado, peeled, pitted, and sliced

¼ cup slivered almonds

3 tablespoons chia seeds

In a large mixing bowl, coat the kale with the olive oil. Massage the leaves with your hands to tenderize them and remove bitterness. Toss the massaged kale with the dressing. Divide the salad among 4 bowls and top each bowl with the avocado, almonds, and chia seeds.

Per Serving: Calories: 370; Fat: 30g; Protein: 9g; Total Carbs: 22g; Fiber: 12g; Net Carbs: 10g; Macros: Fat: 69%; Protein: 9%; Carbs: 22%

Vegan Niçoise Salad

SERVES 4 | PREP TIME: 10 minutes

15 to 20 fresh green beans

3 small heads butter lettuce, coarsely chopped

⅓ cup vinaigrette

1 small cucumber, chopped

1 small tomato, chopped

¼ cup olives

5 radishes, chopped

Pour water into a medium bowl and add a generous amount of ice. Set aside. In a medium saucepan over high heat, bring plenty of water to a boil. Toss the green beans into the pot and blanch them for 3 minutes. Remove the green beans from the water and immediately submerge them in the ice-water bath to preserve their color and crunch. Toss the butter lettuce with the dressing and divide among 4 bowls. Top each bowl with the green beans, cucumber, tomato, olives, and radishes.

Per Serving: Calories: 153; Fat: 13g; Protein: 3g; Total Carbs: 9g; Fiber: 3g; Net Carbs: 6g; Macros: Fat: 71%; Protein: 7%; Carbs: 22%

Japanese Hibachi House Salad

SERVES 6 | PREP TIME: 5 minutes

1-inch knob fresh ginger, peeled and chopped

½ medium carrot

½ celery stalk

Juice of 2 limes

¼ cup liquid aminos

1 teaspoon sesame oil

3 drops liquid stevia

2 heads romaine lettuce, chopped

1 small tomato, diced

½ cup sliced mushrooms

⅓ cup shredded carrots

⅓ cup diced red onion

2 tablespoons sesame seeds

In a high-powered blender, combine the ginger, carrot, celery, lime juice, aminos, sesame oil, and liquid stevia. Divide the lettuce among 6 bowls and top each bowl with a generous portion of dressing. Garnish with the tomato, mushrooms, shredded carrots, onion, and sesame seeds.

Per Serving: Calories: 65; Fat: 3g; Protein: 4g; Total Carbs: 8g; Fiber: 4g; Net Carbs: 4g; Macros: Fat: 36%; Protein: 22%; Carbs: 42%

Ranch Wedge Salad with Coconut "Bacon"

SERVES 6 | PREP TIME: 15 minutes | COOK TIME: 25 minutes

For the coconut "bacon"

Nonstick cooking spray

¼ cup liquid smoke

½ cup tamari

½ cup olive oil

½ cup monk fruit sweetener

1 tablespoon ground paprika

4 cups dried coconut flakes

For the salad

1 head iceberg lettuce, cut into 6 wedges

½ cup keto ranch dressing

1 small tomato, chopped

¼ cup chopped fresh chives

Sea salt

Freshly ground black pepper

Preheat the oven to 375°F, line a baking sheet with parchment paper, and spray with cooking spray. In a large skillet over medium heat, whisk the liquid smoke, tamari, olive oil, monk fruit sweetener, and paprika. Stir the mixture occasionally to melt the sweetener. Once the sweetener is dissolved, toss in the coconut flakes and cook for 5 minutes, allowing the liquid to evaporate. Remove the coconut flakes from the skillet and transfer to the prepared baking sheet, spreading the coconut out evenly. Bake for 20 minutes or until the edges become toasted, then remove the sheet from the oven and set aside to cool. To make the salad: Top the lettuce wedges with the dressing and garnish with the tomato, chives, and coconut "bacon." Season with salt and pepper and serve.

Per Serving: Calories: 500; Fat: 48g; Protein: 8g; Total Carbs: 18g; Fiber: 8g; Net Carbs: 10g; **Macros:** Fat: 81%; Protein: 6%; Carbs: 13%

Spinach Salad with Warm Bacon Dressing

SERVES 6 | PREP TIME: 10 minutes | COOK TIME: 25 minutes

12 bacon slices

5 tablespoons red wine vinegar

1 teaspoon erythritol-based sweetener

1 teaspoon Dijon mustard

¼ teaspoon salt

¼ teaspoon freshly ground black pepper

12 ounces baby spinach

4 hard-boiled eggs, peeled and sliced

6 large button mushrooms, thinly sliced

1 small red onion, very thinly sliced

Cook the bacon, chop, and set aside. Transfer ¼ cup of bacon fat to a small saucepan over low heat. Add the vinegar, sweetener, mustard, salt, and pepper. Whisk vigorously until a vinaigrette is formed and the sweetener is dissolved. Let it sit over low heat to stay warm. In a large salad bowl, gently toss the spinach, eggs, mushrooms, onion, and bacon. When ready to serve, drizzle the hot vinaigrette over the salad and toss again.

Per Serving: Calories: 162; Fat: 11g; Protein: 12g; Total Carbs: 4g; Fiber: 2g; Net Carbs: 2g; **Macros:** Fat: 60%; Protein: 31%; Carbs: 9%

Strawberry Spinach Salad

SERVES 4 | PREP TIME: 15 minutes | COOK TIME: 5 minutes

2 teaspoons butter

2 teaspoons brown erythritol blend

¼ cup chopped pecans

3 tablespoons extra-light olive oil

3 tablespoons white wine vinegar

2 teaspoons granulated erythritol blend

1 teaspoon garlic powder

½ teaspoon minced onion

¼ teaspoon salt

⅛ teaspoon freshly ground black pepper

1 (10-ounce) package fresh baby spinach, torn into bite-size pieces

1 cup strawberries, cored and sliced

½ cup fresh blueberries

½ avocado, peeled, pitted, and cut into bite-size pieces

⅓ cup crumbled blue cheese

Spread a piece of parchment paper on the counter by the stove. In a small pan over medium heat, melt the butter. Add the brown sweetener and pecans. Stir for 3 to 5 minutes, until the pecans are well coated and the sauce has thickened. Spread evenly on the parchment paper, and allow to cool and dry. In a small bowl, whisk the olive oil, vinegar, sweetener, garlic powder, minced onion, salt, and pepper. Set aside. In a large bowl, combine the spinach, strawberries, and blueberries. Add half the dressing and toss to coat. Top the salad with the avocado, candied pecans, and blue cheese.

Per Serving: Calories: 260; Fat: 23g; Protein: 5g; Total Carbs: 15g; Fiber: 5g; Net Carbs: 6g; **Macros:** Fat: 72%; Protein: 7%; Carbs: 21%

Pistachio Pomegranate Salad

SERVES 4 | PREP TIME: 10 minutes | COOK TIME: 10 minutes

1 tablespoon avocado oil

2 shallots, sliced thinly

6 cups spinach

3 tablespoons pomegranate seeds

3 tablespoons pistachios, shelled

2 ounce goat cheese or Manchego cheese (optional)

1 tablespoon Dijon mustard

½ teaspoon salt

¼ teaspoon black pepper

1 garlic clove, minced

¼ cup balsamic vinegar

¾ cup extra-virgin olive oil

In a small skillet, heat the avocado oil over medium heat and add in the shallots. Sauté for 5 to 10 minutes until the shallots are soft, remove from heat and let cool. Make the dressing by combining the mustard, salt, pepper, garlic, and vinegar in a bowl. Slowly pour in the olive oil, whisking vigorously for 1 to 2 minutes. Assemble the salad by placing the spinach, shallots, pomegranate seeds, pistachios, and cheese (if using) in a large bowl. Pour your desired amount of dressing over the salad.

Per Serving: Calories: 460; Fat: 47g; Protein: 3g; Total Carbs: 9g; Fiber: 2g; Net Carbs: 7g; **Macros:** Fat: 90%; Protein: 2%; Carbs: 8%

Bacon and Berry Harvest Salad

SERVES 4 | PREP TIME: 20 minutes

¼ cup spicy brown mustard

¼ cup balsamic vinegar

2 garlic cloves, minced

1 tablespoons fresh thyme

⅔ cup extra-virgin olive oil

6 cups mixed greens

8 bacon slices, cooked and chopped

½ cup pecans, toasted and chopped

4 hard-boiled eggs, chopped

¾ cup blackberries

3 ounces crumbled goat cheese (optional)

Make the dressing by combining the mustard, vinegar, garlic, and thyme in bowl. Slowly pour in the olive oil, whisking vigorously for 1 to 2 minutes. Assemble the salad by placing the greens, followed by the cooked bacon, pecans, hard-boiled eggs, blackberries, and cheese (if using) in a large bowl. Pour your desired amount of dressing over the salad.

Per Serving: Calories: 656; Fat: 63g; Protein: 16g; Total Carbs: 10g; Fiber: 4g; Net Carbs: 6g; **Macros:** Fat: 84%; Protein: 9%; Carbs: 7%

Classic Club Salad

SERVES 4 | PREP TIME: 10 minutes

3 tablespoons sour cream	4 cups coarsely chopped
3 tablespoons mayonnaise	romaine lettuce
¾ teaspoon garlic powder	1 cup diced cucumber
¾ teaspoon onion powder	½ cup halved cherry tomatoes
1 teaspoon dried parsley	4 hard-boiled eggs, chopped
1 tablespoon heavy	4 ounces cheddar
(whipping) cream	cheese, grated

In a small bowl, mix the sour cream, garlic powder, onion powder, and parsley. Stir in the cream and set aside. Build the salad by layering the lettuce, cucumber, tomatoes, eggs, and cheddar cheese. Divide the salad into 4 servings and top with dressing.

Per Serving: Calories: 293; Fat: 24g; Protein: 14g; Total Carbs: 5g; Fiber: 1g; Net Carbs: 4g; **Macros:** Fat: 74%; Protein: 19%; Carbs: 7%

Hemp Cobb Salad

SERVES 2 | PREP TIME: 10 minutes

2 cups fresh spinach leaves	¼ cup hemp seeds
4 hard-boiled eggs, chopped	2 tablespoons diced scallions,
¼ cup diced cucumber	white and green parts
1 avocado, sliced	¼ cup blue cheese
¼ cup diced tomato	4 ounces blue cheese dressing
4 slices cooked bacon, sliced	

Divide the spinach leaves between two bowls. Arrange half the eggs, cucumber, avocado, tomato, and bacon in sections on top of each bowl of spinach. Sprinkle each salad with half the hemp seeds, scallions, and blue cheese. Top each salad with the dressing and serve.

Per Serving: Calories: 858; Fat: 72g; Protein: 32g; Total Carbs: 20g; Fiber: 9g; Net Carbs: 11g; **Macros:** Fat: 76%; Protein: 15%; Carbs: 9%

Mediterranean Salad

SERVINGS 2 | PREP TIME: 10 minutes

3 tablespoons olive oil	1 head romaine lettuce, leaves
2 tablespoons red	torn into small pieces
wine vinegar	½ red onion, sliced
3 garlic cloves, minced	½ cup diced cucumber
½ teaspoon salt	24 Kalamata olives
¼ teaspoon freshly ground	2 small Campari tomatoes,
black pepper	diced and seeded
	1 cup crumbled feta cheese

In a small bowl, mix the olive oil, vinegar, garlic, salt, and pepper. Set aside. In a large bowl, combine the lettuce, onion, cucumber, olives, tomatoes, and feta cheese. Pour the dressing over the salad and toss it well to coat the ingredients. Divide equally between two bowls and serve.

Per Serving: Calories: 515; Fat: 43g; Protein: 13g; Total Carbs: 19g; Fiber: 4g; Net Carbs: 15g; **Macros:** Fat: 75%; Protein: 10%; Carbs: 15%

Italian Garden Salad

SERVES 4 | PREP TIME: 15 minutes

¼ cup olive oil	2 cups chopped
2 tablespoons white vinegar	romaine lettuce
2 tablespoons avocado oil	¼ cup sliced black olives
mayonnaise	2 small Roma tomatoes,
1 teaspoon dried Italian	sliced
seasoning	¼ cup thinly sliced
½ teaspoon garlic powder	red onion
¼ teaspoon sea salt	¼ cup chopped green
⅛ teaspoon freshly ground	bell pepper
black pepper	⅓ cup Parmesan cheese
4 slices low-carb	
bread toasted	

In a medium bowl, whisk the oil, vinegar, mayonnaise, Italian seasoning, garlic powder, salt, and pepper until well combined. Cut the toast into small cubes. In a large bowl, toss the lettuce, olives, tomatoes, onion, and bell pepper. Add the croutons and toss again. Pour in the dressing and toss until the vegetables are completely coated. Stir in the Parmesan cheese. Divide the salad into bowls and serve immediately.

Per Serving: (1 cup): Calories: 309; Fat: 30g; Protein: 6g; Total Carbs: 6g; Fiber: 2g; Net Carbs: 4g; **Macros:** Fat: 85%; Protein: 8%; Carbs: 7%

Avocado and Asparagus Salad

SERVES 4 | PREP TIME: 15 minutes | COOK TIME: 2 minutes

½ pound asparagus, trimmed	⅓ cup olive oil
and halved	1 teaspoon freshly squeezed
4 cups red leaf lettuce	lemon juice
1 cup cherry tomatoes, halved	½ teaspoon Dijon mustard
1 ripe avocado, sliced	Salt
1 cup sliced mozzarella	Freshly ground black pepper
¼ cup fresh basil leaves	

Prepare an ice bath by filling a large bowl with cold water and plenty of ice. Put a pot of water over medium-high heat and bring to a boil. Add the asparagus to the boiling water and cook for 1 to 2 minutes. Immediately drain the asparagus and transfer it to the ice bath to stop the cooking process. Let cool for 5 minutes. Drain the asparagus and pat it dry with paper towels. Layer equal amounts of lettuce, asparagus, tomatoes, avocado, mozzarella, and basil leaves on four serving plates. In a small bowl, combine the olive oil, lemon juice, and Dijon mustard and add salt and pepper as needed. Pour the dressing evenly over the salads and serve.

Per Serving: Calories: 346; Fat: 30g; Protein: 10g; Total Carbs: 9g; Fiber: 5g; Net Carbs: 4g; **Macros:** Fat: 78%; Protein: 12%; Carbs: 10%

Killer Kale Salad

SERVES 4 | PREP TIME: 5 minutes

6 cups roughly chopped kale,	2 tablespoons extra-virgin
tough ribs removed	olive oil
1 garlic clove, very	1 tablespoon white
finely minced	wine vinegar
Sea salt	1 large avocado, pitted, peeled,
Freshly ground black pepper	and diced

Place the kale in a large salad bowl. Add the garlic and season with salt and pepper. Drizzle with the olive oil. Using your hands, massage the oil and garlic into the kale leaves until they become a darker shade of green and lose some of their liquid. Sprinkle with the vinegar and toss gently to coat. Gently fold in the diced avocado and serve immediately.

Per Serving: Calories: 188; Fat: 14g; Protein: 5g; Total Carbs: 15g; Fiber: 7g; Net Carbs: 8g; **Macros:** Fat: 67%; Protein: 11%; Carbs: 22%

Shaved Brussels Sprouts Salad with Avocado Dressing

SERVES 4 | PREP TIME: 15 minutes

½ avocado	Sea salt
5 tablespoons olive oil	Freshly ground black pepper
2 tablespoons chopped fresh cilantro	1 pound Brussels sprouts
	4 hard-boiled eggs, grated
2 tablespoons freshly squeezed lemon juice	¼ red onion, thinly sliced
	¼ cup chopped fresh parsley
½ teaspoon minced garlic	½ cup chopped Brazil nuts

Place the avocado, olive oil, cilantro, lemon juice, and garlic in a blender and pulse until smooth and thick. Season with salt and pepper and set aside. Shave the Brussels sprouts into a large bowl using a mandoline or carrot peeler. Add the eggs, red onion, and parsley and toss to combine. Add the dressing and toss to coat. Serve topped with Brazil nuts.

Per Serving: Calories: 431; Fat: 38g; Protein: 13g; Total Carbs: 15g; Fiber: 7g; Net Carbs: 8g; **Macros:** Fat: 79%; Protein: 15%; Carbs: 6%

Tuscan Kale Salad with Anchovies

SERVES 4 | PREP TIME: 15 minutes, plus 30 minutes to rest

1 large bunch lacinato or dinosaur kale	8 anchovy fillets, roughly chopped
¼ cup toasted pine nuts	2 to 3 tablespoons freshly squeezed lemon juice (from 1 large lemon)
1 cup shaved or coarsely shredded fresh Parmesan cheese	
	2 teaspoons red pepper flakes (optional)
¼ cup extra-virgin olive oil	

Remove the rough center stems from the kale leaves and roughly tear each leaf into about 4-by-1-inch strips. Place the torn kale in a large bowl and add the pine nuts and cheese. In a small bowl, whisk the olive oil, anchovies, lemon juice, and red pepper flakes (if using). Drizzle over the salad and toss to coat well. Let sit at room temperature 30 minutes before serving, tossing again just prior to serving.

Per Serving: Calories: 337; Fat: 25g; Protein: 16g; Total Carbs: 12g; Fiber: 2g; Net Carbs: 10g; **Macros:** Fat: 67%; Protein: 19%; Carbs: 14%

Everyday Caesar Salad

SERVES 4 | PREP TIME: 10 minutes

⅓ cup mayonnaise	1 teaspoon anchovy paste (optional)
2 tablespoons extra-virgin olive oil	
	1 teaspoon Worcestershire sauce
1 tablespoon lemon juice	
1 garlic clove, minced	1 teaspoon Dijon mustard

8 cups chopped romaine lettuce	¼ cup grated Parmesan cheese

In a large bowl, whisk the mayonnaise, olive oil, lemon juice, garlic, anchovy paste (if using), Worcestershire sauce, and mustard. Add the romaine lettuce to the bowl, and using clean hands, toss to coat the lettuce in the dressing. Serve with a sprinkle a tablespoon of Parmesan cheese over each salad.

Per Serving: Calories: 224; Fat: 22g; Protein: 4g; Total Carbs: 4g; Fiber: 2g; Net Carbs: 2g; **Macros:** Fat: 88%; Protein: 7%; Carbs: 5%

Walnut-Fennel Salad with Sherry Vinaigrette

SERVES 4 | PREP TIME: 25 minutes

⅓ cup walnut oil	1 cup shredded romaine
2 tablespoons sherry vinegar	½ cup thinly sliced fennel
1 tablespoon minced shallot	½ avocado, diced
1 teaspoon chopped fresh thyme	½ cup walnuts, chopped
	3 ounces goat cheese, crumbled
2 cups shredded arugula	

In a small bowl, whisk the walnut oil, vinegar, shallot, and thyme. Set aside. In a medium bowl, toss the arugula, romaine, and fennel with the dressing until the ingredients are coated. Arrange the greens and fennel on 4 plates, top each salad evenly with avocado, walnuts, and goat cheese, and serve.

Per Serving: Calories: 384; Fat: 34g; Protein: 16g; Total Carbs: 8g; Fiber: 5g; Net Carbs: 3g; **Macros:** Fat: 76%; Protein: 16%; Carbs: 8%

Traditional Greek Salad

SERVES 4 | PREP TIME: 10 minutes

2 large English cucumbers	1 tablespoon red wine vinegar
4 Roma tomatoes, quartered	1 tablespoon chopped fresh oregano or 1 teaspoon dried oregano
1 green bell pepper, cut into 1- to 1½-inch chunks	
¼ small red onion, thinly sliced	¼ teaspoon freshly ground black pepper
4 ounces pitted Kalamata olives	
	4 ounces crumbled traditional feta cheese
¼ cup extra-virgin olive oil	
2 tablespoons freshly squeezed lemon juice	

Cut the cucumbers in half lengthwise and then into ½-inch-thick half-moons. Place in a large bowl. Add the quartered tomatoes, bell pepper, red onion, and olives. In a small bowl, whisk the olive oil, lemon juice, vinegar, oregano, and pepper. Drizzle over the vegetables and toss to coat. Divide between salad plates and top each with 1 ounce of feta.

Per Serving: Calories: 278; Fat: 22g; Protein: 8g; Total Carbs: 12g; Fiber: 4g; Net Carbs: 8g; **Macros:** Fat: 71%; Protein: 13%; Carbs: 16%

Weeknight Greek Salad

SERVES 4 | PREP TIME: 5 minutes

8 cups roughly chopped romaine lettuce	½ cup Marinated Antipasto Veggies or marinated artichoke hearts
4 ounces feta cheese, crumbled	
	20 pitted Kalamata olives

2 tablespoons chopped fresh oregano or rosemary or 2 teaspoons dried oregano

¼ cup extra-virgin olive oil

Juice of 1 lemon (about 2 tablespoons)

½ teaspoons freshly ground black pepper or red pepper flakes

In a large bowl, combine the lettuce, feta, antipasto veggies, olives, and oregano. Drizzle with olive oil, then lemon juice and pepper. Toss to coat and serve immediately.

Per Serving: Calories: 300; Fat: 27g; Protein: 6g; Total Carbs: 10g; Fiber: 3g; Net Carbs: 7g; **Macros:** Fat: 81%; Protein: 8%; Carbs: 11%

Powerhouse Arugula Salad

SERVES 4 | PREP TIME: 10 minutes

¼ cup extra-virgin olive oil

Zest and juice of 2 clementines or 1 orange (2 to 3 tablespoons)

1 tablespoon red wine vinegar

½ teaspoon salt

¼ teaspoon freshly ground black pepper

8 cups baby arugula

1 cup coarsely chopped walnuts

1 cup crumbled goat cheese

½ cup pomegranate seeds

In a small bowl, whisk the olive oil, zest and juice, vinegar, salt, and pepper and set aside. To assemble the salad for serving, in a large bowl, combine the arugula, walnuts, goat cheese, and pomegranate seeds. Drizzle with the dressing and toss to coat.

Per Serving: Calories: 444; Fat: 40g; Protein: 10g; Total Carbs: 11g; Fiber: 3g; Net Carbs: 8g; **Macros:** Fat: 81%; Protein: 9%; Carbs: 10%

Tuna and Jicama Salad with Mint Cucumber Dressing

SERVES 4 | PREP TIME: 20 minutes | COOK TIME: 10 minutes

1½ cups canned coconut milk

½ English cucumber, cut into chunks

¼ cup mint leaves

2 teaspoons freshly squeezed lemon juice

1 teaspoon Swerve

½ teaspoon ground coriander

2 tablespoons olive oil

¼ pound raw tuna fillet

4 cups mixed greens

1 jicama, peeled and shredded

3 baby bok choy, shredded

2 scallions, white and green parts, thinly sliced

½ cup crumbled goat cheese

Place the coconut milk, cucumber, mint, lemon juice, Swerve, and coriander in a blender and pulse until smooth. Heat the olive oil in a small skillet over medium-high heat. Pan sear the tuna until it is just cooked through, turning once, about 10 minutes. Chop the cooked tuna and set aside. In a large bowl, toss the mixed greens, jicama, and bok choy. Add three-quarters of the dressing to the salad and toss to coat. Arrange the salad on four plates and top with the tuna, scallions, and goat cheese. To serve, equally divide the remaining dressing between the plates, drizzling it over the top.

Per Serving: Calories: 429; Fat: 31g; Protein: 18g; Total Carbs: 21g; Fiber: 11g; Net Carbs: 10g; **Macros:** Fat: 65%; Protein: 17%; Carbs: 18%

Red Radish "Potato" Salad

SERVES 8 | PREP TIME: 15 minutes | COOK TIME: 45 minutes

4 pounds red radishes, leaves and ends trimmed, halved (about 8 bunches)

¼ cup olive oil

1 teaspoon salt

1 teaspoon freshly ground black pepper

1 teaspoon garlic powder

¼ cup heavy (whipping) cream

1 cup mayonnaise

3 tablespoons chopped dill

1 tablespoon white vinegar

3 scallions, chopped

2 teaspoons Dijon mustard

Paprika, for garnish

Preheat the oven to 350°F, and line a baking sheet with parchment paper. In a gallon resealable bag, add the radishes and olive oil. Seal and shake gently to evenly coat. Empty the radishes onto the baking sheet, arrange cut-side up, and season with the salt, pepper, and garlic powder. Roast for 45 minutes, shaking the pan occasionally. Remove from the oven, cool, and then transfer to a large serving bowl. In a small bowl, use a hand mixer to whip the heavy cream, mayonnaise, dill, vinegar, scallions, and Dijon mustard. Pour over the radishes, gently fold into the mixture until incorporated, garnish with paprika, and serve.

Per Serving: Calories: 300; Fat: 30g; Protein: 2g; Total Carbs: 6g; Fiber: 2.5g; Net Carbs: 3.5g; **Macros:** Fat: 90%; Protein: 3%; Carbs: 7%

Tuna Niçoise Salad

SERVES 6 | PREP TIME: 15 minutes

6 cups roughly chopped iceberg lettuce

3 (12-ounce) cans tuna in water, drained

6 large hard-boiled eggs, peeled

2 medium tomatoes, seeded and diced

18 pitted black olives

3 tablespoons red wine vinegar

1 tablespoon Dijon mustard

6 tablespoons extra-virgin olive oil

Place the lettuce in a large bowl. Add the tuna, breaking it up as necessary. Slice, quarter, or halve the eggs, depending on your preference, and add them to the bowl. Add the tomatoes to the salad, followed by the olives. In a small bowl, whisk the vinegar and mustard. Slowly add the oil in a steady stream, whisking constantly, until the dressing has emulsified. Pour the dressing over the salad and serve. You can toss the salad or leave it in layers.

Per Serving: Calories: 223; Fat: 20g; Protein: 7g; Total Carbs: 5g; Fiber: 2g; Net Carbs: 3g; **Macros:** Fat: 79%; Protein: 14%; Carbs: 7%

Creamy Dill and Radish "Potato" Salad

SERVES 6 | PREP TIME: 10 minutes | COOK TIME: 10 minutes, plus 1 hour to overnight for chilling

5 cups red radishes, leaves and ends trimmed, quartered

½ cup mayonnaise

½ cup diced celery

2 dill pickles, diced

⅓ cup minced red onion

3 tablespoons chopped fresh dill or 1 tablespoon dried

2 teaspoons Dijon mustard

Juice of ½ lemon

½ teaspoon salt

½ teaspoon freshly ground black pepper

2 hard-boiled eggs, peeled and chopped

Place the radishes in a shallow pan with just enough to water to cover. Bring to a boil, reduce the heat to low, cover, and simmer for 5 minutes. Drain the radishes and turn out onto folded paper towels to cool and dry completely. In a large bowl, stir the mayonnaise, celery, pickles, onion, dill, mustard, lemon juice, salt, and pepper. Add the radishes and eggs to the bowl and gently fold into the dressing. Serve chilled.

Per Serving: Calories: 174; Fat: 16g; Protein: 3g; Total Carbs: 6g; Fiber: 2g; Net Carbs: 4g; **Macros:** Fat: 81%; Protein: 7%; Carbs: 12%

Simple Egg Salad

MAKES 2 CUPS | PREP TIME: 15 minutes |
COOK TIME: 8 minutes

8 large eggs	1 scallion, chopped
¼ cup mayonnaise	½ teaspoon freshly ground
2 tablespoons coconut oil	black pepper
½ teaspoon Dijon mustard	¼ teaspoon sea salt

Place the eggs in the bottom of a large saucepan, in one layer, and cover the eggs with cold water by about 3-inches. Place the saucepan over high heat, and bring to a boil. Reduce the heat to medium, and boil the eggs for 8 minutes. Remove the saucepan from the heat, and pour out the water. Run cold water over the eggs until they are cool to the touch. Remove the eggs from the water, and peel them. Grate the eggs into a medium bowl, and stir in the mayonnaise, coconut oil, Dijon mustard, scallion, pepper, and salt.

Per Serving: (¼ cup): Calories: 131; Fat: 11g; Protein: 6g; Total Carbs: 2g; Fiber: 0g; Net Carbs: 2g; **Macros:** Fat: 76%; Protein: 18%; Carbs: 6%

Curried Egg Salad

SERVES 4 | PREP TIME: 5 minutes

6 hard-boiled eggs, finely chopped	1½ teaspoons curry powder
1 celery stalk, diced	¼ teaspoon salt
½ cup cashews, finely diced	¼ teaspoon freshly ground black pepper
¼ cup olive oil mayonnaise	8 butter lettuce leaves
1 tablespoon Dijon mustard	

In a medium mixing bowl, combine the eggs with the celery and cashews. Add the mayonnaise, mustard, curry powder, salt, and pepper, and stir until thoroughly combined. Divide the salad into four equal servings and serve on top of the butter lettuce leaves.

Per Serving: Calories: 600; Fat: 50g; Protein: 23g; Total Carbs: 15g; Fiber: 2g; Net Carbs: 13g; **Macros:** Fat: 75%; Protein: 15%; Carbs: 10%

Avocado Egg Salad

SERVES 2 | PREP TIME: 5 minutes

½ avocado, mashed	¼ teaspoon freshly ground black pepper
1 tablespoon freshly squeezed lemon juice	6 hard-boiled eggs, finely chopped
¼ teaspoon salt	2 radishes, sliced

In a medium bowl, combine the avocado with the lemon juice, salt, and pepper. Add the chopped eggs to the avocado mixture and stir gently to combine. Serve topped with the radish slices.

Per Serving: Calories: 272; Fat: 20g; Protein: 18g; Total Carbs: 5g; Fiber: 3g; Net Carbs: 2g; **Macros:** Fat: 66%; Protein: 26%; Carbs: 8%

Turmeric and Avocado Egg Salad

SERVES 2 | PREP TIME: 10 minutes | COOK TIME: 12 minutes plus 1 hour to chill

4 large eggs	½ teaspoon ground turmeric
1 medium avocado, halved and pitted	½ teaspoon salt
2 tablespoons keto mayonnaise	Zest and juice of 1 lime
1 tablespoon diced capers	¼ teaspoon freshly ground black pepper
1 tablespoon finely minced red onion	¼ cup chopped fresh cilantro (optional)

In a medium saucepan, place the eggs and cover with room temperature water. Set a timer for 12 minutes, place the saucepan over high heat, and bring the water to a boil. Reduce the heat to medium and gently boil the eggs until the 12 minutes is up. Remove the eggs from the hot water and soak them in a small bowl of ice water for 3 to 4 minutes, until cool to the touch. While the eggs cool, using a spoon, scoop the avocado flesh into a medium bowl. Mash well with a fork. Add the mayonnaise, capers, onion, turmeric, salt, lime zest and juice, and pepper and stir until well blended. Add the cilantro (if using), and stir to incorporate well. Once the eggs have cooled, peel them and chop well. Add the eggs to the avocado mixture and stir to combine. Allow to chill in the refrigerator for at least 1 hour before eating.

Per Serving: Calories: 328; Fat: 30g; Protein: 8g; Total Carbs: 10g; Fiber: 5g; Net Carbs: 5g; **Macros:** Fat: 82%; Protein: 10%; Carbs: 8%

Chicken, Avocado, and Egg Salad

SERVES 6 | PREP TIME: 10 minutes

1½ pounds cooked chicken, diced (about 6 cups)	6 large hard-boiled eggs, peeled and diced
3 avocados, pitted, peeled, and diced	¾ cup mayonnaise
	Salt
	Freshly ground black pepper

In a large bowl, combine the chicken, avocados, eggs, and mayonnaise. Mix and season with salt and pepper. Spoon the salad into a serving dish and serve at room temperature.

Per Serving: Calories: 621; Fat: 45g; Protein: 43g; Total Carbs: 12g; Fiber: 9g; Net Carbs: 3g; **Macros:** Fat: 64%; Protein: 29%; Carbs: 7%

Deviled Egg Salad with Bacon

SERVES 6 | PREP TIME: 15 minutes | CHILL TIME: 4 hours

8 hard-boiled eggs, peeled and chopped	¼ teaspoon freshly ground black pepper
1 cup diced celery	¼ teaspoon paprika
4 scallions, sliced	¼ teaspoon onion powder
¾ cup mayonnaise	¼ teaspoon garlic powder
2 teaspoon Dijon mustard	8 crispy cooked bacon slices, chopped
¾ teaspoon kosher salt	1 tablespoon chopped fresh parsley
½ teaspoon hot sauce	
½ teaspoon gluten-free Worcestershire sauce	

In a medium bowl, combine the eggs, celery, and scallions. Toss to combine. In a small bowl, whisk the mayonnaise, mustard, salt, hot sauce, Worcestershire sauce, pepper, paprika, onion powder, and garlic powder. Pour the mayonnaise mixture over the eggs and gently stir to combine. Stir in the bacon and parsley. Cover and refrigerate for 2 to 4 hours before serving.

Per Serving: Calories: 413; Fat: 37g; Protein: 17g; Total Carbs: 3g; Fiber: 1g; Net Carbs: 2g; **Macros:** Fat: 81%; Protein: 16%; Carbs: 3%

Cool and Creamy Cucumber Tomato Salad

SERVES 6 | PREP TIME: 15 minutes, plus 1 hour to overnight to chill

¾ cup mayonnaise

2 tablespoons white vinegar

2 teaspoons erythritol-based sweetener

½ teaspoon salt

½ teaspoon freshly ground black pepper

5 large cucumbers, peeled and thinly sliced

1 small red onion, halved and thinly sliced

5 ounces cherry tomatoes, halved

In a large bowl, whisk the mayonnaise, vinegar, sweetener, salt, and pepper. Add the cucumbers, onion, and tomatoes. Gently toss to coat. Chill for at least 1 hour, and preferably overnight. Gently toss again before serving.

Per Serving: Calories: 234; Fat: 21g; Protein: 2g; Total Carbs: 11g; Fiber: 2g; Net Carbs: 9g; **Macros:** Fat: 80%; Protein: 3%; Carbs: 17%

Greek Cottage Cheese Salad

SERVES 1 | PREP TIME: 5 minutes

1 cup 4-percent cottage cheese

⅓ cup halved cherry tomatoes

1 tablespoon chopped scallion, white part only

⅓ cup peeled and diced cucumber

2 tablespoons olive oil

½ cup Kalamata olives

Salt

Freshly ground black pepper

In a serving bowl, mix the cottage cheese, cherry tomatoes, scallion, cucumber, olive oil, and olives, and season with salt and pepper as needed.

Per Serving: Calories: 610; Fat: 51g; Protein: 27g; Total Carbs: 15g; Fiber: 4g; Net Carbs: 11g; **Macros:** Fat: 72%; Protein: 19%; Carbs: 9%

Thai Noodle Salad

SERVES 4 | PREP TIME: 10 minutes

1 cup shredded purple cabbage

1 cup shredded green cabbage

¼ cup chopped scallions

¼ cup chopped fresh cilantro

3 cups shirataki noodles, rinsed and drained

½ cup chopped cashews

2 tablespoons minced garlic

2 tablespoons minced fresh ginger

½ cup water

1 tablespoon freshly squeezed lime juice

1 tablespoon soy sauce

1 tablespoon coconut aminos

⅓ cup creamy natural cashew butter

½ teaspoon salt

Liquid stevia

In a large bowl, combine the purple and green cabbage, scallions, cilantro, noodles, and cashews. In a medium bowl, combine the garlic, ginger, water, lime juice, soy sauce, coconut aminos, cashew butter, and salt. Sweeten with stevia as desired. Mix well with a whisk until thoroughly combined. Pour the dressing over the vegetable and noodle mixture, then toss well.

Per Serving: Calories: 295; Fat: 19g; Protein: 8g; Total Carbs: 23g; Fiber: 6g; Net Carbs: 17g; **Macros:** Fat: 58%; Protein: 11%; Carbs: 31%

Smoked Salmon and Cucumber Noodles

SERVES 4 | PREP TIME: 10 minutes

2 English cucumbers

Salt

Freshly ground black pepper

12 ounces sliced smoked salmon, sliced into thin strips

2 large hard-boiled eggs, peeled and chopped

2 scallions, green and white parts, finely chopped, for garnish

1 lemon, cut into wedges, for serving

Prepare the cucumber noodles using a spiralizer, spiral cutter, or julienne peeler. Remove as much excess liquid from the cucumbers as possible by squeezing the noodles in a colander over the sink or pressing with paper towels. Season the cucumber noodles well with salt and pepper, then divide them among four plates. Arrange the salmon on top of the cucumber noodles. Sprinkle with the chopped eggs. Garnish with the scallions and serve with lemon wedges.

Per Serving: Calories: 160; Fat: 6g; Protein: 20g; Total Carbs: 6g; Fiber: 1g; Net Carbs: 5g; **Macros:** Fat: 35%; Protein: 51%; Carbs: 14%

Classic Chicken Salad

SERVES 6 | PREP TIME: 10 minutes, plus 1 hour to overnight for chilling

3 cups chopped cooked chicken

2 scallions, white and green parts sliced

1 celery stalk, thinly sliced

1 teaspoon Dijon mustard

½ cup plus 2 tablespoons mayonnaise

½ teaspoon salt

½ teaspoon freshly ground black pepper

¼ cup slivered almonds (optional)

Lettuce, for serving (optional)

In a large bowl, combine all the ingredients. Mix well. Refrigerate for at least 1 hour and preferably overnight for best flavor. Serve as-is, in a lettuce cup, or on a bed of salad greens.

Per Serving: Calories: 266; Fat: 20g; Protein: 19g; Total Carbs: 1g; Fiber: 0g; Net Carbs: 1g; **Macros:** Fat: 69%; Protein: 1%; Carbs: 30%

Buffalo Chicken Salad

SERVES 4 | PREP TIME: 10 minutes

4 cups cooked chicken, diced or shredded

½ cup buffalo sauce

6 cups chopped romaine lettuce

2 avocados, pitted, peeled, and diced

2 celery stalks, chopped

½ cup blue cheese crumbles

In a large bowl, combine the chicken and buffalo sauce and stir well. Place the lettuce in a large serving bowl. Add the avocados, celery, and chicken mixture. Toss to combine and sprinkle with the blue cheese.

Per Serving: Calories: 591; Fat: 37g; Protein: 50g; Total Carbs: 15g; Fiber: 10g; Net Carbs: 5g; **Macros:** Fat: 55%; Protein: 36%; Carbs: 9%

Chicken Salad on Romaine Boats

SERVES 4 | PREP TIME: 10 minutes

- 4 (12½-ounce) cans chicken, drained, or 1¾ pounds chopped cooked boneless skinless chicken breasts or rotisserie chicken
- ¼ cup chopped red onion
- 1 teaspoon seasoned salt
- 1 teaspoon freshly ground black pepper
- 1 teaspoon garlic powder
- ½ cup mayonnaise
- ¼ cup sour cream
- 12 whole romaine lettuce leaves
- ¾ cup ranch dressing

In a large bowl, add the chicken. Use a fork to break apart the bigger chunks. Add the red onion, seasoned salt, pepper, and garlic powder, and toss to mix. Add the mayonnaise and sour cream, and mix well. On a plate, lay down three romaine leaves. Spread ¼ cup of chicken salad down the center of each leaf. Drizzle 1 tablespoon of ranch dressing down the center of each chicken salad boat.

Per Serving: (3 boats with ¼ cup chicken salad in each) Calories: 576; Fat: 36g; Protein: 57g; Total Carbs: 6g; Fiber: 2g; Net Carbs: 4g; **Macros:** Fat: 56%; Protein: 40%; Carbs: 4%

Chicken Melon Salad

SERVES 3 | PREP TIME: 20 minutes

- 4 ounces cooked boneless, skinless chicken breast, chopped
- 2 celery stalks, chopped
- ½ cup diced cantaloupe
- ½ red bell pepper, chopped
- ½ cup mayonnaise
- 1 tablespoon chopped basil
- Sea salt
- Freshly ground black pepper
- 4 cups baby spinach
- 1 cup shredded Cheddar cheese
- ½ cup chopped pecans

In a medium bowl, mix the chicken, celery, cantaloupe, bell pepper, mayonnaise, and basil. Season the chicken salad with salt and pepper. Arrange the baby spinach on three plates and top each with a generous scoop of chicken salad. Top with cheese and pecans and serve.

Per Serving: Calories: 621; Fat: 56g; Protein: 22g; Total Carbs: 12g; Fiber: 5g; Net Carbs: 7g; **Macros:** Fat: 81%; Protein: 14%; Carbs: 5%

Lobster BLT Salad

SERVES 4 | PREP TIME: 15 minutes | COOK TIME: 10 to 15 minutes

- 2 (2½-pound) lobsters
- 8 slices bacon (pork, turkey, beef, or salmon)
- 2 tablespoons keto-friendly mayonnaise (spicy or regular)
- 1 tablespoon Dijon mustard
- 1 tablespoon chopped fresh chives
- Salt
- 1 pound butter lettuce, chopped
- 1 large beefsteak tomato, sliced
- 1 avocado, halved, pitted, peeled, and sliced

Bring a pot of water to a boil. Put the lobsters in the pot, cover, and steam for 5 to 7 minutes per pound. Remove the lobsters from the pot and let cool. While lobsters cool, cook the bacon to your desired doneness, about 5 minutes. When lobster is cool enough to handle, use a sharp knife and a claw cracker to get the meat out. Separate the claw and tail meat for this recipe and set aside the remainder for another use. Chop the meat into pieces and put in a medium bowl. Add the mayonnaise, mustard, and chives, season with salt, and mix. Arrange the butter lettuce, tomato, and avocado on plates. Scoop the lobster mixture alongside and serve with the bacon slices either whole or crumbled and sprinkled on top.

Per Serving: Calories: 436; Fat: 28g; Protein: 35g; Total Carbs: 11g; Fiber: 4g; Net Carbs: 7g; **Macros:** Fat: 58%; Protein: 32%; Carbs: 10%

Pecan Chicken Salad

SERVES 12 | PREP TIME: 15 minutes | CHILL TIME: 2 hours

- 4 cups shredded cooked chicken
- 1 cup finely diced celery
- ¾ cup chopped pecans, lightly toasted
- ¼ cup sliced scallion
- 1 to 1½ cups mayonnaise
- 1 tablespoon freshly squeezed lemon juice
- 2 teaspoons celery salt
- 1 teaspoon freshly ground black pepper

In a large bowl, toss the chicken, celery, pecans, and scallion. In a small bowl, stir together the mayonnaise, lemon juice, celery salt, and pepper until thoroughly combined. Pour the mayonnaise mixture over the chicken and toss to combine. Cover and chill for at least 1 to 2 hours before serving.

Per Serving: (½ cup): Calories: 248; Fat: 20g; Protein: 15g; Total Carbs: 2g; Fiber: 1g; Net Carbs: 1g; **Macros:** Fat: 73%; Protein: 24%; Carbs: 3%

Classic Tuna Salad

SERVES 6 | PREP TIME: 10 minutes, plus 1 hour to overnight for chilling

- 3 (5-ounce) cans tuna packed in olive oil, drained
- 2 hard-boiled eggs, peeled and chopped
- 2 scallions, white and green parts sliced
- 1 celery stalk, thinly sliced
- 1 tablespoon sugar-free pickle relish (I like Mt. Olive brand)
- 1 teaspoon Dijon mustard
- ½ cup plus 2 tablespoons mayonnaise
- ½ teaspoon salt
- ½ teaspoon freshly ground black pepper
- 2 to 4 dashes hot sauce (optional)
- Lettuce, for serving (optional)

In a large bowl, combine all the ingredients. Mix well. Refrigerate for 1 hour, or preferably overnight for best flavor. Serve as-is, in a lettuce cup, or on a bed of salad greens.

Per Serving: Calories: 292; Fat: 23g; Protein: 17g; Total Carbs: 2g; Fiber: 0g; Net Carbs: 2g; **Macros:** Fat: 72%; Protein: 26%; Carbs: 2%

Lemony Chicken Salad with Blueberries and Fennel

SERVES 4 | PREP TIME: 5 minutes

½ cup mayonnaise

¼ cup extra-virgin olive oil

Juice and zest of 1 lemon

1 teaspoon fennel seeds, slightly crushed

½ teaspoon salt

¼ teaspoon freshly ground black pepper

2 cups cooked shredded chicken (about 12 to 16 ounces of meat)

2 celery ribs, finely chopped

½ cup fresh or frozen blueberries, halved

½ cup slivered almonds

In a medium bowl, combine the mayo, olive oil, lemon zest and juice, fennel, salt, and pepper and whisk well to combine. Add the chicken, celery, blueberries, and almonds and stir to coat.

Per Serving: Calories: 564; Fat: 51g; Protein: 23g; Total Carbs: 8g; Fiber: 3g; Net Carbs: 5g; **Macros:** Fat: 81%; Protein: 16%; Carbs: 3%

Mayo-Less Tuna Salad

SERVES 1 | PREP TIME: 5 minutes

1 (6-ounce) can tuna, packed in olive oil

5 olives, pitted and chopped

4 sun-dried tomatoes, chopped

1 tablespoon olive oil

1 teaspoon mustard

1 teaspoon dried basil (optional)

Salt

Freshly ground black pepper

1 cup fresh spinach leaves

Sugar-free hot sauce, for serving (optional)

In a medium bowl, combine the tuna and its oil with the olives, sun-dried tomatoes, olive oil, and mustard. Season with the basil (if using), salt, and pepper. Stir everything together until well combined. Arrange the spinach leaves on a plate or in a bowl and top with the tuna salad. If you'd like, sprinkle with some hot sauce.

Per Serving: Calories: 450; Fat: 38g; Protein: 18g; Total Carbs: 9g; Fiber: 4g; Net Carbs: 5g; **Macros:** Fat: 76%; Protein: 16%; Carbs: 8%

Italian Tuna Salad

1 SERVING | PREP TIME: 5 minutes

1 (5-ounce) can tuna packed in olive oil

4 cherry tomatoes, halved

¼ medium red onion, cut into half-inch pieces

4 Kalamata olives, pitted and halved

2 tablespoons Italian vinaigrette

Combine all the ingredients in a bowl; mix gently. Season with salt and freshly ground black pepper to taste.

Per Serving: Calories: 430; Fat: 28g; Protein: 39g; Total Carbs: 10g; Fiber: 2g; Net Carbs: 8g; **Macros:** Fat: 63%; Protein: 27%; Carbs: 10%

Curried Tuna Salad with Pepitas

SERVES 2 | PREP TIME: 10 minutes

1 very ripe avocado, halved and pitted

Juice of 1 lime

1 tablespoon avocado or extra-virgin olive oil

1 teaspoon curry powder

½ teaspoon salt

1 (4-ounce) can oil-packed tuna

2 tablespoons chopped fresh cilantro leaves

2 tablespoons roasted pumpkin seeds

Using a spoon, scoop the avocado flesh into a medium bowl and mash well with a fork. Add the lime juice, oil, curry powder, and salt and mix well. Add the tuna and its oil, cilantro, and pumpkin seeds and mix well with a fork.

Per Serving: Calories: 347; Fat: 26g; Protein: 22g; Total Carbs: 9g; Fiber: 6g; Net Carbs: 3g; **Macros:** Fat: 67%; Protein: 25%; Carbs: 8%

Caprese Stuffed Avocados

SERVES 4 | PREP TIME: 10 minutes

½ cup small mozzarella balls or bocconcini

⅓ cup halved cherry tomatoes

2 tablespoons pesto

2 garlic cloves, minced

1 teaspoon garlic salt

2 avocados, halved

2 tablespoons balsamic vinegar

Freshly ground black pepper

2 tablespoons chopped fresh basil

In a medium bowl, mix the mozzarella, tomatoes, pesto, garlic, and garlic salt. Fill each avocado half with one-fourth of the cheese-and-tomato mixture. Drizzle with the vinegar, season with pepper, and garnish with the basil.

Per Serving: (1 avocado half) Calories: 244; Fat: 20g; Protein: 6g; Total Carbs: 10g; Fiber: 6g; Net Carbs: 4g; **Macros:** Fat: 74%; Protein: 10%; Carbs: 16%

Crab Salad–Stuffed Avocado

SERVES 2 | PREP TIME: 20 minutes

1 avocado, peeled, halved lengthwise, and pitted

½ teaspoon freshly squeezed lemon juice

4½ ounces Dungeness crabmeat

½ cup cream cheese

¼ cup chopped red bell pepper

¼ cup chopped, peeled English cucumber

½ scallion, green part chopped

1 teaspoon chopped cilantro

Pinch sea salt

Freshly ground black pepper

Brush the cut edges of the avocado with the lemon juice and set the halves aside on a plate. In a medium bowl, stir the crabmeat, cream cheese, red pepper, cucumber, scallion, cilantro, salt, and pepper until well mixed. Divide the crab mixture between the avocado halves and serve.

Per Serving: Calories: 389; Fat: 31g; Protein: 19g; Total Carbs: 10g; Fiber: 5g; Net Carbs: 5g; **Macros:** Fat: 70%; Protein: 20%; Carbs: 10%

Tuna-Stuffed Avocado

SERVES 2 | PREP TIME: 5 minutes | COOK TIME: 0 minutes

3 ounces canned tuna packed in water and drained

2 tablespoons mayonnaise

¼ cup minced celery

1 tablespoon minced shallot

Sea salt

Freshly ground black pepper

1 large avocado, halved and pitted

In a small bowl, mix the tuna, mayonnaise, celery, and shallot. Season with salt and pepper. Spoon about half of the tuna mixture into each avocado half. Serve immediately.

Per Serving: Calories: 275; Fat: 24g; Protein: 10g; Total Carbs: 9g; Fiber: 6g; Net Carbs: 3g; Macros: Fat: 78%; Protein: 14%; Carbs: 8%

Turkey-Stuffed Avocados

SERVES 2 TO 4 | PREP TIME: 5 to 10 minutes | COOK TIME: 5 to 10 minutes

4 asparagus spears, trimmed	Salt
1½ cups cubed roasted turkey	Freshly ground black pepper
2 cups fresh spinach, chopped	2 large avocados, halved
¼ cup avocado oil mayonnaise	and pitted

Fill a medium saucepan with ¼-inch of water and bring to a boil over medium-high heat. Add the asparagus, cover, and cook for 2 to 3 minutes, until tender (or to your desired doneness). Meanwhile, in a large bowl, combine the turkey, spinach and mayonnaise and season with salt and pepper. Chop the asparagus into pieces, and add it to the turkey and mix. Scoop out some of the avocado flesh to create bigger hollows and mix it into the turkey mixture before spooning everything into the avocado halves.

Per Serving: Calories: 624; Fat: 48g; Protein: 31g; Total Carbs: 17g; Fiber: 13g; Net Carbs: 4g; Macros: Fat: 70%; Protein: 20%; Carbs: 10%

Chicken Salad–Stuffed Avocados

SERVES 4 | PREP TIME: 25 minutes

2 small avocados, peeled and pitted	1 teaspoon coconut oil
1½ cups chopped cooked chicken	½ teaspoon ground paprika
¼ cup mayonnaise	¼ teaspoon garlic powder
1 tablespoon chopped scallion	¼ teaspoon ground cayenne pepper
1 tablespoon freshly squeezed lemon juice	2 tablespoons Parmesan cheese

Place the avocado halves on a plate, and set aside. In a medium bowl, stir the chicken, Mayonnaise, scallion, lemon juice, coconut oil, paprika, garlic powder, and cayenne until well mixed. Spoon the chicken mixture evenly between the avocado halves, sprinkle each with Parmesan cheese, and serve.

Per Serving: Calories: 361; Fat: 28g; Protein: 19g; Total Carbs: 12g; Fiber: 7g; Net Carbs: 5g; Macros: Fat: 67%; Protein: 20%; Carbs: 13%

Italian Green Bean Salad

SERVES 4 | PREP TIME: 5 minutes | COOK TIME: 5 minutes, plus 15 minutes inactive time

¼ cup extra-virgin olive oil, divided	2 garlic cloves, thinly sliced
1 pound green beans, trimmed	½ cup slivered almonds
2 tablespoons red wine vinegar	¼ cup thinly sliced fresh basil leaves
1 teaspoon salt	2 tablespoons chopped fresh mint
1 teaspoon red pepper flakes	

In a large skillet, heat 2 tablespoons of olive oil over medium-high heat. Sauté the green beans for about 5 minutes, until just tender.

Remove from the heat and place into a large serving bowl. In a small bowl, whisk the remaining 2 tablespoons of olive oil, vinegar, salt, red pepper flakes, and garlic. Pour the dressing over the green beans and toss to coat well. Add the almonds, basil, and mint, and toss well. Serve warm or chill for at least 1 hour to serve cold.

Per Serving: Calories: 238; Fat: 21g; Protein: 5g; Total Carbs: 12g; Fiber: 5g; Net Carbs: 7g; Macros: Fat: 79%; Protein: 8%; Carbs: 13%

Guacamole Salad

SERVES 4 | PREP TIME: 10 minutes

2 ripe avocados, peeled, pitted, and cut into 1-inch chunks	½ cup whole fresh cilantro leaves
4 Roma tomatoes, quartered	¼ cup extra-virgin olive oil
1 green bell pepper, cut into 1-inch chunks	Juice of 2 limes
	1 teaspoon salt
¼ red onion, cut into slivers	½ teaspoon freshly ground black pepper

In a medium bowl, combine the avocado, tomatoes, bell pepper, onion, and cilantro. In a small bowl, whisk the olive oil, lime juice, salt, and pepper and drizzle over the salad. Toss to coat well and serve immediately.

Per Serving: Calories: 258; Fat: 24g; Protein: 2g; Total Carbs: 12g; Fiber: 6g; Net Carbs: 6g; Macros: Fat: 84%; Protein: 3%; Carbs: 13%

Avocado Caprese Lettuce Wraps

SERVES 4 | PREP TIME: 10 minutes

16 large iceberg lettuce leaves	16 fresh basil leaves, finely chopped
2 (8-ounce) balls fresh mozzarella	Salt
4 avocados	Freshly ground black pepper
32 cherry tomatoes, halved	

Rinse the lettuce leaves and pat dry with paper towels. Place the leaves on a platter. Cut each ball of mozzarella into 8 slices (for a total of 16), then halve each slice. Add 2 pieces to each lettuce leaf. Halve the avocados, remove the pits, and cut each half into 4 slices. Add 2 slices to each lettuce leaf. Add 4 tomato halves to each leaf and finish with a sprinkling of basil, salt, and pepper. Serve open-faced and ready to roll into a wrap.

Per Serving: Calories: 732; Fat: 56g; Protein: 33g; Total Carbs: 32g; Fiber: 19g; Net Carbs: 13g; Macros: Fat: 66%; Protein: 18%; Carbs: 16%

Broccoli Salad with Bacon

1 SERVING | PREP TIME: 10 minutes | COOK TIME: 5 minutes, plus 60 minutes

1 tablespoon mayonnaise	1½ cups broccoli florets
1 tablespoon apple cider vinegar	2 bacon slices, cooked and crumbled
½ teaspoon stevia or 4 drops liquid stevia extract (optional)	¼ medium red onion, diced
	¼ cup raw sliced almonds

In a small bowl, mix the mayonnaise, vinegar, and stevia (if using) until well combined. Season the dressing with salt and freshly ground black pepper to taste. In a large bowl, combine the broccoli, bacon, onion, and almonds. Pour the dressing over the broccoli mixture and stir until evenly coated. Cover and refrigerate for at least 1 hour before serving.

Per Serving: Calories: 511; Fat: 39g; Protein: 23g; Total Carbs: 17g; Fiber: 8g; Net Carbs: 9g; Macros: Fat: 69%; Protein: 18%; Carbs: 13%

Creamy Broccoli Salad

SERVES 4 | PREP TIME: 10 minutes | COOK TIME: 10 minutes

2 bacon slices, cut into pieces	Freshly ground black pepper
½ cup mayonnaise	4 cups broccoli florets
Juice of 1 lemon	½ small red onion, thinly sliced
Sea salt	1 cup shredded red cabbage

Cook the bacon in a medium skillet over medium-low heat until the bacon is crisp. Set the cooked bacon aside. In a large salad bowl, whisk the bacon fat, mayonnaise, and lemon juice. Season with salt and pepper. Add the broccoli, onion, and red cabbage to the bowl, and mix well. Sprinkle the bacon pieces over the salad just before serving.

Per Serving: Calories: 251; Fat: 23g; Protein: 5g; Total Carbs: 9g; Fiber: 4g; Net Carbs: 5g; Macros: Fat: 82%; Protein: 8%; Carbs: 10%

Israeli Salad with Nuts and Seeds

SERVES 4 | PREP TIME: 15 minutes

¼ cup pine nuts	½ cup finely chopped fresh flat-leaf Italian parsley
¼ cup shelled pistachios	
¼ cup coarsely chopped walnuts	¼ cup extra-virgin olive oil
¼ cup shelled pumpkin seeds	2 to 3 tablespoons freshly squeezed lemon juice (from 1 lemon)
¼ cup shelled sunflower seeds	
2 large English cucumbers, finely chopped	1 teaspoon salt
1 pint cherry tomatoes, finely chopped	¼ teaspoon freshly ground black pepper
½ small red onion, finely chopped	4 cups baby arugula

In a large dry skillet, toast the pine nuts, pistachios, walnuts, pumpkin seeds, and sunflower seeds over medium-low heat until golden and fragrant, 5 to 6 minutes. Remove from the heat and set aside. In a large bowl, combine the cucumber, tomatoes, red onion, and parsley. In a small bowl, whisk olive oil, lemon juice, salt, and pepper. Pour over the chopped vegetables and toss to coat. Add the toasted nuts and seeds and arugula and toss with the salad to blend well. Serve at room temperature or chilled.

Per Serving: Calories: 414; Fat: 34g; Protein: 10g; Total Carbs: 17g; Fiber: 6g; Net Carbs: 11g; Macros: Fat: 74%; Protein: 10%; Carbs: 16%

Moroccan Cauliflower Salad

SERVES 4 | PREP TIME: 5 minutes | COOK TIME: 25 minutes, plus 15 minutes cooling time

4 cups cauliflower florets, fresh or frozen	1 teaspoon salt, divided
	¼ cup extra-virgin olive oil
2 tablespoons coconut oil, melted	Juice and zest of 1 lemon
	1 teaspoon chili powder

1 teaspoon ground cinnamon	½ cup finely sliced fresh mint leaves
1 teaspoon garlic powder	
½ teaspoon ground turmeric	¼ cup finely sliced red onion
½ teaspoon ground ginger	¼ cup shelled pistachios
2 celery ribs, thinly sliced	

If using frozen cauliflower, thaw to room temperature in a colander, draining off any excess water. Cut larger florets in half into bite-sized pieces. Preheat the oven to 450°F and line a baking sheet with foil. In a medium bowl, toss the cauliflower with coconut oil and ½ teaspoon of salt. Lay out in a single layer on the baking sheet. Roast the cauliflower for 20 to 25 minutes, until lightly browned and crispy. While cauliflower roasts, in the same medium bowl, whisk olive oil, lemon juice and zest, remaining ½ teaspoon of salt, chili powder, cinnamon, garlic powder, turmeric, and ginger. Stir in the celery, mint leaves, and red onion. Remove the cauliflower from the oven and allow to cool for 10 to 15 minutes. Toss warm (but not too hot) cauliflower with dressing until well combined. Add the pistachios and toss to incorporate. Serve warm or chilled.

Per Serving: Calories: 262; Fat: 24g; Protein: 4g; Total Carbs: 11g; Fiber: 4g; Net Carbs: 7g; Macros: Fat: 82%; Protein: 6%; Carbs: 12%

Cucumber and Tomato Feta Salad

SERVES 8 | PREP TIME: 15 minutes

3 medium cucumbers, peeled, cut into ¼-inch-thick slices and then quartered	¼ cup chopped red onion
	½ cup olive oil
2 Roma tomatoes, roughly chopped	3 tablespoons red wine vinegar
	½ teaspoon Dijon mustard
12 pitted Kalamata olives (or your favorite), halved	1 teaspoon garlic salt
	1 teaspoon freshly ground black pepper
8 ounces feta cheese, cut into cubes or crumbled	

In a large serving bowl, combine the cucumbers, tomatoes, olives, feta, and onion. In a small bowl, whisk the olive oil, vinegar, Dijon mustard, garlic salt, and pepper. Add the dressing to the salad, toss all the ingredients, and serve.

Per Serving: Calories: 219; Fat: 18g; Protein: 6g; Total Carbs: 4g; Fiber: 1g; Net Carbs: 3g; Macros: Fat: 74%; Protein: 11%; Carbs: 5%

Cucumber, Tomato, and Avocado Salad

SERVES 4 | PREP TIME: 10 minutes

1 cup halved cherry tomatoes	2 tablespoons extra-virgin olive oil
1 cup diced cucumber	
2 large avocados, pitted, peeled, and cut into ½-inch pieces	2 tablespoons red wine vinegar
	Sea salt
1 shallot, thinly sliced	Freshly ground black pepper

In a medium serving bowl, toss the tomatoes, cucumber, avocados, and shallot. In a separate container, whisk the olive oil, vinegar, salt, and pepper. Pour the dressing over the salad.

Per Serving: Calories: 221; Fat: 20g; Protein: 2g; Total Carbs: 11g; Fiber: 7g; Net Carbs: 4g; Macros: Fat: 78%; Protein: 2%; Carbs: 20%

Goat Cheese Caprese Salad

SERVES 4 | PREP TIME: 10 minutes

1 large ripe tomato
1 teaspoon salt, divided
1 (4-ounce) goat cheese log,
    cut into 4 equal pieces
8 whole fresh basil leaves,
    thinly sliced

¼ cup extra-virgin olive oil
1 tablespoon balsamic vinegar
½ teaspoon freshly ground
    black pepper

Slice the tomato into four thick slices and place them in a single layer on a plate or serving dish. Sprinkle with ½ teaspoon of salt. Place a slice of goat cheese on each tomato slice and, using a knife, spread to cover the tomato. Top each with basil and drizzle each with 1 tablespoon of olive oil and ¼ tablespoon of vinegar. Season with the remaining ½ teaspoon of salt and the pepper. Serve immediately.

Per Serving: Calories: 212; Fat: 21g; Protein: 6g; Total Carbs: 4g; Fiber: 1g; Net Carbs: 3g; **Macros:** Fat: 84%; Protein: 10%; Carbs: 6%

Sausage and Cauliflower Salad

SERVES 4 | PREP TIME: 10 minutes

6 cooked sausages, chopped
4 cups store-bought cau-
    liflower rice, cooked
    according to package
    directions
1 red bell pepper, seeded
    and chopped

¼ cup extra-virgin olive oil
1 tablespoon red wine vinegar
1 teaspoon Italian seasoning
Salt
Freshly ground black pepper
Chopped fresh parsley,
    for garnish

In a large bowl, combine the sausages, cauliflower rice, and bell pepper and set aside. In a small bowl, combine the oil, vinegar, and Italian seasoning and whisk until emulsified, 2 to 3 minutes. Add the dressing to the large bowl, season with salt and black pepper, and mix well to combine. Transfer to a serving bowl and garnish with the parsley.

Per Serving: Calories: 503; Fat: 41g; Protein: 22g; Total Carbs: 12g; Fiber: 3g; Net Carbs: 9g; **Macros:** Fat: 74%; Protein: 18%; Carbs: 8%

Creamy Riced Cauliflower Salad

SERVES 4 | PREP TIME: 10 minutes, plus 30 minutes inactive time

4 ounces crumbled
    feta cheese
½ cup mayonnaise
Juice and zest of 1 lemon
2 tablespoons minced
    red onion
1½ teaspoons dried dill

½ teaspoon salt
½ to 1 teaspoon red pepper
    flakes, to taste
3 cups fresh riced cauliflower
    (not frozen)
½ cup pitted roughly chopped
    Kalamata olives

In a medium bowl, combine the feta, mayonnaise, lemon juice and zest, onion, and dill and with a fork, whisk well until smooth and creamy. Add the riced cauliflower and olives and mix well to combine thoroughly. Refrigerate at least 30 minutes before serving.

Per Serving: Calories: 370; Fat: 37g; Protein: 7g; Total Carbs: 6g; Fiber: 2g; Net Carbs: 4g; **Macros:** Fat: 90%; Protein: 8%; Carbs: 2%

Apple Cabbage Cumin Coleslaw

SERVES 4 | PREP TIME: 5 minutes

¼ cup mayonnaise
½ teaspoon Dijon mustard
½ teaspoon ground cumin
Juice of 1 lemon
½ small head Savoy cabbage,
    shredded

½ red onion, thinly sliced
1 small Granny Smith
    apple, cored and cut into
    matchsticks

In a medium salad bowl, whisk the mayonnaise, mustard, cumin, and lemon juice. Add the cabbage and red onion, and using your hands, mix thoroughly. Fold in the apples and serve immediately.

Per Serving: Calories: 135; Fat: 10 g; Protein: 2g; Total Carbs: 11g; Fiber: 3g; Net Carbs: 8g; **Macros:** Fat: 67%; Protein: 6%; Carbs: 17%

Sesame Ginger Slaw

SERVES 4 | PREP TIME: 10 minutes

2 tablespoons toasted
    sesame oil
2 tablespoons extra-virgin
    olive oil
2 tablespoons low-sodium
    soy sauce
1 tablespoon lime juice
1 teaspoon minced
    fresh ginger
1 teaspoon minced fresh garlic

Pinch red pepper flakes
½ small head Savoy cabbage,
    shredded
¼ cup roughly chopped
    cilantro
¼ cup roughly chopped mint
1 scallion, white and green
    parts thinly sliced
¼ cup sesame seeds

In a medium salad bowl, whisk the sesame oil, olive oil, soy sauce, lime juice, garlic, ginger, and red pepper flakes. Add the cabbage, cilantro, mint, and scallion to the bowl and toss gently to mix. Sprinkle with the sesame seeds before serving.

Per Serving: Calories: 200; Fat: 19g; Protein: 4g; Total Carbs: 8g; Fiber: 4g; Net Carbs: 4g; **Macros:** Fat: 86%; Protein: 8%; Carbs: 6%

Crisp and Creamy Southern Coleslaw

SERVES 6 TO 8 | PREP TIME: 10 minutes |
CHILL TIME: 30 minutes

½ cup mayonnaise
½ cup sour cream
1½ to 2 tablespoons monk
    fruit/erythritol blend
    sweetener
1½ tablespoons apple
    cider vinegar
1½ teaspoons mustard
½ teaspoon kosher salt

¼ teaspoon freshly ground
    black pepper
¼ teaspoon paprika
¼ teaspoon onion powder
⅛ teaspoon garlic powder
1 (14-ounce) package
    shredded cabbage or
    coleslaw mix
1 (12-ounce) package
    broccoli slaw

In a small bowl, whisk the mayonnaise, sour cream, sweetener, vinegar, mustard, salt, pepper, paprika, onion powder, and garlic powder until smooth and the sweetener is dissolved. Set aside. In a large bowl, combine the cabbage and broccoli slaw. Add the dressing and toss to combine. Refrigerate at least 30 minutes before serving to let the flavors mingle.

Per Serving: Calories: 206; Fat: 18g; Protein: 3g; Total Carbs: 9g; Fiber: 4g; Net Carbs: 5g; **Macros:** Fat: 79%; Protein: 4%; Carbs: 17%

Ranch Broccoli Slaw

SERVES 2 | PREP TIME: 5 minutes

1 (12-ounce) bag shredded
  broccoli slaw
1 cup sliced almonds
Store-bought ranch dressing

½ cup sliced radishes
¼ cup dried sugar-free
  cranberries

In a large bowl, combine all the ingredients and toss to coat. Serve immediately.

Per serving: Calories: 546; Fat: 35g; Protein: 20g; Total Carbs: 42g; Fiber: 14g; Net Carbs: 28g; **Macros:** Fat: 58%; Protein: 15%; Carbs: 27%

Turkey and Kale Coleslaw

SERVES 4 | PREP TIME: 25 minutes

1 cup heavy (whipping) cream
2 tablespoons apple
  cider vinegar
1 teaspoon freshly squeezed
  lemon juice
1 teaspoon Swerve
½ teaspoon ground cumin
¼ teaspoon sea salt
2 cups shredded Napa cabbage

1 cup shredded cooked turkey
1 cup shredded kale
1 cup shredded fennel
2 scallions, white and green
  parts, chopped
2 tablespoons chopped
  fresh parsley
½ cup toasted pumpkin seeds

Make the dressing: In a small bowl, whisk the cream, vinegar, lemon juice, Swerve, cumin, and salt. Set aside. Make the slaw: In a large bowl, toss the cabbage, turkey, kale, fennel, scallions, and parsley. Add the dressing and toss to coat. Top with pumpkin seeds and serve.

Per Serving: Calories: 322; Fat: 25g; Protein: 15g; Total Carbs: 11g; Fiber: 3g; Net Carbs: 8g; **Macros:** Fat: 70%; Protein: 19%; Carbs: 11%

Roasted Chicken, Artichoke, and Hearts of Palm Salad

SERVES 2 | PREP TIME: 10 minutes | COOK TIME: 30 minutes

4 skin-on chicken thighs
1 tablespoon avocado oil
½ teaspoon salt
8 cups mixed greens
1 (14 ounce) can of artichokes,
  drained and cut in quarters
1 (14 ounce) can sliced hearts
  of palm, drained

2 avocados, sliced
3 tablespoons red wine vinegar
½ teaspoon dried oregano
½ teaspoon garlic powder
½ teaspoon thyme
⅓ cup extra-virgin olive oil

Preheat the oven to 400°F. Line a baking sheet with parchment paper. Coat the chicken thighs with avocado oil and season with ½ teaspoon salt. Place the chicken on the baking sheet and roast in the oven for 20 to 30 minutes or until the juices run clear. Let cool slightly and dice into 1-inch pieces. Assemble the salad by placing the greens, artichokes, hearts of palm, chicken, and avocado in a large bowl. In a small bowl, vigorously whisk the vinegar, oregano, and a pinch of salt. Slowly pour in the olive oil and continue to whisk until fully combined. Pour the dressing over the salad and toss.

Per Serving: Calories: 1129; Fat: 93g; Protein: 43g; Total Carbs: 30g; Fiber: 16g; Net Carbs: 7g; **Macros:** Fat: 74%; Protein: 15%; Carbs: 11%

Chef Salad

1 SERVING | PREP TIME: 15 minutes

2 cups mixed greens
4 cherry tomatoes, halved
1 scallion, finely sliced
1 hard-boiled egg, peeled and
  quartered

½ avocado, pitted, peeled,
  and diced
1 cooked boneless chicken
  thigh, diced
2 tablespoons balsamic
  vinaigrette

Place the mixed greens on a plate or in a large bowl. Top with the tomatoes, scallion, egg, avocado, and chicken. Drizzle with the simple balsamic vinaigrette.

Per Serving: Calories: 563; Fat: 43g; Protein: 25g; Total Carbs: 19g; Fiber: 10g; Net Carbs: 9g; **Macros:** Fat: 69%; Protein: 18%; Carbs: 13%

Chopped Salad

1 SERVING | PREP TIME: 10 minutes

4 cherry tomatoes, halved
¼ medium red onion, cut into
  half-inch pieces
¼ green bell pepper, cut into
  half-inch pieces
¼ cucumber, peeled and cut
  into half-inch pieces
4 Kalamata olives, pitted
  and halved

2 tablespoons Italian
  vinaigrette, divided
1 cooked boneless
  chicken thigh, cut into
  half-inch pieces
1 tablespoon feta cheese
  (optional)
½ avocado, cut into half-inch
  pieces (optional)

Combine the tomatoes, onion, bell pepper, cucumber, olives, and 1 tablespoon of Italian vinaigrette in a bowl and stir gently, making sure the dressing is distributed evenly. Add the chicken, and drizzle the remaining 1 tablespoon of dressing over the salad. Season with salt and freshly ground black pepper to taste. Add the feta cheese and avocado (if using).

Per Serving: Calories: 371; Fat: 27g; Protein: 17g; Total Carbs: 15g; Fiber: 3g; Net Carbs: 12g; **Macros:** Fat: 65%; Protein: 19%; Carbs: 16%

Zesty Chicken Tender Salad

1 SERVING | PREP TIME: 10 minutes

Juice of 1 lime
1 teaspoon Dijon mustard
1 teaspoon Italian seasoning
1 garlic clove, minced
½ teaspoon pink Hima-
  layan salt

1 tablespoon extra-virgin
  olive oil
2 cups fresh spinach
3 cooked chicken tenderloins

Put the lime juice, mustard, Italian Seasoning, garlic, salt, and oil into a blender; process until smooth. Place the spinach on a plate or in a bowl. Arrange the chicken tenders on top of the spinach, and drizzle with the blended dressing.

Per Serving: Calories: 284; Fat: 16g; Protein: 28g; Total Carbs: 7g; Fiber: 2g; Net Carbs: 5g; **Macros:** Fat: 51%; Protein: 39%; Carbs: 10%

Grilled Chicken Cobb Salad

SERVES 6 | PREP TIME: 15 minutes

6 cups (2 large heads) romaine
  lettuce, chopped into
  bite-size pieces

8 ounces grilled
  chicken, chopped into
  bite-size pieces

8 cherry tomatoes, halved

½ small red onion, thinly sliced

1 avocado, peeled, pitted, and chopped into bite-size pieces

8 strips crispy cooked bacon, coarsely chopped

2 large eggs, hard-boiled, peeled, and coarsely chopped

½ medium cucumber, thinly sliced and cut in halves

¼ cup coarsely chopped pecans

½ cup dressing of choice

In a big serving bowl, evenly distribute the romaine across the bottom. Starting with the chicken, make a row across the bowl, and then follow with rows of tomato, red onion, avocado, bacon, eggs, and cucumber. Sprinkle the pecans evenly over the top of the salad. Toss at the table, serve in bowls, and top with 2 tablespoons dressing, or more or less to taste.

Per Serving: Calories: 279; Fat: 20g; Protein: 18g; Total Carbs: 8g; Fiber: 3.5g; Net Carbs: 4.5g; **Macros:** Fat: 65%; Protein: 26%; Carbs: 6%

Chicken Caesar Salad

SERVES 4 | PREP TIME: 25 minutes

8 cups romaine lettuce

1 cup caesar dressing

9 bacon slices, cooked and chopped

½ cup grated Parmesan cheese

1 cup chopped, cooked chicken

Lemon wedges, for garnish

In a large bowl, toss the romaine lettuce and Traditional Caesar Dressing until the lettuce is well coated. Arrange the dressed romaine on 4 plates, and evenly divide the bacon pieces, Parmesan cheese, and chicken over each salad. Serve with lemon wedges.

Per Serving: Calories: 547; Fat: 45g; Protein: 33g; Total Carbs: 6g; Fiber: 1g; Net Carbs: 5g; **Macros:** Fat: 72%; Protein: 24%; Carbs: 4%

Essential Cobb Salad with Crumbled Bacon

SERVES 4 | PREP TIME: 10 minutes

¼ cup extra-virgin olive oil

1 teaspoon Dijon mustard

2 tablespoons white wine vinegar

Sea salt

Freshly ground black pepper

8 cups roughly chopped butter or romaine lettuce

½ cup crumbled cooked bacon

2 eggs, hard-boiled, peeled, and crumbled

¼ cup blue cheese crumbles

1 large avocado, pitted, peeled, and diced

1 small red onion, halved and thinly sliced

½ pint cherry tomatoes, halved

In a large salad bowl, whisk the olive oil, mustard, and vinegar. Season with salt and pepper. Add the lettuce and toss gently to coat. Divide the salad among the serving bowls. Top each salad with bacon, egg, blue cheese, avocado, red onion, and cherry tomatoes.

Per Serving: Calories: 500; Fat: 44g; Protein: 16g; Total Carbs: 11g; Fiber: 5g; Net Carbs: 6g; **Macros:** Fat: 79%; Protein: 13%; Carbs: 8%

Classic Steak Salad

1 SERVING | PREP TIME: 10 minutes | COOK TIME: 10 minutes

1 (6-ounce) skirt steak

¼ cup coconut aminos

2 tablespoons avocado oil

2 cups mixed greens

4 cherry tomatoes, halved

2 radishes, sliced

2 tablespoons extra-virgin olive oil

Juice of ½ lemon

Marinate the steak in the coconut aminos for 5 minutes. In a skillet, heat the avocado oil over high heat. Cook the marinated steak to your desired level of doneness. Place the steak on a plate, and let it sit for 5 minutes. Prepare the salad by tossing the mixed greens, tomatoes, and radishes in a bowl with the olive oil and lemon juice. Season with salt and freshly ground black pepper to taste. Cut the steak into slices, and arrange them on top of the salad.

Per Serving: Calories: 792; Fat: 68g; Protein: 33g; Total Carbs: 12g; Fiber: 4g; Net Carbs: 8g; **Macros:** Fat: 77%; Protein: 17%; Carbs: 6%

Grilled Steak Salad with Cucumber and Mint

SERVES 2 | PREP TIME: 10 minutes | COOK TIME: 10 minutes

12 ounces skirt steak

2 garlic cloves, minced

3 tablespoons lime juice

1 tablespoon fish sauce

1 tablespoons fresh cilantro, chopped

1 teaspoon pure maple syrup

½ teaspoon salt

¼ cup extra-virgin olive oil

1 tablespoon shallot, thinly sliced

1 cucumber, sliced into thin ribbons

⅔ cups fresh mint leaves

1 avocado, thinly sliced

Heat your grill or grill pan to high heat. Place the steak on the grill for about 10 minutes or until the internal temperature reaches 120 to 125°F, flipping halfway through. Place the steak aside on a plate, and let it rest for 10 minutes before slicing it against the grain. While the steak is resting, prepare the dressing by mixing the garlic, lime juice, fish sauce, cilantro, maple syrup, and salt in a bowl. Slowly whisk in the olive oil until well combined. Next, add in the shallots and mix well. In a salad bowl, mix the cucumber ribbons and mint leaves. Assemble the salad by plating the cucumber and mint first, followed by the steak, then topping with the dressing and sliced avocado.

Per Serving: Calories: 675; Fat: 51g; Protein: 40g; Total Carbs: 14g; Fiber: 6g; Net Carbs: 8g; **Macros:** Fat: 69%; Protein: 24%; Carbs: 7%

Sirloin Steak Salad with Goat Cheese and Pecans

SERVES 4 | PREP TIME: 20 minutes, plus 4 hours to marinate | COOK TIME: 10 minutes

½ pound sirloin steak

Sea salt

Freshly ground black pepper

¼ cup extra-virgin olive oil, divided

1 teaspoon minced garlic, divided

2 tablespoons apple cider vinegar

2 teaspoons Dijon mustard

6 cups spinach

6 ounces goat cheese, crumbled

¾ cup pecan halves, toasted

Season the steak with salt and pepper. Generously rub the steak with 1 tablespoon of olive oil and ½ teaspoon of garlic. Refrigerate the steak for 3 hours, and let it stand at room temperature for 45 minutes before grilling it. While the steak is sitting, in a large bowl, whisk the remaining 3 tablespoons of olive oil with the apple cider vinegar, Dijon mustard, and remaining ½ teaspoon of garlic, and set aside. Preheat a barbecue grill to medium-high or the oven to broil. Cook the steak to medium-rare, about 4 minutes per side on the grill or in the oven. Let the steak rest for 10 minutes before slicing it thinly across the grain. Add the spinach to the bowl with the dressing, and toss to coat. Arrange the spinach on 4 plates, and evenly divide the steak among the plates. Top the salads with the goat cheese and pecans, and serve.

Per Serving: Calories: 505; Fat: 40g; Protein: 33g; Total Carbs: 5g; Fiber: 2g; Net Carbs: 3g; **Macros:** Fat: 70%; Protein: 26%; Carbs: 4%

Ground Beef Taco Salad with Peppers and Ranch

SERVES 4 | PREP TIME: 20 minutes | COOK TIME: 6 minutes

½ pound regular ground beef (25% fat)

2 tablespoons water

2 tablespoons taco seasoning

2 cups romaine lettuce

1 avocado, diced

1 green bell pepper, chopped

1 scallion, chopped

½ cup shredded Cheddar cheese

¼ cup chopped fresh cilantro

1 jalapeño pepper, thinly sliced

½ cup buttermilk ranch dressing

2 chipotle peppers in adobo, chopped

In a large skillet over medium-high heat, brown the ground beef, stirring frequently, until it is cooked through, about 5 minutes. Pour off any grease, and return the skillet to the heat. Stir in the water and taco seasoning. Cook the meat mixture until the water evaporates, about 1 minute. Remove the skillet from the heat, and set aside. Arrange the lettuce on 4 plates, and top each evenly with the seasoned beef. Evenly divide the avocado, bell pepper, scallion, cheese, cilantro, and jalapeño among the salads. In a small bowl, stir the dressing and chipotle peppers. Spoon the dressing over the salads, and serve.

Per Serving: Calories: 401; Fat: 31g; Protein: 21g; Total Carbs: 13g; Fiber: 8g; Net Carbs: 5g; **Macros:** Fat: 67%; Protein: 20%; Carbs: 13%

BLT Salad

SERVES 4 | PREP TIME: 15 minutes

2 tablespoons melted bacon fat

2 tablespoons red wine vinegar

Freshly ground black pepper

4 cups shredded lettuce

1 tomato, chopped

6 bacon slices, cooked and chopped

2 hard-boiled eggs, chopped

1 tablespoon roasted unsalted sunflower seeds

1 teaspoon toasted sesame seeds

1 cooked chicken breast, sliced (optional)

In a medium bowl, whisk the bacon fat and vinegar until emulsified. Season with black pepper. Add the lettuce and tomato to the bowl and toss the vegetables with the dressing. Divide the salad between 4 plates and top each with equal amounts of bacon, egg, sunflower seeds, sesame seeds, and chicken (if using). Serve.

Per serving: Calories: 228; Fat: 18g; Protein: 1g; Total Carbs: 4g; Fiber: 2g; Net Carbs: 2g; **Macros:** Fat: 76%; Protein: 17%; Carbs: 7%

Deluxe Sub Salad

SERVES 6 | PREP TIME: 10 minutes

6 cups romaine lettuce, chopped

12 ounces salami, chopped

1 cup cherry tomatoes, halved

½ cup cucumber, sliced

½ cup black olives

½ cup banana peppers, sliced

For the dressing

3 tablespoons red wine vinegar

½ teaspoon dried oregano

½ teaspoon garlic powder

½ teaspoon thyme

Pinch of salt

⅓ cup extra-virgin olive oil

Assemble the salad by placing the lettuce, salami, tomato, cucumber, olives and banana peppers in a large bowl. In a small bowl, whisk the vinegar, oregano, and salt vigorously. Slowly pour in the olive oil and continue to whisk until fully combined. Pour the vinaigrette over the salad and toss to combine.

Per Serving: Calories: 295; Fat: 27g; Protein: 8g; Total Carbs: 5g; Fiber: 2g; Net Carbs: 3g; **Macros:** Fat: 82%; Protein: 11%; Carbs: 7%

Quick Fiesta Taco Salad

SERVES 4 | PREP TIME: 10 minutes | COOK TIME: 10 minutes

1 tablespoon olive oil

1 pound ground beef

4 ounces shredded iceberg lettuce

8 cherry tomatoes, halved

2 teaspoons dried oregano

2 teaspoons ground cumin

2 teaspoons paprika

¼ cup low-carb salsa

¼ cup shredded Mexican blend cheese

1 avocado, pitted, peeled, and diced

Fresh cilantro leaves, for garnish

1 jalapeño, sliced, for garnish (optional)

Sour cream, for serving (optional)

In a large skillet, heat the oil over medium heat. Add the ground beef and cook, breaking apart with a wooden spoon, for about 10 minutes, or until browned all over. While the meat is cooking, place the lettuce and tomatoes in a large serving bowl. Drain any excess oil from the cooked meat. Stir in the oregano, cumin, paprika, and salsa. Remove from the heat, and spoon the beef over the salad. Top with the cheese, then garnish with the avocado, cilantro, and jalapeño (if using). Toss everything or leave in layers. Serve immediately with sour cream, if using.

Per Serving: Calories: 457; Fat: 36g; Protein: 24g; Total Carbs: 11g; Fiber: 6g; Net Carbs: 5g; **Macros:** Fat: 70%; Protein: 22%; Carbs: 8%

Spinach Salad with Bacon and Soft-Boiled Eggs

SERVES 4 | PREP TIME: 10 minutes | COOK TIME: 12 to 13 minutes

4 large eggs

5 ounces applewood smoked bacon, cut into pieces

2 tablespoons minced red onion or shallots

2 tablespoons extra-virgin olive oil

1 (10-ounce) package fresh spinach

1 teaspoon apple cider vinegar

Sea salt

Freshly ground black pepper

Place the eggs in a small saucepan and cover with fresh water. Bring to a simmer, remove from the heat and cover for 12 minutes. Remove the eggs to an ice-water bath and peel when cool enough to handle. Slice each of the eggs in half lengthwise. Meanwhile, cook the bacon in a large skillet over medium-low heat until the bacon is crisp, about 10 minutes. Transfer it to a separate dish. Add the olive oil and onion or shallots to the skillet and cook for 2 to 3 minutes to soften. Add the spinach to the pan and cook for about 1 minute, just until wilted but not yet losing its liquid. Sprinkle with the vinegar and season generously with salt and pepper. Divide the spinach among the serving plates and top with equal amounts of the cooked bacon. Place two egg halves on top of each salad.

Per Serving: Calories: 352; Fat: 30g; Protein: 16g; Total Carbs: 4g; Fiber: 2g; Net Carbs: 2g; Macros: Fat: 78%; Protein: 18%; Carbs: 4%

Asian Shrimp Salad

SERVES 4 | PREP TIME: 25 minutes

⅓ cup extra-virgin olive oil
Juice of 1 lime
2 tablespoons soy sauce
2 teaspoons sambal oelek
1 teaspoon fish sauce
1 (7g) stevia packet
4 cups shredded
  romaine lettuce
½ cup julienned snow peas
½ cup julienned red
  bell pepper
¼ cup chopped fresh cilantro
½ pound chopped
  cooked shrimp
½ cup chopped peanuts,
  for garnish

In a small bowl, whisk the olive oil, lime juice, soy sauce, sambal oelek, fish sauce, and stevia. Set aside. In a large bowl, toss the romaine, snow peas, red pepper, and cilantro. Add the dressing, and toss to coat. Arrange the salad on 4 plates, and evenly divide the shrimp among the salads. Top each salad with peanuts, and serve.

Per Serving: Calories: 374; Fat: 31g; Protein: 19g; Total Carbs: 8g; Fiber: 3g; Net Carbs: 5g; Macros: Fat: 72%; Protein: 20%; Carbs: 8%

Shrimp & Avocado Salad

1 SERVING | PREP TIME: 10 minutes

2 cups mixed greens
4 cherry tomatoes, halved
1 scallion, finely sliced
1 avocado, pitted, peeled,
  and diced
6 ounces cooked shrimp
2 tablespoons simple balsamic
  vinaigrette

Place the mixed greens in a medium bowl. Top with the tomatoes, scallion, avocado, and shrimp. Drizzle the simple balsamic vinaigrette onto the salad.

Per Serving: Calories: 674; Fat: 42g; Protein: 45g; Total Carbs: 29g; Fiber: 16g; Net Carbs: 13g; Macros: Fat: 56%; Protein: 27%; Carbs: 17%

Crab Salad Lettuce Cups

SERVES 4 | PREP TIME: 25 minutes, plus 15 minutes to marinate | COOK TIME: 20 minutes

1 pound jumbo lump crab
1 large egg
6 tablespoons aioli or avocado
  oil mayonnaise, divided
2 tablespoons Dijon mustard
½ cup almond flour
¼ cup minced red onion
2 teaspoons smoked paprika
1 teaspoon celery salt
1 teaspoon garlic powder
1 teaspoon dried dill (optional)
½ teaspoon freshly ground
  black pepper
¼ cup extra-virgin olive oil
4 large Bibb lettuce leaves,
  thick spine removed

Place the crabmeat in a large bowl and pick out any visible shells, then break apart the meat with a fork. In a small bowl, whisk the

egg, 2 tablespoons aioli, and Dijon mustard. Add to the crabmeat and blend with a fork. Add the almond flour, red onion, paprika, celery salt, garlic powder, dill (if using), and pepper and combine well. Let sit at room temperature for 10 to 15 minutes. Form into 8 small cakes, about 2 inches in diameter. In a large skillet, heat the olive oil over medium-high heat. Fry the cakes until browned, 2 to 3 minutes per side. Cover the skillet, reduce the heat to low, and cook for another 6 to 8 minutes, or until set in the center. Remove from the skillet. To serve, wrap 2 small crab cakes in each lettuce leaf and top with 1 tablespoon aioli.

Per Serving: (2 crab cakes): Calories: 344; Fat: 24g; Protein: 24g; Total Carbs: 8g; Fiber: 2g; Net Carbs: 6g; Macros: Fat: 63%; Protein: 28%; Carbs: 9%

Greek Salad with Shrimp

SERVES 4 | PREP TIME: 10 minutes

¼ cup extra-virgin olive oil
2 tablespoons white
  wine vinegar
1 teaspoon minced
  fresh thyme
1 teaspoon minced
  fresh oregano
1 teaspoon minced garlic
Sea salt
Freshly ground black pepper
8 cups roughly chopped
  romaine lettuce
1 small red onion, halved and
  thinly sliced
1 cup roughly chopped
  tomatoes
1 cup diced, peeled cucumber
½ cup pitted Kalamata olives
4 ounces feta cheese,
  crumbled
1 pound cooked shrimp,
  tails removed

In a small jar, combine the olive oil, vinegar, thyme, oregano, and garlic. Add salt and pepper. Cover tightly with a lid and shake vigorously. In a large bowl, toss the romaine lettuce, onion, tomatoes, cucumber, and olives. Pour the dressing over the salad and mix to coat thoroughly. Divide the salad among the serving plates. Top with the feta cheese and cooked shrimp.

Per Serving: Calories: 382; Fat: 25g; Protein: 30g; Total Carbs: 9g; Fiber: 3g; Net Carbs: 6g; Macros: Fat: 59%; Protein: 31%; Carbs: 10%

Smoked Trout Salad

SERVES 4 | PREP TIME: 25 minutes

½ cup extra-virgin olive oil
¼ cup freshly squeezed
  lemon juice
1 teaspoon chopped chives
Sea salt
Freshly ground black pepper
2 cups watercress
2 cups spinach
½ red bell pepper, chopped
½ cup cherry tomatoes,
  quartered
8 ounces smoked trout
1 avocado, peeled, pitted,
  and sliced
2 tablespoons chopped dill

In a small bowl, whisk the olive oil, lemon juice, and chives. Season the dressing with salt and pepper, and set aside. Arrange the watercress, spinach, red pepper, cherry tomatoes, trout, avocado, and dill on 4 plates. Drizzle the dressing over the salads, and serve.

Per Serving: Calories: 444; Fat: 40g; Protein: 20g; Total Carbs: 5g; Fiber: 3g; Net Carbs: 2g; Macros: Fat: 78%; Protein: 17%; Carbs: 5%

Omega-3 Salad

SERVES 2 | PREP TIME: 10 minutes

6 cups baby arugula or spinach	2 tablespoons minced scallions, both white and green parts, or red onion
1 (4-ounce) can olive oil-packed tuna, mackerel, or salmon	1 medium avocado, thinly sliced
¼ cup minced fresh parsley	¼ cup roasted pumpkin or sunflower seeds
10 green or black olives, pitted and halved	6 tablespoons vinaigrette

Divide the greens between bowls. In a small bowl, combine the can of fish and its oil with the parsley, olives, and onion. Divide the fish mixture evenly on top of greens. Divide the avocado slices and pumpkin seeds between the bowls. Drizzle with 3 tablespoons of dressing and toss to coat.

Per Serving: Calories: 716; Fat: 61g; Protein: 31g; Total Carbs: 16g; Fiber: 11g; Net Carbs: 5g; Macros: Fat: 77%; Protein: 17%; Carbs: 6%

Shrimp Ceviche Salad

SERVES 4 | PREP TIME: 15 minutes, plus 2 hours to marinate

1 pound fresh shrimp, peeled, deveined and halved lengthwise	2 tablespoons freshly squeezed lemon juice
1 small red or yellow bell pepper, cut into ½-inch chunks	2 tablespoons freshly squeezed clementine juice or orange juice
½ English cucumber, peeled and cut into ½-inch chunks	½ cup extra-virgin olive oil
½ small red onion, cut into thin slivers	1 teaspoon salt
¼ cup chopped fresh cilantro or flat-leaf Italian parsley	½ teaspoon freshly ground black pepper
⅓ cup freshly squeezed lime juice	2 ripe avocados, peeled, pitted, and cut into ½-inch chunks

In a large glass bowl, combine the shrimp, bell pepper, cucumber, onion, and cilantro. In a small bowl, whisk the lime, lemon, and clementine juices, olive oil, salt, and pepper. Pour the mixture over the shrimp and veggies and toss to coat. Cover and refrigerate for at least 2 hours, or up to 8 hours. Give the mixture a toss every 30 minutes for the first 2 hours to make sure all the shrimp "cook" in the juices. Add the cut avocado just before serving and toss to combine.

Per Serving: Calories: 497; Fat: 40g; Protein: 25g; Total Carbs: 14g; Fiber: 6g; Net Carbs: 8g; Macros: Fat: 69%; Protein: 21%; Carbs: 10%

Mint-Marinated Artichoke Hearts

SERVES 2 | PREP TIME: 5 minutes | COOK TIME: 0 minutes

1 cup drained jarred artichoke hearts	Zest and juice of 1 lemon
2 tablespoons extra-virgin olive oil	1 garlic clove, finely minced
	Sea salt
1 tablespoon minced fresh mint	Freshly ground black pepper

In a small bowl, toss the artichoke hearts, olive oil, mint, lemon zest and juice, and garlic. Season with salt and pepper. Serve immediately, or cover and refrigerate until ready to serve.

Per Serving: Calories: 212; Fat: 20g; Protein: 1g; Total Carbs: 9g; Fiber: 2g; Net Carbs: 7g; Macros: Fat: 85%; Protein: 1%; Carbs: 14%

Bacon-Wrapped Asparagus Bundles

SERVES 4 | PREP TIME: 5 minutes | COOK TIME: 15 to 17 minutes

1 bunch asparagus, ends trimmed	Sea salt
	Freshly ground black pepper
2 tablespoons extra-virgin olive oil	8 bacon slices

Preheat the oven to 375°F. Line a baking sheet with parchment paper. Coat the asparagus in the olive oil and season generously with salt and pepper. Place 3 to 4 asparagus spears on a slice of bacon and roll the meat around to hold the asparagus together. Place it on the baking sheet. Repeat with the remaining asparagus and bacon. Bake for 15 to 17 minutes, or until the asparagus is wilted and the bacon is crispy.

Per Serving: (2 bundles) Calories: 202; Fat: 17g; Protein: 10g; Total Carbs: 4g; Fiber: 2g; Net Carbs: 3g; Macros: Fat: 76%; Protein: 20%; Carbs: 4%

Prosciutto-Wrapped Asparagus and Lemon Aioli

SERVES 6 | PREP TIME: 10 minutes | COOK TIME: 5 minutes

½ cup mayonnaise	18 asparagus spears, trimmed to the same length
1 tablespoon fresh lemon juice, plus lemon slices, for garnish	2 tablespoons olive oil
1 teaspoon Dijon mustard	9 prosciutto slices, cut in half lengthwise
½ teaspoon garlic powder	½ teaspoon salt
¼ teaspoon salt	¼ teaspoon freshly ground black pepper

In a small bowl, make the aioli by mixing the mayonnaise, lemon juice, Dijon mustard, garlic powder, and salt. Preheat the oven to 425°F, and line a baking sheet with parchment paper. Place the asparagus in a gallon resealable bag. Add the olive oil. Seal and massage the bag to coat each asparagus spear. Empty the asparagus onto the lined baking sheet. Starting at the tip, wrap each asparagus spear with a piece of prosciutto, and place back on the baking sheet with about 2 inches between them. Season with the salt and pepper. Roast for 6 minutes, rotating the baking sheet halfway through and turning the asparagus. Remove from the oven, and plate. Drizzle each serving with a tablespoon of aioli, or serve the aioli as a dip. Garnish each serving with a slice of lemon.

Per Serving: (3 asparagus spears): Calories: 222; Fat: 21g; Protein: 7g; Total Carbs: 3g; Fiber: 1g; Net Carbs: 2g; Macros: Fat: 85%; Protein: 13%; Carbs: 4%

Sautéed Asparagus with Walnuts

SERVES 4 | PREP TIME: 10 minutes | COOK TIME: 5 minutes

1½ tablespoons olive oil
¾ pound asparagus, woody ends trimmed
Sea salt
Freshly ground pepper
¼ cup chopped walnuts

Place a large skillet over medium-high heat and add the olive oil. Sauté the asparagus until the spears are tender and lightly browned, about 5 minutes. Season the asparagus with salt and pepper. Remove the skillet from the heat and toss the asparagus with the walnuts. Serve.

Per serving: Calories: 124; Fat: 12g; Protein: 3g; Total Carbs: 4g; Fiber: 2g; Net Carbs: 2g; **Macros:** Fat: 81%; Protein: 9%; Carbs: 10%

Roasted Asparagus with Goat Cheese

SERVES 4 | PREP TIME: 15 minutes | COOK TIME: 15 minutes

¼ cup extra-virgin olive oil
2 teaspoons minced garlic
Juice and zest of ½ lemon
2 pounds asparagus, trimmed
1 cup goat cheese, crumbled

Preheat the oven to 425°F. In a small saucepan over medium heat, heat the olive oil. Heat the garlic, lemon juice, and lemon zest in the oil until the garlic is lightly caramelized, about 5 minutes. In a large bowl, pour the olive oil mixture over the asparagus, and toss to coat. Arrange the asparagus on a baking sheet, and sprinkle the goat cheese evenly over the vegetables. Roast the asparagus in the oven until tender, about 10 minutes, and serve.

Per Serving: Calories: 284; Fat: 23g; Protein: 14g; Total Carbs: 19g; Fiber: 5g; Net Carbs: 5g; **Macros:** Fat: 61%; Protein: 17%; Carbs: 22%

Citrus Asparagus with Pistachios

SERVES 4 | PREP TIME: 10 minutes | COOK TIME: 15 minutes

5 tablespoons extra-virgin olive oil, divided
Zest and juice of 2 clementines or 1 orange (about ¼ cup juice and 1 tablespoon zest)
Zest and juice of 1 lemon
1 tablespoon red wine vinegar
1 teaspoon salt, divided
¼ teaspoon freshly ground black pepper
½ cup shelled pistachios
1 pound fresh asparagus trimmed
1 tablespoon water

In a small bowl, whisk ¼ cup olive oil, the clementine and lemon juices and zests, vinegar, ½ teaspoon salt, and pepper. Set aside. In a medium dry skillet, toast the pistachios over medium-high heat until lightly browned, 2 to 3 minutes. Transfer to a cutting board and coarsely chop. In a skillet, heat the remaining 1 tablespoon olive oil over medium-high heat. Add the asparagus and sauté for 2 to 3 minutes. Sprinkle with the remaining ½ teaspoon salt and add the water. Reduce the heat to medium-low, cover, and cook until tender, another 2 to 4 minutes. Transfer the cooked asparagus to a serving dish. Add the pistachios to the dressing and whisk to combine. Pour the dressing over the warm asparagus and toss to coat.

Per Serving: Calories: 284; Fat: 24g; Protein: 6g; Total Carbs: 11g; Fiber: 4g; Net Carbs: 7g; **Macros:** Fat: 76%; Protein: 9%; Carbs: 15%

Creamed Broccoli

SERVES 4 | PREP TIME: 5 minutes | COOK TIME: 16 minutes

1 tablespoon olive oil
2 garlic cloves, minced
Pinch red pepper flakes
1 bunch broccoli, broken into florets, stems chopped
½ cup chicken bone broth or low-sodium chicken broth
Sea salt
½ cup heavy (whipping) cream

In a large skillet with a lid, heat the olive oil over medium heat. Add the garlic and red pepper flakes. Cook for about 1 minute, just until fragrant. Add the broccoli and broth. Season with salt. Cover the skillet, and cook until the broccoli is tender, about 15 minutes. Remove the lid, and stir in the heavy cream. Use an immersion blender or a potato masher to break up the broccoli.

Per Serving: Calories: 202; Fat: 17g; Protein: 8g; Total Carbs: 10g; Fiber: 5g; Net Carbs: 5g; **Macros:** Fat: 76%; Protein: 16%; Carbs: 8%

Creamy Broccoli Casserole

SERVES 6 | PREP TIME: 15 minutes | COOK TIME: 6 hours on low

1 tablespoon extra-virgin olive oil
1 pound broccoli, cut into florets
1 pound cauliflower, cut into florets
¼ cup almond flour
2 cups coconut milk
½ teaspoon ground nutmeg
Pinch freshly ground black pepper
1½ cups shredded Gouda cheese, divided

Lightly grease the insert of the slow cooker with the olive oil. Place the broccoli and cauliflower in the insert. In a small bowl, stir the almond flour, coconut milk, nutmeg, pepper, and 1 cup of the cheese. Pour the coconut milk mixture over the vegetables and top the casserole with the remaining ½ cup of the cheese. Cover and cook on low for 6 hours. Serve warm.

Per Serving: Calories: 377; Fat: 32g; Protein: 16g; Total Carbs: 12g; Fiber: 6g; Net Carbs: 6g; **Macros:** Fat: 72%; Protein: 16%; Carbs: 12%

Roasted Broccoli

1 SERVING | PREP TIME: 5 minutes | COOK TIME: 25 minutes

1½ cups broccoli florets
2 tablespoons avocado oil
2 garlic cloves, thinly sliced
Juice of ½ lemon
2 tablespoons raw sliced almonds
1 teaspoon freshly grated Parmesan cheese (optional)

Preheat the oven to 425°F; line a baking sheet with parchment paper. In a large bowl, toss the broccoli, oil, and garlic until well combined. Season with salt and freshly ground black pepper. Spread the broccoli evenly on the baking sheet, drizzling any excess oil on top, and put the baking sheet in the oven. After 15 minutes, drizzle the lemon juice over the broccoli and top with the almonds and cheese (if using). Continue to bake for an additional 5 to 10 minutes, until the florets are crispy and caramelized.

Per Serving: Calories: 192; Fat: 10g; Protein: 7g; Total Carbs: 16g; Fiber: 7g; Net Carbs: 9g; **Macros:** Fat: 52%; Protein: 15%; Carbs: 33%

Sesame-Roasted Broccoli

SERVES 4 | PREP TIME: 5 minutes | COOK TIME: 10 minutes

Extra-virgin olive oil, for
  greasing
4 cups broccoli, cut into
  small florets
3 tablespoons sesame oil

1 teaspoon garlic
1 teaspoon freshly squeezed
  lemon juice
2 teaspoons sesame seeds

Preheat the oven to 425°F. Lightly oil a baking sheet with olive oil. In a large bowl, toss the broccoli florets with the sesame oil and garlic. Transfer the broccoli to the baking sheet, and spread it out in a single layer. Roast the broccoli until tender, about 10 minutes. Transfer the roasted broccoli to a serving bowl, top with the lemon juice and sesame seeds, and serve.

Per Serving: Calories: 131; Fat: 11g; Protein: 3g; Total Carbs: 6g; Fiber: 3g; Net Carbs: 3g; **Macros:** Fat: 73%; Protein: 9%; Carbs: 18%

Broccoli Stir-Fry

SERVES 1 | PREP TIME: 5 minutes | COOK TIME: 10 minutes

1 cup fresh spinach
1 tablespoon coconut oil
½ cup broccoli florets
1 cup frozen cauliflower rice
2 ounces seitan strips or cubes

1 tablespoon toasted
  sesame oil
1 tablespoon soy sauce
½ avocado, sliced

In a dry, nonstick pan over medium heat, wilt the spinach leaves. Remove from the heat and transfer to a serving plate. Turn the temperature up to medium high, and in the same skillet, melt the coconut oil. Add the broccoli and frozen cauliflower rice. Cook for 5 to 6 minutes or until tender. Place the vegetables on the wilted spinach. Top with the seitan. In a small bowl, mix the sesame oil and soy sauce. Pour the dressing over the seitan and vegetables. Top with the avocado slices and enjoy warm.

Per Serving: Calories: 664; Fat: 44g; Protein: 49g; Total Carbs: 18g; Fiber: 13g; Net Carbs: 5g; **Macros:** Fat: 60%; Protein: 30%; Carbs: 10%

Garlicky Broccoli Rabe with Artichokes

SERVES 4 | PREP TIME: 5 minutes | COOK TIME: 10 minutes

2 pounds fresh broccoli rabe
½ cup extra-virgin olive
  oil, divided
3 garlic cloves, finely minced
1 teaspoon salt
1 teaspoon red pepper flakes

1 (14-ounce) can artichoke
  hearts, drained and
  quartered
1 tablespoon water
2 tablespoons red
  wine vinegar
Freshly ground black pepper

Trim away any thick lower stems and yellow leaves from the broccoli rabe and discard. Cut into individual florets with a couple inches of thin stem attached. In a large skillet, heat ¼ cup olive oil over medium-high heat. Add the trimmed broccoli, garlic, salt, and red pepper flakes and sauté for 5 minutes, until the broccoli begins to soften. Add the artichoke hearts and sauté for another 2 minutes. Add the water and reduce the heat to low. Cover and simmer until the broccoli stems are tender, 3 to 5 minutes. In a small bowl, whisk remaining ¼ cup olive oil and the vinegar. Drizzle over the broccoli and artichokes. Season with ground black pepper, if desired.

Per Serving: Calories: 385; Fat: 35g; Protein: 11g; Total Carbs: 18g; Fiber: 10g; Net Carbs: 8g; **Macros:** Fat: 81%; Protein: 8%; Carbs: 11%

Brussels Sprouts Casserole

SERVES 8 | PREP TIME: 15 minutes | COOK TIME: 30 minutes

8 bacon slices
1 pound Brussels sprouts,
  blanched for 10 minutes and
  cut into quarters

1 cup shredded Swiss
  cheese, divided
¾ cup heavy (whipping) cream

Preheat the oven to 400°F. Place a skillet over medium-high heat and cook the bacon until it is crispy, about 6 minutes. Reserve 1 tablespoon of bacon fat to grease the casserole dish and roughly chop the cooked bacon. Lightly oil a casserole dish with the reserved bacon fat and set aside. In a medium bowl, toss the Brussels sprouts with the chopped bacon and ½ cup of cheese and transfer the mixture to the casserole dish. Pour the heavy cream over the Brussels sprouts and top the casserole with the remaining ½ cup of cheese. Bake until the cheese is melted and lightly browned and the vegetables are heated through, about 20 minutes. Serve.

Per serving: Calories: 299; Fat: 11g; Protein: 12g; Total Carbs: 7g; Fiber: 3g; Net Carbs: 4g; **Macros:** Fat: 77%; Protein: 15%; Carbs: 8%

Crispy Brussels Sprouts

1 SERVING | PREP TIME: 5 minutes | COOK TIME: 25 minutes

⅓ pound Brussels sprouts,
  trimmed and thinly sliced
  (about 1½ cups)
2 garlic cloves, minced

2 tablespoons avocado oil
Juice of ½ lemon
1 teaspoon freshly grated
  Parmesan cheese (optional)

Preheat the oven to 400°F; line a baking sheet with parchment paper. Place the Brussels sprouts and garlic on the lined baking sheet. Cover well with the oil, and season with salt and freshly ground black pepper to taste. Using your hands, mix all the ingredients, then spread everything out in one even layer. Roast in the oven for 20 to 25 minutes, stirring every 8 to 10 minutes, until the Brussels sprouts are tender. Transfer to a bowl, drizzle with the lemon juice, and stir to combine. Sprinkle with the cheese (if using).

Per Serving: Calories: 385; Fat: 29g; Protein: 8g; Total Carbs: 23g; Fiber: 10g; Net Carbs: 13g; **Macros:** Fat: 68%; Protein: 8%; Carbs: 24%

Roasted Brussels Sprouts & Poached Eggs

SERVES 2 | PREP TIME: 8 minutes | COOK TIME: 35 minutes

2 cups halved Brus-
  sels sprouts
3 tablespoons olive or
  avocado oil
1 teaspoon garlic powder
1 teaspoon salt

½ teaspoon freshly ground
  black pepper
2 large eggs
Hollandaise (page 306)
¼ teaspoon red pepper flakes
  (optional)

Preheat the oven to 400°F. Put the Brussels sprouts in a bowl, add the oil, and season with garlic powder, salt, and pepper. Stir until the sprouts are evenly coated. Spread the sprouts out evenly on a baking sheet and roast for 30 to 35 minutes, tossing halfway through. When the Brussels sprouts have about 10 more minutes to cook, poach the eggs. Bring a saucepan of water to a boil, then reduce the heat to low. Crack the eggs into a small bowl and carefully pour them into the simmering water. Turn off the heat, cover the pan, and let the eggs cook for about 5 minutes. Remove the Brussels sprouts from the oven arrange them on two plates. Using a slotted spoon, carefully remove the eggs from the water and place on top of the sprouts. Drizzle hollandaise sauce over the top, then sprinkle with the red pepper flakes (if using).

Per Serving: Calories: 310; Fat: 26g; Protein: 9g; Total Carbs: 10g; Fiber: 4g; Net Carbs: 6g; **Macros:** Fat: 75%; Protein: 12%; Carbs: 13%

Brussels Sprouts with Bacon

SERVES 4 | PREP TIME: 5 minutes | COOK TIME: 12 to 13 minutes

4 bacon slices, cut into pieces	Sea salt
1 pound Brussels sprouts, wilted outer leaves and tough stem ends removed	Freshly ground black pepper
	1 tablespoon sherry vinegar or apple cider vinegar

Cook the bacon in a large skillet over medium-low heat until the bacon renders all of its fat and begins to crisp. Transfer the bacon to a separate dish with a slotted spoon. While the bacon is cooking, shred the Brussels sprouts. Increase the heat to medium-high. Cook the shredded Brussels sprouts in the bacon fat for 2 to 3 minutes, until just wilted. Season with salt and pepper, and drizzle with the vinegar just before serving. Top each serving with the cooked bacon pieces.

Per Serving: Calories: 210; Fat: 16g; Protein: 10g; Total Carbs: 9g; Fiber: 3g; Net Carbs: 6g; **Macros:** Fat: 69%; Protein: 17%; Carbs: 14%

Brussels Sprouts with Hazelnuts

SERVES 4 | PREP TIME: 15 minutes | COOK TIME: 15 minutes

¾ pound Brussels sprouts, trimmed and halved lengthwise	4 teaspoons coconut oil, melted
	½ teaspoon ground coriander
	½ cup chopped hazelnuts

Preheat the oven to 400°F. Line a baking sheet with parchment paper. In a large bowl, toss the Brussels sprouts with the coconut oil and coriander until well coated. Spread the Brussels sprouts on a baking sheet, and bake until tender-crisp, about 15 minutes. Remove the Brussels sprouts from the oven, toss with the chopped hazelnuts, and serve.

Per Serving: Calories: 162; Fat: 13g; Protein: 6g; Total Carbs: 9g; Fiber: 5g; Net Carbs: 5g; **Macros:** Fat: 66%; Protein: 20%; Carbs: 14%

Roasted Cabbage "Steaks"

SERVES 4 | PREP TIME: 5 minutes | COOK TIME: 30 to 40 minutes

1 head white or green cabbage, sliced 1-inch thick	Salt
¼ cup olive oil	Freshly ground black pepper
1 teaspoon garlic powder	4 eggs, over-easy, for serving (optional)
1 teaspoon onion powder	

Preheat the oven to 450°F. Put the cabbage pieces on a baking sheet and brush them all over with the olive oil. Sprinkle all over with the garlic and onion powder and season with salt and pepper. Roast for 30 to 40 minutes, flipping the cabbage several times. Serve topped with eggs (if using).

Per Serving: Calories: 194; Fat: 14g; Protein: 3g; Total Carbs: 14g; Fiber: 6g; Net Carbs: 8g; **Macros:** Fat: 65%; Protein: 6%; Carbs: 29%

Sweet-Braised Red Cabbage

SERVES 8 | PREP TIME: 15 minutes | COOK TIME: 7 to 8 hours on low

1 tablespoon extra-virgin olive oil	⅛ teaspoon ground cloves
1 small red cabbage, coarsely shredded (about 6 cups)	2 tablespoons butter
½ sweet onion, thinly sliced	Salt, for seasoning
¼ cup apple cider vinegar	Freshly ground black pepper, for seasoning
3 tablespoons granulated erythritol	½ cup chopped walnuts, for garnish
2 teaspoons minced garlic	½ cup crumbled blue cheese, for garnish
½ teaspoon ground nutmeg	Pink peppercorns, for garnish (optional)

Lightly grease the insert of the slow cooker with the olive oil. Add the cabbage, onion, apple cider vinegar, erythritol, garlic, nutmeg, and cloves to the insert, stirring to mix well. Break off little slices of butter and scatter them on top of the cabbage mixture. Cover and cook on low for 7 to 8 hours. Season with salt and pepper. Serve topped with the walnuts, blue cheese, and peppercorns (if desired).

Per Serving: Calories: 152; Fat: 12g; Protein: 7g; Total Carbs: 4g; Fiber: 1g; Net Carbs: 3g; **Macros:** Fat: 71%; Protein: 18%; Carbs: 12%

Grilled Balsamic Cabbage

SERVES 4 | PREP TIME: 10 minutes | COOK TIME: 17 to 19 minutes

1 small head red cabbage	¼ teaspoon ground cumin
¼ cup extra-virgin olive oil	½ teaspoon sea salt
2 tablespoons balsamic vinegar	¼ teaspoon freshly ground black pepper
1 teaspoon Dijon mustard	

Preheat a gas or charcoal grill to medium-high. Slice the cabbage into 16 wedges. In a small bowl, whisk the olive oil, balsamic vinegar, mustard, cumin, salt, and pepper. Cut 16 small squares of aluminum foil. Place a cabbage wedge onto a square of foil and drizzle with about 1 teaspoon of the balsamic mixture. Fold the foil into a tight package. Repeat with the remaining cabbage. Place the foil packets onto the grill grate and cook for 12 to 15 minutes, until the cabbage is tender. Remove the cabbage from the foil and carefully place them directly onto the grill. Grill on each side for about 2 minutes.

Per Serving: Calories: 169; Fat: 14g; Protein: 3g; Total Carbs: 11g; Fiber: 4g; Net Carbs: 7g; **Macros:** Fat: 75%; Protein: 7%; Carbs: 18%

Asian Cabbage Stir-Fry

SERVES 4 | PREP TIME: 30 minutes | COOK TIME: 15 minutes

2 tablespoons sesame oil	½ cup cashew halves
1 sweet onion, thinly sliced	¼ cup chicken stock
2 celery stalks, thinly sliced	2 tablespoons soy sauce
1 teaspoon minced garlic	½ pound finely shredded green cabbage
½ red bell pepper, cut into thin strips	1 tablespoon sesame seeds
1 cup sliced mushrooms	

In a large skillet over medium heat, heat the sesame oil. Sauté the onion, celery, and garlic until softened, about 5 minutes. Add the red pepper, mushrooms, and cashews, and stir-fry for 3 minutes. Stir in the chicken stock, soy sauce, and cabbage. Cover the skillet, and steam the cabbage until it is tender, about 5 minutes. Top with the sesame seeds, and serve.

Per Serving: Calories: 151; Fat: 12g; Protein: 4g; Total Carbs: 10g; Fiber: 4g; Net Carbs: 6g; **Macros:** Fat: 66%; Protein: 10%; Carbs: 24%

Roasted Cauliflower with Parsley and Pine Nuts

SERVES 4 | PREP TIME: 5 minutes | COOK TIME: 30 minutes

1 small head cauliflower, broken into small florets
4 garlic cloves, minced
Zest and juice of 1 lemon
¼ cup olive oil
Sea salt

Freshly ground black pepper
¼ cup roughly chopped fresh parsley
¼ cup roughly chopped toasted pine nuts

Preheat the oven to 400°F. Spread the cauliflower out on a rimmed baking sheet and add the garlic, lemon zest, and olive oil. Toss to coat, and season with salt and pepper. Roast for 30 minutes, or until the cauliflower is deeply browned on the bottom and soft. Toss with the lemon juice, parsley, and pine nuts before serving.

Per Serving: Calories: 192; Fat: 18g; Protein: 2g; Total Carbs: 7g; Fiber: 3g; Net Carbs: 4g; **Macros:** Fat: 84%; Protein: 4%; Carbs: 12%

Thai-Inspired Peanut Roasted Cauliflower

SERVES 2 | PREP TIME: 10 minutes | COOK TIME: 20 minutes

½ head cauliflower, cut into bite-size florets
1 tablespoon olive oil
Salt
Freshly ground black pepper
½ cup unsweetened full-fat coconut milk

2 tablespoons sugar-free peanut butter
¼ teaspoon red curry paste
1 clove garlic, minced
1 tablespoon chopped fresh or dried parsley

Preheat the oven to 400°F. On a baking sheet, arrange the cauliflower in a single layer. Drizzle with the olive oil and season with salt and pepper. Roast for 20 minutes or until the edges are brown. While the cauliflower is cooking, in a blender, combine the coconut milk, peanut butter, curry paste, and garlic. Process until smooth. Divide the cauliflower between two plates and drizzle the peanut sauce over top. Garnish with the parsley and serve.

Per serving: Calories: 290; Fat: 27g; Protein: 8g; Total Carbs: 9g; Fiber: 3g; Net Carbs: 6g; **Macros:** Fat: 84%; Protein: 11%; Carbs: 5%

Cauliflower Rice

SERVES 4 | PREP TIME: 5 minutes | COOK TIME: 5 minutes

1 large head of cauliflower, broken into florets

1 tablespoon coconut oil
Sea salt

Pulse the cauliflower in a food processor until coarsely ground, about the texture of rice. Heat the coconut oil in a large skillet over medium-high heat and stir-fry the cauliflower for 5 minutes, until just heated through. Season with salt.

Per Serving: Calories: 82; Fat: 4g; Protein: 4g; Total Carbs: 11g; Fiber: 5g; Net Carbs: 6g; **Macros:** Fat: 44%; Protein: 20%; Carbs: 36%

Mexican Cauliflower Rice

1 SERVING | PREP TIME: 5 minutes | COOK TIME: 15 minutes

½ head cauliflower, cut into small florets (about 1½ cups)
1 tablespoon avocado oil
1 garlic clove, minced
¼ cup tomato sauce
¼ cup water or broth

1 teaspoon onion powder
½ teaspoon ground cumin
Juice of ½ lime
1 tablespoon minced fresh cilantro (optional)

Place the cauliflower florets in a food processor, and process until the mixture resembles rice. In a large skillet, heat the oil over medium heat. Add the cauliflower "rice" and garlic to the skillet, and cook for 5 minutes. Stir in the tomato sauce, water, onion powder, and cumin. Season with salt and freshly ground black pepper to taste. Cover and cook for 5 to 10 more minutes, until tender. Uncover, toss with the lime juice, and garnish with the cilantro (if using).

Per Serving: Calories: 219; Fat: 15g; Protein: 4g; Total Carbs: 17g; Fiber: 5g; Net Carbs: 12g; **Macros:** Fat: 62%; Protein: 7%; Carbs: 31%

Nutty Miso Cauliflower Rice

SERVES 4 | PREP TIME: 15 minutes | COOK TIME: 7 minutes

3 cups cauliflower
1 cup fennel
¼ cup walnuts
1 tablespoon extra-virgin olive oil

2 teaspoons white miso
1 teaspoon freshly squeezed lemon juice

In a food processor, pulse the cauliflower, fennel, and walnuts until the mixture resembles coarse crumbs. In a large skillet over medium heat, heat the olive oil. Sauté the cauliflower mixture in the oil until heated through and tender, about 6 minutes. Stir in the miso and lemon juice, and sauté for 1 minute. Remove the "rice" from the heat, and serve.

Per Serving: Calories: 167; Fat: 14g; Protein: 5g; Total Carbs: 8g; Fiber: 5g; Net Carbs: 3g; **Macros:** Fat: 71%; Protein: 11%; Carbs: 18%

Green Goddess Buddha Bowl

SERVES 1 | PREP TIME: 10 minutes | COOK TIME: 5 minutes

2 cups fresh spinach
2 tablespoons avocado oil
4 broccolini spears
⅛ teaspoon salt
⅛ teaspoon freshly ground black pepper
⅓ cup frozen cauliflower rice, thawed

2 tablespoons shredded carrots
½ avocado, sliced
1 tablespoon almond butter, melted
1 tablespoon minced fresh cilantro

Place the spinach in the bottom of a medium serving bowl. In a skillet over medium-high heat, heat the avocado oil. Add the broccolini and sauté for 2 to 3 minutes. Season with the salt and pepper and transfer it to the bowl containing the spinach. Add the cauliflower rice to the skillet and cook for 3 minutes. Add it to the serving bowl. Top with the carrots and avocado. Drizzle with the melted almond butter, sprinkle the cilantro on top, and serve.

Per Serving: Calories: 571; Fat: 51g; Protein: 9g; Total Carbs: 19g; Fiber: 11g; Net Carbs: 8g; **Macros:** Fat: 80%; Protein: 6%; Carbs: 14%

Raw Tabouli

SERVES 4 | PREP TIME: 5 minutes

4 cups cauliflower rice
4 cups chopped fresh parsley
1 cup finely diced tomato
½ cup finely diced yellow onion
2 cups finely diced cucumber

½ cup chopped fresh mint
Juice of 3 lemons
½ cup cold-pressed olive oil
Sea salt
Freshly ground black pepper

In a medium bowl, stir the cauliflower rice, parsley, tomato, onion, cucumber, and mint. Dress with the lemon juice and olive oil, and season with salt and pepper. Place the tabouli in the refrigerator to chill for up to 1 hour to allow the flavors to combine, then serve.

Per Serving: Calories: 317; Fat: 28g; Protein: 5g; Total Carbs: 17g; Fiber: 6g; Net Carbs: 11g; **Macros:** Fat: 74%; Protein: 6%; Carbs: 20%

Mediterranean Cauliflower Tabbouleh

SERVES 6 | PREP TIME: 15 minutes, plus 30 minutes to chill | COOK TIME: 5 minutes

6 tablespoons extra-virgin olive oil, divided
4 cups riced cauliflower
3 garlic cloves, finely minced
1½ teaspoons salt
½ teaspoon freshly ground black pepper
½ large cucumber, peeled, seeded, and chopped
½ cup chopped mint leaves
½ cup chopped Italian parsley

½ cup chopped pitted Kalamata olives
2 tablespoons minced red onion
Juice of 1 lemon (about 2 tablespoons)
2 cups baby arugula or spinach leaves
2 medium avocados, peeled, pitted, and diced
1 cup quartered cherry tomatoes

In a large skillet, heat 2 tablespoons of olive oil over medium-high heat. Add the riced cauliflower, garlic, salt, and pepper and sauté until just tender, 3 to 4 minutes. Remove from the heat and place in a large bowl. Add the cucumber, mint, parsley, olives, red onion, lemon juice, and remaining ¼ cup olive oil and toss well. Place in the refrigerator, uncovered, and refrigerate for at least 30 minutes, or up to 2 hours. Before serving, add the arugula, avocado, and tomatoes and toss to combine well. Season to taste with salt and pepper and serve cold or at room temperature.

Per Serving: Calories: 235; Fat: 21g; Protein: 4g; Total Carbs: 12g; Fiber: 6g; Net Carbs: 6g; **Macros:** Fat: 77%; Protein: 4%; Carbs: 19%

Mashed Cauliflower

SERVES 4 | PREP TIME: 5 minutes | COOK TIME: 10 minutes

1 large head cauliflower, broken into florets
¼ cup heavy (whipping) cream

2 tablespoons butter
Sea salt

Fill a large pot with 1 inch of water and add a steamer basket. Place the cauliflower in the basket, cover the pot, and bring the water to a simmer. Cook for 10 minutes, or until the cauliflower is very tender. Transfer the steamed cauliflower to a food processor along with the heavy cream, butter, and a generous pinch of sea salt. Purée until very smooth.

Per Serving: Calories: 155; Fat: 12g; Protein: 5g; Total Carbs: 11g; Fiber: 5g; Net Carbs: 6g; **Macros:** Fat: 70%; Protein: 13%; Carbs: 17%

Mashed Cauliflower with Yogurt

SERVES 4 | PREP TIME: 15 minutes | COOK TIME: 10 minutes

8 cups cauliflower
2 teaspoons minced garlic
¼ cup Greek yogurt

2 tablespoons extra-virgin olive oil, divided
2 tablespoons butter, divided
½ teaspoon sea salt

In a large saucepan over high heat, bring 3-inches of water to a boil. Place the cauliflower and garlic in a steamer basket or sieve over the water, and steam until the vegetables are very tender, about 10 minutes. Transfer the cauliflower and garlic to a food processor, and add the yogurt, olive oil, 1 tablespoon of butter, and the salt. Purée until the cauliflower is very fluffy, about 2 minutes. Transfer the cauliflower to a serving dish, dot with the remaining 1 tablespoon of butter, and serve.

Per Serving: Calories: 168; Fat: 13g; Protein: 6g; Total Carbs: 11g; Fiber: 6g; Net Carbs: 5g; **Macros:** Fat: 63%; Protein: 13%; Carbs: 24%

Cheesy Mashed Cauliflower

SERVES 4 | PREP TIME: 15 minutes | COOK TIME: 5 minutes

1 head cauliflower, chopped roughly
½ cup shredded Cheddar cheese
¼ cup heavy (whipping) cream

2 tablespoons butter, at room temperature
Sea salt
Freshly ground black pepper

Place a large saucepan filled three-quarters full with water over high heat and bring to a boil. Blanch the cauliflower until tender, about 5 minutes, and drain. Transfer the cauliflower to a food processor and add the cheese, heavy cream, and butter. Purée until very creamy and whipped. Season with salt and pepper. Serve.

Per serving: Calories: 183; Fat: 15g; Protein: 8g; Total Carbs: 6g; Fiber: 2g; Net Carbs: 4g; **Macros:** Fat: 75%; Protein: 14%; Carbs: 11%

Cauliflower-Pecan Casserole

SERVES 6 | PREP TIME: 15 minutes | COOK TIME: 6 hours on low

1 tablespoon extra-virgin olive oil
2 pounds cauliflower florets
10 bacon slices, cooked and chopped
1 cup chopped pecans
4 garlic cloves, sliced
½ teaspoon salt

½ teaspoon freshly ground black pepper
2 tablespoons freshly squeezed lemon juice
4 hard-boiled eggs, shredded, for garnish
1 scallion, white and green parts, chopped, for garnish

Lightly grease the insert of the slow cooker with the olive oil. In a medium bowl, toss the cauliflower, bacon, pecans, garlic, salt, and pepper. Transfer the mixture to the insert and sprinkle the lemon juice over the top. Cover and cook on low for 6 hours. Garnish with hard-boiled eggs and scallion and serve.

Per Serving: Calories: 280; Fat: 23g; Protein: 14g; Total Carbs: 9g; Fiber: 5g; Net Carbs: 4g; **Macros:** Fat: 69%; Protein: 19%; Carbs: 12%

Cheesy Cauliflower Mac 'n' Cheese

SERVES 6 | PREP TIME: 10 minutes | COOK TIME: 30 minutes

Nonstick cooking spray
1 cauliflower head, chopped
   into small florets
8 ounces heavy (whip-
   ping) cream
4 ounces shredded
   Cheddar cheese

4 ounces grated Parme-
   san cheese
2 ounces cream cheese
1 teaspoon salt
¼ teaspoon freshly ground
   black pepper

Preheat the oven to 375°F. Spray an 8-inch-square baking dish with cooking spray. Place the cauliflower in a microwave-safe bowl and cook for 3 minutes on high. Drain any excess liquid. In a small saucepan over medium heat, combine the heavy cream, cheddar cheese, Parmesan cheese, cream cheese, salt, and pepper. Stir until well combined, and then remove from the heat. Pour the cheese sauce over the cauliflower and toss to coat. Transfer the mixture to the prepared baking dish and cook for 25 minutes.

Per Serving: (½ cup) Calories: 324; Fat: 28g; Protein: 13g; Total Carbs: 5g; Fiber: 1g; Net Carbs: 4g; Macros: Fat: 78%; Protein: 16%; Carbs: 6%

Cauliflower Mac and Cheese

SERVES 8 | PREP TIME: 10 minutes |
COOK TIME: 30 minutes | TOTAL TIME: 45 minutes

1 teaspoon salt, divided
1 head fresh cauliflower,
   chopped into small florets
1 cup heavy (whipping) cream
⅓ cup cream cheese, cubed
1 cup shredded Ched-
   dar cheese

½ cup shredded mozza-
   rella cheese
½ teaspoon minced garlic
¼ teaspoon freshly ground
   black pepper
Cooking spray for baking pan
½ cup shredded
   Parmesan cheese

Preheat the oven to 400°F. Bring a large pot of water to a boil. Season with ½ teaspoon of salt. Carefully drop the cauliflower into the boiling water and cook for 5 minutes. Drain thoroughly, and place the florets on paper towels to drain. Put the cauliflower in a large bowl and set aside. To a large skillet over medium heat, add the heavy cream and bring to a simmer. Whisk in the cream cheese until smooth. Add the Cheddar cheese, mozzarella cheese, and garlic. Whisk until the cheeses melt, about 2 minutes. Remove the cheese sauce from heat and pour over the cauliflower. Stir to coat the florets evenly. Sprinkle with the remaining ½ teaspoon of salt and the pepper. Spray an 8-inch-square baking pan with cooking spray. Transfer the cauliflower mixture to the pan. Top with the Parmesan cheese. Place the pan in the preheated oven. Bake for 20 minutes, or until the top is browned. Cool for 5 minutes before serving.

Per Serving: Calories: 198; Fat: 17g; Protein: 10g; Total Carbs: 3g; Fiber: 1g; Net Carbs: 2g; Macros: Fat: 75%; Protein: 20%; Carbs: 5%

Cauliflower Pizza

SERVES 2 | PREP TIME: 10 minutes | COOK TIME: 30 minutes | TOTAL TIME: 40 minutes

¾ teaspoon salt, divided
2 cups cauliflower florets
1 large egg

2½ cups shredded mozzarella
   cheese, divided
½ teaspoon garlic powder

⅛ teaspoon freshly ground
   black pepper

¼ cup sugar-free pizza
   sauce, divided
10 pepperoni slices, divided

Preheat the oven to 450°F. Bring a large pot of water to a boil. Season with ½ teaspoon of salt. Add the cauliflower to the boiling water. Cook for 8 minutes. Drain thoroughly, using paper towels to soak up any excess moisture. Place the drained cauliflower into a food processor. Pulse for 1 minute until the cauliflower is "riced." Transfer the cauliflower to a large bowl. Add the egg, 1 cup of mozzarella cheese, the garlic powder, the remaining ¼ teaspoon of salt, and pepper. Stir until the cheese fully melts. Separate the cauliflower dough into two equal balls. On a parchment-lined baking sheet, spread each ball into an 8-inch crust. The crust should be very thin. Bake for 15 to 20 minutes, or until browned. The edges of the crust should almost be burned. Remove the crusts from the oven. Turn the oven to broil. Spread ⅛ cup of pizza sauce over each crust. Top each crust with ¾ cup of mozzarella cheese and half the pepperoni. Return the sheet to the oven. Bake the pizzas for 2 to 3 minutes, or until the cheese is melted and bubbling. Remove the sheet from the oven and allow the pizzas to cool for 3 to 5 minutes before slicing and serving.

Per Serving: (1 8-inch pizza): Calories: 457; Fat: 31g; Protein: 36g; Total Carbs: 11g; Fiber: 2g; Net Carbs: 9g; Macros: Fat: 60%; Protein: 31%; Carbs: 9%

Roasted Cauliflower Lettuce Cups

SERVES 4 | PREP TIME: 10 minutes | COOK TIME: 20 minutes

Nonstick cooking spray
1 head cauliflower, chopped
1 tablespoon avocado oil
½ teaspoon minced garlic
2 tablespoons curry powder
½ teaspoon salt

¼ teaspoon freshly ground
   black pepper
4 butter lettuce leaves
2 avocados, sliced
¼ cup cashews
¼ cup ranch dressing

Preheat the oven to 425°F. Grease a rimmed baking sheet with cooking spray and put the cauliflower florets on it. Pour the avocado oil on the florets and toss to coat; sprinkle the florets with the garlic, curry powder, salt, and pepper. Roast for about 20 minutes, or until the tops of the florets are slightly browned. Remove from the oven and allow to cool for 5 to 7 minutes. Place a scoop of florets into each butter lettuce cup and top each with ¼ of the avocado slices. Sprinkle each cup with 1 tablespoon of cashews and 1 tablespoon of ranch dressing.

Per Serving: Calories: 349; Fat: 29g; Protein: 5g; Total Carbs: 17g; Fiber: 9g; Net Carbs: 8g; Macros: Fat: 75%; Protein: 6%; Carbs: 19%

Celery Root Purée

SERVES 4 | PREP TIME: 10 minutes | COOK TIME: 30 minutes

4 cups peeled, diced celeriac
½ cup diced onion
1 garlic clove, minced
1 sprig fresh thyme

1 cup vegetable broth or
   chicken bone broth
1 cup heavy (whipping) cream
Sea salt
2 tablespoons butter

Place the celeriac, onion, garlic, thyme, broth, and cream in a large pot. Season generously with salt. Bring to a simmer over medium-low heat. Cover and cook for 30 minutes, until the celeriac is tender. Discard the thyme sprig. Strain the vegetables and transfer to a food processor, reserving the cooking liquid. Purée until smooth, adding some cooking liquid as needed to reach the desired consistency. Stir in the butter.

Per Serving: Calories: 307; Fat: 28g; Protein: 3g; Total Carbs: 13g; Fiber: 2g; Net Carbs: 11g; **Macros:** Fat: 82%; Protein: 3%; Carbs: 15%

Sautéed Swiss Chard

SERVES 4 | PREP TIME: 15 minutes | COOK TIME: 25 minutes

6 bacon slices, chopped
2 tablespoons butter
2 tablespoons chopped
   sweet onion
1 teaspoon minced garlic
8 cups Swiss chard
Sea salt

In a large skillet over medium heat, cook the bacon until crispy, about 5 minutes. Add the butter to the skillet, and melt. Sauté the onion and garlic until the vegetables are softened, about 3 minutes. Stir in the chard, and sauté, stirring occasionally, until the greens wilt, about 20 minutes. Season with salt, and serve.

Per Serving: Calories: 102; Fat: 8g; Protein: 5g; Total Carbs: 4g; Fiber: 2g; Net Carbs: 2g; **Macros:** Fat: 67%; Protein: 19%; Carbs: 14%

Braised Greens with Olives and Walnuts

SERVES 4 | PREP TIME: 5 minutes | COOK TIME: 20 minutes

8 cups fresh greens (such as kale, mustard greens, spinach, or chard)
2 to 4 garlic cloves, finely minced
½ cup roughly chopped pitted green or black olives
½ cup roughly chopped shelled walnuts
¼ cup extra-virgin olive oil
2 tablespoons red wine vinegar
1 to 2 teaspoons freshly chopped herbs such as oregano, basil, rosemary, or thyme

Remove the tough stems from the greens and chop into bite-size pieces. Place in a large rimmed skillet or pot. Turn the heat to high and add the minced garlic and enough water to just cover the greens. Bring to a boil, reduce the heat to low, and simmer until the greens are wilted and tender and most of the liquid has evaporated, adding more if the greens start to burn. Tender greens such as spinach, should take 5 minutes, and tougher greens such as chard up to 20 minutes. Remove from the heat and add the chopped olives and walnuts. In a small bowl, whisk olive oil, vinegar, and herbs. Drizzle over the cooked greens and toss to coat. Serve warm.

Per Serving: Calories: 280; Fat: 20g; Protein: 7g; Total Carbs: 18g; Fiber: 5g; Net Carbs: 13g; **Macros:** Fat: 65%; Protein: 10%; Carbs: 25%

Quick Pickled Cucumbers

SERVES 4 | PREP TIME: 5 minutes, plus 30 minutes to marinate | COOK TIME: 0 minutes

1 English cucumber, cut into ½-inch pieces
¼ cup white wine vinegar
2 tablespoons minced fresh dill
1 teaspoon coriander seeds
¼ teaspoon red pepper flakes
¼ teaspoon sea salt

In a glass mixing bowl, toss all of the ingredients. Cover and refrigerate for at least 30 minutes before serving.

Per Serving: Calories: 13; Fat: 0g; Protein: 1g; Total Carbs: 2g; Fiber: 1g; Net Carbs: 1g; **Macros:** Fat: 0%; Protein: 23%; Carbs: 67%

Spiced Cucumbers

1 SERVING | PREP TIME: 5 minutes, plus 30 minutes to chill

½ cucumber, peeled and diced
1 scallion, finely sliced
½ tablespoon sesame oil
½ tablespoon rice vinegar
½ teaspoon sesame seeds
¼ teaspoon red pepper flakes

Put the diced cucumber in a small bowl. Add the scallion, sesame oil, rice vinegar, sesame seeds, and red pepper flakes; stir to combine. Cover the bowl with plastic wrap, and refrigerate for at least 30 minutes or up to 24 hours.

Per Serving: Calories: 108; Fat: 8g; Protein: 2g; Total Carbs: 7g; Fiber: 2g; Net Carbs: 5g; **Macros:** Fat: 67%; Protein: 7%; Carbs: 26%

Eggplant Lasagna

SERVES 4 | PREP TIME: 10 minutes | COOK TIME: 1 hour 10 minutes

Nonstick cooking spray
1 large eggplant, cut into ⅛-inch-thick slices
Salt
1½ cups ricotta cheese
1 large egg
1 (28-ounce) can whole tomatoes, drained
1 cup grated Parmesan cheese
2 cups shredded mozzarella cheese
2 tablespoons dried parsley

Preheat the oven to 375°F. Grease an 8-inch-square baking dish with cooking spray. Sprinkle the eggplant slices with salt. Allow them to sit for 15 minutes and then blot with a paper towel. In a dry skillet over high heat, cook the eggplant slices for 3 minutes on each side. Remove and set aside. In a medium bowl, combine the ricotta cheese and egg, and stir well. Crush a handful of tomatoes and place them in the bottom of the baking dish. Layer a few slices of eggplant, a layer of cheese sauce, and another layer of crushed tomatoes. Repeat this layering until the dish is full. Sprinkle the Parmesan and mozzarella cheeses on top, followed by the parsley. Cover the dish with aluminum foil and bake for 40 minutes. Remove the foil and bake for an additional 10 minutes. Remove the lasagna from the oven and let it sit for 5 minutes before cutting and serving.

Per Serving: (¼ of dish) Calories: 439; Fat: 27g; Protein: 31g; Total Carbs: 18g; Fiber: 7g; Net Carbs: 11g; **Macros:** Fat: 55%; Protein: 28%; Carbs: 17%

Roasted Eggplant with Mint and Harissa

SERVES 4 | PREP TIME: 10 minutes | COOK TIME: 35 minutes

2 medium eggplants, cut into ½-inch cubes
¼ cup extra-virgin olive oil
1 teaspoon salt
¼ teaspoon freshly ground black pepper
1 cup chopped fresh mint
¼ cup harissa
¼ cup chopped scallions, green part only

Preheat the oven to 425°F. Line a baking sheet with parchment paper. In a large bowl, place the eggplant, olive oil, salt, and pepper and toss to coat well. Place the eggplant on the prepared baking sheet, reserving the bowl, and roast for 15 minutes. Remove from the oven and toss the eggplant pieces to flip. Return to the oven and roast until golden and cooked through, another 15 to 20 minutes.

When the eggplant is cooked, remove from the oven and return to the large bowl. Add the mint, harissa, and scallions and toss to combine.

Per Serving: Calories: 300; Fat: 28g; Protein: 3g; Total Carbs: 15g; Fiber: 8g; Net Carbs: 7g; **Macros:** Fat: 81%; Protein: 2%; Carbs: 17%

Stuffed Eggplant

SERVES 2 TO 4 | PREP TIME: 20 minutes | COOK TIME: 1 hour

1 small eggplant, halved lengthwise

3 tablespoons olive oil

1 onion, diced

12 asparagus spears or green beans, diced

1 red bell pepper, seeded and diced

1 large tomato, chopped

2 garlic cloves, minced

½ block (8 ounces) extra-firm tofu (optional)

3 tablespoons chopped fresh basil leaves

Salt

Freshly ground black pepper

¼ cup water

2 eggs

Chopped fresh parsley, for garnish (optional)

Shredded cheese, for garnish (optional)

Preheat the oven to 350°F. Scoop out the flesh from the halved eggplant and chop it into cubes. Reserve the eggplant skin. In a skillet with a lid, heat the oil over medium-high heat. Add the eggplant, onion, asparagus, bell pepper, tomato, garlic, and tofu (if using) and stir. Stir in the basil, season with salt and pepper, and cook for about 5 minutes. Add the water, cover the pan, reduce the heat to medium, and cook for about 15 minutes longer. Put the eggplant "boats" (the reserved skin) on a baking sheet. Scoop some of the cooked eggplant mixture into each boat. Crack an egg into each eggplant boat then bake for about 40 minutes, or until desired doneness. Remove the eggplant from the oven and, if desired, sprinkle with parsley and cheese. Let the cheese melt and cool for about 5 minutes, then serve them up!

Per Serving: Calories: 380; Fat: 26g; Protein: 12g; Total Carbs: 25g; Fiber: 10g; Net Carbs: 15g; **Macros:** Fat: 62%; Protein: 12%; Carbs: 26%

Caramelized Fennel

SERVES 4 | PREP TIME: 5 minutes | COOK TIME: 30 minutes

2 fennel bulbs

¼ cup extra-virgin olive oil

Sea salt

Freshly ground black pepper

Preheat the oven to 375°F. Remove the fennel stems and fronds. Cut the fennel bulbs into 8 to 12 wedges, keeping the root ends intact. Spread the fennel on a rimmed baking sheet. Drizzle with the olive oil and turn over to coat. Season with salt and pepper. Roast for 30 minutes, or until the fennel is tender and gently browned on the bottom.

Per Serving: Calories: 156; Fat: 14g; Protein: 2g; Total Carbs: 9g; Fiber: 4g; Net Carbs: 5g; **Macros:** Fat: 79%; Protein: 1%; Carbs: 20%

Garlicky Green Beans

SERVES 4 | PREP TIME: 10 minutes | COOK TIME: 10 minutes

1 pound green beans, stemmed

2 tablespoons olive oil

1 teaspoon minced garlic

Sea salt

Freshly ground black pepper

¼ cup freshly grated Parmesan cheese

Preheat the oven to 425°F. Line a baking sheet with aluminum foil and set aside. In a large bowl, toss the green beans, olive oil, and garlic until well mixed. Season the beans lightly with salt and pepper. Spread the beans on the baking sheet and roast them until they are tender and lightly browned, stirring them once, about 10 minutes. Serve topped with the Parmesan cheese.

Per serving: Calories: 104; Fat: 9g; Protein: 4g; Total Carbs: 2g; Fiber: 1g; Net Carbs: 1g; **Macros:** Fat: 77%; Protein: 15%; Carbs: 8%

Southern Green Beans

1 SERVING | PREP TIME: 5 minutes | COOK TIME: 25 minutes

½ pound green beans, trimmed

¼ cup chopped pecans

1 tablespoon butter or ghee

2 garlic cloves, minced

Preheat the oven to 450°F; line a baking sheet with parchment paper. In a medium bowl, mix the green beans, pecans, butter, and garlic. Spread out the mixture in one even layer on the prepared baking sheet. Roast in the oven for 20 to 25 minutes.

Per Serving: Calories: 249; Fat: 17g; Protein: 5g; Total Carbs: 19g; Fiber: 10g; Net Carbs: 9g; **Macros:** Fat: 61%; Protein: 8%; Carbs: 31%

Tofu Green Bean Casserole

SERVES 8 | PREP TIME: 15 minutes | COOK TIME: 25 minutes

Nonstick cooking spray

1 cauliflower head, chopped into florets

2 tablespoons coconut oil

¼ cup chopped onion

14 ounces green beans, trimmed

1 tablespoon salt

¼ teaspoon freshly ground black pepper

¾ cup full-fat coconut milk

10 ounces tofu

2 cups grated Parmesan cheese

1 cup shredded mozzarella cheese

Preheat the oven to 250°F. Grease a 9-by-13-inch casserole dish with cooking spray. Put the cauliflower florets in a microwave-safe dish. Add 1 to 2 tablespoons of water and cover the dish with plastic wrap. Microwave the cauliflower for 8 minutes, or until tender enough to mash. While the cauliflower is cooking, heat a skillet over medium heat and melt the coconut oil. Add the onions and green beans, and cook until slightly tender and bright green. Once the cauliflower is cooked, transfer it to a high-powered blender. Add the salt, pepper, and coconut milk. Pulse until creamy. Spread the cauliflower mash in an even layer in the prepared casserole dish. Place the green beans on top of the mash, and then crumble the tofu on top. Cover with the Parmesan and mozzarella cheeses. Bake the casserole for 15 minutes. For a bubbly cheesy crust, broil the casserole uncovered under a low heat for 1 to 2 minutes.

Per Serving: Calories: 297; Fat: 21g; Protein: 18g; Total Carbs: 9g; Fiber: 3g; Net Carbs: 6g; **Macros:** Fat: 64%; Protein: 24%; Carbs: 12%

Green Bean Casserole

SERVES 6 | PREP TIME: 15 minutes | COOK TIME: 6 hours on low

¼ cup butter, divided

½ sweet onion, chopped

1 cup sliced button mushrooms

1 teaspoon minced garlic

2 pounds green beans, cut into 2-inch pieces

1 cup chicken broth

8 ounces cream cheese

¼ cup grated Parmesan cheese

Lightly grease the insert of the slow cooker with 1 tablespoon of the butter. In a large skillet over medium-high heat, melt the remaining butter. Add the onion, mushrooms, and garlic and sauté until the vegetables are softened, about 5 minutes. Stir the green beans into the skillet and transfer the mixture to the insert. In a small bowl, whisk the broth and cream cheese until smooth. Add the cheese mixture to the vegetables and stir. Top the combined mixture with the Parmesan. Cover and cook on low for 6 hours. Serve warm.

Per Serving: Calories: 274; Fat: 22g; Protein: 9g; Total Carbs: 10g; Fiber: 5g; Net Carbs: 5g; **Macros:** Fat: 72%; Protein: 13%; Carbs: 15%

Smoky Stewed Kale

SERVES 4 | PREP TIME: 5 minutes | COOK TIME: 30 minutes

¼ cup extra-virgin olive oil

½ cup minced onion

2 garlic cloves, minced

Pinch red pepper flakes

1 teaspoon smoked paprika

1 tablespoon tomato paste

6 cups roughly chopped kale

½ cup vegetable broth or chicken bone broth

1 tablespoon red wine vinegar

Heat the olive oil in a large skillet over medium heat. Cook the onion and garlic until they begin to soften, about 5 minutes. Add the red pepper flakes, paprika, and tomato paste, and cook until the onion and garlic begin to caramelize. Add the kale, broth, and red wine vinegar to the skillet, and cook for 20 to 25 minutes, stirring often, until the kale is tender and most of the liquid has evaporated.

Per Serving: Calories: 190; Fat: 15g; Protein: 5g; Total Carbs: 14g; Fiber: 5g; Net Carbs: 9g; **Macros:** Fat: 71%; Protein: 11%; Carbs: 18%

Kale with Bacon

SERVES 8 | PREP TIME: 15 minutes | COOK TIME: 6 hours on low

2 tablespoons bacon fat

2 pounds kale, rinsed and chopped roughly

12 bacon slices, cooked and chopped

2 teaspoons minced garlic

2 cups vegetable broth

Salt, for seasoning

Freshly ground black pepper, for seasoning

Generously grease the insert of the slow cooker with the bacon fat. Add the kale, bacon, garlic, and broth to the insert. Gently toss to mix. Cover and cook on low for 6 hours. Season with salt and pepper, and serve hot.

Per Serving: Calories: 147; Fat: 10g; Protein: 7g; Total Carbs: 7g; Fiber: 3g; Net Carbs: 4g; **Macros:** Fat: 62%; Protein: 21%; Carbs: 19%

Garlicky Kale

1 SERVING | PREP TIME: 5 minutes | COOK TIME: 25 minutes

1 tablespoon avocado oil

4 garlic cloves, sliced

½ bunch kale, stemmed

¼ cup water or chicken broth

In a large skillet, heat the oil over medium heat. Add the garlic and let it cook for 1 to 2 minutes, until it starts to sizzle. Add the kale and toss with tongs to coat it fully in the oil. Add the water, season with salt and freshly ground black pepper, and reduce the heat to low. Cook for 20 minutes, until the kale is tender and most of the liquid has evaporated.

Per Serving: Calories: 192; Fat: 14g; Protein: 4g; Total Carbs: 13g; Fiber: 2g; Net Carbs: 11g; **Macros:** Fat: 63%; Protein: 10%; Carbs: 27%

Kale and Cashew Stir-Fry

SERVES 1 | PREP TIME: 5 minutes | COOK TIME: 5 minutes

1 tablespoon coconut oil

1 cup frozen cauliflower rice (or pearls)

½ cup frozen stir-fry vegetables

1 cup destemmed and torn kale (small pieces)

3 tablespoons tamari sauce or low-sodium soy sauce

⅓ cup chopped cashews

In a skillet over medium heat, melt the coconut oil. Add the cauliflower, stir-fry vegetables, and kale, and cook for 2 to 3 minutes, or until tender but still crisp. Pour in the tamari and toss the vegetables until they are coated with the sauce. Transfer the stir-fry to a serving dish, top with the cashews, and enjoy.

Per Serving: Calories: 523; Fat: 35g; Protein: 18g; Total Carbs: 34g; Fiber: 6g; Net Carbs: 28g; **Macros:** Fat: 60%; Protein: 14%; Carbs: 26%

Slow Cooker Mushrooms

SERVES 8 | PREP TIME: 10 minutes | COOK TIME: 6 hours on low

3 tablespoons extra-virgin olive oil

1 pound button mushrooms, wiped clean and halved

2 teaspoons minced garlic

¼ teaspoon salt

⅛ teaspoon freshly ground black pepper

2 tablespoons chopped fresh parsley

Place the olive oil, mushrooms, garlic, salt, and pepper in the insert of the slow cooker and toss to coat. Cover and cook on low for 6 hours. Serve tossed with the parsley.

Per Serving: Calories: 58; Fat: 5g; Protein: 2g; Total Carbs: 2g; Fiber: 1g; Net Carbs: 1g; **Macros:** Fat: 74%; Protein: 13%; Carbs: 13%

Roasted Mushrooms

1 SERVING | PREP TIME: 5 minutes | COOK TIME: 15 minutes

1 (8-ounce) package sliced cremini mushrooms

1 tablespoon garlic and herb compound butter

Preheat the oven to 375°F; line a baking sheet with parchment paper. In a bowl, combine the mushrooms and the compound butter. Season with salt and freshly ground black pepper to taste. Place the mushrooms in a single layer on the lined baking sheet. Bake for 12 to 15 minutes, tossing occasionally, until browned and tender.

Per Serving: Calories: 168; Fat: 12g; Protein: 6g; Total Carbs: 9g; Fiber: 2g; Net Carbs: 7g; **Macros:** Fat: 64%; Protein: 14%; Carbs: 22%

Pumpkin Seed and Swiss Chard-Stuffed Portabella Mushrooms

SERVES: 4 | Prep time: 10 minutes | COOK TIME: 35 minutes

4 large portabella mushroom caps

5 tablespoons olive oil, divided

1 cup chopped Swiss chard

½ onion, chopped

1 tablespoon minced garlic

2 teaspoons chopped fresh thyme

1½ cups pumpkin seeds

¼ cup store-bought balsamic vinaigrette

Sea salt

Freshly ground black pepper

½ cup shredded Cheddar cheese

Preheat the oven to 350°F. Use a spoon to scoop the black gills out of the mushrooms, then massage 2 tablespoons of olive oil all over them. Place the mushrooms hollow-side up on a baking sheet. Heat the remaining olive oil in a large skillet over medium-high heat. Sauté the Swiss chard, onion, garlic, and thyme until the vegetables are tender, about 10 minutes. Stir in the pumpkin seeds and balsamic vinaigrette and season the filling with salt and pepper. Divide the filling among the mushroom caps and top with shredded Cheddar. Bake until tender, about 25 minutes.

Per Serving: Calories: 517; Fat: 46g; Protein: 19g; Total Carbs: 14g; Fiber: 4g; Net Carbs: 10g; **Macros:** Fat: 79%; Protein: 14%; Carbs: 7%

Mushrooms with Camembert

SERVES 4 | PREP TIME: 5 minutes | COOK TIME: 15 minutes

2 tablespoons butter

2 teaspoons minced garlic

1 pound button mushrooms, halved

4 ounces Camembert cheese, diced

Freshly ground black pepper

Place a large skillet over medium-high heat and melt the butter. Sauté the garlic until translucent, about 3 minutes. Sauté the mushrooms until tender, about 10 minutes. Stir in the cheese and sauté until melted, about 2 minutes. Season with pepper and serve.

Per serving: Calories: 161; Fat: 13g; Protein: 9g; Total Carbs: 4g; Fiber: 1g; Net Carbs: 3g; **Macros:** Fat: 70%; Protein: 21%; Carbs: 9%

Stuffed Mushrooms

SERVES 20 | PREP TIME: 20 minutes | COOK TIME: 25 minutes

40 whole fresh white button mushrooms, stemmed

2 tablespoons olive oil

3 garlic cloves, minced

24 ounces (3 bricks) cream cheese, melted

1 cup grated Parmesan cheese

½ teaspoon freshly ground black pepper

½ teaspoon minced onion

½ teaspoon salt

Preheat the oven to 375°F, and line a baking sheet with parchment paper. Mince the stems, and place the mushroom caps on the baking sheet, stem-side up. In a large skillet over medium heat, heat the olive oil. Place the minced stems in the skillet, and stir for 2 to 3 minutes. Add the garlic, and stir for 30 seconds. Remove from the heat, and stir in the cream cheese, Parmesan, pepper, onion, and salt. With a spoon, fill each mushroom cap with the cheese mixture. Bake for 20 minutes, and serve.

Per Serving: (2 mushrooms): Calories: 145; Fat: 13g; Protein: 4g; Total Carbs: 4g; Fiber: 0g; Net Carbs: 4g; **Macros:** Fat: 80%; Protein: 11%; Carbs: 9%

Herbed Ricotta–Stuffed Mushrooms

SERVES 4 | PREP TIME: 10 minutes | COOK TIME: 30 minutes

6 tablespoons extra-virgin olive oil, divided

4 portabella mushroom caps, cleaned and gills removed

1 cup whole-milk ricotta cheese

⅓ cup chopped fresh herbs (such as basil, parsley, rosemary, oregano, or thyme)

2 garlic cloves, finely minced

½ teaspoon salt

¼ teaspoon freshly ground black pepper

Preheat the oven to 400°F. Line a baking sheet with parchment and drizzle with 2 tablespoons olive oil, spreading evenly. Place the mushroom caps on the baking sheet, gill-side up. In a medium bowl, mix the ricotta, herbs, 2 tablespoons olive oil, garlic, salt, and pepper. Stuff each mushroom cap with one-quarter of the cheese mixture, pressing down if needed. Drizzle with remaining 2 tablespoons olive oil and bake until golden brown and the mushrooms are soft, 30 to 35 minutes, depending on the size of the mushrooms.

Per Serving: Calories: 285; Fat: 25g; Protein: 7g; Total Carbs: 8g; Fiber: 2g; Net Carbs: 6g; **Macros:** Fat: 79%; Protein: 10%; Carbs: 11%

Portabella Mushroom Pizza

SERVES 4 | PREP TIME: 15 minutes | COOK TIME: 5 minutes

4 large portobello mushrooms, stems removed

¼ cup olive oil

1 teaspoon minced garlic

1 medium tomato, cut into 4 slices

2 teaspoons chopped fresh basil

1 cup shredded mozzarella cheese

Preheat the oven to broil. Line a baking sheet with aluminum foil and set aside. In a small bowl, toss the mushroom caps with the olive oil until well coated. Place the mushrooms on the baking sheet gill-side down and broil the mushrooms until they are tender on the tops, about 2 minutes. Flip the mushrooms over and broil 1 minute more. Take the baking sheet out and spread the garlic over each mushroom, top each with a tomato slice, sprinkle with the basil, and top with the cheese. Broil the mushrooms until the cheese is melted and bubbly, about 1 minute. Serve.

Per serving: Calories: 251; Fat: 20g; Protein: 14g; Total Carbs: 7g; Fiber: 3g; Net Carbs: 4g; **Macros:** Fat: 71%; Protein: 19%; Carbs: 10%

Portabella Mushroom Burger with Avocado

SERVES 1 | PREP TIME: 15 minutes | COOK TIME: 10 minutes

Nonstick cooking spray

4 large portabella mushrooms, destemmed and wiped clean

1 tablespoon avocado oil

½ teaspoon salt

¼ teaspoon freshly ground black pepper

1 avocado, mashed

1 tablespoon plain Greek yogurt

1 tablespoon mayonnaise

1 tablespoon freshly squeezed lime juice

¼ teaspoon ground cumin

½ cup broccoli sprouts

Preheat the oven to 400°F. Spray a baking sheet with cooking spray. Brush the tops of the mushrooms with the avocado oil. Place them on the prepared baking sheet (tops up) and sprinkle with the salt and pepper. Cook for 8 to 10 minutes and then flip the mushrooms over and cook for an additional 8 to 10 minutes. Remove from the oven. In a small bowl, combine the avocado, Greek yogurt, mayonnaise, lime juice, and cumin. Stir until well blended. Layer half of the avocado mixture between 2 mushroom "buns" and top with half the broccoli sprouts. Repeat to make the second burger.

Per Serving: (2 burgers) Calories: 638; Fat: 50g; Protein: 13g; Total Carbs: 34g; Fiber: 17g; Net Carbs: 17g; **Macros:** Fat: 71%; Protein: 8%; Carbs: 21%

Wild Mushroom Stroganoff

SERVES 6 | PREP TIME: 15 minutes | COOK TIME: 6 hours on low

3 tablespoons extra-virgin olive oil, divided
2 tablespoons butter
14 ounces mushrooms, sliced
½ sweet onion, diced
2 teaspoons minced garlic
2 cups beef broth

3 tablespoons paprika
1 tablespoon tomato paste
½ cup heavy (whipping) cream
½ cup sour cream
2 tablespoons chopped parsley, for garnish

Lightly grease the insert of the slow cooker with 1 tablespoon of the olive oil. In a large skillet over medium heat, heat the remaining 2 tablespoons of the olive oil and the butter. Add the mushrooms, onion, and garlic and sauté until they are softened, about 5 minutes. Transfer the mushroom mixture to the insert and add the broth, paprika, and tomato paste. Cover and cook on low for 6 hours. Stir in the heavy cream and sour cream Serve topped with the parsley.

Per Serving: Calories: 236; Fat: 20g; Protein: 7g; Total Carbs: 7g; Fiber: 3g; Net Carbs: 4g; **Macros:** Fat: 76%; Protein: 12%; Carbs: 12%

Stuffed Portabella Mushrooms

SERVES 4 | PREP TIME: 25 minutes | COOK TIME: 15 minutes

4 portabella mushrooms
1 tablespoon extra-virgin olive oil
2 teaspoons minced garlic
1 cup shredded kale
1 cup cream cheese, softened
2 teaspoons chopped fresh basil

¼ teaspoon freshly ground black pepper
4 teaspoons almond meal, divided
¼ cup shredded mozzarella, divided

Preheat the oven to 350°F. Remove the stems from the mushroom caps, and use a spoon to scoop out the black gills to form a hollow. Set them aside on a small baking sheet. In a medium skillet, heat the olive oil and sauté the garlic and kale until fragrant and the greens are tender, about 5 minutes. Transfer the kale to a medium bowl, and stir in the cream cheese, basil, and pepper. Mound the cheese mixture into the mushroom caps, and top each with 1 teaspoon of almond meal and 1 tablespoon of mozzarella cheese. Bake the caps until the filling is heated through and the cheese is bubbly and golden, about 15 minutes, and serve.

Per Serving: Calories: 300; Fat: 25g; Protein: 11g; Total Carbs: 9g; Fiber: 3g; Net Carbs: 6g; **Macros:** Fat: 74%; Protein: 14%; Carbs: 12%

Stuffed Cremini Mushrooms

SERVES 4 | PREP TIME: 10 minutes | COOK TIME: 20 to 25 minutes

12 cremini mushrooms, stems removed
6 ounces cream cheese
¼ cup Parmesan cheese
2 garlic cloves, minced

2 teaspoons minced fresh thyme
Sea salt
Freshly ground black pepper

Preheat the oven to 400°F. Line a baking sheet with parchment paper. Place the mushrooms cap-side down on the baking sheet. In a small mixing bowl, mix the cream cheese, Parmesan cheese, garlic, and thyme. Season with salt and pepper. Divide the mixture among the mushroom caps. Bake for 20 to 25 minutes, or until the mushrooms are soft and the tops are golden brown. Allow to rest for 5 minutes before serving.

Per Serving: Calories: 186; Fat: 17g; Protein: 7g; Total Carbs: 4g; Fiber: 1g; Net Carbs: 3g; **Macros:** Fat: 81%; Protein: 14%; Carbs: 5%

Roasted Onions

SERVES 4 | PREP TIME: 15 minutes | COOK TIME: 40 minutes

1 tablespoon extra-virgin olive oil, plus more for greasing
4 sweet onions, cut into ¼-inch slices
Sea salt

Freshly ground black pepper
1 cup heavy (whipping) cream
1 teaspoon apple cider vinegar
¾ cup blue cheese

Preheat the oven to 375°F. Lightly grease a baking sheet with olive oil, and arrange the onion slices on the sheet. Drizzle the onion slices with the olive oil, and season with salt and pepper. Roast the onions until golden, about 15 minutes. While the onions are roasting, in a small saucepan over medium-high heat, whisk the cream and apple cider vinegar. Bring the cream mixture to a simmer, and then remove the saucepan from the heat. Remove the onions from the oven, and increase the oven temperature to 450°F. Transfer the onion to a 9-by-13-inch baking dish, and pour the cream mixture over them. Sprinkle the blue cheese over the onion mixture, and cover the baking dish with foil. Bake the onions in the oven for 15 minutes, remove the foil, and bake for another 10 minutes. Serve.

Per Serving: Calories: 267; Fat: 22g; Protein: 7g; Total Carbs: 11g; Fiber: 3g; Net Carbs: 8g; **Macros:** Fat: 73%; Protein: 11%; Carbs: 16%

Goat Cheese Stuffed Roasted Peppers

SERVES 4 | PREP TIME: 10 minutes | COOK TIME: 15 minutes | TOTAL TIME: 25 minutes

¾ cup goat cheese, at room temperature
1 teaspoon minced garlic
2 teaspoons chopped fresh basil
¼ teaspoon salt

⅛ teaspoon freshly ground black pepper
12 sweet cherry peppers, stemmed and seeded
1 tablespoon olive oil

Preheat the oven to 425°F. In a small bowl, mix the goat cheese, garlic, basil, salt, and pepper. With a spoon, fill the peppers with the goat cheese mixture. Place the peppers on a parchment-lined baking sheet. Drizzle the peppers with the olive oil. Put the baking sheet in the oven. Bake for 15 minutes, or until the peppers are browned and the cheese is bubbling.

Per Serving: (3 stuffed peppers): Calories: 253; Fat: 19g; Protein: 13g; Total Carbs: 5g; Fiber: 2g; Net Carbs: 3g; **Macros:** Fat: 70%; Protein: 21%; Carbs: 9%

Creamy Stuffed Peppers

SERVES 2 | PREP TIME: 10 minutes | COOK TIME: 15 minutes

2 green bell peppers, halved and deseeded	12 ounces ricotta cheese
1 tablespoon olive oil	1 large egg
¼ cup chopped onion	1 teaspoon dried basil
1 teaspoon minced garlic	½ cup grated Parmesan cheese
1 cup fresh spinach	

Preheat the oven to 350°F. Line a baking sheet with aluminum foil. Place the bell peppers on the baking sheet, cut-side up, and bake for 10 minutes. Set aside. While the peppers are baking, set a skillet over medium-high heat and pour in the olive oil. Add the onion, garlic, and spinach and sauté for 2 minutes, or until the spinach is wilted. Transfer the mixture to a mixing bowl. Stir in the ricotta cheese, egg, and basil. Mix well. Fill each pepper half with equal amounts of filling and top with 2 tablespoons of Parmesan cheese. Return the peppers to the oven and bake for an additional 5 minutes. Remove and serve.

Per Serving: (2 pepper halves) Calories: 546; Fat: 38g; Protein: 33g; Total Carbs: 18g; Fiber: 3g; Net Carbs: 15g; **Macros:** Fat: 63%; Protein: 24%; Carbs: 13%

Chiles Rellenos

SERVES 8 | PREP TIME: 15 minutes | COOK TIME: 50 minutes

Nonstick cooking spray	4 cups fresh spinach
8 poblano chiles	½ cup sour cream
1 tablespoon olive oil	½ cup heavy (whipping) cream
½ onion, chopped	16 ounces shredded pepper Jack cheese
2 garlic cloves, minced	
1 cup chopped button mushrooms	

Preheat the oven to 450°F. Spray a baking dish with cooking spray. Cut a slit down the length of each pepper and carefully scoop out and discard all the seeds and membranes. Cut another slit horizontally at the top of the peppers to make an opening for the filling. Place the peppers in the baking dish and cook for about 20 minutes, or until they start to blister. Remove and set aside. While the peppers are in the oven, set a skillet over medium-high heat and pour in the olive oil. Add the onion, garlic, and mushrooms and cook until fragrant, 2 to 3 minutes. Add the spinach and cook until wilted, 4 to 5 minutes. Transfer the mushroom mixture to a medium mixing bowl. Add the sour cream, heavy cream, and pepper Jack cheese, and stir until combined. Remove the peppers from the oven and stuff each one with an equal amount of filling.

Close with a toothpick. Return the peppers to the oven for an additional 15 minutes, or until the cheese is melted. Serve warm.

Per Serving: (1 pepper) Calories: 341; Fat: 29g; Protein: 16g; Total Carbs: 4g; Fiber: 1g; Net Carbs: 3g; **Macros:** Fat: 77%; Protein: 19%; Carbs: 4%

Carrot-Pumpkin Pudding

SERVES 6 | PREP TIME: 15 minutes | COOK TIME: 6 hours on low

1 tablespoon extra-virgin olive oil or ghee	2 large eggs
2 cups finely shredded carrots	1 tablespoon granulated erythritol
2 cups puréed pumpkin	1 teaspoon ground nutmeg
½ sweet onion, finely chopped	½ teaspoon salt
1 cup heavy (whipping) cream	¼ cup pumpkin seeds, for garnish
½ cup cream cheese, softened	

Lightly grease the insert of the slow cooker with the olive oil or ghee. In a large bowl, whisk the carrots, pumpkin, onion, heavy cream, cream cheese, eggs, erythritol, nutmeg, and salt. Cover and cook on low for 6 hours. Serve warm, topped with the pumpkin seeds.

Per Serving: Calories: 239; Fat: 19g; Protein: 6g; Total Carbs: 11g; Fiber: 4g; Net Carbs: 7g; **Macros:** Fat: 72%; Protein: 10%; Carbs: 18%

Herbed Pumpkin

SERVES 6 | PREP TIME: 15 minutes | COOK TIME: 7 to 8 hours on low

3 tablespoons extra-virgin olive oil, divided	1 tablespoon apple cider vinegar
1 pound pumpkin, cut into 1-inch chunks	½ teaspoon chopped thyme
½ cup coconut milk	1 teaspoon chopped oregano
	¼ teaspoon salt
	1 cup Greek yogurt

Lightly grease the insert of the slow cooker with 1 tablespoon of the olive oil. Add the remaining 2 tablespoons of the olive oil with the pumpkin, coconut milk, apple cider vinegar, thyme, oregano, and salt to the insert. Cover and cook on low for 7 to 8 hours. Mash the pumpkin with the yogurt using a potato masher until smooth. Serve warm.

Per Serving: Calories: 158; Fat: 13g; Protein: 5g; Total Carbs: 8g; Fiber: 3g; Net Carbs: 5g; **Macros:** Fat: 69%; Protein: 12%; Carbs: 19%

Radishes with Olive Mayo

SERVES 1 | PREP TIME: 5 minutes | COOK TIME: 0 minutes

4 medium radishes	4 Kalamata olives, pitted and minced
2 tablespoons mayonnaise	⅛ teaspoon balsamic vinegar
1 tablespoon minced shallot or red onion	

Scrub the radishes and remove all but 1 inch of the leaves and stems. Pat the radishes dry with paper towels. In a small bowl, whisk the mayonnaise, shallot, olives, and balsamic vinegar. Serve alongside the radishes as a dip.

Creamed Spinach

1 SERVING | PREP TIME: 5 minutes | COOK TIME: 15 minutes

1 tablespoon avocado oil
1 tablespoon butter or ghee
1/4 medium white onion, diced
2 garlic cloves, minced

1 tablespoon cream cheese
1 teaspoon freshly grated
   Parmesan cheese
6 cups fresh spinach

In a skillet, heat the oil and butter over medium heat. Add the onion and garlic, and sauté for 5 to 7 minutes or until the onion is soft. Whisk in the cream cheese and Parmesan cheese until they are completely melted. Fold in the spinach until evenly combined (add a little water if the mixture seems dry). Season with salt and freshly ground black pepper to taste. Cook for 5 minutes or until the spinach is fully wilted.

Per Serving: Calories: 363; Fat: 31g; Protein: 9g; Total Carbs: 12g; Fiber: 5g; Net Carbs: 7g; **Macros:** Fat: 77%; Protein: 10%; Carbs: 13%

Cheesy Spinach Bake

SERVES 4 | PREP TIME: 10 minutes | COOK TIME: 40 minutes

Nonstick cooking spray
2 tablespoons butter
2 cups chopped onion
2 garlic cloves, minced
2 zucchini, chopped into
   bite-size pieces
2 cups fresh spinach
3 large eggs, beaten

1/4 cup heavy (whipping) cream
1/2 teaspoon salt
1/4 teaspoon freshly ground
   black pepper
1 1/2 cups shredded mozzarella cheese
1/2 cup grated Parme-
   san cheese

Preheat the oven to 350°F. Coat a 9-inch pie plate with cooking spray. In a skillet over medium-high heat, melt the butter. Add the onion and garlic and sauté for 2 minutes. Add the zucchini and cook for another 4 minutes. Add the spinach and stir until wilted. Transfer the mixture to the pie plate and spread it evenly with a spatula. In a small bowl, mix the eggs, cream, salt, and pepper. Pour the mixture over the vegetables. Top with the mozzarella and Parmesan cheeses and bake for 30 to 35 minutes.

Per Serving: Calories: 386; Fat: 30g; Protein: 21g; Total Carbs: 8g; Fiber: 2g; Net Carbs: 6g; **Macros:** Fat: 70%; Protein: 22%; Carbs: 8%

Spinach Soufflé

SERVES 6 | PREP TIME: 15 minutes | COOK TIME: 40 minutes

1/4 cup butter, softened, plus
   more for greasing
8 cups spinach, chopped
16 ounces cottage cheese
8 ounces aged Cheddar
   cheese, cubed

6 large eggs, beaten
2 tablespoons almond flour
1/2 teaspoon sea salt
1/2 teaspoon ground nutmeg

Preheat the oven to 350°F. Lightly grease a 9-by-13-inch casserole dish with butter. Set aside. Place a large saucepan filled with water over high heat, and bring the water to a boil. Blanch the spinach until it is tender, about 2 minutes. Drain the spinach, and squeeze out all the water. Transfer the spinach to a large bowl, and stir in the cottage cheese, Cheddar cheese, eggs, butter, almond flour, salt, and nutmeg. Spoon the mixture into the casserole dish, and bake until the soufflé is set and golden brown, about 35 minutes. Serve.

Per Serving: Calories: 356; Fat: 28g; Protein: 23g; Total Carbs: 4g; Fiber: 1g; Net Carbs: 3g; **Macros:** Fat: 70%; Protein: 26%; Carbs: 4%

Golden Rosti

SERVES 8 | PREP TIME: 15 minutes | COOK TIME: 15 minutes

8 bacon slices, chopped
1 cup shredded acorn squash
1 cup shredded raw celeriac
2 tablespoons grated or
   shredded Parmesan cheese
2 teaspoons minced garlic

1 teaspoon chopped
   fresh thyme
Sea salt
Freshly ground black pepper
2 tablespoons butter

In a large skillet over medium-high heat, cook the bacon until crispy, about 5 minutes. While the bacon is cooking, in a large bowl, mix the squash, celeriac, Parmesan cheese, garlic, and thyme. Season the mixture generously with salt and pepper, and set aside. Remove the cooked bacon with a slotted spoon to the rosti mixture and stir to incorporate. Remove all but 2 tablespoons of bacon fat from the skillet and add the butter. Reduce the heat to medium-low and transfer the rosti mixture to the skillet and spread it out evenly to form a large round patty about 1-inch thick. Cook until the bottom of the rosti is golden brown and crisp, about 5 minutes. Flip the rosti over and cook until the other side is crispy and the middle is cooked through, about 5 minutes more. Remove the skillet from the heat and cut the rosti into 8 pieces. Serve.

Per Serving: Calories: 171; Fat: 15g; Protein: 5g; Total Carbs: 3g; Fiber: 0g; Net Carbs: 3g; **Macros:** Fat: 81%; Protein: 12%; Carbs: 7%

Twice-Baked Spaghetti Squash

SERVES 4 | PREP TIME: 20 minutes | COOK TIME: 55 minutes

Extra-virgin olive oil, for
   drizzling
1 spaghetti squash, halved
1/2 cup heavy (whipping) cream
6 slices cooked pan-
   cetta, chopped
2 tablespoons butter

1 teaspoon minced garlic
1 scallion, chopped
Sea salt
Freshly ground black pepper
1 cup shredded Cheddar
   cheese, divided

Preheat the oven to 350°F. Line a baking sheet with parchment paper. Lightly drizzle the cut sides of the squash with olive oil, and place them cut-side down on the baking sheet. Bake the squash until it is very tender, about 35 minutes. Scoop the cooked squash flesh into a large bowl, and discard the rinds. Stir in the cream, pancetta, butter, garlic, and scallion. Season the squash mixture with salt and pepper. Spoon the squash mixture into 4 (6-ounce) ramekins. Top each ramekin with 1/4 cup of cheese. Bake the squash for 20 minutes, until the Cheddar on top is melted and bubbly, and serve.

Per Serving: Calories: 229; Fat: 18g; Protein: 12g; Total Carbs: 6g; Fiber: 0g; Net Carbs: 6g; **Macros:** Fat: 69%; Protein: 21%; Carbs: 10%

Sautéed Summer Squash

1 SERVING | PREP TIME: 5 minutes | COOK TIME: 10 minutes

1 tablespoon avocado oil
1/2 zucchini, cut into
   half-moons

1/2 yellow summer squash, cut
   into half-moons
1 teaspoon freshly grated
   Parmesan cheese (optional)

In a large skillet, heat the oil over medium heat. Add the zucchini and yellow squash in as even a layer as possible. It should sizzle as it hits the skillet. Sprinkle with salt and freshly ground black pepper. Let the squash sit without stirring or moving for 2 minutes so it can get nice and golden. After 2 minutes, give it a good stir, and then let it continue to cook for an additional 5 minutes, stirring occasionally, until the squash is tender. Transfer to a bowl and sprinkle with the cheese (if using).

Per Serving: Calories: 162; Fat: 14g; Protein: 2g; Total Carbs: 7g; Fiber: 2g; Net Carbs: 5g; **Macros:** Fat: 78%; Protein: 5%; Carbs: 17%

Creamy Spaghetti Squash Bake

SERVES 4 | PREP TIME: 10 minutes | COOK TIME: 30 minutes

Nonstick cooking spray
1 tablespoon butter
5 garlic cloves, minced
½ cup water
1 teaspoon seasoned vegetable base
1 cup heavy (whipping) cream
4 cups cooked and shredded spaghetti squash
½ cup grated Parmesan cheese
½ cup shredded mozzarella cheese
2 tablespoons chopped fresh parsley
1 teaspoon freshly ground black pepper

Preheat the oven to 350°F. Spray an 8-inch-square casserole dish with cooking spray. In a medium saucepan over medium-low heat, melt the butter. Add the garlic and cook until fragrant, 2 to 3 minutes. Add the water, vegetable base, and cream. Cook until well combined, and then remove from the heat. Place the squash in the bottom of the prepared dish. Pour the cream mixture on top, and then top with the Parmesan and mozzarella cheeses, parsley, and pepper. Bake for 20 minutes and serve warm.

Per Serving: Calories: 371; Fat: 31g; Protein: 11g; Total Carbs: 12g; Fiber: 1g; Net Carbs: 11g; **Macros:** Fat: 75%; Protein: 12%; Carbs: 13%

Fakeachini Alfredo

SERVES 1 | PREP TIME: 15 minutes | COOK TIME: 5 minutes

½ tablespoon extra-virgin olive oil
1 teaspoon minced garlic
¼ teaspoon salt
¼ teaspoon garlic powder
1 wedge Laughing Cow Swiss cheese, cubed
1 to 2 tablespoons heavy (whipping) cream
3 tablespoons grated Parmesan cheese
2 ounces seitan strips or cubes
⅓ cup cooked spaghetti squash
1 tablespoon chopped fresh parsley

In a small saucepan over medium-low heat, warm the olive oil. Add the garlic, salt, and garlic powder and stir for 1 to 2 minutes or until fragrant. Add the cubed cheese and stir until melted. Thin the sauce to your desired consistency with the cream. Lower the heat and stir in the Parmesan cheese. Continue to stir until melted. Add the seitan to the sauce. Place the squash in a serving bowl, pour the sauce on top, and sprinkle with the parsley.

Per Serving: Calories: 452; Fat: 24g; Protein: 52g; Total Carbs: 7g; Fiber: 3g; Net Carbs: 4g; **Macros:** Fat: 48%; Protein: 46%; Carbs: 6%

Ratatouille

SERVES 6 | PREP TIME: 15 minutes | COOK TIME: 6 hours on low

3 tablespoons extra-virgin olive oil, divided
2 zucchini, diced
1 red bell pepper, diced
1 yellow bell pepper, diced
1 cup diced pumpkin
½ sweet onion, diced
3 teaspoons minced garlic
¼ teaspoon salt
¼ teaspoon freshly ground black pepper
Pinch red pepper flakes
1 (14-ounce) can diced tomatoes
1 cup crumbled goat cheese, for garnish

Lightly grease the insert of the slow cooker with 1 tablespoon of the olive oil. Add the zucchini, red and yellow bell peppers, pumpkin, onion, garlic, salt, pepper, and red pepper flakes to the insert, and toss to combine. Add the remaining 2 tablespoons of the olive oil and the tomatoes and stir. Cover and cook on low for 6 hours. Serve topped with the goat cheese.

Per Serving: Calories: 232; Fat: 18g; Protein: 7g; Total Carbs: 11g; Fiber: 5g; Net Carbs: 6g; **Macros:** Fat: 69%; Protein: 12%; Carbs: 19%

Zucchini Noodles

SERVES 4 | PREP TIME: 5 minutes, plus 20 minutes inactive time | COOK TIME: 2 to 3 minutes

2 medium zucchini spiralized
Sea salt
2 tablespoons coconut oil

Place the zucchini noodles in a colander and season very generously with salt. Place the colander into the sink and let the zucchini sweat for 20 minutes. Rinse the zucchini with fresh water and wring as much moisture as you can from the noodles, trying not to break them. Heat a large skillet over high heat. When it is hot, add the coconut oil. When the oil is hot, sauté the zucchini noodles for 2 to 3 minutes, or until hot but not browned.

Per Serving: Calories: 75; Fat: 7g; Protein: 1g; Total Carbs: 4g; Fiber: 1g; Net Carbs: 3g; **Macros:** Fat: 84%; Protein: 5%; Carbs: 11%

Avocado Pesto Zoodles

SERVES 2 | PREP TIME: 10 minutes | COOK TIME: 10 minutes

2 avocados, halved
1 tablespoon pine nuts
½ cup fresh basil
2 teaspoons olive oil
4 medium zucchini, spiralized
1 tablespoon minced garlic
¼ cup shredded Parmesan cheese
½ teaspoon salt
½ teaspoon freshly ground black pepper

In the bowl of a food processor, combine the avocados, pine nuts, and basil. Pulse until a paste forms, using a few tablespoons of water to thin the consistency if necessary. Heat a medium skillet over medium-high heat and heat the olive oil. Add the zoodles and garlic and sauté for 5 to 7 minutes. Add the avocado pesto to the skillet and stir until well combined. Cook for an additional 1 to 2 minutes and top with the Parmesan cheese, salt, and pepper.

Per Serving: Calories: 404; Fat: 31g; Protein: 14g; Total Carbs: 27g; Fiber: 14g; Net Carbs: 13g; **Macros:** Fat: 65%; Protein: 11%; Carbs: 24%

Vegetarian Zucchini Noodle Carbonara

SERVES 4 | PREP TIME: 10 minutes | COOK TIME: 15 minutes

24 ounces store-bought
  zucchini noodles
3 large eggs
2 tablespoons heavy
  (whipping) cream

1 teaspoon onion powder
¼ teaspoon freshly ground
  black pepper
1 cup grated Parmesan cheese

Cook the zucchini noodles according to the package directions. In a small bowl, beat the eggs, heavy cream, onion powder, and pepper. Add the mixture to the zucchini noodles in the pan and toss to coat. Stir frequently until the egg is cooked, about 10 minutes. Add the Parmesan, mix well to combine, and serve.

Per Serving: Calories: 215; Fat: 14g; Protein: 14g; Total Carbs: 10g; Fiber: 2g; Net Carbs: 8g; **Macros:** Fat: 57%; Protein: 26%; Carbs: 17%

Greek Stewed Zucchini

SERVES 4 TO 6 | PREP TIME: 5 minutes |
COOK TIME: 40 minutes

¼ cup extra-virgin olive oil
1 small yellow onion, peeled
  and slivered
4 medium zucchini squash, cut
  into ½-inch-thick rounds
4 small garlic cloves, minced
1 to 2 teaspoons
  dried oregano

2 cups chopped tomatoes
½ cup halved and pitted Kalamata olives
¾ cup crumbled feta cheese
¼ cup chopped fresh flat-leaf
  Italian parsley, for garnish
  (optional)

In a large skillet, heat the oil over medium-high heat. Add the onion and sauté until just tender, 6 to 8 minutes. Add the zucchini, garlic, and oregano and sauté another 6 to 8 minutes, or until the zucchini is just tender. Add the tomatoes and bring to a boil. Reduce the heat to low and add the olives. Cover and simmer on low heat for 20 minutes, or until the flavors have developed and the zucchini is very tender. Serve warm topped with feta and parsley (if using).

Per Serving: Calories: 272; Fat: 20g; Protein: 8g; Total Carbs: 15g; Fiber: 5g; Net Carbs: 10g; **Macros:** Fat: 66%; Protein: 12%; Carbs: 22%

Mediterranean Spiralized Zucchini

SERVES 4 | PREP TIME: 15 minutes | COOK TIME: 10 minutes

3 tablespoons olive oil
1 tablespoon butter
1 tablespoon minced garlic
1 cup chopped Swiss chard
½ cup sliced Kalamata olives
2 tablespoons chopped
  fresh basil

3 zucchini, spiralized
Sea salt
Freshly ground black pepper
1 cup shredded fresh mozzarella cheese

Heat the olive oil and butter in a large skillet over medium-high heat. Sauté the garlic until softened, about 2 minutes. Add the Swiss chard, olives, and basil and sauté until the greens are wilted, about 8 minutes. Stir in the zucchini and toss to combine. Season with salt and pepper. Serve topped with mozzarella cheese.

Per Serving: Calories: 281; Fat: 25g; Protein: 11g; Total Carbs: 10g; Fiber: 3g; Net Carbs: 7g; **Macros:** Fat: 80%; Protein: 16%; Carbs: 4%

Sautéed Crispy Zucchini

SERVES 4 | PREP TIME: 15 minutes | COOK TIME: 10 minutes

2 tablespoons butter
4 zucchini, cut into ¼-inch-
  thick rounds

½ cup freshly grated Parmesan cheese
Freshly ground black pepper

Place a large skillet over medium-high heat and melt the butter. Add the zucchini and sauté until tender and lightly browned, about 5 minutes. Spread the zucchini evenly in the skillet and sprinkle the Parmesan cheese over the vegetables. Cook without stirring until the Parmesan cheese is melted and crispy where it touches the skillet, about 5 minutes. Serve.

Per serving: Calories: 94; Fat: 8g; Protein: 4g; Total Carbs: 1g; Fiber: 0g; Net Carbs: 1g; **Macros:** Fat: 76%; Protein: 20%; Carbs: 4%

Pesto Zucchini Noodles

SERVES 4 | PREP TIME: 15 minutes

4 small zucchini, ends trimmed
¾ cup Herb-Kale Pesto

¼ cup grated or shredded
  Parmesan cheese

Use a spiralizer or peeler to cut the zucchini into "noodles" and place them in a medium bowl. Add the pesto and the Parmesan cheese and toss to coat. Serve.

Per serving: Calories: 93; Fat: 8g; Protein: 4g; Total Carbs: 2g; Fiber: 0g; Net Carbs: 2g; **Macros:** Fat: 70%; Protein: 15%; Carbs: 8%

Coconut-Zucchini Noodles

SERVES 4 | PREP TIME: 15 minutes

½ avocado, diced
2 tablespoons water
1 tablespoon freshly squeezed
  lemon juice
1 tablespoon coconut oil
2 tablespoons shredded
  unsweetened coconut

1 tablespoon chopped cilantro
3 zucchini, cut into long
  ribbons with a peeler or
  spiralized
Juice of 1 lime
1 cup blanched asparagus, cut
  into 2-inch pieces

In a blender, blend the avocado, water, lemon juice, and coconut oil until smooth. Pour the avocado mixture into a bowl, and whisk in the coconut and cilantro. Set aside. In a large bowl, toss the zucchini, lime juice, and asparagus. Add the sauce, toss to combine well, and serve.

Per Serving: Calories: 131; Fat: 9g; Protein: 5g; Total Carbs: 10g; Fiber: 6g; Net Carbs: 4g; **Macros:** Fat: 57%; Protein: 15%; Carbs: 28%

Zucchini Lasagna

SERVES 8 | PREP TIME: 15 minutes | COOK TIME: 1 hour

½ cup extra-virgin olive
  oil, divided
4 to 5 medium zucchini squash
1 teaspoon salt
8 ounces frozen spinach,
  thawed and well drained
  (about 1 cup)
2 cups whole-milk
  ricotta cheese
¼ cup chopped fresh basil or
  2 teaspoons dried basil

1 teaspoon garlic powder
½ teaspoon freshly ground
  black pepper
2 cups shredded fresh
  whole-milk mozza-
  rella cheese
1¾ cups shredded Parme-
  san cheese
½ (24-ounce) jar low-sugar
  marinara sauce (less than
  5 grams sugar)

Preheat the oven to 425°F. Line two baking sheets with parchment paper and drizzle each with 2 tablespoons olive oil, spreading evenly. Slice the zucchini lengthwise into ¼-inch-thick long slices and place on the prepared baking sheet in a single layer. Sprinkle them with ½ teaspoon salt per sheet. Bake until softened, but not mushy, 15 to 18 minutes. Remove from the oven and allow to cool slightly before assembling the lasagna. Reduce the oven temperature to 375°F. In a large bowl, combine the spinach, ricotta, basil, garlic powder, and pepper. In a small bowl, mix the mozzarella and Parmesan cheeses. In a medium bowl, combine the marinara sauce and remaining ¼ cup olive oil and stir to fully incorporate the oil into sauce. To assemble the lasagna, spoon a third of the marinara sauce mixture into the bottom of a 9-by-13-inch glass baking dish and spread evenly. Place 1 layer of softened zucchini slices to fully cover the sauce, then add a third of the ricotta-spinach mixture and spread evenly on top of the zucchini. Sprinkle a third of the mozzarella-Parmesan mixture on top of the ricotta. Repeat with 2 more cycles of these layers: marinara, zucchini, ricotta-spinach, then cheese blend. Bake until the cheese is bubbly and melted, 30 to 35 minutes. Turn the broiler to low and broil until the top is golden brown, about 5 minutes. Remove from the oven and allow to cool slightly before slicing.

Per Serving: Calories: 521; Fat: 41g; Protein: 25g; Total Carbs: 13g; Fiber: 3g; Net Carbs: 10g; **Macros:** Fat: 71%; Protein: 19%; Carbs: 10%

Sautéed Zucchini with Mint and Pine Nuts

SERVES 4 | PREP TIME: 5 minutes | COOK TIME: 7 minutes

¼ cup pine nuts	Zest and juice of 1 lemon
2 tablespoons canola oil	2 tablespoons minced mint
2 medium zucchini, cut into ½-inch pieces	Sea salt
2 garlic cloves, minced	Freshly ground black pepper

Heat a large skillet over high heat. Toast the pine nuts until fragrant and beginning to brown, 1 to 2 minutes. Transfer the pine nuts to a cutting board, and chop roughly. Add the canola oil to the same skillet, tilting to coat. When the canola oil is heated, add the zucchini. Sauté for 5 minutes until the zucchini is well browned. Remove the skillet from the heat. Add the garlic, lemon zest and juice, mint, and chopped pine nuts, and toss to mix. Season with salt and pepper.

Per Serving: Calories: 125; Fat: 11g; Protein: 2g; Total Carbs: 6g; Fiber: 2g; Net Carbs: 4g; **Macros:** Fat: 79%; Protein: 6%; Carbs: 15%

Stuffed Zucchini

SERVES 4 | PREP TIME: 20 minutes | COOK TIME: 30 minutes

3 tablespoons olive oil	¼ cup hemp hearts
1 cup finely chopped broccoli	1 tablespoon chopped fresh basil
1 red bell pepper, chopped	
1 cup shredded kale	Sea salt
1 scallion, white and green parts, chopped	Freshly ground black pepper
	4 medium zucchini
½ cup finely chopped pecans	1 cup crumbled goat cheese

Preheat the oven to 350°F. Heat the olive oil in a large skillet over medium-high heat. Sauté the broccoli, bell pepper, kale,

and scallion until tender, 6 to 8 minutes. Stir in the pecans, hemp hearts, and basil. Season the filling with salt and pepper. Cut a thin, lengthwise layer off the zucchini and scoop out the insides of the vegetables, leaving the outer shell intact. (Save the zucchini flesh for another meal.) Spoon the filling into the zucchini shells and top with goat cheese. Bake until the filling is warmed through and the cheese is melted, about 20 minutes.

Per Serving: Calories: 408; Fat: 35g; Protein: 15g; Total Carbs: 16g; Fiber: 7g; Net Carbs: 9g; **Macros:** Fat: 77%; Protein: 15%; Carbs: 8%

Zucchini Fritters

SERVES 4 | PREP TIME: 15 minutes | COOK TIME: 10 minutes

1½ pounds zucchini, grated and the liquid squeezed out	1 large egg, beaten
	Dash freshly ground black pepper
6 tablespoons Parmesan cheese	2 tablespoons extra-virgin olive oil
¼ cup almond flour	
1 teaspoon minced garlic	

In a large bowl, stir the zucchini, Parmesan cheese, almond flour, garlic, egg, and pepper. Roll the mixture into 12 equal balls, flattening them out slightly. In a large skillet over medium-high heat, heat the olive oil. When the olive oil is sizzling, place 6 zucchini fritters in the skillet, and cook until the bottom is golden brown, about 3 minutes. Turn the fritters over, and brown the other side, about 2 minutes. Transfer the fritters to paper towels, and repeat with the remaining fritters. Serve.

Per Serving: Calories: 187; Fat: 15g; Protein: 8g; Total Carbs: 7g; Fiber: 3g; Net Carbs: 4g; **Macros:** Fat: 69%; Protein: 17%; Carbs: 14%

Zucchini Mini Pizzas

SERVES 2 | PREP TIME: 10 minutes |
COOK TIME: 5 minutes | TOTAL TIME: 15 minutes

1 medium zucchini, sliced diagonally (about 8 slices)	¼ cup goat cheese, crumbled
	16 pepperoni slices (optional)
1 teaspoon olive oil	⅛ teaspoon salt
2 tablespoons sugar-free pizza sauce	⅛ teaspoon freshly ground black pepper
¼ cup shredded mozzarella cheese	1 teaspoon Italian seasoning

Preheat the oven to broil. Place the zucchini slices on a baking sheet and drizzle with the olive oil. Broil the zucchini for 2 minutes per side. Remove the baking sheet from the oven. Top each slice with equal amounts of the pizza sauce, mozzarella cheese, and goat cheese. Top each with two slice of pepperoni (if using). Season each slice evenly with the salt, pepper, and Italian seasoning. Place the baking sheet back in the oven. Broil for 2 minutes, or until the cheese browns.

Per Serving: (4 mini pizzas): Calories: 220; Fat: 16g; Protein: 14g; Total Carbs: 7g; Fiber: 1g; Net Carbs: 6g; **Macros:** Fat: 64%; Protein: 25%; Carbs: 11%

Zucchini Pizza Boats

SERVES 1 | PREP TIME: 10 minutes | COOK TIME: 30 minutes

1 medium zucchini, halved lengthwise and deseeded	2 tablespoons olive oil
	2 garlic cloves, minced

1 cup fresh spinach

2 tablespoons low-sugar marinara sauce

8 ounces ricotta cheese

Line a baking sheet with aluminum foil. Place the zucchini, hollow-side up, on the prepared baking sheet. In a small skillet over medium-high heat, warm the olive oil. Add the garlic and stir for 1 to 2 minutes or until fragrant; then add the spinach and stir until it wilts. Divide the spinach mixture evenly between the zucchini halves. Top evenly with the marinara sauce and ricotta cheese. Bake for 20 to 25 minutes, or until the cheese is melted and the zucchini is tender.

Per Serving: Calories: 689; Fat: 57g; Protein: 28g; Total Carbs: 16g; Fiber: 3g; Net Carbs: 14g; **Macros:** Fat: 74%; Protein: 16%; Carbs: 10%

Mexican Zucchini Hash

SERVES 4 | PREP TIME: 5 minutes | COOK TIME: 10 minutes

2 tablespoons avocado oil

½ onion, diced

2 garlic cloves, minced

4 large zucchini, diced

½ teaspoon salt

¼ teaspoon freshly ground black pepper

1 teaspoon ground cumin

1 cup sliced button mushrooms

1 cup queso blanco cheese

2 avocados, diced

2 tablespoons chopped fresh cilantro

In a large skillet over medium-high heat, warm the avocado oil. Add the onion, garlic, and zucchini, and season with the salt, pepper, and cumin. Stir to mix. Add the mushrooms and sauté for 4 to 6 minutes, or until the vegetables are soft. Remove from the heat and top with the queso blanco, diced avocado, and cilantro. Serve warm.

Per Serving: Calories: 401; Fat: 29g; Protein: 12g; Total Carbs: 23g; Fiber: 10g; Net Carbs: 13g; **Macros:** Fat: 65%; Protein: 13%; Carbs: 22%

Vegetable Hash

SERVES 4 | PREP TIME: 15 minutes | COOK TIME: 20 minutes

3 tablespoons avocado oil

1 onion, chopped

1 tablespoon minced garlic

4 cups chopped cauliflower

2 zucchini, diced

2 cups chopped kale

1 cup chopped pecans

2 tablespoons nutritional yeast

1 tablespoon chopped fresh oregano

Freshly ground black pepper

1 avocado, diced

Heat the oil in a large skillet over medium-high heat. Sauté the onion and garlic until softened, about 3 minutes. Add the cauliflower, zucchini, and kale and sauté until the vegetables are tender, about 15 minutes. Stir in the pecans, nutritional yeast, and oregano and sauté for 2 minutes. Remove from the heat and season with pepper. Serve topped with avocado.

Per Serving: Calories: 456; Fat: 39g; Protein: 10g; Total Carbs: 24g; Fiber: 12g; Net Carbs: 12g; **Macros:** Fat: 77%; Protein: 9%; Carbs: 14%

Cayenne Pepper Vegetable Bake

SERVES 12 | PREP TIME: 20 minutes | COOK TIME: 1 hour

1 bunch Brussels sprouts (about 20), stemmed and diced

1 bunch radishes (about 12), diced

2 turnips, peeled and diced

1 tomato, diced

1 yellow onion, diced

6 tablespoons olive oil

2 tablespoons cayenne pepper

2 teaspoons salt

1 teaspoon freshly ground black pepper

Preheat the oven to 400°F. On a large, rimmed baking sheet, combine the Brussels sprouts, radishes, turnips, tomato, and onion. Add the olive oil and toss to coat. Season with the cayenne, salt, and pepper. Bake for 1 hour or until the vegetables are browned and crisp.

Per serving: Calories: 89; Fat: 7g; Protein: 2g; Total Carbs: 6g; Fiber: 2g; Net Carbs: 4g; **Macros:** Fat: 71%; Protein: 9%; Carbs: 20%

Creamed Vegetables

SERVES 6 | PREP TIME: 15 minutes | COOK TIME: 6 hours on low

1 tablespoon extra-virgin olive oil

½ head cauliflower, cut into small florets

2 cups green beans, cut into 2-inch pieces

1 cup asparagus spears, cut into 2-inch pieces

½ cup sour cream

½ cup shredded Cheddar cheese

½ cup shredded Swiss cheese

3 tablespoons butter

¼ cup water

1 teaspoon ground nutmeg

Pinch freshly ground black pepper, for seasoning

Lightly grease the insert of the slow cooker with the olive oil. Add the cauliflower, green beans, asparagus, sour cream, Cheddar cheese, Swiss cheese, butter, water, nutmeg, and pepper to the insert. Cover and cook on low for 6 hours. Serve warm.

Per serving: Calories: 207; Fat: 18g; Protein: 8g; Total Carbs: 5g; Fiber: 2g; Net Carbs: 3g; **Macros:** Fat: 76%; Protein: 15%; Carbs: 9%

Crustless Spanakopita

SERVES 6 | PREP TIME: 15 minutes | COOK TIME: 45 minutes

¾ cup extra-virgin olive oil, divided

1 small yellow onion, diced

1 (32-ounce) bag frozen chopped spinach, thawed, fully drained, and patted dry (about 4 cups)

4 garlic cloves, minced

½ teaspoon salt

½ teaspoon freshly ground black pepper

1 cup whole-milk ricotta cheese

4 large eggs

¾ cup crumbled feta cheese

¼ cup pine nuts

Preheat the oven to 375°F. In a large skillet, heat ¼ cup of olive oil over medium-high heat. Add the onion and sauté until softened, 6 to 8 minutes. Add the spinach, garlic, salt, and pepper and sauté another 5 minutes. Remove from the heat and allow to cool slightly. In a medium bowl, whisk the ricotta and eggs. Add to the cooled spinach and stir to combine. Pour ¼ cup of olive oil in the bottom of a 9-by-13-inch glass baking dish and swirl to coat the bottom and sides. Add the spinach-ricotta mixture and spread into an even layer. Bake for 20 minutes or until the mixture begins to set. Remove from the oven and crumble the feta evenly across the top of the spinach. Add the pine nuts and drizzle with the remaining ¼ cup of olive oil. Return to the oven and bake for an additional 15 to 20 minutes, or until the spinach is fully set and the top is starting to turn golden brown. Allow to cool slightly before cutting to serve.

Konjac Noodles with Spinach Hemp Pesto and Goat Cheese

SERVES 4 | PREP TIME: 15 minutes | COOK TIME: 10 minutes

½ cup Spinach Hemp Pesto (page 306)

2 cups sliced mushrooms

30 ounces konjac noodles, such as NuPasta, drained and rinsed

1 cup crumbled goat cheese

Place a large skillet over medium heat. Add the pesto and mushrooms. Sauté the mushrooms until lightly caramelized, about 8 minutes. Add the noodles to the skillet and toss until they are heated through, about 2 minutes. Serve topped with goat cheese.

Per Serving: Calories: 187; Fat: 14g; Protein: 7g; Total Carbs: 10g; Fiber: 6g; Net Carbs: 4g; **Macros:** Fat: 67%; Protein: 15%; Carbs: 18%

North African Vegetable Stew

SERVES 6 | PREP TIME: 15 minutes | COOK TIME: 7 to 8 hours on low

1 tablespoon extra-virgin olive oil

2 cups diced pumpkin

2 cups chopped cauliflower

1 red bell pepper, diced

½ sweet onion, diced

2 teaspoons minced garlic

2 cups coconut milk

2 tablespoons natural peanut butter

1 tablespoon ground cumin

1 teaspoon ground coriander

¼ cup chopped cilantro, for garnish

Lightly grease the insert of the slow cooker with the olive oil. Add the pumpkin, cauliflower, bell pepper, onion, and garlic to the insert. In a small bowl, whisk the coconut milk, peanut butter, cumin, and coriander until smooth. Pour the coconut milk mixture over the vegetables in the insert. Cover and cook on low for 7 to 8 hours. Serve topped with the cilantro.

Per serving: Calories: 415; Fat: 35g; Protein: 11g; Total Carbs: 14g; Fiber: 7g; Net Carbs: 7g; **Macros:** Fat: 76%; Protein: 11%; Carbs: 13%

Mixed-Vegetable Lasagna

SERVES 6 | PREP TIME: 20 minutes | COOK TIME: 7 to 8 hours on low

3 tablespoons extra-virgin olive oil, divided

1 cup sliced mushrooms

2 cups marinara sauce

2 zucchini, thinly sliced lengthwise

2 cups shredded kale

1 tablespoon chopped basil

8 ounces ricotta cheese

8 ounces goat cheese

2 cups shredded mozzarella cheese

Lightly grease the insert of the slow cooker with 1 tablespoon olive oil. In a large skillet over medium-high heat, heat the remaining 2 tablespoons of the olive oil. Add the mushrooms and sauté until they are softened, about 5 minutes. Stir the marinara sauce into the mushrooms and stir to combine. Pour about one-third of the sauce into the insert. Arrange one-third of the zucchini strips over the sauce. Top with one-third of the kale. Sprinkle half of both the ricotta and goat cheese over the kale. Repeat with the sauce, zucchini, kale, ricotta, and goat cheese to create another layer. Top with the remaining zucchini strips

and the sauce. Sprinkle the mozzarella cheese on top. Cover and cook on low for 7 to 8 hours. Serve warm.

Per serving: Calories: 345; Fat: 25g; Protein: 21g; Total Carbs: 10g; Fiber: 3g; Net Carbs: 7g; **Macros:** Fat: 64%; Protein: 25%; Carbs: 11%

Mediterranean Spaghetti

SERVES 2 | PREP TIME: 10 minutes | COOK TIME: 20 minutes

3 tablespoons olive oil

1 onion, diced

2 garlic cloves, minced

1 cup diced eggplant

2 whole artichoke hearts, quartered

½ (15-ounce) can tomato purée

½ cup olives, pitted and coarsely chopped

2 tablespoons chopped fresh basil leaves

1 tablespoon dried oregano

3 tablespoons capers

1 teaspoon salt

½ teaspoon freshly ground black pepper

½ can tomato paste (optional)

16 ounces cooked spaghetti squash or hearts of palm noodles

Chopped fresh parsley, for serving (optional)

Grated cheese, for serving (optional)

In a large skillet, heat the olive oil over medium-high heat. Add the onion and garlic and cook for 3 to 5 minutes, stirring, then add the eggplant. Reduce the heat to medium, cook for 5 minutes, and add the artichoke hearts. Stir everything together, then add the tomato purée, olives, basil, oregano, capers, salt, and pepper. Cook for another 5 to 8 minutes, adding the tomato paste if you'd like the sauce to be thicker. Add the cooked spaghetti squash and toss to coat with the sauce. Sprinkle with parsley and cheese (if using).

Per Serving: Calories: 430; Fat: 26g; Protein: 9g; Total Carbs: 40g; Fiber: 12g; Net Carbs: 28g; **Macros:** Fat: 55%; Protein: 9%; Carbs: 36%

Moroccan Vegetable Tagine

SERVES 6 | PREP TIME: 20 minutes | COOK TIME: 1 hour

½ cup extra-virgin olive oil

2 medium yellow onions, sliced

6 celery stalks, sliced into ¼-inch crescents

6 garlic cloves, minced

1 teaspoon ground cumin

1 teaspoon ginger powder

1 teaspoon salt

½ teaspoon paprika

½ teaspoon ground cinnamon

¼ teaspoon freshly ground black pepper

2 cups vegetable stock

1 medium eggplant, cut into 1-inch cubes

2 medium zucchini, cut into ½-inch-thick semicircles

2 cups cauliflower florets

1 (14-ounce) can artichoke hearts, drained and quartered

1 cup halved and pitted green olives

½ cup chopped fresh flat-leaf parsley, for garnish

½ cup chopped fresh cilantro leaves, for garnish

Greek yogurt, for garnish (optional)

In a large, thick soup pot or Dutch oven, heat the olive oil over medium-high heat. Add the onion and celery and sauté until softened, 6 to 8 minutes. Add the garlic, cumin, ginger, salt, paprika, cinnamon, and pepper and sauté for another 2 minutes. Add the stock and bring to a boil. Reduce the heat to low and add the eggplant, zucchini, and cauliflower. Simmer on low heat, covered, until the vegetables are tender, 30 to 35 minutes. Add the artichoke hearts and olives, cover, and simmer for another 15 minutes. Serve garnished with parsley, cilantro, and Greek yogurt (if using).

Per Serving: Calories: 309; Fat: 21g; Protein: 6g; Total Carbs: 24g; Fiber: 9g; Net Carbs: 15g; **Macros:** Fat: 61%; Protein: 27%; Carbs: 12%

Pesto Sautéed Vegetables

SERVES 4 | PREP TIME: 5 minutes | COOK TIME: 5 minutes

2 tablespoons canola oil
1 yellow or orange bell pepper, seeds and ribs removed, thinly sliced
1 medium zucchini, cut into ½-inch pieces
1 cup grape tomatoes
½ cup pesto
Sea salt
Freshly ground black pepper

Heat a large skillet over high heat. When the skillet is hot, add the canola oil, tilting the pan to coat. Allow the oil to get hot. Add the pepper and zucchini to the skillet, and sauté for 3 minutes until the vegetables are beginning to brown. Add the tomatoes and cook until hot but not bursting, about 2 minutes. Remove the pan from the heat and add the pesto. Stir to coat the vegetables in the pesto, and season with salt and pepper.

Per Serving: Calories: 239; Fat: 21g; Protein: 3g; Total Carbs: 9g; Fiber: 2g; Net Carbs: 7g; **Macros:** Fat: 79%; Protein: 6%; Carbs: 15%

Green Vegetable Stir-Fry with Tofu

SERVES 2 | PREP TIME: 15 minutes | COOK TIME: 15 minutes

3 tablespoons avocado oil, divided
1 cup halved Brussels sprouts
½ onion, diced
½ leek, white and light green parts, diced
½ head green cabbage, diced
¼ cup water, plus more if needed
½ cup kale, coarsely chopped
1 cup spinach, coarsely chopped
8 ounces tofu, diced
2 teaspoons garlic powder
Salt
Freshly ground black pepper
½ avocado, pitted, peeled, and diced
MCT oil (optional)

In a large skillet with a lid, heat 2 tablespoons of avocado oil over medium-high heat. Add the Brussels sprouts, onion, leek, and cabbage and stir. Add the water, cover, lower the heat to medium, and cook for about 5 minutes. Toss in the kale and spinach and cook for 3 minutes, stirring constantly, until the onion, leek, and cabbage are caramelized. Add the tofu to the stir-fry, then season with the garlic, salt, pepper, and the remaining tablespoon of avocado oil. Turn the heat back up to medium-high and cook for about 10 minutes, stirring constantly, until the tofu is nice and caramelized on all sides. Divide the stir-fry between two plates and top with diced avocado. Drizzle MCT oil over the top (if using).

Per Serving: Calories: 473; Fat: 33g; Protein: 17g; Total Carbs: 27g; Fiber: 12g; Net Carbs: 15g; **Macros:** Fat: 63%; Protein: 15%; Carbs: 22%

Vegetable Vindaloo

SERVES 6 | PREP TIME: 15 minutes | COOK TIME: 6 hours on low

1 tablespoon extra-virgin olive oil
4 cups cauliflower florets
1 carrot, diced
1 zucchini, diced
1 red bell pepper, diced
2 cups coconut milk
½ sweet onion, chopped
1 dried chipotle pepper, chopped
1 tablespoon grated fresh ginger
2 teaspoons minced garlic
2 teaspoons ground cumin
1 teaspoon ground coriander
½ teaspoon turmeric
¼ teaspoon cayenne pepper
¼ teaspoon cardamom
1 cup Greek yogurt, for garnish
2 tablespoons chopped cilantro, for garnish

Lightly grease the insert of the slow cooker with the olive oil. Place the cauliflower, carrot, zucchini, and bell pepper in the insert. In a small bowl, whisk the coconut milk, onion, chipotle pepper, ginger, garlic, cumin, coriander, turmeric, cayenne pepper, and cardamom until well blended. Pour the coconut milk mixture into the insert and stir to combine. Cover and cook on low for 6 hours. Serve each portion topped with the yogurt and cilantro.

Per serving: Calories: 299; Fat: 23g; Protein: 9g; Total Carbs: 14g; Fiber: 5g; Net Carbs: 9g; **Macros:** Fat: 69%; Protein: 12%; Carbs: 19%

Summer Vegetable Mélange

SERVES 6 | PREP TIME: 15 minutes | COOK TIME: 6 hours on low

½ cup extra-virgin olive oil
¼ cup balsamic vinegar
1 tablespoon dried basil
1 teaspoon dried thyme
¼ teaspoon salt
2 cups cauliflower florets
2 zucchini, diced into 1-inch pieces
1 yellow bell pepper, cut into strips
1 cup halved button mushrooms

In a large bowl, whisk the oil, vinegar, basil, thyme, and salt, until blended. Add the cauliflower, zucchini, bell pepper, and mushrooms, and toss to coat. Transfer the vegetables to the insert of a slow cooker. Cover and cook on low for 6 hours. Serve.

Per Serving: (1 cup) Calories: 189; Fat: 18g; Protein: 1g; Total Carbs: 5g; Fiber: 1g; Net Carbs: 4g; **Macros:** Fat: 87%; Protein: 2%; Carbs: 11%

FISH & SEAFOOD

Chili Fish Stew

SERVES 6 | PREP TIME: 15 minutes | COOK TIME: 35 minutes

¼ cup coconut oil
1 onion, chopped
2 celery stalks, chopped
1 tablespoon minced garlic
½ fennel bulb, thinly sliced
1 sweet potato, diced
1 carrot, diced
1 (15-ounce) can low-sodium diced tomatoes
1 cup low-sodium chicken broth
1 cup coconut milk
¼ teaspoon red pepper flakes
12 ounces firm fish, cut into 1-inch chunks (salmon, halibut, haddock)
2 tablespoons chopped fresh cilantro, for garnish

Heat the coconut oil in a large stockpot over medium-high heat. Sauté the onion, celery, and garlic until softened, about 4 minutes. Add the fennel, sweet potato, and carrot and sauté for 4 minutes more. Stir in the tomatoes, broth, coconut milk, and red pepper flakes and bring the stew to a boil. Reduce the heat to low and simmer until the vegetables are tender, about 15 minutes. Stir in the fish and simmer until it is cooked through, about 10 minutes. Serve topped with the cilantro.

Per Serving: Calories: 277; Fat: 21g; Protein: 14g; Total Carbs: 7g; Fiber: 3g; Net Carbs: 4g; **Macros:** Fat: 70%; Protein: 20%; Carbs: 10%

Nut-Crusted Baked Fish

SERVES 4 | PREP TIME: 10 minutes | COOK TIME: 20 minutes

½ cup extra-virgin olive oil, divided
1 pound flaky white fish (such as cod, haddock, or halibut), skin removed
½ cup shelled finely chopped pistachios
½ cup ground flaxseed

Zest and juice of 1 lemon, divided
1 teaspoon ground cumin
1 teaspoon ground allspice
½ teaspoon salt (use 1 teaspoon if pistachios are unsalted)
¼ teaspoon freshly ground black pepper

Preheat the oven to 400°F. Line a baking sheet with parchment paper and drizzle 2 tablespoons olive oil over the sheet, spreading to evenly coat the bottom. Cut the fish into 4 equal pieces and place on the prepared baking sheet. In a small bowl, combine the pistachios, flaxseed, lemon zest, cumin, allspice, salt, and pepper. Drizzle in ¼ cup olive oil and stir well. Divide the nut mixture evenly atop the fish pieces. Drizzle the lemon juice and remaining 2 tablespoons oil over the fish and bake until cooked through, 15 to 20 minutes, depending on the thickness of the fish.

Per Serving: Calories: 509; Fat: 41g; Protein: 26g; Total Carbs: 9g; Fiber: 6g; Net Carbs: 3g; **Macros:** Fat: 72%; Protein: 20%; Carbs: 8%

Easy Oven-Fried Catfish

SERVES 4 | PREP TIME: 10 minutes, plus 3 hours to soak | COOK TIME: 30 minutes

4 catfish fillets
2 teaspoons baking soda
Avocado oil
½ cup almond flour
¼ cup crushed pork rinds

¼ teaspoon paprika
¼ teaspoon garlic powder
¼ teaspoon kosher salt
⅛ teaspoon cayenne pepper
2 eggs, lightly beaten

Place the catfish in a large bowl of cold water, add the baking soda, and stir to combine. Let the fish soak in the refrigerator for a few hours to overnight. Preheat the oven to 350°F. Line a baking sheet with parchment paper and brush it liberally with avocado oil. Drain the catfish, rinse it, and pat it dry with a paper towel. In a shallow pie plate, stir the almond flour, pork rinds, paprika, garlic powder, salt, and cayenne. In another shallow dish, whisk the beaten eggs and 1 tablespoon water to combine. Coat each catfish fillet in the egg mixture and dredge it in the almond flour mixture, coating both sides well. Place the fillets, not touching, on the baking sheet. Bake for 25 to 30 minutes, or until the fish is cooked through and flaky, turning the fish halfway through the baking time. Serve with tartar sauce.

Per Serving: Calories: 308; Fat: 20g; Protein: 30g; Total Carbs: 2g; Fiber: 1g; Net Carbs: 1g; **Macros:** Fat: 60%; Protein: 36%; Carbs: 4%

Halibut Curry

SERVES 4 | PREP TIME: 5 minutes | COOK TIME: 35 minutes

1 tablespoon avocado oil
½ cup finely chopped celery
½ cup frozen butternut squash cubes
1 cup full-fat canned coconut milk
½ cup seafood stock
1½ tablespoons curry powder

1 tablespoon dried cilantro
½ tablespoon garlic powder
½ tablespoon ground turmeric
1 teaspoon ground ginger
1 pound skinless halibut fillet, cut into chunks
Cooked cauliflower rice, for serving (optional)

In a large saucepan with a lid, heat the avocado oil over medium-high heat. Add the celery and cook for about 3 minutes. Add the squash and cook for 5 minutes. Add the coconut milk and seafood stock and cook, stirring, for 3 minutes. Stir in the curry powder, cilantro, garlic, turmeric, and ginger. Add the halibut to the pot, reduce the heat to medium, cover, and cook for 15 to 20 minutes, or until the fish is completely white and flakes easily with a fork. Serve the halibut curry over cauliflower rice if you'd like, or just eat it by itself!

Per Serving: Calories: 362; Fat: 22g; Protein: 33g; Total Carbs: 8g; Fiber: 3g; Net Carbs: 5g; **Macros:** Fat: 55%; Protein: 36%; Carbs: 9%

Pecan-Crusted Catfish

SERVES 4 | PREP TIME: 20 minutes | COOK TIME: 25 minutes

4 (4-ounce) catfish fillets, rinsed and patted dry
2 cups chopped pecans
1½ teaspoons gluten-free Worcestershire sauce
1¼ teaspoons garlic powder
1¼ teaspoons paprika
1 teaspoon kosher salt, plus more for seasoning

½ teaspoon freshly ground black pepper, plus more for seasoning
¼ teaspoon onion powder
¼ teaspoon cayenne pepper (optional)
2 eggs, lightly beaten
1 teaspoon hot sauce
Chopped fresh parsley, for serving
Lemon wedges, for serving

Preheat the oven to 375°F. Line a baking sheet with parchment paper. Set aside. In a food processor, combine the pecans, Worcestershire sauce, garlic powder, paprika, salt, black pepper, onion powder, and cayenne. Pulse until the pecans are finely chopped. Pour the mixture into a shallow pie plate and set aside. In a separate shallow dish, whisk the eggs and hot sauce. Dip each catfish fillet into the egg, coating it on both sides, and dredge in the pecan mixture, pressing the pecan coating onto the fish as needed to make sure the top of the fillet is well coated. Place the fillets onto the baking sheet. Bake for 20 to 25 minutes, or until done and the pecan crust is golden brown and fragrant. The thickest part of the fish should flake easily and will be opaque all the way through. Cooking time will vary depending on the size and thickness of the fish fillets. Sprinkle with parsley and serve with lemon wedges for squeezing.

Per Serving: Calories: 647; Fat: 55g; Protein: 27g; Total Carbs: 11g; Fiber: 7g; Net Carbs: 4g; **Macros:** Fat: 77%; Protein: 17%; Carbs: 6%

Fish Tacos

SERVES 4 | PREP TIME: 15 minutes | COOK TIME: 20 minutes

1 large egg, beaten
½ cup coconut flour, divided
1 teaspoon salt
1 teaspoon ground cumin
¼ teaspoon paprika
⅛ teaspoon chili powder

1 pound skinless boneless
   cod, cut into 1-inch pieces,
   patted dry
8 large butter lettuce leaves
½ cup coleslaw, divided
1 sliced avocado
¼ cup pico de gallo, divided
1 lime, quartered

Preheat the oven to 400°F. Line a baking sheet with parchment paper. Pour the egg into a small bowl. Pour ¼ cup of coconut flour into a medium bowl. In a second medium bowl, thoroughly combine the remaining ¼ cup of coconut flour, salt, cumin, paprika, and chili powder. Dip the cod pieces first into the plain coconut flour, then the egg, and finally the seasoned flour. Lay the cod on the prepared baking sheet in a single layer. Bake for 10 minutes, flip, and then bake for another 10 minutes. Let cool for 2 minutes. To assemble the tacos, lay out the lettuce leaves and top with equal amounts of cod, coleslaw, avocado, and pico de gallo. Squeeze lime juice on top. Serve immediately.

Per Serving: (2 tacos): Calories: 344; Fat: 22g; Protein: 25g; Total Carbs: 19g; Fiber: 9g; Net Carbs: 10g; Macros: Fat: 57%; Protein: 29%; Carbs: 14%

Crispy Fried Cod

SERVES 4 | PREP TIME: 15 minutes | COOK TIME: 15 minutes

1 cup crushed pork rinds
¼ cup grated Parmesan cheese
½ cup heavy (whipping) cream
1 large egg
4 (4-ounce) cod fillets,
   patted dry

Extra-virgin olive oil, for frying
1 (10-ounce) can original
   Ro-Tel (drained)
2 tablespoons lemon juice
   (optional)

In a small bowl, combine the pork rinds and grated Parmesan. In another bowl, whisk the heavy cream and egg. Dip each cod fillet completely in the egg mixture, then dip on both sides into the pork rind mixture, making sure the entire fillet is covered. Place the fillets on a plate and refrigerate while the oil heats. In a large skillet over medium heat, heat 2 to 3 inches of oil. Heat the oil to 365°F. Working in batches if necessary, fry each fillet for about 2 minutes on each side or until the outside is golden brown. Drain on a paper towel if needed, then plate and serve, topping each fillet with one-quarter of the can of Ro-Tel.

Per Serving: (1 fillet): Calories: 375; Fat: 28g; Protein: 36g; Total Carbs: 6g; Fiber: 0g; Net Carbs: 6g; Macros: Fat: 60%; Protein: 34%; Carbs: 6%

Mustard-Crusted Cod with Roasted Broccoli

SERVES 4 | PREP TIME: 5 minutes | COOK TIME: 10 minutes

1 pound broccoli, cut
   into florets
2 tablespoons olive oil
Salt
½ cup Dijon mustard

4 skinless cod fillets
   (4 ounces each)
¾ cup pork rind crumbs
Parsley leaves, for garnish

Preheat the oven to 400°F. Line a large baking sheet with parchment paper. In a medium bowl, combine the broccoli, oil, and ½ teaspoon salt and toss to combine. Spread the broccoli in a single layer on one side of the baking sheet. Roast for 15 minutes. Meanwhile, spread the mustard onto one side of each fillet. Press the pork rind crumbs onto the mustard. Place the cod on the empty side of the baking sheet. Roast for 8 to 10 minutes, until the fish is opaque and flakes easily with a fork. Season the broccoli with salt to taste. Serve the broccoli with the cod, garnished with the parsley.

Per Serving: Calories: 337; Fat: 17g; Protein: 37g; Total Carbs: 9g; Fiber: 4g; Net Carbs: 5g; Macros: Fat: 45%; Protein: 44%; Carbs: 11%

Cod with Parsley Pistou

SERVES 4 | PREP TIME: 15 minutes | COOK TIME: 10 minutes

1 cup packed roughly
   chopped fresh flat-leaf
   Italian parsley
1 to 2 small garlic
   cloves, minced
Zest and juice of 1 lemon
1 teaspoon salt

½ teaspoon freshly ground
   black pepper
1 cup extra-virgin olive
   oil, divided
1 pound cod fillets, cut into
   4 equal-sized pieces

In a food processor, pulse the parsley, garlic, lemon zest and juice, salt, and pepper. While the food processor is running, slowly stream in ¾ cup olive oil until well combined. In a large skillet, heat the remaining ¼ cup olive oil over medium-high heat. Add the cod fillets, cover, and cook for 4 to 5 minutes on each side, or until cooked through. Remove from the heat and keep warm. Add the pistou to the skillet and heat over medium-low heat. Return the cooked fish to the skillet, flipping to coat in the sauce. Serve warm, covered with pistou.

Per Serving: Calories: 581; Fat: 55g; Protein: 21g; Total Carbs: 3g; Fiber: 1g; Net Carbs: 2g; Macros: Fat: 84%; Protein: 15%; Carbs: 1%

Roasted Cod with Garlic Butter and Bok Choy

SERVES 2 | PREP TIME: 5 minutes | COOK TIME: 20 minutes

2 (8-ounce) cod fillets
¼ cup (½ stick) butter,
   thinly sliced
1 tablespoon minced garlic
½ pound baby bok choy,
   halved lengthwise

¼ teaspoon salt
¼ teaspoon freshly ground
   black pepper

Preheat the oven to 400°F. Make a large pouch from aluminum foil and place the cod inside. Top with slices of butter and the garlic, evenly divided. Tuck the bok choy around the fillets. Season with the salt and pepper. Close the pouch with the two ends of the foil meeting at the top, so the butter remains in the pouch. Place the sealed pouches in a baking dish. Bake for 15 to 20 minutes, depending on the thickness of the fillets. Serve immediately.

Per Serving: Calories: 317; Fat: 24g; Protein: 23g; Total Carbs: 4g; Fiber: 1g; Net Carbs: 3g; Macros: Fat: 67%; Protein: 28%; Carbs: 5%

Poached Cod over Brothy Veggie Noodles

SERVES 2 | PREP TIME: 15 minutes | COOK TIME: 15 minutes

1 teaspoon olive oil
1 garlic clove, smashed
1 small shallot, thinly sliced
1½ cups chicken broth

2 (6-ounce) fillets cod
Salt
Freshly ground black pepper
1 large turnip, spiralized

1 large zucchini, spiralized

3 or 4 radishes, spiralized

1 to 2 tablespoons chopped fresh parsley, for garnish

Lemon wedges, for serving

In a small saucepan (big enough to hold the fish) over medium heat, heat the olive oil. Add the garlic and shallot. Sauté for 2 to 3 minutes, or until fragrant. Pour in the chicken broth and bring to a simmer. Season the fish with salt and pepper and gently add to the broth. Cover the pan and cook for about 10 minutes, or until the flesh is opaque and flakes easily with a fork. Assemble the bowls by dividing the turnip, zucchini, and radish noodles evenly between them. Top each with cooked fish and ladle the broth over each bowl. Serve topped with parsley and with a lemon wedge on the side for squeezing.

Per Serving: Calories: 203; Fat: 4g; Protein: 29g; Total Carbs: 14g; Fiber: 4g; Net Carbs: 10g; **Macros:** Fat: 16%; Protein: 58%; Carbs: 26%

Cod Cakes

SERVES 2 | PREP TIME: 5 minutes | COOK TIME: 20 minutes

2 tablespoons plus 1 teaspoon extra-virgin olive oil, divided

¼ medium onion, chopped

1 garlic clove, minced

1 cup cauliflower rice

1 pound cod fillets

½ cup almond flour

1 large egg

2 tablespoons chopped fresh parsley

2 tablespoons ground flaxseed

1 tablespoon freshly squeezed lemon juice

1 teaspoon dried dill

½ teaspoon ground cumin

½ teaspoon pink Himalayan sea salt

¼ teaspoon freshly ground black pepper

Tartar sauce

In a medium skillet, heat 1 tablespoon of olive oil over medium heat. Add the onion and garlic and cook for about 7 minutes, until tender. Add the cauliflower rice and continue to stir for 5 to 7 minutes, until warmed through and tender. Transfer to a large bowl. In the same skillet, heat 1 teaspoon of olive oil over medium-high heat. Cook the cod for 4 to 5 minutes on each side, until cooked through. Let the cod cool for a couple of minutes. Add the almond flour, egg, parsley, flaxseed, lemon juice, dill, cumin, salt, and pepper to the bowl with the cauliflower rice. Mix until the ingredients are well combined. Add the fish to the bowl and mix well. In the skillet, heat the remaining 1 tablespoon of olive oil over medium heat. Using a ½ cup measuring cup, form 4 fish cakes by packing the mixture into the cup, then slipping the cake out of the cup onto a plate. Place the fish cakes in the hot oil and cook for about 5 minutes per side, flipping once, until golden brown on both sides. Place the cod cakes on serving plates, and serve with tartar sauce.

Per Serving: Calories: 531; Fat: 34g; Protein: 45g; Total Carbs: 12g; Fiber: 6g; Net Carbs: 6g; **Macros:** Fat: 57%; Protein: 34%; Carbs: 9%

Baked Halibut with Herb Sauce

SERVES 4 | PREP TIME: 15 minutes | COOK TIME: 18 minutes

4 (5-ounce) halibut fillets

1 tablespoon extra-virgin olive oil

Sea salt

Freshly ground black pepper

½ cup plain Greek yogurt

¼ cup mayonnaise

2 tablespoons sour cream

Juice and zest of 1 lemon

1 tablespoon chopped fresh dill

1 teaspoon chopped fresh basil

1 teaspoon chopped fresh chives

Preheat the oven to 400°F. Line a baking sheet with parchment paper. Pat the fish dry with paper towels, and lightly oil with the olive oil. Season both sides of the fish with salt and pepper. Place the fillets on the baking sheet, and bake until cooked through, about 15 to 18 minutes. While the fish is cooking, in a small bowl, stir the yogurt, mayonnaise, sour cream, lemon juice, lemon zest, dill, basil, and chives. Serve the fish with a generous dollop of sauce.

Per Serving: Calories: 374; Fat: 25g; Protein: 33g; Total Carbs: 2g; Fiber: 0g; Net Carbs: 2g; **Macros:** Fat: 62%; Protein: 36%; Carbs: 2%

Pesto Flounder with Bok Choy

SERVES 6 | PREP TIME: 10 minutes | COOK TIME: 10 minutes

2 pounds bok choy (about 1 large head)

6 skinless flounder fillets (4 ounces each)

6 tablespoons pesto

6 tablespoons finely grated Parmesan cheese

Freshly ground black pepper

2 tablespoons olive oil

1 garlic clove, minced

Salt

Preheat the broiler to high. Line a baking sheet with aluminum foil. Trim off the thick root end of the bok choy. Slice each stalk into quarters, then cut into rough chunks. Pat the fish dry with paper towels and place on the prepared baking sheet. Spread 1 tablespoon of pesto over each fillet. Sprinkle 1 tablespoon of Parmesan over the pesto on each fillet. Season with pepper. Cook the flounder under the broiler for 5 to 7 minutes, until it has reached an internal temperature of 145°F and is opaque. Meanwhile, in a large skillet, heat the olive oil over medium-high heat. Add the bok choy and garlic and cook, stirring frequently, for 5 minutes. Remove the flounder from the broiler and transfer to serving plates. Add the bok choy and season with salt.

Per Serving: Calories: 264; Fat: 17g; Protein: 19g; Total Carbs: 10g; Fiber: 4g; Net Carbs: 6g; **Macros:** Fat: 57%; Protein: 29%; Carbs: 14%

Coconut Milk Baked Haddock

SERVES 4 | PREP TIME: 10 minutes | COOK TIME: 27 minutes

2 tablespoons olive oil

1 onion, thinly sliced

1 tablespoon minced garlic

4 (3-ounce) haddock fillets

2 cups canned coconut milk

1 teaspoon ground coriander

½ teaspoon ground cumin

Sea salt

Freshly ground black pepper

2 tablespoons chopped fresh cilantro

Preheat the oven to 350°F. Heat the olive oil in a large ovenproof skillet over medium-high heat. Sauté the onion and garlic until lightly caramelized, about 7 minutes. Add the fish to the skillet and brown, turning once, about 8 minutes in total. Add the coconut milk, coriander, and cumin, stirring carefully. Cover and bake until the fish flakes with a fork, about 12 minutes. Season with salt and pepper and serve topped with cilantro.

Per Serving: Calories: 381; Fat: 29g; Protein: 23g; Total Carbs: 6g; Fiber: 1g; Net Carbs: 5g; **Macros:** Fat: 69%; Protein: 24%; Carbs: 7%

Cheesy Golden Fried Haddock

SERVES 4 | **PREP TIME:** 15 minutes | **COOK TIME:** 12 minutes

1 pound boneless haddock fillets, cut into 4 equal pieces
¼ cup almond flour, divided
1 large egg
1 tablespoon water
½ cup Parmesan cheese

¼ cup flaxseed meal
¼ teaspoon freshly ground black pepper
Pinch ground cayenne pepper
½ cup extra-virgin olive oil
Lemon wedges, for garnish

Pat the fish dry with paper towels, and set aside. Put 2 tablespoons of almond flour in a small bowl, and set it next to the fish. In another small bowl, stir the eggs and water, and set the mixture next to the almond flour. In a medium bowl, stir the remaining 2 tablespoons of almond flour with the Parmesan cheese, flaxseed meal, black pepper, and cayenne pepper. Set the bowl next to the egg mixture. Dredge the fish pieces in the almond flour, the egg mixture, and the flour mixture, in that order, until all 4 pieces are coated. In a large skillet over medium-high heat, heat the olive oil. When the oil is hot, fry the fish, turning once, until both sides are golden and crispy and the fish is cooked through, about 6 minutes per side, depending on the thickness of the fish. Transfer the fish to a paper towel-lined plate, and use paper towels to blot off the excess oil. Serve with the lemon wedges.

Per Serving: Calories: 349; Fat: 25g; Protein: 27g; Total Carbs: 4g; Fiber: 3g; Net Carbs: 1g; **Macros:** Fat: 64%; Protein: 31%; Carbs: 5%

Crispy "Breaded" Haddock

SERVES 4 | **PREP TIME:** 20 minutes | **COOK TIME:** 12 minutes

16 ounces boneless, skinless haddock fillet, cut into 4 pieces
1 cup almond flour
½ teaspoon paprika
⅛ teaspoon ground cardamom

⅛ teaspoon sea salt
Pinch freshly ground black pepper
½ cup heavy (whipping) cream
¼ cup coconut oil

Rinse the fillets in cold water and pat them completely dry with paper towels. In a medium bowl, stir the almond flour, paprika, cardamom, salt, and pepper until well blended. Pour the cream into another medium bowl and set it beside the almond flour mixture. Dredge one fish fillet in the flour mixture, shaking off the excess. Then dip the fillet into the cream, shaking off the excess liquid. Finally, dredge the fish in the flour again to coat completely and set aside. Repeat with the remaining fillets. Place a large skillet over medium-high heat and add the oil. When the oil is hot, place the fillets in the skillet and fry until the fish is golden and crispy, turning once, about 12 minutes total.

Per Serving: Calories: 475; Fat: 39g; Protein: 28g; Total Carbs: 7g; Fiber: 3g; Net Carbs: 4g; **Macros:** Fat: 74%; Protein: 24%; Carbs: 2%

Balsamic Teriyaki Halibut

SERVES 1 | **PREP TIME:** 5 minutes | **COOK TIME:** 15 minutes

1 tablespoon balsamic vinegar
1 tablespoon coconut aminos
1 teaspoon grated ginger root
1 tablespoon avocado oil
1 (6-ounce) halibut fillet

Pink Himalayan salt
Freshly ground black pepper

In a small saucepan, heat the balsamic vinegar, coconut aminos, and grated ginger until it is bubbling. Reduce the heat to low and simmer for 5 minutes. Transfer to a bowl and set aside. In a medium sauté pan or skillet, heat the avocado oil over medium-high heat. Season the halibut with salt and pepper and add the fish to the skillet. Sear for about 3 minutes and then flip and sear the other side for 3 more minutes. Flip once more and brush 1 tablespoon of teriyaki sauce over the top and sides of the fish. Reduce the heat to medium and cook for another 2 minutes on each side, or until the center is opaque. Remove the halibut from the skillet and top with them remaining sauce before serving.

Per Serving: Calories: 393; Fat: 19g; Protein: 45g; Total Carbs: 5g; Fiber: 0g; Net Carbs: 5g; **Macros:** Fat: 44%; Protein: 46%; Carbs: 10%

Baked Nutty Halibut

SERVES 4 | **PREP TIME:** 20 minutes | **COOK TIME:** 15 minutes

½ cup heavy (whipping) cream
½ cup finely chopped pecans
¼ cup finely chopped almonds
4 (4-ounce) boneless halibut fillets

Sea salt
Freshly ground black pepper
2 tablespoons extra-virgin olive oil

Preheat the oven to 400°F. Line a baking sheet with parchment. Pour the heavy cream into a bowl and set it on your work surface. In another bowl, stir the pecans and almonds and set beside the cream. Pat the halibut fillets dry with paper towels and lightly season with salt and pepper. Dip the fillets in the cream, shaking off the excess; then dredge the fish in the nut mixture so that both sides of each piece are thickly coated. Place the fish on the prepared baking sheet and brush both sides of the pieces generously with olive oil. Bake the fish until the topping is golden and the fish flakes easily with a fork, 12 to 15 minutes. Serve.

Per Serving: Calories: 392; Fat: 31g; Protein: 26g; Total Carbs: 3g; Fiber: 2g; Net Carbs: 1g; **Macros:** Fat: 70%; Protein: 27%; Carbs: 3%

Halibut in Tomato Basil Sauce

SERVES 4 | **PREP TIME:** 10 minutes | **COOK TIME:** 20 minutes

½ cup extra-virgin olive oil, divided
2 large garlic cloves, minced
1 pint grape tomatoes, halved
¼ cup dry white wine
Juice of 1 lemon

½ cup roughly chopped fresh basil
Sea salt
Freshly ground black pepper
1¼ pounds halibut, cut into 4 (5-ounce) fillets

Heat 6 tablespoons of the olive oil in a small saucepan over medium heat. Cook the garlic for about 30 seconds, until fragrant. Add the tomatoes and cook for 10 minutes, until they partially break down. Stir in the wine and simmer for 1 to 2 minutes to cook off the alcohol. Stir in the basil and lemon juice and season generously with salt and pepper. While the sauce is cooking, heat the remaining 2 tablespoons of olive oil in a large skillet over medium-high heat. Season the halibut fillets liberally with salt and pepper. Sear on each side for 3 to 4 minutes, or until the fish flakes easily with a fork.

Per Serving: Calories: 467; Fat: 31g; Protein: 38g; Total Carbs: 5g; Fiber: 0g; Net Carbs: 5g; **Macros:** Fat: 60%; Protein: 33%; Carbs: 7%

Blackened Redfish with Spicy Crawfish Cream Sauce

SERVES 4 | PREP TIME: 10 minutes | COOK TIME: 20 minutes

For the blackened redfish

1 tablespoon paprika

2 teaspoons kosher salt

1 teaspoon onion powder

1 teaspoon garlic powder

1 teaspoon freshly ground black pepper

½ teaspoon dried thyme

½ teaspoon dried oregano

¼ teaspoon cayenne pepper

4 (4-ounce) redfish fillets, skinned and boned

2 tablespoons butter

3 tablespoons butter, melted, divided

For the cream sauce

2 tablespoons butter

¼ cup sliced scallion

2 garlic cloves, finely minced

⅓ cup chicken broth

2 tablespoons white wine

1 cup heavy (whipping) cream

1 pound crawfish tails, thawed if frozen

In a small bowl, stir the paprika, salt, onion powder, garlic powder, black pepper, thyme, oregano, and cayenne. Set aside. Place the fillets on paper towels and pat dry. Place the 3 tablespoons melted butter in a shallow dish. Dredge each fillet in the melted butter, coating each side well. Liberally sprinkle both sides of the fillets with the blackening seasoning. Reserve ½ teaspoon of seasoning. Preheat a large heavy skillet over medium to medium-high heat for 2 to 3 minutes. Add the remaining 2 tablespoons of butter to the pan to melt. Quickly add the fillets to the hot pan and sear for 2 to 3 minutes per side, or until done. The thickest part of the fish should flake easily and will be opaque all the way through. Remove the fillets from the pan. Return the skillet to the heat and reduce the heat to medium. Add the butter, scallion, garlic, and reserved ½ teaspoon of seasoning. Sauté for 1 to 2 minutes. Add the chicken broth and wine. Cook for 3 to 4 minutes until reduced by half, stirring constantly to pick up the browned bits left on the bottom of the pan. Add the heavy cream and simmer the sauce for 3 to 4 minutes, stirring constantly until thickened. Add the crawfish tails and stir until heated through. Serve the sauce over the blackened fillets.

Per Serving: Calories: 670; Fat: 46g; Protein: 58g; Total Carbs: 6g; Fiber: 1g; Net Carbs: 5g; Macros: Fat: 62%; Protein: 35%; Carbs: 3%

Macadamia-Crusted Halibut with Mango Coulis

SERVES 4 | PREP TIME: 10 minutes | COOK TIME: 10 minutes

½ cup finely chopped macadamia nuts

½ teaspoon sea salt

¼ teaspoon freshly ground black pepper

¼ teaspoon garlic powder

½ teaspoon onion powder

1¼ pounds halibut, cut into 4 (5-ounce) fillets

2 tablespoons coconut oil

½ cup diced mango

1 tablespoon lime juice

½ cup full-fat coconut milk

4 sprigs fresh cilantro, for garnish

Preheat the oven to 425°F. Line a rimmed baking sheet with parchment paper. In a shallow dish, mix the macadamia nuts, salt, pepper, garlic powder, and onion powder. Coat the halibut fillets in the coconut oil and then dredge in the nut mixture. Place the fillets onto the baking sheet, and bake for 12 minutes, or until the fish flakes easily with a fork. While the halibut is cooking, in a

blender, purée the mango, lime juice, and coconut milk until very smooth. Drizzle a few tablespoons of the mango coulis over each plate and then top with the baked halibut and a sprig of cilantro.

Per Serving: Calories: 423; Fat: 27g; Protein: 40g; Total Carbs: 6g; Fiber: 2g; Net Carbs: 4g; Macros: Fat: 57%; Protein: 38%; Carbs: 5%

Mackerel Escabeche

SERVES 4 | PREP TIME: 10 minutes | COOK TIME: 20 minutes, plus 15 minutes to rest

1 pound wild-caught mackerel fillets, cut into 4 pieces

1 teaspoon salt

½ teaspoon freshly ground black pepper

½ cup extra-virgin olive oil, divided

1 bunch asparagus, trimmed and cut into 2-inch pieces

1 (14-ounce) can artichoke hearts, drained and quartered

4 large garlic cloves, peeled and crushed

2 bay leaves

¼ cup red wine vinegar

½ teaspoon smoked paprika

Sprinkle the fillets with salt and pepper and let sit at room temperature for 5 minutes. In a large skillet, heat 2 tablespoons of olive oil over medium-high heat. Add the fish, skin-side up, and cook for 5 minutes. Flip and cook for 5 minutes on the other side, until browned and cooked through. Transfer to a serving dish, pour the cooking oil over the fish, and cover to keep warm. Heat the remaining 6 tablespoons of olive oil in the same skillet over medium heat. Add the asparagus, artichokes, garlic, and bay leaves and sauté until the vegetables are tender, 6 to 8 minutes. Using a slotted spoon, top the fish with the cooked vegetables, reserving the oil in the skillet. Add the vinegar and paprika to the oil and whisk to combine well. Pour the vinaigrette over the fish and vegetables and let sit at room temperature for at least 15 minutes, or marinate in the refrigerator for up to 24 hours for a deeper flavor. Remove the bay leaf before serving.

Per Serving: Calories: 578; Fat: 50g; Protein: 26g; Total Carbs: 13g; Fiber: 5g; Net Carbs: 8g; Macros: Fat: 76%; Protein: 18%; Carbs: 6%

Turmeric Coconut Mahi-Mahi

SERVES 1 | PREP TIME: 5 minutes | COOK TIME: 25 minutes

1 tablespoon coconut oil

1 teaspoon ground turmeric

½ teaspoon smoked paprika

1 (6-ounce) mahi-mahi fillet

Pink Himalayan salt

Freshly ground black pepper

Preheat the oven to 425°F. Line a baking sheet with parchment paper. In a small bowl, combine the coconut oil, turmeric, and paprika. Place the mahi-mahi on the prepared baking sheet. Season with salt and pepper to taste. Rub the mahi-mahi with the coconut oil mixture and evenly coat. Roast for 20 to 25 minutes, or until the mahi-mahi is cooked through.

Per Serving: Calories: 308; Fat: 16g; Protein: 40g; Total Carbs: 2g; Fiber: 1g; Net Carbs: 1g; Macros: Fat: 47%; Protein: 52%; Carbs: 1%

Baked Mackerel with Kale and Asparagus

SERVES 4 | PREP TIME: 20 minutes | COOK TIME: 15 minutes

2 cups chopped kale

1 cup asparagus, cut into 1-inch pieces

¼ onion, thinly sliced

2 teaspoons chopped fresh basil

4 (3-ounce) mackerel fillets
Sea salt
Freshly ground black pepper
¼ cup olive oil
1 lemon, cut into thin slices

Preheat the oven to 400°F. Lay out 4 sheets of aluminum foil, each about 12-inches long. Place ½ cup kale, ¼ cup asparagus, a quarter of the onion slices, and ½ teaspoon of basil in the middle of each piece of foil. Place a fillet on the vegetables and season the fish with salt and pepper. Drizzle the fish with olive oil and arrange lemon slices on top. Fold the foil up to form loose packets. Set the packets on a baking sheet and bake until the fish is opaque, about 15 minutes. Open the packets carefully and serve.

Per Serving: Calories: 327; Fat: 26g; Protein: 18g; Total Carbs: 9g; Fiber: 3g; Net Carbs: 6g; **Macros:** Fat: 72%; Protein: 22%; Carbs: 6%

Garlic Parmesan Crusted Salmon

SERVES 8 | PREP TIME: 15 minutes | COOK TIME: 15 minutes

4 pounds salmon
    fillets, skin on
½ cup (1 stick) butter, melted
3 garlic cloves, minced
1 teaspoon salt
½ teaspoon freshly ground
    black pepper
½ cup finely crushed
    pork skins
½ cup grated Parme-
    san cheese
1 lemon, for squeezing
    (optional)

Preheat the oven to 350°F, and line a baking sheet with parchment paper. Place the salmon fillets, skin-side down, on the lined baking sheet. In a small bowl, mix the butter and minced garlic. Spread or brush over the salmon. Season the fillets with the salt and pepper, and then sprinkle with the crushed pork skins and Parmesan. Bake for 15 minutes, remove from the oven, and squeeze lemon over the top (if using).

Per Serving: Calories: 532; Fat: 32g; Protein: 56g; Total Carbs: 1g; Fiber: 0g; Net Carbs: 1g; **Macros:** Fat: 54%; Protein: 42%; Carbs: 1%

Salmon in Cream Sauce

SERVES 4 | PREP TIME: 10 minutes | COOK TIME: 10 minutes

4 (5- to 6-ounce) fillets, about
    an inch thick, patted dry
1 tablespoon olive oil
¼ teaspoon salt
⅛ teaspoon freshly ground
    black pepper
⅓ cup sour cream
⅓ cup mayonnaise
½ teaspoon Dijon mustard
½ cup heavy (whipping) cream

Heat a large nonstick skillet over medium-high heat. Drizzle each fillet with olive oil, and season both sides with the salt and pepper. Place each fillet, skin-side up, in the hot pan, and allow to sear, undisturbed, for about 4 minutes. Flip, and cook another 3 minutes, or until cooked through. Transfer the fillets to a serving plate. Meanwhile, in a small bowl, whisk the sour cream, mayonnaise, and Dijon mustard. In a medium bowl with a hand mixer on high, beat the heavy cream until soft peaks form, about 1 minute, and fold into the sour cream mixture. Pour the sauce into the skillet and warm over low heat for 1 to 2 minutes. Serve the salmon topped with the cream sauce.

Per Serving: (1 fillet) Calories: 530; Fat: 42g; Protein: 34g; Total Carbs: 2g; Fiber: 0g; Net Carbs: 2g; **Macros:** Fat: 71%; Protein: 26%; Carbs: 2%

Whole Roasted Sea Bass

SERVES 4 | PREP TIME: 15 minutes | COOK TIME: 25 minutes

2 whole sea bass (about
    2 pounds), cleaned
    and scaled
2 tablespoons olive or
    avocado oil
Salt
Freshly ground black pepper
1 red onion, cut into
    ¼-inch slices
3 lemons, sliced into rounds
1 large leek, white and
    light green parts, sliced
    into rounds
8 dried bay leaves
3 tablespoons fresh oregano
Nut-free pesto, for serving
    (optional)

Preheat the oven to 425°F. Put the fish in a shallow baking dish and brush the fish with the oil. Season with salt and pepper. Fill the cavity of each fish with the onion, lemon, and leek slices, and the bay leaves and oregano. Roast the fish in the oven for about 25 minutes, or until the skin is crispy and the fish is flaky. To serve, remove the head and tail, then cut the fish into 4 equal-size fillets. Serve with nut-free pesto, if desired.

Per Serving: Calories: 307; Fat: 19g; Protein: 26g; Total Carbs: 8g; Fiber: 3g; Net Carbs: 5g; **Macros:** Fat: 56%; Protein: 34%; Carbs: 10%

Ginger Scallion Steamed Fish

SERVES 4 | PREP TIME: 5 minutes | COOK TIME: 25 minutes

4 scallions, white part
    chopped, green part cut in
    2- to 3-inch pieces and sliced
    lengthwise in half
2 garlic cloves, minced
1½ thumb-size pieces fresh
    ginger, thinly sliced
1 (4- to 5-pound) (or 2 smaller)
    head-on tilapia (or sea bass,
    catfish, flounder, or other
    white-fleshed fish), scaled,
    gutted, and patted dry
1 tablespoon soy sauce
2 teaspoons rice wine vinegar
2 teaspoons sesame oil

Preheat the oven to 400°F, and place parchment paper in a baking dish large enough to hold the fish, with a little extra room for the foil on the ends and sides. Lay a piece of aluminum foil, large enough to fold over the fish and seal, on top of the parchment paper. Place one-third of the green and white scallions, garlic, and ginger across the bottom of the foil, and then place the fish on top. Open the fish cavity, and place another third of the scallions, garlic, and ginger inside. Close the fish, and top with the remaining garlic and ginger, reserving the remaining scallions for garnish. In a small bowl, whisk the soy sauce, vinegar, and sesame oil, and drizzle over the fish. Fold the foil over and roll the edges a couple of times to seal the foil pouch. Bake for 25 minutes. Remove the foil, plate the fish, and sprinkle the remaining scallions on top.

Per Serving: Calories: 272; Fat: 7g; Protein: 51g; Total Carbs: 3g; Fiber: 1g; Net Carbs: 2g; **Macros:** Fat: 22%; Protein: 75%; Carbs: 3%

Sesame Salmon

SERVES 4 | PREP TIME: 15 minutes | COOK TIME: 15 minutes

Olive oil, for greasing
2 tablespoons soy sauce
2 tablespoons rice vinegar
4 teaspoons sesame oil
4 (5-ounce) boneless
    salmon fillets
Sea salt
Freshly ground black pepper
¼ cup sesame seeds
2 teaspoons chopped
    fresh thyme

Preheat the oven to 425°F. Lightly oil a 9-by-13-inch baking dish with olive oil, and set aside. In a small bowl, whisk the soy sauce, rice vinegar, and sesame oil. Pat the salmon dry with paper towels, and lightly season both sides of the fillets with salt and pepper. Place the salmon in the baking dish. Pour the soy mixture over the salmon, and bake the fish in the oven until it is just cooked through, about 13 to 15 minutes. Top the salmon with sesame seeds and chopped thyme, and serve.

Per Serving: Calories: 303; Fat: 19g; Protein: 30g; Total Carbs: 3g; Fiber: 1g; Net Carbs: 2g; **Macros:** Fat: 56%; Protein: 40%; Carbs: 4%

Teriyaki Salmon with Spicy Mayo and Asparagus

SERVES 2 | PREP TIME: 20 minutes | COOK TIME: 25 minutes

For the spicy mayo

2 teaspoons minced garlic	1 tablespoon cayenne pepper
1 tablespoon freshly squeezed lemon juice	⅛ teaspoon freshly ground black pepper
1 large egg	½ cup olive oil
½ teaspoon salt	

For salmon and asparagus

12 asparagus spears trimmed	¼ cup sugar-free teriyaki sauce
½ teaspoon minced fresh ginger	
2 teaspoons olive oil, divided	2 (8-ounce) salmon fillets
½ teaspoon rice wine vinegar	Sliced scallions, for garnish
¼ teaspoon freshly ground black pepper	

In a food processor, mix the garlic and lemon juice until smooth. Add the egg, salt, cayenne pepper, and black pepper to the garlic and lemon juice purée. While puréeing, slowly add the olive oil until the mayo forms. Refrigerate while the fillets cook. Preheat the oven to 400°F. In a medium bowl, mix the ginger, 1 teaspoon of olive oil, rice wine vinegar, pepper, and the teriyaki sauce. Add the salmon and cover completely with the sauce. Line a baking dish with aluminum foil. Transfer the salmon from the sauce to the dish. Pour any remaining sauce over the fillets. Tuck the asparagus around the fillets and drizzle them with the remaining teaspoon of olive oil. Bake for 15 to 20 minutes, depending on the thickness of the fillets. Remove the dish from the oven and check the fillets for doneness. Serve immediately with half of the spicy mayo. Garnish with the scallions.

Per Serving: Calories: 577; Fat: 42g; Protein: 42g; Total Carbs: 13g; Fiber: 3g; Net Carbs: 10g; **Macros:** Fat: 63%; Protein: 28%; Carbs: 9%

Salmon Poke

SERVES 2 | PREP TIME: 5 minutes

½ pound sushi-grade salmon, chopped into ½-inch cubes	½ teaspoon olive oil
¼ red onion, finely chopped	Juice of ½ small lemon
1 tablespoon dried chives	Salt
½ tablespoon capers	Freshly ground black pepper
1 tablespoon dried basil	1 cucumber, sliced into rounds, for serving (optional)
1 teaspoon Dijon mustard	

In a medium bowl, mix the salmon, red onion, and chives, capers, basil, mustard, olive oil, and lemon juice and season with salt and pepper. If desired, spoon the poke onto cucumber rounds.

Per Serving: Calories: 177; Fat: 9g; Protein: 23g; Total Carbs: 1g; Fiber: 0g; Net Carbs: 1g; **Macros:** Fat: 50%; Protein: 52%; Carbs: 8%

Charred Alaskan Salmon with Garlic Green Beans

SERVES 4 | PREP TIME: 15 minutes | COOK TIME: 25 minutes

For the rub

2 tablespoons stevia, or other sugar substitute	½ tablespoon ground cumin
	½ tablespoon paprika
1 tablespoon chili powder	½ tablespoon salt
1 teaspoon freshly ground black pepper	¼ teaspoon dry mustard
	Dash cinnamon

For the salmon

¼ cup coconut oil	¼ cup Dijon mustard, divided
4 (4- to 6-ounce) salmon fillets	

For the green beans

3 tablespoons butter	½ teaspoon salt
1 tablespoon olive oil	¼ teaspoon freshly ground black pepper
4 garlic cloves, minced	
1 pound green beans	

In a medium bowl, combine the stevia, chili powder, black pepper, cumin, paprika, salt, dry mustard, and cinnamon. In a large skillet over medium heat, heat the coconut oil for about 5 minutes. Liberally coat each salmon fillet with 1 tablespoon of mustard. Season each fillet, on both sides, with an equal amount of the rub. Set aside. Once the coconut oil has heated, increase the heat to medium-high. Add the salmon and sear for about 2 minutes. Flip and reduce the heat to medium. Cook for 6 to 8 minutes more, until the fish is opaque. In another large skillet over medium heat, heat the butter and olive oil. Add the garlic and cook until fragrant, about 1 minute. Add the green beans, salt, and pepper. Cover and reduce the heat to medium-low. Cook for 10 to 12 minutes, stirring occasionally. Serve immediately alongside the salmon.

Per Serving: Calories: 539; Fat: 42g; Protein: 31g; Total Carbs: 12g; Fiber: 6g; Net Carbs: 6g; **Macros:** Fat: 69%; Protein: 23%; Carbs: 8%

Sushi

SERVES 2 TO 4 | PREP TIME: 15 minutes | COOK TIME: 3 to 5 minutes

4 cups cauliflower rice	1 small cucumber (or any other vegetable you'd like), thinly sliced
2 tablespoons gelatin	
1 tablespoon apple cider vinegar	Sesame seeds, for topping (optional)
1 teaspoon salt	Coconut aminos or tamari, wasabi, sugar-free pickled ginger, sliced avocado, and/or avocado oil mayonnaise mixed with sugar-free hot sauce, for serving (optional)
2 to 4 nori sheets	
½ pound sushi-grade fish, thinly sliced	
1 small avocado, halved, pitted, peeled, and thinly sliced	

In a shallow saucepan with a lid, combine the cauliflower with 3 tablespoons of water. Turn the heat to medium, cover, and steam for 3 to 5 minutes. Drain the cauliflower and transfer to a medium bowl. Stir in the gelatin, vinegar, and salt until the mixture is smooth and sticky. Set aside. Fold a dish towel in half lengthwise and place it on your counter. Cover the towel in plastic wrap. Place a nori sheet on top of the plastic wrap, then spread with a layer of the cauliflower rice. Layer slices of fish, avocado, and cucumber over the cauliflower on the end of the nori sheet closest to you. Starting at the end closest to you, gently roll the nori sheet over all the ingredients, using the towel as your rolling aid. When you're done rolling, remove the towel and plastic wrap as you slide the roll onto a plate or cutting board. Using a sharp knife, cut the roll into equal pieces. Repeat with the remaining nori and filling ingredients. Sprinkle sesame seeds on top of your sushi, if desired.

Per Serving: Calories: 295; Fat: 15g; Protein: 30g; Total Carbs: 10g; Fiber: 8g; Net Carbs: 2g; **Macros:** Fat: 46%; Protein: 41%; Carbs: 13%

Smoked Salmon Avocado Sushi Roll

SERVES 4 | PREP TIME: 15 minutes | COOK TIME: 20 minutes

14 ounces smoked salmon

1 tablespoon wasabi paste (optional)

¾ cup cream cheese, at room temperature

½ avocado, sliced

1 tablespoon sesame seeds

On a cutting board, lay out a large piece of plastic wrap. Place the salmon pieces on the plastic wrap, overlapping, to create a large rectangle 6 to 7 inches long and 4 inches wide. In a small bowl, mix the wasabi paste (if using) and the cream cheese. Spread the cream cheese evenly over the entire smoked salmon rectangle. Arrange the avocado over the cream cheese, in the center of the rectangle. Grabbing the plastic wrap at one end, lift and carefully begin to roll the salmon. Hold the plastic wrap tightly over the roll as you go to apply pressure to hold it together. Unwrap the plastic wrap from the sushi roll. Cover the sushi roll in sesame seeds, patting them into the outer layer. Refrigerate the roll for 15 to 20 minutes. With a very sharp knife, slice into pieces and serve.

Per Serving: Calories: 539; Fat: 42g; Protein: 31g; Total Carbs: 12g; Fiber: 6g; Net Carbs: 6g; **Macros:** Fat: 69%; Protein: 22%; Carbs: 9%

Moroccan Salmon with Cauliflower Rice Pilaf

SERVES 4 | PREP TIME: 5 minutes | COOK TIME: 10 minutes

1 medium head of cauliflower, riced

3 tablespoons coconut oil, melted, divided

1 tablespoon extra-virgin olive oil

1 teaspoon white wine vinegar

1 tablespoon minced preserved lemons (optional)

¼ cup roughly chopped mint

¼ cup roughly chopped pistachios

½ teaspoon coarse sea salt, plus more for seasoning pilaf, divided

Freshly ground black pepper

4 (5-ounce) salmon fillets

1 teaspoon ground cumin

1 teaspoon ground coriander

1 teaspoon ground ginger

1 teaspoon paprika

Heat 1 tablespoon of the coconut oil in a large skillet over medium-high heat. Stir-fry the cauliflower for 5 minutes, until just heated through. Sprinkle in the olive oil, white wine vinegar, preserved lemons (if using), mint, and pistachios, and toss gently to mix. Season with salt and pepper. Set aside. Heat a separate large skillet over medium-high heat until hot. In a small bowl, combine the salt, cumin, coriander, ginger, and paprika. Coat the salmon fillets with the remaining 2 tablespoons of coconut oil and season with the spice mixture, ½ teaspoon salt, and pepper. Sear the salmon for about 2 minutes on each side, until it flakes easily with a fork but is still a deeper shade of pink on the inside. Serve each salmon fillet alongside a serving of the cauliflower rice.

Per Serving: Calories: 409; Fat: 24g; Protein: 41g; Total Carbs: 10g; Fiber: 5g; Net Carbs: 5g; **Macros:** Fat: 53%; Protein: 40%; Carbs: 7%

Pepper-Crusted Salmon with Wilted Kale

SERVES 4 | PREP TIME: 5 minutes | COOK TIME: 5 minutes

4 (6-ounce) salmon fillets

2 tablespoons coconut oil, melted

1 tablespoon freshly ground black pepper

½ teaspoon coarse sea salt, divided

1 bunch kale, tough ribs removed and roughly chopped

2 tablespoons extra-virgin olive oil

1 teaspoon red wine vinegar

¼ cup roughly chopped hazelnuts

½ cup fresh blueberries (optional)

Preheat a large skillet over medium-high heat. Coat the salmon fillets with the oil and then season liberally with the pepper and salt. In the hot skillet, sear the salmon for about 2 minutes on each side, until it flakes easily with a fork but is still a deeper shade of pink on the inside. While the salmon is cooking, place the kale in a large bowl, season with a generous pinch of sea salt, and drizzle with the olive oil. Using your hands, massage the oil and salt into the kale until it releases some of its liquid and becomes soft. Season with the red wine vinegar. Divide the kale among the serving plates and top with equal amounts of the hazelnuts and blueberries (if using). Serve the salmon fillets alongside the kale.

Per Serving: Calories: 442; Fat: 29g; Protein: 37g; Total Carbs: 8g; Fiber: 3g; Net Carbs: 5g; **Macros:** Fat: 60%; Protein: 33%; Carbs: 7%

Sheet Pan Salmon With Lemon Green Beans

SERVES 4 | PREP TIME: 10 minutes | COOK TIME: 25 minutes

3 tablespoons butter

3 garlic cloves, finely chopped

1½ tablespoons freshly squeezed lemon juice

¾ teaspoon kosher salt, plus more for seasoning

½ teaspoon paprika

½ teaspoon garlic powder

¼ teaspoon onion powder

4 (4-ounce) salmon fillets

12 ounces fresh green beans, trimmed

2 tablespoons olive oil

Freshly ground black pepper

Lemon wedges, for serving

Preheat the oven to 400°F. Line a baking sheet with parchment paper. Set aside. In a small microwave-safe bowl, combine the butter, garlic, lemon juice, salt, paprika, garlic powder, and onion powder. Microwave for 30 to 45 seconds until the butter melts. Brush the skin side of the salmon with the butter mixture and place the fish, skin-side down, on the baking sheet. Brush the butter mixture on the other side of the fish. In a medium bowl, toss the green beans and olive oil. Season with salt and pepper. Spread the green beans in a single layer on the baking sheet around the salmon. Bake for 12 minutes. Flip the salmon over and stir the green beans. Bake for 10 minutes more, or until the salmon is cooked to your desired doneness. Cooking time will depend on the thickness of your fillet. To crisp the skin, broil the salmon for 2 to 3 minutes before removing it from the oven. Serve immediately with lemon wedges for squeezing.

Per Serving: Calories: 408; Fat: 32g; Protein: 21g; Total Carbs: 9g; Fiber: 4g; Net Carbs: 5g; **Macros:** Fat: 71%; Protein: 21%; Carbs: 8%

Salmon with Spinach Hemp Pesto

SERVES 4 | PREP TIME: 5 minutes | COOK TIME: 20 minutes

4 (3-ounce) skinless
salmon fillets

½ cup Spinach Hemp Pesto
(page 306)

½ lemon, cut into 4 wedges

Preheat the oven to 350°F. Line a small baking sheet with aluminum foil. Place the salmon fillets on the baking sheet and spread 2 tablespoons of pesto on each piece of fish. Bake until the fish is opaque, 17 to 20 minutes. Serve with lemon wedges.

Per Serving: Calories: 244; Fat: 19g; Protein: 18g; Total Carbs: 1g; Fiber: 1g; Net Carbs: 0g; **Macros:** Fat: 70%; Protein: 30%; Carbs: 0%

Salmon in Lime Caper Brown Butter Sauce

SERVES 4 | PREP TIME: 10 minutes | COOK TIME: 15 minutes

½ cup butter, cut into pieces

Juice and zest of 1 lime

1 tablespoon capers

Sea salt

Freshly ground black pepper

4 (4-ounce) salmon fillets

Sea salt

Freshly ground black pepper

2 tablespoons coconut oil

Place a small saucepan over medium heat and melt the butter. Continue to heat the butter, stirring occasionally, until it is golden brown and very fragrant, about 4 minutes. Remove the brown butter from the heat and stir in the lime zest, lime juice, and capers. Season with salt and pepper and set aside. Pat the fish dry and season lightly with salt and pepper. Heat the coconut oil in a large skillet over medium-high heat. When the oil is hot, add the salmon and panfry until crispy and golden on both sides, turning once, 6 to 7 minutes per side. Transfer the fish to a serving plate, drizzle with the sauce, and serve.

Per Serving: Calories: 485; Fat: 44g; Protein: 23g; Total Carbs: 0g; Fiber: 0g; Net Carbs: 0g; **Macros:** Fat: 82%; Protein: 18%; Carbs: 0%

Roasted Salmon with Black Olive Salsa

SERVES 4 | PREP TIME: 25 minutes | COOK TIME: 16 minutes

½ cup sliced black olives

½ English cucumber, chopped

¼ cup chopped sun-dried
tomatoes packed in oil

1 scallion, white and green
parts, chopped

¼ cup avocado oil

1 teaspoon chopped
fresh basil

1 teaspoon chopped
fresh oregano

4 (4-ounce) salmon fillets

2 tablespoons olive oil

Sea salt

Freshly ground black pepper

In a medium bowl, mix the olives, cucumber, sun-dried tomatoes, scallion, avocado oil, basil, and oregano. Preheat the oven

to 350°F. Line a small baking sheet with aluminum foil. Place the fish fillets on the sheet and drizzle them with olive oil. Season the fish lightly with salt and pepper. Bake the fish until it is opaque, turning once, about 5 minutes per side or until the fish flakes easily with a fork. Serve the fish topped with salsa.

Per Serving: Calories: 457; Fat: 39g; Protein: 24g; Total Carbs: 4g; Fiber: 1g; Net Carbs: 3g; **Macros:** Fat: 77%; Protein: 21%; Carbs: 2%

Lemon Salmon and Asparagus

1 SERVING | PREP TIME: 5 minutes | COOK TIME: 15 minutes

2 tablespoons avocado
oil, divided

2 garlic cloves, minced

1 (6-ounce) salmon fillet

Juice of ½ lemon

6 asparagus spears, woody
ends removed

Half a lemon, sliced thinly

Preheat the oven to 425°F; line a baking sheet with parchment paper. Combine 1 tablespoon of avocado oil and the garlic in a bowl. Place the salmon on the baking sheet. Rub the salmon with the garlic and oil mixture until it is evenly coated. Squeeze the lemon juice over the salmon, and season with salt and pepper. Arrange the asparagus around the salmon in a single layer, drizzle the spears with the remaining 1 tablespoon of avocado oil, and place the lemon slices over them. Roast for 12 to 15 minutes, until the salmon is cooked through.

Per Serving: Calories: 527; Fat: 39g; Protein: 36g; Total Carbs: 8g; Fiber: 3g; Net Carbs: 5g; **Macros:** Fat: 67%; Protein: 27%; Carbs: 6%

Pan-Seared Dijon-Ginger Salmon

SERVES 1 | PREP TIME: 10 minutes | COOK TIME: 10 minutes

1 teaspoon Dijon mustard

1 teaspoon coconut aminos

1 teaspoon avocado oil

1 garlic clove, minced

¼ teaspoon freshly grated
ginger root

1 (6-ounce) salmon fillet

Combine mustard, oil, garlic, and ginger to make a marinade. Drizzle over the salmon, and allow it to sit for 10 minutes. Heat a skillet over medium-high heat. Place the salmon in the skillet; discard any leftover marinade. Cook for 4 to 5 minutes, depending on the thickness of the fish. Turn the salmon carefully with a spatula, then cook for another 4 to 5 minutes or until it is cooked through to your liking.

Per Serving: Calories: 355; Fat: 23g; Protein: 34g; Total Carbs: 3g; Fiber: 0g; Net Carbs: 3g; **Macros:** Fat: 60%; Protein: 37%; Carbs: 3%

Glazed Salmon

SERVES 4 | PREP TIME: 10 minutes | COOK TIME: 15 minutes

Nonstick cooking spray

2 tablespoons sugar-free
maple syrup

2 tablespoons Dijon mustard

2 teaspoons melted
coconut oil

4 (6-ounce) skinless salmon
fillets, rinsed and patted dry

1 teaspoon sea salt

¼ teaspoon freshly ground
black pepper

Preheat the oven to 400°F. Line a baking sheet with aluminum foil and lightly spray with cooking spray. In a small bowl, whisk together the sugar-free maple syrup, mustard, and coconut oil. Season the salmon with the salt and pepper. Spoon half the sauce evenly over each fillet. Place the salmon skin-side down on the foil. Bake for 8 minutes. Spoon the remaining sauce evenly over each fillet, and then bake for another 3 to 4 minutes or until the fish flakes easily.

Per Serving: Calories: 230; Fat: 9g; Protein: 33g; Total Carbs: 2g; Fiber: 2g; Net Carbs: 0g; **Macros:** Fat: 60%; Protein: 37%; Carbs: 3%

Grilled Salmon Foil Packets

SERVES 4 | PREP TIME: 10 minutes | COOK TIME: 21 minutes

1½ pounds salmon, skin removed

Extra-virgin olive oil, for greasing

1 small bunch fresh dill, divided

1 medium lemon, thinly sliced, divided

2 tablespoons unsalted butter, melted

3 garlic cloves, minced

¾ teaspoon kosher salt

¼ teaspoon freshly ground black pepper

Let the salmon stand at room temperature for 10 minutes while you prepare the other ingredients. Preheat an outdoor grill to medium heat, about 375°F. Line a baking sheet with aluminum foil and lightly grease it with oil. Arrange half of the dill sprigs down the middle of the baking sheet, add half of the lemon slices, and place the salmon on top. Drizzle the salmon with the melted butter and sprinkle it with the garlic, salt, and pepper. Top with the remaining half of the dill and the remaining lemon slices. Fold the foil's sides up and over the top of the salmon until the fish is completely enclosed. If the piece of foil is not large enough, place a second piece on top and fold the edges under so that it forms a sealed packet. Carefully slide the wrapped salmon onto the grill. Close the lid and grill the salmon for 14 to 18 minutes, or until the salmon is almost cooked through at the thickest part. Then carefully open the foil so that the top of the fish is uncovered. Close the grill and continue grilling until the fish is cooked through, about 3 minutes more. To serve, cut the salmon into 4 portions.

Per Serving: Calories: 308; Fat: 18g; Protein: 34g; Total Carbs: 2g; Fiber: 0g; Net Carbs: 2g; **Macros:** Fat: 51%; Protein: 47%; Carbs: 2%

Salmon Gratin

SERVES 4 | PREP TIME: 5 minutes, plus 10 minutes to marinate | COOK TIME: 10 minutes

1 pound skinless salmon fillets, cut into 1-inch cubes

Grated zest and juice of 1 lemon

¾ cup heavy (whipping) cream

2 tablespoons chopped fresh tarragon

1 teaspoon onion powder

1 teaspoon minced garlic

Salt

Freshly ground black pepper

½ cup shredded Swiss cheese

Preheat the broiler to high. Place an oven rack about a third of the way down in the oven. Place the salmon in a 7-by-11-inch broiler-safe baking dish and add the lemon zest and juice. Cover and let marinate for 10 minutes, stirring halfway through. Meanwhile, in a medium bowl, combine the heavy cream, tarragon, onion powder, garlic, and salt and pepper to taste. Mix well. Drain the juice from the salmon and return it to the baking dish. Pour the cream mixture over the salmon. Top with the Swiss cheese.

Broil for about 10 minutes, or until the cheese has melted and has turned golden brown.

Per Serving: Calories: 375; Fat: 28g; Protein: 27g; Total Carbs: 4g; Fiber: 0g; Net Carbs: 4g; **Macros:** Fat: 65%; Protein: 31%; Carbs: 4%

Salmon with Tarragon-Dijon Sauce

SERVES 4 | PREP TIME: 5 minutes | COOK TIME: 15 minutes, plus 10 minutes to rest

1¼ pounds salmon fillet (skin on or removed), cut into 4 equal pieces

¼ cup avocado oil mayonnaise

¼ cup Dijon or stone-ground mustard

Zest and juice of ½ lemon

2 tablespoons chopped fresh tarragon or 1 to 2 teaspoons dried tarragon

½ teaspoon salt

¼ teaspoon freshly ground black pepper

¼ cup extra-virgin olive oil, for serving

Preheat the oven to 425°F. Line a baking sheet with parchment paper. Place the salmon pieces, skin-side down, on a baking sheet. In a small bowl, whisk the mayonnaise, mustard, lemon zest and juice, tarragon, salt, and pepper. Top the salmon evenly with the sauce mixture. Bake until lightly browned on top and slightly translucent in the center, 10 to 12 minutes, depending on the thickness of the salmon. Remove from the oven and leave on the baking sheet for 10 minutes. Drizzle each fillet with 1 tablespoon olive oil before serving.

Per Serving: Calories: 387; Fat: 28g; Protein: 29g; Total Carbs: 4g; Fiber: 1g; Net Carbs: 3g; **Macros:** Fat: 64%; Protein: 31%; Carbs: 5%

Pecan-Crusted Salmon

SERVES 4 | PREP TIME: 5 minutes | COOK TIME: 15 minutes

1 tablespoon butter, melted, plus more for greasing the pan

12 ounces salmon fillet (skin-on)

½ cup finely chopped pecans

¼ cup grated Parmesan cheese

2 tablespoons cream cheese, at room temperature

1 teaspoon garlic salt

1 teaspoon freshly ground black pepper

Preheat the oven to 425°F. Lightly grease a 13-by-9-inch baking dish. Place the salmon skin-side down in the dish. In a small bowl, mix the pecans, Parmesan cheese, cream cheese, melted butter, garlic salt, and pepper, and spread evenly over the top of the salmon. Bake for about 15 minutes or until the salmon flakes easily with a fork.

Per Serving: (3 ounces) Calories: 303; Fat: 24g; Protein: 21g; Total Carbs: 3g; Fiber: 1g; Net Carbs: 2g; **Macros:** Fat: 69%; Protein: 27%; Carbs: 4%

Pan-Seared Lemon-Garlic Salmon

SERVES 2 | PREP TIME: 5 minutes | COOK TIME: 10 minutes

1 tablespoon extra-virgin olive oil

2 (8-ounce) salmon fillets

1 lemon, halved

Pink Himalayan sea salt

Freshly ground black pepper

2 tablespoons butter

1 tablespoon chopped fresh parsley

2 garlic cloves, minced

In a medium skillet, heat the olive oil over medium-high heat. Squeeze the juice from a lemon half over the fillets. Season the salmon with salt and pepper. Place the salmon skin-side up in the skillet. Cook for 4 to 5 minutes, then flip the fish and cook for an additional 2 to 3 minutes on the other side. Add the butter, the juice from the other lemon half, the parsley, and garlic to the pan. Toss to combine. Allow the fish to cook for 2 to 3 more minutes, until the flesh flakes easily with a fork. Transfer the fish to a serving plate, then top with the butter sauce and serve.

Per Serving: Calories: 489; Fat: 33g; Protein: 45g; Total Carbs: 1g; Fiber: 0g; Net Carbs: 1g; **Macros:** Fat: 62%; Protein: 37%; Carbs: 1%

Salmon Oscar

SERVES 2 | PREP TIME: 5 minutes | COOK TIME: 20 minutes

¼ cup (½ stick) butter
1 tablespoon finely minced onion
1½ teaspoons white wine vinegar
1 teaspoon freshly squeezed lemon juice
½ teaspoon dried tarragon
¼ teaspoon dried parsley
1 large egg yolk

2 tablespoons heavy whipping cream
1 tablespoon extra-virgin olive oil
2 (8-ounce) salmon fillets
Pink Himalayan sea salt
Freshly ground black pepper
1 (6- to 8-ounce) container lump crab meat

In a small saucepan, melt the butter over medium heat. Add the onion and cook for 3 to 5 minutes, until it begins to turn translucent. Add the vinegar, lemon juice, tarragon, and parsley. Stir to combine. In a small bowl, whisk the egg yolk and cream. Once the mixture in the saucepan starts to simmer, remove it from the heat and slowly add the egg mixture, whisking while you pour. Continue to whisk for 2 to 3 minutes, until the sauce thickens. Cover and set aside. Season the salmon fillets with salt and pepper. In a medium skillet, heat the olive oil over medium-high heat. Place the fillets skin-side up in the skillet. Cook for 4 to 5 minutes, then turn and cook for an additional 4 to 5 minutes on the other side, until the flesh flakes easily with a fork. Transfer the salmon to a serving plate, then place the crab in the skillet and quickly heat it, stirring gently. Top the salmon fillets with the crab, then drizzle on the sauce.

Per Serving: Calories: 741; Fat: 53g; Protein: 62g; Total Carbs: 1g; Fiber: 0g; Net Carbs: 1g; **Macros:** Fat: 63%; Protein: 36%; Carbs: 1%

Roasted Herb-Crusted Salmon with Asparagus and Tomatoes

SERVES 4 | PREP TIME: 10 minutes | COOK TIME: 15 minutes

¼ cup chopped fresh parsley
¼ cup chopped fresh chives
¼ cup fresh oregano leaves
2 tablespoons mayonnaise
4 (3- to 4-ounce) salmon fillets

20 asparagus spears, ends trimmed
16 cherry tomatoes, halved
2 tablespoons olive oil
Salt
Freshly ground black pepper

Preheat the oven to 400°F. Line a large baking sheet with aluminum foil. In a medium bowl, combine the parsley, chives, oregano, and mayonnaise. Lay the salmon fillets in the middle of the baking sheet and spread the herb mixture over the salmon. Surround the salmon with the asparagus and tomatoes. Drizzle the oil over the vegetables and season everything with salt and pepper. Cook for about 12 minutes.

Per Serving: Calories: 258; Fat: 18g; Protein: 19g; Total Carbs: 6g; Fiber: 3g; Net Carbs: 3g; **Macros:** Fat: 61%; Protein: 30%; Carbs: 9%

Salmon Cakes

SERVES 4 | PREP TIME: 10 minutes | COOK TIME: 15 minutes

1 (16-ounce) can pink salmon, drained and bones removed
¼ cup almond flour
¼ cup crushed pork rinds
2 scallions, diced
1 large egg

3 tablespoons mayonnaise
1 teaspoon garlic salt
1 teaspoon freshly ground black pepper
2 tablespoons extra-virgin olive oil

Line a plate with paper towels and set aside. In a bowl, combine the salmon, almond flour, pork rinds, scallions, egg, mayonnaise, garlic salt, and pepper, and mix well. Form 8 small patties or 4 large patties. In a skillet over medium heat, heat the oil. Cook the patties for 4 to 5 minutes on each side, until crispy. Larger patties may need to cook a little longer. Transfer the patties to the lined plate to drain.

Per Serving: (2 small patties or 1 large patty) Calories: 313; Fat: 21g; Protein: 26g; Total Carbs: 5g; Fiber: 0g; Net Carbs: 5g; **Macros:** Fat: 60%; Protein: 33%; Carbs: 7%

Curried Salmon Fish Cakes

SERVES 4 | PREP TIME: 5 minutes, plus 1 hour to chill | COOK TIME: 25 minutes

1 pound skinless salmon fillets, roughly chopped
2 large eggs
2 tablespoons chopped fresh cilantro

4 scallions, green and white parts, roughly chopped
1 teaspoon Thai red curry paste
2 tablespoons olive oil

Place parchment paper on a large plate and set aside. In a food processor or blender, combine the salmon, eggs, cilantro, scallions, and curry paste and process until smooth. Divide the mixture into 8 portions and place 4 on the lined plate. Flatten them into patties and place another layer of paper on top. Spoon out the remaining 4 portions, flatten, and top with paper. Cover everything with plastic wrap and refrigerate for at least 1 hour. In a large skillet, heat the oil over medium heat. Cook the fish cakes on one side for 5 minutes, flip, and cook for another 5 minutes, or until cooked through.

Per Serving: Calories: 305; Fat: 21g; Protein: 26g; Total Carbs: 2g; Fiber: 1g; Net Carbs: 1g; **Macros:** Fat: 62%; Protein: 36%; Carbs: 2%

Coconut Ginger Salmon Burgers

SERVES 4 | PREP TIME: 15 minutes, plus time to chill | COOK TIME: 20 minutes

12 ounces fresh salmon, chopped
1 egg, beaten
2 tablespoons coconut flour
1 scallion, white and green parts, finely chopped
Juice of 1 lemon
2 teaspoons peeled, grated fresh ginger

½ teaspoon ground coriander
Pinch sea salt
Pinch freshly ground black pepper
¼ cup coconut oil
¼ cup mayonnaise

In a large bowl, combine the salmon, egg, coconut flour, scallion, lemon juice, ginger, coriander, salt, and pepper until well mixed. Form the salmon mixture into 8 equal patties, each ½-inch thick. Chill the salmon patties in the refrigerator until firm, about 1 hour. Heat the oil in a large skillet over medium-high heat. Panfry the salmon burgers, turning once, until cooked through and lightly browned, about 10 minutes per side. Serve 2 burgers per person topped with mayonnaise.

Per Serving: Calories: 369; Fat: 31g; Protein: 20g; Total Carbs: 4g; Fiber: 2g; Net Carbs: 2g; **Macros:** Fat: 76%; Protein: 22%; Carbs: 2%

Salmon Cakes with Avocado

SERVES 4 | PREP TIME: 15 minutes, plus 15 minutes to rest | COOK TIME: 15 minutes

1 (14.5-ounce) can red salmon or 1 pound wild-caught salmon fillet, skin removed
½ cup minced red onion
1 large egg
2 tablespoons avocado oil mayonnaise, plus more for serving
1 very ripe avocado, pitted, peeled, and mashed

½ cup almond flour
1 to 2 teaspoons dried dill
1 teaspoon garlic powder
1 teaspoon salt
½ teaspoon paprika
½ teaspoon freshly ground black pepper
Zest and juice of 1 lemon
¼ cup extra-virgin olive oil

Remove the spine, large bones, and pieces of skin from the salmon. Place the salmon and red onion in a large bowl and using a fork, break up any lumps. Add the egg, mayonnaise, and avocado and combine well. In a small bowl, whisk the almond flour, dill, garlic powder, salt, paprika, and pepper. Add the dry ingredients and lemon zest and juice to the salmon and combine well. Form into 8 small patties, about 2 inches in diameter and place on a plate. Let rest for 15 minutes. In a large skillet, heat the olive oil over medium heat. Fry the patties until browned, 2 to 3 minutes per side. Cover the skillet, reduce heat to low, and cook for another 6 to 8 minutes, or until the cakes are set in the center. Remove from the skillet and serve warm with additional mayonnaise or aioli.

Per Serving: Calories: 343; Fat: 26g; Protein: 23g; Total Carbs: 5g; Fiber: 1g; Net Carbs: 4g; **Macros:** Fat: 66%; Protein: 28%; Carbs: 6%

Snapper Veracruz

SERVES 4 | PREP TIME: 10 minutes | COOK TIME: 22 minutes

¼ cup extra-virgin olive oil
¼ cup diced yellow onion
2 teaspoons roughly chopped garlic
Pinch red pepper flakes
2 tablespoons minced fresh parsley
1 teaspoon minced oregano
¼ cup pitted green olives
2 tablespoons drained capers

1 cup canned plum tomatoes with juices, hand crushed
1 tablespoon red wine vinegar
1¼ pounds red snapper, cut into 4 (5-ounce) fillets
3 tablespoons cold butter, cut into pieces
Sea salt
Freshly ground black pepper

Heat the olive oil in a large skillet over medium heat. Cook the onion, garlic, and red pepper flakes until beginning to soften,

about 5 minutes. Add the parsley, oregano, olives, capers, tomatoes, and vinegar to the skillet and cook for 10 minutes, until the sauce has reduced somewhat and the tomatoes are pulpy. Season the fish generously on both sides with salt and pepper, then add the fillets to the pan, spooning some of the sauce over the fish. Cook for about 3 minutes on each side, or until the fish flakes easily with a fork. Transfer the cooked fish to a serving platter. Remove the pan from the heat and whisk the cold butter into the tomato mixture one tablespoon at a time. Pour the sauce over the cooked fish and serve immediately.

Per Serving: Calories: 434; Fat: 27g; Protein: 38g; Total Carbs: 8g; Fiber: 2g; Net Carbs: 6g; **Macros:** Fat: 58%; Protein: 35%; Carbs: 7%

Rosemary-Lemon Snapper Baked in Parchment

SERVES 4 | PREP TIME: 15 minutes | COOK TIME: 15 minutes

1¼ pounds fresh red snapper fillet, cut into two equal pieces
2 lemons, thinly sliced
6 to 8 sprigs fresh rosemary, stems removed or 1 to 2 tablespoons dried rosemary

½ cup extra-virgin olive oil
6 garlic cloves, thinly sliced
1 teaspoon salt
½ teaspoon freshly ground black pepper

Preheat the oven to 425°F. Place two large sheets of parchment (about twice the size of each piece of fish) on the counter. Place 1 piece of fish in the center of each sheet. Top the fish pieces with lemon slices and rosemary leaves. In a small bowl, combine the olive oil, garlic, salt, and pepper. Drizzle the oil over each piece of fish. Top each piece of fish with a second large sheet of parchment and starting on a long side, fold the paper up to about 1 inch from the fish. Repeat on the remaining sides, going in a clockwise direction. Fold in each corner once to secure. Place both parchment pouches on a baking sheet and bake until the fish is cooked through, 10 to 12 minutes.

Per Serving: Calories: 390; Fat: 29g; Protein: 29g; Total Carbs: 3g; Fiber: 0g; Net Carbs: 3g; **Macros:** Fat: 66%; Protein: 32%; Carbs: 2%

Sole with Cucumber Radish Salsa

SERVES 4 | PREP TIME: 15 minutes | COOK TIME: 8 minutes

½ English cucumber, chopped
½ avocado, diced
4 radishes, finely chopped
½ scallion, white and green parts, finely chopped
⅓ cup avocado oil, divided
Juice of ½ lemon

1 teaspoon chopped fresh thyme
Sea salt
Freshly ground black pepper
4 (3-ounce) sole fillets
½ cup almond flour

In a small bowl, stir the cucumber, avocado, radish, scallion, 2 tablespoons oil, lemon juice, and thyme. Season with salt and pepper and set aside. Dredge the sole fillets in almond flour. Heat the remaining oil in a large skillet over medium-high heat. Panfry the fish until golden, crispy, and cooked through, turning once, about 8 minutes total. Serve immediately with the cucumber salsa.

Sole Meunière

SERVES 4 | PREP TIME: 15 minutes | COOK TIME: 10 minutes

4 (4-ounce) sole fillets	Juice and zest of 3 lemons
Sea salt	½ cup chopped fresh parsley
Freshly ground black pepper	1 teaspoon fresh
½ cup almond flour	chopped thyme
½ cup butter, divided	

Pat the fish almost dry with paper towels, and season both sides with salt and pepper. On a large plate, dredge the sole in the almond flour. In a large skillet over medium-high heat, heat 6 tablespoons of butter. Swirl the skillet until the butter starts to foam and brown flecks appear, about 1 minute. Reduce the heat to medium-low, and add the fish fillets to the skillet. Fry the fish until browned on both sides, turning once, about 6 minutes in total. Remove the fish from the skillet, and transfer them to plates. Stir in the remaining butter, lemon juice, lemon zest, parsley, and thyme. Whisk over the heat for 2 minutes, and then serve the fish with the buttery sauce.

Swordfish in Tarragon-Citrus Butter

SERVES 4 | PREP TIME: 5 minutes | COOK TIME: 20 minutes

1 pound swordfish steaks, cut into 2-inch pieces	2 tablespoons unsalted butter
1 teaspoon salt	Zest and juice of 2 clementines
¼ teaspoon freshly ground black pepper	Zest and juice of 1 lemon
¼ cup extra-virgin olive oil, plus 2 tablespoons, divided	2 tablespoons chopped fresh tarragon

In a bowl, toss the swordfish with salt and pepper. In a large skillet, heat ¼ cup olive oil over medium-high heat. Add the swordfish chunks to the hot oil and sear on all sides, 2 to 3 minutes per side, until they are golden brown. Using a slotted spoon, remove the fish from the skillet and keep warm. Add the remaining 2 tablespoons olive oil and butter to the oil already in the skillet and return the heat to medium-low. Once the butter has melted, whisk in the clementine and lemon zests and juices, along with the tarragon. Season with salt. Return the fish pieces to the pan and toss to coat in the butter sauce.

Parmesan-Crusted Tilapia with Sautéed Spinach

SERVES 2 | PREP TIME: 15 minutes | COOK TIME: 15 minutes

½ cup grated Parmesan cheese	2 tilapia fillets
2 tablespoons almond flour	2 tablespoons olive oil, divided
1 teaspoon paprika	1½ cups spinach
¼ teaspoon salt	½ teaspoon garlic powder
⅛ teaspoon freshly ground black pepper	1 tablespoon chopped fresh parsley

Preheat the oven to 400°F. In a medium bowl, mix the Parmesan cheese, almond flour, paprika, salt, and pepper. Place the tilapia fillets on a plate and drizzle with 1 tablespoon of olive oil. Massage the oil into the fish, and then dredge them in the Parmesan mix, coating thoroughly. Line a baking dish with aluminum foil. Place the fillets inside. Put the dish in the preheated oven and bake for 10 to 15 minutes, depending on the thickness of the fillets. While the fillets cook, add the remaining tablespoon of olive oil to a large skillet and heat over medium-high heat. Add the spinach and sauté until tender, about 6 minutes. Add the garlic powder. Cover, and reduce the heat to medium-low. Cook for 3 to 5 minutes. Remove the baking dish from the oven. Check the fillets for doneness. Plate the spinach with the fillets on top and serve immediately, garnished with the parsley.

Brown Butter–Lime Tilapia

SERVES 4 | PREP TIME: 10 minutes | COOK TIME: 15 minutes

½ cup unsalted butter	Sea salt
¼ cup chopped fresh dill	Freshly ground black pepper
Juice of 1 lime	4 teaspoons coconut oil
4 (4-ounce) tilapia fillets	

In a small saucepan over medium-high heat, heat the butter until it starts to foam up and fizz. Swirl the saucepan until tiny brown specks form and the butter smells nutty, about 1 minute. Remove from the heat, and set aside. In a blender, purée the dill and lime juice until a paste forms. Slowly pour the brown butter into the blender while it is running until an emulsified sauce forms and all the butter is used. Rinse the tilapia fillets, and pat them dry with paper towels. Season the fish lightly with salt and pepper on both sides. In a large skillet over medium-high heat, heat the coconut oil. Brown the fish on both sides, turning once, for about 10 minutes total. Serve with the brown butter sauce.

Pan-Fried Tilapia

SERVES 6 | PREP TIME: 5 minutes | COOK TIME: 25 minutes

6 large tilapia fillets (fresh, or thawed if frozen)	2 tablespoons olive oil
½ teaspoon salt	½ cup oat fiber or coconut flour
½ teaspoon freshly ground black pepper	3 tablespoons butter
	2 garlic cloves, minced

Preheat the oven to 250°F or its lowest temperature. Line a baking sheet with paper towels. Season the fillets on both sides with the salt and pepper. In a large skillet over medium-high heat, heat the olive oil. Pour the oat fiber onto a shallow plate. Dredge the fillets in the oat fiber, covering both sides, and shake to remove the excess. Add the fillets to the pan, 1 or 2 at a time so they're not crowded. Pan-fry for 3 to 4 minutes per side or until the fish flakes easily with a fork. Use a spatula to transfer the cooked fish to the baking sheet and place in the oven to keep warm while you fry the remaining fillets. Turn the heat under the skillet to low, wipe out any excess oil, and add the butter and garlic. Stir until the butter is melted and the garlic is fragrant, 1 to 2 minutes. Serve the fish with the garlic butter spooned over the top.

Per Serving: Calories: 263; Fat: 13g; Protein: 30g; Total Carbs: 6g; Fiber: 1g; Net Carbs: 5g; **Macros:** Fat: 45%; Protein: 45%; Carbs: 10%

Garlic Herb Marinated Tilapia

SERVES 4 | PREP TIME: 10 minutes, plus 30 minutes to marinate | COOK TIME: 18 minutes

1 cup Garlic Herb Marinade (page 305)	4 (4-ounce) tilapia fillets Lime wedges

Place the marinade in a medium bowl and add the tilapia, turning to coat. Place the bowl, covered, in the refrigerator for 30 minutes. Preheat the oven to 350°F. Line a 9-by-9-inch baking dish with aluminum foil. Arrange the fillets in the baking dish. Pour the marinade over the fish. Bake the fish until it is just cooked through and flaky, 15 to 18 minutes. Serve the tilapia garnished with lime wedges.

Per Serving: Calories: 354; Fat: 30g; Protein: 23g; Total Carbs: 2g; Fiber: 1g; Net Carbs: 1g; **Macros:** Fat: 75%; Protein: 74%; Carbs: 1%

Parmesan Baked Tilapia

SERVES 4 | PREP TIME: 10 minutes | COOK TIME: 15 minutes

¼ cup butter, melted	4 (4-ounce) tilapia fillets, patted dry
2 teaspoons garlic salt	
1 teaspoon freshly ground black pepper	4 ounces grated Parmesan cheese
	4 ounces crushed pork rinds

Preheat the oven to 400°F. Line a baking sheet with parchment paper and set aside. In a small bowl, mix the melted butter, garlic salt, and pepper. Place the tilapia fillets on the prepared baking sheet, then drizzle or brush the butter mixture across each fillet. Sprinkle each fillet with Parmesan cheese and crushed pork rinds. Bake for about 13 minutes, and then turn the oven up to broil and broil for 2 more minutes.

Per Serving: Calories: 372; Fat: 24g; Protein: 38g; Total Carbs: 1g; Fiber: 0g; Net Carbs: 1g; **Macros:** Fat: 58%; Protein: 41%; Carbs: 1%

Cream-Poached Trout

SERVES 4 | PREP TIME: 10 minutes | COOK TIME: 20 minutes

4 (4-ounce) skinless trout fillets	1 leek, white and green parts, halved lengthwise, thinly sliced, and thoroughly washed
Sea salt	
Freshly ground black pepper	
3 tablespoons butter	1 teaspoon minced garlic
1 teaspoon chopped fresh parsley, for garnish	1 cup heavy (whipping) cream
	Juice of 1 lemon

Preheat the oven to 400°F. Pat the trout fillets dry with paper towels and lightly season with salt and pepper. Place them in a 9-inch-square baking dish in one layer. Set aside. Place a medium saucepan over medium-high heat and melt the butter. Sauté the leek and garlic until softened, about 6 minutes. Add the heavy cream and lemon juice to the saucepan and bring to

a boil, whisking. Pour the sauce over the fish and bake until the fish is just cooked through, 10 to 12 minutes. Serve topped with the parsley.

Per Serving: Calories: 449; Fat: 37g; Protein: 24g; Total Carbs: 5g; Fiber: 1g; Net Carbs: 4g; **Macros:** Fat: 74%; Protein: 21%; Carbs: 5%

Rainbow Trout with Cream Leek Sauce

SERVES 4 | PREP TIME: 15 minutes | COOK TIME: 17 minutes

2 tablespoons olive oil	4 (3-ounce) rainbow trout fillets
2 leeks, white and light green parts, thinly sliced and thoroughly washed	2 teaspoons chopped fresh thyme
1½ cups canned coconut milk	Sea salt
	Freshly ground black pepper

Heat the olive oil in a large skillet over medium-high heat. Add the leeks and sauté until they are tender, about 7 minutes. Stir in the coconut milk and bring the mixture to a boil. Place the trout in one layer in the liquid and reduce the heat to medium. Simmer until the fish is just cooked through, about 10 minutes. Remove the fillets and place onto 4 plates. Stir the thyme into the leek cream sauce. Season the sauce with salt and pepper. Spoon the leek sauce over the trout and serve.

Per Serving: Calories: 337; Fat: 28g; Protein: 14g; Total Carbs: 9g; Fiber: 1g; Net Carbs: 8g; **Macros:** Fat: 75%; Protein: 17%; Carbs: 8%

Roasted Trout with Swiss Chard

SERVES 4 | PREP TIME: 30 minutes | COOK TIME: 15 minutes

1 teaspoon salt, divided	2 pounds Swiss chard, cleaned and leaves separated from stems
½ teaspoon freshly ground black pepper, divided	
4 (8-ounce) trout, cleaned	¼ cup olive oil, divided
4 fresh dill sprigs	¼ cup butter, divided
4 fresh fennel sprigs	1 lemon, quartered
	¼ cup dry vermouth, or white wine, divided

Preheat the oven to 450°F. Using ½ teaspoon of salt and ¼ teaspoon of pepper, season the insides of the trout. Place 1 dill sprig and 1 fennel sprig inside each trout. Cut the Swiss chard stems into 2-inch pieces. Cut the leaves crosswise into 1½-inch strips. Cut four large pieces of aluminum foil into oval shapes large enough to fit one trout and one-quarter of the Swiss chard, with room enough to be sealed. Using ¾ tablespoon of olive oil, brush the trout. Place one trout in the center of each piece of foil. Top each trout with one-quarter of the Swiss chard. Season the trout with the remaining ½ teaspoon of salt, ¼ teaspoon of pepper, and 3¼ tablespoons of olive oil. Top each trout with 1 tablespoon of butter. Squeeze a lemon quarter over each Swiss chard and trout bundle. Spoon 1 tablespoon of vermouth over each. Close and seal the foil pouches tightly. Place the foil packets on a baking sheet. Bake for 10 to 12 minutes, depending on the thickness of the fish. Remove from the oven and allow the packets to cool for 1 to 2 minutes before opening. Serve in the foil packet.

Per Serving: Calories: 556; Fat: 36g; Protein: 44g; Total Carbs: 11g; Fiber: 4g; Net Carbs: 7g; **Macros:** Fat: 60%; Protein: 32%; Carbs: 8%

Grandma Bev's Ahi Poke

SERVES 6 | PREP TIME: 10 minutes

3 scallions, both white and green parts diced

½ cup soy sauce

2 teaspoons sesame oil

1 tablespoon sesame seeds

¼ teaspoon ground ginger

1 teaspoon garlic powder

1 teaspoon salt

2 pounds fresh ahi tuna, cut into ½-inch cubes

In a medium bowl, mix the scallions, soy sauce, sesame oil, sesame seeds, ginger, garlic powder, and salt. Combine the soy sauce mixture with the tuna, and toss well. Serve immediately.

Per Serving: Calories: 241; Fat: 9g; Protein: 38g; Total Carbs: 2g; Fiber: 1g; Net Carbs: 1g; **Macros:** Fat: 34%; Protein: 63%; Carbs: 3%

Tuna Slow-Cooked in Olive Oil

SERVES 4 | PREP TIME: 5 minutes | COOK TIME: 45 minutes

1 cup extra-virgin olive oil, plus more if needed

4 (3- to 4-inch) sprigs fresh rosemary

8 (3- to 4-inch) sprigs fresh thyme

2 large garlic cloves, thinly sliced

2 (2-inch) strips lemon zest

1 teaspoon salt

½ teaspoon freshly ground black pepper

1 pound fresh tuna steaks (about 1 inch thick)

Combine the olive oil, rosemary, thyme, garlic, lemon zest, salt, and pepper over medium-low heat and cook until warm and fragrant, 20 to 25 minutes. Remove from the heat and allow to cool for 25 to 30 minutes, until warm but not hot. Add the tuna to the bottom of the pan, adding additional oil if needed so that tuna is fully submerged, and return to medium-low heat. Cook for 5 to 10 minutes, or until the oil heats back up and is warm and fragrant but not smoking. Lower the heat if it gets too hot. Remove the pot from the heat and let the tuna cook in warm oil for 4 to 5 minutes, to your desired level of doneness. For a tuna that is rare in the center, cook for 2 to 3 minutes. Remove from the oil and serve warm, drizzling 2 to 3 tablespoons seasoned oil over the tuna. When both have cooled, remove the herb stems with a slotted spoon and pour the cooking oil over the tuna.

Per Serving: Calories: 363; Fat: 28g; Protein: 27g; Total Carbs: 1g; Fiber: 0g; Net Carbs: 1g; **Macros:** Fat: 68%; Protein: 31%; Carbs: 1%

Sesame-Crusted Tuna with Sweet Chili Vinaigrette

SERVES 4 | PREP TIME: 10 minutes | COOK TIME: 5 minutes

1 tablespoon Thai chili sauce, such as sambal

1 tablespoon rice wine vinegar

¼ cup light olive oil or canola oil

4 to 6 drops liquid stevia

4 (6-ounce) ahi tuna steaks

2 tablespoons toasted sesame oil

Sea salt

Freshly ground black pepper

½ cup sesame seeds

4 packed cups mixed spring greens

In a small bowl, combine the chili sauce, vinegar, oil, and stevia. Preheat a large skillet over medium-high heat. Pat the tuna steaks dry with paper towels. Coat each side of the steaks with the sesame oil, and season with the salt and pepper. Spread the sesame seeds in a shallow dish. Press the tuna steaks into the seeds to coat them on both sides. Immediately place the tuna steaks into the hot skillet. Sear on each side for 1½ minutes for rare. Divide the greens among the serving plates and drizzle each salad with the chili vinaigrette. Transfer the tuna to a cutting board and slice each steak on an angle into ½-inch pieces. It will still be dark and barely warm in the center. Place equal portions of the tuna on each serving plate.

Per Serving: Calories: 475; Fat: 32g; Protein: 41g; Total Carbs: 11g; Fiber: 3g; Net Carbs: 8g; **Macros:** Fat: 60%; Protein: 32%; Carbs: 8%

Seared Tuna with Steamed Turnips, Broccoli, and Green Beans

SERVES 4 | PREP TIME: 10 minutes | COOK TIME: 20 minutes

1 large turnip, peeled and cut into 1-inch cubes

10 ounces broccoli florets

1 pound green beans, trimmed

Salt

Freshly ground black pepper

½ teaspoon onion powder

½ teaspoon garlic powder

4 (6-ounce) tuna steaks

2 tablespoons olive oil

Fill a large saucepan with about 1 inch of water and place it over medium heat. Insert a steamer basket. Place the turnip in the basket. Place the broccoli on top of the turnip and the green beans on the top of the broccoli. Cover and cook for 10 to 15 minutes, until the vegetables are tender. Season with salt and pepper. Meanwhile, in a small dish, mix the onion powder, garlic powder, and 1 teaspoon pepper. Press the tuna steaks into the spice mixture, coating both sides In a large skillet, heat the oil over medium-high heat. Cook the tuna for 3 to 4 minutes per side for medium-rare (internal temperature of 115°F, slightly pink in the center) or longer to desired doneness. Transfer the tuna to serving plates with the vegetables.

Per Serving: Calories: 319; Fat: 8g; Protein: 46g; Total Carbs: 16g; Fiber: 6g; Net Carbs: 10g; **Macros:** Fat: 23%; Protein: 59%; Carbs: 18%

Tuna Casserole

SERVES 6 | PREP TIME: 20 minutes | COOK TIME: 40 minutes

3 cups zucchini noodles

1½ teaspoons salt, divided

Cooking spray

1 tablespoon avocado oil

¼ cup diced white onion

½ cup thinly sliced baby portabella mushroom caps

1 garlic clove, minced

¼ teaspoon freshly ground black pepper

2 (6-ounce) cans solid white albacore tuna in water, drained

½ cup avocado oil mayonnaise

2 teaspoons Dijon mustard

1 teaspoon freshly squeezed lemon juice

½ cup shredded cheddar cheese

½ cup shredded mozzarella cheese

Lay paper towels on top of a baking sheet. Spread the zoodles onto the paper towels, sprinkle with 1 teaspoon salt, and cover with another layer of paper towels. Lightly press down on the zoodles to draw out the water. Allow the zoodles to sit, covered in paper towels, and set aside. Preheat the oven to 350°F. Spray a 9-by-13-inch casserole dish with cooking spray. In a large skillet over medium heat, warm the avocado oil. Add the onion and mushrooms and cook, stirring frequently, for 4 to 5 minutes or until the onion becomes translucent and the mushrooms begin to brown. Stir in the garlic and cook for 1 more minute. Add the zoodles, remaining ½ teaspoon of salt, and the pepper. Cook, stirring frequently, for about 3 more minutes. The zoodles should be cooked but still al dente. Remove from the heat. In a large bowl, use a fork to mix the tuna, mayonnaise, mustard, and lemon juice until well combined. Add the cooked vegetables and stir to coat. Pour the mixture into the prepared dish. Cover with the cheddar and mozzarella. Bake for 25 to 30 minutes or until the cheese is golden and bubbly. Let the casserole sit for 2 to 3 minutes.

Per Serving: (⅙ of recipe): Calories: 310; Fat: 26g; Protein: 17g; Total Carbs: 7g; Fiber: 2g; Net Carbs: 5g; **Macros:** Fat: 71%; Protein: 21%; Carbs: 8%

Crab Cakes with Spicy Tartar Sauce

SERVES 8 | PREP TIME: 15 minutes | COOK TIME: 25 minutes

For the spicy tartar sauce

½ cup mayonnaise

1 small garlic clove, grated

2 teaspoons whole-grain mustard

1½ teaspoons freshly squeezed lemon juice

1 teaspoon dill relish

½ teaspoon gluten-free Worcestershire Sauce

¼ teaspoon paprika

¼ teaspoon kosher salt

2 or 3 dashes hot sauce

⅛ teaspoon cayenne pepper

For the crab cakes

3 tablespoons mayonnaise

1 tablespoon freshly squeezed lemon juice

1 tablespoon whole-grain mustard

1½ teaspoons Old Bay seasoning

1 teaspoon gluten-free Worcestershire sauce

¼ teaspoon freshly ground black pepper

2 or 3 dashes hot sauce

Pinch kosher salt

1 pound lump crabmeat

3 tablespoons sliced scallion

2 tablespoons chopped fresh parsley

1 egg, lightly beaten

3½ tablespoons coconut flour

¼ cup butter, divided

Lemon wedges, for serving

In a small bowl, stir the mayonnaise, garlic, mustard, lemon juice, relish, Worcestershire sauce, paprika, salt, and hot sauce. Add cayenne to taste and stir to combine. Refrigerate while preparing the crab cakes. In a medium bowl, stir the mayonnaise, lemon juice, mustard, Old Bay seasoning, Worcestershire sauce, black pepper, hot sauce, and salt. Add the crab, scallion, and parsley, and gently toss to coat in the mayonnaise mixture. Gently stir in the egg and coconut flour. Let rest for 5 minutes. Divide the crab mixture into 8 portions and form each into a patty about ½-inch thick. In a large sauté pan or skillet over medium heat, melt 2 tablespoons of butter. Place 2 or 3 crab cakes in the pan and cook for 3 to 4 minutes per side, or until golden. Repeat with the remaining patties. Serve with lemon wedges for squeezing and spicy tartar sauce.

Per Serving: Calories: 219; Fat: 15g; Protein: 11g; Total Carbs: 10g; Fiber: 4g; Net Carbs: 6g; **Macros:** Fat: 62%; Protein: 20%; Carbs: 18%

"Spaghetti" with Clams

SERVES 2 | PREP TIME: 10 minutes | COOK TIME: 10 minutes

1 tablespoon olive oil

1 garlic clove, minced

½ cup chicken broth

2 large zucchini, spiralized

Salt

Freshly ground black pepper

1 (6-ounce) can clams, drained and minced

Juice of ½ lemon

2 tablespoons chopped fresh parsley, for garnish

In a large skillet over medium heat, heat the olive oil. Add garlic and sauté for just under 1 minute. Add the chicken stock and bring to a simmer. Add the zucchini noodles and gently toss to combine. Taste and season with salt and pepper. Stir in the clams and lemon juice. Toss again to combine and cook for 2 to 3 minutes to warm through. Serve immediately topped with fresh parsley.

Per Serving: Calories: 214; Fat: 9g; Protein: 20g; Total Carbs: 16g; Fiber: 3g; Net Carbs: 13g; **Macros:** Fat: 37%; Protein: 36%; Carbs: 27%

Crab Cakes with Cilantro Crema

SERVES 4 | PREP TIME: 10 minutes | COOK TIME: 15 to 18 minutes

¼ cup almond flour

1 egg, whisked

1 scallion, minced

1 garlic clove, minced

½ teaspoon sea salt

Pinch cayenne pepper

1 pound lump crabmeat, picked over for shells

1 tablespoon coconut oil

½ cup sour cream

½ cup mayonnaise

1 tablespoon freshly squeezed lime juice

2 tablespoons minced cilantro

Preheat the oven to 375°F. Line a baking sheet with parchment paper. In a medium bowl, whisk the almond flour, egg, scallion, garlic, sea salt, and cayenne pepper. Fold in the crabmeat. Divide the mixture into 8 cakes and place them on the baking sheet. Brush with the oil. Bake for 15 to 18 minutes until the cakes are gently browned and set. While the crab cakes bake, whisk the sour cream, mayonnaise, lime juice, and cilantro in a jar to make the cilantro crema. Serve alongside the crab cakes.

Per Serving: Calories: 455; Fat: 36g; Protein: 30g; Total Carbs: 4g; Fiber: 1g; Net Carbs: 3g; **Macros:** Fat: 71%; Protein: 26%; Carbs: 3%

Classic Crab Cakes

SERVES 6 | PREP TIME: 25 minutes | COOK TIME: 10 minutes

1 large egg, separated

½ cup avocado oil mayonnaise

1 tablespoon Dijon mustard

1 teaspoon Old Bay seasoning

1 teaspoon dried parsley

1 pound jumbo lump crab meat, picked over for shell pieces

⅓ cup crushed pork rinds

2 tablespoons avocado oil, divided

Lemon wedges, for serving (optional)

Line a baking sheet with parchment paper. In a large bowl, whisk the egg yolk, mayonnaise, mustard, Old Bay seasoning, and parsley until well combined. Gently fold in the crab, being careful to leave large lumps of crab meat. In a large bowl, beat the egg white until soft peaks form. Gently fold the egg whites into the crab mixture, keeping as many large lumps of crab meat as possible. Gently fold in the pork rinds. Divide the crab mixture into 6 equal portions and form into patties. Place the patties on the prepared baking sheet and refrigerate for 15 minutes. Heat 1 tablespoon of avocado oil in a large skillet over medium heat. Place 3 crab cakes in the skillet and cook for 3 to 4 minutes per side, just until golden and cooked through. Repeat with the remaining tablespoon of avocado oil and 3 crab cakes. Serve immediately with lemon wedges (if using).

Per Serving: (1 crab cake): Calories: 262; Fat: 23g; Protein: 16g; Total Carbs: 0g; Fiber: 0g; Net Carbs: 0g; **Macros:** Fat: 74%; Protein: 26%; Carbs: 0%

Spicy Crab Cakes

SERVES 4 | PREP TIME: 20 minutes, plus 1 hour to chill | COOK TIME: 20 minutes

1 pound crab	1 teaspoon Dijon mustard
½ cup almond flour, plus additional for dusting	1 teaspoon Worcestershire sauce
½ red bell pepper, minced	1 teaspoon chopped fresh dill
¼ cup mayonnaise	Splash Tabasco sauce
3 tablespoons minced red onion	3 tablespoons extra-virgin olive oil

In a large bowl, stir the crab, almond flour, red pepper, Mayonnaise, red onion, Dijon mustard, Worcestershire sauce, dill, and Tabasco sauce until the mixture holds together when pressed. Form the crab mixture into 12 patties, and refrigerate them on a plate, covered, for 1 hour. Dust with additional almond flour. In a large skillet over medium-high heat, heat the olive oil. Cook the crab cakes in batches, until golden brown and heated through, about 10 minutes per side. Serve.

Per Serving: Calories: 349; Fat: 29g; Protein: 16g; Total Carbs: 6g; Fiber: 2g; Net Carbs: 4g; **Macros:** Fat: 75%; Protein: 18%; Carbs: 7%

Crab Cakes with Garlic Aioli

SERVES 4 | PREP TIME: 15 minutes | COOK TIME: 15 minutes

For the crab cakes

½ pound jumbo lump crabmeat	¼ cup finely chopped bell pepper
½ pound lump crabmeat	1 tablespoon finely chopped fresh parsley
¼ cup mayonnaise	¼ teaspoon salt
1 large egg, beaten	¼ teaspoon freshly ground black pepper
¼ cup coconut flour	
1 teaspoon mustard	1 cup shredded Parmesan cheese
1 teaspoon seafood seasoning	
¼ teaspoon paprika	3 tablespoons butter
1 teaspoon minced garlic	
¼ cup finely chopped onion	

For the aioli

2 teaspoons minced garlic	½ teaspoon salt
1 tablespoon freshly squeezed lemon juice	⅛ teaspoon freshly ground black pepper
1 large egg	½ cup olive oil

In a large bowl, combine the jumbo lump crabmeat, lump crabmeat, mayonnaise, egg, coconut flour, mustard, seafood

seasoning, paprika, garlic, onion, bell pepper, parsley, salt, and pepper. Mix well. Mix in the Parmesan cheese. Divide the crabmeat mixture into six equal portions. Form each into a patty. Refrigerate to firm up while making the aioli. In a food processor, mix the garlic and lemon juice until smooth. Add the egg, salt, and pepper. Purée, while slowly adding the olive oil until the aioli forms. Heat a large skillet over medium-high heat. Add the butter. Cook for 1 minute. Gently add the crab cakes to the pan. Cook for 7 minutes, being careful not to burn the butter. Reduce the heat to medium. Flip the cakes. Cook for 5 to 7 minutes more, or until done. Transfer the crab cakes to paper towels to drain. Serve immediately with half of the aioli.

Per Serving: Calories: 576; Fat: 46g; Protein: 32g; Total Carbs: 11g; Fiber: 3g; Net Carbs: 8g; **Macros:** Fat: 71%; Protein: 22%; Carbs: 7%

Crab Cakes with Green Goddess Dressing

SERVES 4 | PREP TIME: 15 minutes, plus 1 hour to chill | COOK TIME: 17 minutes

5 tablespoons avocado oil, divided	¾ pound real crab meat, shredded
½ red bell pepper, finely chopped	¼ cup almond meal
1 scallion, white and green parts, finely chopped	1 egg
	1 teaspoon Dijon mustard
¼ jalapeño pepper, finely chopped	Sea salt
	Freshly ground black pepper
	½ cup green goddess dressing

Heat 2 tablespoons of avocado oil in a large skillet over medium-high heat. Sauté the bell pepper, scallion, and jalapeño until softened, about 5 minutes. Transfer the cooked vegetables to a large bowl and add the crab, almond meal, egg, and mustard, mixing until the ingredients are well combined and hold together. Form the crab mixture into 12 patties and place them on a plate, cover with plastic wrap, and chill in the refrigerator to firm for up to 1 hour. Wipe the skillet out and heat the remaining oil over medium-high heat. Panfry the crab cakes until cooked through, about 12 minutes per side, turning once. Season with salt and pepper and top the crab cakes with the dressing and serve.

Per Serving: Calories: 358; Fat: 28g; Protein: 20g; Total Carbs: 4g; Fiber: 2g; Net Carbs: 2g; **Macros:** Fat: 70%; Protein: 22%; Carbs: 8%

Crab au Gratin

SERVES 4 | PREP TIME: 10 minutes | COOK TIME: 35 minutes

½ cup (1 stick) butter	1 teaspoon pink Himalayan sea salt
1 (8-ounce) container crab claw meat	½ teaspoon freshly ground black pepper
2 ounces cream cheese	½ teaspoon onion powder
½ cup heavy (whipping) cream	1 cup shredded cheddar cheese, divided
2 tablespoons freshly squeezed lemon juice	1 (12-ounce) package cauliflower rice, cooked and drained
1 tablespoon white wine vinegar	

Preheat the oven to 350°F. In a medium sauté pan or skillet, melt the butter over medium heat. Add the crab and cook until warmed through. Add the cream cheese, cream, lemon juice, vinegar, salt, pepper, and onion powder. Keep stirring until the cream cheese fully melts into the sauce. Add ½ cup of cheddar cheese and stir it into the sauce. Spread the cauliflower rice on the bottom of an 8-inch square baking dish. Pour the crab and sauce over, then sprinkle with the remaining ½ cup of cheddar cheese. Bake for 25 to 30 minutes, until the sauce is bubbling. Turn the broiler on to high. Broil for an additional 2 to 3 minutes, until the cheese topping is slightly browned. Allow to cool for 5 to 10 minutes, then serve.

Per Serving: Calories: 555; Fat: 49g; Protein: 23g; Total Carbs: 7g; Fiber: 2g; Net Carbs: 5g; Macros: Fat: 79%; Protein: 16%; Carbs: 5%

Crab-Stuffed Portabella Mushrooms

SERVES 4 | PREP TIME: 5 minutes | COOK TIME: 20 minutes

8 portabella mushroom caps

Nonstick cooking spray

4 (6-ounce) cans crab-meat, drained

8 ounces cream cheese

¼ cup sour cream

4 scallions, green and white parts, finely chopped

2 tablespoons chopped fresh parsley

Salt

Freshly ground black pepper

Preheat the oven to 375°F. Line a large baking sheet with aluminum foil. Place the mushrooms on the prepared baking sheet, stem-side up, and coat with cooking spray. Bake for 15 minutes. Meanwhile, in a large bowl, combine the crab, cream cheese, sour cream, scallions, and parsley. Stir well and season with salt and pepper to taste. Remove the mushrooms from the oven and pat dry with paper towels. Return to the baking sheet, stem-side up, and divide the crab mixture evenly among them. Return to the oven and bake for about 5 minutes, or until the crab is warmed through.

Per Serving: Calories: 456; Fat: 26g; Protein: 46g; Total Carbs: 12g; Fiber: 3g; Net Carbs: 9g; Macros: Fat: 49%; Protein: 41%; Carbs: 10%

Spicy Italian Sausage and Mussels

SERVES 4 | PREP TIME: 10 minutes | COOK TIME: 18 to 20 minutes

2 tablespoons extra-virgin olive oil

8 ounces spicy Italian sausage, casings removed

1 medium onion, halved and thinly sliced

4 garlic cloves, smashed

½ cup dry red wine

2 tablespoons tomato paste

1 cup chicken bone broth or low-sodium chicken broth

2 pounds fresh mussels, scrubbed and debearded

Sea salt

Freshly ground black pepper

2 tablespoons cold butter, cut into pieces

Heat the olive oil in a large pot over medium heat. Cook the sausage and onion for 7 to 8 minutes, until the sausage is gently browned and the onion begins to soften. Add the garlic and cook for 30 seconds. Add the wine and tomato paste and scrape the pan with a wooden spoon to remove the bits stuck to the bottom. Simmer for 2 minutes to burn off some of the alcohol. Add the chicken broth and the mussels to the pot. Season with salt and pepper. Toss well, cover, and steam for 8 to 10 minutes, until all of the mussels have opened. Discard

any that have not opened after 10 minutes. Remove cooked mussels, vegetables, and sausage to a serving dish. Return the pot to the stove and simmer the cooking liquid until reduced to about 1 cup. Whisk in the butter 1 tablespoon at a time. Pour the broth over the mussels, vegetables, and sausage.

Per Serving: Calories: 486; Fat: 29g; Protein: 36g; Total Carbs: 13g; Fiber: 1g; Net Carbs: 12g; Macros: Fat: 59%; Protein: 30%; Carbs: 11%

Crab Fried Rice

SERVES 4 | PREP TIME: 10 minutes | COOK TIME: 12 minutes

¼ cup avocado oil

½ yellow onion, diced

4 garlic cloves, minced

2 large eggs, beaten

6 cups cauliflower rice

¼ cup coconut aminos

1 tablespoon sesame oil

1 (8-ounce) container lump crabmeat, drained

8 cherry tomatoes, halved

Pink Himalayan salt

Freshly ground black pepper

Fresh chopped cilantro, for garnish (optional)

Sliced scallions, for garnish (optional)

Sesame seeds, for garnish (optional)

In a large sauté pan or skillet, heat the avocado oil over medium-high heat. Add the onions and garlic and cook for 3 to 4 minutes, or until soft. Push the onions and garlic to one side of the skillet and pour the eggs into the other side. Let the eggs set for 30 seconds or so. Add the cauliflower rice, coconut aminos, and sesame oil, tossing everything together and breaking up the eggs. Cook the cauliflower rice for about 5 minutes, stirring frequently until the cauliflower softens. Add in the crab and tomatoes and season with salt and pepper. Cook for 2 more minutes and top with cilantro, scallions, and sesame seeds.

Per Serving: Calories: 302; Fat: 21g; Protein: 16g; Total Carbs: 13g; Fiber: 4g; Net Carbs: 9g; Macros: Fat: 63%; Protein: 21%; Carbs: 16%

Steamed Mussels with Garlic and Thyme

SERVES 8 | PREP TIME: 25 minutes | COOK TIME: 20 minutes

4 pounds mussels, cleaned, scrubbed, and debearded

½ cup butter

3 tablespoons olive oil

½ cup diced onion

4 garlic cloves, minced

½ cup diced tomato

1 tablespoon fresh thyme

½ cup white wine

1 cup chicken or seafood broth

2 tablespoons freshly squeezed lemon juice

½ teaspoon salt

¼ teaspoon freshly ground black pepper

Place the cleaned mussels in a large bowl. Cover with cool water. Set aside. In a large, heavy pot over medium heat, heat the butter and olive oil for about 1 minute. Add the onions. Cook for 3 to 5 minutes, until translucent. Add the garlic and cook for 1 to 2 minutes more. Add the tomato, thyme, white wine, broth, lemon juice, salt, and pepper. Increase the heat and bring the mixture to a boil. Add the mussels and cover the pot. Cook for 8 to 10 minutes, shaking the pot at various intervals to allow the mussels to cook evenly. Pour the steaming mussels into a bowl. Discard any that are unopened. Serve immediately.

Per Serving: Calories: 374; Fat: 23g; Protein: 28g; Total Carbs: 12g; Fiber: 0g; Net Carbs: 12g; Macros: Fat: 56%; Protein: 31%; Carbs: 13%

Coconut Saffron Mussels

SERVES 4 | PREP TIME: 15 minutes | COOK TIME: 12 minutes

¼ cup low-sodium vegetable or chicken stock

Pinch saffron

3 tablespoons coconut oil

1 scallion, white and green parts, thinly sliced

2 teaspoons minced garlic

1 teaspoon peeled, grated fresh ginger

1 cup canned coconut milk

Juice and zest of 1 lime

1½ pounds fresh mussels, scrubbed and debearded

2 tablespoons chopped fresh cilantro

Put the stock in a small bowl and sprinkle in the saffron. Set aside for 15 minutes. Heat the oil in a large skillet and sauté the scallions, garlic, and ginger until softened, about 3 minutes. Stir in the coconut milk, saffron and liquid, lime juice, and lime zest and bring to a boil. Add the mussels, cover, and steam until the shells are open, about 8 minutes. Discard any unopened shells and take the skillet off the heat. Stir in the cilantro. Serve immediately with the sauce.

Per Serving: Calories: 245; Fat: 22g; Protein: 7g; Total Carbs: 7g; Fiber: <1g; Net Carbs: 6g; **Macros:** Fat: 80%; Protein: 11%; Carbs: 9%

Pan-Fried Scallops

SERVES 1 | PREP TIME: 5 minutes | COOK TIME: 5 minutes

½ tablespoon avocado oil

1 tablespoon butter or ghee

6 ounces scallops, rinsed with cold water and patted dry

In a large skillet, heat the oil and butter over high heat until it begins to smoke. Generously season the scallops with salt and pepper. Gently add the scallops to the skillet, making sure they are not touching. Sear the scallops for 90 seconds on each side. The scallops should have a nice golden crust on each side and be translucent in the center.

Per Serving: Calories: 304; Fat: 20g; Protein: 29g; Total Carbs: 4g; Fiber: 0g; Net Carbs: 4g; **Macros:** Fat: 60%; Protein: 38%; Carbs: 2%

Sea Scallops with Curry Sauce

SERVES 4 | PREP TIME: 12 minutes | COOK TIME: 18 minutes

¾ pound sea scallops, washed, cleaned, and thoroughly dried

Sea salt

Freshly ground black pepper

3 tablespoons olive oil

1 tablespoon peeled, grated fresh ginger

1 to 1½ tablespoons Thai red curry paste

1½ cups canned coconut milk

1 tablespoon chopped fresh cilantro

Zest and juice of 1 lime

Season the scallops with salt and pepper. Heat the olive oil in a large skillet over medium-high heat. Pan sear the scallops until browned, about 3 minutes; turn and brown the other side for 3 minutes. Transfer the scallops to a plate, cover loosely with foil, and set aside. Return the skillet to the heat and sauté the ginger until softened, about 2 minutes. Stir in the curry paste, coconut milk, cilantro, lime juice, and lime zest and bring to a simmer for 10 minutes. Reduce the heat to low and return the scallops to the skillet, along with any juices on the plate. Turn the scallops with tongs to coat in the sauce and serve.

Per Serving: Calories: 334; Fat: 27g; Protein: 16g; Total Carbs: 6g; Fiber: 0g; Net Carbs: 6g; **Macros:** Fat: 73%; Protein: 19%; Carbs: 8%

Sea Scallops with Bacon Cream Sauce

SERVES 4 | PREP TIME: 15 minutes | COOK TIME: 20 minutes

6 bacon slices, chopped

½ small onion, chopped fine

1 teaspoon minced garlic

¼ cup dry white wine

1 cup heavy (whipping) cream

1 teaspoon chopped fresh thyme

1 tablespoon extra-virgin olive oil

1 pound sea scallops, washed, cleaned, and dried thoroughly

Sea salt

Freshly ground black pepper

In a saucepan over medium-high heat, cook the bacon, stirring, until it is crispy, about 5 minutes. Using a slotted spoon, remove the cooked bacon to a plate. Sauté the onions and garlic in the bacon fat until softened, about 3 minutes. Add the white wine, and deglaze the saucepan, stirring to scrape up the browned bits from the bottom. Whisk in the heavy cream and reserved bacon, and bring the mixture to a simmer. Simmer until the sauce thickens, about 5 minutes. Remove the sauce from the heat, and stir in the thyme. Set aside. In a large nonstick skillet over medium-high heat, heat the olive oil. Season the scallops with salt and pepper. Cook the scallops undisturbed until the bottoms are browned and crisped, about 3 minutes. Using tongs, carefully turn the scallops, and sear the other side until they are also browned and crisped, 3 minutes longer. Transfer the seared scallops to a plate, and serve with the sauce.

Per Serving: Calories: 410; Fat: 32g; Protein: 25g; Total Carbs: 5g; Fiber: 0g; Net Carbs: 5g; **Macros:** Fat: 71%; Protein: 25%; Carbs: 4%

Pan-Seared Butter Scallops

SERVES 4 | PREP TIME: 5 minutes | COOK TIME: 5 minutes

¼ cup butter

2 tablespoons extra-virgin olive oil

1 pound large scallops

Sea salt

Freshly ground black pepper

2 teaspoons roughly chopped garlic

¼ cup roughly chopped fresh parsley

Heat a large skillet over high heat. Melt the butter and add the olive oil. Pat the scallops dry with paper towels and season generously with salt and pepper. When the butter and oil are hot, place the scallops in the pan, being sure not to crowd them. Tilt the pan slightly and pick up a spoonful of the melted butter. Drizzle this over the scallops as they cook. Sear for about 2 minutes on the first side. Carefully flip and sear on the second side for 2 more minutes, or until the scallops are cooked through and opaque in the center. During the last minute of cooking, add the garlic and parsley, and spoon the flavored oil and butter over the scallops.

Per Serving: Calories: 324; Fat: 21g; Protein: 29g; Total Carbs: 5g; Fiber: 1g; Net Carbs: 4g; **Macros:** Fat: 59%; Protein: 36%; Carbs: 5%

Bacon-Wrapped Scallops and Broccolini

SERVES 3 | PREP TIME: 15 minutes | COOK TIME: 15 minutes

5 bacon slices

1 pound scallops (about 10)

½ teaspoon salt, divided

¼ teaspoon freshly ground black pepper, divided

¼ cup (½ stick) butter, divided

15 broccolini pieces

1 teaspoon minced garlic

2 tablespoons dry white wine

2 teaspoons olive oil

Cut the bacon slices in half crosswise, creating 10 small slices. Wrap one slice around each scallop, securing with a toothpick. Season with ¼ teaspoon of salt and ⅛ teaspoon of pepper. Heat a medium skillet over medium-high heat. Add 3 tablespoons of butter and heat for 2 minutes. Add the broccolini, garlic, and wine. Sauté for 2 minutes. Cover and reduce the heat to medium-low. Heat a large skillet over medium-high heat. Add the remaining tablespoon of butter and the olive oil and heat for 2 minutes. Increase the heat under the large skillet to high. Add the scallops. Sear for 1½ minutes per side. Roll the scallops onto their sides so the bacon crisps. Cook for about 1 minute on each side. Check the broccolini for doneness. Season with the remaining ¼ teaspoon of salt and ⅛ teaspoon of pepper. Plate immediately with the scallops, saucing with any excess garlic butter from the pan.

Per Serving: (3 bacon-wrapped scallops): Calories: 510; Fat: 35g; Protein: 42g; Total Carbs: 9g; Fiber: 1g; Net Carbs: 8g; Macros: Fat: 61%; Protein: 32%; Carbs: 7%

Salt-and-Pepper Scallops and Calamari

SERVES 4 | PREP TIME: 5 minutes, plus 15 minutes to rest | COOK TIME: 10 minutes

8 ounces calamari, cut into ½-inch-thick strips or rings
8 ounces sea scallops
1½ teaspoons salt, divided
1 teaspoon freshly ground black pepper
1 teaspoon garlic powder
⅓ cup extra-virgin olive oil
2 tablespoons butter

Place the calamari and scallops on several layers of paper towels and pat dry. Sprinkle with 1 teaspoon salt and allow to sit for 15 minutes at room temperature. Pat dry with additional paper towels. Sprinkle with the pepper and garlic powder. In a deep medium skillet, heat the olive oil and butter over medium-high heat. When the oil is hot but not smoking, add the scallops and calamari in a single layer to the skillet and sprinkle with the remaining ½ teaspoon salt. Cook 2 to 4 minutes on each side, depending on the size of the scallops, until just golden but still slightly opaque in center. Using a slotted spoon, remove from the skillet and transfer to a serving platter. Allow the cooking oil to cool slightly and drizzle over the seafood before serving.

Per Serving: Calories: 309; Fat: 25g; Protein: 18g; Total Carbs: 3g; Fiber: 0g; Net Carbs: 3g; Macros: Fat: 71%; Protein: 25%; Carbs: 4%

Seafood Coconut Stew

SERVES 4 | PREP TIME: 15 minutes | PREP TIME: 30 minutes

¼ cup olive oil
1 onion, chopped
1 yellow bell pepper, chopped
1 cup sliced mushrooms
1 tablespoon minced garlic
2 teaspoons peeled, grated fresh ginger
2 cups low-sodium chicken stock
1 cup canned coconut milk
2 teaspoons ground turmeric
½ pound salmon fillets, diced
½ pound shrimp, peeled, deveined, and each cut into 4 pieces
1 cup cauliflower florets
Sea salt
Freshly ground black pepper
1 cup shredded kale

Heat the olive oil in a large stockpot over medium-high heat. Sauté the onion, bell pepper, mushrooms, garlic, and ginger until the vegetables are softened, about 5 minutes. Add the chicken stock, coconut milk, and turmeric and bring the soup to a boil. Add the fish, shrimp, and cauliflower and reduce the heat to low. Simmer the soup until the fish is cooked through, about 5 minutes. Season with salt and pepper. Stir in the kale and simmer 4 more minutes. Serve immediately.

Per Serving: Calories: 426; Fat: 32g; Protein: 25g; Total Carbs: 12g; Fiber: 3g; Net Carbs: 9g; Macros: Fat: 68%; Protein: 23%; Carbs: 9%

Sheet Pan Seafood Boil

SERVES 6 | PREP TIME: 15 minutes | COOK TIME: 35 minutes

1½ pounds turnips, peeled and cut into ½-inch pieces
Kosher salt
¾ cup (1½ sticks) butter, melted, plus more for serving
1½ tablespoons Old Bay seasoning
1½ tablespoon freshly squeezed lemon juice
1 tablespoon minced garlic
1 teaspoon gluten-free Worcestershire sauce
2 pounds medium raw shrimp, rinsed
1 pound mussels or clams, cleaned (frozen will work as well)
1 pound andouille sausage or kielbasa, cut into 2-inch pieces
1 pound asparagus, woody ends trimmed
1 small onion, peeled and cut into 8 wedges
Lemon wedges, for serving

Preheat the oven to 475°F. Line 2 large sheet pans with parchment paper. Set aside. In a medium saucepan, combine the turnips, a pinch of salt, and enough water to cover. Place the pan over high heat and bring to a boil. Cook for 12 to 15 minutes, or until fork-tender. Drain and set aside. In a small bowl, stir the melted butter, Old Bay seasoning, lemon juice, garlic, and Worcestershire sauce. Evenly divide the shrimp, mussels, sausage, cooked turnips, asparagus, and onion between the prepared sheet pans. Drizzle half the butter mixture over each baking sheet. Toss the seafood and vegetables with the butter to coat. Tightly cover each pan with aluminum foil. Bake for 15 to 20 minutes, or until the shrimp are pink and done, and the shellfish are opened. Discard any shellfish that have not opened. Serve family style with fresh lemon wedges for squeezing and melted butter for dipping.

Per Serving: Calories: 588; Fat: 40g; Protein: 42g; Total Carbs: 15g; Fiber: 5g; Net Carbs: 10g; Macros: Fat: 61%; Protein: 29%; Carbs: 10%

Creamy Shrimp and Grits Casserole

SERVES 6 | PREP TIME: 15 minutes | COOK TIME: 40 minutes

For the grits

3 tablespoons butter, plus more for preparing the baking dish
½ teaspoon minced garlic
¾ cup almond flour
1½ tablespoons coconut flour
¾ cup almond milk
3 tablespoons heavy (whipping) cream
¼ teaspoon kosher salt
⅛ teaspoon freshly ground black pepper
½ cup shredded Cheddar cheese
1 large egg, lightly beaten

For the shrimp

6 thick-cut bacon slices, diced	½ teaspoon kosher salt
½ cup diced onion	½ teaspoon freshly ground
⅓ cup diced green bell pepper	black pepper
2 garlic cloves, finely chopped	⅛ teaspoon cayenne pepper
¼ cup white wine	1½ pounds medium raw shrimp,
¼ cup chicken stock or	peeled and deveined
bone broth	¾ cup heavy (whipping) cream
1 teaspoon dried parsley	3 scallions, sliced
½ teaspoon dried thyme	

Preheat the oven to 350°F. Coat an 8-inch-square baking dish with butter. Set aside. In a medium saucepan over medium heat, melt the butter. Add the garlic and sauté for 1 to 2 minutes. Stir in the almond and coconut flours. Add the almond milk, heavy cream, salt, and pepper. Bring the mixture to a simmer. Cook, stirring constantly, for 2 to 3 minutes until thickened. Remove from the heat and stir in the Cheddar cheese. Whisk the egg into the mixture and pour the grits into the prepared baking dish. Bake for 12 to 15 minutes, or until golden around the edges and set in the center. In a large sauté pan or skillet over medium-high heat, cook the bacon for 7 to 10 minutes until crispy. Using a slotted spoon, transfer the bacon to paper towels to drain, leaving the fat in the skillet. Return the skillet to the heat and add the onion and green bell pepper to the bacon drippings. Sauté for 3 to 5 minutes until softened. Add the garlic and cook for 1 minute more, stirring constantly. Add the wine and chicken stock. Simmer for 3 to 4 minutes until reduced by about half. Add the parsley, thyme, salt, black pepper, and cayenne. Cook for 1 to 2 minutes more. Add the shrimp and heavy cream. Simmer for 3 to 5 minutes until the sauce is thickened and the shrimp are cooked through and opaque. Pour the shrimp mixture over the baked grits. Garnish with scallions and reserved crispy bacon. Serve immediately.

Per Serving: Calories: 581; Fat: 45g; Protein: 34g; Total Carbs: 10g; Fiber: 5g; Net Carbs: 5g; **Macros:** Fat: 70%; Protein: 23%; Carbs: 7%

Seafood Fideo

SERVES 6 TO 8 | PREP TIME: 15 minutes |
COOK TIME: 20 minutes

2 tablespoons extra-virgin olive oil, plus ½ cup, divided	4 ounces crabmeat
	½ cup crumbled goat cheese
6 cups zucchini noodles, roughly chopped (2 to 3 medium zucchini)	½ cup crumbled feta cheese
	1 (28-ounce) can chopped tomatoes, with their juices
1 pound shrimp, peeled, deveined and roughly chopped	1 teaspoon salt
	1 teaspoon garlic powder
	½ teaspoon smoked paprika
6 to 8 ounces canned chopped clams, drained (about 3 to 4 ounces drained)	½ cup shredded Parmesan cheese
	¼ cup chopped fresh flat-leaf Italian parsley, for garnish

Preheat the oven to 375°F. Pour 2 tablespoons of olive oil in the bottom of a 9-by-13-inch baking dish and swirl to coat the bottom. In a large bowl, combine the zucchini noodles, shrimp, clams, and crabmeat. In another bowl, combine the goat cheese,

feta, and ¼ cup olive oil and stir to combine well. Add the canned tomatoes and their juices, salt, garlic powder, and paprika and combine well. Add the mixture to the zucchini and seafood mixture and stir to combine. Pour the mixture into the prepared baking dish, spreading evenly. Spread shredded Parmesan over top and drizzle with the remaining ¼ cup olive oil. Bake until bubbly, 20 to 25 minutes. Serve warm, garnished with chopped parsley.

Per Serving: Calories: 434; Fat: 31g; Protein: 29g; Total Carbs: 12g; Fiber: 3g; Net Carbs: 9g; **Macros:** Fat: 63%; Protein: 27%; Carbs: 10%

Seafood Ceviche

SERVES 3 | PREP TIME: 10 minutes, plus 1 hour to chill

4 ounces shrimp, peeled and chopped	¼ teaspoon freshly ground black pepper
1 (4-ounce) white fish fillet, chopped into bite-size pieces	3 or 4 limes
	½ medium cucumber, peeled and chopped
4 ounces bay or other small scallops	½ avocado, slightly firm, chopped
¼ small red onion, chopped	⅓ cup grape tomatoes, halved
½ jalapeño pepper, seeded and finely chopped	3 tablespoons chopped fresh cilantro
1 garlic clove, minced	2 teaspoons extra-virgin olive oil
½ teaspoon pink Himalayan sea salt	Firm lettuce leaves, for wraps

In a large bowl, combine the shrimp, fish, and scallops. Add the red onion, jalapeño, garlic, salt, and pepper. Using a wooden spoon, stir to mix the ingredients. Squeeze the juice into the bowl and stir well. Cover the bowl with plastic wrap, and place in the refrigerator for 45 minutes to 1 hour. Add the cucumber, avocado, tomatoes, and cilantro to the bowl. Gently mix, trying not to smash the avocado. Drizzle the ceviche with the olive oil, then serve with the lettuce to make wraps.

Per Serving: Calories: 211; Fat: 9g; Protein: 21g; Total Carbs: 13g; Fiber: 4g; Net Carbs: 9g; **Macros:** Fat: 40%; Protein: 42%; Carbs: 18%

Shrimp and "Grits"

SERVES 4 | PREP TIME: 20 minutes | COOK TIME: 25 minutes

1 pound medium peeled, deveined shrimp	3 cups cauliflower rice
	½ cup shredded Cheddar cheese
1 teaspoon salt, divided	
¼ teaspoon freshly ground black pepper, divided	¼ cup shredded Parmesan cheese
	½ cup heavy (whipping) cream
⅛ teaspoon chili powder	
4 bacon slices	2 scallions, green parts, thinly sliced
2 tablespoons butter	

Line two plates with paper towels. In a large bowl, toss the shrimp, ½ teaspoon of salt, ⅛ teaspoon of pepper, and the chili powder. Cover and refrigerate. In a large skillet over medium heat, fry the bacon until crisp. Transfer to one of the prepared plates. Set the skillet aside, reserving 2 tablespoons of bacon fat. In a medium saucepan on medium-low heat, melt the butter. Add the cauliflower rice and stir to coat. Cook for 3 minutes, stirring frequently. Slowly stir in the cheeses until well combined. Stir in the cream and remaining salt and pepper. Increase the heat to medium high and simmer, stirring frequently, until the rice becomes soft and smooth, about 10 minutes. Heat the reserved bacon grease in the skillet over medium heat. Add the shrimp and sauté until pink and cooked through, 3 to 5 minutes. Use a slotted spoon to transfer the shrimp to the second prepared plate. Serve the cauliflower rice mixture in bowls, topped with the shrimp, crumbled bacon, and scallions.

Per Serving: (¼ recipe): Calories: 369; Fat: 26g; Protein: 28g; Total Carbs: 6g; Fiber: 2g; Net Carbs: 4g; **Macros:** Fat: 63%; Protein: 30%; Carbs: 7%

Popcorn Shrimp

SERVES 2 | PREP TIME: 15 minutes | COOK TIME: 8 minutes

½ cup coconut oil
2 large eggs
1 crushed chicken bouillon cube
⅓ cup coconut flour

½ teaspoon chili powder (optional)
½ pound small peeled, deveined shrimp

Line a plate with paper towels. Melt the oil in a medium saucepan over medium heat. The oil should be ½ inch deep. In a large bowl, beat the eggs. In another large bowl, whisk the bouillon cube, coconut flour, and chili powder (if using). Drop ¼ cup of shrimp at a time first into the eggs and then the flour mixture until each shrimp is completely coated. Add the coated shrimp, ¼ cup at a time, to the oil, making sure each shrimp is submerged in the oil (adding more oil if necessary). Fry until golden, about 2 minutes per side. Use a slotted spoon to transfer the fried shrimp to the prepared plate. Repeat with the remaining shrimp, cooking in ¼-cup batches. Serve immediately.

Per Serving: (½ recipe): Calories: 452; Fat: 35g; Protein: 22g; Total Carbs: 12g; Fiber: 7g; Net Carbs: 5g; **Macros:** Fat: 70%; Protein: 19%; Carbs: 11%

Shrimp Veracruz

SERVES 6 | PREP TIME: 10 minutes | COOK TIME: 15 minutes

1½ pounds shrimp, peeled and deveined
Kosher salt
Freshly ground black pepper
Garlic powder, for seasoning
Chili powder, for seasoning
3 tablespoons ghee or avocado oil, divided
½ cup diced onion
½ cup diced green bell pepper
4 garlic cloves, finely minced
3 large ripe tomatoes, seeded and diced

1 tablespoon finely diced jalapeño pepper
½ teaspoon ground cumin
½ cup water or chicken stock
Chopped fresh cilantro, for garnish
Sliced scallion, for garnish
Steamed cauliflower rice or zucchini noodles, for serving
Lime wedges, for serving

Pat the shrimp dry with paper towels and lightly season both sides with salt, pepper, garlic powder, and chili powder. Preheat a large heavy skillet over medium-high heat. Add 2 tablespoons of ghee to melt. Add the shrimp and cook for about 2 minutes per side until

golden brown. Remove from the skillet and set aside. Return the skillet to the heat and add the remaining 1 tablespoon of ghee, the onion, and green bell pepper. Sauté for 2 to 3 minutes until the onion is translucent, scraping up any browned bits from the bottom of the pan. Add the garlic, tomatoes, jalapeño, ½ teaspoon of salt, ¼ teaspoon of garlic powder, and the cumin. Cook for 1 to 2 minutes more, stirring constantly. Add the water to the skillet and simmer for about 3 minutes until the sauce has thickened. Add the shrimp to the pan and cook for 2 minutes more, just until the shrimp are cooked and heated through. Garnish with cilantro and scallion. Serve over cauliflower rice with lime wedges for squeezing.

Per Serving: Calories: 221; Fat: 9g; Protein: 25g; Total Carbs: 10g; Fiber: 4g; Net Carbs: 6g; **Macros:** Fat: 37%; Protein: 45%; Carbs: 18%

Sheet-Pan Shrimp

SERVES 4 | PREP TIME: 15 minutes | COOK TIME: 10 minutes

½ cup (1 stick) butter, melted
4 ounces cream cheese, at room temperature
1 teaspoon garlic salt

1 pound shrimp, any size, peeled, deveined, tails off, patted dry
Juice of 1 lemon
2 scallions, white and green parts thinly sliced

Preheat the oven to 400°F. Line a rimmed baking sheet with parchment paper and set aside. In a medium bowl, mix the melted butter, cream cheese, and garlic salt until well combined. Drop the shrimp into the butter mixture and fold gently to coat all the shrimp. Pour the shrimp mixture onto the prepared baking sheet and spread out the shrimp so none overlap. Bake for 8 to 10 minutes. Squeeze the lemon juice across the top of the shrimp, garnish with the scallions, and serve immediately.

Per Serving: (¼ recipe) Calories: 420; Fat: 35g; Protein: 25g; Total Carbs: 3g; Fiber: 0g; Net Carbs: 3g; **Macros:** Fat: 74%; Protein: 23%; Carbs: 3%

Bacon-Wrapped Shrimp

SERVES 2 | PREP TIME: 5 minutes | COOK TIME: 20 minutes

1 teaspoon granulated erythritol
½ teaspoon chili powder
¼ teaspoon pink Himalayan sea salt

¼ teaspoon freshly ground black pepper
¼ teaspoon onion powder
12 extra-jumbo shrimp, peeled, tails on
6 bacon slices

Preheat the oven to 400°F. Line a baking sheet with aluminum foil. In a small bowl, combine the erythritol, chili powder, salt, pepper, and onion powder. In a medium bowl, combine the shrimp with the spice mixture, tossing to evenly distribute the seasoning. Cut the bacon strips in half crosswise. Wrap each shrimp with one of the pieces, using the slight overlap to hold it together. Place the bacon-wrapped shrimp on the baking sheet seam-side down. Bake for 18 to 20 minutes, until the bacon is crisp. Allow the shrimp to cool for about 5 minutes, then serve.

Per Serving: Calories: 194; Fat: 13g; Protein: 17g; Total Carbs: 2g; Fiber: 0g; Net Carbs: 2g; **Macros:** Fat: 61%; Protein: 35%; Carbs: 4%

Roasted Shrimp and Veggies

SERVES 1 | PREP TIME: 5 minutes | COOK TIME: 20 minutes

½ zucchini, cut into
　half-moons
¼ red onion, cut into
　half-inch pieces
¼ red bell pepper, cut into
　half-inch pieces
2 garlic cloves, minced, divided

¼ teaspoon paprika, divided
2 tablespoons butter or ghee,
　melted, divided
6 ounces peeled shrimp
½ lemon, cut into wedges,
　for garnish

Preheat the oven to 425°F; line a baking sheet with parchment paper. Place the zucchini, onion, and bell pepper in a large bowl, and sprinkle with half the garlic and half the paprika. Add 1 tablespoon of the butter. Spread the vegetables onto the prepared baking sheet, and bake for 12 to 15 minutes. Put the shrimp in the same large bowl, and mix in the remaining garlic, paprika, and butter. Combine to completely coat the shrimp. Add the shrimp to the baking sheet with the vegetables, and bake for 5 additional minutes, until the shrimp are pink. Spoon the shrimp and vegetables into a bowl; garnish with the lemon wedges.

Per Serving: Calories: 421; Fat: 25g; Protein: 39g; Total Carbs: 10g; Fiber: 3g; Net Carbs: 7g; **Macros:** Fat: 53%; Protein: 37%; Carbs: 10%

Shrimp Coconut Pad Thai

SERVES 4 | PREP TIME: 20 minutes | COOK TIME: 17 minutes

1 cup canned coconut milk
¼ cup natural peanut butter
2 tablespoons fish sauce
2 tablespoons apple
　cider vinegar
2 tablespoons Swerve
1 tablespoon soy sauce
1 tablespoon sriracha
　hot sauce

¼ cup coconut oil
½ pound shrimp, peeled,
　deveined, and chopped
1 cup bean sprouts
3 zucchini, spiralized
1 scallion, white and green
　parts, thinly sliced on a bias

In a medium bowl, whisk the coconut milk, peanut butter, fish sauce, vinegar, Swerve, soy sauce, and sriracha until smooth. Set the sauce aside. Heat the oil in a large skillet over medium-high heat. Sauté the shrimp until just cooked through, about 10 minutes. Add the bean sprouts and sauté 4 minutes. Add the sauce, tossing to coat, and cook until the sauce is heated through, about 3 minutes. Remove from the heat and stir in the zucchini noodles. Serve topped with scallion.

Per Serving: Calories: 405; Fat: 34g; Protein: 18g; Total Carbs: 10g; Fiber: 2g; Net Carbs: 8g; **Macros:** Fat: 76%; Protein: 18%; Carbs: 6%

Chimichurri Shrimp

SERVES 4 | PREP TIME: 10 minutes | COOK TIME: 2 to 3 minutes

½ cup plus 1 tablespoon
　extra-virgin olive oil, divided
½ cup roughly chopped parsley
½ cup roughly chopped
　cilantro
1 tablespoon fresh oregano
3 garlic cloves, smashed
1 shallot, peeled and diced

½ teaspoon sea salt
¼ teaspoon red pepper flakes
2 tablespoons red
　wine vinegar
1½ pounds large shrimp,
　peeled and deveined

In a blender, pulse ½ cup of the olive oil, parsley, cilantro, oregano, garlic, shallot, sea salt, and red pepper flakes until nearly smooth. Stir in the red wine vinegar. Heat the remaining tablespoon of olive oil in a large skillet over medium-high heat. Sauté the shrimp for 2 to 3 minutes, or until barely cooked through. Pour the chimichurri sauce into the pan to briefly warm it for about 30 seconds, and then remove from the heat.

Per Serving: Calories: 459; Fat: 33g; Protein: 35g; Total Carbs: 4g; Fiber: 1g; Net Carbs: 3g; **Macros:** Fat: 65%; Protein: 31%; Carbs: 4%

Oregano Shrimp with Tomatoes and Feta

SERVES 4 | PREP TIME: 5 minutes | COOK TIME: 25 minutes

1 (15-ounce) can diced
　tomatoes
1 tablespoon minced garlic
2 teaspoons dried oregano
1 teaspoon onion powder
1 pound raw medium shrimp,
　peeled and deveined

½ cup crumbled feta cheese
Salt
Freshly ground black pepper
Chopped fresh parsley,
　for garnish

Preheat the oven to 375°F. In a large oven-safe skillet, combine the tomatoes, garlic, oregano, and onion powder. Cook over medium-high heat for 5 minutes to allow some of the liquid to reduce. Add the shrimp and stir well. Sprinkle with the feta, then place in the oven for 10 to 15 minutes, until the shrimp has cooked through. Season with salt and pepper to taste, garnish with the parsley, and serve.

Per Serving: Calories: 153; Fat: 5g; Protein: 19g; Total Carbs: 7g; Fiber: 2g; Net Carbs: 5g; **Macros:** Fat: 31%; Protein: 52%; Carbs: 17%

Cajun Shrimp and Cauliflower Rice

SERVES 4 | PREP TIME: 10 minutes | COOK TIME: 15 minutes

2 tablespoons olive oil
2 tablespoons Cajun
　seasoning
1 cup chicken broth or sea-
　food stock

1 pound raw large shrimp,
　peeled and deveined
Fresh parsley leaves,
　for garnish
4 cups cauliflower rice

In a large stockpot or Dutch oven, heat the oil over medium heat. Add the cauliflower rice and Cajun seasoning. Stir well to combine, then add the broth. Bring to a boil, then reduce to a simmer and cook for 10 minutes, or until the cauliflower is tender. Add the shrimp and cook until they are pink and opaque. Using a fine-mesh ladle or slotted spoon, transfer the shrimp and cauliflower to serving bowls and garnish with parsley.

Per Serving: Calories: 190; Fat: 9g; Protein: 19g; Total Carbs: 9g; Fiber: 2g; Net Carbs: 7g; **Macros:** Fat: 42%; Protein: 41%; Carbs: 17%

Basil Butter Grilled Shrimp

SERVES 4 | PREP TIME: 10 minutes | COOK TIME: 5 minutes

½ cup butter, at room
　temperature
½ cup roughly chopped
　fresh basil

Zest and juice of 1 lime
1 pound large EZ-peel
　shrimp

In a small bowl, mix the butter, basil, and lime zest. Spoon the butter mixture into each shrimp between the meat and the shell. Thread the shrimp onto four bamboo skewers, about four shrimp per skewer. Place them on a hot grill and cook for 1 to 2 minutes per side, until gently charred.

Per Serving: Calories: 328; Fat: 25g; Protein: 23g; Total Carbs: 2g; Fiber: 0g; Net Carbs: 2g; **Macros:** Fat: 70%; Protein: 28%; Carbs: 2%

Shrimp with Creamy Tomato-and-Spinach Sauce

SERVES 4 | PREP TIME: 5 minutes | COOK TIME: 15 minutes

2 tablespoons (1 ounce) unsalted butter
1 pound raw large shrimp, peeled and deveined
1 tablespoon minced garlic
½ cup heavy (whipping) cream
¼ cup tomato sauce
¼ cup chicken broth or seafood stock
10 ounces baby spinach
Salt
Freshly ground black pepper
Fresh parsley, for garnish

In a large saucepan or deep skillet, melt the butter over medium heat. Add the shrimp and garlic and cook for 2 to 3 minutes, until the shrimp are pink and opaque. Use a slotted spoon to transfer the shrimp to a plate. Add the heavy cream, tomato sauce, broth, and spinach to the skillet. Increase the heat to medium-high and cook for 10 minutes, or until the spinach has fully wilted and the sauce has thickened. Return the shrimp to the pan, stir well, and season with salt and pepper to taste. Garnish with parsley before serving.

Per Serving: Calories: 279; Fat: 18g; Protein: 26g; Total Carbs: 5g; Fiber: 2g; Net Carbs: 3g; **Macros:** Fat: 57%; Protein: 37%; Carbs: 6%

Shrimp and Sausage Jambalaya

SERVES 4 | PREP TIME: 10 minutes | COOK TIME: 18 to 20 minutes

1 head cauliflower
¼ cup extra-virgin olive oil
½ cup diced yellow onion
½ cup diced green bell pepper
¼ cup diced celery stalk
1 teaspoon minced garlic
½ cup canned diced plum tomatoes, drained
1 pound andouille sausage
1 to 2 teaspoons Cajun seasoning
½ pound large shrimp, peeled and deveined
Sea salt
Freshly ground black pepper
2 tablespoons minced fresh parsley

In a food processor, pulse the cauliflower until coarsely ground, about the texture of rice. In a large skillet, heat the olive oil over medium heat. Cook the onion, bell pepper, celery, and garlic until soft, about 10 minutes. Add the tomatoes, and cook until most of the liquid has evaporated, about 2 minutes. Add the sausage to the pan, and cook for 2 minutes. Add the cauliflower and Cajun seasoning to the pan and sauté for 2 to 3 minutes. Add the shrimp and continue cooking until the shrimp is cooked through, another 2 to 3 minutes. Season with salt and pepper and garnish with parsley before serving.

Per Serving: Calories: 392; Fat: 26g; Protein: 30g; Total Carbs: 13g; Fiber: 5g; Net Carbs: 7g; **Macros:** Fat: 60%; Protein: 31%; Carbs: 9%

Shrimp Scampi with Zucchini Noodles

SERVES 3 | PREP TIME: 20 minutes | COOK TIME: 10 minutes

2 tablespoons olive oil
1 tablespoon minced garlic
1 pound shrimp, peeled and deveined
¼ cup dry white wine
2 tablespoons freshly squeezed lemon juice
1 tablespoon butter
3 tablespoons heavy (whipping) cream
2½ cups zucchini noodles
¼ teaspoon salt
¼ teaspoon freshly ground black pepper
1 tablespoon chopped fresh parsley

Heat a large skillet over medium heat. Add the olive oil and heat for about 1 minute. Add the garlic. Cook for 1 minute. Add the shrimp to the pan. Cook on all sides, turning, about 4 minutes. Remove the shrimp from the skillet. Set aside, leaving the liquid in the pan. To the skillet with the reserved liquid, add the white wine and lemon juice. Scrape the bottom of the pan to incorporate any solids with the liquid, stirring constantly for 2 minutes. Add the butter and heavy cream. Cook for 1 minute. Add the zucchini noodles to the pan. Cook, stirring occasionally, for about 2 minutes or until the zucchini is al dente (noodle-like) in texture. Return the shrimp to the pan. Season with the salt and pepper. Stir to incorporate all ingredients. Plate and garnish with fresh parsley. Serve immediately.

Per Serving: Calories: 384; Fat: 22g; Protein: 36g; Total Carbs: 8g; Fiber: 1g; Net Carbs: 7g; **Macros:** Fat: 53%; Protein: 39%; Carbs: 8%

Grilled Shrimp with Avocado Salad

SERVES 3 | PREP TIME: 20 minutes | COOK TIME: 5 minutes

1 pound shrimp, peeled and deveined
2 tablespoons olive oil
½ teaspoon garlic powder
½ teaspoon salt, divided
⅛ teaspoon freshly ground black pepper
1 avocado, peeled, pitted, and diced
¼ cup chopped bell pepper
¼ cup chopped tomato
¼ cup chopped onion
1 teaspoon freshly squeezed lime juice

Heat a griddle over medium-high heat. In a large bowl, combine the shrimp, olive oil, garlic powder, ¼ teaspoon of salt, and pepper. Mix until the shrimp are coated thoroughly. In a medium bowl, mix the avocado, bell pepper, tomato, onion, and lime juice. Sprinkle with the remaining ¼ teaspoon of salt and refrigerate. Place the shrimp on the hot griddle, on their sides. Cook for 2 to 3 minutes. Flip, and cook for another 1 to 2 minutes. Remove the shrimp from the griddle. Plate with the avocado salad to serve.

Per Serving: Calories: 409; Fat: 25g; Protein: 36g; Total Carbs: 11g; Fiber: 5g; Net Carbs: 6g; **Macros:** Fat: 54%; Protein: 35%; Carbs: 11%

Vietnamese Shrimp Cakes

SERVES 4 | PREP TIME: 10 minutes | COOK TIME: 5 minutes

1 pound large shrimp, peeled and deveined
1 tablespoon coconut flour
½ teaspoon sea salt
1 tablespoon minced lemongrass
1 teaspoon minced garlic
1 teaspoon minced red chile
¼ cup coconut oil

In a food processor, blend the shrimp, coconut flour, salt, lemongrass, garlic, and red chile until the mixture is thick but still slightly chunky. Heat the coconut oil in a large skillet over medium-high heat until hot. Form the shrimp mixture into small cakes, about 2 tablespoons each. Fry for 2 to 3 minutes on each side, until golden brown and cooked through.

Per Serving: Calories: 246; Fat: 16g; Protein: 23g; Total Carbs: 3g; Fiber: 1g; Net Carbs: 2g; **Macros:** Fat: 59%; Protein: 37%; Carbs: 4%

Bang Bang Shrimp

SERVES 4 | PREP TIME: 10 minutes | COOK TIME: 10 minutes

For the shrimp

½ cup coconut flour

¼ cup shredded pepper Jack cheese

1 teaspoon baking powder

½ teaspoon kosher salt

¼ teaspoon freshly ground black pepper

1 large egg

1 pound small shrimp (51/60 count), peeled and deveined

Olive oil, for frying

For the sauce

¼ cup mayonnaise

3 tablespoons chili sauce

1 teaspoon sriracha

¼ teaspoon freshly squeezed lime juice

In a food processor, blend the coconut flour, cheese, baking powder, salt, and pepper until the mixture resembles fine bread crumbs, then transfer it to a shallow bowl. In a small bowl, beat the egg. Dip each shrimp into the egg, then coat it with the breading mixture. Repeat with the remaining shrimp and set aside. In a large skillet, heat 1 inch of oil over medium-high heat until it reaches 375°F. Fry the shrimp for about 1 minute per side, then transfer them to a paper towel–lined plate to soak up the excess oil. In a medium bowl, combine the mayo, chili sauce, sriracha, and lime juice and mix well. Place the breaded shrimp on a serving dish, drizzle with the sauce, and serve.

Per Serving: Calories: 302; Fat: 18g; Protein: 22g; Total Carbs: 13g; Fiber: 6g; Net Carbs: 7g; **Macros:** Fat: 54%; Protein: 29%; Carbs: 17%

Shrimp and Vegetable Kebabs with Chipotle Sour Cream Sauce

SERVES 2 | PREP TIME: 20 minutes | COOK TIME: 10 minutes

¾ pound shrimp, peeled and deveined

2 tablespoons olive oil

2 tablespoons freshly squeezed lime juice

½ teaspoon garlic powder, divided

½ teaspoon onion powder, divided

¼ cup chopped fresh cilantro

¼ teaspoon salt

¼ teaspoon freshly ground black pepper

½ teaspoon liquid smoke (optional)

½ cup roughly chopped bell pepper

⅓ cup roughly chopped onion

¼ cup sour cream

1 teaspoon chipotle pepper powder

Heat a grill, or griddle, to medium-high heat. In a large bowl, combine the shrimp, olive oil, lime juice, ¼ teaspoon garlic powder, ¼ teaspoon onion powder, cilantro, salt, and pepper. If cooking indoors, add the liquid smoke (if using). Mix until the shrimp

are coated thoroughly. In a small bowl, mix the sour cream, chipotle powder, the remaining ¼ teaspoon garlic powder, and the remaining ¼ teaspoon onion powder and refrigerate. Skewer the shrimp, alternating with the bell peppers and onions. Place the kebabs on the preheated grill. Cook for 3 to 5 minutes. Flip, and cook for 3 to 5 minutes more. Remove from the grill. Check the shrimp for doneness. The shrimp is done when firm in texture, opaque, and tinged with its signature pink-orange color. Remove the shrimp and vegetables from the kebabs. Serve with the chipotle sour cream sauce.

Per Serving: Calories: 410; Fat: 23g; Protein: 40g; Total Carbs: 10g; Fiber: 1g; Net Carbs: 9g; **Macros:** Fat: 51%; Protein: 39%; Carbs: 10%

Shrimp Fried Rice

SERVES 4 | PREP TIME: 20 minutes | COOK TIME: 15 minutes

2 tablespoons coconut oil, divided

1 pound peeled and deveined shrimp

½ teaspoon sea salt

⅛ teaspoon freshly ground black pepper

3 cups cauliflower rice

¼ cup diced red bell pepper

¼ cup chopped broccoli florets

2 tablespoons diced white onion

2 garlic cloves, minced

2 large eggs

2 tablespoons coconut aminos

Heat 1 tablespoon of oil in a large skillet over high heat. Add the shrimp and season with the salt and pepper. Sauté the shrimp until pink, about 3 minutes. Transfer to a plate and set aside. In the same skillet over medium-high heat, heat the remaining 1 tablespoon of oil. Add the cauliflower rice and cook, stirring frequently, until most of its water has evaporated, 5 to 7 minutes. Stir in the bell pepper, broccoli, and onion. Cook, stirring frequently, until the onions are translucent, about 3 minutes. Stir in the garlic and cook for 1 more minute. Move the veggies toward the outer edges of the skillet. Crack the eggs into the middle of the pan and allow to cook untouched for 1 minute. Mix the veggies into the egg, scrambling the egg as you go. Cook for another minute, until the eggs are cooked through. Add the shrimp and coconut aminos. Stir thoroughly to fully incorporate.

Per Serving: (¼ recipe): Calories: 217; Fat: 12g; Protein: 20g; Total Carbs: 10g; Fiber: 2g; Net Carbs: 8g; **Macros:** Fat: 49%; Protein: 37%; Carbs: 14%

Shrimp, Bamboo Shoot, and Broccoli Stir-Fry

SERVES 2 | PREP TIME: 15 minutes | COOK TIME: 15 minutes

2 tablespoons olive oil

¾ pound shrimp, peeled and deveined

1 tablespoon minced garlic

1 cup sliced bamboo shoots

¼ cup chopped onion

1 cup broccoli florets

½ teaspoon sesame oil

3 tablespoons soy sauce

½ teaspoon unsweetened rice wine vinegar

½ teaspoon Chinese five-spice powder

¼ teaspoon freshly ground black pepper

Heat a large skillet over medium-high heat. Add the olive oil and heat for 1 minute. Add the shrimp and garlic to the skillet. Cook for 2 to 3 minutes, or until the shrimp are mostly cooked. Remove the shrimp from the skillet. Lower the heat to medium. Add the bamboo shoots, onion, and broccoli and sauté for 5 to

8 minutes, or until room temperature. Add the sesame oil, soy sauce, rice wine vinegar, Chinese five-spice powder, and black pepper. Mix to combine. Add the shrimp back to the skillet, and cook for another 1 to 2 minutes. Serve immediately.

Per Serving: Calories: 394; Fat: 18g; Protein: 44; Total Carbs: 14g; Fiber: 4g; Net Carbs: 10g; Macros: Fat: 41%; Protein: 45%; Carbs: 14%

Shrimp in Creamy Pesto over Zoodles

SERVES 4 | PREP TIME: 10 minutes | COOK TIME: 10 minutes

1 pound peeled and deveined fresh shrimp
Salt
Freshly ground black pepper
2 tablespoons extra-virgin olive oil
½ small onion, slivered
8 ounces store-bought jarred pesto

¾ cup crumbled goat or feta cheese, plus more for serving
6 cups zucchini noodles (from about 2 large zucchini), for serving
¼ cup chopped flat-leaf Italian parsley, for garnish

In a bowl, season the shrimp with salt and pepper and set aside. In a large skillet, heat the olive oil over medium-high heat. Sauté the onion until just golden, 5 to 6 minutes. Reduce the heat to low and add the pesto and cheese, whisking to combine and melt the cheese. Bring to a low simmer and add the shrimp. Reduce the heat back to low and cover. Cook until the shrimp is cooked through and pink, another 3 to 4 minutes. Serve warm over zucchini noodles, garnishing with chopped parsley and additional crumbled cheese, if desired.

Per Serving: Calories: 491; Fat: 35g; Protein: 29g; Total Carbs: 15g; Fiber: 4g; Net Carbs: 11g; Macros: Fat: 65%; Protein: 25%; Carbs: 10%

Coconut Shrimp

SERVES 6 | PREP TIME: 15 minutes | COOK TIME: 15 minutes

For the coconut shrimp

Oil for frying
1 cup unsweetened shredded coconut
½ cup unsweetened flaked coconut
¼ cup unsweetened coconut milk
½ cup mayonnaise

2 large egg yolks
¼ teaspoon salt
⅛ teaspoon freshly ground black pepper
½ teaspoon garlic powder
1 pound shrimp, peeled and deveined, tails left on

For the aioli

½ cup mayonnaise
2 tablespoons chili sauce, such as Huy Fong Foods brand

2 teaspoons freshly squeezed lime juice
1 teaspoon red pepper flakes

In a large pot, heat 2 inches of oil to 350°F for deep-frying. In a medium bowl, thoroughly mix the shredded coconut, flaked coconut, coconut milk, mayonnaise, egg yolks, salt, pepper, and garlic powder. Using 1 to 2 tablespoons of batter, carefully form it around each shrimp, leaving the tails exposed. Immediately drop the battered shrimp into the preheated oil. Repeat with 2 to 3 more shrimp. Cook for 4 to 6 minutes, until golden brown. Remove the shrimp from the oil. Set aside to cool on a paper-towel-lined plate. Repeat the process with the remaining shrimp. In a small bowl, thoroughly combine the mayonnaise,

chili sauce, lime juice, and red pepper flakes. Serve immediately with the coconut shrimp.

Per Serving: Calories: 466; Fat: 41g; Protein: 19g; Total Carbs: 6g; Fiber: 2g; Net Carbs: 4g; Macros: Fat: 79%; Protein: 16%; Carbs: 5%

Garlicky Shrimp with Mushrooms

SERVES 4 | PREP TIME: 10 minutes | COOK TIME: 15 minutes

1 pound peeled and deveined fresh shrimp
1 teaspoon salt
1 cup extra-virgin olive oil
8 large garlic cloves, thinly sliced

4 ounces sliced mushrooms (shiitake, baby bella, or button)
½ teaspoon red pepper flakes
¼ cup chopped fresh flat-leaf Italian parsley

Rinse the shrimp and pat dry. Place in a small bowl and sprinkle with the salt. In a large skillet, heat the olive oil over medium-low heat. Add the garlic and heat until very fragrant, 3 to 4 minutes, reducing the heat if the garlic starts to burn. Add the mushrooms and sauté for 5 minutes, until softened. Add the shrimp and red pepper flakes and sauté until the shrimp begins to turn pink, another 3 to 4 minutes. Remove from the heat and stir in the parsley. Serve.

Per Serving: Calories: 620; Fat: 56g; Protein: 24g; Total Carbs: 4g; Fiber: 0g; Net Carbs: 4g; Macros: Fat: 81%; Protein: 15%; Carbs: 4%

Garlic and Herb Baked Shrimp with Cauliflower Rice

SERVES 6 | PREP TIME: 10 minutes | COOK TIME: 15 minutes

6 tablespoons olive oil
1 tablespoon minced garlic
¼ cup fresh flat-leaf parsley leaves
4 scallions, white and green parts, roughly chopped

½ cup dry white wine
1½ pounds raw large shrimp, peeled and deveined
4 cups cauliflower rice, cooked according to package directions

Preheat the oven to 375°F. In a food processor or blender, combine the oil, garlic, parsley, and scallions. Blend until smooth. Stir in the wine. Place the shrimp in a 9-by-13-inch baking dish and pour the oil mixture over top. Turn to coat. Transfer to the oven and bake for 15 minutes, or until the shrimp have cooked through. Serve over the cauliflower rice.

Per Serving: Calories: 241; Fat: 15g; Protein: 17g; Total Carbs: 7g; Fiber: 2g; Net Carbs: 5g; Macros: Fat: 58%; Protein: 31%; Carbs: 11%

Greek Stuffed Squid

SERVES 4 | PREP TIME: 15 minutes | COOK TIME: 30 minutes

8 ounces frozen spinach, thawed and drained (about 1½ cups)
4 ounces crumbled goat cheese
½ cup chopped pitted olives
½ cup extra-virgin olive oil, divided
¼ cup chopped sun-dried tomatoes

¼ cup chopped fresh flat-leaf Italian parsley
2 garlic cloves, finely minced
¼ teaspoon freshly ground black pepper
2 pounds baby squid, cleaned and tentacles removed

Preheat the oven to 350°F. In a medium bowl, combine the spinach, goat cheese, olives, ¼ cup olive oil, sun-dried tomatoes, parsley, garlic, and pepper. Pour 2 tablespoons of olive oil in the bottom of an 8-inch-square baking dish and spread to coat the bottom. Stuff each cleaned squid with 2 to 3 tablespoons of the cheese mixture, depending on the size of the squid, and place in the prepared baking dish. Drizzle the tops with the remaining 2 tablespoons olive oil and bake until the squid are cooked through, 25 to 30 minutes.

Per Serving: Calories: 469; Fat: 37g; Protein: 24g; Total Carbs: 10g; Fiber: 3g; Net Carbs: 7g; **Macros:** Fat: 71%; Protein: 20%; Carbs: 9%

POULTRY

Chicken Vegetable Hash

SERVES 4 | PREP TIME: 15 minutes | COOK TIME: 40 minutes

¼ cup coconut oil	½ cup shredded cabbage
14 ounces boneless, skinless chicken thighs, diced	1 teaspoon chopped fresh thyme
1 onion, chopped	Sea salt
1 red bell pepper, diced	Freshly ground black pepper
2 teaspoons minced garlic	1 cup pumpkin seeds
1 cup diced raw or frozen pumpkin	½ cup shredded kale

Heat the oil in a large skillet over medium-high heat. Sauté the chicken until it is cooked through, about 15 minutes. Transfer the chicken to a plate using a slotted spoon. Add the onion, bell pepper, and garlic and sauté until softened, about 5 minutes. Stir in the pumpkin, cabbage, and thyme and sauté until the vegetables are tender, about 15 minutes. Place the chicken back in the skillet and season with salt and pepper. Add the pumpkin seeds and kale and sauté until the greens are wilted, about 5 minutes.

Per Serving: Calories: 443; Fat: 33g; Protein: 26g; Total Carbs: 14g; Fiber: 5g; Net Carbs: 9g; **Macros:** Fat: 67%; Protein: 23%; Carbs: 10%

Chicken Cutlets with Garlic Cream Sauce

SERVES 4 | PREP TIME: 20 minutes, plus time to chill | COOK TIME: 25 minutes

¾ cup canned coconut milk	¾ cup unsweetened shredded coconut
Juice and zest of 1 lime	
1 tablespoon Swerve	¼ cup almond meal
2 teaspoons minced garlic	4 (3-ounce) boneless, skinless chicken breasts, pounded to about ⅓-inch thick
1 teaspoon soy sauce	
½ cup almond flour	
2 large eggs, beaten	3 tablespoons olive oil

Stir the coconut milk, lime juice, lime zest, Swerve, garlic, and soy sauce in a small saucepan over medium heat. Bring the sauce to a boil, then reduce the heat to low and simmer until thickened, about 5 minutes. Remove the sauce from the heat, pour into a container, and refrigerate until chilled, about 2 hours. Preheat the oven to 350°F. Line a baking sheet with parchment paper. Put the almond flour in a small bowl. Put the beaten eggs in another small bowl. In a third bowl, stir the coconut and almond meal. Line up the bowls with the almond flour, eggs, then the coconut. Pat the chicken dry with paper towels and dredge each piece in the almond flour, then the egg mixture, and finally the coconut mixture to coat. Place the coated chicken on the baking sheet. Brush the cutlets carefully with the olive oil. Bake the chicken until golden brown and cooked through, turning once, about 20 minutes in total. Serve with chilled dipping sauce.

Per Serving: Calories: 508; Fat: 43g; Protein: 26g; Total Carbs: 10g; Fiber: 4g; Net Carbs: 6g; **Macros:** Fat: 76%; Protein: 20%; Carbs: 4%

Loaded Chicken and Cauliflower Nachos

SERVES 4 | PREP TIME: 10 minutes | COOK TIME: 25-minutes

¼ cup olive oil	Freshly ground black pepper
1 tablespoon onion powder	1 cup cooked chicken, diced or shredded
1 teaspoon paprika	
1 teaspoon ground cumin	¾ cup shredded Mexican blend cheese
1 large head cauliflower (about 1 pound)	
	¼ cup low-carb salsa
Salt	

Preheat the oven to 375°F. Line a baking sheet with aluminum foil. In a large bowl, combine the oil, onion powder, paprika, and cumin. Set aside. Cut the cauliflower into quarters and remove any leaves and thick stem. Cut the quarters crosswise into even ½-inch-thick slices. Add the cauliflower to the bowl with the spice mixture and turn to coat. Transfer the cauliflower to the prepared baking sheet and spread in a single layer. Season with salt and pepper. Roast for 20 minutes, then remove from the oven. Top with the chicken and cheese and return to the oven for 5 to 10 minutes, until the cheese has melted. Remove from the oven, top with the salsa, and serve.

Per Serving: Calories: 297; Fat: 22g; Protein: 16g; Total Carbs: 9g; Fiber: 3g; Net Carbs: 6g; **Macros:** Fat: 67%; Protein: 22%; Carbs: 11%

Shredded Chicken

MAKES 6 CUPS | PREP TIME: 5 minutes |
COOK TIME: 8 minutes, plus 10 minutes to come to pressure
MAKES ABOUT 6 CUPS | RELEASE: Natural, 10 minutes

1 cup chicken broth	4 large boneless, skinless chicken breasts (about 6 ounces each)
¼ cup tomato sauce	
1 teaspoon salt	

Pour the broth, tomato sauce, and salt into an electric pressure cooker and stir to mix. Add the chicken breasts and cover in the sauce. Lock the pressure cooker lid in place with the steam vent set to Sealing. Select high pressure and set the timer for 8 minutes. After cooking, allow a 10-minute natural pressure release. Open the pressure release valve and let out any remaining steam. Carefully open the pressure cooker and use two forks to shred the chicken into the broth. Let sit for 5 minutes, then use a slotted spoon to remove the chicken.

Per Serving (1 cup): Calories: 140; Fat: 2g; Protein: 26g; Total Carbs: 2g; Fiber: 0g; Net Carbs: 2g; **Macros:** Fat: 15%; Protein: 80%; Carbs: 5%

Roast Chicken with Cilantro Mayonnaise

SERVES 6 | PREP TIME: 10 minutes | COOK TIME: 1 hour and 30 minutes

1 (3-pound) whole
   roasting chicken
Sea salt, for seasoning
1 onion, cut into 8 wedges
¼ cup olive oil

Freshly ground black pepper
½ mayonnaise
1 tablespoon chopped fresh
   cilantro

Preheat the oven to 350°F. Wash the chicken in cold water, inside and out, and pat it completely dry with paper towels. Place the chicken in a baking dish and lightly salt the cavity. Place the onion in the cavity. Brush the chicken skin all over with olive oil and season the skin with the salt and pepper. Roast the chicken until it is golden brown and cooked through (to an internal temperature of 185°F), about 90 minutes. Remove the chicken from the oven and let it sit for 15 minutes. In a small bowl, stir the mayonnaise and cilantro. Carve the chicken and serve with the mayonnaise.

Per Serving: Calories: 578; Fat: 45g; Protein: 43g; Total Carbs: 4g; Fiber: 1g; Net Carbs: 3g; Macros: Fat: 70%; Protein: 30%; Carbs: 0%

Buffalo Chicken Wings

SERVES 4 | PREP TIME: 15 minutes | COOK TIME: 50 minutes

1 tablespoon olive oil
1 teaspoon salt, divided
½ teaspoon freshly ground
   black pepper, divided
2 pounds chicken wings
¼ cup hot sauce

1 tablespoon butter, melted
¼ teaspoon cayenne pepper
1 cup blue cheese sauce or
   ranch dressing, or purchased bottled dressing

Preheat the oven to 400°F. In a large bowl, mix the olive oil, ½ teaspoon of salt, and ¼ teaspoon of black pepper. Add the wings and stir to coat. Evenly divide the wings between two baking sheets. Place the sheets in the oven. Bake for 45 to 50 minutes, or until the outer skin is crispy. In another large bowl, mix the hot sauce, butter, cayenne pepper, the remaining ½ teaspoon of salt, and remaining ¼ teaspoon of black pepper. Add the cooked wings. Toss them in the sauce for 1 minute to coat. Serve with bleu cheese sauce or ranch dressing.

Per Serving: Calories: 507; Fat: 23g; Protein: 67g; Total Carbs: 4g; Fiber: 0g; Net Carbs: 4g; Macros: Fat: 42%; Protein: 55%; Carbs: 3%

Chicken Tenders

SERVES 4 | PREP TIME: 10 minutes | COOK TIME: 25 to 30 minutes

2 cups crushed pork rinds
¼ cup grated Parmesan
   cheese
1 teaspoon garlic powder
1 teaspoon freshly ground
   black pepper

1 large egg
½ cup heavy (whipping) cream
1 pound boneless skinless
   chicken tenderloins (10 to
   12 tenderloins), patted dry

Preheat the oven to 425°F. Line a baking sheet with parchment paper and set aside. In a shallow bowl, mix the pork rinds, Parmesan cheese, garlic powder, and pepper. In a separate bowl, whisk the egg and heavy cream. Dip a tenderloin entirely in the

egg mixture, then lay the tenderloin in the pork rind mixture, turning to coat both sides. Lay the coated tenderloin on the prepared baking sheet and repeat with the remaining tenderloins. Bake for 25 to 30 minutes.

Per Serving: (3 tenderloins) Calories: 460; Fat: 32g; Protein: 41g; Total Carbs: 2g; Fiber: 0g; Net Carbs: 2g; Macros: Fat: 63%; Protein: 36%; Carbs: 1%

Almond Meal–Crusted Chicken Fingers

SERVES 4 | PREP TIME: 10 minutes | COOK TIME: 20 minutes

Nonstick cooking spray
1 cup almond meal
1 teaspoon garlic powder
½ teaspoon ground cumin
½ teaspoon paprika
¼ teaspoon cayenne pepper
2 large eggs
1½ tablespoon olive oil,
   to brush on the fingers
   before basting

1 pound boneless, skinless
   chicken tenders
Fresh spinach leaves, for
   serving (optional)
Sugar-free ketchup, barbecue
   sauce, or sugar-free hot
   sauce, for serving (optional)

Preheat the oven to 425°F. Line a baking sheet with aluminum foil and coat with nonstick spray. In a shallow bowl, combine the almond meal, garlic powder, cumin, paprika, and cayenne. Beat the eggs into another shallow bowl. Working one at a time, dip the chicken tenders into the egg mixture, letting the excess drip off. Dredge in the almond meal mixture to fully coat, then place on the prepared baking sheet. Bake the chicken tenders for about 20 minutes, checking them periodically and flipping about halfway through. Serve on a bed of spinach.

Per Serving: Calories: 206; Fat: 14g; Protein: 17g; Total Carbs: 3g; Fiber: 2g; Net Carbs: 1g; Macros: Fat: 62%; Protein: 33%; Carbs: 5%

Garlic Parmesan Wings

SERVES 5 | PREP TIME: 5 minutes | COOK TIME: 1 hour

2½ pounds chicken wing
   pieces (20 to 22 wings),
   patted dry ½ cup
1 stick butter, melted

1 tablespoon garlic salt or
   1 tablespoon minced garlic
½ cup grated Parme-
   san cheese

Preheat the oven to 375°F. Line a baking sheet with parchment paper. Place the chicken wings on the parchment paper. Bake for 1 hour, flipping the wings halfway through the cooking time. Remove the chicken wings from the oven and place them in a large bowl. Gently toss the wings in the butter and garlic salt. Top with the grated Parmesan cheese.

Per Serving: (4 chicken wings) Calories: 469; Fat: 40g; Protein: 26g; Total Carbs: 1g; Fiber: 0g; Net Carbs: 1g; Macros: Fat: 77%; Protein: 22%; Carbs: 1%

Chicken Paprikash

SERVES 4 | PREP TIME: 15 minutes | COOK TIME: 30 minutes

¼ cup olive oil, divided
¾ pound boneless, skinless
   chicken breasts, cut into
   ½-inch strips
1 medium onion, sliced

1 red bell pepper, diced
1 tablespoon minced garlic
½ cup low-sodium
   chicken stock
½ cup canned coconut milk

¼ cup no-salt-added
  tomato paste
3 tablespoons
  smoked paprika
½ cup sour cream

Sea salt
Freshly ground black pepper
2 tablespoons chopped
  fresh parsley

Heat 2 tablespoons of olive oil in a large skillet over medium-high heat. Brown the chicken until cooked through, about 10 minutes, and transfer to a plate using a slotted spoon. Add the remaining olive oil and sauté the onion, bell pepper, and garlic until softened, about 4 minutes. Stir in the reserved cooked chicken, chicken stock, coconut milk, tomato paste, and paprika. Cover the skillet and simmer, stirring occasionally, until the chicken and vegetables are very tender, about 15 minutes. Stir in the sour cream and simmer an additional 1 minute. Season with salt and pepper and serve topped with parsley.

Per Serving: Calories: 378; Fat: 28g; Protein: 21g; Total Carbs: 14g; Fiber: 4g; Net Carbs: 10g; **Macros:** Fat: 67%; Protein: 22%; Carbs: 11%

Paprika Chicken with Broccoli

SERVES 6 | PREP TIME: 5 minutes, plus 30 minutes to marinate | COOK TIME: 40 minutes

6 boneless, skinless chicken
  breasts (6 ounces each)
6 tablespoons mayonnaise
2 tablespoons paprika

2 teaspoons onion powder
Salt
Freshly ground black pepper
1 pound broccoli florets

Preheat the oven to 375°F. Line a baking sheet with aluminum foil. Meanwhile, in a large resealable bag or a bowl, combine the chicken, mayonnaise, paprika, and onion powder and massage the spices into the meat. Let marinate in the refrigerator for 30 minutes. Transfer the chicken to the prepared baking sheet and season with salt and pepper. Discard the remaining marinade. Cook for 40 minutes, or until the chicken has reached an internal temperature of 165°F. While the chicken cooks, bring a large saucepan of water to a boil. Add the broccoli. Cook for 6 to 8 minutes, until tender. Drain, season with salt and pepper to taste, and serve with the chicken.

Per Serving: Calories: 421; Fat: 27g; Protein: 38g; Total Carbs: 7g; Fiber: 3g; Net Carbs: 4g; **Macros:** Fat: 57%; Protein: 38%; Carbs: 5%

Chicken Parmesan

SERVES 6 | PREP TIME: 20 minutes | COOK TIME: 35 minutes

3 large boneless chicken
  breasts, halved
¾ cup grated Parmesan
  cheese, divided
½ cup almond flour
1 teaspoon Italian seasoning
½ teaspoon garlic powder
¼ teaspoon salt

⅛ teaspoon freshly ground
  black pepper
1 large egg
¼ cup olive oil
6 tablespoons sugar-free
  pasta sauce, divided
1 cup shredded mozzarella
  cheese, divided

Preheat the oven to 350°F. Place the chicken between two pieces of plastic wrap. Pound the chicken and flatten until all pieces are about ½ inch thick. In a medium bowl, mix ½ cup of Parmesan cheese, the almond flour, Italian seasoning, garlic powder, salt, and pepper. In another bowl, beat the egg. Set up a "breading"

station: Line up the egg wash, then the Parmesan coating. Dip each piece of chicken into the egg wash, then thoroughly coat in the "breading." Set aside. In a large skillet over medium-high heat, heat the olive oil for about 2 minutes. Add the "breaded" chicken. Cook for 5 to 7 minutes, or until browned on each side. Remove from the skillet and place on a parchment-lined baking sheet. Top with 1 tablespoon of pasta sauce and divide the 1 cup of mozzarella cheese among the chicken. Sprinkle each with the remaining Parmesan cheese. Place the baking sheet in the oven. Bake for 20 minutes, until the cheese is thoroughly melted.

Per Serving: (½ chicken breast with sauce and cheese): Calories: 469; Fat: 30g; Protein: 44g; Total Carbs: 4g; Fiber: 1g; Net Carbs: 3g; **Macros:** Fat: 58%; Protein: 38%; Carbs: 4%

Stuffed Chicken Breasts

SERVES 4 | PREP TIME: 30 minutes, plus 30 minutes to chill | COOK TIME: 30 minutes

1 tablespoon butter
¼ cup chopped sweet onion
½ cup goat cheese, at room
  temperature
¼ cup Kalamata
  olives, chopped
¼ cup chopped roasted
  red pepper

2 tablespoons chopped
  fresh basil
4 (5-ounce) chicken
  breasts, skin-on
2 tablespoons extra-virgin
  olive oil

Preheat the oven to 400°F. In a small skillet over medium heat, melt the butter and add the onion. Sauté until tender, about 3 minutes. Transfer the onion to a medium bowl and add the cheese, olives, red pepper, and basil. Stir until well blended, then refrigerate for about 30 minutes. Cut horizontal pockets into each chicken breast, and stuff them evenly with the filling. Secure the two sides of each breast with toothpicks. Place a large ovenproof skillet over medium-high heat and add the olive oil. Brown the chicken on both sides, about 10 minutes in total. Place the skillet in the oven and roast until the chicken is just cooked through, about 15 minutes. Remove the toothpicks and serve.

Per Serving: Calories: 389; Fat: 30g; Protein: 25g; Total Carbs: 3g; Fiber: 0g; Net Carbs: 3g; **Macros:** Fat: 70%; Protein: 28%; Carbs: 2%

Coconut Chicken

SERVES 4 | PREP TIME: 15 minutes | COOK TIME: 25 minutes

2 tablespoons olive oil
4 (4-ounce) boneless
  chicken breasts, cut into
  2-inch chunks
½ cup chopped sweet onion

1 cup coconut milk
1 tablespoon curry powder
1 teaspoon ground cumin
1 teaspoon ground coriander
¼ cup chopped fresh cilantro

Place a large saucepan over medium-high heat and add the olive oil. Sauté the chicken until almost cooked through, about 10 minutes. Add the onion and sauté for an additional 3 minutes. In a medium bowl, whisk the coconut milk, curry powder, cumin, and coriander. Pour the sauce into the saucepan with the chicken and bring the liquid to a boil. Reduce the heat and simmer until the chicken is tender and the sauce has thickened, about 10 minutes. Serve the chicken with the sauce, topped with cilantro.

Per Serving: Calories: 382; Fat: 31g; Protein: 23g; Total Carbs: 5g; Fiber: 1g; Net Carbs: 4g; **Macros:** Fat: 70%; Protein: 26%; Carbs: 4%

Breaded Chicken Strip Lettuce Wraps

SERVES 1 | PREP TIME: 5 minutes | COOK TIME: 5 minutes

1 large egg
1 teaspoon Italian seasoning
1 tablespoon avocado oil
2 boneless chicken thighs, cut into thin strips
2 Bibb lettuce leaves

In a medium bowl, whisk the egg and Italian seasoning. Season with a little salt and freshly ground black pepper. In a large skillet, heat the oil over medium heat. Coat the chicken strips in the egg mixture. Add the chicken to the skillet and cook for 5 minutes, turning occasionally, until fully cooked. Wrap the chicken in the lettuce leaves.

Per Serving: Calories: 544; Fat: 44g; Protein: 36g; Total Carbs: 1g; Fiber: 0g; Net Carbs: 1g; **Macros:** Fat: 73%; Protein: 26%; Carbs: 1%

Chopped Chicken-Avocado Lettuce Wraps

SERVES 4 | PREP TIME: 10 minutes

½ avocado, peeled and pitted
⅓ cup mayonnaise
1 teaspoon freshly squeezed lemon juice
2 teaspoons chopped fresh thyme
1 (6-ounce) cooked chicken breast, chopped
Sea salt
Freshly ground black pepper
8 large lettuce leaves
¼ cup chopped walnuts

In a medium bowl, mash the avocado with the mayonnaise, lemon juice, and thyme until well combined. Stir in the chopped chicken and season the filling with salt and pepper. Spoon the chicken salad into the lettuce leaves and top with the walnuts. Serve 2 lettuce wraps per person.

Per Serving: Calories: 264; Fat: 20g; Protein: 12g; Total Carbs: 9g; Fiber: 3g; Net Carbs: 6g; **Macros:** Fat: 70%; Protein: 16%; Carbs: 14%

BBQ Chicken Wraps

SERVES 4 | PREP TIME: 10 minutes

2 cups cooked chicken, diced or shredded
½ cup low-carb barbecue sauce
8 (8-inch) low-carb tortillas
1 cup chopped or shredded iceberg lettuce

In a large bowl, mix the chicken and barbecue sauce. Divide the mixture among the tortillas, then add the lettuce. Roll up the tortillas and place them on a serving plate, seam-side down.

Per Serving: Calories: 340; Fat: 8g; Protein: 26g; Total Carbs: 41g; Fiber: 31g; Net Carbs: 10g; **Macros:** Fat: 21%; Protein: 31%; Carbs: 48%

BBQ Chicken Skewers

SERVES 4 | PREP TIME: 10 minutes, plus 30 minutes to marinate | COOK TIME: 20 minutes

4 boneless, skinless chicken breasts (6 ounces each)
1 cup low-carb barbecue sauce, divided
1 red bell pepper cut into 2-inch chunks
2 medium zucchini cut into ½-inch rounds
1 (8-ounce) package white mushrooms, stems removed
Salt
Freshly ground black pepper

Cut the chicken into even 2-inch pieces. Set ¼ cup of barbecue sauce aside for basting. Combine the remaining ¾ cup of barbecue sauce and the chicken in a resealable bag. Seal and place in the refrigerator for at least 30 minutes. Preheat the grill to medium-high. When ready to cook, remove the chicken from the marinade (discard the marinade). Thread each skewer, alternating the ingredients. Each skewer should have 3 pieces of chicken, 1 slice of zucchini, 1 or 2 mushrooms, and 1 or 2 pieces of bell pepper. Season with salt and black pepper. Cook the skewers on the grill, turning occasionally, for about 20 minutes, or until the chicken has reached an internal temperature of 165°F. Brush the cooked skewers with the reserved ¼ cup of barbecue sauce before serving.

Per Serving (3 skewers): Calories: 360; Fat: 16g; Protein: 41g; Total Carbs: 13g; Fiber: 4g; Sugar Alcohols: 6g; Net Carbs: 9g; **Macros:** Fat: 40%; Protein: 46%; Carbs: 14%

Bacon-Wrapped Jalapeño Chicken

SERVES 4 | PREP TIME: 30 minutes | COOK TIME: 20 minutes

4 (4-ounce) boneless chicken breasts
¾ cup cream cheese, at room temperature
4 jalapeño peppers, halved
1 teaspoon onion powder
2 garlic cloves, minced
8 bacon slices
¼ teaspoon salt
⅛ teaspoon freshly ground black pepper
2 tablespoons olive oil

Preheat the oven to 400°F. On a flat surface, cut each chicken breast in half horizontally. Do not cut all the way through the other side. Open the breasts flat. Spread an equal amount of cream cheese over each of the butterflied breasts. Top each with two jalapeño halves. Sprinkle with onion powder and garlic. Fold the breasts closed. Wrap each breast with two bacon slices. Secure with toothpicks. Season the outside of the breasts with the salt and pepper. Place the bacon-wrapped chicken in a baking pan. Drizzle with the olive oil. Bake the chicken for 20 minutes, or until the internal temperature is 165°F. Remove the pan from the oven. Allow the chicken to rest for 2 to 3 minutes. Remove the toothpicks from the meat and serve.

Per Serving: Calories: 586; Fat: 42g; Protein: 47g; Total Carbs: 4g; Fiber: 1g; Net Carbs: 3g; **Macros:** Fat: 65%; Protein: 32%; Carbs: 3%

Chicken Breast Tenders with Riesling Cream Sauce

SERVES 4 | PREP TIME: 10 minutes | COOK TIME: 28 to 30 minutes

4 (about 6-ounce) boneless, skinless chicken breasts
½ cup almond flour
2 tablespoons coconut flour
1 teaspoon garlic powder
Sea salt
Freshly ground black pepper
2 tablespoons canola oil
½ cup Riesling or Sauvignon Blanc
½ cup chicken bone broth
½ cup heavy (whipping) cream
4 cups mixed greens

Preheat the oven to 250°F. Slice the chicken into 4-by-2-inch pieces. In a shallow dish, mix the almond flour, coconut flour, garlic powder, salt, and pepper. Dredge the chicken pieces in the flour mixture. Heat the canola oil in a large skillet over medium-high heat. Sear the chicken pieces for 2 to 3 minutes on each side until well browned. Transfer to a baking dish and place in the oven to keep warm. Add the Riesling to the skillet and cook until reduced to about ¼ cup, about 3 minutes. Add the broth and heavy cream, and cook over medium-low heat to thicken the sauce for 5 minutes. Place the chicken onto serving plates and garnish with the mixed greens. Serve the Riesling cream sauce on the side.

Per Serving: Calories: 475; Fat: 30g; Protein: 43g; Total Carbs: 7g; Fiber: 4g; Net Carbs: 3g; Macros: Fat: 57%; Protein: 36%; Carbs: 7%

Curried Chicken Salad

SERVES 4 | PREP TIME: 10 minutes

½ cup mayonnaise
1 tablespoon lemon juice
1 teaspoon curry powder
Sea salt
Freshly ground black pepper

16 ounces shredded cooked chicken, light and dark meat
¼ cup roughly chopped toasted cashews
1 celery stalk, minced
¼ cup diced red onion

In a medium bowl, whisk the mayonnaise, lemon juice, and curry powder. Season with salt and pepper. Fold in the chicken, cashews, celery, and red onion. Serve immediately or refrigerate until ready to serve.

Per Serving: Calories: 379; Fat: 28g; Protein: 27g; Total Carbs: 4g; Fiber: 1g; Net Carbs: 3g; Macros: Fat: 67%; Protein: 29%; Carbs: 4%

Crispy Chicken Paillard

SERVES 4 | PREP TIME: 10 minutes | COOK TIME: 10 minutes

½ cup grated Parmesan cheese
¼ cup almond flour
1 teaspoon garlic powder
½ teaspoon sea salt

½ teaspoon freshly ground black pepper
4 (6-ounce) boneless chicken breasts
2 tablespoons canola oil

Mix the Parmesan cheese, almond flour, garlic powder, salt, and pepper in a shallow dish. Place the chicken breasts one at a time between two sheets of parchment paper. Pound with the flat side of a meat mallet until the chicken is about ½-inch thick. Heat the canola oil in a large skillet over medium-high heat. Lightly coat the chicken pieces in the Parmesan and flour mixture, and sear for 5 minutes on each side, or until just cooked through.

Per Serving: Calories: 362; Fat: 19g; Protein: 45g; Total Carbs: 2g; Fiber: 1g; Net Carbs: 1g; Macros: Fat: 48%; Protein: 50%; Carbs: 2%

Chicken Kebabs with Spicy Almond Sauce

SERVES 4 | PREP TIME: 15 minutes, plus time to marinate | COOK TIME: 12 minutes

½ cup almond butter
1 tablespoon soy sauce
1 tablespoon finely chopped fresh cilantro

1 teaspoon Swerve
1 teaspoon minced garlic
Juice of 1 lime
Pinch red pepper flakes

Juice of 1 lime
¼ cup olive oil
2 tablespoons soy sauce
1 tablespoon minced garlic

¾ pound boneless, skinless chicken breast, cut into strips

Whisk the almond butter, soy sauce, cilantro, Swerve, garlic, lime juice, and red pepper flakes in a small bowl until well combined. Set aside, covered, in the refrigerator. In a medium bowl, stir the lime juice, olive oil, soy sauce, garlic, and chicken until well mixed. Marinate at least 1 hour and up to 24 hours, covered, in the refrigerator. Preheat the oven to broil. Remove the chicken strips from the marinade and thread them onto wooden skewers that have been soaked in water. Arrange the kebabs on a baking sheet and broil, turning once, until the meat is cooked through but still juicy, 10 to 12 minutes total. Serve with almond butter sauce.

Per Serving: Calories: 409; Fat: 33g; Protein: 23g; Total Carbs: 9g; Fiber: 3g; Net Carbs: 6g; Macros: Fat: 73%; Protein: 22%; Carbs: 5%

Chicken Pot Pie

SERVES 6 | PREP TIME: 15 minutes | COOK TIME: 1 hour 5 minutes

3 tablespoons olive oil
1½ pounds boneless, skinless chicken thighs, cut into 1-inch pieces
¼ cup diced white onion
⅓ cup diced zucchini
⅓ cup diced celery
1 garlic clove, minced
1 teaspoon sea salt

½ teaspoon dried thyme
½ teaspoon dried parsley
1 cup low-sodium chicken broth
¼ cup heavy (whipping) cream
¼ teaspoon cream of tartar
Cooking spray
Formed into 2 balls, chilled
1 large egg, beaten (optional)

In a large skillet over medium heat, warm the olive oil until shimmering. Add the chicken and cook until browned, about 3 minutes per side. Drop the heat to medium and add the onion, zucchini, and celery. Cook, stirring frequently, until the onions and celery are soft and the zucchini is beginning to brown, about 7 minutes. Stir in the garlic, salt, thyme, and parsley. Cook for 1 more minute. Pour in the broth and scrape the bottom of the pan to release any brown bits. Bring to a boil and then reduce the heat to low and simmer for 20 minutes or until the liquid reduces and the mixture thickens. Slowly pour in the cream and sprinkle in the cream of tartar, whisking constantly. Simmer for another 5 to 10 minutes, until thickened. Preheat the oven to 350°F. Spray a 9-inch pie dish with cooking spray. Remove the dough from the refrigerator. Place 1 dough ball at a time between 2 pieces of parchment paper and roll out to ⅛-inch-thick circles. Lay 1 dough circle in the bottom of the pie dish. Pour the pie filling into the dish and then top with the remaining dough circle. Crimp the edges of the dough and use a fork to poke holes all over the top of the dough. Brush the dough with the egg (if using), for a darker pie crust. Bake until the dough is just golden on top, 20 to 25 minutes. Let cool for 5 minutes. Serve immediately.

Per Serving: (⅙ recipe) Calories: 639; Fat: 51g; Protein: 39g; Total Carbs: 10g; Fiber: 3g; Net Carbs: 7g; Macros: Fat: 72%; Protein: 24%; Carbs: 4%

Chicken and Dumplings

SERVES 4 | PREP TIME: 15 minutes | COOK TIME: 15 minutes

1 tablespoon avocado oil
⅓ cup diced white onion
¼ cup chopped carrots
½ cup chopped celery
2 garlic cloves, minced

1½ cups shredded cooked
   chicken breast
1 teaspoon dried thyme
4 cups low-sodium
   chicken broth

Heat the oil in a large saucepan over medium heat. Add the onion, carrots, and celery. Cook, stirring frequently, until the onion is translucent, 5 to 6 minutes. Stir in the garlic and cook until fragrant, 1 to 2 minutes. Stir in the chicken and thyme. Pour in the broth and bring to a boil. Reduce the heat to low and simmer while you make the dumplings. Roll the dough into a square ¼ inch thick. Slice the dough into long pieces and then tear into roughly 1-inch chunks. Drop the dumpling pieces into the simmering soup and stir to incorporate. Cook, stirring frequently so the dumplings don't bind together, for another 3 to 5 minutes or until the dumplings are cooked through. Serve immediately.

Per Serving: (1¼ cups): Calories: 454; Fat: 31g; Protein: 35g; Total Carbs: 10g; Fiber: 3g; Net Carbs: 7g; **Macros:** Fat: 61%; Protein: 31%; Carbs: 8%

Chicken Enchiladas

SERVES 4 | PREP TIME: 10 minutes, plus 30 minutes to marinate | COOK TIME: 20 minutes

4 cups cooked chicken, diced
   or shredded
½ cup low-carb salsa
1 cup tomato sauce
1 teaspoon paprika

1 teaspoon onion powder
1 teaspoon dried oregano
4 (8-inch) low-carb tortillas
½ cup shredded Mexican
   blend cheese

Preheat the oven to 350°F. In a resealable bag, combine the chicken and salsa. Massage the bag to blend, seal, and refrigerate for 30 minutes to marinate. In a bowl, mix the tomato sauce, paprika, onion powder, and oregano. Spread half the mixture on the bottom of a 9-by-13-inch baking dish. Place the tortillas on a large cutting board. Divide the chicken mixture evenly among them. Roll each tortilla up and place them in the dish, seam-side down. Cover the enchiladas with the remaining tomato sauce mixture, then sprinkle the cheese on top. Cook uncovered for 15 to 20 minutes, until the meat is fully warmed through and the cheese has melted.

Per Serving: Calories: 368; Fat: 12g; Protein: 40g; Total Carbs: 25g; Fiber: 17g; Net Carbs: 8g; **Macros:** Fat: 29%; Protein: 43%; Carbs: 28%

Chicken Fajitas

SERVES 4 | PREP TIME: 10 minutes | COOK TIME: 15 to 20 minutes

1 pound boneless, skinless
   chicken breasts and/or
   thighs, sliced into thin strips
1 teaspoon salt

1 teaspoon dried oregano
1 teaspoon garlic powder
½ teaspoon freshly ground
   black pepper

1 teaspoon ground cumin
½ teaspoon red pepper flakes
½ teaspoon paprika
¼ teaspoon ground cinnamon
2 tablespoons avocado oil or
   butter, divided
½ white onion, sliced
½ red bell pepper, sliced
   into strips
½ green bell pepper, sliced
   into strips

2 tablespoons chicken broth
   (optional)
2 to 4 coconut or almond flour
   wraps, or grain-free chips
1 cup shredded
   romaine lettuce
Sugar-free salsa, Guacamole,
   sour cream, and shred-
   ded cheese, for serving
   (optional)

In a large bowl, combine the chicken with the salt, oregano, garlic powder, pepper, cumin, red pepper flakes, paprika, cinnamon, and 1 tablespoon of oil. Heat the remaining tablespoon of oil in a large skillet over medium-high heat. Sauté the onion for 3 to 5 minutes, until translucent. Add the bell peppers and sauté for 5 minutes, until tender. Add the chicken mixture and sauté for 2 to 3 minutes, then reduce the heat to medium, cover, and cook for about 5 minutes, or until the chicken is cooked through. Let the chicken mixture cool a bit. Divide the wraps or chips among plates, sprinkle the shredded romaine on top, and spoon the chicken fajita mixture on top of the lettuce. Serve the fajitas with salsa, Guacamole, sour cream, and cheese, if desired.

Per Serving: Calories: 235; Fat: 13g; Protein: 25g; Total Carbs: 5g; Fiber: 2g; Net Carbs: 3g; **Macros:** Fat: 50%; Protein: 43%; Carbs: 7%

Chicken Cacciatore

SERVES 4 | PREP TIME: 10 minutes | COOK TIME: 1 hour 10 minutes

4 large bone-in, skin-on
   chicken thighs
   (6 ounces each)
Salt
Freshly ground black pepper
2 tablespoons olive oil
2 bell peppers (any
   color), diced
¼ cup diced onion
1 tablespoon minced garlic

1 (8-ounce) package white
   mushrooms, sliced
¼ cup dry red wine
1 (14.5-ounce) can diced
   tomatoes with liquid
1½ cups chicken or
   vegetable broth
1 tablespoon dried oregano
3 ounces pitted black
   olives, sliced

Season the chicken on both sides with salt and black pepper. In a Dutch oven, heat the oil over medium-high heat. Add the chicken and cook for about 3 minutes on each side. Transfer to a plate and set aside. Add the bell peppers, onion, and garlic to the pot and cook for 5 minutes. Add the mushrooms and cook for another 5 minutes. Stir in the wine, scraping up any browned bits from the bottom of the pot. Add the tomatoes and their juices, the broth, and oregano. Bring to a boil, then reduce to a simmer. Season with salt and pepper to taste. Return the chicken to the pot, cover, and cook for 45 minutes to 1 hour, until the chicken has reached an internal temperature of 165°F and is cooked through. Stir in the olives and serve.

Per Serving: Calories: 502; Fat: 35g; Protein: 30g; Total Carbs: 17g; Fiber: 5g; Net Carbs: 12g; **Macros:** Fat: 63%; Protein: 24%; Carbs: 13%

Creamy Chicken and Spinach Bake

SERVES 4 | PREP TIME: 10 minutes | COOK TIME: 30 minutes

Nonstick cooking spray

1 pound boneless, skinless chicken breasts, cubed

10 ounces baby spinach

8 ounces cream cheese, at room temperature

¾ cup shredded mozzarella cheese, divided

¼ cup sour cream

2 teaspoons minced garlic

Salt

Freshly ground black pepper

Preheat the oven to 400°F. Coat a 9-by-13-inch baking dish with cooking spray. Spread out the chicken in the dish. Layer the spinach over the top, keeping it as flat as possible. In a medium bowl, combine the cream cheese, ¼ cup of mozzarella, the sour cream, and garlic. Season with salt and pepper to taste. Spoon the mixture on top of the spinach. Cover with aluminum foil and bake for 20 minutes. Remove from the oven, uncover, and top with the remaining ½ cup of mozzarella. Bake for another 10 to 15 minutes, until the chicken has reached an internal temperature of 165°F.

Per Serving: Calories: 491; Fat: 31g; Protein: 46g; Total Carbs: 6g; Fiber: 2g; Net Carbs: 4g; **Macros:** Fat: 56%; Protein: 39%; Carbs: 5%

Caprese Balsamic Chicken

SERVES 4 | PREP TIME: 10 minutes | COOK TIME: 25 minutes

3 tablespoons balsamic vinegar

1 tablespoon butter

2 (6-ounce) boneless, skinless chicken breasts, halved lengthwise

Sea salt

Freshly ground black pepper

1 tablespoon extra-virgin olive oil

¼ cup herb pesto, divided

1 tomato, cut into 4 slices

1 cup shredded mozzarella cheese

Preheat the oven to 400°F. In a small saucepan over medium heat, bring the balsamic vinegar and butter to a boil; then reduce the heat to low and simmer until thickened, about 5 minutes. Set aside. Season the chicken breasts with salt and pepper. In a medium skillet over medium heat, heat the olive oil. Cook the chicken, turning once, until just cooked through, about 10 minutes total. Place the cooked chicken in a 9-by-13-baking dish. Spread 1 tablespoon of pesto over each piece of chicken, top each with tomato slices, and evenly divide the cheese between the pieces. Bake in the oven until the cheese is melted and golden, about 5 minutes. Serve with a drizzle of the reduced balsamic vinegar.

Per Serving: Calories: 375; Fat: 25g; Protein: 35g; Total Carbs: 3g; Fiber: 0g; Net Carbs: 3g

Caprese-Stuffed Chicken Breasts

SERVES 4 | PREP TIME: 20 minutes | COOK TIME: 40 minutes

½ cup extra-virgin olive oil, divided

2 boneless, skinless chicken breasts (about 6 ounces each)

4 ounces frozen spinach, thawed and drained well

1 cup shredded fresh mozzarella cheese

¼ cup chopped fresh basil

2 tablespoons chopped sun-dried tomatoes (preferably marinated in oil)

1 teaspoon salt, divided

1 teaspoon freshly ground black pepper, divided

½ teaspoon garlic powder

1 tablespoon balsamic vinegar

Preheat the oven to 375°F. Drizzle 1 tablespoon olive oil in a small deep baking dish and swirl to coat the bottom. Make a deep incision about 3 to 4 inches long along the length of each chicken breast to create a pocket. Using your knife or fingers, carefully increase the size of the pocket without cutting through the chicken breast. In a medium bowl, combine the spinach, mozzarella, basil, sun-dried tomatoes, 2 tablespoons olive oil, ½ teaspoon salt, ½ teaspoon pepper, and the garlic powder and combine well with a fork. Stuff half of the filling mixture into the pocket of each chicken breast. Press the opening together and secure with toothpicks. In a medium skillet, heat 2 tablespoons of olive oil over medium-high heat. Carefully sear the chicken breasts until browned, 3 to 4 minutes per side. Transfer to the prepared baking dish, incision-side up. Scrape up any filling that fell out in the skillet and add it to the baking dish. Cover the pan with foil and bake until the chicken is cooked through, 30 to 40 minutes, depending on the thickness of the breasts. Remove from the oven and rest, covered, for 10 minutes. Meanwhile, in a small bowl, whisk the remaining 3 tablespoons olive oil, balsamic vinegar, ½ teaspoon salt, and ½ teaspoon pepper. To serve, remove the toothpicks cut each chicken breast in half, widthwise, and serve a half chicken breast drizzled with oil and vinegar.

Per Serving: Calories: 434; Fat: 35g; Protein: 27g; Total Carbs: 3g; Fiber: 1g; Net Carbs: 2g; **Macros:** Fat: 71%; Protein: 26%; Carbs: 3%

Chicken Milanese

SERVES 4 | PREP TIME: 30 minutes | COOK TIME: 40 minutes

2 tablespoons butter

½ scallion, chopped, green part only

¼ cup dry white wine

½ cup chicken stock

½ cup heavy (whipping) cream

1 teaspoon thyme

1 teaspoon freshly squeezed lemon juice

2 (8-ounce) boneless chicken breasts, halved lengthwise

¾ cup almond flour

¼ cup Parmesan cheese

1 large egg

1 tablespoon water

¼ cup extra-virgin olive oil

¼ cup chopped fresh parsley

In a medium saucepan over medium-high heat, melt the butter. Sauté the scallion until it is bright green, about 2 minutes. Add the wine, chicken stock, and cream. Bring the sauce to a boil, reduce the heat to low, and simmer until the sauce reduces to about 1 cup, about 20 minutes. Remove the sauce from the heat, and stir in the thyme and lemon juice. Use a mallet to pound the chicken pieces out thin without ripping through. Pat the pieces dry with paper towels. In a large bowl, stir the almond flour and Parmesan cheese together. In another small bowl, stir the egg and water together. Dip the chicken pieces in the egg mixture, and then dredge them in the almond-cheese mixture to coat. In a large skillet over medium heat, heat the olive oil. In a large skillet, cook the breaded chicken pieces until the bottom is golden brown, about 3 minutes. Turn the cutlets over, and cook until the chicken is cooked through and the second side is golden brown, about 4 minutes. Top the cutlets with the parsley, and serve with the sauce.

Per Serving: Calories: 542; Fat: 41g; Protein: 32g; Total Carbs: 6g; Fiber: 3g; Net Carbs: 3g; **Macros:** Fat: 71%; Protein: 25%; Carbs: 4%

Bacon Ranch Cheesy Chicken Breasts

SERVES 4 | PREP TIME: 10 minutes | COOK TIME: 55 minutes

Cooking spray for the
  baking dish
3 tablespoons olive oil
4 boneless chicken breasts
½ teaspoon salt
¼ teaspoon freshly ground
  black pepper
1 tablespoon garlic powder
8 bacon slices sliced into
  ½-inch pieces

¼ cup butter
¼ cup ranch dressing, or purchased bottled dressing
½ cup shredded Cheddar
  cheese, divided
½ cup shredded mozza-
  rella cheese
½ cup grated Parme-
  san cheese
½ teaspoon dried parsley

Preheat the oven to 350°F and prepare a baking dish with cooking spray. In a large skillet over medium-high heat, heat the olive oil for about 1 minute. Season the chicken breasts with the salt, pepper, and garlic powder. Add them to the skillet. Sear each breast for 5 minutes per side. Place the chicken into the prepared dish. Spread 1 tablespoon of butter and 1 tablespoon of ranch dressing over each breast. Top the chicken with the bacon, covering each breast completely. Place the dish in the preheated oven. Bake for 30 minutes. Remove from the oven. Sprinkle equal amounts of the Cheddar, mozzarella, and Parmesan cheeses over the bacon-topped breasts. Season with the dried parsley. Return the dish to the oven. Bake for another 10 to 12 minutes, or until the cheese melts.

Per Serving: Calories: 674; Fat: 52g; Protein: 47g; Total Carbs: 4g; Fiber: 0g; Net Carbs: 4g; Macros: Fat: 70%; Protein: 28%; Carbs: 2%

Chicken Fajita Stuffed Bell Peppers

SERVES 6 | PREP TIME: 10 minutes | COOK TIME: 50 minutes

½ cup butter, divided
1 pound boneless
  chicken thighs
½ cup chopped onion
1½ cups cauliflower rice
¼ cup chopped scallions
½ cup chicken broth
2 teaspoons chili powder
1 teaspoon paprika
1 teaspoon salt

½ teaspoon cumin
½ teaspoon garlic powder
¼ teaspoon dried oregano
¼ teaspoon cayenne pepper
  (optional)
6 bell peppers, tops removed
  and seeded
1 cup shredded Mexican
  cheese blend

Preheat the oven to 350°F. In a large skillet over medium-high heat, heat 6 tablespoons of butter. Add the chicken. Sear for 3 to 4 minutes on each side. Cover. Reduce the heat to medium-low. Cook for another 10 to 12 minutes. Check the chicken for doneness. Set aside to cool. Once cooled, shred the chicken into small pieces. Set aside. In a large skillet over medium-high heat, melt the remaining 2 tablespoons of butter. Add the onion. Cook for 3 to 4 minutes, until translucent. Add the cauliflower "rice," shredded chicken, scallions, chicken broth, chili powder, paprika, salt, cumin, garlic powder, dried oregano, and cayenne pepper (if using). Slice a thin piece from the bottom of each bell pepper so it will not tip over. Place the peppers open-side up on a baking sheet. Fill each bell pepper with an equal amount of the chicken mixture. Top evenly with the Mexican cheese blend. Place the sheet in the oven. Bake for about 30 minutes, or until the cheese browns.

Per Serving: Calories: 419; Fat: 28g; Protein: 29g; Total Carbs: 12g; Fiber: 4g; Net Carbs: 8g; Macros: Fat: 61%; Protein: 28%; Carbs: 11%

Curried Chicken with Bamboo Shoots

SERVES 4 | PREP TIME: 10 minutes | COOK TIME: 25 minutes

¼ cup coconut oil
¼ cup diced onion
1 cup bamboo shoots
1 pound boneless chicken
  thighs, diced
1 teaspoon minced
  fresh ginger

1 tablespoon curry powder
1 tablespoon paprika
1¼ cups coconut milk
¼ cup heavy (whipping) cream
¼ teaspoon salt
⅛ teaspoon freshly ground
  black pepper

In a large skillet over medium-high heat, heat the coconut oil for about 1 minute. Add the onion, bamboo shoots, and chicken meat. Cook for 5 minutes. Stir in the ginger, curry powder, and paprika. Continue cooking for 2 to 3 minutes more. Add the coconut milk and heavy cream. Reduce the heat to medium-low. Simmer for about 15 minutes. Season with salt and pepper. Serve over cauliflower "rice" or zucchini noodles.

Per Serving: Calories: 582; Fat: 52g; Protein: 24g; Total Carbs: 9g; Fiber: 4g; Net Carbs: 5g; Macros: Fat: 78%; Protein: 16%; Carbs: 6%

Basil Chicken Zucchini "Pasta"

SERVES 1 | PREP TIME: 10 minutes | COOK TIME: 15 minutes

1 tablespoon butter or ghee
2 boneless chicken
  thighs, cubed
¼ medium white onion, diced
2 garlic cloves, minced

½ zucchini, peeled into thin
  ribbons or spiralized
1 teaspoon avocado oil
¼ cup basil pesto
4 cherry tomatoes, halved

Melt the butter in a large skillet over medium-high heat. Add the chicken and onion, and cook for several minutes, until the chicken begins to brown. Add the garlic and cook for another 2 to 3 minutes, until the chicken is cooked through. Turn the heat down to low. In a medium bowl, coat the zucchini in the oil. Add the zucchini to the skillet and cook for 1 minute, stirring occasionally. Transfer the mixture to a medium bowl, and toss with the pesto and tomatoes.

Per Serving: Calories: 875; Fat: 74g; Protein: 37g; Total Carbs: 15g; Fiber: 8g; Net Carbs: 7g; Macros: Fat: 76%; Protein: 17%; Carbs: 7%

Lemon-Rosemary Spatchcock Chicken

SERVES 6 TO 8 | PREP TIME: 20 minutes | COOK TIME: 45 minutes

½ cup extra-virgin olive
  oil, divided
1 (3- to 4-pound) roasting
  chicken, spatchcocked
8 garlic cloves,
  roughly chopped

2 to 4 tablespoons chopped
  fresh rosemary
2 teaspoons salt, divided
1 teaspoon freshly ground
  black pepper, divided
2 lemons, thinly sliced

Preheat the oven to 425°F. Pour 2 tablespoons of olive oil in the bottom of a 9-by-13-inch baking dish and swirl to coat the bottom. Place the chicken in the baking dish. Loosen the skin over the breasts and thighs by cutting a small incision and sticking one or two fingers inside to pull the skin away from the meat without removing it. In a small bowl, combine ¼ cup olive oil, garlic, rosemary, 1 teaspoon salt, and ½ teaspoon pepper and whisk. Rub the garlic-herb oil evenly under the skin of each breast and each thigh. Add the lemon slices evenly to the same areas. Whisk the remaining 2 tablespoons olive oil, 1 teaspoon salt, and ½ teaspoon pepper and rub over the outside of the chicken. Place in the oven, uncovered, and roast for 45 minutes, or until cooked through and golden brown. Allow to rest 5 minutes before carving to serve.

Per Serving: Calories: 435; Fat: 34g; Protein: 28g; Total Carbs: 2g; Fiber: 0g; Net Carbs: 2g; **Macros:** Fat: 70%; Protein: 28%; Carbs: 2%

Moroccan Chicken and Vegetable Tagine

SERVES 6 | PREP TIME: 10 minutes | COOK TIME: 1 hour

½ cup extra-virgin olive oil, divided

1½ pounds boneless skinless chicken thighs, cut into 1-inch chunks

1½ teaspoons salt, divided

½ teaspoon freshly ground black pepper

1 small red onion, chopped

1 red bell pepper, cut into 1-inch squares

1 cup water

2 medium tomatoes, chopped or 1½ cups diced canned tomatoes

2 medium zucchini, sliced into ¼-inch-thick half moons

1 cup pitted halved olives (Kalamata or Spanish green work nicely)

¼ cup chopped fresh cilantro or flat-leaf Italian parsley

Riced cauliflower or sautéed spinach, for serving

In a Dutch oven or large rimmed skillet, heat ¼ cup olive oil over medium-high heat. Season the chicken with 1 teaspoon salt and pepper and sauté until just browned on all sides, 6 to 8 minutes. Add the onions and peppers and sauté until wilted, another 6 to 8 minutes. Add the chopped tomatoes and water, bring to a boil, and reduce the heat to low. Cover and simmer over low heat until the meat is cooked through and very tender, 30 to 45 minutes. Add the remaining ¼ cup olive oil, zucchini, olives, and cilantro, stirring to combine. Continue to cook over low heat, uncovered, until the zucchini is tender, about 10 minutes. Serve warm over riced cauliflower or atop a bed of sautéed spinach.

Per Serving: Calories: 358; Fat: 25g; Protein: 25g; Total Carbs: 8g; Fiber: 3g; Net Carbs: 5g; **Macros:** Fat: 63%; Protein: 29%; Carbs: 8%

Chicken Shawarma

SERVES 6 | PREP TIME: 5 minutes (plus 2 to 24 hours of marinating time) | COOK TIME: 30 minutes

1½ pounds boneless, skinless chicken breast

1 pound skinless chicken thighs

5 tablespoons olive oil, divided

2 teaspoons paprika

1 teaspoon allspice

¾ teaspoon ground turmeric

¼ teaspoon garlic powder

¼ teaspoon ground cinnamon

Pinch cayenne pepper

Salt

Freshly ground black pepper

Leafy greens, for serving (optional)

Cooked cauliflower rice, for serving (optional)

Put the chicken breast and thighs in a large resealable plastic bag and add 4 tablespoons of the olive oil, paprika, allspice, turmeric,

garlic powder, cinnamon, cayenne, salt, and pepper, seal, and shake to make sure the chicken is evenly coated. Let marinate in the refrigerator for at least 2 hours or up to 24 hours. The longer you marinate the chicken, the more flavorful it becomes. When there are 15 to 20 minutes of marinating left, preheat the oven to 400°F and line a 9-by-13-inch baking dish with aluminum foil. Remove the chicken from the marinade and place in the baking dish, making sure the pieces don't touch. Bake the chicken, flipping at least once, until no longer pink inside, 15 to 20 minutes. Remove the chicken from the oven and slice into thin strips. Heat the remaining 1 tablespoon of olive oil in a skillet over medium-high heat and add the chicken strips. Cook for 5 to 7 minutes, or until crispy. If desired, serve on a bed of leafy greens, paired with some cauliflower rice.

Per Serving: Calories: 410; Fat: 30g; Protein: 35g; Total Carbs: 0g; Fiber: 0g; Net Carbs: 0g; **Macros:** Fat: 66%; Protein: 34%; Carbs: 0%

Balsamic Chicken with Asparagus and Tomatoes

SERVES 1 | PREP TIME: 5 minutes | COOK TIME: 15 minutes

1 teaspoon balsamic vinegar

2 tablespoons avocado oil, divided

1 teaspoon Dijon mustard

1 garlic clove, minced

Pinch red pepper flakes

2 boneless chicken thighs

4 asparagus spears, woody ends removed

4 cherry tomatoes, halved

In a small bowl, combine the vinegar, 1 tablespoon of oil, the mustard, garlic, and red pepper flakes. Whisk until fully combined, and set aside. In a large skillet over medium heat, add the remaining 1 tablespoon of oil. Thoroughly season the chicken thighs with salt and freshly ground black pepper, and add them to the skillet, searing each side for 3 minutes or until golden. Remove the chicken from the skillet, and set it on a plate. Next, add the asparagus and tomatoes to the same skillet, season with more salt and pepper to taste, and cook for about 5 minutes, until the asparagus is bright green and the tomatoes are slightly wilted. Move the vegetables to one side of the skillet, and return the chicken to the skillet. Pour the balsamic mixture over the chicken and vegetables. Toss everything together, and cook for about 5 minutes more, until the chicken is fully cooked through and the vinaigrette has thickened.

Per Serving: Calories: 650; Fat: 54g; Protein: 33g; Total Carbs: 8g; Fiber: 5g; Net Carbs: 3g; **Macros:** Fat: 75%; Protein: 20%; Carbs: 5%;

Bacon Barbecued Chicken

SERVES 8 | PREP TIME: 15 minutes | COOK TIME: 15 minutes

8 (6-ounce) skinless boneless chicken breasts

½ cup brown erythritol blend

½ cup soy sauce

3 tablespoons olive oil

1 teaspoon garlic powder

½ teaspoon freshly ground black pepper

16 bacon slices

Preheat the grill to medium-high heat. Soak 16 toothpicks in water. Place a chicken breast between two large pieces of plastic wrap and use a rolling pin or mallet to pound to ¼-inch thickness. Repeat with the remaining chicken breasts. In a small bowl, mix the brown sweetener, soy sauce, olive oil, garlic powder, and pepper. Rub or brush half of the mixture onto both sides of the breasts. Roll up a chicken breast and wrap with two slices of bacon, end to end, secured with toothpicks. Brush more of the soy sauce mixture on the bacon, and repeat with the remaining breasts. Place the chicken on the grill, seam-side down, and grill for 6 to 8 minutes on each side, or until cooked through. Remove from grill, let sit for a few minutes, and then serve.

Per Serving: Calories: 487; Fat: 28g; Protein: 54g; Total Carbs: 14g; Fiber: 0g; Net Carbs: 2g; **Macros:** Fat: 52%; Protein: 44%; Carbs: 2%

Bacon-Wrapped Chicken

SERVES 1 | PREP TIME: 5 minutes | COOK TIME: 25 minutes

2 garlic cloves, minced
1 tablespoon avocado oil
2 boneless chicken thighs
4 bacon slices

Preheat the oven to 400°F; line a baking sheet with parchment paper. Mix the garlic and oil in a bowl. Coat the chicken thighs in the garlic mixture, and wrap each thigh in 2 slices of bacon. Place the chicken on the prepared baking sheet, and bake for about 25 minutes, flipping the pieces halfway through, until the bacon is crisp.

Per Serving: Calories: 887; Fat: 71g; Protein: 59g; Total Carbs: 3g; Fiber: 0g; Net Carbs: 3g; **Macros:** Fat: 72%; Protein: 27%; Carbs: 1%

Cilantro Chili Chicken Skewers

SERVES 4 | PREP TIME: 15 minutes | COOK TIME: 10 minutes

1 cup fresh cilantro leaves, chopped
2 tablespoons olive oil
¼ cup red chili paste
2 tablespoons soy sauce
2 garlic cloves, minced
1 teaspoon onion powder
1 teaspoon minced fresh ginger
¼ teaspoon freshly ground black pepper
1 pound boneless chicken thighs, cut into 1-inch cubes
1 onion, roughly chopped
2 red bell peppers, roughly chopped

Preheat the oven to broil. In a large bowl, combine the cilantro, olive oil, red chili paste, soy sauce, garlic, onion powder, ginger, and black pepper. Add the thigh meat. Toss to coat. Refrigerate for 15 minutes to marinate. Skewer the chicken cubes, alternating with the onions and peppers between each piece. Place a foil-lined baking sheet on the lowest oven rack. Lay the chicken skewers directly on the middle rack above the baking sheet, perpendicular to the rack. Cook for 3 minutes. Turn the skewers over and cook for 3 minutes more. Turn the skewers again, and cook for 4 minutes more. When it reaches 165°F, remove from the oven to cool.

Per Serving: Calories: 355; Fat: 25g; Protein: 22g; Total Carbs: 11g; Fiber: 2g; Net Carbs: 9g; **Macros:** Fat: 63%; Protein: 25%; Carbs: 13%

Carne Asada Chicken Bowls

SERVES 4 | PREP TIME: 10 minutes | COOK TIME: 25 minutes

¼ cup extra-virgin olive oil, divided
2 tablespoons low-sodium soy sauce
2 tablespoons lime juice
½ cup minced fresh cilantro
2 garlic cloves, minced
1 teaspoon ground cumin
1 teaspoon smoked paprika
¼ teaspoon cayenne pepper

1 pound boneless, skinless chicken thighs
1 small head cauliflower, riced
1 tablespoon coconut oil
1 avocado, pitted, peeled, and sliced
½ cup sour cream
4 radishes, thinly sliced

Preheat the oven to 350°F. In a small baking dish, mix 3 tablespoons of the olive oil, soy sauce, lime juice, cilantro, garlic, cumin, paprika, and cayenne. Add the chicken to the dish and coat thoroughly in the mixture. Bake for 25 minutes, or until the chicken is cooked through. Use a fork to shred the chicken. Heat the remaining tablespoon of oil in a large skillet over medium-high heat, and stir-fry the cauliflower for 5 minutes, until just heated through. Divide the cauliflower rice among the serving dishes. Place equal portions of the cooked chicken along with some of the pan juices over the rice. Top each serving with a quarter of the avocado slices, sour cream, and radish slices.

Per Serving: Calories: 422; Fat: 31g; Protein: 28g; Total Carbs: 9g; Fiber: 5g; Net Carbs: 4g; **Macros:** Fat: 66%; Protein: 27%; Carbs: 7%

Crispy Chicken Thighs with Radishes and Mushrooms

SERVES 4 | PREP TIME: 5 minutes | COOK TIME: 35 minutes

4 large bone-in, skin-on chicken thighs (6 ounces each)
Salt
Freshly ground black pepper
3 tablespoons olive oil
1 pound radishes, halved
1 (8-ounce) container white mushrooms, sliced
Chopped fresh parsley, for garnish

Preheat the oven to 375°F. Season the chicken with salt and pepper. In a large oven-safe skillet, heat the oil over medium heat. Cooking in batches if needed, place the chicken in the skillet, skin-side down. Cook for 10 minutes, until the skin is golden brown and crispy. Remove the chicken and set aside. Add the radishes and mushrooms to the skillet. Cook, stirring frequently, for 5 minutes. Return the chicken to the skillet, place it in the oven, and roast for 15 minutes, or until it has reached an internal temperature of at least 165°F or the juices run clear from a cut into the thickest part of the thigh. Garnish with the parsley and serve.

Per Serving: Calories: 433; Fat: 34g; Protein: 26g; Total Carbs: 6g; Fiber: 2g; Net Carbs: 4g; **Macros:** Fat: 70%; Protein: 25%; Carbs: 5%

Chicken Tenderloin Packets with Broccoli, Radishes, and Parmesan

SERVES 4 | PREP TIME: 10 minutes | COOK TIME: 20 minutes

2 pounds chicken tenderloins
14 ounces broccoli, cut into florets (about 2 small heads)
8 ounces radishes, halved
¼ cup (2 ounces) unsalted butter
¼ cup grated Parmesan cheese
Salt
Freshly ground black pepper
¼ cup olive oil

Preheat the oven to 400°F. Cut four 12-inch squares of aluminum foil. Divide the chicken, broccoli, and radishes evenly among the foil squares. Add 1 tablespoon each of butter and Parmesan to each packet. Season well with salt and pepper.

Fold up the edges to create a bowl shape. Add 1 tablespoon of oil to each packet and seal the top by pinching the foil together. Place the packets on a baking sheet and bake for 20 minutes, or until the chicken has reached an internal temperature of at least 165°F or the juices run clear.

Per Serving: Calories: 537; Fat: 33g; Protein: 51g; Total Carbs: 9g; Fiber: 4g; Net Carbs: 5g; **Macros:** Fat: 54%; Protein: 39%; Carbs: 7%

Chicken Thigh Chili with Avocado

SERVES 4 | PREP TIME: 15 minutes | COOK TIME: 40 minutes

3 tablespoons olive oil, divided
1 pound boneless, skinless chicken thighs, diced
1 onion, chopped
2 jalapeño peppers, minced
1 tablespoon minced garlic
2 cups diced raw or frozen pumpkin
1 cup low-sodium chicken stock
1 cup canned coconut milk
3 tablespoons no-salt-added tomato paste
3 tablespoons chili powder
Juice of 1 lime
1 avocado, diced

Heat 2 tablespoons of olive oil in a large skillet over medium-high heat. Sauté the chicken until just cooked through, 10 to 12 minutes. Transfer the chicken to a plate using a slotted spoon. Add the remaining olive oil and sauté the onion, jalapeños, and garlic until softened, about 5 minutes. Stir in the cooked chicken, pumpkin, chicken stock, coconut milk, tomato paste, chili powder, and lime juice. Bring the chili to a boil, then reduce the heat to low and simmer until the chicken and vegetables are tender, about 20 minutes. Serve topped with avocado.

Per Serving: Calories: 461; Fat: 36g; Protein: 20g; Total Carbs: 18g; Fiber: 7g; Net Carbs: 11g; **Macros:** Fat: 70%; Protein: 17%; Carbs: 13%

Tomato Basil Chicken Zoodle Bowls

SERVES 4 | PREP TIME: 20 minutes | COOK TIME: 7 to 10 minutes

2 medium zucchini, spiralized
Sea salt
Freshly ground black pepper
¼ cup extra-virgin olive oil, divided
1 pound boneless chicken thighs, cut into 1-inch pieces
½ cup roughly chopped fresh basil
1 pint grape tomatoes, halved
1 garlic clove, minced
8 ounces fresh mozzarella, cut into ½-inch pieces

Place the zucchini noodles into a colander and season very generously with salt. Place the colander into the sink and let the zucchini sweat for 20 minutes. Rinse the zucchini with fresh water and wring as much moisture as you can from the noodles, trying not to break them. Heat a large skillet over high heat. Season the chicken generously with salt and pepper. When the skillet is hot, add 2 tablespoons of the olive oil. Cook the chicken for 5 to 7 minutes, or until browned and cooked through. Transfer to a large serving dish. In the same skillet, sauté the zucchini noodles for 2 to 3 minutes, or until hot but not browned. Transfer the cooked zucchini to the serving dish along with the basil, tomatoes, garlic, and fresh mozzarella. Give everything a good toss, drizzle with the remaining olive oil, and season with salt and pepper.

Per Serving: Calories: 456; Fat: 31g; Protein: 37g; Total Carbs: 6g; Fiber: 1g; Net Carbs: 5g; **Macros:** Fat: 61%; Protein: 32%; Carbs: 7%

Spaghetti Squash Chicken Bowls

SERVES 4 | PREP TIME: 10 minutes | COOK TIME: 30 minutes

1 small spaghetti squash
2 tablespoons canola oil, divided
1½ pounds boneless, skinless chicken thighs, cut into 2-inch pieces
Sea salt
Freshly ground black pepper
1 teaspoon minced ginger
1 teaspoon minced garlic
Pinch red pepper flakes
2 tablespoons toasted sesame oil
¼ cup low-sodium soy sauce
Juice of 1 lime
¼ cup roasted cashews

Preheat the oven to 375°F. Slice the spaghetti squash into 1-inch-thick rings, and scoop out the strings and seeds. Place the squash rings onto a rimmed baking sheet and brush with 1 tablespoon of the canola oil. Roast for 30 minutes, until the squash is tender. While the squash is roasting, heat the remaining tablespoon of oil in a large skillet. Season the chicken with salt and pepper. Sear the chicken in the pan, and cook for 5 to 7 minutes, or until it is well browned and cooked through. Add the ginger, garlic, and red pepper flakes to the pan and cook for 30 seconds. Remove the pan from the heat. When the spaghetti squash rings are cool enough to handle, use a fork to shred the flesh into long, thin strands. Divide the squash among the serving bowls, and top with equal portions of the cooked chicken. In a small measuring cup, whisk the sesame oil, soy sauce, and lime juice. Pour the sauce over the spaghetti squash bowls and top with the roasted cashews.

Per Serving: Calories: 440; Fat: 25g; Protein: 40g; Total Carbs: 13g; Fiber: 2g; Net Carbs: 11g; **Macros:** Fat: 51%; Protein: 36%; Carbs: 13%

Chicken Teriyaki

SERVES 4 | PREP TIME: 5 minutes (plus 1 to 24 hours of marinating time) | COOK TIME: 35 minutes

2 pounds boneless, skin-on chicken breasts and thighs
2 tablespoons olive oil
⅓ cup erythritol
¼ cup tamari
1 teaspoon freshly squeezed lemon juice
½ teaspoon garlic powder
¼ teaspoon ground ginger
⅓ cup water
2 tablespoons psyllium husk powder (optional but recommended)
Cooked cauliflower rice, for serving (optional)

Place the chicken pieces in a large resealable plastic bag and add the olive oil, erythritol, tamari, lemon juice, garlic, ginger, water, and psyllium husk powder (if using), seal, and shake to make sure the chicken is evenly coated. Let marinate in the refrigerator for at least 1 hour or up to 24 hours. The longer you marinate the chicken, the more flavorful it becomes. When there is 15 to 20 minutes of marinating left, preheat the oven to 400°F and line a 9-by-13-inch baking dish with aluminum foil. Remove the chicken from the marinade (discard the marinade) and place in the baking dish, making sure the pieces don't touch. Roast the chicken for about 30 minutes, flipping halfway through, until cooked all the way through—internal temperature of 165°F. Serve with cauliflower rice and/or cucumber salad, if desired.

Per Serving: Calories: 452; Fat: 32g; Protein: 40g; Total Carbs: 1g; Fiber: 0g; Net Carbs: 1g; **Macros:** Fat: 64%; Protein: 35%; Carbs: 1%

Chicken Cordon Bleu

SERVES 4 | PREP TIME: 5 minutes | COOK TIME: 25 minutes

1 tablespoon butter	4 ounces prosciutto or deli
1 pound boneless, skinless	ham, roughly chopped
chicken thighs	4 ounces sliced Swiss cheese
2 teaspoons Dijon mustard	½ cup almond flour
Sea salt	½ cup grated Parmesan
Freshly ground black pepper	cheese

Preheat the oven to 400°F. Coat the interior of an 8-inch-square baking dish with butter. Coat the chicken thighs with the mustard, and season with salt and pepper. Place the chicken into the baking dish. Top the chicken with the prosciutto. Spread the Swiss cheese slices over the prosciutto layer. In a bowl, mix the almond flour, Parmesan cheese, and paprika. Sprinkle this mixture over the cheese and season with salt and pepper. Bake for 25 minutes or until the chicken is cooked through and the top is browned and bubbling.

Per Serving: Calories: 476; Fat: 31g; Protein: 45g; Total Carbs: 5g; Fiber: 2g; Net Carbs: 3g; **Macros:** Fat: 59%; Protein: 37%; Carbs: 4%

Thai Chicken Lettuce Cups

SERVES 4 | PREP TIME: 10 minutes | COOK TIME: 10 minutes

2 tablespoons toasted	Freshly ground black pepper
sesame oil	3 tablespoons low-sodium soy
2 tablespoons canola oil	sauce, divided
1 pound boneless, skinless	Juice of 1 lime
chicken thighs, finely diced	⅓ cup natural peanut butter
8 ounces button mushrooms,	Pinch red pepper flakes
finely diced	8 to 12 butter lettuce leaves
2 teaspoons minced	¼ cup roughly chopped
ginger, divided	roasted peanuts
2 teaspoons minced	¼ cup grated carrot
garlic, divided	1 scallion, white and green
Sea salt	parts thinly sliced

Heat the sesame oil and canola oil in a large skillet over medium-high heat. Add the chicken and mushrooms, and sauté until cooked through and well-browned, about 10 minutes. Add 1 teaspoon each of the ginger and garlic and cook for another 30 seconds. Stir in 1 tablespoon of soy sauce. Remove the pan from the heat. Season with salt and pepper. Meanwhile, combine the remaining 1 teaspoon of ginger, remaining 1 teaspoon of garlic, remaining 2 tablespoons of soy sauce, peanut butter, lime juice, and red pepper flakes in a small jar. Cover tightly with a lid and shake vigorously. Thin with 2 to 3 tablespoons of water until it reaches the desired consistency. To serve, place a spoonful of the chicken mushroom mixture into each lettuce cup. Top with a pinch of peanuts, carrot, and scallion. Serve with the peanut sauce.

Per Serving: Calories: 490; Fat: 34g; Protein: 35g; Total Carbs: 12g; Fiber: 3g; Net Carbs: 9g; **Macros:** Fat: 62%; Protein: 29%; Carbs: 9%

Chicken with Mushrooms, Port, and Cream

SERVES 4 | PREP TIME: 10 minutes | COOK TIME: 20 minutes

2 tablespoons canola oil	1 shallot, minced
8 boneless, skinless	8 ounces mushrooms, sliced
chicken thighs	¼ cup port wine
Sea salt	½ cup heavy (whipping) cream
Freshly ground black pepper	

Heat the canola oil in a large skillet over medium-high heat. Pat the chicken thighs dry with paper towels and season generously with salt and pepper. Sear the chicken thighs on each side until well browned and cooked through to an internal temperature of 165°F, about 8 minutes. Transfer them to a dish. Add the shallot and mushrooms to the pan and cook for 10 minutes, until the mushrooms are browned and most of the moisture has evaporated from the pan. Add the port and cook until reduced to just a couple of tablespoons, about 2 minutes. Stir in the heavy cream and bring to the barest simmer. Return the chicken thighs to the pan, basting with the cream sauce. Season with salt and pepper.

Per Serving: Calories: 389; Fat: 24g; Protein: 30g; Total Carbs: 6g; Fiber: 1g; Net Carbs: 5g; **Macros:** Fat: 61% ; Protein: 33%; Carb: 6%

Chicken Cordon Bleu Casserole

SERVES 6 | PREP TIME: 10 minutes | COOK TIME: 5 hours on low

Nonstick cooking spray	Cheese Sauce using
2¼ pounds boneless, skinless	Swiss cheese
chicken breasts, cubed	2 tablespoons Dijon mustard
8 ounces deli ham, cut into	Freshly ground black pepper
1-inch cubes	½ cup pork rind crumbs

Coat the bowl of a slow cooker with cooking spray. Add the chicken, ham, cheese sauce, and mustard. Season with pepper and mix well. Sprinkle the pork rinds over the top, close the lid, and cook on low for 5 hours, or until the chicken has reached an internal temperature of 165°F.

Per Serving: Calories: 597; Fat: 41g; **Macros:** Fat: 62%; Protein: 36%; Carbs: 2%

Chicken Tikka Masala

SERVES 4 | PREP TIME: 10 minutes | COOK TIME: 20 minutes, plus 10 minutes to come to pressure | RELEASE: Quick:

1 tablespoon olive oil	1 teaspoon ground cumin
1½ pounds boneless, skinless	1 teaspoon paprika
chicken thighs, diced	½ teaspoon ground turmeric
1 cup tomato sauce	Salt
1 tablespoon onion powder	2 tablespoons heavy
2 teaspoons minced garlic	(whipping) cream
2 teaspoons garam masala	

In a large skillet, heat the oil over medium heat. Add the chicken and cook for about 10 minutes, or until the outsides are browned. Use a slotted spoon to transfer the chicken from the skillet into a pressure cooker bowl. Add the tomato sauce, onion powder, garlic, garam masala, cumin, paprika, turmeric, and ½ teaspoon salt. Stir well. Lock the pressure cooker lid in place with the steam vent set to Sealing. Select high pressure and set the timer for 10 minutes. After cooking, quick release the pressure. Open the lid and stir in the heavy cream and season with salt to taste. Serve warm.

Per Serving: Calories: 459; Fat: 35g; Protein: 29g; Total Carbs: 7g; Fiber: 2g; Net Carbs: 5g; **Macros:** Fat: 68%; Protein: 27%; Carbs: 5%

Tandoori Vegetable Chicken Skewers

SERVES 4 | PREP TIME: 10 minutes, plus 15 minutes to marinate | COOK TIME: 15 minutes

½ cup yogurt

2 tablespoons lemon juice

1 tablespoon minced garlic

1 teaspoon ground turmeric

1 teaspoon ground coriander

1 teaspoon ground cumin

1 teaspoon garam masala

¼ teaspoon cayenne pepper

1½ pounds boneless, skinless chicken thighs, cut into 2-inch pieces

2 tablespoons canola oil

1 green bell pepper, seeds and ribs removed, cut into 2-inch pieces

1 yellow bell pepper, seeds and ribs removed, cut into 2-inch pieces

1 red onion

Sea salt

Freshly ground black pepper

2 tablespoons white wine vinegar

¼ cup extra virgin olive oil

4 cups arugula

1 cup grape tomatoes, halved

1 tablespoon sesame seeds

Preheat an outdoor grill or a grill pan to medium-high. In a large glass bowl, whisk the yogurt, lemon juice, garlic, turmeric, coriander, cumin, garam masala, and cayenne pepper. Add the chicken thighs to the yogurt mixture and toss to coat. Allow the chicken to marinate for at least 15 minutes. Slice the onion in half and then slice each half into four pieces, reserving two for the salad. Thread the chicken, green and yellow peppers, and red onion onto bamboo or wooden skewers. Brush the vegetables with the canola oil (some will get onto the chicken, and that's okay). Season generously with salt and pepper. Grill the skewers for about 15 minutes total, turning the skewers as you go so the chicken and vegetables are gently browned on all sides. Meanwhile, whisk the white wine vinegar and olive oil in a large mixing bowl. Slice the remaining red onion into thin pieces and toss with the arugula and tomatoes in the vinaigrette. Divide the salad and grilled chicken skewers among the serving plates, and sprinkle each with an equal portion of the sesame seeds.

Per Serving: Calories: 463; Fat: 30g; Protein: 39g; Total Carbs: 8g; Fiber: 1g; Net Carbs: 7g; **Macros:** Fat: 58%; Protein: 37%; Carbs: 5%

Kung Pao Chicken

SERVES 4 | PREP TIME: 5 minutes | COOK TIME: 15 minutes

½ teaspoon ground Sichuan peppercorns

2 tablespoons low-sodium soy sauce

2 tablespoons Chinese black vinegar or balsamic vinegar

1 tablespoon rice wine or dry sherry

1 teaspoon toasted sesame oil

3 tablespoons canola oil

1½ pounds boneless, skinless chicken thighs, cut into 2-inch pieces

Sea salt

Freshly ground black pepper

1 red bell pepper, seeds and ribs removed, cut into 1-inch pieces

4 scallions, white and pale green parts, thinly sliced

1 teaspoon minced garlic

1 teaspoon minced ginger

¼ teaspoon red pepper flakes

½ cup peanuts

In a small bowl, whisk the Sichuan pepper, soy sauce, vinegar, rice wine or sherry, and sesame oil. Heat the canola oil in a large skillet over medium-high heat. Season the chicken generously with salt and pepper. Sauté the chicken in the hot oil until just cooked through to an internal temperature of 165°F, about 10 minutes. Transfer the chicken to a separate dish. Cook the bell pepper and scallions in the same skillet for 3 minutes, or until crisp-tender. Add the scallions, garlic, ginger, and red pepper flakes to the skillet and cook for 30 seconds, just until fragrant. Return the cooked chicken and any accumulated juices to the pan and add the Sichuan pepper sauce. Cook for 1 minute to allow the flavors to come together. Garnish each portion with a quarter of the peanuts.

Per Serving: Calories: 451; Fat: 27g; Protein: 42g; Total Carbs: 10g; Fiber: 3g; Net Carbs: 7g; **Macros:** Fat: 54%; Protein: 37%; Carbs: 9%

Chicken Piccata

SERVES 4 | PREP TIME: 10 minutes | COOK TIME: 15 minutes

1 pound boneless chicken thighs

¼ teaspoon salt

⅛ teaspoon freshly ground black pepper

¼ cup olive oil

½ cup dry white wine

1 tablespoon freshly squeezed lemon juice

1 garlic clove, minced

1 tablespoon capers, chopped

3 tablespoons chopped fresh parsley

On a flat surface, flatten the chicken thighs with a meat tenderizer until they are ¼ inch thick. Season with the salt and pepper. In a large skillet over medium heat, heat the olive oil for about 1 minute. Place two chicken thighs in the pan. Cook for about 4 minutes per side. Remove to a plate. Repeat, two at a time, with the remaining thighs. Set aside. Using the same skillet, increase the heat to high. Add the white wine, lemon juice, garlic, and capers. Stir the sauce, scraping any browned bits from the bottom of the pan. Bring to a boil. Cook for 1 minute. Add the chicken back into the pan. Heat in the sauce for 1 minute. Add the parsley and stir to incorporate before serving.

Per Serving: Calories: 377; Fat: 30g; Protein: 20g; Total Carbs: 1g; Fiber: 0g; Net Carbs: 1g; **Macros:** Fat: 76%; Protein: 22%; Carbs: 2%

Baked Chicken Tenders

SERVES 4 | PREP TIME: 15 minutes | COOK TIME: 20 minutes

2 large eggs

½ cup pork rinds, ground

½ cup shredded Parmesan cheese

1 teaspoon garlic powder

1 teaspoon onion powder

¼ teaspoon salt

⅛ teaspoon freshly ground black pepper

1 pound boneless chicken thighs, halved

Preheat the oven to 400°F. Line a baking sheet with parchment paper. In a medium bowl, beat the eggs. In another medium bowl, combine the pork rinds, Parmesan cheese, garlic powder, onion powder, salt, and pepper. Create a "breading" station: Line up the egg wash, then the pork rind mixture, then the baking sheet. Take one thigh half and dredge thoroughly in the egg wash, then coat in the pork rind mixture, pressing the "breading" into the meat so it adheres. Place the "breaded" thigh on the baking sheet. Repeat with the remaining thigh halves. Place the baking sheet in the preheated oven. Cook for 18 to 20 minutes, or until golden brown.

Per Serving: Calories: 489; Fat: 33g; Protein: 46g; Total Carbs: 2g; Fiber: 0g; Net Carbs: 2g; **Macros:** Fat: 61%; Protein: 38%; Carbs: 1%

Chicken Nuggets

MAKES 20 | PREP TIME: 15 minutes | COOK TIME: 30 minutes

Nonstick cooking spray	¾ cup finely crushed
1 pound ground chicken	pork rinds
1 large beaten egg	3 tablespoons Parmesan
¼ cup almond flour	cheese
½ teaspoon sea salt	¾ teaspoon dried oregano
¼ teaspoon onion powder	½ teaspoon garlic powder
⅛ teaspoon freshly ground	½ teaspoon paprika
black pepper	

Preheat the oven to 350°F. Line a baking sheet with parchment paper and spray with cooking spray. In a large bowl, mix the chicken, egg, flour, salt, onion powder, and pepper until well combined. In a medium bowl, combine the pork rinds, Parmesan, oregano, garlic powder, and paprika. Scoop the chicken mixture 1 tablespoon at a time and form into your chosen shape. Completely coat in the pork rind mixture and place on the prepared baking sheet. Bake for 15 minutes, flip, and bake for an additional 15 minutes until golden. Serve immediately.

Per Serving: (5 nuggets): Calories: 275; Fat: 17g; Protein: 28g; Total Carbs: 3g; Fiber: 1g; Net Carbs: 2g; **Macros:** Fat: 56%; Protein: 41%; Carbs: 3%

Harissa Chicken and Brussels Sprouts with Yogurt Sauce

SERVES 4 | PREP TIME: 10 minutes | COOK TIME: 1 hour

½ cup extra-virgin olive	1 pound Brussels sprouts,
oil, divided	ends trimmed and halved
2 tablespoons harissa	½ cup plain Greek yogurt
1½ teaspoons salt, divided	1 garlic clove, finely minced
½ teaspoon ground cumin	Zest and juice of 1 lemon
4 skin-on, bone-in chicken	½ cup chopped mint leaves,
thighs (or a combination of	for serving
thighs and drumsticks)	½ cup chopped cilantro
	leaves, for serving

Preheat the oven to 425°F. Line a rimmed baking sheet with aluminum foil. In a small bowl, whisk 6 tablespoons olive oil, the harissa oil, 1 teaspoon salt, and cumin. Place the chicken in a large bowl and drizzle half of the harissa mixture over top. Toss to combine well. Place the chicken in a single layer on the prepared baking sheet and roast for 20 minutes. While the chicken roasts, place the Brussels sprouts in a large bowl and drizzle with the remaining harissa mixture. Toss to combine well. After the chicken has roasted for 20 minutes, remove from the oven and add the Brussels sprouts to the baking sheet in a single layer around the chicken. Return to the oven and continue to roast until the chicken is cooked through and the Brussels sprouts

are golden and crispy, another 20 to 25 minutes. In a small bowl, combine the yogurt, remaining 2 tablespoons olive oil, garlic, lemon zest and juice, and remaining ½ teaspoon salt and whisk to combine. Remove the chicken and veggies from the oven and cool for 10 minutes. Drizzle with yogurt sauce and sprinkle with mint and cilantro. Toss to combine and serve warm.

Per Serving: Calories: 607; Fat: 52g; Protein: 25g; Total Carbs: 13g; Fiber: 5g; Net Carbs: 8g; **Macros:** Fat: 76%; Protein: 16%; Carbs: 8%

Spinach and Bacon Stuffed Chicken Thighs

SERVES 4 | PREP TIME: 15 minutes | COOK TIME: 35 minutes

5 bacon slices	1 pound boneless
2 tablespoons butter	chicken thighs
1½ cups spinach	¼ cup shredded Swiss
1 teaspoon minced garlic	cheese, divided
¾ cup cream cheese, at room	¼ teaspoon salt
temperature	¼ teaspoon freshly ground
	black pepper

Preheat the oven to 425°F. On a baking sheet, place the bacon slices about ½ inch apart. Cook for 10 to 15 minutes, or until crispy. Set aside to cool. In a large skillet over medium-high heat, melt the butter. Add the spinach and garlic. Cook until the spinach wilts, about 2 minutes. Remove the spinach from the skillet. Set aside. Chop the cooled bacon into small pieces. In a large bowl, mix the cream cheese, sautéed spinach, and chopped bacon. On a flat surface, lay out the chicken thighs. Spread the meat open so the thighs lay flat. Place an equal portion of the cream cheese mixture on each piece of chicken. Top each with the Swiss cheese, equally divided. Close the thighs. Secure with toothpicks. Season with the salt and pepper. Place the chicken thighs in a baking dish. Bake for about 18 minutes. With a meat thermometer, check the internal temperature. It should reach 165°F before serving.

Per Serving: Calories: 527; Fat: 44g; Protein: 29g; Total Carbs: 2g; Fiber: 0g; Net Carbs: 2g; **Macros:** Fat: 76%; Protein: 22%; Carbs: 2%

Chicken Piccata with Mushrooms

SERVES 4 | PREP TIME: 25 minutes | COOK TIME: 25 minutes

1 pound thinly sliced	2 cups sliced mushrooms
chicken breasts	½ cup dry white wine or
1½ teaspoons salt, divided	chicken stock
½ teaspoon freshly ground	¼ cup freshly squeezed
black pepper	lemon juice
¼ cup ground flaxseed	¼ cup roughly
2 tablespoons almond flour	chopped capers
½ cup extra-virgin olive	Zucchini Noodles, for serving
oil, divided	¼ cup chopped fresh flat-leaf
¼ cup butter, divided	Italian parsley, for garnish

Season the chicken with 1 teaspoon salt and the pepper. On a plate, combine the ground flaxseed and almond flour and dredge each chicken breast in the mixture. In a large skillet, heat ¼ cup olive oil and 1 tablespoon butter over medium-high heat. Working in batches if necessary, brown the chicken, 3 to 4 minutes per side. Remove from the skillet and keep warm. Add the remaining ¼ cup olive oil and 1 tablespoon butter to the skillet along with mushrooms and sauté over medium heat until just tender, 6 to 8 minutes. Add the white wine, lemon juice, capers, and remaining ½ teaspoon salt to the skillet and bring to a boil, whisking to incorporate any little browned bits that have stuck to the bottom of the skillet. Reduce the heat to low and whisk in the final 2 tablespoons butter. Return the browned chicken to the skillet, cover, and simmer over low heat until the chicken is cooked through and the sauce has thickened, 5 to 6 more minutes. Serve chicken and mushrooms warm over Zucchini Noodles, spooning the mushroom sauce over top and garnishing with chopped parsley.

Per Serving: Calories: 538; Fat: 44g; Protein: 30g; Total Carbs: 8g; Fiber: 3g; Net Carbs: 5g; **Macros:** Fat: 74%; Protein: 22%; Carbs: 4%

Greek Chicken Souvlaki

SERVES 4 | PREP TIME: 10 minutes, plus 1 hour to marinate | COOK TIME: 15 minutes

½ cup extra-virgin olive oil, plus extra for serving	½ teaspoons salt
¼ cup dry white wine (optional; add extra lemon juice instead, if desired)	½ teaspoon freshly ground black pepper
	1 pound boneless, skinless chicken thighs, cut into 1½-inch chunks
6 garlic cloves, finely minced	
Zest and juice of 1 lemon	1 cup tzatziki or Greek yogurt, for serving
1 tablespoon dried oregano	
1 teaspoon dried rosemary	

In a large glass bowl or resealable plastic bag, combine the olive oil, white wine (if using), garlic, lemon zest and juice, oregano, rosemary, salt, and pepper and whisk or shake to combine well. Add the chicken to the marinade and toss to coat. Cover or seal and marinate in the refrigerator for at least 1 hour, or up to 24 hours. In a bowl, submerge wooden skewers in water and soak for at least 30 minutes before using. To cook, heat the grill to medium-high heat. Thread the marinated chicken on the soaked skewers, reserving the marinade. Grill until cooked through, flipping occasionally so that the chicken cooks evenly, 5 to 8 minutes. Remove and keep warm. Bring the reserved marinade to a boil in a small saucepan. Reduce the heat to low and simmer 3 to 5 minutes. Serve chicken skewers drizzled with hot marinade, adding more olive oil if desired, and tzatziki.

Per Serving: Calories: 677; Fat: 61g; Protein: 26g; Total Carbs: 8g; Fiber: 0g; Net Carbs: 8g; **Macros:** Fat: 80%; Protein: 15%; Carbs: 5%

Feta and Olive Stuffed Chicken Thighs

SERVES 4 | PREP TIME: 15 minutes | COOK TIME: 20 minutes

1 cup crumbled feta cheese	1 pound boneless chicken thighs
¼ cup shredded Swiss cheese	
1 teaspoon minced garlic	¼ teaspoon salt
1 tablespoon olive oil	¼ teaspoon freshly ground black pepper
¼ cup olives, chopped	

Preheat the oven to 425°F. In a large bowl, mix the feta cheese, Swiss cheese, garlic, olive oil, and olives. On a flat surface, lay out the chicken thighs. Spread the meat open so the thighs lay flat. Place an equal portion of the feta mixture on each piece of chicken. Close the thighs. Secure with toothpicks. Season with

the salt and pepper. Place the chicken in a baking dish. Put the dish into the preheated oven and bake for about 18 minutes or when the internal temperature reaches 165°F.

Per Serving: Calories: 407; Fat: 31g; Protein: 27g; Total Carbs: 3g; Fiber: 0g; Net Carbs: 3g; **Macros:** Fat: 70%; Protein: 27%; Carbs: 3%

Lemon Butter Chicken

SERVES 4 | PREP TIME: 10 minutes | COOK TIME: 40 minutes

4 bone-in, skin-on chicken thighs	2 teaspoons minced garlic
	½ cup chicken stock
Sea salt	½ cup heavy (whipping) cream
Freshly ground black pepper	Juice of ½ lemon
2 tablespoons butter, divided	

Preheat the oven to 400°F. Lightly season the chicken thighs with salt and pepper. Place a large ovenproof skillet over medium-high heat and add 1 tablespoon of butter. Brown the chicken thighs until golden on both sides, about 6 minutes in total. Remove the thighs to a plate and set aside. Add the remaining 1 tablespoon of butter and sauté the garlic until translucent, about 2 minutes. Whisk in the chicken stock, heavy cream, and lemon juice. Bring the sauce to a boil and then return the chicken to the skillet. Place the skillet in the oven, covered, and braise until the chicken is cooked through, about 30 minutes.

Per Serving: Calories: 294; Fat: 26g; Protein: 12g; Total Carbs: 4g; Fiber: 1g; Net Carbs: 3g; **Macros:** Fat: 78%; Protein: 17%; Carbs: 5%

Lemon Chicken and Asparagus Stir-Fry

SERVES 4 | PREP TIME: 5 minutes | COOK TIME: 25 minutes

2 tablespoons olive oil	¼ cup chicken broth
1½ pounds boneless, skinless chicken breasts, cut into 1-inch cubes	2 tablespoons soy sauce
	Juice of 1 lemon
	Salt
1 pound asparagus, ends trimmed, cut into 2-inch pieces	Freshly ground black pepper

In a large skillet, heat the oil over medium heat. Add the chicken. Cook, stirring frequently, for 10 minutes, or until browned all over. Add the asparagus and cook, stirring frequently, for another 5 minutes. Add the broth and soy sauce and mix well. Cook for 10 minutes, or until the asparagus is tender but still crisp. Stir in the lemon juice and season with salt and pepper.

Per Serving: Calories: 293; Fat: 11g; Protein: 41g; Total Carbs: 6g; Fiber: 3g; Net Carbs: 3g; **Macros:** Fat: 35%; Protein: 59%; Carbs: 6%

Sesame Broiled Chicken Thighs

SERVES 4 | PREP TIME: 5 minutes | COOK TIME: 20 minutes

4 bone-in, skin-on chicken thighs	1 tablespoon sesame oil
	1 teaspoon minced garlic
¼ teaspoon salt	1 teaspoon red wine vinegar
¼ teaspoon freshly ground black pepper	½ teaspoon crushed red pepper flakes
2 tablespoons soy sauce	
2 tablespoons sugar-free maple syrup	

Season the chicken with the salt and pepper. Set aside. In a bowl large enough to hold the chicken, combine the soy sauce, maple syrup, sesame oil, garlic, vinegar, and red pepper flakes. Reserve about one-quarter of the sauce. Add the chicken thighs to the bowl, skin-side up. Submerge in the soy sauce. Refrigerate to marinate for at least 15 minutes. Preheat the oven to broil. Remove the chicken from the refrigerator. Place the thighs skin-side down in the baking dish. Place the dish in the preheated oven, about 6 inches from the broiler. Broil for 5 to 6 minutes with the oven door slightly ajar. Turn the chicken skin-side up. Broil for about 2 minutes more. Turn the chicken again so it is now skin-side down. Move the baking dish to the bottom rack of the oven. Close the oven door and broil for another 6 to 8 minutes. Turn the chicken again to skin-side up. Baste with the reserved sauce. Close the oven door and broil for 2 minutes more. Remove the chicken from the oven. When it reaches 165°F internal temperature.

Per Serving: Calories: 360; Fat: 26g; Protein: 27g; Total Carbs: 2g; Fiber: 0g; Net Carbs: 2g; **Macros:** Fat: 67%; Protein: 31%; Carbs: 2%

Roasted Chicken Thighs and Zucchini with Wine Reduction

SERVES 4 | PREP TIME: 10 minutes | COOK TIME: 30 to 32 minutes

2 tablespoons coconut oil
8 bone-in, skin-on chicken thighs
Sea salt
Freshly ground black pepper
2 medium zucchini, halved lengthwise and cut into 1-inch pieces
1 teaspoon minced fresh thyme
½ cup dry red wine
3 tablespoons cold butter, cut into pieces

Preheat the oven to 400°F. Heat a large ovenproof skillet over medium-high heat. Melt the coconut oil in the skillet. Pat the chicken thighs dry with paper towels. Season generously with salt and pepper. Place the chicken thighs skin-side down in the skillet, and cook for 5 to 7 minutes, until a crispy skin develops. Flip the chicken, and add the zucchini and thyme to the skillet. Transfer the skillet to the oven and bake for 20 minutes, or until the chicken is cooked through to an internal temperature of 165°F. Transfer the chicken and zucchini to individual serving plates. Using potholders, return the skillet to the stove top. Pour the red wine into the skillet and simmer over medium heat until reduced by half, about 5 minutes. Remove the skillet from the heat. Whisk in the cold butter 1 tablespoon at a time. The sauce will become thick and glossy. Drizzle the sauce around the chicken and zucchini.

Per Serving: Calories: 490; Fat: 34g; Protein: 36g; Total Carbs: 5g; Fiber: 1g; Net Carbs: 4g; **Macros:** Fat: 64%; Protein: 32%; Carbs: 4%

Chicken Thighs with Lemon Cream Sauce

SERVES 4 | PREP TIME: 15 minutes | COOK TIME: 20 minutes

1 tablespoon butter
1 tablespoon minced shallots
1 cup sour cream
2 tablespoons freshly squeezed lemon juice
½ teaspoon salt, divided
¼ teaspoon freshly ground black pepper, divided
1 pound bone-in chicken thighs

Preheat the oven to 425°F. In a large skillet over medium-low heat, melt the butter. Add the shallots. Cook for 3 to 4 minutes, or until tender. Decrease the heat to low. Add the sour cream, lemon juice, ¼ teaspoon of salt, and ⅛ teaspoon of pepper. Mix well to combine. Refrigerate until ready to serve. Season the chicken with the remaining ¼ teaspoon of salt and ⅛ teaspoon of pepper. Place the chicken into an 9-inch-square baking dish. Bake for about 18 minutes or it reaches 165°F. Plate the chicken, spooning an equal amount of lemon cream sauce on each thigh.

Per Serving: Calories: 393; Fat: 32g; Protein: 22g; Total Carbs: 3g; Fiber: 0g; Net Carbs: 3g; **Macros:** Fat: 74%; Protein: 23%; Carbs: 3%

Chorizo, Chicken, and Salsa Verde

SERVES 4 | PREP TIME: 20 minutes | COOK TIME: 40 to 43 minutes

2 tablespoons canola oil
1 pound bone-in, skin-on chicken thighs
1 tablespoon good-quality chili powder
Sea salt
Freshly ground black pepper
8 ounces chorizo
1 onion, roughly chopped
1 cup canned plum tomatoes, hand crushed
2 cups chicken bone broth
1 jalapeño pepper
1 cup minced fresh cilantro
¼ cup extra-virgin olive oil
2 tablespoons lime juice
¼ teaspoon sea salt
1 bay leaf

Preheat the oven to 400°F. Heat a large ovenproof skillet over medium-high heat. Heat the canola oil. Pat the chicken pieces dry with paper towels and season with the chili powder, salt, and pepper. Place the chicken skin-side down in the skillet and sear for 7 to 10 minutes, until it gets a nice, brown crust. Flip the chicken and sear for about 3 minutes on the bottom side. Transfer the partially cooked chicken to a dish. Add the chorizo to the skillet and cook until just browned. Transfer it to the dish with the chicken. Add the onion and garlic to the skillet and cook for 10 minutes, until soft. Add the plum tomatoes, chicken broth, and bay leaf. Bring to a simmer. Return the chicken pieces and chorizo to the skillet and transfer to the oven. Bake for 20 minutes, or until the chicken is cooked through to an internal temperature of 165°F. Remove and discard the bay leaf. While the chicken is baking, combine the cilantro, jalapeño, olive oil, lime juice, and salt in a blender. Purée until the mixture is mostly smooth. To serve, scoop a quarter of the tomato and onion mixture into four serving bowls. Top with a piece of chicken and drizzle with the salsa verde.

Per Serving: Calories: 661; Fat: 52g; Protein: 40g; Total Carbs: 8g; Fiber: 2g; Net Carbs: 6g; **Macros:** Fat: 71%; Protein: 24%; Carbs: 5%

Herb-Infused Chicken

SERVES 4 | PREP TIME: 15 minutes | COOK TIME: 35 minutes

3 tablespoons extra-virgin olive oil, divided
4 (7-ounce) bone-in chicken thighs
½ cup green olives
Juice of 2 lemons
1 teaspoon lemon zest
1 teaspoon minced garlic
1 teaspoon chopped fresh tarragon

1 teaspoon chopped fresh thyme	1 teaspoon chopped fresh rosemary

Preheat the oven to 450°F. In a large ovenproof skillet over medium heat, heat 1 tablespoon of olive oil. Sear the chicken thighs for 4 minutes per side. Remove the skillet from the heat, and use a fork to prick the chicken thighs all over. In a small bowl, stir the remaining 2 tablespoons of olive oil with the green olives, lemon juice, lemon zest, garlic, tarragon, thyme, and rosemary. Add the olive oil mixture to the chicken, cover the skillet, and place it in the oven. Braise the chicken thighs until they are cooked through and tender, about 25 minutes, and serve.

Per Serving: Calories: 435; Fat: 36g; Protein: 26g; Total Carbs: 2g; Fiber: 1g; Net Carbs: 1g; **Macros:** Fat: 74%; Protein: 24%; Carbs: 2%

Mustard Shallot Chicken Drumsticks

SERVES 4 | **PREP TIME:** 15 minutes | **COOK TIME:** 20 minutes

1½ pounds chicken drumsticks	¼ cup dry white wine
¼ teaspoon salt	1 teaspoon Worcestershire sauce
¼ teaspoon freshly ground black pepper	½ cup chicken broth
2 tablespoons butter	2 teaspoons tomato paste
3 tablespoons finely chopped shallots	½ cup heavy (whipping) cream
2 fresh thyme sprigs	1 tablespoon Dijon mustard
1 tablespoon balsamic vinegar	2 tablespoons finely chopped fresh parsley

Season the drumsticks with the salt and pepper. Set aside. In a large skillet over medium-high heat, melt the butter. Add the drumsticks, and cook for 6 to 7 minutes, until browned. Turn the drumsticks on their sides. Cook for 2 minutes more. Turn the drumsticks again to the remaining uncooked side. Cook for 3 to 4 minutes more until the chicken reaches 165°F. Transfer the cooked chicken to a serving dish. Keep warm. Add the shallots and thyme to the skillet. Cook for 1 minute, until the shallots are tender. Add the vinegar, white wine, and Worcestershire sauce. Bring the mixture to a boil. Stir in the chicken broth. Return the mixture to a boil. Add the tomato paste. Stir to combine. Cook for 5 to 6 minutes, or until the mixture reduces by half. Once reduced, add the heavy cream. Bring to a boil again. Whisk in the mustard. You will have about 1 cup of sauce. Pour the sauce over the drumsticks. Allow the drumsticks to rest for 2 minutes. Garnish with the chopped parsley, and serve.

Per Serving: Calories: 420; Fat: 21g; Protein: 48g; Total Carbs: 3g; Fiber: 0g; Net Carbs: 3g; **Macros:** Fat: 48%; Protein: 49%; Carbs: 3%

Jamaican Jerk Chicken

SERVES 4 | **PREP TIME:** 10 minutes plus 4 hours to marinate | **COOK TIME:** 1 hour

1 onion, finely chopped	2 teaspoons chopped fresh thyme
½ cup finely chopped scallions	2 teaspoons Splenda, or other sugar substitute
3 tablespoons soy sauce	1 teaspoon liquid smoke
1 tablespoon apple cider vinegar	1 teaspoon salt
1 tablespoon olive oil	1 teaspoon allspice

1 teaspoon cayenne pepper	½ teaspoon nutmeg
1 teaspoon freshly ground black pepper	½ teaspoon cinnamon
	1 whole chicken, quartered

In a medium bowl, mix the onion, scallion, soy sauce, cider vinegar, olive oil, thyme, Splenda, liquid smoke, salt, allspice, cayenne pepper, black pepper, nutmeg, and cinnamon. In a large baking dish, place the chicken pieces skin-side down. Pour the marinade over it. Marinate covered, in the refrigerator, for at least 4 hours. When ready to cook, preheat the oven to 425°F. Cook for 30 minutes. Remove the baking dish from the oven. Turn the chicken skin-side up. Return the pan to the oven. Cook for 20 to 30 minutes more, or until the internal temperature reaches 165°F.

Per Serving: Calories: 557; Fat: 36g; Protein: 43g; Total Carbs: 4g; Fiber: 1g; Net Carbs: 3g; **Macros:** Fat: 63%; Protein: 34%; Carbs: 3%

Herb Roasted Whole Chicken with Jicama

SERVES 4 | **PREP TIME:** 15 minutes | **COOK TIME:** 1¼ hours

1 shallot, minced	1 (5-pound) chicken
2 fresh thyme sprigs, chopped	¼ cup olive oil
2 fresh rosemary sprigs, chopped	1 cup roughly chopped jicama
2 garlic cloves, minced	½ teaspoon salt
2 fresh sage sprigs, chopped	¼ teaspoon freshly ground black pepper
2 tablespoons chopped fresh parsley	

Preheat the oven to 425°F. To a food processor or blender, add the shallot, thyme, rosemary, and garlic. Pulse to chop. Add the sage and parsley. Pulse lightly until mixed. On a flat surface, place the chicken breast-side up. Carefully slide your fingers under the skin of each breast to separate the skin from the meat, creating a pocket. Do not remove the skin from the chicken. Turn the chicken onto its side. Repeat the process of lifting up the skin on the thighs. Stuff an equal amount of the herb mixture under the skin of the breasts and thighs. Place the chicken into a baking dish. Pour the olive oil over the herbed chicken. Massage it into the skin. If any herb mixture is left, spread it over the outside of the chicken. Place the baking dish in the preheated oven. Bake for 15 minutes. Remove the pan from the oven. Arrange the jicama around the chicken, and season with salt and pepper. Return the pan to the oven. Reduce the heat to 375°F. Cook the chicken for 1 hour, or until the internal temperature reaches 165°F. Remove the chicken from the oven. Rest for at least 15 minutes before carving.

Per Serving: Calories: 604; Fat: 49g; Protein: 39g; Total Carbs: 3g; Fiber: 2g; Net Carbs: 1g; **Macros:** Fat: 72%; Protein: 26%; Carbs: 2%

Fried Chicken

SERVES 8 | **PREP TIME:** 15 minutes | **COOK TIME:** 45 minutes

3 cups lard, coconut oil, or avocado oil, for frying	1 teaspoon freshly ground black pepper
8 chicken thighs, bone-in, skin-on (about 3 pounds)	1 teaspoon baking powder
2 teaspoons salt, divided	1 teaspoon baking soda
1½ cups whey protein isolate, unflavored	½ cup buttermilk
1 teaspoon garlic powder	½ cup almond milk
	3 large eggs

Preheat the oven to 325°F, and place a cooling rack on top of a baking sheet. Place a large skillet on the stove, and fill it with the lard or oil. Season the chicken thighs with 1 teaspoon of salt. Put two shallow bowls on the counter beside the stove. In one bowl, combine the whey protein, garlic powder, remaining teaspoon of salt, and pepper, and mix well. In the other bowl, combine the baking powder and baking soda, and mix. Add the buttermilk, almond milk, and eggs. Whisk well with a fork. Over medium heat, heat the oil to 350°F. Dredge one of the thighs in the whey protein mixture, then dredge the thigh in the egg mixture, coating both sides, and then back over to the whey protein mixture until fully coated. Pick up the thigh, and carefully lay in the hot oil. When the edges around the thigh are golden brown, use tongs to turn the thigh over and cook 2 or 3 minutes, until golden brown. Transfer the thigh onto the cooling rack on the baking sheet. One at a time, repeat coating and frying with each thigh, and then place the baking sheet in oven to finish cooking for 15 to 20 minutes. Remove from the oven and serve.

Per Serving: (1 thigh): Calories: 418; Fat: 24g; Protein: 49g; Total Carbs: 2g; Fiber: 0g; Net Carbs: 2g; **Macros:** Fat: 52%; Protein: 46%; Carbs: 2%

Chicken Adobo

SERVES 4 | PREP TIME: 5 minutes | COOK TIME: 33 to 36 minutes

2 tablespoons canola oil
4 bone-in, skin-on chicken leg and thighs
Sea salt
Freshly ground black pepper
6 garlic cloves, smashed
½ cup rice vinegar
⅓ cup low-sodium soy sauce
½ cup chicken bone broth or low-sodium chicken broth
2 bay leaves
1 scallion, white and green parts thinly sliced

Preheat the oven to 400°F. Heat a large ovenproof skillet over medium-high heat. Heat the oil until it shimmers. Pat the chicken pieces dry with paper towels and season generously with salt and pepper. Place the chicken skin-side down into the pan and sear for 7 to 10 minutes, until it gets a nice, brown crust. Flip the chicken. Add the garlic to the pan, and cook for 1 minute. Stir in the rice vinegar, soy sauce, chicken broth, and bay leaves, and bring to a simmer. Transfer the pan to the oven and cook for another 25 minutes until the chicken is cooked through to an internal temperature of 165°F. Garnish with scallions just before serving.

Per Serving: Calories: 392; Fat: 25g; Protein: 36g; Total Carbs: 3g; Fiber: 0g; Net Carbs: 3g; **Macros:** Fat: 58%; Protein: 37%; Carbs: 5%

Southern Oven-Fried Chicken

SERVES 8 | PREP TIME: 20 minutes | CHILL TIME: 4 hours | COOK TIME: 50 minutes

½ cup sour cream
¼ cup unsweetened almond milk
2 teaspoons hot sauce
8 bone-in, skin-on chicken thighs
Avocado oil
1 cup almond flour
1 cup crushed pork rinds
⅓ cup grated Parmesan cheese
1 teaspoon paprika
1 teaspoon kosher salt
½ teaspoon garlic powder
½ teaspoon freshly ground black pepper
¼ teaspoon cayenne pepper
2 eggs, lightly beaten

In a gallon-size, zip-top bag, combine the sour cream, almond milk, and hot sauce. Add the chicken thighs, seal the bag, and shake until the chicken is thoroughly coated. Refrigerate for at least 4 hours, and up to 24 hours. Preheat the oven to 400°F. Line a baking sheet with parchment paper, brush with avocado oil, and set aside. In a shallow dish, stir the almond flour, pork rinds, Parmesan cheese, paprika, salt, garlic powder, black pepper, and cayenne. Place the eggs in another shallow bowl. Remove the chicken from the bag, place it on paper towels, and pat dry. Dip the chicken into the egg and dredge it in the almond flour mixture, coating all sides. Place the coated chicken, skin-side down, on the baking sheet. Bake for 35 minutes. Flip the chicken and bake for 15 minutes more, or until the chicken reaches 165°F on an instant-read thermometer. Serve warm.

Per Serving: Calories: 395; Fat: 31g; Protein: 26g; Total Carbs: 3g; Fiber: 1g; Net Carbs: 2g; **Macros:** Fat: 71%; Protein: 26%; Carbs: 3%

Roasted Herb Chicken

SERVES 6 | PREP TIME: 15 minutes | COOK TIME: 1 hour 30 minutes

½ cup (1 stick) butter, room temperature
2 tablespoons olive oil or avocado oil
3 garlic cloves, minced
1 tablespoon rosemary
1 tablespoon thyme
1 teaspoon garlic salt
1 teaspoon freshly ground black pepper
Juice of ½ lemon
5- to 6-pound whole chicken, room temperature, patted dry, and giblets and neck removed
Chopped parsley, for garnish

Preheat the oven to 425°F, and line a roasting pan with aluminum foil. In a small bowl, mix the butter, oil, garlic, rosemary, thyme, garlic salt, pepper, and lemon juice. Gently loosen the skin on the chicken, and rub the mixture under each area as far as you can reach and all over the outer skin and bottom. Tie the chicken legs together with string. Set a rack in the roasting pan and the chicken, breast-side up, on top of the rack. Roast for 90 minutes, basting every 30 minutes using the juices in the bottom of the pan. If it starts to brown too much toward the end, lay a piece of foil loosely over the top. The chicken should be 165°F internal temperature. Garnish with chopped parsley, and serve.

Per Serving: Calories: 549; Fat: 37g; Protein: 54g; Total Carbs: 0g; Fiber: 0g; Net Carbs: 0g; **Macros:** Fat: 61%; Protein: 39%; Carbs: 0%

Avocado Chicken Burger

SERVES 4 | PREP TIME: 5 minutes | COOK TIME: 15 minutes

1 pound ground chicken
½ cup almond flour
2 garlic cloves, minced
1 teaspoon onion powder
¼ teaspoon salt
⅛ teaspoon freshly ground black pepper
1 avocado, diced
2 tablespoons olive oil
4 low-carb buns or lettuce wraps (optional)

In a large bowl, mix the ground chicken, almond flour, garlic, onion powder, salt, and pepper. Add the avocado, gently incorporating into the meat while forming four patties. Set aside. In a large skillet over medium heat, heat the olive oil for about 1 minute. Add the patties to the skillet. Cook for about 8 minutes per side, or until golden brown and cooked through. Serve on a low-carb bun, in a lettuce wrap (if using), or on its own.

Per Serving: Calories: 413; Fat: 26g; Protein: 34g; Total Carbs: 8g; Fiber: 5g; Net Carbs: 3g; **Macros:** Fat: 58%; Protein: 33%; Carbs: 9%

Lettuce-Wrapped Chicken Burger

1 SERVING | PREP TIME: 5 minutes | COOK TIME: 10 minutes

1 tablespoon avocado oil

6 ounces ground chicken

1 avocado, pitted, peeled, and sliced

4 Bibb lettuce leaves

In a large skillet, heat the oil over medium heat. Form the ground chicken into a patty and season with salt and freshly ground black pepper. Add the chicken patty to the skillet and cook until it is nicely browned on each side and no longer pink in the center, 3 to 5 minutes on each side. Top the patty with the sliced avocado, and wrap it in the lettuce leaves.

Per Serving: Calories: 682; Fat: 54g; Protein: 33g; Total Carbs: 16g; Fiber: 12g; Net Carbs: 4g; **Macros:** Fat: 71%; Protein: 19%; Carbs: 10%

Chicken Bacon Burgers

SERVES 6 | PREP TIME: 10 minutes | COOK TIME: 25 minutes

1 pound ground chicken

8 bacon slices, chopped

¼ cup ground almonds

1 teaspoon chopped fresh basil

¼ teaspoon sea salt

Pinch freshly ground black pepper

2 tablespoons coconut oil

4 large lettuce leaves

1 avocado, peeled, pitted, and sliced

Preheat the oven to 350°F. Line a baking sheet with parchment paper and set aside. In a medium bowl, combine the chicken, bacon, ground almonds, basil, salt, and pepper until well mixed. Form the mixture into 6 equal patties. Place a large skillet over medium-high heat and add the coconut oil. Pan sear the chicken patties until brown on both sides, about 6 minutes in total. Place the browned patties on the baking sheet and bake until completely cooked through, about 15 minutes. Serve on the lettuce leaves, topped with the avocado slices.

Per Serving: Calories: 374; Fat: 33g; Protein: 18g; Total Carbs: 3g; Fiber: 2g; Net Carbs: 1g; **Macros:** Fat: 78%; Protein: 20%; Carbs: 2%

White Chili

SERVES 12 | PREP TIME: 15 minutes | COOK TIME: 6 hours

½ cup butter

2 cups chopped onion

2 cups peeled, cubed turnips

1½ cups diced red bell pepper

½ cup diced orange or yellow bell pepper

1 (3-ounce) can diced green chiles

4 garlic cloves, minced

2 pounds ground chicken

5 cups chicken broth

2 teaspoons chili powder (or to taste)

2 teaspoons cumin

2 teaspoons oregano

1 teaspoon cayenne pepper

1 teaspoon salt

1 teaspoon freshly ground black pepper

16 ounces sour cream

2 cups shredded Cheddar cheese

In a large stockpot over medium-high heat, melt the butter. Add the onion. Sweat for 8 to 10 minutes, stirring occasionally. Add the turnips, red bell pepper, orange bell pepper, green chiles, and garlic. Sauté for 5 to 6 minutes. Add the ground chicken. Stir to break up the meat, browning on all sides for 6 to 8 minutes. Pour in the chicken broth. Stir to combine. Add the chili powder, cumin, oregano, and cayenne pepper. Bring to a boil. Reduce the heat to low. Cook the chili for 6 to 8 hours, until reduced and thickened. Season with the salt and black pepper. Serve with the sour cream and Cheddar cheese.

Per Serving: Calories: 413; Fat: 28g; Protein: 31g; Total Carbs: 8g; Fiber: 2g; Net Carbs: 6g; **Macros:** Fat: 61%; Protein: 30%; Carbs: 9%

Spicy Kung Pao Chicken

SERVES 6 | PREP TIME: 20 minutes, plus 10 minutes to marinate | COOK TIME: 10 minutes

1½ pounds boneless skinless chicken breast, cut into bite-size pieces

6 tablespoons soy sauce

4 teaspoons sesame oil

3 teaspoons sriracha sauce

2 teaspoons granulated erythritol blend

1 teaspoon fish sauce

1 teaspoon apple cider vinegar

½ teaspoon minced fresh ginger

1 medium red pepper, chopped

1 medium zucchini, cut into ½-inch half moons

2 tablespoons olive oil

½ teaspoon xanthan gum

2 ounces (20 to 25) cashews, halved

1 tablespoon sesame seeds, for garnish

2 scallions, chopped, for garnish

Place the chicken in a medium bowl. In a small bowl, whisk the soy sauce, sesame oil, sriracha, sweetener, fish sauce, vinegar, and ginger. Pour 2 tablespoons of the soy sauce mixture over the chicken, stir, cover, and marinate for at least 10 minutes or up to overnight. In a large skillet over medium heat, heat the olive oil. Place the chicken in the skillet, and cook, stirring occasionally, for 3 to 5 minutes, until cooked through. Add the red pepper and zucchini, and stir for another 2 or 3 minutes. Stir in the remainder of the sauce. Add the xanthan gum, and mix well with the sauce; then add the cashews. Stir for 2 to 3 minutes as the sauce thickens, and then remove from heat. Sprinkle with the sesame seeds and scallions, and serve.

Per Serving: Calories: 287; Fat: 15g; Protein: 29g; Total Carbs: 9g; Fiber: 1.5g; Net Carbs: 6g; **Macros:** Fat: 47%; Protein: 40%; Carbs: 13%

Chicken Potstickers

MAKES 12 | PREP TIME: 15 minutes | COOK TIME: 50 minutes

For the potstickers

1 large head cabbage

1 pound ground chicken

2 garlic cloves, minced

1 tablespoon soy sauce

1 teaspoon sesame oil

1 teaspoon sriracha sauce

2 tablespoons olive oil

For the sauce

¼ cup soy sauce	1 teaspoon sesame oil
2 tablespoons peanut butter	1 teaspoon sriracha sauce
1 teaspoon rice wine vinegar	

In a large pot over medium heat, add enough water to fill the pot halfway. When the water begins boiling, place the head of cabbage in the water, core-side down, cover, and cook for 15 minutes. Remove the cabbage, and when cool enough to handle, scoop or cut out the core. Carefully peel off the leaves. Choose 12 of the best leaves, and place on paper towels. Cut ½ inch off the cupped part (part of the leaf close to the core), and use the knife to shave across the rib/vein (without cutting the leaf in half) so it's easier to roll. In a medium bowl, stir the chicken, garlic, soy sauce, 1 teaspoon of sesame oil, and sriracha. Scoop a spoonful of the mixture into the cupped part of one of the leaves. Roll over once, fold in the edges, and continue rolling up. Repeat with the remaining mixture and leaves. Add a couple inches of water to the large pot. Lightly grease a steamer, and set it in the pot of water. When the water is hot, place the rolls in the steamer, cover, and steam over medium-low heat for 25 minutes. Place a plate lined with paper towels by the stove. In a nonstick pan over medium-high heat, heat the olive oil. When the oil is hot, add 2 or 3 rolls and panfry for 2 to 3 minutes, rolling them back and forth occasionally to get a good char on each side, and then transfer to the paper towel–lined plate. Repeat with the remaining rolls. In a small bowl, mix the soy sauce, peanut butter, vinegar, 1 teaspoon of sesame oil, and sriracha. Serve the sauce with the rolls.

Per Serving: (2 potstickers with sauce): Calories: 229; Fat: 10g; Protein: 22g; Total Carbs: 15g; Fiber: 5.5g; Net Carbs: 9.5g; **Macros:** Fat: 39%; Protein: 38%; Carbs: 23%

Chicken Quesadillas

SERVES 4 | PREP TIME: 10 minutes | COOK TIME: 10 minutes

2 tablespoons butter	½ cup grated mozzarella cheese
2 tablespoons cream cheese	
2 low-carb tortillas	2 teaspoons taco seasoning
6 ounces grilled chicken, chopped (or canned or rotisserie)	½ cup sour cream
	½ avocado, peeled, pitted, and chopped
½ cup grated Cheddar cheese	

In a large skillet over medium heat, melt the butter. Spread the cream cheese evenly on one side of the tortillas. Place one tortilla in the skillet, cream cheese–side up. Add the chicken, cheddar, and mozzarella evenly over the tortilla, and season with the taco seasoning. Place the other tortilla on top of the chicken, cream cheese–side down, and cook for 3 to 4 minutes, or until the bottom is golden brown. Carefully flip the tortilla and cook another 3 to 4 minutes, until golden brown. Remove from heat, and allow to cool for a couple of minutes. Slice the quesadilla into 8 wedges, and serve with sour cream and avocado.

Per Serving: (2 wedges): Calories: 384; Fat: 27g; Protein: 21g; Total Carbs: 15g; Fiber: 7g; Net Carbs: 8g; **Macros:** Fat: 63%; Protein: 22%; Carbs: 15%

Smothered Sour Cream Chicken Thighs

SERVES 4 | PREP TIME: 15 minutes | COOK TIME: 45 minutes

4 bone-in, skin-on chicken thighs	8 ounces sliced cremini mushrooms or white button mushrooms
Kosher salt	
Freshly ground black pepper	⅓ cup diced onion
Paprika, for seasoning	¼ cup sherry or white wine
Garlic powder, for seasoning	1 cup chicken stock
	½ cup heavy (whipping) cream
	⅓ cup sour cream

Preheat the oven to 375°F. Season both sides of the chicken thighs with salt, pepper, paprika, and garlic powder. Heat a large ovenproof skillet over medium-high heat. Place the chicken in the skillet, skin-side down. Cook for 5 to 7 minutes and turn the chicken over. Place the skillet in the oven and roast the chicken for 35 to 40 minutes until the internal temperature reaches 165°F on an instant-read thermometer. Remove the chicken from the skillet and set aside. Remove all but 2 to 3 tablespoons of fat from the pan. Add the mushrooms, onion, and ¼ teaspoon of salt to the skillet. Cook for 5 to 7 minutes until the mushrooms and onion are tender and the mushrooms begin to caramelize. Add the sherry and chicken stock. Simmer for 10 minutes, stirring occasionally and scraping up any bits from the bottom of the pan. Stir in the heavy cream and simmer for 2 to 3 minutes more. Stir in the sour cream and return the chicken thighs to the pan to warm.

Per Serving: Calories: 406; Fat: 34g; Protein: 20g; Total Carbs: 5g; Fiber: 1g; Net Carbs: 4g; **Macros:** Fat: 75%; Protein: 20%; Carbs: 5%

Chicken and Cheese Quesadillas

SERVES 4 | PREP TIME: 5 minutes | COOK TIME: 15 minutes

1 tablespoon olive oil	2 jalapeños, seeded and sliced (optional)
2 cups cooked chicken, diced or shredded	
4 (8-inch) low-carb tortillas	4 teaspoons hot sauce (optional)
1 cup shredded Mexican blend cheese	

In a large skillet, heat the oil over medium heat. Spoon ½ cup of chicken onto one side of a tortilla. Top with ¼ cup of cheese. Add some jalapeños and/or hot sauce, if using. Fold the empty side of the tortilla over the full side. Add to the skillet and cook for 2 minutes, pressing down lightly. Flip and cook for another 2 minutes, or until warmed through and the cheese has melted. Place the cooked quesadilla on a plate and cover with aluminum foil to keep warm. Repeat with the remaining tortillas.

Per Serving: Calories: 383; Fat: 23g; Protein: 25g; Total Carbs: 19g; Fiber: 15g; Net Carbs: 4g; **Macros:** Fat: 54%; Protein: 26%; Carbs: 20%

Green-Chile Chicken Enchilada Casserole

SERVES 8 | PREP TIME: 30 minutes | COOK TIME: 45 minutes

3 cups chicken broth	1 cup sour cream
1½ pounds boneless chicken thighs	2 cups shredded Monterey Jack cheese
2 cups chopped fresh roasted green chiles, or canned	½ cup diced onion
	1 tablespoon minced garlic

½ teaspoon salt

½ teaspoon freshly ground black pepper

¼ teaspoon cayenne pepper

1 tablespoon olive oil

1 bunch fresh cilantro, chopped

2 low-carb tortillas cut into ½-inch-wide strips

Preheat the oven to 400°F. To a large pot over high heat, bring the chicken broth to a boil. Reduce the heat to a simmer. Add the chicken thighs. Cook for 12 minutes. Remove the thighs and set aside to cool. Once cooled, shred the chicken into bite-size pieces. Transfer to a large bowl. To the shredded chicken, add the green chiles, sour cream, Monterey Jack cheese, onion, garlic, salt, black pepper, and cayenne pepper. Mix thoroughly to combine. In a medium skillet over medium-high heat, heat the olive oil for 1 minute. Add the tortilla strips and crisp for 2 to 3 minutes. Transfer the chicken mixture to a large baking dish. Apply the cilantro liberally to the top of the chicken mixture, then add the tortilla strips. Place the dish in the preheated oven. Cook for 15 to 20 minutes, or until golden brown. Remove from the oven. Cool the casserole for 5 minutes before serving.

Per Serving: Calories: 413; Fat: 27g; Protein: 33g; Total Carbs: 8g; Fiber: 2g; Net Carbs: 6g; Macros: Fat: 60%; Protein: 32%; Carbs: 8%

Potluck Chicken Spaghetti Squash Casserole

SERVES 8 | PREP TIME: 30 minutes | COOK TIME: 50 minutes

Olive oil

1 spaghetti squash (about 3 pounds) halved lengthwise and seeded

Kosher salt

5 tablespoons butter

1 cup diced celery

½ cup diced onion

1 cup diced green bell pepper

½ cup diced poblano pepper

4 garlic cloves, minced

1 (10-ounce) can diced tomatoes and green chilies (like Ro-Tel), drained

⅓ cup chicken stock

1 cup heavy (whipping) cream

5 ounces cream cheese, at room temperature

1 teaspoon ground cumin

½ teaspoon garlic powder

¼ teaspoon freshly ground black pepper

1½ cups shredded Colby cheese

4 cups shredded cooked chicken

Preheat the oven to 400°F. Line a baking sheet with parchment paper. Coat a 9-by-13-inch baking pan with olive oil. Set aside. Pierce the squash several times with a fork. Microwave the whole squash for 5 to 7 minutes to soften it slightly. Drizzle the cut sides of the squash with olive oil and season lightly with salt. Place the squash, cut-side down, on the baking sheet. Roast for 30 minutes. While the squash roasts, in a large skillet over medium-high heat, melt the butter. Add the celery, onion, green bell pepper, and poblano. Cook for about 7 minutes, or until softened. Throw in garlic and cook for 1 to 2 minutes more. Stir in the tomatoes and green chilies and chicken stock. Cook for about 4 minutes until reduced by half. You should have about 3 tablespoons of liquid left. Add the heavy cream to the veggies and simmer for 3 to 4 minutes until reduced and thickened. Remove from the heat and transfer the veggie mixture to a large bowl. Stir in the cream cheese, cumin, garlic powder, pepper, and season with salt. Stir until combined and the cream cheese is melted. Remove the squash from the oven and carefully flip it

over. It should be tender on top but not completely done all the way through. Using a fork, scrape across the spaghetti squash to create strands. Lower the oven temperature to 350°F. Gently mix the squash into the veggie mixture. Stir in ½ cup of Colby cheese and the chicken. Transfer the mixture to the prepared baking pan. Top with the remaining 1 cup of Colby cheese. Bake for 20 minutes, or until warmed through and the cheese is melted and bubbly.

Per Serving: Calories: 530; Fat: 38g; Protein: 30g; Total Carbs: 17g; Fiber: 3g; Net Carbs: 14g; Macros: Fat: 65%; Protein: 23%; Carbs: 12%

Calabacitas Con Pollo

SERVES 6 | PREP TIME: 15 minutes | COOK TIME: 40 minutes

1½ pounds boneless, skinless chicken thighs

Kosher salt

Freshly ground black pepper

Garlic powder, for seasoning

2 tablespoons avocado oil, olive oil, or ghee

1 green bell pepper, seeded and diced

½ medium onion, diced

3 garlic cloves, finely minced

2½ teaspoons chili powder

1 teaspoon ground cumin

1 (10-ounce) can diced tomatoes and green chilies (like Ro-Tel)

1 (8-ounce) can tomato sauce

1 cup chicken stock or bone broth

4 Mexican squash or calabacitas, halved lengthwise and sliced

1 large yellow squash, halved lengthwise and sliced

Sliced avocado, for garnish

Season the chicken with salt, pepper, and garlic powder. In a large sauté pan or skillet, over medium-high heat, heat the avocado oil. Add the chicken and cook for 2 to 3 minutes per side until golden in color. Remove the chicken and set aside to cool. When cooled, dice into bite-size pieces and set aside. Return the skillet to the heat and add the green bell pepper and onion. Sauté for 3 to 5 minutes, or until the onion is translucent. Add the garlic, chili powder, 1½ teaspoons salt, and cumin. Sauté for 1 minute, stirring constantly. Reduce the heat to medium and add the tomatoes and green chilies, tomato sauce, chicken stock, Mexican squash, yellow squash, and chicken. Stir to combine. Simmer, uncovered, for 20 to 25 minutes, or until the sauce is thickened and the squash is tender. Serve topped with avocado.

Per Serving: Calories: 299; Fat: 15g; Protein: 26g; Total Carbs: 15g; Fiber: 6g; Net Carbs: 9g; Macros: Fat: 45%; Protein: 35%; Carbs: 20%

Cheesy Chicken and Rice Skillet Casserole

SERVES 4 | PREP TIME: 10 minutes | COOK TIME: 20 minutes

2 tablespoons olive oil

1 pound boneless, skinless chicken breasts, diced

4 cups store-bought cauliflower rice

¾ cup chicken or vegetable broth

8 ounces baby spinach

½ cup heavy (whipping) cream

1 cup shredded cheddar cheese

Salt

Freshly ground black pepper

In a large skillet, heat the oil over medium heat. Add the chicken and cook, turning occasionally, for 5 minutes. Add the cauliflower rice and broth. Bring the liquid to a boil, then reduce to a simmer. Add the spinach and cook for about 10 minutes, or until the spinach has wilted and the cauliflower is tender. To finish, stir in the heavy cream and cheddar. Season with salt and pepper to taste. Continue cooking for another 5 minutes, or until the sauce thickens a little, then serve.

Per Serving: Calories: 444; Fat: 31g; Protein: 34g; Total Carbs: 9g; Fiber: 4g; Net Carbs: 5g; Macros: Fat: 62%; Protein: 31%; Carbs: 7%

Jalapeño Popper Chicken Casserole

SERVES 6 | PREP TIME: 10 minutes | COOK TIME: 20 minutes

4 cups diced or shredded cooked chicken (about 1 pound)
1 (8-ounce) package cream cheese, at room temperature
3 large jalapeños (about 6 ounces total), seeded and diced

1 cup shredded Cheddar cheese, divided
¼ cup heavy (whipping) cream
¼ cup chicken broth
1 teaspoon paprika
½ cup pork rind crumbs

Preheat the oven to 375°F. In a large bowl, mix the chicken, cream cheese, jalapeños, ½ cup of cheddar, the heavy cream, broth, and paprika. Spoon the mixture into a 9-by-13-inch baking dish. In a medium bowl, combine the remaining ½ cup of cheddar and the pork rind crumbs. Mix then spread over the chicken mixture. Bake uncovered for 20 minutes, or until bubbling and golden brown on top.

Per Serving: Calories: 386; Fat: 27g; Protein: 32g; Total Carbs: 3g; Fiber: 0g; Net Carbs: 3g; Macros: Fat: 63%; Protein: 35%; Carbs: 2%

Golden Chicken Asiago

SERVES 4 | PREP TIME: 15 minutes | COOK TIME: 15 minutes

2 large eggs
2 tablespoons heavy (whipping) cream
1 cup almond flour, divided
1 cup grated Asiago cheese

4 (4-ounce) boneless, skinless chicken breasts, pounded to a ½-inch thickness
¼ cup extra-virgin olive oil
½ cup mayonnaise
1 tablespoon hot sauce

In a small bowl, whisk the eggs and heavy cream and set aside. Place ½ cup of almond flour in another bowl and set beside the egg mixture. In a third bowl, stir the remaining ½ cup of almond flour and the Asiago cheese. Dredge one piece of chicken in the almond flour, then in the egg mixture, and then the cheese mixture. Repeat with the remaining chicken. Heat the olive oil in a large skillet over medium-high heat and pan-fry the chicken until cooked through and browned on both sides, turning once, about 15 minutes in total. In a small bowl, stir the mayonnaise and hot sauce. Serve the chicken with the sauce.

Per Serving: Calories: 532; Fat: 39g; Protein: 36g; Total Carbs: 8g; Fiber: 2g; Net Carbs: 6g; Macros: Fat: 65%; Protein: 29%; Carbs: 6%

Chicken & Waffles

SERVES 2 | PREP TIME: 15 minutes | COOK TIME: 20 minutes

4 large eggs, divided
3 tablespoons heavy (whipping) cream
¾ cup almond flour

1 tablespoon plus ½ teaspoon kosher salt, divided
1¼ teaspoons freshly ground black pepper, divided

½ teaspoon chili powder
2 (4-ounce) boneless, skinless chicken breasts, pounded ¼-inch thick
Extra-virgin olive oil, for frying

1 cup shredded Cheddar cheese
2 tablespoons sugar-free maple syrup, for serving

Preheat the oven to 350°F. Set up a breading station. In a small bowl, whisk 2 eggs and the heavy cream. In another medium bowl, combine the almond flour, 1 tablespoon of salt, 1 teaspoon of pepper, and the chili powder. Coat the chicken in the flour mixture, then in the egg mixture, and then again in the flour mixture. In a large, deep saucepan, heat 2 inches of oil until it reaches 375°F. Once the oil is hot, fry the chicken until browned and it reaches an internal temperature of 165°F, about 4 to 5 minutes per side. Remove the chicken and place it on a rack set on top of a baking sheet. Preheat the waffle maker according to manufacturer instructions. In a small bowl, mix the remaining 2 eggs, the cheese, the remaining ½ teaspoon of salt, and the remaining ¼ teaspoon of pepper. Pour half of the batter into the waffle maker and cook for 4 to 5 minutes, or until golden brown. Repeat with the remaining batter. Place the chicken on top of the waffles, drizzle with the maple syrup, and serve.

Per Serving: Calories: 785; Fat: 58g; Protein: 57g; Total Carbs: 8g; Fiber: 3g; Net Carbs: 5g; Macros: Fat: 66%; Protein: 30%; Carbs: 4%

Tuscan Chicken

SERVES 6 | PREP TIME: 5 minutes | COOK TIME: 23 minutes

2 tablespoons extra-virgin olive oil
6 (4-ounce) boneless, skinless chicken breasts, thinly sliced
Kosher salt
Freshly ground black pepper
1 cup heavy (whipping) cream
½ cup chicken stock

¼ cup grated Parmesan cheese
1 teaspoon garlic powder
1 teaspoon Italian seasoning
½ cup chopped fresh baby spinach
¼ cup julienned sun-dried tomatoes

In a large skillet, heat the oil over medium-high heat. Season the chicken to taste with salt and pepper. Add it to the skillet and cook for 3 to 5 minutes per side, or until cooked through and no longer pink. Add the heavy cream, chicken stock, Parmesan cheese, garlic powder, and Italian seasoning. Whisk until the mixture starts to thicken, about 10 minutes. Add the spinach and sun-dried tomatoes and let simmer until the spinach starts to wilt, about 3 minutes. Remove from the heat and serve.

Per Serving: Calories: 338; Fat: 23g; Protein: 28g; Total Carbs: 3g; Fiber: 0g; Net Carbs: 3g; Macros: Fat: 61%; Protein: 35%; Carbs: 4%

Chicken Salad–Stuffed Peppers

SERVES 2 | PREP TIME: 10 minutes | COOK TIME: 26 minutes

2 (6-ounce) boneless, skinless chicken breasts
1 teaspoon extra-virgin olive oil
1½ teaspoons kosher salt, plus more for seasoning
½ teaspoon freshly ground black pepper, plus more for seasoning

6 bacon slices
½ cup olive oil mayonnaise
2 teaspoons dried parsley
1 teaspoon garlic powder
1 teaspoon minced onion
2 bell peppers, any color, halved and seeded

Preheat the oven to 400°F. Line a baking sheet with foil. Toss the chicken breasts with the oil and season with salt and pepper. Place the chicken on one half of the baking sheet and bake for 6 minutes. After the chicken has cooked for 6 minutes, lay the bacon in a single layer on the other half of the baking sheet and continue baking for 16 to 20 minutes more, or until the internal temperature of the chicken reaches 165°F. Let the chicken rest for 5 minutes before dicing. Drain the bacon on a paper towel–lined plate, then crumble it. In a medium bowl, mix the chicken, bacon, mayo, parsley, salt, pepper, garlic powder, and minced onion together until combined. Fill each pepper half with the chicken salad and serve.

Per Serving: Calories: 815; Fat: 60g; Protein: 54g; Total Carbs: 14g; Fiber: 2g; Net Carbs: 12g; **Macros:** Fat: 63%; Protein: 26%; Carbs: 11%

California Chicken Bake with Guacamole

SERVES 4 | PREP TIME: 5 minutes | COOK TIME: 25 minutes

For the chicken

4 (4-ounce) chicken breasts	1 tablespoon extra-virgin
1 teaspoon kosher salt	olive oil
½ teaspoon freshly ground	
black pepper	

For the guacamole

4 bacon slices	½ teaspoon chili powder
1 avocado, chopped	½ teaspoon garlic powder
1 large tomato, diced	½ cup shredded
½ onion, diced	Cheddar cheese
1 teaspoon freshly squeezed	
lime juice	

Season the chicken with the salt and pepper. In a large skillet heat the oil over medium-high heat. Add the chicken breasts and cook for 6 to 8 minutes per side, or until the internal temperature reaches 165°F. Preheat the oven to 400°F. Line a large baking sheet with foil. Lay the bacon in a single layer on the baking sheet. Bake until the desired crispiness is reached, about 20 minutes. Drain on a paper towel–lined plate, then crumble. Meanwhile, in a medium bowl, combine the avocado, tomato, onion, lime juice, chili powder, and garlic powder. When the chicken has finished cooking, transfer it to a 9-by-13-inch oven-safe baking dish. Top with the guacamole, cheese, and bacon. Cook until the cheese is melted, about 5 minutes. Remove from the oven and serve.

Per Serving: Calories: 385; Fat: 23g; Protein: 35g; Total Carbs: 10g; Fiber: 5g; Net Carbs: 5g; **Macros:** Fat: 52%; Protein: 38%; Carbs: 10%

Chicken Tamale Pie

SERVES 8 | PREP TIME: 15 minutes | COOK TIME: 35 minutes

For the muffins

Nonstick cooking spray	½ teaspoon garlic powder
1 cup coconut flour	4 large eggs
¼ cup flaxseed meal	¼ cup heavy (whipping) cream
½ teaspoon baking powder	¼ cup buttermilk

For the chicken

1½ pounds shredded chicken

1 (10-ounce) can red enchilada	¼ cup heavy (whipping) cream
sauce (mild, medium, or hot	1 teaspoon taco seasoning
to taste)	1 cup grated Cheddar cheese
4 ounces (½ brick)	2 scallions, green part only
cream cheese	chopped, for garnish
1 (4-ounce) can chopped	
green chiles	

Preheat the oven to 350°F, and grease 8 holes of a standard muffin pan with nonstick cooking spray. In a medium bowl, stir the flour, flaxseed, baking powder, and garlic powder. In a small bowl, whisk the eggs, cream, and buttermilk. Pour the egg mixture into the flour mixture, and stir. Spoon evenly into 8 muffin holes, and bake for 25 to 30 minutes. Leaving the oven on, remove the muffins, chop them up, and spread on the bottom of a medium cast-iron skillet or 1½-quart baking dish. In a large skillet over medium heat, combine the chicken, enchilada sauce, cream cheese, green chiles, cream, and taco seasoning. Cook until heated through. Pour over the muffins, top evenly with the cheddar cheese, and return to the oven for about 5 minutes to melt the cheese. Garnish with the scallions, and serve.

Per Serving: Calories: 423; Fat: 28g; Protein: 29g; Total Carbs: 15g; Fiber: 7.5g; Net Carbs: 7.5g; **Macros:** Fat: 60%; Protein: 30%; Carbs 10%

Mezze Cake

SERVES 2 TO 4 | PREP TIME: 10 minutes |
COOK TIME: 35 minutes

Nonstick cooking spray	½ (14-ounce) can quartered
2 coconut wraps (one of them	artichoke hearts
is optional)	½ cup cauliflower rice
1 small eggplant, thinly sliced	¼ cup black olives, pitted and
lengthwise	coarsely chopped
Salt	2 cooked sugar-free
1 zucchini, thinly sliced	chicken sausages, cut into
lengthwise	bite-size pieces
1 (8-ounce) jar sun-dried	1 tablespoon dried oregano or
tomatoes packed in olive oil	marjoram
(do not discard oil), chopped	½ tablespoon garlic powder
or whole	Freshly ground black pepper

Preheat the oven to 350°F. Coat a baking dish with nonstick spray and place a coconut wrap in the bottom. Sprinkle the eggplant with ½ teaspoon of salt and let sit for 5 minutes. Wipe off the salt and excess water from the eggplant with a clean kitchen towel. Lay the eggplant slices on top of the coconut wrap, then top with the zucchini slices. Add the sun-dried tomatoes and drizzle with the olive oil from the jar. Add the artichoke hearts and cauliflower rice. Scatter the olives and sausage on top, and season with the oregano, garlic powder, salt, and pepper. Place another coconut wrap over the top, if desired, and bake for about 25 minutes, or until the vegetables are a bit wilted. Turn the oven to broil and cook for another 5 minutes, or until the top is crisp. Remove from the oven and let cool before slicing and serving.

Per Serving: Calories: 510; Fat: 38g; Protein: 17g; Total Carbs: 25g; Fiber: 12g; Net Carbs: 13g; **Macros:** Fat: 67%; Protein: 13%; Carbs: 20%

Roast Turkey

SERVES 8 | **PREP TIME:** 15 minutes | **COOK TIME:** 3 hours

10- to 12-pound turkey (with no added ingredients)
1 cup (2 sticks) butter
2 tablespoons chopped thyme
2 tablespoons chopped sage
1 teaspoon salt
1 teaspoon freshly ground black pepper

The night before cooking, remove the packaging and allow the turkey to sit uncovered in the refrigerator overnight to dry out. In the morning, remove the neck, giblets, and liver from the cavity, and discard. Preheat the oven to 350°F, and place a rack in a roasting pan. Melt the butter in the microwave, and mix with the thyme and sage. Rub half the mixture all over the skin of the bird, lifting the skin to rub as much on the underside of the skin as possible. Season all over with the salt and pepper. Place on the roasting rack, breast-side up, cover with aluminum foil, and roast for 2 hours (add 15 minutes per pound for a larger turkey). Remove the foil, increase the oven temperature to 425°F, baste with the remaining butter, and place back in the oven for another hour. Allow to rest for 30 minutes before carving.

Per Serving: Calories: 447; Fat: 21g; Protein: 66g; Total Carbs: 0g; Fiber: 0g; Net Carbs: 0g; **Macros:** Fat: 42%; Protein: 58%; Carbs: 0%

Marinara Turkey Meatballs

SERVES 1 | **PREP TIME:** 5 minutes | **COOK TIME:** 30 minutes

1 large egg
6 ounces ground turkey
¼ cup almond flour
1 tablespoon Italian seasoning
½ cup marinara sauce

Preheat the oven to 425°F; line a baking sheet with parchment paper. In a small bowl, beat the egg. Add the ground turkey, almond flour, and Italian Seasoning to the egg. Mix with your hands until fully combined. Form into three meatballs, and place them on the prepared baking sheet. Bake for 30 minutes. Place the meatballs in a bowl, and top with the marinara sauce.

Per Serving: Calories: 382; Fat: 22g; Protein: 39g; Total Carbs: 7g; Fiber: 3g; Net Carbs: 4g; **Macros:** Fat: 52%; Protein: 41%; Carbs: 7%

Turkey Meatloaf

SERVES 6 | **PREP TIME:** 10 minutes | **COOK TIME:** 35 minutes

1 tablespoon olive oil
½ sweet onion, chopped
1½ pounds ground turkey
⅓ cup heavy (whipping) cream
¼ cup freshly grated Parmesan cheese
1 tablespoon chopped fresh parsley
Pinch sea salt
Pinch freshly ground black pepper

Heat the oven to 450°F. Place a small skillet over medium heat and add the olive oil. Sauté the onion until it is tender, about 4 minutes. Transfer the onion to a large bowl and add the turkey, heavy cream, Parmesan cheese, parsley, salt, and pepper. Stir until the ingredients are combined and hold together. Press the mixture into a 9-by-5-inch loaf pan. Bake until cooked through, about 30 minutes. Let the meatloaf rest for 10 minutes and serve.

Per Serving: Calories: 216; Fat: 19g; Protein: 15g; Total Carbs: 1g; Fiber: 0g; Net Carbs: 1g; **Macros:** Fat: 69%; Protein: 29%; Carbs: 2%

Turkey Meatloaf Muffins

SERVES 2 TO 4 | **PREP TIME:** 10 minutes | **COOK TIME:** 40 minutes

Nonstick cooking spray
1 to 2 tablespoons olive oil
½ cup chopped onions
1 teaspoon garlic powder
¼ cup shredded carrots
½ cup chopped mushrooms
½ cup chopped green bell pepper
1 pound ground turkey (the fattier, the better)
1 large egg
1 teaspoon dried thyme
1 teaspoon dried rosemary
1 teaspoon mustard
Sugar-free ketchup, for spreading

Preheat the oven to 350°F. Coat a muffin tin with nonstick spray. Heat the olive oil in a large skillet over medium-high heat. Add the onions and season with the garlic powder. Add the carrots, mushrooms, and bell pepper and cook for 3 to 5 minutes, or until the onion is translucent. Put the ground turkey in a medium bowl and add the vegetable mixture. Add the egg thyme, rosemary, and mustard. Mix until well combined. Divide the turkey mixture evenly among the muffin cups and bake for about 15 minutes. Remove the muffins from the oven and slather each with 1 teaspoon of ketchup. Bake for another 15 minutes, or until the meat is no longer pink.

Per Serving: Calories: 346; Fat: 26g; Protein: 22g; Total Carbs: 6g; Fiber: 1g; Net Carbs: 5g; **Macros:** Fat: 68%; Protein: 25%; Carbs: 7%

Turkey and Cauliflower Rice–Stuffed Bell Peppers

SERVES 4 | **PREP TIME:** 15 minutes | **COOK TIME:** 35 minutes

2 tablespoons olive oil
1 pound ground turkey
1 tablespoon paprika
2 cups store-bought cauliflower rice
4 red, orange, or yellow bell peppers
1 cup shredded Cheddar cheese
Salt
Freshly ground black pepper

Preheat the oven to 350°F. In a large skillet, heat the oil over medium heat. Add the ground turkey and cook, breaking apart with a wooden spoon, for about 10 minutes, or until browned all over. Add the paprika and cauliflower rice. Continue to cook, stirring occasionally, for another 10 minutes, or until the cauliflower is tender. Meanwhile, slice the tops off the bell peppers, then remove the seeds and ribs. When the filling is cooked, stir in the cheddar and season with salt and black pepper to taste. Carefully spoon the mixture into the bell peppers. Place the stuffed peppers on a baking sheet and bake for 10 to 15 minutes.

Per Serving: Calories: 411; Fat: 26g; Protein: 32g; Total Carbs: 16g; Fiber: 4g; Net Carbs: 12g; **Macros:** Fat: 56%; Protein: 30%; Carbs: 14%

Turkey Rissoles

SERVES 4 | **PREP TIME:** 10 minutes | **COOK TIME:** 25 minutes

1 pound ground turkey
1 scallion, white and green parts, finely chopped
1 teaspoon minced garlic
Pinch sea salt

| Pinch freshly ground | 1 cup ground almonds |
| black pepper | 2 tablespoons olive oil |

Preheat the oven to 350°F. Line a baking sheet with aluminum foil and set aside. In a medium bowl, mix the turkey, scallion, garlic, salt, and pepper until well combined. Shape the turkey mixture into 8 patties and flatten them out. Place the ground almonds in a shallow bowl and dredge the turkey patties in the ground almonds to coat. Place a large skillet over medium heat and add the olive oil. Brown the turkey patties on both sides, about 10 minutes in total. Transfer the patties to the baking sheet and bake them until cooked through, flipping them once, about 15 minutes in total.

Per Serving: Calories: 440; Fat: 34g; Protein: 27g; Total Carbs: 7g; Fiber: 4g; Net Carbs: 3g; **Macros:** Fat: 70%; Protein: 25%; Carbs: 5%

Turkey Burgers

SERVES 4 | PREP TIME: 10 minutes | COOK TIME: 10 minutes

20 ounces ground turkey	2 tablespoons almond flour
1 teaspoon salt	1 large egg, beaten
¾ teaspoon paprika	1 large Hass avocado, cut
¾ teaspoon ground cumin	into cubes
½ teaspoon dried oregano	1 tablespoon avocado oil
¼ teaspoon garlic powder	4 large lettuce leaves
⅛ teaspoon freshly ground	
black pepper	

In a large bowl, combine the turkey, salt, paprika, cumin, oregano, garlic powder, pepper, flour, and egg. Mix until thoroughly combined. Gently fold the avocado chunks into the mixture. Form the mixture into 4 equal patties no more than ½ inch thick. Heat the oil in a skillet over medium-high heat. Cook the burgers for 5 minutes per side, or until they are browned and crisped and the middle of each burger feels firm (not rock solid) to the touch. Serve each burger wrapped inside a large lettuce leaf.

Per Serving: (1 burger): Calories: 522; Fat: 39g; Protein: 39g; Total Carbs: 6g; Fiber: 4g; Net Carbs: 2g; **Macros:** Fat: 67%; Protein: 30%; Carbs: 3%

Avocado Turkey "Toast"

SERVES 1 TO 2 | PREP TIME: 10 minutes | COOK TIME: 20 minutes

1 tablespoon avocado oil	¼ teaspoon salt
8 ounces ground turkey	1 small avocado, halved
½ teaspoon dried thyme	and pitted
½ teaspoon dried rosemary	Freshly squeezed lime juice
½ teaspoon dried sage	(optional)
¼ teaspoon garlic powder	Everything bagel spice, for
½ teaspoon freshly ground	serving (optional)
black pepper	Cherry tomatoes, halved, for
¼ teaspoon paprika	serving (optional)

Preheat the oven to 400°F. Coat a baking sheet with the avocado oil. In a large bowl, combine the ground turkey, thyme, rosemary, sage, garlic powder, pepper, paprika, and salt. Mix everything until well combined. Place the ground turkey mixture onto the baking sheet and press as flat as you can. Bake for 20 minutes, flipping halfway through, until the meat is no longer

pink. Meanwhile, scoop the avocado flesh into a medium bowl, season with salt, pepper, and a squeeze of lime juice (if using), and mash with a fork until smooth. Remove the turkey from the oven and, cut it into toast-like squares. Spread the mashed avocado over the top of the turkey "toast" and, if desired, serve seasoned with "everything bagel" spice and topped with halved cherry tomatoes.

Per Serving: Calories: 466; Fat: 38g; Protein: 22g; Total Carbs: 9g; Fiber: 6g; Net Carbs: 3g; **Macros:** Fat: 73%; Protein: 19%; Carbs: 8%

Turkey Enchilada Skillet

SERVES 4 | PREP TIME: 5 minutes | COOK TIME: 25 minutes

2 tablespoons olive oil	2 teaspoons ground cumin
1½ pounds ground turkey	2 teaspoons dried oregano
2 teaspoons onion powder	1 cup shredded Mexican
2 red bell peppers, seeded	blend cheese
and diced	Chopped fresh cilantro,
2 teaspoons paprika	for garnish

In a large skillet, heat the oil over medium heat. Add the ground turkey and onion powder. Cook, breaking the turkey apart with a wooden spoon, for about 10 minutes, until browned all over. Add the bell peppers, paprika, cumin, and oregano. Continue to cook, stirring occasionally, for about 10 minutes, or until the bell peppers have softened. Sprinkle the cheese on top of the meat mixture and continue cooking until melted. Remove from the heat and top with the cilantro before serving.

Per Serving: Calories: 443; Fat: 28g; Protein: 41g; Total Carbs: 6g; Fiber: 2g; Net Carbs: 4g; **Macros:** Fat: 57%; Protein: 37%; Carbs: 6%

Turkey Thyme Burgers

SERVES 4 | PREP TIME: 20 minutes | COOK TIME: 25 minutes

1 pound ground turkey	1 teaspoon chopped
½ cup ground pumpkin seeds	fresh thyme
½ cup shredded unsweet-	¼ teaspoon freshly ground
ened coconut	black pepper
1 celery stalk, minced	¼ teaspoon sea salt
1 scallion, white and green	¼ cup coconut oil
parts, finely chopped	4 lettuce leaves
1 teaspoon minced garlic	2 tablespoons mayonnaise

Preheat the oven to 350°F. In a large bowl, combine the turkey, pumpkin seeds, coconut, celery, scallion, garlic, thyme, pepper, and salt until uniformly mixed. Form the turkey mixture into 4 patties and flatten them out, so they are about ¾-inch thick. Heat the oil in a large ovenproof skillet over medium-high heat. Brown the turkey burgers, turning once, about 4 minutes per side. Transfer the skillet to the oven and finish cooking until the turkey is cooked through, 15 to 17 minutes. Serve the burgers on lettuce leaves topped with mayo.

Per Serving: Calories: 474; Fat: 39g; Protein: 28g; Total Carbs: 7g; Fiber: 3g; Net Carbs: 4g; **Macros:** Fat: 74%; Protein: 24%; Carbs: 2%

Turkey Egg Roll in a Bowl

SERVES 4 | PREP TIME: 10 minutes | COOK TIME: 20 minutes

| 2 tablespoons sesame oil, plus | 1 (8-ounce) package mush- |
| more for drizzling | rooms, sliced |

1 tablespoon minced garlic	4 scallions, green and white
1 tablespoon minced	parts, finely chopped
fresh ginger	3 tablespoons soy sauce
1 pound ground turkey	1 tablespoon rice vinegar or
1 (14-ounce) bag coleslaw mix	cider vinegar

In a Dutch oven, warm the sesame oil over medium heat. Add the mushrooms, garlic, and ginger and cook, stirring frequently, for 5 minutes. Add the ground turkey and cook, breaking apart with a wooden spoon, for about 10 minutes, or until browned all over. Add the coleslaw, scallions, soy sauce, and vinegar. Stir well to combine and cook for another 5 minutes, or until the cabbage starts to wilt slightly. Scoop into individual serving bowls. Drizzle with additional sesame oil, if desired.

Per Serving: Calories: 282; Fat: 16g; Protein: 27g; Total Carbs: 10g; Fiber: 4g; Net Carbs: 6g; Macros: Fat: 51%; Protein: 36%; Carbs: 13%

Turkey Pilaf

SERVES 4 | PREP TIME: 15 minutes | COOK TIME: 30 minutes

¼ cup coconut oil	¼ cup chopped fresh parsley
¾ pound ground turkey	2 tablespoons butter
½ onion, chopped	1 teaspoon chopped
1 red bell pepper, diced	fresh thyme
1 zucchini, diced	Sea salt
2 teaspoons minced garlic	Freshly ground black pepper
4 cups finely chopped	1 cup shredded
cauliflower	Cheddar cheese

Heat the oil in a large ovenproof skillet over medium-high heat. Sauté the ground turkey until cooked through, 12 to 15 minutes. Transfer the meat to a plate using a slotted spoon. Sauté the onion, bell pepper, zucchini, and garlic until softened, about 6 minutes. Stir in the cauliflower, parsley, and cooked turkey and sauté until the cauliflower is tender, about 10 minutes. Preheat the oven to broil. Stir the butter and thyme into the skillet and season everything with salt and pepper. Top the pilaf with the cheese and place the skillet under the broiler until the cheese is melted and bubbly, about 2 minutes.

Per Serving: Calories: 448; Fat: 35g; Protein: 26g; Total Carbs: 11g; Fiber: 4g; Net Carbs: 7g; Macros: Fat: 70%; Protein: 23%; Carbs: 7%

Turkey Florentine Bake

SERVES 4 | PREP TIME: 5 minutes | COOK TIME: 35 minutes

1 tablespoon olive oil	1 cup shredded Cheddar
1 pound ground turkey	cheese, divided
4 ounces cream cheese	Salt
6 ounces baby spinach	Freshly ground black pepper
1 large egg, beaten	

Preheat the oven to 375°F. In a Dutch oven, heat the oil over medium heat. Add the ground turkey and cook, breaking apart with a wooden spoon, for about 10 minutes, or until fully browned. Drain off any excess liquid. Add the cream cheese and spinach and continue to cook, stirring frequently, until the cream cheese has melted and the spinach has wilted. Stir in the egg and ½ cup of cheddar. Season with salt and pepper

and stir well. Sprinkle the remaining ½ cup of cheddar over the turkey. Transfer to the oven and bake for 20 minutes.

Per Serving: Calories: 437; Fat: 33g; Protein: 33g; Total Carbs: 3g; Fiber: 1g; Net Carbs: 2g; Macros: Fat: 67%; Protein: 31%; Carbs: 2%

Turkey Bacon Ranch Casserole

SERVES 6 | PREP TIME: 15 minutes | COOK TIME: 25 minutes

1 tablespoon butter	10 ounces frozen
1 pound ground turkey	spinach, thawed and thor-
¾ teaspoon sea salt	oughly drained
¼ teaspoon freshly ground	1 garlic clove, minced
black pepper	½ cup ranch dressing
4 bacon slices, cooked	½ cup shredded mozzarella
and chopped	cheese, divided
	½ cup shredded cheddar
	cheese, divided

Preheat the oven to 375°F. In a large skillet over medium heat, melt the butter. Add the turkey and season with the salt and pepper. Cook, breaking up the turkey with a spoon, until it is browned. Set aside. In a large bowl, combine the turkey, bacon, spinach, garlic, ranch dressing, ¼ cup of mozzarella, and ¼ cup of cheddar. Pour into an 8-inch-square casserole dish. Top the mixture with the remaining cheeses and bake for 15 to 18 minutes, until the cheese is bubbling and slightly browned.

Per Serving: Calories: 400; Fat: 32g; Protein: 27g; Total Carbs: 3g; Fiber: 1g; Net Carbs: 2g; Macros: Fat: 72%; Protein: 27%; Carbs: 1%

Turkey Tetrazzini

SERVES 4 | PREP TIME: 25 minutes | COOK TIME: 30 minutes

1 tablespoon avocado oil	½ teaspoon dried parsley
¼ cup diced white onion	¼ teaspoon freshly ground
1 cup sliced mushrooms	black pepper
1 garlic clove, minced	¾ cup heavy (whipping) cream
2 cups chopped	¼ teaspoon cream of tartar
cooked turkey	1 cup spiralized zucchini
1 teaspoon sea salt	½ cup shredded mozza-
½ teaspoon dried basil	rella cheese

Preheat the oven to 400°F. Heat the oil in a large oven-safe skillet over medium heat. Add the onion and mushrooms and cook until the onions are translucent and the mushrooms begin to brown, 5 to 6 minutes. Stir in the garlic and cook for 1 more minute. Add the turkey and season everything with the salt, basil, parsley, and pepper. Reduce the heat to medium-low and slowly stir in the cream. Bring to a boil and then reduce the heat to a simmer for 2 minutes. Remove from the heat and whisk in the cream of tartar until thoroughly combined. Return the skillet to low heat. Squeeze any remaining water from the zoodles and stir into the turkey mixture until completely combined. Spread the mozzarella cheese evenly on top. Bake for 15 to 20 minutes, until the cheese browns and bubbles.

Per Serving: (1 heaping cup): Calories: 326; Fat: 25g; Protein: 21g; Total Carbs: 6g; Fiber: 1g; Net Carbs: 5g; Macros: Fat: 69%; Protein: 26%; Carbs: 5%

Unstuffed Bell Pepper Skillet

SERVES 6 | PREP TIME: 20 minutes | COOK TIME: 20 minutes

2 tablespoons butter or
  avocado oil
1¼ pounds 85% lean
  ground turkey
1½ cups diced green
  bell pepper
½ cup diced onion
2 teaspoons kosher
  salt, divided
1 teaspoon freshly ground
  black pepper, divided
1 teaspoon garlic
  powder, divided

1 (14-ounce) can diced
  tomatoes
⅓ cup heavy (whipping) cream
2 tablespoons tomato paste
1½ tablespoons Worcester-
  shire sauce
1 (10- or 12-ounce) package
  frozen cauliflower rice,
  cooked according to the
  package directions
1 cup shredded Colby or
  Cheddar cheese, divided
¼ cup grated Parme-
  san cheese

Preheat the oven to 400°F. In a large ovenproof skillet over medium-high heat, melt the butter. Add the ground turkey, green bell pepper, onion, 1 teaspoon of salt, ½ teaspoon of pepper, and ½ teaspoon of garlic powder. Cook for about 8 minutes until the turkey is brown and the vegetables are tender. Stir in the tomatoes, heavy cream, tomato paste, Worcestershire sauce, and remaining 1 teaspoon of salt, ½ teaspoon of pepper, and ½ teaspoon of garlic powder. Cook for 1 to 2 minutes. Stir in the cauliflower rice, ½ cup of Colby cheese, and the Parmesan cheese until fully incorporated. Top with the remaining ½ cup of Colby cheese and place the skillet in the oven. Bake for 7 to 10 minutes, or until bubbly and the cheese is melted.

Per Serving: Calories: 387; Fat: 27g; Protein: 26g; Total Carbs: 10g; Fiber: 3g; Net Carbs: 7g; **Macros:** Fat: 63%; Protein: 26%; Carbs: 11%

Weeknight Texas Turkey Chili

SERVES 4 | PREP TIME: 15 minutes | COOK TIME: 40 minutes

1 tablespoon avocado oil
1¼ pounds 85% lean
  ground turkey
½ cup chopped onion
½ cup chopped green
  bell pepper
2 garlic cloves, minced
1 teaspoon kosher salt
1½ tablespoons chili powder
2 teaspoons paprika
1 teaspoon garlic powder

½ teaspoon dried Mexi-
  can oregano
½ teaspoon ground cumin
1 (14-ounce) can diced
  tomatoes
1½ cups water or
  chicken stock
1 tablespoon tomato paste
Shredded cheese, for garnish
Sour cream, for garnish
Diced avocado, for garnish
Sliced scallion, for garnish

In a Dutch oven over medium-high heat, heat the avocado oil. Add the ground turkey, onion, green bell pepper, garlic, and salt. Cook for about 8 minutes until the turkey is brown and cooked through, crumbling it while cooking. Stir in the chili powder, paprika, garlic powder, oregano, and cumin. Cook for 1 minute. Stir in the tomatoes, water, and tomato paste. Simmer, uncovered, for 30 minutes. Serve topped with shredded cheese, sour cream, avocado, and scallion.

Per Serving: Calories: 540; Fat: 40g; Protein: 32g; Total Carbs: 13g; Fiber: 6g; Net Carbs: 7g; **Macros:** Fat: 67%; Protein: 24%; Carbs: 9%

Bacon-Wrapped Cajun Turkey Tenderloins with Roasted Brussels Sprouts

SERVES 6 | PREP TIME: 20 minutes |
CHILL TIME: 4 hours | COOK TIME: 45 minutes

2 turkey tenderloins (about
  1¼ pounds total), large ten-
  dons removed, if needed
3 teaspoons Cajun seasoning,
  plus more as needed
2 teaspoons garlic
  powder, divided
2 teaspoons kosher
  salt, divided

8 bacon slices
1½ pounds Brussels
  sprouts, washed, trimmed,
  and halved
3 tablespoons bacon drip-
  pings or avocado oil
½ teaspoon freshly ground
  black pepper

Season the turkey tenderloins on both sides with the Cajun seasoning, 1 teaspoon of garlic powder, and 1 teaspoon of salt. Place them in a zip-top bag and refrigerate for at least 4 hours. Preheat the oven to 400°F. Line a baking sheet with parchment paper. Set aside. Wrap each tenderloin with 4 bacon strips and secure with toothpicks, if needed. Place the wrapped tenderloins on the baking sheet and sprinkle with additional Cajun seasoning, if desired. In a medium bowl, toss the Brussels sprouts, bacon drippings, the remaining 1 teaspoon each of salt and garlic powder, and the pepper. Place the Brussels sprouts on the baking sheet around the turkey. Bake for about 40 minutes, or until the internal temperature of the turkey reaches 160°F. Broil for 2 to 3 minutes to crisp the bacon, if needed. Let rest for 10 minutes before slicing.

Per Serving: Calories: 355; Fat: 19g; Protein: 35g; Total Carbs: 11g; Fiber: 4g; Net Carbs: 7g; **Macros:** Fat: 48%; Protein: 39%; Carbs: 13%

MEAT

Breaded Pork Chops

SERVES 2 | PREP TIME: 5 minutes | COOK TIME: 20 minutes

2 (8-ounce) boneless pork
  loin chops
¼ cup pork panko crumbs
  (fried pork rinds, crushed)
1 teaspoon extra-virgin
  olive oil
1 teaspoon grated
  Parmesan cheese
¼ teaspoon pink Himalayan
  sea salt

¼ teaspoon onion powder
¼ teaspoon paprika
¼ teaspoon garlic powder
⅛ teaspoon freshly ground
  black pepper
⅛ teaspoon dried parsley
⅛ teaspoon dried basil
⅛ teaspoon dried oregano
Pinch of cayenne pepper

Preheat the oven to 425°F. Place a baking rack on a small baking sheet. Pat the chops dry with a paper towel. In a food processor, combine the pork crumbs, olive oil, Parmesan, salt, onion powder, paprika, garlic powder, pepper, parsley, basil, oregano, and cayenne and run on high until the mixture forms a uniform, fine powder. Transfer the mixture to a resealable 1-gallon plastic bag. Add the chops to the bag, one at a time, shaking to coat them in the breading. Transfer the chops to the rack and bake for 20 minutes, until an instant-read thermometer registers 160°F or the juices run clear when the meat is pierced.

Per Serving: Calories: 435; Fat: 23g; Protein: 57g; Total Carbs: 0g; Fiber: 0g; Net Carbs: 0g; **Macros:** Fat: 48%; Protein: 52%; Carbs: 0%

Smothered Pork Chops with Onion Gravy

SERVES 4 | PREP TIME: 15 minutes | COOK TIME: 30 minutes

- 1 teaspoon kosher salt
- ½ teaspoon freshly ground black pepper
- ½ teaspoon garlic powder
- ½ teaspoon paprika
- 4 (8-ounce) center cut, ½-inch thick, bone-in pork chops, patted dry
- 3 tablespoons butter or ghee
- 1 onion, sliced
- ¾ cup chicken stock, beef stock, or bone broth
- 2 tablespoons sherry or dry white wine
- 1 garlic clove, finely minced
- 1 teaspoon Dijon mustard
- ¼ teaspoon dried thyme
- ¾ cup heavy (whipping) cream
- Chopped fresh parsley, for garnish

In a small bowl, stir the salt, pepper, garlic powder, and paprika. Season the pork chops on both sides with the spices. In a large cast-iron skillet, over medium-high heat, melt the butter. Add the pork chops and sear for 2 to 3 minutes per side, or until browned. Remove the browned pork chops from the skillet and set aside. Turn the heat to medium-low and add the onion to the skillet. Cook for about 5 minutes, or until the onion begins to turn translucent. Stir in the chicken stock, sherry, garlic, mustard, and thyme. Cook for 3 to 5 minutes more, until the onion is soft and the liquid is reduced. Add the heavy cream and return the pork chops to the skillet. Simmer for 10 to 15 minutes, or until the pork chops are cooked through—at least 145°F. Remove from the heat. Carefully transfer the pan juices/cream mixture and the onions from the skillet into a blender. Blend until smooth. Pour the gravy over the pork chops and garnish with parsley.

Per Serving: Calories: 675; Fat: 51g; Protein: 49g; Total Carbs: 5g; Fiber: 1g; Net Carbs: 4g; **Macros:** Fat: 68%; Protein: 29%; Carbs: 3%

Pork Chops Smothered in Caramelized Onions & Leeks

SERVES 2 | PREP TIME: 5 to 10 minutes | COOK TIME: 20 minutes

- 2 bone-in free-range pork chops
- 1 teaspoon salt
- 1 teaspoon freshly ground black pepper
- 2 tablespoons avocado oil, divided
- 1 tablespoon butter or butter-flavored coconut oil
- 1 red onion, thinly sliced
- 1 leek, white and light green parts thinly sliced

Season the pork chops with the salt and pepper. Heat 1 tablespoon of avocado oil in a large skillet over medium-high heat. Add the butter and pork chops and cook until golden brown, about 3 minutes, flip, and cook on the other side for 3 to 5 minutes, until cooked through and golden brown. In medium skillet, heat the remaining avocado oil over medium-high heat. Add the onion and leek and cook until translucent, 5 to 8 minutes. Transfer the pork chops to plates and top with the sautéed onion and leek.

Per Serving: Calories: 480; Fat: 32g; Protein: 36g; Total Carbs: 12g; Fiber: 3g; Net Carbs: 9g; **Macros:** Fat: 60%; Protein: 30%; Carbs: 10%

Breaded Pork Chops with Creamy Mashed Cauliflower

SERVES 4 | PREP TIME: 5 minutes | COOK TIME: 20 minutes

- ½ cup pork rind crumbs
- ½ cup grated Parmesan cheese
- 4 (5-ounce) bone-in pork chops
- 1 tablespoon olive oil
- 1¼ pounds fresh or frozen cauliflower florets
- 2 ounces cream cheese
- Salt
- Freshly ground black pepper
- 2 tablespoons chopped fresh parsley, for garnish

Preheat the oven to 400°F. Line a large baking sheet with a silicone baking mat or aluminum foil. On a large plate, mix the pork rind crumbs and Parmesan. Brush each pork chop on both sides with oil, then press them into the mixture to coat. Place the pork chops on the prepared baking sheet and bake, flipping halfway through, for 18 to 20 minutes. Meanwhile, place the cauliflower in a large saucepan and cover with water. Cook over medium-high heat for 10 minutes, or until soft. Drain the cooked cauliflower and transfer to a bowl. Add the cream cheese and mash. Season with salt and pepper to taste. Spoon the mashed cauliflower onto serving plates and add the pork chops. Serve garnished with the parsley.

Per Serving: Calories: 406; Fat: 26g; Protein: 39g; Total Carbs: 9g; Fiber: 3g; Net Carbs: 6g; **Macros:** Fat: 62%; Protein: 32%; Carbs: 6%

Spiced Pork Chops

SERVES 4 | PREP TIME: 10 minutes | COOK TIME: 10 minutes

- 4 center-cut, bone-in, ¾-inch-thick pork chops
- ½ teaspoon brown sugar substitute
- ½ teaspoon ground cinnamon
- ¼ teaspoon salt
- ⅛ teaspoon freshly ground black pepper
- ⅛ teaspoon ground nutmeg
- ⅛ teaspoon ground ginger
- 2 tablespoons coconut oil

Pat the pork chops dry. In a small bowl, combine the brown sugar substitute, cinnamon, salt, pepper, nutmeg, and ginger. Rub both sides of each pork chop with the spice mixture. In a large skillet over medium-high heat, melt the coconut oil. Place the chops in the skillet and cook for 4 to 5 minutes per side, until golden and cooked through.

Per Serving: (1 chop): Calories: 252; Fat: 17g; Protein: 23g; Total Carbs: <1g; Fiber: <1g; Net Carbs: <1g; **Macros:** Fat: 61%; Protein: 38%; Carbs: <1%

Cracked Pepper Fried Pork Chops

SERVES 4 | PREP TIME: 5 minutes | COOK TIME: 10 minutes

- 1 cup coconut oil
- 2 (1¾ ounces) bags pork rinds (crushed)
- 2 tablespoons coconut flour
- ½ teaspoon cracked black pepper
- ½ teaspoon cayenne pepper
- ¼ teaspoon paprika
- ¼ teaspoon garlic powder
- Pinch of salt
- 1 large egg
- 1 tablespoon coconut milk

4 pork chops, patted dry and
  seasoned with salt and
  cracked black pepper
1 tablespoon horseradish
2 tablespoons sugar-free
  barbecue sauce
2 tablespoons avocado-oil
  mayonnaise
2 teaspoons chopped fresh
  parsley (optional)

In a large skillet, heat the coconut oil over medium heat. In a shallow dish, combine the pork rinds, coconut flour, pepper, cayenne, paprika, garlic powder, and salt. In another shallow dish, whisk the egg and coconut milk. Dip the pork into the egg mixture, then into the pork rind mixture, firmly pressing the crumbs onto all sides. Place the breaded pork chops in the skillet and fry for 3 to 4 minutes on each side or until they are golden brown. Transfer the cooked pork chops to a wire rack to cool slightly. In a small bowl, prepare the sauce by mixing the horseradish and barbeque sauce. Top the fried pork chops with the sauce and garnish with the parsley.

Per Serving: Calories: 469; Fat: 35g; Protein: 33g; Total Carbs: 6g; Fiber: 3g; Net Carbs: 3g; Macros: Fat: 68%; Protein: 27%; Carbs: 5%

Pan-Fried Pork Chops with Peppers and Onions

SERVES 4 | PREP TIME: 5 minutes | COOK TIME: 25 minutes

4 (4-ounce) pork chops,
  untrimmed
1½ teaspoons salt, divided
1 teaspoon freshly ground
  black pepper, divided
½ cup extra-virgin olive
  oil, divided
1 red or orange bell pepper,
  thinly sliced
1 green bell pepper, thinly sliced
1 small yellow onion,
  thinly sliced
2 teaspoons dried Italian
  herbs (such as oregano,
  parsley, or rosemary)
2 garlic cloves, minced
1 tablespoon balsamic vinegar

Season the pork chops with 1 teaspoon salt and ½ teaspoon pepper. In a large skillet, heat ¼ cup olive oil over medium-high heat. Fry the pork chops in the oil until browned and almost cooked through but not fully cooked, 4 to 5 minutes per side, depending on the thickness of chops. Remove from the skillet and cover to keep warm. Pour the remaining ¼ cup olive oil in the skillet and sauté the peppers, onions, and herbs over medium-high heat until tender, 6 to 8 minutes. Add the garlic, stirring to combine, and return the pork to the skillet. Cover, reduce the heat to low, and cook for another 2 to 3 minutes, or until the pork is cooked through. Transfer the pork, peppers, and onions to a serving platter. Add the vinegar to the oil in the skillet and whisk to combine well. Drizzle the vinaigrette over the pork and serve warm.

Per Serving: Calories: 508; Fat: 40g; Protein: 31g; Total Carbs: 8g; Fiber: 2g; Net Carbs: 6g; Macros: Fat: 71%; Protein: 24%; Carbs: 5%

Pork Chops with Mushroom Sauce

SERVES 4 | PREP TIME: 15 minutes | COOK TIME: 45 minutes

4 (4-ounce) pork rib chops
Sea salt
Freshly ground black pepper
3 tablespoons olive oil
1 onion, chopped
1 tablespoon minced garlic
4 cups sliced mushrooms
2 cups canned coconut milk
2 teaspoons chopped
  fresh basil

Season the pork chops with salt and pepper. Heat the olive oil in a large skillet over medium-high heat. Pan sear the pork chops on both sides, about 5 minutes per side. Remove the pork chops from the skillet and set aside on a plate. Sauté the onion and garlic until softened, for 3 minutes. Stir in the mushrooms and sauté until they are lightly caramelized, about 10 minutes. Stir in the coconut milk and basil and add the pork chops back to the skillet. Cover the skillet, reduce the heat, and braise until the pork is tender and cooked through, about 20 minutes.

Per Serving: Calories: 521; Fat: 41g; Protein: 28g; Total Carbs: 8g; Fiber: 1g; Net Carbs: 7g; Macros: Fat: 71%; Protein: 21%; Carbs: 8%

Nut-Stuffed Pork Chops

SERVES 4 | PREP TIME: 20 minutes | COOK TIME: 30 minutes

3 ounces goat cheese
½ cup chopped walnuts
¼ cup toasted
  chopped almonds
1 teaspoon chopped
  fresh thyme
4 center-cut pork chops,
  butterflied
Sea salt
Freshly ground black pepper
2 tablespoons olive oil

Preheat the oven to 400°F. In a small bowl, make the filling by stirring the goat cheese, walnuts, almonds, and thyme until well mixed. Season the pork chops inside and outside with salt and pepper. Stuff each chop, pushing the filling to the bottom of the cut section. Secure the stuffing with toothpicks through the meat. Place a large skillet over medium-high heat and add the olive oil. Pan sear the pork chops until they're browned on each side, about 10 minutes in total. Transfer the pork chops to a baking dish and roast the chops in the oven until cooked through, about 20 minutes. Serve after removing the toothpicks.

Per Serving: Calories: 481; Fat: 38g; Protein: 29g; Total Carbs: 5g; Fiber: 3g; Net Carbs: 2g; Macros: Fat: 70%; Protein: 25%; Carbs: 5%

Ham-Stuffed Pork Chops

SERVES 4 | PREP TIME: 15 minutes | COOK TIME: 40 minutes

4 (4-ounce) center-cut pork
  chops, about 1 inch thick
4 slices Swiss cheese
4 slices black forest ham
¾ cup almond flour
½ cup Parmesan cheese
1 large egg
1 tablespoon water
2 tablespoons extra-virgin
  olive oil

Preheat the oven to 350°F. Cut the pork chops horizontally throughout the middle without cutting right through, to create a pocket. Stuff each pork chop with a slice of Swiss cheese and a slice of ham. Seal the edges of the meat with toothpicks. In a large bowl, dredge the pork chops in the almond flour. Add the Parmesan cheese to the almond flour left in the bowl, and stir to combine. In another large bowl, stir the egg and water, and dip the pork chops in the egg mixture, shaking off the excess. Dredge the meat in the almond flour-cheese mixture to completely coat. In a large skillet over medium heat, heat the olive oil. Brown the pork chops on both sides until golden brown, about 4 minutes per side. Place the pork chops in a baking dish, and bake until cooked through, about 30 to 35 minutes. Serve.

Per Serving: Calories: 491; Fat: 33g; Protein: 38g; Total Carbs: 6g; Fiber: 3g; Net Carbs: 3g; Macros: Fat: 63%; Protein: 32%; Carbs: 5%

Cheese-Stuffed Pork Chops

SERVES 2 | PREP TIME: 15 minutes | COOK TIME: 20 minutes

2 tablespoons olive oil, divided
1 teaspoon minced garlic
3 tablespoons finely chopped onion
⅓ cup spinach
2 ounces Muenster cheese, shredded
1 large egg, beaten
2 (6- to 8-ounce) bone-in pork chops
½ teaspoon salt
¼ teaspoon black pepper

In a large oven-safe skillet over medium-high heat, heat 1 tablespoon of olive oil for 1 minute. Add the garlic and sauté until fragrant, about 1 minute. Add the onion and spinach. Lower the heat to medium and cook for 2 to 3 minutes. Transfer the mixture to a small bowl to cool. Once cooled, add the Muenster cheese and the egg. Mix well to combine. Preheat the oven to 375°F. On a flat surface, cut the pork chops through the middle horizontally to the bone. Open the meat up like a butterfly. Stuff half of the spinach mixture into each pork chop. Fold the chop over the stuffing and secure the edges with toothpicks, if necessary. Season with the salt and pepper. In the large oven-safe skillet, heat the remaining tablespoon of olive oil over medium-high heat. Place the chops into the skillet and sear each side for 2 minutes. Once seared, place the skillet into the preheated oven. Bake for 15 minutes, or until the internal temperature reaches 150°F. Serve with your preferred side dishes.

Per Serving: Calories: 591; Fat: 44.5g; Total Carbs: 4g; Net Carbs: 2.6g; Fiber: 1.4g; Protein: 45.5g; **Macros:** Fat: 67%; Protein: 30%; Carbs: 3%

Pork Pumpkin Ragout

SERVES 6 | PREP TIME: 15 minutes | COOK TIME: 45 minutes

2 tablespoons extra-virgin olive oil
1 pound pork center loin chops, cut into 1½-inch chunks
2 cups cubed pumpkin (1-inch chunks)
1 red bell pepper, diced
½ onion, halved and sliced
1 tablespoon minced garlic
1½ cups low-sodium chicken broth
1½ cups coconut milk
2 teaspoons chopped fresh thyme
½ cup heavy (whipping) cream
Salt
Freshly ground black pepper
8 slices cooked bacon, chopped

Heat the olive oil in a large stockpot over medium-high heat and sauté the pork until it is cooked through, about 7 minutes. Add the pumpkin, bell pepper, onion, and garlic and sauté until the vegetables are softened, about 10 minutes. Stir in the chicken broth, coconut milk, and thyme and bring the mixture to a boil. Reduce the heat to low and simmer until the vegetables and meat are tender, about 25 minutes. Stir in the heavy cream and season with salt and pepper. Serve topped with the bacon.

Per Serving: Calories: 526; Fat: 42g; Protein: 27g; Total Carbs: 10g; Fiber: 3g; Net Carbs: 7g; **Macros:** Fat: 71%; Protein: 21%; Carbs: 8%

Pork Fried Rice

SERVES 1 | PREP TIME: 10 minutes | COOK TIME: 15 minutes

1 tablespoon avocado oil
½ head cauliflower riced
1 (6-ounce) pork tenderloin, cut into thin strips
1 tablespoon butter or ghee
1 scallion, finely sliced (green and white parts divided)
1 teaspoon peeled and minced ginger root
1 garlic clove, minced
1 egg, beaten
1 tablespoon coconut aminos
1 teaspoon sesame oil

In a large skillet, heat the oil over medium heat. Sauté the pork strips for 4 to 5 minutes, then transfer them to a plate and set aside. In the same skillet, combine the butter, cauliflower "rice," and the white parts of the scallion, and cook for about 5 minutes or until the cauliflower begins to soften slightly. Add the ginger and garlic, and stir for about 30 seconds. Add the beaten egg and cook, stirring continuously. Add the pork and coconut aminos, and cook for another 2 minutes, stirring continuously. Remove from the heat, and stir in the sesame oil and green parts of the scallion.

Per Serving: Calories: 565; Fat: 41g; Protein: 39g; Total Carbs: 10g; Fiber: 4g; Net Carbs: 6g; **Macros:** Fat: 65%; Protein: 28%; Carbs: 7%

Lemongrass Pork Noodle Bowls

SERVES 4 | PREP TIME: 10 minutes | COOK TIME: 30 minutes

1 tablespoon minced lemongrass
1 serrano pepper, minced
2 teaspoons minced garlic
2 tablespoons low-sodium soy sauce
2 tablespoons lime juice
¼ cup canola oil
1 (1¼-pound) pork tenderloin
2 zucchini spiralized
2 carrots spiralized
½ cup fresh basil leaves
½ cup fresh cilantro
½ cup fresh mint leaves

Preheat the oven to 400°F. Line a baking dish with parchment paper. In a glass measuring cup, whisk the lemongrass, chile, garlic, soy sauce, lime juice, and oil. Pour half of the mixture over the pork tenderloin, turning to coat. Place the pork in the baking dish and roast for 30 minutes, or until cooked to an internal temperature of 145°F. Set aside on a cutting board to rest. Place the spiralized veggies in a large salad bowl and toss them with the remaining dressing. Just before serving, toss the noodles with the basil, cilantro, and mint, and then divide among the serving bowls. Thinly slice the pork tenderloin and place equal portions on top of each noodle serving.

Per Serving: Calories: 446; Fat: 25g; Protein: 44g; Total Carbs: 9g; Fiber: 3g; Net Carbs: 6g; **Macros:** Fat: 50%; Protein: 39%; Carbs: 11%

Pork Pho with Shirataki Noodles

SERVES 2 | PREP TIME: 15 minutes | COOK TIME: 1 hour

5 cups beef broth
4 lemongrass stalks, tough outer leaves and bulb removed
1 small white onion, minced
2 teaspoons minced anchovies
1 tablespoon minced peeled fresh ginger
1 teaspoon garlic powder
½ cinnamon stick
½ tablespoon tamari
½ teaspoon erythritol
Red pepper flakes (optional)
8 ounces pork shoulder
1 tablespoon avocado oil
8 ounces shirataki noodles
⅓ cup fresh cilantro, coarsely chopped
Bean sprouts (optional)
Juice of ½ lime
Sugar-free hot sauce (optional)

Pour the beef broth into a large stockpot and add the lemongrass, onion, anchovies, ginger, garlic, cinnamon stick, tamari, erythritol, and red pepper flakes (if using). Bring to a boil over medium-high heat, cover, reduce the heat to low, and let simmer for about 1 hour. When you have about 15 minutes left for your pho broth, in a large skillet over medium-high heat, sear the pork in the avocado oil for 4 to 5 minutes per side. Remove the pork from the skillet and slice thinly. Divide the shirataki noodles between two soup bowls. Strain the pho broth and discard the solids. Divide the broth between the bowls, then add some of the pork slices, cilantro, and bean sprouts (if using) to each bowl. Garnish with lime juice and sprinkle with some hot sauce!

Per Serving: Calories: 461; Fat: 33g; Protein: 34g; Total Carbs: 7g; Fiber: 1g; Net Carbs: 6g; **Macros:** Fat: 65%; Protein: 29%; Carbs: 6%

Rosemary Balsamic Pork Medallions

SERVES 3 | PREP TIME: 15 minutes | COOK TIME: 20 minutes

1 (1-pound) pork tenderloin, sliced into 1½-inch-thick medallions	1 garlic clove, minced
¼ teaspoon salt	1 shallot, minced
¼ teaspoon freshly ground black pepper	3 tablespoons balsamic vinegar
2 tablespoons olive oil	1 teaspoon soy sauce
¼ cup butter, divided	4 fresh rosemary sprigs
	4 fresh thyme sprigs

Preheat the oven to 475°F. Season each medallion with the salt and pepper. In a large oven-safe skillet over medium-high heat, heat the olive oil and 1 tablespoon of butter for 1 minute. Add the garlic and shallot and sauté until fragrant, about 1 minute. Add the pork medallions to the skillet. Sear on each side for about 2 minutes. Add the balsamic vinegar, soy sauce, rosemary, thyme, and the remaining 3 tablespoons of butter to the skillet. Stir to combine. Spoon the balsamic mixture over the pork. Bring to a simmer and cook for about 2 minutes. Remove the skillet from the heat and place it into the preheated oven. Bake for 5 minutes. Flip the medallions and spoon the balsamic mixture over each piece. Continue baking for an additional 5 minutes, or until the internal temperature reaches 150°F. Remove from the oven and allow the pork to rest for 2 to 3 minutes before serving.

Per Serving: Calories: 458; Fat: 30.7g; Total Carbs: 4.8g; Net Carbs: 2.5g; Fiber: 2.3g; Protein: 40.4g; **Macros:** Fat: 61%; Protein: 35%; Carbs: 4%

Pork Medallions with Blue Cheese Sauce

SERVES 6 | PREP TIME: 10 minutes | COOK TIME: 25 minutes

2 tablespoons olive oil	1 cup chicken or vegetable broth
2 (1-pound) pork tenderloins, cut into 1-inch-thick medallions	1 cup heavy (whipping) cream
Salt	5 ounces blue cheese, cubed
Freshly ground black pepper	2 tablespoons chopped fresh parsley

In a large deep skillet, heat the oil over medium-high heat. Working in batches, place the pork in the skillet, season with salt and pepper, and cook on one side for 5 minutes. Flip, season again with salt and pepper, and cook for another 5 minutes. Transfer to a plate. Repeat with the remaining pork. Pour the broth into the skillet and deglaze, scraping up any browned bits at the bottom. Stir in the heavy cream and blue cheese. Simmer for 5 minutes to allow the cheese to melt and the sauce to thicken. Return the pork to the skillet and continue to cook, stirring occasionally, for about 10 minutes, or until the pork has reached an internal temperature of at least 145°F and is opaque with only a slight pink tinge. Serve garnished with the parsley.

Per Serving: Calories: 289; Fat: 23g; Protein: 17g; Total Carbs: 4g; Fiber: 2g; Net Carbs: 2g; **Macros:** Fat: 70%; Protein: 25%; Carbs: 5%

Glazed Pork Tenderloin

SERVES 6 TO 8 | PREP TIME: 5 minutes | COOK TIME: 25 minutes

2 pounds pork tenderloin	2 tablespoons coconut aminos
2 teaspoons salt	1 tablespoon balsamic vinegar
2 teaspoons fresh thyme	1 teaspoon fish sauce
1½ teaspoons ground cinnamon	2 garlic cloves, minced
1½ teaspoons garlic powder	1 tablespoons chopped fresh cilantro (optional)

Preheat the oven to 375°F. Line a baking sheet with parchment paper. Place the pork tenderloin on the baking sheet. In a small bowl, mix all the spices. Rub the spice mixture all over the pork. Place the pork in the oven and bake for 15 minutes. Meanwhile, prepare the glaze by mixing the coconut aminos, vinegar, fish sauce, and garlic. After 15 minutes, remove the pork from the oven and pour the glaze over it and fully coat. Place the pork back in the oven to continue baking for another 10 minutes or until the internal temperature reaches 130 to 145°F. Slice the pork and garnish with cilantro.

Per Serving: Calories: 181; Fat: 5g; Protein: 31g; Total Carbs: 2g; Fiber: 0g; Net Carbs: 2g; **Macros:** Fat: 27%; Protein: 72%; Carbs: 1%

Balsamic–Thyme Pork Tenderloin

SERVES 4-6 | PREP TIME: 5 minutes | COOK TIME: 25 minutes

2 tablespoons balsamic vinegar	1 (2-pound) pork tenderloin
2 tablespoons avocado oil	Pink Himalayan salt
2 thyme sprigs, leaves stripped and finely chopped	Freshly ground black pepper

Preheat the oven to 475°F. Line a baking sheet with parchment paper. In a small bowl, whisk the balsamic vinegar, avocado oil, and thyme. Place the pork tenderloin on the lined baking sheet and season with salt and pepper. Fully coat the pork with the vinegar mixture on all sides. Roast for 20 to 25 minutes. Remove the pork from the oven, transfer to a cutting board, and cover loosely with foil. Let the tenderloin rest for 5 minutes before slicing.

Per Serving: Calories: 525; Fat: 26g; Protein: 67g; Total Carbs: 1g; Fiber: 0g; Net Carbs: 1g; **Macros:** Fat: 45%; Protein: 51%; Carbs: 4%

Stuffed Pork Loin with Sun-Dried Tomato and Goat Cheese

SERVES 6 | PREP TIME: 15 minutes | COOK TIME: 30 to 40 minutes

1 (1- to 1½-pound) pork tenderloin

1 cup crumbled goat cheese

4 ounces frozen spinach, thawed and well drained

2 tablespoons chopped sun-dried tomatoes

2 tablespoons extra-virgin olive oil (or seasoned oil marinade from sun-dried tomatoes), plus ¼ cup, divided

½ teaspoon salt

½ teaspoon freshly ground black pepper

Preheat the oven to 350°F. Cut cooking twine into eight (6-inch) pieces. Cut the pork tenderloin in half lengthwise, leaving about an inch border, being careful to not cut all the way through. Open the tenderloin like a book to form a large rectangle. Place it between two pieces of parchment paper or plastic wrap and pound to about ¼-inch thickness with a meat mallet. In a small bowl, combine the goat cheese, spinach, sun-dried tomatoes, 2 tablespoons olive oil, salt, and pepper and mix to incorporate well. Spread the filling over the surface of the pork, leaving a 1-inch border from one long edge and both short edges. To roll, start from the long edge with filling and roll towards the opposite edge. Tie cooking twine around the pork to secure it closed, evenly spacing each of the eight pieces of twine along the length of the roll. In a Dutch oven or large oven-safe skillet, heat ¼ cup olive oil over medium-high heat. Add the pork and brown on all sides. Remove from the heat, cover, and bake until the pork is cooked through, 45 to 75 minutes, depending on the thickness of the pork. Remove from the oven and let rest for 10 minutes at room temperature. To serve, remove the twine, slice the pork into medallions, and serve.

Per Serving: Calories: 270; Fat: 21g; Protein: 20g; Total Carbs: 2g; Fiber: 1g; Net Carbs: 1g; **Macros:** Fat: 67%; Protein: 31%; Carbs: 2%

Bacon-Wrapped Pork Tenderloin

SERVES 4 | PREP TIME: 10 minutes | COOK TIME: 45 minutes

1 teaspoon salt

1 teaspoon garlic powder

1 teaspoon onion powder

½ teaspoon smoked paprika

½ teaspoon dried basil

½ teaspoon dried thyme

½ teaspoon dried rosemary

½ teaspoon dried sage

½ teaspoon freshly ground black pepper

¼ teaspoon cayenne pepper

¼ teaspoon cumin

⅛ teaspoon cinnamon

⅛ teaspoon nutmeg

⅛ teaspoon cloves

1 (2-pound) pork tenderloin

2 tablespoons olive oil

8 to 12 bacon slices

In a medium bowl, combine the salt, garlic powder, onion powder, paprika, basil, thyme, rosemary, sage, black pepper, cayenne pepper, cumin, cinnamon, nutmeg, and cloves. Stir to combine. Preheat the oven to 425°F. Trim any excess fat or silverskin (a thin layer of connective tissue) from the pork. Coat the pork with the olive oil. Liberally apply the rub to the pork, covering the entire loin. Set aside. On a cutting board, lay out the bacon pieces side by side. Place the pork in the center of the bacon

strips. Starting at one end, pull the edge of the bacon up and over the tenderloin diagonally. Repeat with the other side of the slice, crossing it over the first side. Repeat the process with the remaining bacon slices, tucking the free ends under the crisscrossed bacon slices as you go. Secure with toothpicks as needed. Put the bacon-wrapped pork in a baking dish and bake for 20 minutes. Lower the heat to 300°F and bake for another 20 minutes. Once it reaches 135°F, increase the heat to broil and crisp the bacon for 3 to 5 minutes. Remove the pork from the oven. Cover with aluminum foil. Allow the meat to rest for at least 10 minutes so the juices set. Slice and serve with your preferred sides.

Per Serving: Calories: 518; Fat: 29.9g; Total Carbs: 1.9g; Net Carbs: 1.9g; Fiber: 0g; Protein: 57.3g; **Macros:** Fat: 53%; Protein: 45%; Carbs: 2%

Jerk Pork Tenderloin

SERVES 6 | PREP TIME: 15 minutes | COOK TIME: 20 minutes

1 tablespoon granulated erythritol

½ tablespoon garlic powder

½ tablespoon ground allspice

½ tablespoon dried thyme

1 teaspoon ground cinnamon

¼ teaspoon salt

¼ teaspoon freshly ground black pepper

⅛ teaspoon cayenne pepper

1 (1-pound) pork tenderloin, cut into 1-inch medallions

¼ cup extra-virgin olive oil

½ cup sour cream

2 tablespoons chopped fresh cilantro, for garnish

In a medium bowl, stir the erythritol, garlic powder, allspice, thyme, cinnamon, salt, pepper, and cayenne. Rub the pork pieces generously on all sides with the seasoning mixture. Heat the olive oil in a large skillet over medium-high heat. Pan-fry the pork until just cooked through, turning once, about 20 minutes in total. Serve topped with the sour cream and cilantro.

Per Serving: Calories: 287; Fat: 23g; Protein: 17g; Total Carbs: 3g; Fiber: 1g; Net Carbs: 2g; **Macros:** Fat: 72%; Protein: 24%; Carbs: 4%

Spice-Rubbed Roasted Pork with Cilantro Pesto

SERVES 8 | PREP TIME: 15 minutes, plus 15 minutes to rest | COOK TIME: 1 hour

¾ cup extra-virgin olive oil, divided

2 teaspoons ground cumin

1 teaspoon chili powder

1 teaspoon garlic powder

2 teaspoons salt, divided

1 (2-pound) pork loin roast, untrimmed

1 packed cup fresh cilantro leaves

2 garlic cloves, peeled and smashed

Juice and zest of 1 lime

Preheat the oven to 375°F. In a small bowl, combine 2 tablespoons of the oil, cumin, chili powder, garlic powder, and 1 teaspoon of salt to form a paste. Rub the pork with the seasoning and let it sit for 15 minutes. In a large ovenproof skillet or Dutch oven, heat 2 tablespoons of oil over medium-high heat. Add the pork and brown on all sides, for 3 to 4 minutes per side. Cover and roast for 40 to 45 minutes, until the internal temperature reaches 150°F. Remove the roast from the oven, and let sit, covered for 10 minutes to bring the internal temperature to 165°F before slicing. In the bowl of a food processor or blender, place the cilantro, garlic, and lime juice and zest and blend until well chopped. With the processor running, stream in the remaining ½ cup of the olive oil and blend until smooth. Serve the pork drizzled with the cilantro pesto.

Per Serving: Calories: 374; Fat: 30g; Protein: 24g; Total Carbs: 2g; Fiber: <1g; Net Carbs: 2g; **Macros:** Fat: 72%; Protein: 26%; Carbs: 2%

Roasted Pork Loin with Grainy Mustard Sauce

SERVES 8 | PREP TIME: 10 minutes | COOK TIME: 70 minutes

1 (2-pound) boneless pork loin roast

Sea salt

Freshly ground black pepper

3 tablespoons olive oil

1½ cups heavy (whipping) cream

3 tablespoons grainy mustard, such as Pommery

Preheat the oven to 375°F. Season the pork roast all over with sea salt and pepper. Place a large skillet over medium-high heat and add the olive oil. Brown the roast on all sides in the skillet, about 6 minutes in total, and place the roast in a baking dish. Roast until a meat thermometer inserted in the thickest part of the roast reads 155°F, about 1 hour. When there is approximately 15 minutes of roasting time left, place a small saucepan over medium heat and add the heavy cream and mustard. Stir the sauce until it simmers, then reduce the heat to low. Simmer the sauce until it is very rich and thick, about 5 minutes. Remove the pan from the heat and set aside. Let the pork rest for 10 minutes before slicing and serve with the sauce.

Per serving: Calories: 368; Fat: 29g; Protein: 25g; Total Carbs: 2g; Fiber: 0g; Net Carbs: 2g; **Macros:** Fat: 70%; Protein: 25%; Carbs: 5%

BBQ Baby Back Ribs

SERVES 4 | PREP TIME: 10 minutes | COOK TIME: 3 hours

2 teaspoons smoked paprika

¾ teaspoon ground cumin

1 teaspoon onion powder

1 teaspoon garlic powder

1 (1½-pound) rack of pork ribs

Sea salt

Freshly ground black pepper

½ cup apple cider vinegar

2 tablespoons ketchup

2 to 3 drops liquid stevia

¼ cup minced cilantro

1 scallion, white and green parts roughly chopped

Preheat the oven to 250°F. Mix the paprika, cumin, onion powder, and garlic powder in a small mixing bowl. Season the ribs with salt and pepper and half of the spice blend. Place the ribs into a roasting pan or Dutch oven fitted with a lid. Alternatively, cover the baking dish tightly with foil. Bake for 2½ hours. While the ribs cook, mix the vinegar, ketchup, and the remaining spice blend in a small saucepan over medium heat. Simmer for 10 minutes, until reduced slightly. Sweeten with a few drops of liquid stevia. Transfer the barbecue sauce to a blender along with the cilantro and scallion. Remove the pork from the oven and transfer the cooked ribs to a separate dish momentarily. Carefully remove ½ cup of the accumulated pan juices from the roasting pan. Add it to the blender and purée until smooth. Discard the remaining pan juices and then return the ribs to the pan. Pour the barbecue sauce over the ribs and roast uncovered for 30 minutes.

Per Serving: Calories: 654; Fat: 51g; Protein: 42g; Total Carbs: 6g; Fiber: 1g; Net Carbs: 5g; **Macros:** Fat: 70%; Protein: 26%; Carbs: 4%

Pork Ribs

SERVES 3 | PREP TIME: 15 minutes | COOK TIME: 2 hours 5 minutes

2 tablespoons avocado oil

1 tablespoon Dijon mustard

2½ tablespoons brown sugar substitute

2 tablespoons paprika

1 tablespoon sea salt

½ tablespoon chili powder

2 teaspoons freshly ground black pepper

3 pounds baby back pork ribs, membranes removed

Preheat the oven to 300°F. Line a baking sheet with aluminum foil. In a bowl, whisk the oil, mustard, brown sugar substitute, paprika, salt, chili powder, and pepper. Massage the spice mixture evenly over the front and back of the ribs, covering them completely. Place the ribs on the prepared baking sheet bone-side down. Cover with another layer of foil and bake for 1 hour. Flip the ribs, cover again, and roast for another hour. Remove from the oven and turn the heat to broil. Uncover the ribs and discard the top layer of foil. Flip the ribs back over so the meat side is up. Broil for 4 to 5 minutes, just until the top of the meat begins to crisp. Let the ribs cool slightly before serving. To serve, turn so the ribs are bone-side up and cut between each bone.

Per Serving: (1 pound; about 7 ribs): Calories: 754; Fat: 43g; Protein: 86g; Total Carbs: 15g; Fiber: 3g; Net Carbs: 2g; **Macros:** Fat: 51%; Protein: 46%; Carbs: 3%

Oven-Baked Country-Style Pork Ribs

SERVES 8 | PREP TIME: 20 minutes, plus 3 hours to chill | COOK TIME: 2 hours, 45 minutes

1½ tablespoons monk fruit/erythritol blend sweetener

1 tablespoon paprika

2 teaspoons kosher salt

2 teaspoons garlic powder

1 teaspoon freshly ground black pepper

1 teaspoon chili powder

1 teaspoon onion powder

½ teaspoon cayenne pepper

½ teaspoon dry mustard

1 small onion, sliced

5 pounds country-style, bone-in ribs

Sugar-free barbecue sauce, for serving

In a small bowl, stir the sweetener, paprika, salt, garlic powder, black pepper, chili powder, onion powder, cayenne, and dry mustard. Sprinkle the rub over the ribs, coating both sides well. Place the ribs in a zip-top bag and refrigerate for at least 3 hours. Preheat the oven to 275°F. Cover a baking sheet with aluminum foil and line it with parchment paper. Place the ribs on the baking sheet in a single layer. Place the onion over the ribs. Tightly cover everything with foil. Bake for 2 hours. Remove the ribs from the oven and remove the foil. Increase the oven temperature to 350°F. Return the ribs to the oven for 30 to 45 minutes more, or until the ribs are pull-apart tender, basting occasionally with the pan juices.

Per Serving: Calories: 529; Fat: 33g; Protein: 55g; Total Carbs: 3g; Fiber: 1g; Net Carbs: 2g; **Macros:** Fat: 56%; Protein: 42%; Carbs: 2%

Dry Rub Ribs

SERVES 2 | PREP TIME: 10 minutes | COOK TIME: 3 hours

1 tablespoon smoked paprika

½ tablespoon kosher salt

1 teaspoon chili powder

1 teaspoon ground cumin

1 teaspoon garlic powder

½ teaspoon freshly ground
black pepper

½ teaspoon ground mustard

½ teaspoon onion powder

¼ teaspoon cayenne pepper

1 (3½-pound) rack baby back
or spare ribs

Preheat the oven to 325°F. Line a baking sheet with foil. In a small bowl, mix the paprika, salt, chili powder, cumin, garlic powder, black pepper, mustard, onion powder, and cayenne pepper. Place the ribs on the baking sheet and coat both sides with the seasoning mixture. Bake for 3 hours. Remove the ribs from the oven and let rest for 5 to 10 minutes. Serve.

Per Serving: Calories: 1,393; Fat: 113g; Protein: 93g; Total Carbs: 1g; Fiber: 0g; Net Carbs: 1g; **Macros:** Fat: 73%; Protein: 27%; Carbs: 0%

Barbecue Pork Ribs

SERVES 5 | PREP TIME: 4½ hours | COOK TIME: 1 hour

¼ cup olive oil

2 garlic cloves, minced

1 shallot, minced

1 teaspoon cumin

1 teaspoon paprika

1 teaspoon chili powder

1 teaspoon salt

½ teaspoon cayenne pepper

½ teaspoon freshly ground
black pepper

¼ teaspoon ground ginger

2 pounds baby back pork
rib racks

Sugar-free barbecue sauce
(optional)

In a blender or food processor, add the olive oil, garlic, shallot, cumin, paprika, chili powder, salt, cayenne pepper, black pepper, and ginger. Mix until thoroughly incorporated. On a flat surface, cut the rib racks into quarters and arrange on a baking sheet. Cover the ribs evenly with the rub, massaging it into the meat. Refrigerate the ribs to marinate for at least 4 hours. Preheat the oven to 300°F. Place the ribs in the oven. Cook for 1 hour, 10 minutes. Remove the ribs from the oven. Allow them to cool for 2 to 3 minutes before slicing.

Per Serving: Calories: 612; Fat: 53.7g; Total Carbs: 2.3g; Net Carbs: 1.8g; Fiber: 0.5g; Protein: 29.4g; **Macros:** Fat: 80%; Protein: 19%; Carbs: 1%

Smoked Ribs

SERVES 8 | PREP TIME: 20 minutes, plus 5 hours to chill | COOK TIME: 5 hours

¼ cup brown erythritol blend

1 tablespoon paprika

1 tablespoon Lawry's
seasoned salt

1 tablespoon garlic powder

1 tablespoon freshly ground
black pepper

4 racks (8 to 10 pounds)
St. Louis–style pork
ribs, trimmed

¼ cup (½ stick) butter, melted

In a small bowl, combine the brown sweetener, paprika, seasoned salt, garlic powder, and pepper. Set aside. Using a spoon, sprinkle the rub on the ribs, and then, using the back of the spoon as a mallet, slowly and gently pound the rub all over each rack so it sticks. Wrap each rack in plastic wrap and refrigerate for at least 5 to 6 hours or up to overnight. Preheat a grill or smoker to 180°F. Unwrap and lay each rack directly on the racks, meaty-side up, and cook for 2 hours. Remove the ribs, and increase heat to 250°F. Place each rack on a large sheet

of aluminum foil. Pour the melted butter over each rack, wrap tightly in the foil, and place back in the heat for 3 more hours. Serve warm.

Per Serving: (½ rack): Calories: 903; Fat: 79g; Protein: 49g; Total Carbs: 6g; Fiber: 0g; Net Carbs: 0g; **Macros:** Fat: 79%; Protein: 21%; Carbs: 0%

Pork and Sauerkraut

SERVES 6 | PREP TIME: 10 minutes | COOK TIME: 5 hours 35 minutes

¼ cup butter

1 small white onion, sliced

32 ounces sauerkraut in liquid

2 pounds boneless pork
shoulder

1½ teaspoons sea salt

¾ teaspoon freshly ground
black pepper

1 tablespoon avocado oil

Preheat the oven to 250°F. In a large saucepan over medium heat, melt the butter. Add the onion and cook, stirring frequently, until soft and golden. Pour in the sauerkraut and liquid. Stir to thoroughly combine. Drop the heat to medium low and simmer for 15 minutes. While the onions and sauerkraut are simmering, cut the pork into 4 pieces. Season with the salt and pepper. In a large skillet over medium-high heat, brown all sides of the pork. Transfer to a roasting dish. Pour the onion and sauerkraut mixture over the pork. Cover with aluminum foil. Bake for 2 hours and 45 minutes; then rotate the pan and bake for another 2 hours and 30 minutes. Use two forks to shred the pork into the sauerkraut mixture. Serve immediately.

Per Serving: (4 ounces pork + 1 cup sauerkraut): Calories: 492; Fat: 39g; Protein: 28g; Total Carbs: 8g; Fiber: 5g; Net Carbs: 3g; **Macros:** Fat: 71%; Protein: 23%; Carbs: 6%

Spicy Barbecued Pork Wings

SERVES 2 | PREP TIME: 10 minutes | COOK TIME: 2½ to 3½ hours

4 pork wings or trimmed
pork shanks

¼ cup water

1 teaspoon extra-virgin
olive oil

¼ cup sugar-free barbe-
cue sauce

2 tablespoons butter

1 teaspoon hot sauce
of choice

Cayenne pepper

If the wings did not come already cooked, preheat the oven to 300°F. Place the wings in an 8-inch-square baking pan and add the water. Seal the pan with aluminum foil. Bake for 2 to 3 hours, until the meat is tender. In a medium sauté pan or skillet, heat the olive oil over medium-high heat. Add the wings and crisp for 2 to 3 minutes on each side. Transfer the pork to a platter. Lower the heat to medium and add the barbecue sauce, butter, and hot sauce to the skillet. Season to taste with cayenne. Stir the sauce until it starts to simmer, then put the wings back in the skillet and coat with the sauce. Simmer until the sauce has thickened and sticks to the wings, about 2 minutes.

Per Serving: Calories: 458; Fat: 35g; Protein: 34g; Total Carbs: 2g; Fiber: 1g; Net Carbs: 1g; **Macros:** Fat: 69%; Protein: 29%; Carbs: 2%

Roasted Pork Belly and Asparagus

SERVES 4 | PREP TIME: 5 minutes | COOK TIME: 2 hours, 45 minutes

2½ pounds pork belly
1 tablespoon canola oil
Sea salt

Freshly ground black pepper
1 pound asparagus, woody stems removed

Preheat the oven to 325°F. Place an oven-safe rack inside a roasting pan. Place the pork skin-side up on the rack and coat with the oil. Season liberally with salt. Roast uncovered for 2 hours. Increase the heat to 400°F and cook the pork for another 30 minutes to crisp up the skin. Carefully transfer the pork to a cutting board to rest. Remove the rack from the pan. Scatter the asparagus in the roasting pan in the rendered pork fat. Season with salt and pepper. Roast for 15 minutes until crisp tender. Serve with the roasted asparagus.

Per Serving: Calories: 616; Fat: 60g; Protein: 13g; Total Carbs: 6g; Fiber: 3g; Net Carbs: 3g; **Macros:** Fat: 87%; Protein: 8%; Carbs: 5%

Crispy Bourbon Pork Belly

SERVES 4 | PREP TIME: 10 minutes | COOK TIME: 3 hours

For the pork belly

1 pound pork belly, skin removed, cut into 1-inch cubes
Pink Himalayan sea salt

Freshly ground black pepper
1½ ounces (3 tablespoons) Kentucky bourbon

For the sauce

1½ ounces (3 tablespoons) Kentucky bourbon
2 tablespoons sugar-free ketchup
1 tablespoon granulated erythritol

2 teaspoons coconut aminos
¼ teaspoon freshly ground black pepper
Dash of liquid smoke
Pinch pink Himalayan sea salt

Preheat the oven to 300°F. Season the pork belly with salt and pepper. Place the pork in an 8-inch square baking pan and pour over the bourbon. Cover the pan tightly with aluminum foil and bake for 2 hours and 30 minutes. Remove the foil and drain the juices from the pan. Turn the oven up to 425°F and bake the pork for 20 minutes more, until crispy. If it's not crisp enough for your liking, place it under the broiler for a few minutes. In a small saucepan over medium heat, combine the bourbon, ketchup, erythritol, coconut aminos, pepper, liquid smoke, and salt. Simmer for 5 to 7 minutes, stirring occasionally, until the sauce reduces by half. Add the sauce to the pork in the pan and turn the meat to coat with the sauce. Bake for an additional 5 minutes, then serve.

Per Serving: Calories: 638; Fat: 60g; Protein: 11g; Total Carbs: 0g; Fiber: 0g; Net Carbs: 0g; **Macros:** Fat: 92%; Protein: 8%; Carbs: 0%

Sriracha Pork Belly

SERVES 4 | PREP TIME: 10 minutes, plus 3 hours to marinate | COOK TIME: 3 hours

¼ cup sriracha hot sauce
¼ cup no-salt-added tomato paste
2 tablespoons soy sauce

1 tablespoon minced garlic
1 teaspoon Swerve
¾ pound boneless pork belly, with the skin scored

In a small bowl, mix the sriracha, tomato paste, soy sauce, garlic, and Swerve until well combined. Rub half the marinade into the meat part of the pork belly, cover, and marinate for at least 3 hours or overnight. Preheat the oven to 350°F. Place the pork belly skin-side up in a roasting pan, on a wire rack if possible. Roast until the meat is very tender, about 2½ hours. Place the remaining marinade in a small saucepan and cook over medium heat until thick, about 5 minutes. Remove the pork from the oven and lift the crackling (skin) away from the meat. Brush the meat with the glaze and roast for an additional 30 minutes.

Per Serving: Calories: 475; Fat: 45g; Protein: 9g; Total Carbs: 7g; Fiber: 1g; Net Carbs: 6g; **Macros:** Fat: 85%; Protein: 8%; Carbs: 7%

Honey Glazed Ham

SERVES 8 | PREP TIME: 15 minutes | COOK TIME: 1 hour 30 minutes

1 cup water
1 (4- to 6-pound) fully cooked spiral bone-in ham, patted dry
½ cup brown erythritol blend

½ cup sugar-free apricot preserves
2 tablespoons butter, room temperature

Preheat the oven to 300°F and line a large roasting pan with heavy aluminum foil. Pour 1 cup of water into the pan, and lay the ham on its side in the pan. In a small bowl, mix the brown sweetener, apricot preserves, and butter into a paste. Rub half of the paste over the ham, especially in between the spiral cuts. Cover with foil, and bake for 1 hour. Carefully remove the ham from the oven. Spoon out about ¼ cup of juice from the bottom of the pan and mix it with the remaining brown sugar paste. Using half of the mixture, baste the ham and place back in the oven, uncovered, for another 25 minutes. Carefully remove the ham from the oven and increase the temperature to broil. Baste the ham with the remaining mixture, return to the oven, and broil for 3 to 5 minutes, watching so it doesn't burn. Remove from the oven and let sit for at least 15 to 20 minutes before serving.

Per Serving: Calories: 239; Fat: 10g; Protein: 33g; Total Carbs: 11g; Fiber: 2g; Net Carbs: 3g; **Macros:** Fat: 38%; Protein: 55%; Carbs: 7%

Spicy Sausage and Cabbage Casserole

SERVES 4 | PREP TIME: 15 minutes | COOK TIME: 35 minutes

1 tablespoon olive oil, plus more for greasing the baking dish
½ yellow onion, spiralized
1 garlic clove, minced
1 pound ground Italian sausage
Salt

Freshly ground black pepper
2 tablespoons tomato paste
½ teaspoon red pepper flakes (or more, if you like it spicy)
1 head cabbage, spiralized
¼ cup heavy (whipping) cream
½ cup shredded mozzarella cheese, divided

Preheat the oven to 350°F. Coat a 9-by-13-inch baking dish with olive oil. In a large skillet over medium heat, heat 1 tablespoon of olive oil. Add the onion and sauté for 2 to 3 minutes. Add the garlic and cook for 1 to 2 minutes more. Add the sausage to the skillet and season with salt and pepper to taste. Cook, stirring frequently to break up the meat, for 5 to 6 minutes, or until the sausage has browned. Stir in the tomato paste and red pepper flakes. Add the cabbage. Turn the heat to medium and stir in the heavy cream and ¼ cup of mozzarella cheese. Transfer the mixture to the prepared baking dish. Top with the remaining ¼ cup of mozzarella. Bake for 15 to 20 minutes, or until the cheese has melted and is slightly browned. Let cool for 10 minutes before serving.

Per Serving: Calories: 573; Fat: 48g; Protein: 22g; Total Carbs: 15g; Fiber: 5g; Net Carbs: 10g; **Macros:** Fat: 75%; Protein: 16%; Carbs: 9%

Fried Ham "Rice"

SERVES 4 | PREP TIME: 15 minutes | COOK TIME: 12 minutes

- 3 tablespoons toasted sesame oil
- 2 scallions, white and green parts chopped
- 1 tablespoon grated fresh ginger
- 1 teaspoon minced garlic
- ½ cup ham, diced
- 3 large whole eggs, beaten
- 4 cups cauliflower rice
- ¼ cup soy sauce
- 4 teaspoons toasted sesame seeds
- 1 tablespoon chopped fresh cilantro

In a large skillet over medium-high heat, heat the sesame oil. Sauté the scallions, ginger, and garlic until softened, about 2 minutes. Add the ham, and sauté for 1 minute. Pour the beaten eggs into the skillet, and scramble them with the vegetables and ham until the eggs are cooked, about 3 minutes. Stir in the cauliflower rice and soy sauce. Sauté until all the ingredients are evenly mixed and heated through, about 5 minutes. Topped with the sesame seeds and cilantro, and serve.

Per Serving: Calories: 246; Fat: 19g; Protein: 12g; Total Carbs: 11g; Fiber: 5g; Net Carbs: 6g; **Macros:** Fat: 65%; Protein: 18%; Carbs: 17%

Ham-Broccoli-Cauliflower Casserole

SERVES 4 | PREP TIME: 20 minutes | COOK TIME: 30 minutes

- 3 cups broccoli florets
- 3 cups cauliflower florets
- 1 cup cream cheese
- 2 tablespoons coconut oil, melted
- 1 teaspoon minced garlic
- ¾ cup diced lean ham
- ½ cup shredded Cheddar cheese

Preheat the oven to 400°F. Place a large saucepan filled with water on high heat, and bring the water to a boil. Lightly blanch the broccoli and cauliflower until tender-crisp, about 3 minutes. Drain the vegetables, and transfer them to a large bowl. In a small bowl, whisk the cream cheese, coconut oil, garlic, and ham. Stir the cream cheese mixture into the broccoli and cauliflower until the vegetables are well coated. Spoon the mixture into an 8-cup casserole dish, and top with the Cheddar cheese. Bake the casserole until heated through, about 20 minutes, and serve.

Per Serving: Calories: 388; Fat: 32g; Protein: 18g; Total Carbs: 10g; Fiber: 4g; Net Carbs: 6g; **Macros:** Fat: 72%; Protein: 18%; Carbs: 10%

Cold Front Kielbasa and Cabbage Skillet

SERVES 8 | PREP TIME: 15 minutes | COOK TIME: 45 minutes

- 2 tablespoons lard or bacon fat
- 1½ pounds Polish smoked sausage, cut into ½-inch pieces
- ½ cup diced onion
- 3 garlic cloves, finely chopped
- 1 (28- or 32-ounce) jar sauerkraut
- 1 small head green cabbage, washed, cored, and chopped
- 1 tablespoon gluten-free Worcestershire sauce
- ½ teaspoon garlic powder
- ½ tablespoon dried parsley
- Kosher salt
- Freshly ground black pepper

In a large, deep cast-iron skillet or Dutch oven over medium heat, melt the lard. Add the sausage and cook for 3 to 5 minutes. Add the onion and cook for 3 to 4 minutes, until the sausage begins to caramelize. Add the garlic and cook for 1 minute more. Add the undrained sauerkraut to the sausage and stir to combine, scraping up any brown bits from the bottom of the pan. Stir in the cabbage, Worcestershire sauce, garlic powder, parsley, ½ teaspoon of salt, and ¼ teaspoon of pepper. Cover the pan and reduce the heat to medium-low. Cook for 25 minutes, or until the cabbage is tender, stirring often to prevent burning. Turn the heat to medium and cook, uncovered, stirring often, for 10 minutes more, or until any liquid is reduced and the cabbage begins to caramelize.

Per Serving: Calories: 338; Fat: 26g; Protein: 13g; Total Carbs: 13g; Fiber: 5g; Net Carbs: 8g; **Macros:** Fat: 70%; Protein: 15%; Carbs: 15%

Keto Lasagna with Deli Meat "Noodles"

SERVES 8 | PREP TIME: 15 minutes | COOK TIME: 1 hour, 5 minutes

- Nonstick cooking spray
- 1 cup whole-milk ricotta cheese
- 1 large egg
- ¼ cup shredded Parmesan cheese
- 3 teaspoons Italian seasoning, divided
- ½ teaspoon garlic powder
- ½ teaspoon onion powder
- ½ teaspoon salt
- ½ teaspoon freshly ground black pepper
- 2 tablespoons olive oil
- ½ medium white onion, diced
- 3 garlic cloves, minced
- 2 pounds mild Italian sausage, casings removed
- 2 cups sugar-free marinara sauce
- 1 pound deli chicken breast, sliced thinly
- 3 cups shredded mozzarella cheese

Preheat the oven to 357°F. Spray a large casserole dish with cooking spray. In a medium bowl, combine the ricotta, egg, Parmesan, 1 teaspoon of Italian seasoning, garlic powder, onion powder, salt, and pepper. Mix well and set aside. In a large skillet over medium heat, heat the oil. Add the onion and sauté until the onion is translucent, about 6 minutes. Add the garlic and remaining 2 teaspoons of Italian seasoning. Cook until fragrant, about 2 minutes. Add the sausage and cook, breaking it up with a spoon, until browned, about 8 minutes. Add the marinara sauce and continue cooking for 10 minutes, uncovered, to thicken. Set aside. Place one-third of the chicken slices in the bottom of the casserole dish. Use a rubber spatula to spread one-third of the ricotta mixture over the chicken. Spoon one-third of the meat mixture on top of the ricotta and spread evenly. Evenly sprinkle one-third of the mozzarella on top of the meat. Repeat the layers two more times. Bake, uncovered, for about 40 minutes or until the cheese on top is browned and the sides are slightly bubbling. Serve with a side salad.

Per Serving: Calories: 708; Fat: 55g; Protein: 42g; Total Carbs: 11g; Fiber: 1g; Net Carbs: 10g; **Macros:** Fat: 70%; Protein: 24%; Carbs: 6%

Creole Sausage and Rice

SERVES 4 | PREP TIME: 10 minutes | COOK TIME: 30 minutes

1 teaspoon extra-virgin
    olive oil
1 pound cooked Ital-
    ian sausage
1 (10-ounce) bag frozen cauli-
    flower rice, thawed, rinsed,
    and patted dry

3 tablespoons chopped
    red onion
2 scallions, thinly sliced
1 cup chicken broth or
    bone broth
2 teaspoons Creole seasoning

In a skillet over medium heat, heat the oil. Brown the cooked sausage for a few minutes. Add the cauliflower rice, red onion, scallions, broth, and Creole seasoning to the skillet with the sausage and mix to incorporate all the ingredients. Cook and stir until heated through. Serve hot.

Per Serving: (¼ skillet) Calories: 426; Fat: 32g; Protein: 24g; Total Carbs: 10g; Fiber: 2g; Net Carbs: 8g; **Macros:** Fat: 68%; Protein: 23%; Carbs: 9%

Sausage, Zucchini, and Green Bean Packets

SERVES 4 | PREP TIME: 10 minutes | COOK TIME: 25 minutes

Nonstick cooking spray
14 ounces cooked sau-
    sages, chopped
4 medium zucchini, sliced into
    ½-inch-thick coins

1 pound green beans, trimmed
4 teaspoons Italian seasoning
Salt
Freshly ground black pepper

Preheat the oven to 375°F. Lightly coat four 12-inch squares of aluminum foil with cooking spray. Divide the sausage, zucchini, and green beans among the foil squares, centered in the foil. Sprinkle each packet with 1 teaspoon of Italian seasoning and season well with salt and pepper. Bring all the sides of each piece of foil into the center and press the edges together to form a sealed packet. Place the packets on a baking sheet and cook for 25 minutes, or until the vegetables are tender.

Per Serving: Calories: 410; Fat: 28g; Protein: 23g; Total Carbs: 15g; Fiber: 5g; Net Carbs: 10g; **Macros:** Fat: 62%; Protein: 23%; Carbs: 15%

Rich Sausage and Spaghetti Squash Casserole

SERVES 4 | PREP TIME: 15 minutes | COOK TIME: 40 minutes

Butter, for greasing
½ pound pork sausage meat
2 cups cooked spa-
    ghetti squash
1 tomato, chopped
1 jalapeño pepper, minced

4 large eggs, beaten
½ cup shredded aged
    Cheddar cheese
¼ cup chopped cilantro

Preheat the oven to 350°F. Lightly grease an 8-cup casserole dish with butter, and set aside. In a large skillet over medium heat, sauté the sausage meat until cooked through. Add the squash, tomato, and jalapeño to the skillet, and stir. Sauté the mixture until most of the liquid has evaporated, about 10 minutes. Remove the skillet from the heat, and stir in the eggs. Transfer the mixture to the casserole dish, and sprinkle with the cheese. Bake

until the casserole is set and the top is golden and bubbly, about 30 minutes. Top with the cilantro, and serve.

Per Serving: Calories: 307; Fat: 24g; Protein: 18g; Total Carbs: 5g; Fiber: 0g; Net Carbs: 4g; **Macros:** Fat: 70%; Protein: 23%; Carbs: 7%

Pork with Sesame Slaw

SERVES 4 | PREP TIME: 5 minutes | COOK TIME: 15 minutes

2 tablespoons sesame oil
½ cup yellow onion, diced
2 garlic cloves, minced
2 teaspoons grated
    fresh ginger
1½ pounds ground pork
1 teaspoon salt
¼ teaspoon freshly ground
    black pepper

1 (12-ounce) bag of
    coleslaw mix
1 tablespoon sriracha
3 tablespoons coconut aminos
1 tablespoon rice wine vinegar
    or white wine vinegar
1 teaspoon pure maple syrup
    (optional)

In a large skillet, heat the sesame oil over medium heat. Add in the onion, garlic, and ginger and sauté for 2 to 3 minutes. Then add in the pork, salt, and pepper. Continue cooking for 10 minutes. Once the pork is just about done cooking, stir in the slaw, sriracha, coconut aminos, vinegar, and maple syrup (if using). Cook for another 3 to 5 minutes until the slaw has softened slightly but is still crisp.

Per Serving: Calories: 539; Fat: 43g; Protein: 30g; Total Carbs: 8g; Fiber: 3g; Net Carbs: 5g; **Macros:** Fat: 72%; Protein: 22%; Carbs: 6%

Pork Larb Lettuce Wraps

SERVES 2 | PREP TIME: 8 minutes | COOK TIME: 20 minutes

1 pound ground pork
¼ medium onion,
    finely chopped
1 fresh long red chile,
    thinly sliced
2 garlic cloves, minced
Juice of 1 lime
2 tablespoons chopped
    fresh basil
1 tablespoon chopped fresh
    cilantro or dried coriander

1 tablespoon fish sauce
1 teaspoon granulated
    erythritol
1 teaspoon dried mint
1 tablespoon extra-virgin
    olive oil
Pink Himalayan sea salt
Freshly ground black pepper
4 large, firm leaves of iceberg
    or butterhead lettuce
4 lime wedges, for garnish

In a large bowl, combine the pork, onion, chile, and garlic. In a small bowl, combine the lime juice, basil, cilantro, fish sauce, erythritol, and mint. In a large sauté pan or skillet, heat the olive oil over medium-high heat. Add the pork mixture and cook for 8 to 10 minutes, until no pink remains. Add the sauce and cook for 5 to 8 minutes more, until most of the sauce is reduced. Season with salt and pepper. Divide the meat mixture among the 4 lettuce leaves, fold into wraps, and serve with a wedge of lime.

Per Serving: Calories: 675; Fat: 55g; Protein: 39g; Total Carbs: 5g; Fiber: 0g; Net Carbs: 5g; **Macros:** Fat: 73%; Protein: 25%; Carbs: 2%

Baked Sausage and Shrimp with Turnips and Green Peppers

SERVES 4 | PREP TIME: 15 minutes | COOK TIME: 20 minutes

1 pound turnips (2 or 3 large),
    peeled and diced

3 tablespoons olive oil
1 teaspoon paprika

1 teaspoon dried thyme	Salt
1 teaspoon onion powder	Freshly ground black pepper
1 green bell pepper, seeded and sliced into strips	½ pound raw large shrimp, peeled and deveined
1 pound cooked sausage links, sliced into ½-inch-thick coins	Chopped fresh parsley, for garnish

Preheat the oven to 400°F. Place the turnips on a large baking sheet and drizzle with the oil. Roast for 5 minutes. In a small bowl, mix the paprika, thyme, and onion powder. Remove the baking sheet from the oven and add the bell pepper, sausage, and seasoning blend. Mix gently so everything is well coated. Season with salt and black pepper. Roast for another 5 minutes. Add the shrimp and stir to mix. Return to the oven for another 12 to 15 minutes, until the shrimp are opaque and cooked through. Garnish with the parsley and serve.

Per Serving: Calories: 340; Fat: 20g; Protein: 27g; Total Carbs: 12g; Fiber: 3g; Net Carbs: 9g; **Macros:** Fat: 54%; Protein: 32%; Carbs: 14%

Spicy Pork and Eggplant Stir-Fry

SERVES 4 | PREP TIME: 5 minutes | COOK TIME: 20 minutes

2 tablespoons olive oil	2 tablespoons hot sauce
1 medium unpeeled eggplant (about 1 pound), cut into cubes	1 teaspoon rice vinegar or white wine vinegar
1 pound ground pork	4 scallions, sliced, white and green parts for garnish
2 tablespoons soy sauce	

In a large skillet, heat the oil over medium heat. Add the eggplant and cook, stirring frequently, for 5 minutes. Use a slotted spoon to transfer the eggplant to a medium bowl. Add the ground pork to the pan and cook, stirring occasionally, for about 10 minutes, or until fully browned. Meanwhile, in a small bowl, combine the soy sauce, hot sauce, and vinegar and stir to blend. Return the eggplant to the pan and add the sauce. Cook for 5 minutes to allow the flavors to combine. Plate the stir-fry, top with the scallions, and serve.

Per Serving: Calories: 399; Fat: 31g; Protein: 21g; Total Carbs: 9g; Fiber: 4g; Net Carbs: 5g; **Macros:** Fat: 70%; Protein: 22%; Carbs: 8%

Brussels Sprout Ground Pork Hash

SERVES 4 | PREP TIME: 15 minutes | COOK TIME: 30 minutes

3 tablespoons extra-virgin olive oil, divided	1 sweet potato, diced
8 ounces ground pork	Juice of 1 lemon
4 bacon slices, chopped	1 teaspoon chopped fresh parsley
½ onion, chopped	Sea salt
1 tablespoon minced garlic	Freshly ground black pepper
8 ounces Brussels sprouts, trimmed and sliced	

Heat 1 tablespoon of olive oil in a large skillet over medium-high heat. Sauté the pork and bacon until cooked through, about 7 minutes. With a slotted spoon, remove the meat to a plate and set aside. Add the remaining 2 tablespoons of olive oil to

the skillet and sauté the onion and garlic until softened, about 3 minutes. Stir in the Brussels sprouts and sweet potato and sauté until the vegetables are tender, 18 to 20 minutes. Stir in the reserved pork and bacon, lemon juice, and parsley. Season with salt and pepper and serve.

Per Serving: Calories: 353; Fat: 26g; Protein: 20g; Total Carbs: 12g; Fiber: 4g; Net Carbs: 8g; **Macros:** Fat: 65%; Protein: 23%; Carbs: 12%

Spaghetti Squash & Ground Pork Stir-Fry with Kale

SERVES 3 TO 4 | PREP TIME: 10 minutes | COOK TIME: 1 hour 25 minutes

1 medium spaghetti squash, halved lengthwise and seeded	1 bunch kale, stems removed, leaves chopped (2 to 3 cups)
2 tablespoons avocado oil, divided	1 teaspoon garlic powder
	1 teaspoon onion powder
	1 teaspoon dried parsley
1 pound ground free-range pork	½ teaspoon dry mustard powder
Salt	½ teaspoon dried rosemary
Freshly ground black pepper	½ teaspoon dried oregano

Preheat the oven to 400°F. Line a baking sheet with aluminum foil. Brush the cut sides of the spaghetti squash with 1 tablespoon of the oil. Place it cut-side down on the baking sheet and roast for 45 minutes to 1 hour, or until tender when pierced with a fork. Remove from the oven and let sit until cool enough to handle. In a large skillet, heat the oil over medium-high heat. Add the ground pork and season with salt and pepper. Cook for about 5 minutes. Shred the squash strands into the skillet using a fork and stir to combine with the meat. Reserve the spaghetti squash shells for serving if you'd like. Add the kale, garlic and onion powders, parsley, dry mustard powder, rosemary, oregano, salt, and pepper. Cook for 10 minutes, or until the meat is no longer pink and the kale is wilted. To serve, scoop the pork mixture into the reserved spaghetti squash shells or into bowls.

Per Serving: Calories: 355; Fat: 23g; Protein: 23g; Total Carbs: 14g; Fiber: 6g; Net Carbs: 8g; **Macros:** Fat: 60%; Protein: 25%; Carbs: 15%

Egg Roll in a Bowl

SERVES 1 | PREP TIME: 10 minutes | COOK TIME: 10 minutes

6 ounces ground pork	1 teaspoon coconut aminos
2 cups cabbage coleslaw mix or shredded cabbage	1 scallion, white and green parts finely sliced
1 garlic clove, minced	1 teaspoon sesame oil
1 teaspoon minced fresh ginger	

Heat a large skillet over medium heat. Add the ground pork and cook, stirring often to crumble it, until it is cooked through. Add the cabbage, garlic, ginger, and coconut aminos, and cook for 3 to 4 minutes or until the cabbage softens. Transfer to a plate, sprinkle with the scallion, and drizzle with the sesame oil.

Per Serving: Calories: 463; Fat: 35g; Protein: 26g; Total Carbs: 11g; Fiber: 5g; Net Carbs: 6g; **Macros:** Fat: 69%; Protein: 22%; Carbs: 9%

Pork Spring Rolls

SERVES 1 TO 2 | PREP TIME: 15 minutes | COOK TIME: 15 to 20 minutes

2½ tablespoons avocado oil, divided

½ pound ground free-range pork

½ medium jicama, peeled and grated

1 small carrot, peeled and grated

1 small summer squash, grated

1½ cups fresh spinach, coarsely chopped

2½ tablespoons pickled ginger, finely chopped

1 large egg

Salt

Freshly ground black pepper

2 coconut flour wraps

Coconut aminos, or tamari, for dipping (optional)

In a large skillet, heat 1¼ tablespoons of avocado oil over medium-high heat. Add the ground meat and cook 8 to 10 minutes, until cooked through. Transfer to a large bowl. Mix in the jicama, carrot, summer squash, spinach, pickled ginger, and egg, and season with salt and pepper. Lay the wraps on a cutting board and brush them with a little water to make them pliable. Place half of the meat mixture on one side of each wrap and fold up like a burrito. In a large skillet, heat the remaining 1¼ tablespoons of avocado oil over medium-high heat. Add the spring rolls and fry on each side for 3 to 5 minutes, or until the wraps start to char and are nicely crisped. Eat plain or serve with dipping sauce.

Per Serving: Calories: 513; Fat: 33g; Protein: 27g; Total Carbs: 27g; Fiber: 14g; Net Carbs: 13g; **Macros:** Fat: 60%; Protein: 20%; Carbs: 20%

Beef and Broccoli Stir-fry

SERVES 4 | PREP TIME: 10 minutes | COOK TIME: 12 minutes

2 tablespoons toasted sesame oil

3 tablespoons canola oil

1 pound boneless sirloin, cut in paper-thin slices

Sea salt

Freshly ground black pepper

2 tablespoons minced ginger

2 teaspoons minced garlic

Pinch red pepper flakes

1 head broccoli, cut into florets and stalks, diced

¼ cup low-sodium soy sauce

2 tablespoons dry sherry

Heat the sesame oil and canola oil in a large wok or skillet over medium-high heat until very hot. Season the sirloin generously with salt and pepper. Stir-fry the sirloin until just cooked through, about 5 minutes. Add the ginger, garlic, and red pepper flakes and cook for 1 minute, just until fragrant. Transfer the beef to a separate dish with a slotted spoon. Add the broccoli to the pan and stir-fry for 5 minutes, until bright green and crisp tender. Return the beef and any accumulated juices to the pan, and add the soy sauce and sherry. Simmer for 2 minutes until the liquid has reduced and the beef and broccoli are coated in the sauce.

Per Serving: Calories: 472; Fat: 29g; Protein: 41g; Total Carbs: 12g; Fiber: 5g; Net Carbs: 7g; **Macros:** Fat: 55%; Protein: 35%; Carbs: 10%

Steak with Drunken Broccoli Noodles

SERVES 4 | PREP TIME: 15 minutes | COOK TIME: 15 minutes

1 tablespoon olive oil, peanut oil, or vegetable oil

½ white onion, spiralized

2 garlic cloves, minced

1 Thai chile, seeded and very finely chopped

1 pound thinly sliced steak

2 teaspoons fish sauce

4 heads broccoli, florets removed, stems peeled and spiralized

¼ cup soy sauce

2 tablespoons oyster sauce

2 scallions, cut into 1- to 2-inch pieces

Salt

Freshly ground black pepper

½ cup Thai basil leaves

In a large skillet over medium-high heat, heat the olive oil. Add the onion noodles and sauté for 2 to 3 minutes. Add the garlic and chile and cook for just under 1 minute. Add the beef to the skillet and stir-fry for 4 to 5 minutes. Add the fish sauce, broccoli florets, and broccoli noodles. Cook, stirring frequently, for 3 to 4 minutes. In a small bowl, whisk the soy sauce and oyster sauce to combine. Pour the sauce into the skillet and add the scallions. Toss to combine. Cook for 1 to 2 minutes. Taste and season with salt and pepper, as needed. Remove the skillet from the heat and add the basil, tossing until slightly wilted from the heat. Serve immediately.

Per Serving: Calories: 355; Fat: 17g; Protein: 33g; Total Carbs: 21g; Fiber: 7g; Net Carbs: 14g; **Macros:** Fat: 43%; Protein: 35%; Carbs: 22%

Ginger Pork Meatballs

SERVES 4 | PREP TIME: 10 minutes | COOK TIME: 15 minutes

1 large egg, whisked

¼ cup almond flour

1 teaspoon minced fresh ginger

1 teaspoon minced garlic

½ teaspoon sea salt

¼ teaspoon freshly ground black pepper

¼ cup minced cilantro

1 cup roughly chopped spinach

1 scallion, white and green parts thinly sliced

1 pound ground pork

2 tablespoons coconut oil

Whisk the egg, almond flour, ginger, garlic, salt, and pepper in a large bowl. Stir in the cilantro, spinach, and scallion. Add the pork, and using your hands, mix the ingredients until combined. Shape the pork mixture into 8 to 12 meatballs. Heat a large skillet over medium-high heat. Melt the coconut oil. When it is hot, sear the meatballs on all sides until well browned and cooked through to an internal temperature of 160°F, about 15 minutes.

Per Serving: Calories: 460; Fat: 35g; Protein: 33g; Total Carbs: 3g; Fiber: 1g; Net Carbs: 2g; **Macros:** Fat: 68%; Protein: 29%; Carbs: 3%

Beef Fajitas

SERVES 4 | PREP TIME: 20 minutes, plus time to marinate | COOK TIME: 22 minutes

¼ cup olive oil, divided

1 tablespoon freshly squeezed lime juice

1 teaspoon ground cumin

1 teaspoon chili powder

1 teaspoon paprika

¼ teaspoon cayenne pepper

Pinch sea salt

Pinch freshly ground black pepper

1 pound boneless rib eye steak

1 red onion, thinly sliced

1 red bell pepper, cut into thin strips

1 green bell pepper, cut into thin strips

2 tablespoons chopped fresh cilantro

½ cup sour cream

Put 2 tablespoons of the olive oil, the lime juice, cumin, chili powder, paprika, cayenne, salt, and black pepper in a large resealable plastic bag and shake to combine. Pierce the steak all over with a fork and place the meat in the bag with the marinade. Squeeze out as much air as possible and seal the bag. Marinate the steak for 1 hour in the refrigerator, turning the bag over once. Heat the remaining olive oil in a large skillet over medium-high heat. Pan sear the steak until medium-rare, turning once, 6 to 7 minutes per side. Remove the steak from the heat and let rest for 10 minutes. While the meat rests, sauté the onion and peppers until they are lightly caramelized, about 5 minutes. Remove the vegetables from the heat and stir in the cilantro. Slice the steak thinly on a bias across the grain and serve the meat topped with the vegetable mixture and sour cream.

Per Serving: Calories: 435; Fat: 32g; Protein: 24g; Total Carbs: 11g; Fiber: 2g; Net Carbs: 9g; **Macros:** Fat: 66%; Protein: 22%; Carbs: 12%

Beef Stroganoff

SERVES 4 | PREP TIME: 20 minutes | COOK TIME: 30 minutes

2 tablespoons extra-virgin olive oil	1 cup beef broth
¾ pound top sirloin steak, cut into thin strips	1 cup heavy (whipping) cream
	½ cup sour cream
1 sweet onion, chopped	2 tablespoons chopped fresh parsley
2 teaspoons minced garlic	Sea salt
1 cup sliced button mushrooms	Freshly ground black pepper

In a large skillet over medium-high heat, heat the olive oil. Sauté the beef until lightly browned, about 2 minutes. Using a slotted spoon, remove the beef from the skillet and set aside on a plate. Add the onion and garlic to the skillet, and sauté until the vegetables are softened, about 3 minutes. Stir in the mushrooms, and sauté until they are lightly browned, about 5 minutes. Add the beef broth, cream, and the beef with any accumulated juices. Bring the mixture to a boil, reduce the heat to low, and simmer until the beef is very tender, about 15 minutes. Stir in the sour cream and parsley, season with salt and pepper, and serve.

Per Serving: Calories: 410; Fat: 31g; Protein: 29g; Total Carbs: 6g; Fiber: 1g; Net Carbs: 5g; **Macros:** Fat: 67%; Protein: 28%; Carbs: 5%

Southwest-Style Fajita Bowls

SERVES 6 | PREP TIME: 15 minutes | COOK TIME: 25 minutes

For the marinade

⅓ cup olive oil	½ teaspoon freshly ground black pepper
½ cup freshly squeezed lime juice	½ teaspoon red pepper flakes
2 garlic cloves, minced	½ teaspoon dried oregano
1 teaspoon salt	½ teaspoon ground cumin
1 teaspoon chili powder	1 or 2 dashes hot sauce (optional)
½ teaspoon onion powder	
½ teaspoon garlic powder	

For the cauliflower rice

1 pound frozen riced cauliflower	¼ cup chopped fresh cilantro (optional)
1 tablespoon olive oil	1 teaspoon salt
2 tablespoons lime juice	½ teaspoon ground cumin

For the fajitas

2 pounds stir-fry beef or thinly sliced sirloin
3 bell peppers (red or green), sliced
1 medium white onion, halved and sliced

For the garnish

Lime wedges	Sour cream
1 avocado, sliced	2 or 3 scallions, sliced

Combine all the ingredients in a large measuring cup or medium bowl. Reserve half of the marinade. In a large bowl, combine the steak slices and half the marinade. Toss to coat the steak well and allow to sit, covered, for 15 to 20 minutes while you prepare the rice. In a skillet over medium-high heat, sauté the cauliflower in the oil for about 8 minutes or until the cauliflower is the texture of rice. Remove from the heat and add the lime juice, cilantro, salt, and cumin. Mix well. Transfer to a bowl and set aside. Wipe out the skillet and heat it over medium-high heat. When the skillet is hot, put the marinated steak and any marinade left in the bowl into the skillet. Cook, stirring frequently, for 6 to 8 minutes until the steak is cooked through. Transfer to a bowl and set aside. In the same skillet, combine the peppers and onion with 2 tablespoons of reserved marinade. Sauté for about 6 minutes or until the peppers are soft and the onion is translucent. To assemble, divide the cauliflower rice among 6 wide bowls or plates. Top the rice with the steak and vegetables. Spoon a bit of reserved marinade on top. Garnish with lime wedges for squeezing, avocado, a dollop of sour cream, and scallions.

Per Serving: Calories: 499; Fat: 34g; Protein: 34g; Total Carbs: 16g; Fiber: 6g; Net Carbs: 10g; **Macros:** Fat: 60%; Protein: 28%; Carbs: 12%

Chicken-Fried Steak Fingers with Gravy

SERVES 6 | PREP TIME: 15 minutes | COOK TIME: 20 minutes

For the chicken-fried steak

1 cup almond flour	½ teaspoon freshly ground black pepper, plus more for seasoning
1 cup crushed pork rinds	
⅓ cup grated Parmesan cheese	
1 teaspoon paprika	2 large eggs, lightly beaten
1 teaspoon kosher salt, plus more for seasoning	2 tablespoons unsweetened almond milk (not vanilla)
½ teaspoon garlic powder	1½ pounds (about 4 steaks) cubed beef steak, cut into 1½-inch strips
	Lard or tallow, for frying

For the gravy

2 tablespoons pan drippings	1¼ cups heavy (whipping) cream
2 tablespoons finely diced onion	
4 ounces cream cheese	Kosher salt
1 cup unsweetened almond milk	Freshly ground black pepper

Make the chicken-fried steak. In a shallow dish, stir the almond flour, pork rinds, Parmesan cheese, paprika, salt, garlic powder, and pepper. In another shallow dish, whisk the eggs and almond milk well. Place the steak strips on a layer of paper towels and pat dry. Lightly season with salt and pepper. One at a time, dip the strips into the egg mixture. Then dredge the strips in the almond flour mixture In a large sauté pan or skillet over medium heat, melt the lard and heat it to 375°F. This will take 3 to 5 minutes. You need about 1½ inches of fat in the pan. Fry the steak strips for 2 to 3 minutes per side, or until golden brown. Drain on paper towels, reserving 2 tablespoons of pan drippings. Serve with the gravy or sugar-free ketchup. Make the gravy. In a medium sauté pan or skillet over medium heat, combine the reserved pan drippings and onion. Sauté for 2 to 3 minutes. Add the cream cheese and almond milk and cook, stirring, until smooth and the cream cheese is melted. Stir in the heavy cream and simmer the gravy for 3 to 5 minutes, or until thick. Season with salt and pepper, and serve immediately.

Per Serving: Calories: 643; Fat: 51g; Protein: 40g; Total Carbs: 6g; Fiber: 2g; Net Carbs: 4g; **Macros:** Fat: 71%; Protein: 25%; Carbs: 4%

Garlic Steak Bites

SERVES 2 | PREP TIME: 5 minutes | COOK TIME: 15 minutes

1 tablespoon beef tallow
1 pound boneless chuck steak, cut into 1-inch cubes
Pink Himalayan sea salt
Freshly ground black pepper
3 tablespoons butter
2 garlic cloves, minced
½ teaspoon dried rosemary

In a large skillet, melt the tallow over medium-high heat. Season the steak cubes with salt and pepper on all sides. Add the steak cubes to the pan. Cook on all sides, turning and stirring, for 30 seconds to 1 minute per side. Transfer the meat to a bowl; leave the drippings in the skillet. Add the butter, garlic, and rosemary to the drippings. Cook over medium heat for 2 to 3 minutes, until the garlic starts to brown. Return the steak to the skillet, and cook, stirring occasionally, for 5 to 10 minutes, until the pieces reach your desired doneness.

Per Serving: Calories: 730; Fat: 62g; Protein: 43g; Total Carbs: 1g; Fiber: 0g; Net Carbs: 1g; **Macros:** Fat: 76%; Protein: 23%; Carbs: 1%

Soy-Ginger Veggie Noodle Steak Roll-Ups

SERVES 4 | PREP TIME: 15 minutes | COOK TIME: 35 minutes

3 tablespoons olive oil, divided
½ red onion, spiralized
2 garlic cloves, minced, divided
1 bell pepper, any color, spiralized
1 large zucchini, spiralized
Salt
Freshly ground black pepper
1 teaspoon minced peeled fresh ginger
¼ cup soy sauce
1 pound flank steak

Preheat the oven to 350°F. In a large ovenproof skillet over medium-high heat, heat 1 tablespoon of olive oil. Add the red onion and sauté for 2 to 3 minutes. Add 1 clove of garlic and cook for 1 minute more, then add the bell pepper and zucchini. Season with salt and pepper to taste. Cook for 4 to 5 minutes, then transfer to a bowl and let cool slightly. Return the skillet to the heat and add 1 tablespoon of olive oil and the remaining 1 clove of garlic. Sauté for 1 to 2 minutes and stir in the ginger and the soy sauce. Bring the sauce to a simmer. While the sauce simmers, place the flank steak on a work surface and season with salt and pepper. Spread the veggie noodle mixture over the steak and, starting from one side, roll it tightly, using toothpicks to secure the roll. Pour the soy-ginger sauce into a ramekin and set aside. Return the skillet to the stovetop and turn the heat to high. Add the remaining 1 tablespoon of olive oil to heat. Carefully transfer the steak roll-ups to the skillet and sear for 1 minute per side,

brushing the soy-ginger sauce over the steak as you sear it. Move the pan to the oven and bake for 10 to 15 minutes, until the roll-ups are browned and cooked through when cut into. Remove and let rest for about 5 minutes before slicing and serving.

Per Serving: Calories: 319; Fat: 20g; Protein: 27g; Total Carbs: 8g; Fiber: 2g; Net Carbs: 6g; **Macros:** Fat: 56%; Protein: 35%; Carbs: 9%

Flank Steak with Kale Chimichurri

SERVES 4 | PREP TIME: 15 minutes | COOK TIME: 12 minutes

½ cup olive oil
½ cup finely chopped kale
2 tablespoons finely chopped fresh parsley
2 tablespoons freshly squeezed lime juice
1 tablespoon minced garlic
1 tablespoon finely chopped fresh chili pepper
½ teaspoon sea salt, plus more for seasoning
½ teaspoon freshly ground black pepper, plus more for seasoning
1 pound flank steak

In a medium bowl, stir the olive oil, kale, parsley, lime juice, garlic, chili pepper, salt, and pepper until well combined. Set aside. Preheat the barbecue to medium-high heat. Lightly season both sides of the steak with salt and pepper. Grill the steak 5 to 6 minutes per side for medium-rare. If you do not have a barbecue, preheat the oven to broil and broil the steak until it is the desired doneness, 5 to 6 minutes per side for medium-rare. Let the steak rest for 10 minutes before slicing it thinly across the grain. Serve with the chimichurri.

Per Serving: Calories: 426; Fat: 35g; Protein: 25g; Total Carbs: 2g; Fiber: 0g; Net Carbs: 2g; **Macros:** Fat: 74%; Protein: 23%; Carbs: 3%

Flank Steak with Orange-Herb Pistou

SERVES 4 | PREP TIME: 10 minutes | COOK TIME: 20 minutes

1 pound flank steak
½ cup extra-virgin olive oil, divided
2 teaspoons salt, divided
1 teaspoon freshly ground black pepper, divided
½ cup chopped fresh flat-leaf Italian parsley
¼ cup chopped fresh mint leaves
2 garlic cloves, roughly chopped
Zest and juice of 1 orange or 2 clementines
1 teaspoon red pepper flakes (optional)
1 tablespoon red wine vinegar

Heat the grill to medium-high heat or, if using an oven, preheat to 400°F. Rub the steak with 2 tablespoons of olive oil and sprinkle with 1 teaspoon salt and 1/2 teaspoon pepper. Let sit at room temperature while you make the pistou. In a food processor, combine the parsley, mint, garlic, orange zest and juice, remaining 1 teaspoon salt, red pepper flakes (if using), and remaining 1/2 teaspoon pepper. Pulse until finely chopped. With the processor running, stream in the red wine vinegar and remaining 6 tablespoons olive oil until well combined. This pistou will be more oil-based than traditional basil pesto. Cook the steak on the grill, 6 to 8 minutes per side. Remove from the grill and allow to rest for 10 minutes on a cutting board. If cooking in the oven, heat a large oven-safe skillet (cast iron works great) over high heat. Add the steak and sear, 1 to 2 minutes per side, until browned. Transfer the skillet to the oven and cook 10 to 12 minutes, or until the steak reaches your desired temperature. To serve, slice the steak and drizzle with the pistou.

Per Serving: Calories: 441; Fat: 36g; Protein: 25g; Total Carbs: 3g; Fiber: 0g; Net Carbs: 3g; **Macros:** Fat: 73%; Protein: 24%; Carbs: 3%

Tandoori Beef Fajitas

SERVES 2 | PREP TIME: 5 to 10 minutes (plus 2 to 24 hours marinating time) | COOK TIME: 10 to 15 minutes

½ cup sugar-free Greek yogurt (optional)
2 tablespoons avocado oil
½ teaspoon garlic powder
½ teaspoon ground cumin
½ teaspoon paprika
½ teaspoon ground coriander
¼ teaspoon ground cinnamon
¼ teaspoon ground turmeric
¼ teaspoon cayenne pepper
¼ teaspoon ground ginger
¼ teaspoon erythritol "brown sugar"
Salt
1 pound sirloin or flank steak, sliced into strips

1 tablespoon butter or butter-flavored coconut oil
2 medium bell peppers (any color), sliced
1 medium red onion, sliced
4 ounces button mushrooms, sliced (optional)
8 asparagus spears, trimmed and chopped (optional)
2 to 4 coconut or almond flour wraps or grain-free chips
1 cup shredded romaine lettuce
Sugar-free salsa, sour cream, Guacamole, and shredded cheese, for serving (optional)

In a large resealable plastic bag, combine the Greek yogurt (if using), avocado oil, garlic, cumin, paprika, coriander, cinnamon, turmeric, cayenne, ginger, erythritol and salt. Add the steak, seal the bag tightly, and massage the marinade into the meat. Marinate in the refrigerator for at least 2 hours or up to 24 hours. In a large skillet over medium-high heat, melt the butter. Sauté the bell peppers, onion, mushrooms (if using), and asparagus (if using) for 5 to 8 minutes, or until the onion is translucent. Add the beef strips and marinade to the skillet and stir-fry for 5 to 8 minutes, or until the meat is cooked through. Be sure the marinade boils for at least 1 full minute to kill off any harmful bacteria. Place the wraps or chips on plates and top with shredded lettuce. Top with the beef fajita mixture, then salsa, sour cream, Guacamole, and cheese (if using).

Per Serving: Calories: 655; Fat: 43g; Protein: 51g; Total Carbs: 16g; Fiber: 4g; Net Carbs: 12g; **Macros:** Fat: 60%; Protein: 30%; Carbs: 10%

Pan-Seared Hanger Steak with Easy Herb Cream Sauce

SERVES 4 | PREP TIME: 5 minutes | COOK TIME: 1 hour

1 head garlic
1 pint heavy (whipping) cream
2 to 4 fresh herb sprigs (e.g., tarragon, rosemary)
2 teaspoons salt, divided

1½ pounds hanger steak
1 teaspoon freshly ground black pepper
2 tablespoons olive oil
2 tablespoons unsalted butter

Separate the garlic cloves and crush them with a knife. In a small saucepan, combine the garlic, cream, herbs, and 1 teaspoon of salt. Simmer, uncovered, on low heat for 1 hour, stirring

occasionally. Strain to remove the herbs and garlic. While the sauce is simmering, allow the steak to come to room temperature. Cook the steak when the cream sauce is almost ready. Heat a large, heavy skillet over medium-high heat. Season both sides of the steak with the pepper and the remaining 1 teaspoon of salt. Pour the oil into the hot skillet, then add the steak. Allow it to cook for 4 minutes without lifting or moving it. Turn the steak and add the butter to the pan. Cook the steak for 4 minutes while continuously spooning the melted butter over the top. Transfer to a plate when a thermometer reads 125°F (for medium rare) in the thickest part of the steak. Cover lightly with aluminum foil and allow to rest for 8 to 10 minutes. Thinly slice the steak against the grain. Spoon the cream sauce over the sliced steak.

Per Serving: Calories: 884; Fat: 80g; Protein: 37g; Total Carbs: 5g; Fiber: 0g; Net Carbs: 5g; **Macros:** Fat: 81%; Protein: 17%; Carbs: 2%

Essential New York Strip Steak

SERVES 4 | PREP TIME: 5 minutes | COOK TIME: 10 to 12 minutes

1 tablespoon coconut oil
4 (6-ounce) New York strip steaks
Sea salt
Freshly ground black pepper

¼ cup butter, at room temperature
1 tablespoon minced shallots
1 tablespoon minced rosemary

Preheat the oven to 350°F. Heat a large skillet over medium-high heat. Add the coconut oil. Pat the steaks dry with paper towels and season generously with salt and pepper. Sear the steaks for about 5 minutes, then flip and sear for another 2 minutes before transferring the skillet to the oven. Continue cooking in the oven for about 3 minutes for medium-rare or 5 minutes for medium. While the steak is cooking, make a simple compound butter by mashing together the butter, shallots, and rosemary. To serve, top each steak with a tablespoon of the compound butter.

Per Serving: Calories: 473; Fat: 36g; Protein: 38g; Total Carbs: 1g; Fiber: 0g; Net Carbs: 1g 68%; **Macros:** Fat: 32%; Protein: <1%; Carbs

Grilled Hanger Steak with Cilantro Crema

SERVES 3 | PREP TIME: 15 minutes | COOK TIME: 20 minutes

For the cilantro crema

¼ cup sliced scallions
¼ cup fresh cilantro, chopped
1 garlic clove
1 teaspoon grated lime rind

1½ teaspoons freshly squeezed lime juice
3 tablespoons mayonnaise
3 tablespoons sour cream
¼ teaspoon salt

For the rub

1 teaspoon onion powder
¾ teaspoon salt
½ teaspoon freshly ground black pepper

½ teaspoon garlic powder
¼ teaspoon cumin
¼ teaspoon paprika
⅛ teaspoon ginger

For the steak

1 (1- to 1½-pound) hanger steak

¼ cup butter

In a food processor, add the scallions, cilantro, garlic, lime rind, and lime juice. Pulse until the scallions and cilantro emulsify. Add the mayonnaise, sour cream, and salt. Pulse until combined. Refrigerate until ready to serve. In a small bowl, mix the onion powder, salt, pepper, garlic powder, cumin, paprika, and ginger. Liberally coat the steak with the rub. In a large skillet over medium high heat, heat the butter for about 2 minutes, being careful not to burn it. Add the seasoned steak to the skillet. Sear for 3 minutes on each side for rare; 4 minutes per side for medium-rare. Remove the steak from the pan and tent with aluminum foil. Allow the steak to cool for 7 to 10 minutes before slicing. Serve the sliced steak with the cilantro crema on the side.

Per Serving: Calories: 672; Fat: 51g; Protein: 43g; Total Carbs: 9g; Fiber: 1g; Net Carbs: 8g; **Macros:** Fat: 69%; Protein: 26%; Carbs: 5%

Grilled Sirloin Steak with Herbed Butter

SERVES 4 | PREP TIME: 10 minutes |
COOK TIME: 15 minutes, plus 5 minutes to rest

½ cup (4 ounces) unsalted butter, at room temperature	2 teaspoons minced garlic
	Salt
¼ cup chopped fresh parsley leaves	Freshly ground black pepper
	4 (6-ounce) sirloin steaks

Place the butter in a medium bowl. Add the parsley and garlic. Season with salt and pepper. Mash everything with a fork until well combined. Scoop the herb-butter mixture onto a piece of plastic wrap and shape it into a log about 3 inches long. Wrap the butter securely and twist the ends of the plastic wrap tightly. Place in the refrigerator. Preheat the grill to medium or place a grill pan over medium heat. Season the steaks on both sides with salt and pepper. Grill on one side for 4 to 5 minutes, flip, and grill for another 3 to 5 minutes for medium-rare (internal temperature of 135°F), 5 to 7 minutes for medium (140°F), or 8 to 10 minutes for medium-well (150°F). Let rest for 5 minutes. To serve, slice the hardened butter into ⅓-inch-thick coins and place on the meat.

Per Serving: Calories: 549; Fat: 45g; Protein: 35g; Total Carbs: 1g; Net Carbs: 1g; **Macros:** Fat: 72%; Protein: 28%; Carbs: 0%

Sirloin with Blue Cheese Compound Butter

SERVES 4 | PREP TIME: 10 minutes, plus 1 hour to chilling |
COOK TIME: 12 minutes

6 tablespoons butter, at room temperature	4 (5-ounce) beef sirloin steaks
	1 tablespoon olive oil
4 ounces blue cheese, such as Stilton or Roquefort	Sea salt
	Freshly ground black pepper

Place the butter in a blender and pulse until the butter is whipped, about 2 minutes. Add the cheese and pulse until just incorporated. Spoon the butter mixture onto a sheet of plastic wrap and roll it into a log about 1½ inches in diameter by twisting both ends of the plastic wrap in opposite directions. Refrigerate the butter until completely set, about 1 hour. Slice the butter into ½-inch disks and set them on a plate in the refrigerator until you are ready to serve the steaks. Preheat a

barbecue to medium-high heat. Let the steaks come to room temperature. Rub the steaks all over with the olive oil and season them with salt and pepper. Grill the steaks until they reach your desired doneness, about 6 minutes per side for medium. If you do not have a barbecue, broil the steaks in a preheated oven for 7 minutes per side for medium. Let the steaks rest for 10 minutes. Serve each topped with a disk of the compound butter.

Per Serving: Calories: 544; Fat: 44g; Protein: 35g; Total Carbs: 0g; Fiber: 0g; Net Carbs: 0g; **Macros:** Fat: 72%; Protein: 28%; Carbs: 0%

Sheet Pan Sirloin Steak with Eggplant and Zucchini

SERVES 4 | PREP TIME: 10 minutes | COOK TIME: 10 minutes

1½ pounds sirloin steak, sliced against the grain into 1-inch-thick strips	3 medium zucchini, sliced into ½-inch-thick half-moons
	3 tablespoons olive oil
1 small eggplant (about 12 ounces), cubed	1 teaspoon paprika
	Salt
	Freshly ground black pepper

Preheat the oven to 400°F. Line a large baking sheet with aluminum foil. Place the steak, eggplant, and zucchini on the baking sheet. Drizzle with the oil and sprinkle with the paprika. Season well with salt and pepper. Roast for about 10 minutes for medium-rare (internal temperature of 135°F), 12 to 13 minutes for medium (140°F), or 15 minutes for well-done (165°F).

Per Serving: Calories: 459; Fat: 30g; Protein: 38g; Total Carbs: 10g; Fiber: 4g; Net Carbs: 6g; **Macros:** Fat: 58%; Protein: 34%; Carbs: 8%

Grilled Sirloin Steak, Roasted Red Pepper, and Mozzarella Lettuce Boats

SERVES 6 | PREP TIME: 5 minutes | COOK TIME: 20 minutes, plus 5 minutes to rest

Nonstick cooking spray	1 or 2 roasted red peppers, chopped
6 (6-ounce) sirloin steaks	
Salt	3 scallions white and white parts, chopped
Freshly ground black pepper	
¾ cup shredded mozzarella cheese	12 large romaine lettuce leaves

Coat the grill with cooking spray and preheat to medium-high. Season the steaks with salt and black pepper on both sides. Grill for 4 to 5 minutes, flip, and grill for another 3 to 5 minutes for medium-rare (internal temperature of 135°F), 5 to 7 minutes for medium (140°F), or 8 to 10 minutes for medium-well (150°F). Transfer the steaks to a cutting board and let rest for 5 minutes. Cut into slices, fanning them out so they overlap slightly. Sprinkle the mozzarella over the steak slices and use a wide spatula to return them to the grill. Cook just until the cheese has melted, then transfer to serving plates. In a small serving bowl, combine the roasted red peppers and scallions. Set out the lettuce and red pepper mixture for everyone to make their own wraps.

Per Serving: Calories: 420; Fat: 28g; Protein: 38g; Total Carbs: 3g; Fiber: 1g; Net Carbs: 2g; **Macros:** Fat: 60%; Protein: 38%; Carbs: 2%

Butter-Basted Rib Eye Steaks

SERVES 4 | PREP TIME: 10 minutes, plus 30 minutes to marinate | COOK TIME: 15 minutes

2 (¾-pound) bone-in rib eye steaks	¼ cup butter
Sea salt	1 teaspoon chopped fresh thyme
Freshly ground black pepper	4 garlic cloves, crushed
1 tablespoon olive oil	

Season the rib eye steaks with salt and pepper. Let the steaks sit at room temperature for 30 minutes. Heat the olive oil in a large skillet, over high heat. Pan sear the steaks until brown and crusty on the bottom, 5 to 6 minutes. Flip the steaks and add the butter, thyme, and garlic to the skillet. Cook the steaks, basting with the melted butter, garlic, and herbs, until the steaks are medium-rare, 6 to 8 minutes more. Let the steaks rest 10 minutes on a cutting board and slice them across the grain.

Per Serving: Calories: 474; Fat: 44g; Protein: 39g; Total Carbs: 1g; Fiber: 0g; Net Carbs: 1g; **Macros:** Fat: 84%; Protein: 33%; Carbs: 1%

Cast-Iron Blackened Rib Eye with Parmesan Roasted Radishes

SERVES 4 | PREP TIME: 20 minutes | COOK TIME: 1 hour

For the roasted radishes

3 (6-ounce) bags fresh radishes, trimmed and halved	¼ teaspoon freshly ground black pepper
3 tablespoons avocado oil or bacon drippings	½ cup shredded Parmesan cheese, plus more for garnish
1 teaspoon kosher salt	
½ teaspoon garlic powder	Chopped fresh parsley, for garnish
¼ teaspoon paprika	

For the steaks

2 (1-pound) 1½-inch-thick rib eye steaks, at room temperature	2 teaspoons garlic powder
	1½ teaspoons kosher salt
	3 tablespoons butter
2 to 4 tablespoons blackening seasoning	

Preheat the oven to 400°F. Line a baking sheet with parchment paper. Add the radishes, avocado oil, salt, garlic powder, paprika, and pepper and toss to coat. Spread into an even layer. Roast for 30 to 35 minutes, stirring once halfway through. Evenly sprinkle the radishes with the Parmesan cheese. Roast for 5 minutes more. Transfer to a serving dish and top with more Parmesan cheese and garnish with parsley. Set aside. Leave the oven on. Liberally season both sides of the steaks with blackening seasoning, garlic powder, and salt. Let rest for 10 minutes. While the steaks rest, preheat a large heavy cast-iron skillet over medium-high heat and turn on your overhead vent. In the hot skillet, melt the butter. As soon as it melts, put the steaks in the skillet. Cook for 2 to 3 minutes on the first side until browned. Flip the steaks and transfer the skillet to the oven. Cook to your desired doneness. For rare, cook for 5 to 7 minutes to an internal temperature of 125°F. For medium-rare, cook for 8 to 9 minutes to an internal temperature of 130°F to 135°F. For medium to medium-well, cook for 8 to 10 minutes to an internal

temperature of 145°F to 150°F. Remove the steaks from the pan, cover loosely with aluminum foil, and let rest for 10 minutes. Serve with the roasted radishes.

Per Serving: Calories: 852; Fat: 72g; Protein: 46g; Total Carbs: 5g; Fiber: 2g; Net Carbs: 3g; **Macros:** Fat: 76%; Protein: 22%; Carbs: 2%

Rib Eye Steaks with Garlic-Thyme Butter

SERVES 4 | PREP TIME: 15 minutes, plus 30 minutes to marinate | COOK TIME: 10 minutes

4 (6-ounce) rib eye steaks, about 1 inch thick	Freshly ground black pepper
	2 tablespoons salted butter
2 tablespoons extra-virgin olive oil	2 teaspoons minced garlic
	2 teaspoons chopped fresh thyme
Sea salt	

Preheat the barbecue or grill pan to medium-high. Rub the steaks all over with the olive oil, and season the meat on both sides with salt and pepper. Set aside for 30 minutes at room temperature. Grill the steaks for 4 minutes per side for medium rare, or until desired doneness is reached. Remove the steaks to a plate, and let them rest for 10 minutes. While the steaks are resting, in a small skillet over medium-high heat, melt the butter. Sauté the garlic and thyme for 2 minutes. Top the steaks topped with the butter sauce and serve.

Per Serving: Calories: 581; Fat: 45g; Protein: 30g; Total Carbs: 2g; Fiber: 0g; Net Carbs: 2g; **Macros:** Fat: 76%; Protein: 22%; Carbs: 2%

Chipotle Coffee-Crusted Bone-In Rib Eye

SERVES 2 | PREP TIME: 5 minutes | COOK TIME: 20 minutes

1 teaspoon finely ground coffee	¼ teaspoon salt
	¼ teaspoon freshly ground black pepper
¾ teaspoon chipotle powder	
½ teaspoon unsweetened cocoa powder	⅛ teaspoon ground cinnamon
	1 (12- to 14-ounce) bone-in rib eye steak
¼ teaspoon onion powder	
¼ teaspoon garlic powder	2 tablespoons butter

In a medium bowl, mix the coffee, chipotle powder, cocoa powder, onion powder, garlic powder, salt, pepper, and cinnamon. On a parchment-covered cutting board, coat the steak completely with the rub, being sure to get the rub deep into the meat. Wrap the steak in the parchment paper and refrigerate to marinate for at least 1 hour. In a large oven-safe skillet over medium-high heat, melt the butter for 90 seconds. Add the steak to the skillet and sear it for 5 to 7 minutes per side for medium-rare. Remove the steak from the skillet and rest for at least 5 minutes.

Per Serving: Calories: 666; Fat: 59.9g; Total Carbs: 1.6g; Net Carbs: 0.9g; Fiber: 0.7g; Protein: 27.5g; **Macros:** Fat: 82%; Protein: 17%; Carbs: 1%

Rib Eye Steak with Anchovy Compound Butter

SERVES 4 | PREP TIME: 15 minutes, plus time to chill time | COOK TIME: 10 minutes

¼ cup unsalted butter, at room temperature	4 anchovies packed in oil, drained and minced
	1 teaspoon minced garlic

½ teaspoon freshly squeezed lemon juice

4 (4-ounce) rib eye steaks

Sea salt

Freshly ground black pepper

In a small bowl, stir the butter, anchovies, garlic, and lemon juice until well blended. Chill the butter in the refrigerator until you are ready to use it. Let the steaks come to room temperature. Season the steaks with salt and pepper. Preheat the grill to medium-high heat. Grill the steak until the desired doneness, 5 minutes per side for medium-rare. Let the steaks rest for 10 minutes and serve topped with the anchovy butter.

Per Serving: Calories: 446; Fat: 38g; Protein: 26g; Total Carbs: 0g; Fiber: 0g; Net Carbs: 0g; **Macros:** Fat: 76%; Protein: 24%; Carbs: 0%

Classic Prime Rib au Jus

SERVES 8 | PREP TIME: 15 minutes, plus overnight to chill | COOK TIME: 2 hours 40 minutes

For the meat

6-pound bone-in beef rib roast, tied, untrimmed

1 teaspoon salt

½ teaspoon freshly ground black pepper

For the horseradish sauce

1½ cups sour cream

⅓ cup prepared horseradish

5 teaspoons Dijon mustard

½ teaspoon salt

¼ teaspoon freshly ground black pepper

Chives, for garnish

For the jus

¼ cup red wine

2 tablespoons Worcestershire sauce

2 cups beef bone broth

The night before cooking, unpackage the meat, place it on a baking sheet lined with parchment paper, and place the sheet in the refrigerator, uncovered, to dry out overnight. A half hour before you plan to cook your prime rib, remove it from the refrigerator. Season it with salt and pepper, and allow it to come to room temperature. In a small bowl, combine the sour cream, horseradish, Dijon mustard, salt, and pepper. Cover and place in the refrigerator. Preheat the oven to 500°F. Place the prime rib on a rack in a roasting pan, fat-side up. To figure out how long to roast your meat, multiply the weight of your prime rib by 5, and this will be the roasting time. So for a 6-pound roast, you'll want to cook it for 30 minutes. Place the pan in the oven, and set the timer for the roasting time. When the timer goes off, turn off the oven, and don't open the oven door for at least 2 hours. After 2 hours, remove the meat from the oven to let it rest while you make the jus. Take the horseradish sauce out of the refrigerator, and allow it to come to room temperature. Garnish with the chives. Pour the drippings and browned bits from the pan into a medium saucepan over medium heat. Bring it to a simmer and whisk in the wine and Worcestershire sauce. Return to a simmer, and pour in the beef broth. Return to a simmer once again, stirring; then turn down the heat, and let it reduce, stirring occasionally, for a few minutes, until reduced by about half. Remove from heat and pour it through a strainer into a bowl, using the back of a spoon

to help mash it through. Carve the prime rib, and serve with jus and horseradish sauce.

Per Serving: (6 ounces meat and jus and horseradish sauce): Calories: 386; Fat: 16g; Protein: 53g; Total Carbs: 5g; Fiber: 0g; Net Carbs: 5g; **Macros:** Fat: 37%; Protein: 55%; Carbs: 8%

Garlic Studded Prime Rib with Thyme au Jus

SERVES 6-8 | PREP TIME: 10 minutes | COOK TIME: 2 hours

1 (6- to 7-pound) bone-in prime rib

8 garlic cloves, thinly sliced

2 tablespoons salt

¼ cup red wine vinegar

4 cups beef broth

1 tablespoon fresh thyme, chopped

Bring the prime rib to room temperature. Preheat the oven to 350°F. Make small slits in the prime rib and stuff each slit with a slice of garlic. Season the prime rib liberally with salt and place it on a rack that is set inside of a roasting pan. Roast the prime rib for about 2 hours or until the internal temperature reaches 130°F. Remove the prime rib to a large platter and tent it with foil to keep it warm while you make the au jus. Place the roasting pan with the rack removed over two stove burners set to high heat. Add the vinegar to the drippings in the pan and cook over high heat, scraping the bottom of the pan with a wooden spoon until the sauce is reduced. Add the stock and cook until it is reduced by half. Whisk in the thyme and season the sauce with salt to taste. Pour the au jus over the beef.

Bacon-Wrapped Beef Tenderloin

SERVES 4 | PREP TIME: 10 minutes | COOK TIME: 20 minutes

4 (4-ounce) beef tenderloin steaks

Sea salt

Freshly ground black pepper

12 bacon slices

2 tablespoons extra-virgin olive oil

Preheat the oven to 450°F. Pat the steaks dry with paper towels, and season them on all sides with salt and pepper. Wrap each steak with 3 slices of bacon around the edges, overlapping the strips, and secure the bacon with toothpicks. In a large skillet over medium-high heat, heat the olive oil. Sear the steaks on each side for 4 minutes. Place the steaks on a baking tray, and roast them in the oven for 5 to 6 minutes for medium doneness. Remove the steaks from the oven, and let the meat rest for 10 minutes. Remove the toothpicks, and serve.

Per Serving: Calories: 396; Fat: 25g; Protein: 40g; Total Carbs: 0g; Fiber: 0g; Net Carbs: 0g; **Macros:** Fat: 58%; Protein: 42%; Carbs: 0%

Rosemary Roasted Beef Tenderloin

SERVES 4 | PREP TIME: 5 minutes | COOK TIME: 30 to 35 minutes

1 (1¼-pound) beef tenderloin

Sea salt

Freshly ground black pepper

2 sprigs fresh rosemary

1 tablespoon coconut oil

Preheat the oven to 350°F. Heat a large ovenproof skillet over medium-high heat until hot, about 2 minutes. While the pan heats, season the beef generously on all sides with salt and pepper. Place the rosemary sprigs on the beef and secure them with kitchen twine. Add the oil to the skillet and tilt to coat the pan in the oil. Sear the tenderloin until it is browned on all sides, about 10 minutes. Transfer the pan to the oven and finish roasting for 20 to 25 minutes until the beef is cooked through to an internal temperature of 145°F for medium-rare. For medium, cook an additional 3 to 5 minutes. For medium-well, cook an additional 8 to 10 minutes. Allow to rest for 10 minutes after you remove it from the oven.

Per Serving: Calories: 382; Fat: 30g; Protein: 28g; Total Carbs: 0g; Fiber: 0g; Net Carbs: 0g; **Macros:** Fat: 71%; Protein: 29%; Carbs: 4%

Beef Stew

SERVES 6 | PREP TIME: 10 minutes | COOK TIME: 2 hours 25 minutes

1 tablespoon olive oil	1 garlic clove, minced
2 pounds beef stew meat	1 teaspoon dried thyme
1½ teaspoons sea salt, divided	4 cups beef broth
¼ teaspoon freshly ground black pepper	1 bay leaf
	1½ cups chopped cauliflower florets
⅓ cup diced white onion	1 cup sliced zucchini
1 cup sliced celery	

Heat the oil in a large stockpot over medium-high heat. Season the beef with 1 teaspoon of salt and the pepper. Add half the meat to the pot and brown on all sides. Transfer to a bowl. Repeat with the remaining meat. Set aside. Keeping the beef fat in the pot, stir in the onion and celery. Cook for 5 to 6 minutes until the onion is translucent. Stir in the garlic, remaining ½ teaspoon of salt, and the thyme and cook for 1 more minute. Add the beef, broth, and bay leaf. Scrape the bottom of the pot to loosen the browned bits. Bring the mixture to a boil and then reduce the heat to low. Cover and cook, stirring occasionally, for 90 minutes or until the beef is tender. Add the cauliflower and zucchini. Stir well to incorporate. Cover and cook, stirring occasionally, for another 30 minutes. Remove and discard the bay leaf. Ladle ½ cup of broth with vegetables into a blender. Blend on high until smooth. Return it to the stew and cook for an additional 5 minutes. Serve immediately.

Per Serving: (1 cup): Calories: 549; Fat: 42g; Protein: 38g; Total Carbs: 4g; Fiber: 1g; Net Carbs: 3g; **Macros:** Fat: 69%; Protein: 28%; Carbs: 3%

Beef Bourguignon Stew

SERVES 6 | PREP TIME: 20 minutes | COOK TIME: 2 hours

8 ounces bacon, cut into 1-inch pieces	3 cups beef broth or bone broth
3 pounds beef chuck, cut into 1-inch cubes	2 cups red wine
	½ teaspoon xanthan gum
2 medium carrots, thinly sliced (¼-inch thick)	2 tablespoons butter
1 small white onion, chopped	1 cup sliced white button mushrooms, cut in half
3 garlic cloves, minced	Chopped chives, for garnish
2 teaspoons tomato paste	

Preheat the oven to 375°F. In a large Dutch oven or ovenproof pot over medium heat, cook the bacon until crispy. Transfer to paper towels to drain, reserving the grease in the pan. Increase the heat to medium-high, and place a plate lined with paper towels next to the stove. Working in small batches, place the chuck cubes in the Dutch oven with the bacon grease, and sear on each side. Transfer to the plate with the paper towels. Reduce the heat to medium, add the carrots and onion to the pot, and cook, stirring, for 3 minutes. If the bottom of the pan is dark or crusty, add a tablespoon or two of water, and scrape up the bits. Stir in the garlic and tomato paste, and then add the broth, wine, and xanthan gum. Stir for 2 minutes, and add the bacon and beef back to the pot. Cover and place in the oven for 1½ hours, stirring every 30 minutes. About 15 minutes before the stew is done, in a small skillet over medium heat, melt the butter. Add the mushrooms, sauté for about 5 minutes, or until soft, and then set aside. Serve the stew topped with the mushrooms and chives.

Per Serving: (1½ cups): Calories: 582; Fat: 30g; Protein: 56g; Total Carbs: 8.5g; Fiber: 1g; Net Carbs: 7.5g; **Macros:** Fat: 51%; Protein: 42%; Carbs: 7%

Beef Taco Stew

SERVES 4 | PREP TIME: 5 minutes | COOK TIME: 25 minutes

1 tablespoon olive oil	1 cup tomato sauce
1 pound ground beef	2 teaspoons paprika
2 cups beef broth	2 teaspoons ground cumin
4 ounces cream cheese	1 teaspoon onion powder
1 orange bell pepper, seeded and finely chopped	Salt
	Freshly ground black pepper

In a stockpot, heat the oil over medium heat. Add the ground beef and cook, breaking apart with a wooden spoon, for about 10 minutes, or until browned all over. Drain off any excess fat to prevent the soup from being oily. Add the broth, cream cheese, bell pepper, tomato sauce, paprika, cumin, and onion powder. Stir well, then bring to a boil. Reduce to a simmer and cook for 10 minutes, or until the cream cheese is thoroughly melted and the soup has thickened. Season with salt and black pepper to taste. Pour the soup into bowls and serve with garnishes of choice.

Per Serving: Calories: 423; Fat: 31g; Protein: 27g; Total Carbs: 10g; Fiber: 2g; Net Carbs: 8g; **Macros:** Fat: 65%; Protein: 26%; Carbs: 9%

Beef Pot Roast

SERVES 6 | PREP TIME: 15 minutes | COOK TIME: 5 hours

3 tablespoons olive oil, divided	1 cup quartered radishes
½ tablespoon sea salt, plus 2 teaspoons, divided	1 cup large cauliflower florets
	3 cups beef broth
1 teaspoon dried thyme	1 tablespoon Worcestershire sauce
1 teaspoon onion powder	
½ teaspoon freshly ground black pepper	3 garlic cloves, minced
	¼ cup heavy (whipping) cream
3 pounds beef chuck roast, fat untrimmed	1 tablespoon Dijon mustard
½ small white onion, quartered	¼ teaspoon cream of tartar
2 celery stalks, quartered	

Preheat the oven to 425°F. Place a skillet over high heat. In a small bowl, combine 2 tablespoons of oil, ½ tablespoon of salt, thyme, onion powder, and pepper. Coat the roast all over with the mixture. Place the roast in the hot skillet and sear until lightly browned on all sides, about 4 minutes per side. Set aside. In a roasting dish, toss the onion, celery, radishes, and cauliflower with the remaining 2 teaspoons of salt and 1 tablespoon of oil. Place the roast directly on top of the vegetables. In another bowl, whisk the broth, Worcestershire, and garlic. Pour the mixture over the meat and vegetables. Cover the roasting dish with enough aluminum foil so none of the meat or vegetables are visible. Roast for 30 minutes. Remove the roast and reduce the heat to 300°F. Keep it covered in foil. When the temperature is 300°F, return the roast to the oven and cook for 4 hours. The meat is done when it is tender enough to be shredded with a fork. Let the roast sit at room temperature while you prepare the gravy. Ladle 2 cups of cooking liquid into a large saucepan over medium-high heat. Whisk in the cream and then the mustard. Sprinkle in the cream of tartar and whisk vigorously. Bring to a boil; then reduce the heat to medium low and simmer for 6 to 7 minutes or until reduced and thickened. To serve, transfer the roast and vegetables to a large platter and slice the meat. Pour the gravy directly on top of the meat and vegetables.

Per Serving: (⅙ recipe): Calories: 663; Fat: 50g; Protein: 46g; Total Carbs: 4g; Fiber: 1g; Net Carbs: 3g; **Macros:** Fat: 68%; Protein: 28%; Carbs: 4%

Pot Roast with Turnips and Radishes

SERVES 6 | PREP TIME: 35 minutes | COOK TIME: 7 hours

1 (4- to 5-pound) bottom round rump roast	3 cups beef stock, divided
¾ teaspoon salt	2 garlic cloves
½ teaspoon freshly ground black pepper	2 fresh thyme sprigs
3 tablespoons olive oil	2 turnips, peeled, roughly chopped
1 onion, quartered	2 cups radishes, halved
	¼ cup heavy (whipping) cream

Preheat the oven to 475°F. Season the roast with the salt and pepper. In a large Dutch oven over medium-high heat, heat the olive oil for 1 minute. Brown the roast on all sides, about 3 minutes per side. Once browned, remove it and set aside. Add the onion to the pot and brown for about 3 minutes, stirring. Remove the onion. Set them aside with the roast. Pour ½ cup of beef stock into the pot, scraping the bottom of the pan to loosen any browned bits. Add the remaining 2½ cups of beef stock, the garlic, and thyme to the pot. Whisk to combine. Add the roast and onion back into the pot. Place the turnips and radishes in the pot, surrounding the roast. Place the pot, uncovered, into the preheated oven. Immediately reduce the heat to 400°F and cook for 6 to 6½ hours, or until the internal temperature reaches 130°F. Remove the roast from the oven and allow it to cool for 2 to 3 minutes. Transfer the roast and vegetables to a dish. Into a large saucepan over medium-high heat, pour the remaining liquid from the Dutch oven. Add the heavy cream. Bring the liquid to a boil. Reduce the heat to medium and let the sauce

reduce for 4 to 5 minutes. Serve with the reduced sauce and vegetables.

Per Serving: Calories: 521; Fat: 25g; Protein: 69g; Total Carbs: 6g; Fiber: 2g; Net Carbs: 4g; **Macros:** Fat: 43%; Protein: 53%; Carbs: 4%

Spiced-Up Sunday Pot Roast and Sautéed Squash

SERVES 8 | PREP TIME: 20 minutes | COOK TIME: 4 hours

For the roast

2 teaspoons chili powder	1 green bell pepper, diced
1½ teaspoons kosher salt	3 garlic cloves, smashed
1 teaspoon ground cumin	1 canned chipotle pepper in adobo, seeded and finely diced
1 teaspoon garlic powder	
½ teaspoon freshly ground black pepper	5 tablespoons adobo sauce, from the can
1 (3½-pound) boneless chuck roast	½ cups beef stock or bone broth
2 tablespoons avocado oil	
1 onion, diced	

For the squash

3 tablespoons butter	1 teaspoon kosher salt
⅓ cup diced purple onion	½ teaspoon ground cumin
2 garlic cloves, finely chopped	¼ teaspoon paprika
4 Mexican calabacitas or zucchini, diced	Crumbled queso fresco cheese, for garnish

Preheat the oven to 325°F. In a small bowl, stir the chili powder, salt, cumin, garlic powder, and pepper. Rub the roast all over with the spices. In a large Dutch oven over medium-high heat, heat the avocado oil. Add the roast and cook for about 3 minutes per side until browned. Add the onion, bell pepper, garlic, chipotle pepper, adobo sauce, and beef stock. Tightly cover the pan. Bake for 3½ to 4 hours, or until tender. Remove the roast from the pan. Carefully transfer the pan juices and vegetables into a saucepan. Skim off the fat, if desired, and simmer over medium-low heat for 10 to 12 minutes until reduced. Carefully pour the reduced juices into a blender and blend until smooth. In a large sauté pan or skillet over medium-high heat, melt the butter. Add the onion and sauté for about 5 minutes, or until translucent. Add the garlic and cook for 1 minute more. Add the squash, salt, cumin, and paprika. Reduce the heat to medium and sauté for 5 to 7 minutes, or until tender. Serve the roast over the squash and top with gravy and queso fresco.

Per Serving: Calories: 410; Fat: 22g; Protein: 43g; Total Carbs: 10g; Fiber: 3g; Net Carbs: 7g; **Macros:** Fat: 48%; Protein: 42%; Carbs: 10%

Braised Beef Short Ribs

SERVES 4 | PREP TIME: 10 minutes | COOK TIME: 2 hours, 15 minutes

1 tablespoon coconut oil	1 onion, diced
4 beef short ribs (about 1¼ pounds)	2 garlic cloves, minced
	4 ounces red wine
Sea salt	4 cups beef bone broth
Freshly ground pepper	1 tablespoon minced fresh oregano
2 carrots, diced	
2 celery stalks, diced	

| 2 tablespoons minced fresh parsley | Zest of 1 lemon |
| 1 scallion, white and green parts minced | 2 packed cups leafy greens, such as lettuce |

Preheat the oven to 325°F. Heat a large ovenproof skillet over medium-high heat. Add the coconut oil. Pat the short ribs dry with paper towels. Season generously with salt and pepper. When the oil is hot, season the short ribs liberally with salt and pepper. Sear them on all sides in the pan until well browned, about 10 minutes. Deglaze the pan with the red wine, scraping up any browned bits. Add the carrots, celery, onion, garlic, and beef broth, and bring to a simmer. Return the short ribs to the pan, and cover with a lid. Transfer to the oven and bake for 2 hours, until the meat is meltingly tender. While the meat cooks, in a small dish, mix the oregano, parsley, scallion, and lemon zest. Set aside. Transfer the vegetables to serving dishes. Carefully return the skillet to the stove and simmer the sauce over medium heat until reduced to about 1 cup of liquid, about 5 minutes. Remove the bones from the short ribs and place the meat on top of the vegetables. Pour the pan sauce over the top. Garnish with the fresh lettuce and the lemon herb mixture.

Per Serving: Calories: 774; Fat: 65g; Protein: 30g; Total Carbs: 10g; Fiber: 4g; Net Carbs: 6g; **Macros:** Fat: 81%; Protein: 15%; Carbs: 4%

Slow-Cooked Shredded Beef

SERVES 4 TO 5 | PREP TIME: 10 minutes | COOK TIME: 6 hours

2 pounds beef chuck roast	1 teaspoon paprika
2 teaspoons salt	1 teaspoon oregano
1 teaspoon freshly ground black pepper	3 tablespoons avocado oil
1 teaspoon garlic powder	1 onion, quartered
1 teaspoon onion powder	2 garlic cloves, peeled
	1½ cups beef broth

Preheat the oven to 275°F. Put the beef chuck roast in a large bowl and add the salt, pepper, garlic and onion powders, paprika, and oregano. Massage with your hands to coat the roast completely with the seasonings. In an oven-safe Dutch oven, heat the oil over medium-high heat. Add the roast and brown on all sides, 3 to 5 minutes per side. Add the onion, garlic, and broth, cover the Dutch oven, transfer to the oven, and cook for about 6 hours, or until fork-tender. Remove the roast from the pot, transfer to a cutting board, and use two forks to shred the meat. Transfer the meat back to the pot and toss with the broth.

Per Serving: Calories: 480; Fat: 36g; Protein: 34g; Total Carbs: 5g; Fiber: 1g; Net Carbs: 4g; **Macros:** Fat: 68%; Protein: 28%; Carbs: 4%

Garlic Braised Short Ribs

SERVES 4 | PREP TIME: 10 minutes | COOK TIME: 2 hours, 20 minutes

4 (4-ounce) beef short ribs	½ cup dry red wine
Sea salt	3 cups beef stock
Freshly ground black pepper	
1 tablespoon olive oil	
2 teaspoons minced garlic	

Preheat the oven to 325°F. Season the beef ribs on all sides with salt and pepper. Place a deep ovenproof skillet over medium-high heat and add the olive oil. Sear the ribs on all sides until browned, about 6 minutes in total. Transfer the ribs to a plate. Add the garlic to the skillet and sauté until translucent, about 3 minutes. Whisk in the red wine to deglaze the pan. Be sure to scrape all the browned bits from the meat from the bottom of the pan. Simmer the wine until it is slightly reduced, about 2 minutes. Add the beef stock, ribs, and any accumulated juices on the plate back to the skillet and bring the liquid to a boil. Cover the skillet and place it in the oven to braise the ribs until the meat is fall-off-the-bone tender, about 2 hours. Serve the ribs with a spoonful of the cooking liquid drizzled over each serving.

Per Serving: Calories: 481; Fat: 38g; Protein: 29g; Total Carbs: 5g; Fiber: 3g; Net Carbs: 2g; **Macros:** Fat: 70%; Protein: 25%; Carbs: 5%

Brisket Nachos

SERVES 4 | PREP TIME: 20 minutes | COOK TIME: 2 hours

1 pound beef brisket	¾ cup beef bone broth
3 tablespoons avocado oil, divided	1 medium celery root, or rutabaga, sliced into ¼-inch-thick rounds
1½ teaspoons red pepper flakes	1 medium onion, sliced into strips
1½ teaspoons salt	Fresh spinach leaves, for serving (optional)
1½ teaspoons garlic powder	Sugar-free barbecue sauce, shredded Cheddar cheese, and diced avocado, for topping (optional)
1½ teaspoons onion powder	
1½ teaspoons erythritol brown sugar	
1 teaspoon freshly ground black pepper	
1 teaspoon mustard	

Preheat the oven to 350°F. Rub the brisket all over with 1 tablespoon of oil and season with the red pepper flakes, salt, garlic powder, onion powder, erythritol, pepper, and mustard. Place the meat in a roasting pan with a rack and roast for 30 minutes. Remove the brisket from the oven and add the bone broth. Cover with aluminum foil, return to the oven, and continue to roast for 1 hour and 30 minutes, or until the meat is fork-tender. Meanwhile, make your "chips." Put the celery root on a baking sheet and rub with 1 tablespoon of avocado oil. Roast in the oven for about 35 minutes, turning once, until browned on both sides. When the brisket has about 10 minutes left to cook, in a large skillet, heat the remaining 1 tablespoon of avocado oil over medium-high heat. Add the onion and sauté for about 5 minutes, or until translucent. Slice the brisket into thin strips. Put the vegetable chips on a serving plate. Top with some spinach leaves (if using) and the brisket. If desired, drizzle with barbecue sauce and top with cheese and diced avocado.

Per Serving: Calories: 326; Fat: 22g; Protein: 25g; Total Carbs: 7g; Fiber: 2g; Net Carbs: 5g; Erythritol: 2g; **Macros:** Fat: 61%; Protein: 30%; Carbs: 9%

Bacon and Egg Cheeseburgers

SERVES 8 | PREP TIME: 15 minutes, plus 2 hours to chill | COOK TIME: 25 minutes

4 pounds ground beef

1 teaspoon salt

1 teaspoon freshly ground black pepper

2 tablespoons olive oil, for brushing the burgers

8 large (deli-sliced) slices cheddar cheese

Butter or nonstick cooking spray, for greasing

8 large eggs

8 bacon slices cooked until crispy

Paprika, for garnish

In a large bowl, mix the ground beef, salt, and pepper. Divide the ground beef into 8 sections, roll each into a ball and pat into a ³/₄-inch-thick patty. Press your thumb in the middle of each patty to make a divot, and place on a tray. Cover with plastic wrap or foil, and refrigerate for at least 2 hours or up to overnight. When ready to cook, heat the grill to high. Brush the burgers with the olive oil on both sides. Cook on the first side for 3 minutes, and then flip and cook 4 more minutes. Add the slices of cheese, and then cook another minute. For medium-rare, cook 1 minute less, and for well done, cook 1 minute more. While the burgers are cooking, generously grease a standard muffin pan with butter or nonstick spray, and crack an egg into 8 of the muffin holes. Place the muffin pan on the grill after you flip the burger and cook for 2 minutes; then remove from heat. Plate the cheeseburgers, and top each one with a slice of crispy bacon. Use a spoon to scoop the eggs out of the muffin pan, and place one on top of each burger. Garnish with paprika, and serve.

Per Serving: Calories: 616; Fat: 42g; Protein: 55g; Total Carbs: 0g; Fiber: 0g; Net Carbs: 0g; **Macros:** Fat: 63%; Protein: 37%; Carbs: 0%

Beef Burgers with Bacon

SERVES 2 TO 4 | PREP TIME: 10 minutes | COOK TIME: 30 minutes

2 sugar-free bacon slices

1 pound ground beef

½ teaspoon onion powder

½ teaspoon garlic powder

½ teaspoon nutmeg

½ teaspoon dried sage

¼ teaspoon dried oregano or marjoram

Salt

Freshly ground black pepper

4 to 8 thick cabbage leaves

Sliced cheese, for serving (optional)

Sliced tomato and raw or grilled onion slices, for serving (optional)

2 to 4 fried eggs, for serving (optional)

Chipotle-lime or plain mayonnaise (optional)

In a large skillet over medium-high heat, fry the bacon to your desired doneness, flipping once, 5 to 8 minutes. Remove the bacon from the skillet, let cool, then chop. In a large bowl, combine the ground beef with the bacon pieces, onion and garlic powders, nutmeg, sage, and oregano. Season with salt and pepper. Mix until well combined, then form into burger patties. Place the large skillet over medium-high heat, cook the burgers to your desired doneness, 3 to 4 minutes per side for medium-rare. Place a thick piece of cabbage or two on each serving plate, then top with a burger. Top with cheese, tomato, and onion slices. Top your burger with a fried egg, if desired. Slather

the remaining cabbage leaves with mayonnaise (if using), then sandwich everything together and enjoy.

Per Serving: Calories: 413; Fat: 33g; Protein: 26g; Total Carbs: 3g; Fiber: 1g; Net Carbs: 2g; **Macros:** Fat: 72%; Protein: 25%; Carbs: 3%

Loaded Burgers

SERVES 4 | PREP TIME: 5 minutes | COOK TIME: 20 minutes

1 tablespoon canola oil

1 yellow onion, halved and thinly sliced

Pinch salt

¼ cup mayonnaise

2 tablespoons ketchup

1 teaspoon adobo sauce from canned chipotles

1 pound ground beef

Sea salt

Freshly ground black pepper

1 head iceberg or butter lettuce

1 beefsteak tomato, cut into 4 thick slices

Heat the canola oil in a large skillet over medium heat. Cook the onion with a pinch of salt until soft and browned, about 20 minutes. While the onion cooks, whisk the mayonnaise, ketchup, and adobo sauce in a small measuring cup. Preheat an outdoor grill or a grill pan to medium heat. Shape the ground beef into 4 patties. Season generously with salt and pepper. Grill for 4 minutes on each side for medium-rare, or longer depending on your desired level of doneness. Break apart the lettuce into 8 large leaves. Top each leaf with a burger patty, followed by a spoonful of the chipotle mayonnaise, a slice of tomato, and the caramelized onions. Top with the remaining lettuce leaf.

Per Serving: Calories: 425; Fat: 35g; Protein: 21g; Total Carbs: 8g; Fiber: 1g; Net Carbs: 7g; **Macros:** Fat: 74%; Protein: 20%; Carbs: 6%

Grilled Burgers with Basil Aioli

SERVES 4 | PREP TIME: 10 minutes | COOK TIME: 10 minutes

For the basil aioli

½ cup avocado-oil mayonnaise

2 tablespoons basil pesto

For the burgers

⅓ cup balsamic vinegar

½ cup avocado oil

2 garlic cloves, minced

4 portabella mushroom caps, stems and gills removed, caps cleaned with damp paper towel

1 pound ground beef

1 avocado, sliced

In a small bowl, mix the mayonnaise and basil pesto until well combined. Set aside. In a large bowl, whisk the balsamic vinegar, oil, and garlic. Add the mushroom caps to the bowl and gently toss to coat fully in the marinade. Let sit for 10 minutes. Form the ground beef into 4 patties. Heat a grill or grill pan to medium heat. Grill the burger patties and mushroom caps for 5 minutes on one side, then flip and grill for another 5 minutes. Spread 1 teaspoon of aioli on each grilled mushroom cap then place the burgers on top. Divide the remaining aioli on each burger patty and top with sliced avocado.

Per Serving: Calories: 613; Fat: 49g; Protein: 33g; Total Carbs: 10g; Fiber: 4g; Net Carbs: 6g; **Macros:** Fat: 72%; Protein: 22%; Carbs: 6%

Classic Meatloaf

SERVES 6 | PREP TIME: 20 minutes | COOK TIME: 1 hour 10 minutes

⅓ cup tomato sauce

2 tablespoons brown sugar alternative

1 tablespoon avocado oil

1 teaspoon Dijon mustard

1 tablespoon olive oil

⅓ cup chopped white onion

1 garlic clove, minced

20 ounces ground beef

1 teaspoon sea salt

1 teaspoon dried parsley

¼ teaspoon freshly ground black pepper

1 large egg, beaten

2 tablespoons melted butter

2 teaspoons Worcestershire sauce

¾ cup crushed pork rinds

¼ cup grated Parmesan cheese

Preheat the oven to 350°F. Line a baking sheet with parchment paper. In a small bowl, whisk the tomato sauce, brown sugar alternative, avocado oil, and mustard. Heat the olive oil in a large skillet over medium heat. Add the onion and cook until translucent, 3 to 5 minutes. Stir in the garlic and cook for 1 more minute. Set aside. In a large bowl, combine the beef, salt, parsley, pepper, egg, butter, Worcestershire, and cooked onion and garlic. Add the pork rinds and Parmesan and gently combine. Transfer the mixture to the prepared baking sheet. Shape it into a loaf and slightly flatten the top. Bake for 40 minutes, remove from the oven, and spoon the tomato sauce mixture on top. Bake for an additional 20 to 25 minutes. Let cool for 5 minutes before serving. Refrigerate leftovers for up to 5 days.

Per Serving: (1 slice): Calories: 376; Fat: 27g; Protein: 29g; Total Carbs: 7g; Fiber: <1g; Net Carbs: 6g; Macros: Fat: 65%; Protein: 31%; Carbs: 4%

Italian Beef Burgers

SERVES 4 | PREP TIME: 10 minutes | COOK TIME: 12 minutes

1 pound 75-percent lean ground beef

¼ cup ground almonds

2 tablespoons chopped fresh basil

1 teaspoon minced garlic

¼ teaspoon sea salt

1 tablespoon olive oil

1 tomato, cut into 4 thick slices

¼ sweet onion, sliced thinly

In a medium bowl, mix the ground beef, ground almonds, basil, garlic, and salt until well mixed. Form the beef mixture into four equal patties and flatten them to about ½ inch thick. Place a large skillet on medium-high heat and add the olive oil. Panfry the burgers until cooked through, flipping them once, about 12 minutes in total. Pat away any excess grease with paper towels and serve the burgers with a slice of tomato and onion.

Per Serving: Calories: 441; Fat: 37g; Protein: 22g; Total Carbs: 4g; Fiber: 1g; Net Carbs: 3g; Macros: Fat: 76%; Protein: 21%; Carbs: 3%

Mozzarella-Stuffed Burgers

SERVES 4 | PREP TIME: 5 minutes | COOK TIME: 15 minutes

1 pound ground beef

4 ounces frozen spinach, thawed and well-drained

2 tablespoons chopped fresh basil

1 teaspoon garlic powder

1 teaspoon salt

½ teaspoon freshly ground black pepper

1 (4-ounce) ball fresh mozzarella cheese, quartered to form 1-inch cubes

4 keto sandwich rounds or lettuce leaves

½ cup mayonnaise or aioli

Heat the grill to medium-high heat. In a large bowl, combine the beef, spinach, basil, garlic powder, salt, and pepper and, using your hands, mix well. Form into 4 balls. Sticking your thumb into the center of each ball, create a pocket and stuff 1 cheese cube into the center, and form into a patty shape. Cook the burgers on the hot grill until browned and cooked through to desired doneness, 5 to 8 minutes per side. Serve the burgers on sandwich rounds, each topped with 2 tablespoons of aioli.

Per Serving: (1 burger; keto round; and 2 tablespoons aioli): Calories: 909; Fat: 78g; Protein: 40g; Total Carbs: 8g; Fiber: 3g; Net Carbs: 5g; Macros: Fat: 77%; Protein: 18%; Carbs: 5%

Double Bacon Cheeseburger

SERVES 4 | PREP TIME: 10 minutes | COOK TIME: 20 minutes

1 pound 80-percent lean ground beef

1 shallot, minced

1 teaspoon minced garlic

1 tablespoon Worcestershire sauce

½ teaspoon salt

¼ teaspoon freshly ground black pepper

4 (1-ounce) slices thick-cut bacon, cooked, grease reserved and cooled

1 tablespoon butter

4 (1-ounce) slices American cheese

4 low-carb buns or lettuce wraps (optional)

In a large bowl, mix the ground beef, shallot, garlic, Worcestershire sauce, salt, pepper, and reserved bacon grease. Divide the mixture into 4 equal portions and form into patties. In a large cast iron skillet over medium-high heat, heat the butter for 1 minute. Add the patties to the skillet and cook for 3 to 4 minutes. Flip and cook 2 to 3 minutes more for medium-rare. Lower the heat to medium-low. Place 1 slice of cheese on each patty. Cover the skillet and melt the cheese for 1 to 2 minutes. Remove the patties from the skillet. Top each with 1 slice of bacon. Serve with your favorite condiments, on a low-carb bun, or with a lettuce wrap (if using).

Per Serving: (1 bacon-and-cheese-topped patty): Calories: 585; Fat: 42.8g; Total Carbs: 3.3g; Net Carbs: 3.3g; Fiber: 0g; Protein: 42.5g; Macros: Fat: 68%; Protein: 30%; Carbs: 2%

Mini Burger Sliders

SERVES 1 | PREP TIME: 5 minutes | COOK TIME: 15 minutes

6 ounces ground beef

1 zucchini, cut into 8 half-inch-thick slices

1 cheddar cheese slice, cut into 4 squares (optional)

1 avocado

Preheat the oven to 400°F; line a baking sheet with parchment paper. In a medium bowl, season the ground beef with salt and freshly ground black pepper, and mix thoroughly. Form four small, slider-size patties, and place them on the prepared baking sheet. Arrange the zucchini slices around the patties on the baking sheet. Bake the patties and zucchini slices for about 5 minutes, flip them, and then continue to bake for another 5 minutes. Place one square of cheddar cheese (if using), on top of each patty during the last minute of baking. Watch carefully so the cheese does not burn. Remove the sliders from the oven, and place them on a plate. Slice or mash the avocado, and place some on top of each patty. Assemble the sliders, using the zucchini slices as buns.

Per Serving: Calories: 950; Fat: 78g; Protein: 40g; Total Carbs: 22g; Fiber: 14g; Net Carbs: 8g; **Macros:** Fat: 74%; Protein: 17%; Carbs: 9%

Oven Burgers

SERVES 4 | PREP TIME: 10 minutes | COOK TIME: 25 minutes

20 ounces ground beef	1 large egg, beaten
1 teaspoon sea salt	¼ cup creamy almond butter
1 teaspoon paprika	8 bacon slices, cooked
1 teaspoon garlic powder	½ cup shredded
¾ teaspoon dried parsley	cheddar cheese
½ teaspoon freshly ground black pepper	

Preheat the oven to 400°F. In a large bowl, combine the beef, salt, paprika, garlic power, parsley, pepper, egg, and almond butter. Gently work the mixture with your hands until the ingredients are thoroughly combined. Press the beef mixture into an 8-inch-square baking dish. Bake for 22 minutes. Remove from the oven and set the oven to broil. Lay the bacon on top of the oven burger. Top it evenly with the cheddar. Broil for 1 to 2 minutes or until the cheese browns and bubbles. Let cool slightly before cutting into 4 squares and serving. Refrigerate for up to 4 days.

Per Serving: (1 burger): Calories: 610; Fat: 43g; Protein: 50g; Total Carbs: 5g; Fiber: 2g; Net Carbs: 3g; **Macros:** Fat: 63%; Protein: 33%; Carbs: 4%

Cheeseburger Meatloaf

SERVES 1 | PREP TIME: 5 minutes | COOK TIME: 45 minutes

6 ounces ground beef	¼ cup cubed cheddar cheese
1 large egg, beaten	2 tablespoons tomato paste
¼ medium white onion, diced	1 tablespoon yellow mustard
1 teaspoon pink Himalayan salt	1 tablespoon coconut aminos
1 teaspoon garlic powder	

Preheat the oven to 350°F; line a baking sheet with parchment paper. In a large bowl, combine the ground beef, egg, onion, salt, garlic, and cheese. Using your hands, gently mix the ingredients. Place the mixture on the prepared baking sheet, and form it into a meat loaf shape. Bake for 30 minutes. In a small bowl, whisk the tomato paste, mustard, and coconut aminos until fully combined. Remove the meatloaf from the oven, and spread the sauce mixture over the top evenly with a spoon. Place the meat loaf back in the oven, and bake for another 15 minutes or until cooked through and browned on top.

Per Serving: Calories: 737; Fat: 57g; Protein: 42g; Total Carbs: 14g; Fiber: 4g; Net Carbs: 10g; **Macros:** Fat: 70%; Protein: 23%; Carbs: 7%

Zucchini Meatloaf

SERVES 7 | PREP TIME: 20 minutes | COOK TIME: 1 hour

1 pound 80-percent lean ground beef	3 tablespoons tomato paste
½ pound bacon, chopped	2 large eggs
1 zucchini, finely chopped	1 tablespoon Dijon mustard
1 onion, finely chopped	¼ teaspoon paprika
	¼ teaspoon salt

¼ teaspoon freshly ground black pepper	1¼ cups almond flour
	Cooking spray for loaf pan

Preheat the oven to 350°F. In a large bowl, combine the ground beef, bacon, zucchini, and onion. Add the tomato paste, eggs, mustard, paprika, salt, and pepper. Mix thoroughly to combine. Add the almond flour and mix again, making sure there are no clumps. Transfer the beef mixture to a loaf pan coated with cooking spray. Cover with aluminum foil and place in the preheated oven. Cook for 1 hour. Take the loaf from the oven and remove the foil. Return the loaf to the oven. Increase the heat to broil. Cook for 10 minutes, or until the top is browned. Remove the pan from the oven. Allow the meatloaf to cool in the pan for 5 minutes. Slice into 7 equal slices and serve.

Per Serving: Calories: 517; Fat: 36.9g; Protein: 32g; Total Carbs: 8g; Fiber: 3.2g; Net Carbs: 4.8g; **Macros:** Fat: 68%; Protein: 26%; Carbs: 6%

Southwest Meatloaf with Lime Guacamole

SERVES 6 | PREP TIME: 15 minutes | COOK TIME: 1 hour

1 pound ground beef	1 tablespoon Southwest seasoning
½ cup almond meal	¼ teaspoon freshly ground black pepper
½ cup chopped onion	
½ cup canned coconut milk	2 cups guacamole
1 tablespoon minced garlic	

Preheat the oven to 350°F. In a large bowl, mix the ground beef, almond meal, onion, coconut milk, garlic, Southwest seasoning, and pepper until very well combined. Pack the meat mixture into a 9-by-4-inch loaf pan. Bake until cooked through and browned, about 1 hour. Let the meatloaf sit for 10 minutes and pour off any accumulated grease. Serve with guacamole.

Per Serving: Calories: 396; Fat: 33g; Protein: 17g; Total Carbs: 10g; Fiber: 5g; Net Carbs: 5g; **Macros:** Fat: 75%; Protein: 17%; Carbs: 8%

Herbed Meatloaf

SERVES 8 | PREP TIME: 15 minutes | COOK TIME: 1 hour

1 tablespoon canola oil	2 tablespoons tomato paste
1 cup minced onion	1 large egg, whisked
1 teaspoon minced garlic	1 teaspoon sea salt
1 teaspoon minced rosemary	1 teaspoon freshly ground black pepper
¼ cup roughly chopped parsley	
½ cup diced tomatoes, fresh or canned	1 pound ground beef
	1 pound ground pork
½ cup almond flour	4 bacon slices

Preheat the oven to 350°F. Heat the canola oil in a skillet over medium heat. Cook the onion, garlic, rosemary, and parsley for 8 to 10 minutes, until soft. Stir in the tomatoes. Remove the skillet from the heat. In a large bowl, whisk the almond flour, tomato paste, egg, salt, and pepper until a thick paste is formed. Add the beef and pork to the cooked onions. Using your hands, mix the ingredients until just combined; do not overmix. Transfer the meat mixture to a loaf pan, and top with the bacon slices. Bake for 1 hour or until the meatloaf is cooked through to an internal temperature of 160°F, being careful not to overbake. Slice the loaf into eight thick slices to serve.

Per Serving: Calories: 437; Fat: 34g; Protein: 28g; Total Carbs: 5g; Fiber: 1g; Net Carbs: 4g; **Macros:** Fat: 70%; Protein: 26%; Carbs: 4%

Cheeseburger Casserole

SERVES 6 | PREP TIME: 10 minutes | COOK TIME: 40 minutes

1 pound 75-percent lean ground beef

½ cup chopped sweet onion

2 teaspoons minced garlic

1½ cups shredded aged Cheddar, divided

½ cup heavy (whipping) cream

1 large tomato, chopped

1 teaspoon minced fresh basil

¼ teaspoon sea salt

⅛ teaspoon freshly ground black pepper

Preheat the oven to 350°F. Place a large skillet over medium-high heat and add the ground beef. Brown the beef until cooked through, about 6 minutes, and spoon off any excess fat. Stir in the onion and garlic and cook until the vegetables are tender, about 4 minutes. Transfer the beef and vegetables to an 8-inch-square casserole dish. In a medium bowl, stir 1 cup of shredded cheese and the heavy cream, tomato, basil, salt, and pepper until well combined. Pour the cream mixture over the beef mixture and top the casserole with the remaining ½ cup of shredded cheese. Bake until the casserole is bubbly and the cheese is melted and lightly browned, about 30 minutes. Serve.

Per Serving: Calories: 410; Fat: 33g; Protein: 20g; Total Carbs: 3g; Fiber: 0g; Net Carbs: 3g; **Macros:** Fat: 75%; Protein: 22%; Carbs: 3%

Simple Reuben Casserole

SERVES 4 | PREP TIME: 25 minutes | COOK TIME: 20 minutes

Butter, for greasing

½ pound corned beef, diced

1 (32-ounce) jar sauerkraut, drained

1 cup shredded Swiss cheese, divided

8 ounces cream cheese, softened

½ teaspoon caraway seeds

Preheat the oven to 350°F. Lightly butter an 8-cup casserole dish, and set aside. In a large bowl, stir the corned beef, sauerkraut, and ½ cup of the Swiss cheese. Stir in the cream cheese and caraway seeds. Spoon the mixture into the baking dish, and sprinkle the reserved ½ cup of cheese evenly on top. Bake until the mixture is bubbling and the cheese is melted, about 20 minutes. Serve.

Per Serving: Calories: 436; Fat: 34g; Protein: 21g; Total Carbs: 12g; Fiber: 7g; Net Carbs: 5g; **Macros:** Fat: 71%; Protein: 19%; Carbs: 10%

Beefy Stuffed Cornbread Casserole

SERVES 9 | PREP TIME: 20 minutes | COOK TIME: 1 hour

For the casserole

2 tablespoons butter, plus more for preparing the baking dish

1 green bell pepper, diced

½ onion, diced

2 pounds ground beef

1½ tablespoons chili powder

1 tablespoon garlic powder

1 tablespoon kosher salt

½ teaspoon paprika

1 (14.5-ounce) can diced tomatoes

2½ tablespoons tomato paste

1½ cups grated Cheddar cheese

For the cornbread topping

1 cup almond flour

2½ tablespoons coconut flour

2½ teaspoons baking powder

1 teaspoon monk fruit/erythritol blend sweetener

½ teaspoon kosher salt

¼ teaspoon baking soda

¼ teaspoon garlic powder

¼ teaspoon onion powder

5 large eggs

5 tablespoons butter, melted

2 tablespoons sour cream, plus more for serving

2 scallions, sliced

Preheat the oven to 350°F. Coat a 9-by-9-inch baking dish with butter. Set aside. In a large sautépan or skillet over medium-high heat, melt the butter. Add the green bell pepper and onion. Sauté for 3 to 4 minutes. Add the ground beef and cook for about 5 minutes until browned. Stir in the chili powder, garlic powder, salt, paprika, tomatoes, and tomato paste. Bring to simmer and cook for 5 minutes. Pour the filling into the prepared pan. Top with the Cheddar cheese. Set aside. In a medium bowl, stir the almond and coconut flours, baking powder, sweetener, salt, baking soda, garlic powder, and onion powder. Add the eggs, melted butter, and sour cream. Whisk until thoroughly incorporated. Stir in the scallions. Spoon the batter over the meat filling and spread it evenly to the edges. Bake for 30 to 35 minutes until golden brown. Serve warm topped with sour cream.

Per Serving: Calories: 434; Fat: 30g; Protein: 30g; Total Carbs: 11g; Fiber: 4g; Net Carbs: 7g; **Macros:** Fat: 62%; Protein: 28%; Carbs: 10%

Cheesy Beef and Spinach Casserole

SERVES 4 | PREP TIME: 5 minutes | COOK TIME: 30 minutes

1 tablespoon olive oil

1 pound ground beef

1 teaspoon onion powder

1 teaspoon paprika

12 ounces frozen spinach, thawed and drained

8 ounces cream cheese, at room temperature

¼ cup heavy (whipping) cream

½ cup shredded Parmesan cheese

Salt

Freshly ground black pepper

Preheat the oven to 375°F. In a Dutch oven, heat the oil over medium heat. Add the ground beef and cook, breaking apart with a wooden spoon, for about 10 minutes, or until browned all over. Drain off any excess liquid. Add the onion powder, paprika, spinach, cream cheese, and heavy cream. Continue to cook, stirring frequently, until the cream cheese is fully melted and incorporated. Add the Parmesan and stir well. Season with salt and pepper to taste. Transfer to the oven and bake uncovered for 15 to 20 minutes, until bubbling and golden brown on top. Let cool for 5 minutes before serving.

Per Serving: Calories: 600; Fat: 49g; Protein: 31g; Total Carbs: 9g; Fiber: 3g; Net Carbs: 6g; **Macros:** Fat: 73%; Protein: 22%; Carbs: 5%

Southern-Style Shepherd's Pie

SERVES 8 | PREP TIME: 20 minutes | COOK TIME: 1 hour

For the topping

1 pound small turnips, peeled and diced

Kosher salt

¼ cup butter

2 ounces cream cheese

2 to 3 tablespoons heavy (whipping) cream

Freshly ground black pepper

For the filling

1½ pounds ground beef

½ cup diced onion

1½ teaspoons kosher salt

2 teaspoons garlic
  powder, divided
1 teaspoon freshly ground
  black pepper, divided
4 cups chopped frozen greens
  (collard, turnip, or chard)
½ cup beef broth or
  beef stock

2 tablespoons tomato paste
1 tablespoon gluten-free
  Worcestershire sauce
¼ teaspoon dried thyme
3 ounces cream cheese
¾ cup shredded Parmesan
  cheese, divided

In a medium saucepan, combine the turnips, 1 teaspoon of salt, and enough water to cover. Place the pan over medium-high heat and bring to a boil. Cook the turnips for 12 to 15 minutes until tender. Drain. Return the turnips to the pan and let them sit on the warm burner (turned off) for 2 to 3 minutes to help eliminate excess water. Add the butter, cream cheese, and heavy cream to the turnips. Using a potato masher, mash until smooth. Taste and add more salt or pepper, as needed. Set aside. Preheat the oven to 375°F. In a large ovenproof skillet over medium-high heat, combine the ground beef, onion, salt, 1 teaspoon of garlic powder, and ½ teaspoon of pepper. Cook for 5 to 7 minutes until the beef is brown and the onion is translucent. Add the greens, beef broth or stock, tomato paste, Worcestershire sauce, thyme, and the remaining 1 teaspoon of garlic powder and ½ teaspoon of pepper. Cook for about 5 minutes until the greens are tender. Stir in the cream cheese until melted and the sauce is thickened. Gently stir in ½ cup of Parmesan cheese and remove the skillet from the heat. Spoon the mashed turnips over the meat filling and spread it evenly. Top with the remaining ¼ cup of Parmesan cheese. Bake for 20 to 25 minutes, or until golden brown. Let sit for 5 to 10 minutes before serving.

Per Serving: Calories: 386; Fat: 30g; Protein: 22g; Total Carbs: 7g; Fiber: 2g; Net Carbs: 5g; **Macros:** Fat: 70%; Protein: 23%; Carbs: 7%

Cottage Pie

SERVES 4 | PREP TIME: 20 minutes | COOK TIME: 30 minutes

For the pie

2 tablespoons extra-virgin
  olive oil
2 celery stalks, chopped
½ medium onion, chopped
2 garlic cloves, minced
1 pound 80-percent lean
  ground beef
¼ cup chicken broth

1 tablespoon tomato paste
1 teaspoon pink Himalayan
  sea salt
1 teaspoon freshly ground
  black pepper
½ teaspoon ground
  white pepper

For the topping

2 (12-ounce) packages
  cauliflower rice, cooked
  and drained
1 cup shredded low-moisture
  mozzarella cheese
2 tablespoons heavy
  (whipping) cream
2 tablespoons butter

½ teaspoon pink Himalayan
  sea salt
½ teaspoon freshly ground
  black pepper
¼ teaspoon ground
  white pepper
¼ teaspoon garlic powder

Preheat the oven to 400°F. In a large skillet, heat the olive oil over medium heat. Add the celery and onion and cook for 8 to 10 minutes, until the onion is tender. Add the garlic and cook for another minute, until fragrant. Add the ground beef, breaking it

up with a wooden spoon or spatula. Continue to cook the beef for 7 to 10 minutes, until fully browned. Stir in the broth and tomato paste and stir to coat the meat. Sprinkle in the salt, black pepper, and white pepper. Transfer the meat mixture to a 9-by-13-inch baking dish. In a food processor, combine the cauliflower rice, mozzarella, cream, butter, salt, black pepper, white pepper, and garlic powder. Puree on high speed until the mixture is smooth, scraping down the sides of the bowl as necessary. Spread the cauliflower mash over the top of the meat and smooth the top. Bake for 10 minutes, until the topping is just lightly browned. Let cool for 5 minutes, then serve.

Per Serving: Calories: 564; Fat: 44g; Protein: 30g; Total Carbs: 13g; Fiber: 4g; Net Carbs: 7g; **Macros:** Fat: 70%; Protein: 21%; Carbs: 9%

Broccoli and Beef Casserole

SERVES 4 | PREP TIME: 15 minutes | COOK TIME: 30 minutes

1 pound ground beef
1 (16-ounce) bag frozen broccoli baby florets
1 (8-ounce) brick
  cream cheese
¼ cup ranch dressing
¼ cup mayonnaise

1 cup shredded
  mozzarella cheese
1 teaspoon Italian seasoning
1 tablespoon garlic salt
1 teaspoon freshly ground
  black pepper
¼ cup Parmesan cheese

In a large skillet over medium heat, cook the ground beef, breaking up any big pieces. Drain the grease. Meanwhile, microwave the broccoli according to the package directions. Drain the liquid, pat the broccoli dry, and chop the broccoli into bite-size chunks. Add the broccoli, cream cheese, ranch dressing, mayonnaise, mozzarella cheese, Italian seasoning, garlic salt, and pepper to the skillet with the meat, mix, reduce the heat to low, and cook for about 20 minutes, stirring occasionally. Sprinkle the Parmesan on top and serve.

Per Serving: Calories: 607; Fat: 51g; Protein: 28g; Total Carbs: 9g; Fiber: 3g; Net Carbs: 6g; **Macros:** Fat: 76%; Protein: 18%; Carbs: 6%

Cottage Pie Muffins

SERVES 2 TO 4 | PREP TIME: 10 minutes | COOK TIME: 35 to 40 minutes

2 tablespoons coconut
  oil, divided
½ medium onion, diced
1 cup diced cremini
  mushrooms
½ cup diced celery
¼ cup diced carrot
Salt
Freshly ground black pepper
1 pound ground
  free-range pork
½ teaspoon garlic powder

½ teaspoon dried oregano
½ teaspoon dried thyme
½ head cauliflower, chopped
  into bite-size florets
½ cup chicken bone broth
1 tablespoon full-fat coconut milk or regular milk
  (optional)
Shredded Cheddar cheese
  (optional)
Chopped fresh tarragon or
  dill, for serving (optional)

Preheat the oven to 380°F. Coat a muffin tin with 1 tablespoon of coconut oil. In a large skillet, heat the remaining 1 tablespoon of coconut oil over medium-high heat. Add the onion, mushrooms, celery, and carrot, season with salt and pepper, and sauté for about 10 minutes, until the veggies are tender. Add the meat, season with the garlic powder, oregano, and thyme, and cook for 3 to 5 minutes. Transfer the meat and vegetable mixture to a large bowl and let rest while you prepare the cauliflower. In a medium saucepan over medium-high heat, bring $\frac{1}{4}$ inch of water to a boil. Add the cauliflower and steam for 3 to 4 minutes. Drain the cauliflower and transfer to a blender along with the bone broth. Blend until it is creamy and smooth. Add the milk if needed. Fill the prepared muffin tin with the meat mixture. Use a spatula to "frost" the muffins with the cauliflower. Season with salt and pepper and bake for about 15 minutes, sprinkling with cheese (if using) in the last 5 minutes. Remove the muffins from the oven and let cool, then sprinkle with dill or tarragon.

Per Serving: Calories: 266; Fat: 18g; Protein: 23g; Total Carbs: 3g; Fiber: 1g; Net Carbs: 2g; **Macros:** Fat: 61%; Protein: 35%; Carbs: 4%

Moussaka

SERVES 6 | PREP TIME: 25 minutes | COOK TIME: 1 hour 25 minutes

1 eggplant, cut into 1-inch rounds	2 large eggs
3 tablespoons olive oil, divided	½ teaspoon sea salt
1 pound ground beef	½ teaspoon freshly ground black pepper
1 onion, chopped	3 tablespoons melted butter
2 teaspoons minced garlic	1 cup canned coconut milk
1 cup no-sugar-added tomato sauce	1 cup shredded mozzarella cheese, divided
¼ cup low-sodium beef stock	¼ teaspoon ground nutmeg
¼ cup almond meal	
2 tablespoons chopped fresh parsley	

Preheat the oven to 375°F. Place the eggplant in a single layer on a large baking sheet and brush with 2 tablespoons of the olive oil. Roast the eggplant in the oven until softened, about 10 minutes. Remove from the oven and let cool. Heat the remaining olive oil in a large skillet over medium-high heat. Brown the beef until completely cooked through, 12 to 15 minutes. Add the onion and garlic and sauté for 3 minutes. Stir in the tomato sauce and beef stock and bring the sauce to a boil. Reduce the heat to low and simmer for 10 minutes. Let the sauce cool for 15 minutes, then stir in the almond meal, parsley, eggs, salt, and pepper. In a medium saucepan over medium heat, whisk the butter, coconut milk, ½ cup of the cheese, and nutmeg. Stir until the cheese is melted and the sauce is thick, about 4 minutes. Place half the eggplant rounds in a 9-by-13-inch baking dish and top with the meat sauce. Layer the remaining eggplant rounds on top of the meat sauce and pour the cheese sauce over them. Sprinkle the remaining mozzarella cheese on top and bake until bubbly and heated through, about 45 minutes.

Per Serving: Calories: 513; Fat: 42g; Protein: 24g; Total Carbs: 14g; Fiber: 4g; Net Carbs: 10g; **Macros:** Fat: 74%; Protein: 19%; Carbs: 7%

Cheesy Triple Meat Baked "Spaghetti"

SERVES 8 | PREP TIME: 30 minutes | COOK TIME: 1½ hours

1 large spaghetti squash (yields 5 cups)	½ pound 80-percent lean ground beef
½ cup butter	½ pound Italian sausage

½ pound chicken sausage	4 ounces ricotta cheese, divided
½ cup red wine	4 ounces mozzarella cheese, divided
1 large onion, diced	8 ounces grated Parmesan cheese, divided
5 garlic cloves, minced	
½ pound mushrooms, sliced	
1 (6-ounce) can tomato paste	½ teaspoon salt
1 (18-ounce) can diced tomatoes	½ teaspoon freshly ground black pepper
1 tablespoon Italian seasoning	

Preheat the oven to 350°F. Place the spaghetti squash in a large microwaveable bowl and use the tip of a sharp knife to pierce the shell all around. Microwave on high for 15 to 20 minutes, depending on the size of your squash. Remove from the microwave. Set aside to cool. Heat a large skillet over medium-high heat. Add the butter and melt for 1 to 2 minutes. Add the ground beef, Italian sausage, and chicken sausage to the pan. Sauté for about 10 minutes. Add the red wine and lower the heat to medium, letting the wine reduce with the meat for 3 to 5 minutes. Add the onion and garlic. Cook until tender, about 4 minutes. Add the mushrooms and stir, cooking for an additional 8 to 9 minutes. Add the tomato paste, diced tomatoes with the juices, and Italian seasoning to the mixture. Stir well to combine. Cook for 10 to 15 minutes, until reduced by half. Return to the spaghetti squash. Cut it in half lengthwise. Clean it, removing the inner seeds, and scoop out the flesh with a fork. In a large baking dish with a lid, spread half of the spaghetti squash in the bottom. Top with 2 ounces of ricotta, 2 ounces of mozzarella, and 4 ounces of Parmesan. Cover with the tomato sauce. Top with the remaining half of the spaghetti squash. Finish with the remaining 2 ounces of ricotta, 2 ounces of mozzarella, and 4 ounces of Parmesan cheese. Cover the pan and bake for 20 minutes. Remove the dish from the oven and carefully remove the lid. Return the uncovered dish to the oven and bake for another 15 to 20 minutes. Finish with 2 to 3 minutes under the broiler for a crispy, browned top. Cool for 10 to 15 minutes before serving.

Per Serving: Calories: 493; Fat: 33g; Protein: 34g; Total Carbs: 15g; Fiber: 6g; Net Carbs: 9g; **Macros:** Fat: 60%; Protein: 28%; Carbs: 12%

Zucchini Lasagna

SERVES 6 | PREP TIME: 5 minutes | COOK TIME: 45 minutes

1 pound 80-percent lean ground beef	½ teaspoon freshly ground black pepper
3 garlic cloves, minced	5 zucchini, cut lengthwise into ¼-inch slices
1 (24-ounce) jar low-carb pasta sauce	1 pound shredded mozzarella cheese
15 ounces ricotta cheese	Preheat the oven to 375°F.
1 large egg yolk	
1 teaspoon kosher salt	

In a medium skillet, heat the ground beef and garlic over medium-high heat. Cook until the meat is browned, about 10 minutes. Drain the excess grease. Stir in the pasta sauce, reduce the heat to low, and simmer for about 10 minutes. In a small bowl, mix the ricotta cheese, egg yolk, salt, and pepper. To assemble the lasagna, layer the bottom of a 9-inch square baking dish with ¼ of the zucchini slices, ¼ of the ricotta mixture, and ¼ of the meat sauce. Top with ¼ of the mozzarella cheese. Repeat the layers until all the ingredients are used up, ending with a layer of mozzarella cheese. Bake for 20 to 25 minutes, until the cheese is melted and bubbly. Allow the lasagna to sit for about 10 to 15 minutes before serving.

Per Serving: Calories: 602; Fat: 43g; Protein: 41g; Total Carbs: 14g; Fiber: 4g; Net Carbs: 10g; **Macros:** Fat: 64%; Protein: 28%; Carbs: 8%

Beef Taco Lasagna

SERVES 4 | PREP TIME: 5 minutes | COOK TIME: 30 minutes

Nonstick cooking spray	Freshly ground black pepper
1 tablespoon olive oil	4 (8-inch) low-carb tortillas
1 pound lean ground beef	1 cup shredded Mexican
1 cup low-carb salsa	blend cheese
Salt	

Preheat the oven to 350°F. Coat a 7-by-11-inch baking dish with cooking spray and set aside. In a large pan, heat the oil. Add the ground beef and cook, breaking apart with a wooden spoon, for about 10 minutes, or until browned all over. Drain off any excess liquid. Add the salsa and cook for another 10 minutes, or until most of the liquid has evaporated. Season with salt and pepper to taste. Cover the bottom of the prepared baking dish with the tortillas, cutting them to fit as needed. Layer the meat mixture on top of the tortillas and sprinkle the cheese over the top. Cook for 10 to 15 minutes, until the cheese is melted and golden brown.

Per Serving: Calories: 441; Fat: 32g; Protein: 34g; Total Carbs: 5g; Fiber: 1g; Net Carbs: 4g; **Macros:** Fat: 65%; Protein: 31%; Carbs: 4%

Philly Cheesesteak Stuffed Peppers

SERVES 4 | PREP TIME: 15 minutes | COOK TIME: 25 minutes

4 green bell peppers, seeded, tops reserved, plus ¼ cup thinly sliced green bell pepper from reserved tops	½ teaspoon paprika
	½ teaspoon ground coriander
	¼ teaspoon dill
	¼ teaspoon crushed red pepper flakes
3 tablespoons butter	½ teaspoon garlic powder
¼ cup chopped onion	½ teaspoon onion powder
1 pound shaved beefsteak	8 slices pepper Jack cheese, divided
1 garlic clove, minced	
1 teaspoon salt	2½ tablespoons mayonnaise
1 teaspoon freshly ground black pepper	

Preheat the oven to 400°F. Slice a thin piece from the bottom of each whole bell pepper so it will not tip over. Place the 4 peppers on a baking sheet and into the preheated oven. Bake for 10 to 15 minutes. In a large skillet over medium-high heat, heat the butter for 1 minute. Add the onions and sliced green bell peppers. Cook for 3 minutes. Add the steak, garlic, salt, black pepper, paprika, coriander, dill, red pepper flakes, garlic powder, and onion powder. Cook for 6 to 7 minutes until the meat browns completely, breaking up the meat as it cooks. Lower the heat to medium-low. Remove the whole bell peppers from the oven. Place 1 slice of cheese in each pepper. Transfer the steak mixture to a medium bowl and continue to shred the meat. Add the mayonnaise and mix well to combine. Stuff each pepper with an equal amount of the meat mixture. Top each pepper with 1 of the

remaining 4 cheese slices. Place the stuffed peppers back in the oven. Cook for 5 to 7 minutes, or until the cheese melts. Remove from the oven. Serve immediately.

Per Serving: Calories: 585; Fat: 43g; Protein: 38g; Total Carbs: 12g; Fiber: 3g; Net Carbs: 9g; **Macros:** Fat: 66%; Protein: 26%; Carbs: 8%

Beef-Stuffed Red Peppers

SERVES 4 | PREP TIME: 20 minutes | COOK TIME: 30 minutes

4 red bell peppers, tops cut off and seeded	½ sweet onion, minced
	2 teaspoons chopped fresh oregano
2 tablespoons extra-virgin olive oil	1 teaspoon minced garlic
½ pound 75-percent lean ground beef	1 teaspoon chopped fresh basil
2 ounces grated Parmesan cheese	¼ teaspoon chopped fresh thyme

Preheat the oven to 350°F. Rub the red peppers all over generously with the olive oil, and place them open-side up in a 9-by-13-inch baking dish. In a medium bowl, stir the beef, Parmesan, onion, oregano, garlic, basil, and thyme until well mixed. Evenly divide the meat mixture among the four red peppers, spooning it into the hollows. Cover with foil, and bake the stuffed red peppers until the meat mixture is cooked through and the peppers are tender, about 30 minutes. Serve.

Per Serving: Calories: 308; Fat: 22g; Protein: 20g; Total Carbs: 8g; Fiber: 3g; Net Carbs: 5g; **Macros:** Fat: 64%; Protein: 26%; Carbs: 10%

Moroccan Stuffed Peppers

SERVES 4 | PREP TIME: 10 minutes | COOK TIME: 30 minutes

¼ cup, plus 2 tablespoons extra-virgin olive oil, divided	1 teaspoon salt
	1 teaspoon ground allspice
2 large red bell peppers halved lengthwise and seeded	½ teaspoon freshly ground black pepper
	½ cup chopped fresh flat-leaf Italian parsley
1 pound ground beef	
1 small onion, finely chopped	½ cup chopped baby arugula leaves
2 garlic cloves, minced	
2 tablespoons chopped fresh sage or 2 teaspoons dried sage	½ cup chopped walnuts
	1 tablespoon freshly squeezed orange juice

Preheat the oven to 425°F. Drizzle 1 tablespoon olive oil in a rimmed baking sheet and swirl to coat the bottom. Place cut-side down on the prepared baking sheet and roast until just softened, 5 to 8 minutes. Remove from the oven and allow to cool. Meanwhile, in a large skillet, heat 1 tablespoon olive oil over medium-high heat. Add the beef and onions and sauté until the meat is browned and cooked through, 8 to 10 minutes. Add the garlic, sage, salt, allspice, and pepper and sauté for 2 more minutes. Remove from the heat and cool slightly. Stir in the parsley, arugula, walnuts, orange juice, and remaining ¼ cup olive oil and mix well. Stuff the filling into each pepper half. Return to the oven and cook for 5 minutes. Serve warm.

Per Serving: Calories: 521; Fat: 44g; Protein: 25g; Total Carbs: 9g; Fiber: 3g; Net Carbs: 6g; **Macros:** Fat: 75%; Protein: 19%; Carbs: 6%

Chili con Carne

SERVES 4 | PREP TIME: 10 minutes **| COOK TIME:** 35 minutes

1 tablespoon avocado oil
1 pound ground beef
¼ cup diced white onion
½ small green bell pepper, chopped
1 garlic clove, minced
1½ cups canned diced tomatoes with liquid

1 cup plain tomato sauce
1 tablespoon chili powder
1 teaspoon sea salt
1 teaspoon ground cumin
½ teaspoon paprika
½ teaspoon freshly ground black pepper
1 large Hass avocado, sliced

Heat the oil in a large stockpot over medium heat. Crumble in the beef. Stir in the onion, bell pepper, and garlic. Cook, stirring frequently, until the beef browns, about 5 minutes. Pour in the tomatoes with their liquid, tomato sauce, chili powder, salt, cumin, paprika, and pepper. Stir to thoroughly combine. Bring the mixture to a boil and then reduce to a simmer over medium-low heat. Cover and cook for 25 minutes until thickened to a stew-like consistency. Serve 1 cup of chili with 2 slices of avocado.

Per Serving: (1 cup): Calories: 453; Fat: 30g; Protein: 32g; Total Carbs: 15g; Fiber: 7g; Net Carbs: 8g; **Macros:** Fat: 60%; Protein: 28%; Carbs: 12%

Five-Alarm Beef Chili

SERVES 12 | PREP TIME: 30 minutes **| COOK TIME:** 2 hours

For the chili

3 tablespoons olive oil
2 cups diced onion
5 garlic cloves, minced
2 green bell peppers, diced
2 poblano peppers, diced
3 serrano peppers, minced
3 jalapeño peppers, diced
2 to 3 habanero peppers, minced (adjust for heat level; optional)
3 pounds 80-percent lean ground beef
1 cup tomato paste
2¼ cups crushed tomatoes

1½ cups diced tomatoes
2 cups dark beer
1½ tablespoons dark chili powder
½ teaspoon paprika
1 teaspoon salt
1 teaspoon freshly ground black pepper
½ teaspoon cumin
2 cups shredded Cheddar cheese
1 cup sour cream
Chopped fresh cilantro, for garnish (optional)

In a large stockpot over medium heat, heat the olive oil for 1 minute. Add the onion and garlic. Cook for 3 minutes until tender. Add the bell peppers, poblano peppers, serrano peppers, jalapeño peppers, and habanero peppers (if using) to the pot. Mix well. Cook for 3 to 4 minutes. Add the ground beef to the peppers and onions. Crumble with the back of a spoon while browning for 4 minutes. Add the tomato paste, crushed tomatoes, and diced tomatoes to the pot. Mix well. Add the beer. Increase the heat to high and bring the mixture to a boil. Once the chili boils, cover and lower the heat to medium-low. Cook for 1½ hours. Add the chili powder, paprika, salt, pepper, and cumin. Stir to incorporate. Cook for 5 more minutes, stirring occasionally. Serve the chili with the shredded cheese and sour cream. Garnish with cilantro (if using).

Per Serving: Calories: 532; Fat: 33.9g; Protein: 38.8g; Total Carbs: 14.9g; Fiber: 3.9g; Net Carbs: 11g; **Macros:** Fat: 59%; Protein: 30%; Carbs: 11%

Classic Beef Chili

SERVES 6 | PREP TIME: 15 minutes **| COOK TIME:** 1 hour 30 minutes

¼ cup olive oil
1 pound ground beef
1 onion, chopped
1 green bell pepper, chopped
1 tablespoon minced garlic
3 tablespoons ancho chili powder

2 teaspoons ground cumin
1 teaspoon ground coriander
1 teaspoon smoked paprika
2 cups low-sodium beef stock
½ cup no-salt-added tomato paste
1 cup sour cream

Heat the olive oil in a large stockpot over medium-high heat. Sauté the beef until it is cooked through, about 15 minutes. Add the onion, bell pepper, and garlic and sauté until softened, about 6 minutes. Stir in the chili powder, cumin, coriander, and paprika and sauté for 4 minutes. Stir in the beef stock and tomato paste and bring the mixture to a boil. Simmer until the sauce thickens and the flavors have mellowed, about 1 hour. Serve topped with 2½ tablespoons sour cream.

Per Serving: Calories: 410; Fat: 32g; Protein: 18g; Total Carbs: 14g; Fiber: 3g; Net Carbs: 11g; **Macros:** Fat: 70%; Protein: 18%; Carbs: 12%

Texas-Style Beef Chili

SERVES 6 | PREP TIME: 20 minutes **| COOK TIME:** 1 hour 45 minutes

3 tablespoons ground chipotle chili powder
2 tablespoons ground cumin
1 tablespoon dried oregano
½ teaspoon ground cinnamon
¼ cup olive oil
2 pounds beef chuck roast, cut into 1-inch cubes
1 onion, diced

2 jalapeño peppers, finely chopped
1 tablespoon minced garlic
6 cups low-sodium beef stock
½ cup no-salt-added tomato paste
1 tablespoon unsweetened cocoa powder
1 cup sour cream

In a small bowl, mix the chili powder, cumin, oregano, and cinnamon until well combined. Set aside. Heat the olive oil in a large saucepan over medium-high heat. Sauté the beef until browned, about 10 minutes, and transfer to a plate using a slotted spoon. Sauté the onion, jalapeños, and garlic until softened, about 4 minutes. Add the beef back to the pot, along with any accumulated juices on the plate, and the spice mixture. Stir to evenly coat. Stir in the beef stock, tomato paste, and cocoa powder. Bring the chili to a boil, cover, and reduce the heat to low. Simmer until the sauce is thickened and the beef is very tender, stirring occasionally, about 1½ hours. Serve topped with sour cream.

Per Serving: Calories: 683; Fat: 55g; Protein: 35g; Total Carbs: 12g; Fiber: 4g; Net Carbs: 8g; **Macros:** Fat: 72%; Protein: 20%; Carbs: 8%

Zoodles Bolognese

SERVES 4 | PREP TIME: 5 minutes | COOK TIME: 20 minutes

2 tablespoons extra-virgin
  olive oil
1 pound ground beef or bison
1 teaspoon salt

½ teaspoon freshly ground
  black pepper
4 cups no-sugar-added marinara sauce
4 cups raw spiralized zucchini

In a skillet, heat the olive oil over medium heat. Sauté the beef, salt, and pepper for 4 to 5 minutes to brown the meat. Add the marinara sauce and bring to a simmer. Reduce the heat to low, cover, and cook for 15 minutes. Serve the meat sauce over the zucchini noodles, tossing to coat. Garnish with shredded Parmesan cheese, if desired.

Per Serving: Calories: 526; Fat: 38g; Protein: 27g; Total Carbs: 22g; Fiber: 6g; Net Carbs: 16g; **Macros:** Fat: 65%; Protein: 21%; Carbs: 14%

Quick and Easy Dirty Rice Skillet

SERVES 4 | PREP TIME: 15 minutes | COOK TIME: 20 minutes

3 tablespoons bacon drip-
  pings or avocado oil
1 pound 80-percent lean
  ground beef
1½ teaspoons kosher
  salt, divided
1 teaspoon garlic
  powder, divided
¼ teaspoon freshly ground
  black pepper
1 cup diced celery
1 cup diced green bell pepper

½ cup diced onion
2 garlic cloves, finely minced
1 teaspoon paprika
¼ teaspoon dried oregano
¼ teaspoon dried thyme
¼ teaspoon cayenne pepper
1 (12-ounce) package frozen
  cauliflower rice
¼ cup chicken stock or
  bone broth
Sliced scallion, for garnish

In a cast-iron skillet over medium-high heat, heat the bacon drippings. Add the ground beef, 1 teaspoon of salt, ½ teaspoon of garlic powder, and the black pepper. Cook, breaking the meat apart with a spoon, for 5 to 7 minutes until the meat browns and begins to caramelize. Reduce the heat to medium. Add the celery, green bell pepper, and onion. Cook for about 5 minutes, or until the vegetables are tender and the onion is translucent. Add the garlic, paprika, oregano, thyme, and cayenne. Cook for 1 minute more. Add the frozen cauliflower rice, chicken stock, remaining ½ teaspoon of salt, and remaining ½ teaspoon of garlic powder. Stir to combine, scraping up any browned bits stuck to the bottom of the pan. Continue to cook for about 5 minutes, stirring often, until the cauliflower rice is tender and there is no liquid left in the pan. Serve garnished with scallion.

Per Serving: Calories: 388; Fat: 28g; Protein: 24g; Total Carbs: 10g; Fiber: 5g; Net Carbs: 5g; **Macros:** Fat: 65%; Protein: 25%; Carbs: 10%

Ground Beef Cauli-Fried Rice

SERVES 1 TO 2 | PREP TIME: 5 to 10 minutes | COOK TIME: 15 to 20 minutes

1 tablespoon avocado or
  sesame oil
6 asparagus spears, trimmed
  and finely chopped

5 scallions, finely chopped
1 (12-ounce) bag frozen cauliflower rice
1 cup beef bone broth

1 large egg
½ pound 80% lean
  ground beef
1 tablespoon tamari or
  coconut aminos

1 teaspoon minced
  pickled ginger
Garlic powder
Fresh spinach leaves, for
  serving (optional)

Heat the oil in a large skillet over medium-high heat. Add the asparagus and scallions and cook for 2 to 3 minutes. Add the cauliflower rice, and cook for another 3 to 5 minutes. Add the bone broth and egg and stir. Add the ground beef and cook for 3 to 5 minutes, or until the meat is browned. Season with the tamari, ginger, and garlic powder to taste, then stir and cook for another 3 minutes. Serve on a bed of spinach.

Per Serving: Calories: 502; Fat: 34g; Protein: 32g; Total Carbs: 17g; Fiber: 7g; Net Carbs: 10g; **Macros:** Fat: 62%; Protein: 25%; Carbs: 13%

Salisbury Steak

SERVES 4 | PREP TIME: 10 minutes | COOK TIME: 25 minutes

1 pound 80-percent lean
  ground beef
1 teaspoon kosher salt
1 teaspoon garlic powder
1 teaspoon onion powder
½ teaspoon freshly ground
  black pepper
½ medium white onion,
  thinly sliced

2 ounces baby bella mush-
  rooms, thinly sliced
2 cups beef stock
1 tablespoon
  reduced-sugar ketchup
1 tablespoon Worcester-
  shire sauce
¼ teaspoon xanthan gum

In a large bowl, mix the ground beef, salt, garlic powder, onion powder, and pepper. Form the meat into 4 equal oval patties. In a large skillet, heat the patties over medium-high heat. Cook for 4 to 5 minutes per side until fully cooked through and crispy on the outside. Remove from the skillet and set aside. Reduce the heat to medium-low and add the onion and mushrooms to the skillet. Cook for 3 to 5 minutes until tender. Add the beef stock, ketchup, and Worcestershire sauce and stir to combine. Bring the sauce to a boil and cook for 3 to 5 minutes. Add the xanthan gum and whisk to combine. Increase the heat to medium and add the cooked patties back into the gravy mixture. Cook for an additional 5 minutes to heat through, then serve.

Per Serving: Calories: 302; Fat: 23g; Protein: 20g; Total Carbs: 3g; Fiber: 0g; Net Carbs: 3g; **Macros:** Fat: 68%; Protein: 28%; Carbs: 4%

Meatza

SERVES 1 TO 2 | PREP TIME: 5 to 10 minutes | COOK TIME: 25 minutes

2 tablespoons avocado
  oil, divided
½ pound ground beef
½ cup cauliflower rice
¼ cup minced carrots
Salt
Freshly ground black pepper
3 tablespoons
  no-sugar-added
  tomato sauce

2 tablespoons chopped
  white onion
Chopped zucchini, egg-
  plant, or leeks, for topping
  (optional)
Shredded cheese, for topping
  (optional)

Preheat the oven to 360°F. Line a baking sheet with aluminum foil and grease with 1 tablespoon of oil. In a mixing bowl, combine the ground beef, cauliflower, and carrots. Season with salt and pepper and mix until well combined. Transfer the meat mixture to the baking sheet and press into a round pizza shape. Bake for 10 to 12 minutes, until the meat is browned. Top the crust with tomato sauce, leaving a ½-inch border. Sprinkle with the onion, any other chopped veggies, and shredded cheese (if using). Put the meatza back in the oven and cook for another 10 minutes, until the vegetables are tender. Remove from the oven and let cool.

Per Serving: Calories: 349; Fat: 21g; Protein: 25g; Total Carbs: 15g; Fiber: 6g; Net Carbs: 9g; **Macros:** Fat: 55%; Protein: 29%; Carbs: 16%

Texas Taco Hash

SERVES 5 | PREP TIME: 15 minutes | COOK TIME: 20 minutes

2 tablespoons avocado oil
1½ pounds 80-percent lean ground beef
½ cup diced onion
½ cup diced green bell pepper
1½ tablespoons chili powder
1 teaspoon garlic powder
1 teaspoon paprika
1 teaspoon kosher salt
½ teaspoon onion powder
½ teaspoon ground cumin
1 (14-ounce) can diced tomatoes with green chilies (like Ro-Tel)
2 cups frozen cauliflower rice

3 tablespoons heavy (whipping) cream
3 tablespoons sour cream
1 cup shredded Colby cheese
Shredded lettuce, for topping (optional)
Chopped fresh tomato, for topping (optional)
Diced avocado, for topping (optional)
Sliced scallion, for topping (optional)
Black olives, for topping (optional)

Preheat the oven to 400°F. In a large ovenproof skillet over medium-high heat, heat the avocado oil. Add the ground beef, onion, and green bell pepper. Cook for 5 to 7 minutes until the beef is browned and the vegetables are tender. Stir in the chili powder, garlic powder, paprika, salt, onion powder, and cumin. Cook for 1 minute. Stir in the tomatoes and cauliflower rice. Cook 3 to 5 minutes, stirring often, until the cauliflower rice is tender. Stir in the heavy cream and sour cream, and remove the skillet from the heat. Top with the Colby cheese. Bake for 5 to 7 minutes, or until bubbly and the cheese is melted. Serve garnished, as desired.

Per Serving: Calories: 550; Fat: 42g; Protein: 33g; Total Carbs: 10g; Fiber: 3g; Net Carbs: 7g; **Macros:** Fat: 69%; Protein: 24%; Carbs: 7%

Ground Beef Taco Salad

SERVES 4 | PREP TIME: 30 minutes |
COOK TIME: 20 minutes

2 tablespoons olive oil
½ cup diced onion
2 garlic cloves, minced
1 green bell pepper, diced
1 jalapeño pepper, diced
6 ounces diced tomatoes, divided

1 pound 80-percent lean ground beef
½ teaspoon cumin
½ teaspoon paprika
¼ teaspoon salt
¼ teaspoon freshly ground black pepper

1 avocado, diced
½ cup shredded Cheddar cheese

¼ cup sour cream
Chopped fresh cilantro

In a large skillet over medium-high heat, heat the olive oil for about 1 minute. Add the onion and garlic. Cook for 2 minutes, until tender. Add the bell pepper, jalapeño pepper, and 3 ounces of diced tomatoes to the skillet. Cook for 3 to 4 more minutes. Transfer the mixture to a large bowl. Set aside. Reserve any liquid left in the skillet and place back over the heat. Add the ground beef to the skillet. Cook for 8 to 10 minutes, crumbling the meat, until browned. Add the cumin, paprika, salt, and pepper. Stir to combine. Transfer the beef to the large bowl with the onion and pepper mixture. Toss to combine. Mix in the remaining 3 ounces of tomatoes. Gently stir in the avocado. Do not overmix. Plate each serving of taco salad with a portion of the Cheddar cheese, sour cream, and cilantro toppings.

Per Serving: Calories: 587; Fat: 45g; Protein: 37g; Total Carbs: 11g; Fiber: 5g; Net Carbs: 6g; **Macros:** Fat: 68%; Protein: 25%; Carbs: 7%

Cilantro Lime Taco Bowls

SERVES 2 | PREP TIME: 10 minutes | COOK TIME: 10 minutes

For the taco bowl

2 tablespoons avocado oil
½ pound ground beef
½ teaspoon garlic powder
½ teaspoon onion powder
½ teaspoon dried oregano

6 cups romaine lettuce, chopped
¼ cup pickled red onions
2 avocados, diced

For the cilantro lime sauce

¼ cup avocado oil
¼ cup lime juice

½ cup fresh cilantro
¼ teaspoon salt

In a large skillet, heat the avocado oil over medium heat. Add the ground beef to the skillet and use a wooden spoon to break it into small crumbles. Sprinkle the spices onto the meat and stir to combine. Let the meat continue to cook for 10 minutes until it is no longer pink. Make the cilantro sauce by placing all ingredients to a food processor or blender; process until smooth. Divide the romaine lettuce among 4 bowls, top with the ground beef, red onions, avocado, and the cilantro sauce.

Per Serving: Calories: 840; Fat: 78g; Protein: 27g; Total Carbs: 18g; Fiber: 11g; Net Carbs: 7g; **Macros:** Fat: 81%; Protein: 12%; Carbs: 7%

Beef Tacos

SERVES 4 | PREP TIME: 10 minutes | COOK TIME: 10 minutes

1 cup shredded cheddar cheese, divided
1 pound 80-percent lean ground beef
1 teaspoon sea salt
½ teaspoon ground cumin
½ teaspoon ground coriander
½ teaspoon paprika
¼ teaspoon garlic powder
¼ teaspoon dried oregano

⅛ teaspoon chili powder
⅛ teaspoon ground black pepper
½ cup water
Optional topping
Shredded lettuce
Sour cream
Shredded cheese
Avocado

Preheat the oven to 375°F. Line a baking sheet with parchment paper. Place ¼ cup of cheese at a time onto the baking sheet and form into circles. Bake for 5 to 7 minutes, checking the cheese frequently to prevent burning. While the cheese bakes, create a taco mold by positioning two equal-size glasses across from one another with a wooden spoon resting on top. Remove the cheese circles from the oven and let them cool for 1 minute. With a spatula, transfer each circle to hang over the wooden spoon. While the cheese shells are hardening, place a large saucepan over medium heat. Cook the ground beef until browned, about 5 minutes. Remove from the heat, drain the fat, and put the pan back on the heat. Add the salt, cumin, coriander, paprika, garlic powder, oregano, chili powder, and black pepper and stir well to combine. Pour in the water and stir again. Bring to a boil; then reduce the heat to medium-low and simmer until the water is gone, 5 to 6 more minutes. To serve, fill each taco shell with one-fourth of the ground beef and top with your desired toppings.

Per Serving: (2 tacos): Calories: 402; Fat: 28g; Protein: 36g; Total Carbs: 2g; Fiber: <1g; Net Carbs: 2g; **Macros:** Fat: 61%; Protein: 37%; Carbs: 2%

Meatballs in Creamy Almond Sauce

SERVES 4-6 | PREP TIME: 15 minutes | COOK TIME: 35 minutes

8 ounces ground beef
8 ounces ground veal or pork
½ cup finely minced onion, divided
1 large egg, beaten
¼ cup almond flour
1½ teaspoons salt, divided
1 teaspoon garlic powder
½ teaspoon freshly ground black pepper
½ teaspoon ground nutmeg

2 teaspoons chopped fresh flat-leaf Italian parsley, plus ¼ cup, divided
½ cup extra-virgin olive oil, divided
¼ cup slivered almonds
1 cup dry white wine or chicken broth
¼ cup unsweetened almond butter

In a large bowl, combine the beef, veal, ¼ cup onion, and the egg and mix well with a fork. In a small bowl, whisk the almond flour, 1 teaspoon salt, garlic powder, pepper, and nutmeg. Add to the meat mixture along with 2 teaspoons chopped parsley and incorporate well. Form the mixture into small meatballs, about 1 inch in diameter, and place on a plate. Let sit for 10 minutes at room temperature. In a large skillet, heat ¼ cup oil over medium-high heat. Add the meatballs to the hot oil and brown on all sides, cooking in batches if necessary, 2 to 3 minutes per side. Remove from the skillet and keep warm. In the hot skillet, sauté the remaining ¼ cup minced onion in the remaining ¼ cup olive oil for 5 minutes. Reduce the heat to medium-low and add the slivered almonds. Sauté until the almonds are golden, another 3 to 5 minutes. In a small bowl, whisk the white wine, almond butter, and remaining ½ teaspoon salt. Add to the skillet and bring to a boil, stirring constantly. Reduce the heat to low, return the meatballs to the skillet, and cover. Cook until the meatballs are cooked through, another 8 to 10 minutes. Serve the meatballs warm and drizzled with almond sauce.

Per Serving: Calories: 449; Fat: 42g; Protein: 16g; Total Carbs: 3g; Fiber: 1g; Net Carbs: 2g; **Macros:** Fat: 83%; Protein: 15%; Carbs: 2%

Swedish Meatballs

SERVES 4 | PREP TIME: 10 minutes | COOK TIME: 25 minutes

2 tablespoons canola oil, divided
1 cup minced onion
1 teaspoon minced garlic
1 large egg, whisked
¼ cup almond flour
⅛ teaspoon ground allspice
¼ teaspoon ground nutmeg
½ teaspoon sea salt

½ teaspoon freshly ground black pepper
½ pound ground beef
½ pound ground pork
1 cup beef bone broth or low-sodium beef broth
¼ cup white wine
2 tablespoons cold butter
½ cup sour cream

Heat 1 tablespoon of the canola oil in a large skillet over medium heat. Add the onion and garlic and cook until soft, about 5 minutes. In a mixing bowl, mix the egg, almond flour, allspice, nutmeg, salt, and pepper. Add the beef, pork, and cooked onion mixture. Using your hands, mix the ingredients until combined. Form the mixture into 8 to 12 meatballs. In the same skillet, heat the remaining tablespoon of canola oil and sear the meatballs on all sides until well browned and cooked through to an internal temperature of 160°F, about 15 minutes. Transfer the meatballs to a separate dish. Deglaze the pan with the white wine, scraping up any browned bits from the bottom of the pan. Add the beef broth and bring to a simmer until reduced to about ½ cup of liquid. Whisk in the butter until melted. Stir in the sour cream and return the meatballs to the pan. Simmer gently over low heat until the meatballs are heated through, about 2 minutes, or until ready to serve.

Per Serving: Calories: 509; Fat: 42g; Protein: 29g; Total Carbs: 3g; Fiber: 1g; Net Carbs: 1g; **Macros:** Fat: 74%; Protein: 23%; Carbs: 3%

Meatballs with Spaghetti Squash

SERVES 4 | PREP TIME: 20 minutes | COOK TIME: 30 minutes

1 large spaghetti squash
3 tablespoons water
2 tablespoons olive oil, divided
½ cup chopped fresh parsley, divided
½ pound 80-percent lean ground beef
½ pound ground pork
½ cup shredded Parmesan cheese, divided

2 tablespoons chopped fresh basil
2 tablespoons chopped fresh oregano
½ teaspoon onion powder
½ teaspoon minced garlic
¼ teaspoon salt
¼ teaspoon freshly ground black pepper
1 cup sugar-free pasta sauce

Cut the spaghetti squash in half lengthwise and remove the seeds. Place each half facedown in a microwave-safe dish. Add the water. Microwave on high for 12 minutes. Using a fork, scoop the squash from the shells. In a large skillet over medium-high heat, heat 1 tablespoon of olive oil for about 1 minute. Add the squash to the skillet, stirring to allow any moisture to dissipate. Cook for about 7 minutes, until the squash begins to brown. Remove it from the heat. Transfer the squash to a large bowl. Add ¼ cup of parsley to the bowl and set aside. In a medium bowl, mix the remaining ¼ cup of parsley, beef, pork, ¼ cup of Parmesan cheese, basil, oregano, onion powder, garlic, salt, and pepper. Form the mixture into 12 meatballs. In a large skillet over medium-high heat, heat the remaining tablespoon of olive oil for about 1 minute. Add the meatballs. Brown for 1 to 2 minutes on each side until fully browned, about 5 minutes total. Add the pasta sauce to the pan. Stir to coat the meatballs thoroughly. Reduce the heat to low. Cover the skillet. Cook for 10 to 15 minutes, or until the meatballs are cooked through. Plate 3 meatballs and ¼ cup of sauce over one-quarter of the spaghetti squash per person. Sprinkle the remaining ¼ cup of Parmesan cheese evenly over the plated servings.

Per Serving: (3 meatballs; ¼ cup sauce; ¼ of squash): Calories: 460; Fat: 28g; Total Carbs: 10.9g; Net Carbs: 9.6g; Fiber: 1.3g; Protein: 43.4g; **Macros:** Fat: 54%; Protein: 37%; Carbs: 9%

Italian Meatballs

SERVES 4 | PREP TIME: 20 minutes | COOK TIME: 20 minutes

¾ pound 75-percent lean ground beef
¾ cup grated Parmesan cheese
½ cup almond flour
1 large egg
¼ sweet onion, minced
1 teaspoon minced garlic
1 teaspoon dried basil
½ teaspoon dried oregano
Pinch ground allspice
2 tablespoons extra-virgin olive oil

Preheat the oven to 350°F. Line a baking sheet with parchment, and set aside. In a large bowl, mix the ground beef, Parmesan, almond flour, egg, onion, garlic, basil, oregano, and allspice until well blended. Roll the beef mixture into 1½-inch balls. In a large skillet over medium-high heat, heat the oil. Brown the meatballs in the skillet all over, for about 10 minutes, and transfer them to the baking sheet. Bake the meatballs until just cooked through, about 10 minutes.

Per Serving: Calories: 480; Fat: 38g; Protein: 34g; Total Carbs: 6g; Fiber: 2g; Net Carbs: 4g; **Macros:** Fat: 68%; Protein: 27%; Carbs: 5%

Baked Cheesy Meatballs

SERVES 3 | PREP TIME: 20 minutes | COOK TIME: 40 minutes

8 ounces 80-percent lean ground beef
8 ounces ground pork
½ cup grated Parmesan cheese
¼ cup almond flour
2 tablespoons water
1 tablespoon minced garlic
½ teaspoon salt
¼ teaspoon freshly ground black pepper
1 tablespoon olive oil
2 tablespoons butter
1½ cups pasta sauce, or purchased sugar-free marinara
¾ cup shredded mozzarella cheese
Fresh parsley for garnish

Preheat the oven to 400°F. In a large bowl, combine the ground beef, pork, Parmesan cheese, almond flour, water, garlic, salt, and pepper. Mix thoroughly. Form the meat into about 10 small meatballs. In a large skillet over medium-high heat, heat the olive oil and butter for about 1 minute. Add the meatballs to the skillet. Brown on all sides, about 2 minutes per side. Remove from the skillet. Set aside. In an oven-safe dish, arrange the meatballs to fill the dish with no large empty space. Cover the meatballs with the pasta sauce. Top the meatballs evenly with the mozzarella. Place the dish into the preheated oven. Bake for 15 to 20 minutes, until the cheese browns and the internal temperature of the meatballs is 170°F. Garnish with the parsley, and serve.

Per Serving: (about 3 meatballs): Calories: 672; Fat: 40g; Protein: 62g; Total Carbs: 10g; Fiber: 2g; Net Carbs: 8g; **Macros:** Fat: 56%; Protein: 38%; Carbs: 6%

Beef Stroganoff Meatballs over Zoodles

SERVES 4 | PREP TIME: 15 minutes | COOK TIME: 30 minutes

1 pound ground beef or bison
¼ cup, plus 2 tablespoons almond flour, divided
2 tablespoons finely minced onion
1 teaspoon salt
1 teaspoon dried thyme
½ teaspoon garlic powder
¼ teaspoon freshly ground black pepper
1 large egg, beaten
¼ cup extra-virgin olive oil
2 cups cream of mushroom soup
⅓ cup sour cream
4 cups raw spiralized zucchini

In a large bowl, combine the ground beef, ¼ cup of almond flour, onion, salt, thyme, garlic powder, and pepper and mix well with a fork. Mix in the egg until well combined. Using your hands, form the mixture into 1-inch round meatballs and set aside. In a shallow dish, place the remaining 2 tablespoons of almond flour and roll the meatballs in the flour. In a large skillet, heat the olive oil over medium-high heat. Sauté the meatballs for 6 to 8 minutes, turning to brown on all sides. Add the soup, bring to a boil, reduce heat to low, cover and cook for 15 to 20 minutes, until the meatballs are cooked through. Remove from the heat and stir in the sour cream until well blended. To serve, top the raw zucchini noodles with the hot meatballs and sauce and toss to combine.

Per Serving: Calories: 580; Fat: 46g; Protein: 30g; Total Carbs: 13g; Fiber: 3g; Net Carbs: 10g; **Macros:** Fat: 71%; Protein: 21%; Carbs: 8%

Cheese-Stuffed Italian Meatballs

SERVES 4 | PREP TIME: 10 minutes | COOK TIME: 30 minutes

For the meatballs

1 pound ground beef (80/20)
½ cup grated Parmesan cheese
1 large egg
2 teaspoons dried Italian seasoning
½ teaspoon pink Himalayan sea salt
½ teaspoon freshly ground black pepper
1 cup shredded low-moisture mozzarella cheese
Extra-virgin olive oil, for greasing

For the sauce

1 cup tomato puree
1 garlic clove, minced
½ teaspoon pink Himalayan sea salt
½ teaspoon Italian seasoning

Preheat the oven to 350°F. In a large bowl, combine the ground beef, Parmesan, egg, Italian seasoning, salt, and pepper. Using your hands, mix the meat with the ingredients until well blended. Divide the meat mixture into 4 equal portions, about 5 ounces each. Flatten each portion into a square and fill the center of each with ¼ cup of the mozzarella. Fold the meat up and around the cheese to seal it well. Coat an 8-inch-square baking dish with some olive oil. Place the meatballs in the dish and bake for 30 minutes. In a medium bowl, mix the tomato puree, garlic, salt, and Italian seasoning. Top the meatballs in the baking pan with the sauce, then bake for an additional 8 to 10 minutes, until the sauce is heated through and coating the meatballs.

Per Serving: Calories: 478; Fat: 34g; Protein: 32g; Total Carbs: 9g; Fiber: 1g; Net Carbs: 8g; **Macros:** Fat: 65%; Protein: 28%; Carbs: 7%

Bison Burgers in Lettuce Wraps

SERVES 4 | PREP TIME: 15 minutes | COOK TIME: 20 minutes

1 pound ground bison

4 ounces feta cheese, crumbled

2 tablespoons extra-virgin olive oil

2 teaspoons ground cumin

1 teaspoon salt

1 teaspoon ground cinnamon

1 teaspoon ground ginger

½ to 1 teaspoon red pepper flakes

4 large Bibb or Romaine lettuce leaves, for serving

1 cup guacamole, for serving

Heat the grill or grill pan to medium-high heat. In a large bowl, combine the bison, feta, olive oil, cumin, salt, cinnamon, ginger, and red pepper flakes and, using your hands, mix well. Form the mixture into 4 burgers and cook for 5 to 8 minutes per side, until browned and cooked through to desired doneness. Serve the burgers wrapped in lettuce leaves and topped with ¼ cup of guacamole per burger.

Per Serving: Calories: 468; Fat: 35g; Protein: 35g; Total Carbs: 8g; Fiber: 5g; Net Carbs: 3g; **Macros:** Fat: 67%; Protein: 30%; Carbs: 3%

Ground Bison Chile Rellenos with Ranchero Sauce

SERVES 4 | PREP TIME: 30 minutes | COOK TIME: 1 hour

4 large whole poblano peppers

2 medium ripe tomatoes, quartered

1 medium red bell pepper, quartered

1 small jalapeño, stemmed and halved (remove seeds for less heat)

1 small red onion, quartered

8 garlic cloves, peeled

½ cup extra-virgin olive oil, divided

2 teaspoons salt, divided

8 ounces ground bison

1 teaspoon ground cumin

1 teaspoon ground coriander

1 teaspoon chili powder

1 teaspoon fennel seed

1 teaspoon garlic powder

4 ounces frozen spinach, thawed and well-drained

4 ounces goat cheese

1 small bunch fresh cilantro, leaves only

Juice and zest of 1 lime

1 large ripe avocado, peeled pitted and thinly sliced, for serving

1 lime, cut into wedges, for serving

2 tablespoons roasted pumpkin seeds, for serving

Preheat the oven to 425°F. Line a baking sheet with foil and place whole poblano peppers in a single layer on the baking sheet. Place in the oven and roast for 20 to 25 minutes, depending on size of pepper until just tender and wilted, but not blackened. Remove from the oven and allow to cool on the foil. Meanwhile, in a large glass baking dish, place the tomatoes, bell peppers, jalapeño, onion, and garlic. Drizzle with ¼ cup of olive oil and 1 teaspoon of salt and toss to coat. Roast for 40 to 45 minutes, stirring once halfway through, until soft and lightly browned. Remove from the oven and let cool. Meanwhile, in a medium skillet, heat 2 tablespoons of olive oil over medium-high heat. Cook the bison for 4 to 5 minutes, stirring occasionally, until

browned. Add the cumin, coriander, chili powder, fennel, garlic powder, and remaining 1 teaspoon of salt. Mix well and sauté for 1 to 2 minutes. Remove from the heat and stir in spinach and goat cheese and mix well. To make the ranchero sauce, transfer the cooled roasted vegetables to a blender or food processor. Add the cilantro and lime juice and zest and blend until smooth. Set aside. To stuff the poblanos, carefully cut a slit in the roasted poblano peppers from stem to end and using your fingers, gently remove the seeds and membrane. Stuff each pepper with the bison and spinach mixture. Spread half of the sauce on the bottom of a glass baking dish. Place the peppers in a single layer on top of sauce and spread remaining sauce evenly over the peppers. Drizzle with remaining 2 tablespoons of olive oil and cover with foil. Bake for 20 minutes. Remove the foil and bake for another 5 minutes, or until bubbly. Serve warm with avocado, lime juice, and pumpkin seeds.

Per Serving: Calories: 605; Fat: 50g; Protein: 24g; Total Carbs: 22g; Fiber: 9g; Net Carbs: 13g; **Macros:** Fat: 74%; Protein: 16%; Carbs: 10%

Rack of Lamb with Kalamata Tapenade

SERVES 4 | PREP TIME: 15 minutes | COOK TIME: 25 minutes

For the tapenade

1 cup pitted Kalamata olives

2 tablespoons chopped fresh parsley

2 tablespoons extra-virgin olive oil

2 teaspoons minced garlic

2 teaspoons freshly squeezed lemon juice

For the lamb chops

2 (1-pound) racks French-cut lamb chops (8 bones each)

Sea salt

Freshly ground black pepper

1 tablespoon olive oil

Place the olives, parsley, olive oil, garlic, and lemon juice in a food processor and process until the mixture is puréed but still slightly chunky. Transfer the tapenade to a container and store sealed in the refrigerator until needed. Preheat the oven to 450°F. Season the lamb racks with salt and pepper. Place a large ovenproof skillet over medium-high heat and add the olive oil. Pan sear the lamb racks on all sides until browned, about 5 minutes in total. Arrange the racks upright in the skillet, with the bones interlaced, and roast them in the oven until they reach your desired doneness, about 20 minutes for medium-rare or until the internal temperature reaches 125°F. Let the lamb rest for 10 minutes and then cut the lamb racks into chops. Top with the Kalamata tapenade.

Per serving: Calories: 348; Fat: 28g; Protein: 21g; Total Carbs: 2g; Fiber: 1g; Net Carbs: 1g; **Macros:** Fat: 72%; Protein: 25%; Carbs: 3%

Herb-Crusted Lamb Chops

SERVES 3 | PREP TIME: 15 minutes | COOK TIME: 15 minutes

1 pound lamb chops

2 tablespoons Dijon mustard

4 fresh rosemary sprigs, chopped

4 fresh thyme sprigs, chopped

3 tablespoons almond flour

4 garlic cloves, minced

1 teaspoon onion powder

¼ teaspoon salt

¼ teaspoon freshly ground black pepper

¼ cup olive oil, divided

Preheat the oven to 350°F. Coat the lamb chops with the mustard. Set aside. To a blender or food processor, add the rosemary, thyme, almond flour, garlic, onion powder, salt, and pepper. Pulse until finely chopped. Slowly add about 2 tablespoons of olive oil to form a thick paste. Press the herb paste firmly around the edges of the mustard-coated chops, creating a crust. In a large oven-safe skillet over medium heat, heat the remaining 2 tablespoons of olive oil for 2 minutes. Add the chops to the skillet on their sides to brown. Cook, undisturbed, for 2 to 3 minutes so the crust adheres properly to the meat. Turn and cook on the opposite edge for 2 to 3 minutes more. Transfer the chops to a baking sheet. Place the sheet in the preheated oven. Cook for 7 to 8 minutes, for medium. Remove the sheet from the oven. Serve immediately.

Per Serving: Calories: 486; Fat: 32g; Protein: 43g; Total Carbs: 4g; Fiber: 1g; Net Carbs: 3g; Macros: Fat: 61%; Protein: 36%; Carbs: 3%

Broiled Lamb Chops with Mint Gremolata and Pan-Fried Zucchini

SERVES 4 | PREP TIME: 5 minutes | COOK TIME: 20 minutes, plus 5 minutes to rest

8 (4-ounce) bone-in lamb chops	4 medium zucchini, sliced into ½-inch-thick coins
Salt	½ cup fresh mint leaves
Freshly ground black pepper	Grated zest of 1 lemon
2 tablespoons olive oil	2 teaspoons minced garlic

Preheat the broiler to high. Season the lamb chops on both sides with salt and pepper and place on a baking sheet. Broil for 4 minutes on each side for rare, 5 minutes on each side for medium-rare, 7 minutes on each side for medium, and 9 minutes on each side for well-done. Let rest for 5 minutes. Meanwhile, in a large skillet, heat the oil over medium heat. Add the zucchini and cook, stirring frequently, for 10 minutes, or to desired tenderness. Finely chop the mint and place in a medium bowl. Add the lemon zest and garlic and mix well. You can also pulse all the ingredients in a food processor until finely minced. Spoon the mint gremolata over the lamb chops and serve with the zucchini.

Per Serving: Calories: 564; Fat: 40g; Protein: 45g; Total Carbs: 7g; Fiber: 2g; Net Carbs: 5g; Macros: Fat: 64%; Protein: 31%; Carbs: 5%

Grilled Moroccan Spiced Lamb Chops

SERVES 4 | PREP TIME: 5 minutes | COOK TIME: 10 minutes

½ teaspoon cumin	¼ teaspoon garlic powder
¼ teaspoon cardamom	⅛ teaspoon black pepper
¼ teaspoon ground ginger	8 lamb chops (about 2 pounds)
¼ teaspoon cayenne pepper	
¼ teaspoon ground cinnamon	1 tablespoon chopped fresh cilantro (optional)
¼ teaspoon salt	

In a small bowl, mix the cumin, cardamom, ginger, cayenne, cinnamon, salt, garlic powder, and pepper. Sprinkle both sides of the lamb chops with the seasoning mixture. Heat your grill or grill pan to high heat and grill the lamb on each side for a total of 6 to 8 minutes or until the internal temperature reaches 130 to 135°F. Set aside. Garnish with fresh cilantro and serve.

Per Serving: Calories: 354; Fat: 24g; Protein: 31g; Total Carbs: 1g; Fiber: 0g; Net Carbs: 1g; Macros: Fat: 62%; Protein: 37%; Carbs: 1%

Rosemary-Garlic Lamb Racks

SERVES 4 | PREP TIME: 10 minutes, plus 1 hour to marinate | COOK TIME: 25 minutes

¼ cup extra-virgin olive oil	Pinch sea salt
2 tablespoons finely chopped fresh rosemary	2 (1-pound) racks French-cut lamb chops (8 bones each)
2 teaspoons minced garlic	

In a small bowl, whisk the olive oil, rosemary, garlic, and salt. Place the racks in a sealable freezer bag and pour the olive oil mixture into the bag. Massage the meat through the bag so it is coated with the marinade. Press the air out of the bag and seal it. Marinate the lamb racks in the refrigerator for 1 to 2 hours. Preheat the oven to 450°F. Place a large ovenproof skillet over medium-high heat. Take the lamb racks out of the bag and sear them in the skillet on all sides, about 5 minutes in total. Arrange the racks upright in the skillet, with the bones interlaced, and roast them in the oven until they reach your desired doneness, about 20 minutes for medium-rare or until the internal temperature reaches 125°F. Let the lamb rest for 10 minutes and then cut the racks into chops. Serve 4 chops per person.

Per Serving: Calories: 354; Fat: 30g; Protein: 21g; Total Carbs: 0g; Fiber: 0g; Net Carbs: 0g; Macros: Fat: 70%; Protein: 30%; Carbs: 0%

Herb Mustard Lamb Racks

SERVES 4 | PREP TIME: 20 minutes | COOK TIME: 20 minutes

2 frenched lamb racks, 8 bones each	1 tablespoon chopped fresh rosemary
Sea salt	¼ teaspoon salt
Freshly ground black pepper	¼ teaspoon freshly ground black pepper
¼ cup olive oil, divided	
½ cup almond meal	2 tablespoons Dijon mustard
1 tablespoon minced garlic	

Preheat the oven to 450°F. Season the lamb racks with salt and pepper. Heat 2 tablespoons of olive oil in a large ovenproof skillet. Sear the lamb racks on all sides, including the bottom, about 5 minutes total. Remove the skillet from the heat. In a medium bowl, stir the almond meal, garlic, rosemary, salt, and pepper until well blended. Add the remaining olive oil to the almond mixture, tossing to mix. Spread the mustard on the lamb racks and roll them in the almond mixture. Place the racks back in the skillet bone-side down, and roast until the lamb is the desired doneness, 15 to 18 minutes for medium-rare (125°F to 130°F internal temperature). Let the lamb rest 10 minutes.

Per Serving: Calories: 739; Fat: 63g; Protein: 35g; Total Carbs: 7g; Fiber: 2g; Net Carbs: 5g; Macros: Fat: 77%; Protein: 19%; Carbs: 4%

Leg of Lamb with Sun-dried Tomato Pesto

SERVES 8 | PREP TIME: 15 minutes | COOK TIME: 70 minutes

For the pesto

1 cup sun-dried tomatoes packed in oil, drained	2 tablespoons extra-virgin olive oil
¼ cup pine nuts	

2 tablespoons chopped
  fresh basil

2 teaspoons minced garlic

For the leg of lamb

1 (2-pound) boneless
  leg of lamb

Sea salt

Freshly ground black pepper

2 tablespoons olive oil

Place the sun-dried tomatoes, pine nuts, olive oil, basil, and garlic in a blender or food processor; process until smooth. Set aside until needed. Preheat the oven to 400°F. Season the lamb leg all over with salt and pepper. Place a large ovenproof skillet over medium-high heat and add the olive oil. Sear the lamb on all sides until nicely browned, about 6 minutes in total. Spread the sun-dried tomato pesto all over the lamb and place the lamb on a baking sheet. Roast until the meat reaches your desired doneness, about 1 hour for medium.

Per Serving: Calories: 352; Fat: 29g; Protein: 17g; Total Carbs: 5g; Fiber: 2g; Net Carbs: 3g; **Macros:** Fat: 74%; Protein: 20%; Carbs: 6%

Lamb Meatball Salad with Yogurt Dressing

SERVES 4 | PREP TIME: 10 minutes | COOK TIME: 20 minutes

¼ cup almond flour

¼ cup minced red onion

1 teaspoon minced garlic

1 large egg, whisked

2 tablespoons minced
  fresh parsley

1 tablespoon minced
  fresh oregano

½ teaspoon sea salt, plus
  more for seasoning

½ teaspoon freshly ground
  black pepper, plus more for
  seasoning

1 pound ground lamb

½ cup plain yogurt

¼ cup full-fat mayonnaise

1 teaspoon minced fresh dill

1 teaspoon minced fresh garlic

1 cup fresh mint leaves

2 cups baby spinach

4 cups hand-torn
  romaine lettuce

4 roasted red bell peppers,
  sliced into 2-inch pieces

½ cup diced peeled
  cucumbers

½ cup assorted pitted olives

Preheat the oven to 400°F. In a medium bowl, mix the almond flour, onion, garlic, egg, parsley, oregano, ½ teaspoon salt, and ½ teaspoon pepper. Add the lamb to the bowl, and using your hands, mix the ingredients until combined. Shape the mixture into 16 small meatballs. Place the meatballs on a rimmed baking sheet and bake for 20 minutes, or until gently browned and cooked through. While the meatballs bake, make the yogurt dressing. In a small bowl, mix the yogurt, mayonnaise, dill, and garlic. Season to taste with salt and pepper. To serve, place the mint, spinach, lettuce, bell peppers, cucumbers, and olives on a large serving platter. Top with the cooked lamb meatballs and pour the yogurt dressing over the salad. Season with more freshly ground pepper.

Per Serving: Calories: 568; Fat: 47g; Protein: 26g; Total Carbs: 11g; Fiber: 3g; Net Carbs: 8g; **Macros:** Fat: 74%; Protein: 18%; Carbs: 8%

Lamb Chili

SERVES 4 | PREP TIME: 15 minutes | COOK TIME: 45 minutes

¼ cup olive oil

1 pound ground lamb

1 onion, chopped

½ fennel bulb, diced

1 red bell pepper, chopped

1 tablespoon minced garlic

3 tablespoons chili powder

1 teaspoon ground cumin

1 teaspoon ground coriander

¼ teaspoon red pepper flakes

2 cups low-sodium
  chicken stock

1 cup canned coconut milk

2 tablespoons chopped fresh
  cilantro

Heat the olive oil in a large stockpot over medium-high heat. Sauté the lamb until it is cooked through, about 15 minutes. Add the onion, fennel, bell pepper, and garlic and sauté until softened, about 6 minutes. Stir in the chili powder, cumin, coriander, and red pepper flakes and sauté 4 minutes. Stir in the chicken stock and coconut milk and bring the mixture to a boil. Simmer until the vegetables are tender and the flavors have mellowed, about 20 minutes. Serve topped with cilantro.

Per Serving: Calories: 600; Fat: 52g; Protein: 22g; Total Carbs: 12g; Fiber: 4g; Net Carbs: 8g; **Macros:** Fat: 78%; Protein: 15%; Carbs: 7%

Simple Lamb Sausage

SERVES 4 | PREP TIME: 10 minutes | COOK TIME: 30 minutes

1 pound ground lamb

½ onion, finely chopped

1 tablespoon chopped
  fresh parsley

2 teaspoons minced garlic

1 teaspoon dried basil

1 teaspoon paprika

¼ teaspoon sea salt

¼ teaspoon fennel seed

⅛ teaspoon freshly ground
  black pepper

Pinch ground cloves

2 tablespoons olive oil, divided

In a large bowl, stir the lamb, onion, parsley, garlic, basil, paprika, salt, fennel seed, pepper, and cloves until very well mixed. Divide the mixture into 8 equal portions and form them into ½-inch-thick patties. Heat 1 tablespoon of olive oil in a large skillet over medium-high heat and panfry the patties 4 at a time, turning once, until cooked through and golden, about 15 minutes total. Transfer the patties to a plate and repeat with the remaining patties and remaining olive oil.

Per Serving: Calories: 390; Fat: 34g; Protein: 19g; Total Carbs: 2g; Fiber: 1g; Net Carbs: 1g; **Macros:** Fat: 78%; Protein: 20%; Carbs: 2%

Savory Lamb Stew

SERVES 4 | PREP TIME: 20 minutes | COOK TIME: 35 minutes

¼ cup olive oil

1 pound ground lamb

1 onion, chopped

2 cups halved mushrooms

1 tablespoon minced garlic

1 teaspoon peeled, grated
  fresh ginger

½ teaspoon ground turmeric

½ teaspoon ground cinnamon

¼ teaspoon ground cloves

2 cups diced raw or
  frozen pumpkin

2 cups low-sodium beef stock

1 tablespoon chopped
  fresh thyme

Sea salt

Freshly ground black pepper

Heat the olive oil in a large stockpot on medium-high heat. Brown the lamb until cooked through, stirring occasionally, about 10 minutes. Add the onion, mushrooms, garlic, ginger, turmeric, cinnamon, and cloves. Sauté until the vegetables are softened, about 5 minutes. Stir in the pumpkin, beef stock, and thyme and bring the stew to a boil. Reduce the heat to low and simmer until the pumpkin is tender, about 20 minutes. Season with salt and pepper and serve.

Per Serving: Calories: 489; Fat: 40g; Protein: 23g; Total Carbs: 9g; Fiber: 2g; Net Carbs: 7g; **Macros:** Fat: 74%; Protein: 19%; Carbs: 7%

Lamb Kofte with Yogurt Sauce

SERVES 4 | PREP TIME: 30 minutes, plus 10 minutes to rest | COOK TIME: 15 minutes

1 pound ground lamb	1 teaspoon ground cinnamon
½ cup finely chopped fresh mint, plus 2 tablespoons	1 teaspoon ground ginger
¼ cup almond or coconut flour	½ teaspoon ground nutmeg
¼ cup finely chopped red onion	½ teaspoon freshly ground black pepper
¼ cup toasted pine nuts	1 cup plain Greek yogurt
2 teaspoons ground cumin	2 tablespoons extra-virgin olive oil
1½ teaspoons salt, divided	Zest and juice of 1 lime

Heat the oven broiler to the low setting. You can also bake these at high heat (450 to 475°F) if you happen to have a very hot broiler. Soak 4 wooden skewers in water for 10 minutes. In a large bowl, combine the lamb, ½ cup mint, almond flour, red onion, pine nuts, cumin, 1 teaspoon salt, cinnamon, ginger, nutmeg, and pepper and, using your hands, mix well. Form the mixture into 12 egg-shaped patties and let sit for 10 minutes. Thread 3 patties onto each skewer, and place on a broiling pan or wire rack on top of a baking sheet lined with aluminum foil. Broil on the top rack until golden and cooked through, 8 to 12 minutes, flipping once halfway through cooking. While the meat cooks, in a small bowl, combine the yogurt, olive oil, remaining 2 tablespoons chopped mint, remaining ½ teaspoon salt, and lime zest and juice and whisk to combine well. Serve with yogurt sauce.

Per Serving: Calories: 500; Fat: 42g; Protein: 23g; Total Carbs: 9g; Fiber: 2g; Net Carbs: 7g; **Macros:** Fat: 75%; Protein: 19%; Carbs: 6%

Greek Meatball Lettuce Wraps

SERVES 2 | PREP TIME: 15 minutes | COOK TIME: 20 minutes

½ pound ground lamb	1 teaspoon dried oregano
2 tablespoons fresh parsley, finely chopped	3 teaspoons avocado oil
½ teaspoon fresh mint, finely chopped	2 Bibb lettuce leaves
1 garlic clove, minced	1 avocado, peeled and sliced
	2 tablespoons tzatziki (optional)

Preheat the oven to 350°F. Line a baking sheet with parchment paper. In a large bowl, mix the lamb, parsley, mint, garlic, and oregano until well combined. Roll the meat mixture into 1½-inch balls. In a medium skillet, heat the avocado oil on high heat. Place the meatballs in the skillet and sear on all sides for 5 to 10 minutes. Transfer the seared meatballs to the baking sheet and bake for about 5 minutes or until the internal temperature reaches about 130°F. Prepare the lettuce wraps by placing 2 to 3 meatballs inside each lettuce leaf and topping them with the avocado and tzatziki, if using.

Per Serving: Calories: 530; Fat: 48g; Protein: 20g; Total Carbs: 7g; Fiber: 5g; Net Carbs: 2g; **Macros:** Fat: 81%; Protein: 16%; Carbs: 5%

Grilled Venison Loin with Dijon Cream Sauce

SERVES 4 | PREP TIME: 10 minutes, plus 2 hours to marinate | COOK TIME: 15 minutes

1 pound venison loin, trimmed of all silver skin	½ teaspoon chopped fresh rosemary
Sea salt	1½ cups heavy (whipping) cream
Freshly ground black pepper	2 tablespoons grainy mustard
2 tablespoons extra-virgin olive oil	½ teaspoon apple cider vinegar
1 teaspoon chopped fresh thyme	1 teaspoon chopped fresh chives

Season the venison all over with the salt and pepper. In a small bowl, stir the olive oil, thyme, and rosemary, and rub the meat all over with the oil mixture. Place the meat in a sealed freezer bag, and refrigerate for 2 hours. Preheat the barbecue or grill pan to medium-high. In a medium saucepan over medium heat, bring the cream to a simmer. Reduce the heat to low, and simmer until the cream is reduced by half into a thick, creamy sauce, about 5 minutes. Remove the cream from the heat, and stir in the mustard, vinegar, and chives. Grill the venison, 4 to 5 minutes per side, turning to get all the surfaces browned. Let the meat rest for 10 minutes, and serve with the sauce.

Per Serving: Calories: 394; Fat: 28g; Protein: 34g; Total Carbs: 2g; Fiber: 0g; Net Carbs: 2g; **Macros:** Fat: 64%; Protein: 34%; Carbs: 2%

Venison Pot Roast

SERVES 4 | PREP TIME: 15 minutes | COOK TIME: 2 hours 10 minutes

1 (1-pound) venison roast	½ cup chopped sweet onion
Sea salt	1 teaspoon minced garlic
Freshly ground black pepper	1 cup beef broth
¼ cup extra-virgin olive oil	2 bay leaves
1 celery stalk, chopped	1 teaspoon dried thyme

Preheat the oven to 275°F. Season the roast with salt and pepper. In a large, ovenproof skillet over medium-high heat, heat the olive oil. Sear the roast on all sides until lightly browned, about 5 minutes total. Remove the roast to a plate. Add the celery, onion, and garlic to the skillet, and sauté until softened, about 3 minutes. Return the roast to the skillet with any accumulated juices on the plate, and stir in the beef broth, bay leaves, and thyme. Cook the roast in the oven for 2 hours, turning it occasionally. Remove the skillet from the oven, and take out the bay leaves. Let the roast rest for 10 minutes before serving it with the pan drippings.

Per Serving: Calories: 342; Fat: 20g; Protein: 40g; Total Carbs: 2g; Fiber: 0g; Net Carbs: 2g; **Macros:** Fat: 52%; Protein: 46%; Carbs: 2%

Pressure Cooker Sloppy Joes

SERVES 4 | PREP TIME: 5 minutes | COOK TIME: 15 minutes, plus 5 minutes to come to pressure | RELEASE: Quick

Nonstick cooking spray
1 pound ground beef
1 cup tomato sauce
2 tablespoons store-bought low-carb ketchup
½ red bell pepper, seeded and diced

1 tablespoon Worcestershire sauce
1 teaspoon mustard powder
1 teaspoon onion powder
Salt
Freshly ground black pepper
Garlic Cloud Bread

Coat a pressure cooker bowl with cooking spray. Put the ground beef in the bowl. Set the electric pressure cooker to Sautè and cook, stirring frequently, until the meat is browned all over. Press Cancel to stop the Sautè function. Drain the excess liquid. Add the tomato sauce, ketchup, bell pepper, Worcestershire sauce, mustard powder, and onion powder. Season with salt and pepper. Stir well to mix. Lock the pressure cooker lid in place with the steam vent set to Sealing. Select low pressure and set the timer for 5 minutes. After cooking, quick release the pressure. Carefully open the pressure cooker and transfer the sloppy joes to a serving bowl. Serve with cloud bread.

Per Serving: Calories: 550; Fat: 42g; Protein: 32g; Total Carbs: 11g; Fiber: 1g; Net Carbs: 10g; Macros: Fat: 69%; Protein: 23%; Carbs: 8%

Pressure Cooker Pot Roast with Sour-Cream Gravy

SERVES 6 | PREP TIME: 10 minutes | COOK TIME: 1 hour 5 minutes, plus 15 minutes to come to pressure | RELEASE: Natural, 10 minutes, then Quick

3 pounds boneless beef chuck roast
Salt
Freshly ground black pepper
1 teaspoon garlic powder
2 tablespoons olive oil
2 cups beef broth
¼ cup chopped onion
1 tablespoon tomato paste

1½ pounds turnips, peeled and diced
1 (8-ounce) package whole white mushrooms
1 orange bell pepper, seeded and diced
2 celery stalks, chopped
½ cup sour cream

Season the meat all over with salt, pepper, and the garlic powder. In a large skillet, heat the oil over medium-high heat. Sear the meat for 5 minutes to brown all sides. Transfer the meat to a pressure cooker. Add the broth, onion, and tomato paste. Lock the pressure cooker lid in place with the steam vent set to Sealing. Select high pressure and set the timer for 60 minutes. Allow the pressure to release naturally for 10 minutes, then quick release any remaining pressure. Open the lid and add the turnips, mushrooms, bell pepper, and celery. Replace the lid, turn the valve to Sealing again, and pressure cook on high for 5 minutes. Carefully quick release the pressure and remove the lid. Transfer the beef to a cutting board and use two forks to shred it into chunks. Remove the vegetables with a slotted spoon. Stir the sour cream into the gravy in the cooker until well combined. Drizzle each serving of roast with about ¼ cup of the gravy from the cooker.

Per Serving: Calories: 566; Fat: 37g; Protein: 48g; Total Carbs: 13g; Fiber: 3g; Net Carbs: 10g; Macros: Fat: 58%; Protein: 33%; Carbs: 9%

Pressure Cooker Pork-and-Beef Meatloaf

SERVES 4 | PREP TIME: 5 minutes | COOK TIME: 30 minutes, plus 10 minutes to come to pressure | RELEASE: Quick

1 pound ground pork or sausage
1 pound ground beef
2 large eggs, beaten
¾ cup pork rind crumbs
1 tablespoon Worcester-shire sauce
1 tablespoon onion powder

1 teaspoon garlic powder
½ teaspoon salt
¼ teaspoon freshly ground black pepper
¼ cup store-bought low-carb ketchup
2 cups water

In a large bowl, mix the ground pork, beef, eggs, pork rind crumbs, Worcestershire sauce, onion powder, garlic powder, salt, and pepper. Form the mixture into a loaf shape and place it on a piece of aluminum foil. Fold the sides of the foil up so it forms a shallow bowl. Spread the ketchup over the top of the meatloaf. Add the water to the electric pressure cooker pot and insert the trivet. Carefully place the meatloaf on the trivet using the sides of the foil. Lock the pressure cooker lid in place with the steam vent set to Sealing. Select high pressure and set the timer for 30 minutes. After cooking, quick release the pressure and check that the center of the meat loaf is at least 165°F. Slice and serve.

Per Serving: Calories: 599; Fat: 43g; Protein: 44g; Total Carbs: 5g; Fiber: 0g; Net Carbs: 5g; Macros: Fat: 65%; Protein: 31%; Carbs: 4%

Lemon-Thyme Asparagus

SERVES 4 | PREP TIME: 5 minutes | COOK TIME: 4 to 8 minutes | TEMPERATURE: 400°F

1 pound asparagus, woody ends trimmed off
1 tablespoon avocado oil
½ teaspoon dried thyme or ½ tablespoon chopped fresh thyme

Sea salt
Freshly ground black pepper
2 ounces goat cheese, crumbled
Zest and juice of 1 lemon
Flaky sea salt, for serving

In a medium bowl, toss the asparagus, avocado oil, and thyme, and season with sea salt and pepper. Place the asparagus in the air fryer basket in a single layer. Set the air fryer to 400°F and cook for 4 to 8 minutes, to your desired doneness. Transfer to a serving platter. Top with the goat cheese, lemon zest, and lemon juice. If desired, season with a pinch of flaky salt.

Per Serving: Calories: 103; Fat: 7g; Protein: 5g; Total Carbs: 7g; Fiber: 3g; Net Carbs: 4g; Macros: Fat: 61%; Protein: 19%; Carbs: 20%

Parmesan-Rosemary Radishes

SERVES 4 | PREP TIME: 5 minutes | COOK TIME: 15 to 20 minutes | TEMPERATURE: 375°F

1 bunch radishes, stemmed, trimmed, and quartered
1 tablespoon avocado oil
2 tablespoons finely grated fresh Parmesan cheese

1 tablespoon chopped fresh rosemary
Sea salt
Freshly ground black pepper

Place the radishes in a medium bowl and toss them with the avocado oil, Parmesan cheese, rosemary, salt, and pepper. Set the air fryer to 375°F. Arrange the radishes in a single layer in the air fryer basket. Cook for 15 to 20 minutes, until golden brown and tender. Let cool for 5 minutes before serving.

Per Serving: Calories: 47; Fat: 4g; Protein: 1g; Total Carbs: 1g; Fiber: <1g; Net Carbs: 1g; **Macros:** Fat: 77%; Protein: 9%; Carbs: 14%

Bacon-Wrapped Jalapeño Poppers

SERVES 12 | PREP TIME: 15 minutes | COOK TIME: 17 to 22 minutes | TEMPERATURE: 400°F

12 jalapeño peppers
8 ounces cream cheese, at room temperature
2 tablespoons minced onion
1 teaspoon garlic powder
½ teaspoon smoked paprika
Sea salt
Freshly ground black pepper
12 strips bacon

Slice the jalapeños in half lengthwise, then seed them and remove any remaining white membranes to make room for the filling. Set the air fryer to 400°F. Place the jalapeños in a single layer, cut-side down, in the air fryer basket. Cook for 7 minutes. Remove the peppers from the air fryer and place them on a paper towel, cut-side up. Allow them to rest until they are cool enough to handle. While the jalapeños are cooking, in a medium bowl, stir the cream cheese, minced onion, garlic powder, and smoked paprika. Season to taste with salt and pepper. Spoon the cream cheese filling into the jalapeños. Cut the bacon strips in half, and wrap 1 piece around each stuffed jalapeño half. Place the bacon-wrapped jalapeños, cut-side up, in a single layer in the air fryer basket. Cook for 10 to 15 minutes, until the bacon is crispy.

Per Serving: Calories: 116; Fat: 10g; Protein: 4g; Total Carbs: 2g; Fiber: 1g; Net Carbs: 1g; **Macros:** Fat: 78%; Protein: 21%; Carbs: 1%

Smoky Zucchini Chips

SERVES 6 | PREP TIME: 15 minutes | COOK TIME: 8 to 10 minutes | TEMPERATURE: 400°F

2 large eggs
1 cup almond flour
½ cup Parmesan cheese
1½ teaspoons sea salt
1 teaspoon garlic powder
½ teaspoon smoked paprika
¼ teaspoon freshly ground black pepper
2 zucchini, cut into ¼-inch-thick slices
Avocado oil spray

Beat the eggs in a shallow bowl. In another bowl, stir the almond flour, Parmesan cheese, salt, garlic powder, smoked paprika, and black pepper. Dip the zucchini slices in the egg mixture, then coat them with the almond flour mixture. Set the air fryer to 400°F. Place the zucchini chips in a single layer in the air fryer basket, working in batches if necessary. Spray the chips with oil and cook for 4 minutes. Flip the chips and spray them with more oil. Cook for 4 to 6 minutes more.

Per Serving: Calories: 181; Fat: 14g; Protein: 11g; Total Carbs: 7g; Fiber: 3g; Net Carbs: 4g; **Macros:** Fat: 70%; Protein: 24%; Carbs: 6%

Lemon-Garlic Mushrooms

SERVES 6 | PREP TIME: 10 minutes | COOK TIME: 10 to 15 minutes | TEMPERATURE: 375°F

12 ounces sliced mushrooms
1 tablespoon avocado oil
Sea salt
Freshly ground black pepper
3 tablespoons unsalted butter
1 teaspoon minced garlic
1 teaspoon freshly squeezed lemon juice
½ teaspoon red pepper flakes
2 tablespoons chopped fresh parsley

Place the mushrooms in a medium bowl and toss with the oil. Season to taste with salt and pepper. Place the mushrooms in a single layer in the air fryer basket. Set your air fryer to 375°F and cook for 10 to 15 minutes, until the mushrooms are tender. While the mushrooms cook, melt the butter in a small pot or skillet over medium-low heat. Stir in the garlic and cook for 30 seconds. Remove the pot from the heat and stir in the lemon juice and red pepper flakes. Toss the mushrooms with the lemon-garlic butter and garnish with the parsley before serving.

Per Serving: Calories: 80; Fat: 8g; Protein: 1g; Total Carbs: 1g; Fiber: <1g; Net Carbs: 1g; **Macros:** Fat: 90%; Protein: 5%; Carbs: 5%

Spicy Roasted Broccoli

SERVES 6 | PREP TIME: 8 minutes | COOK TIME: 10 to 14 minutes | TEMPERATURE: 375°F

1 head broccoli, cut into bite-size florets
1 tablespoon avocado oil
2 teaspoons minced garlic
⅛ teaspoon red pepper flakes
Sea salt
Freshly ground black pepper
1 tablespoon freshly squeezed lemon juice
½ teaspoon lemon zest

In a large bowl, toss the broccoli, avocado oil, garlic, red pepper flakes, salt, and pepper. Set the air fryer to 375°F. Arrange the broccoli in a single layer in the air fryer basket, working in batches if necessary. Cook for 10 to 14 minutes, until the broccoli is lightly charred. Place the florets in a medium bowl and toss with the lemon juice and lemon zest. Serve.

Per Serving: Calories: 52; Fat: 3g; Protein: 3g; Total Carbs: 6g; Fiber: 3g; Net Carbs: 3g; **Macros:** Fat: 52%; Protein: 23%; Carbs: 25%

Buttery Green Beans

SERVES 6 | PREP TIME: 5 minutes | COOK TIME: 8 to 10 minutes | TEMPERATURE: 400°F

1 pound green beans, trimmed
1 tablespoon avocado oil
1 teaspoon garlic powder
Sea salt
Freshly ground black pepper
¼ cup unsalted butter, melted
¼ cup freshly grated Parmesan cheese

In a large bowl, toss the green beans, avocado oil, and garlic powder and season with salt and pepper. Set the air fryer to 400°F. Arrange the green beans in a single layer in the air fryer basket. Cook for 8 to 10 minutes, tossing halfway through. Transfer the beans to a large bowl and toss with the melted butter. Top with the Parmesan cheese and serve warm.

Per Serving: Calories: 134; Fat: 11g; Protein: 3g; Total Carbs: 6g; Fiber: 3g; Net Carbs: 3g; **Macros:** Fat: 74%; Protein: 9%; Carbs: 17%

Sweet and Spicy Pecans

SERVES 8 | PREP TIME: 7 minutes | COOK TIME: 15 minutes | TEMPERATURE: 275°F

3 tablespoons unsalted butter, melted

¼ cup brown sugar substitute, such as Swerve or Sukrin Gold

1½ teaspoons Maldon sea salt (or regular sea salt if you like)

¼ teaspoon cayenne pepper, more or less to taste

2 cups pecan halves

Line your air fryer basket with parchment paper or an air fryer liner. Place the melted butter in a small pot and whisk in the brown sugar substitute, sea salt, and cayenne pepper. Stir until well combined. Place the pecans in a medium bowl and pour the butter mixture over them. Toss to coat. Set the air fryer to 275°F. Place the pecans in the air fryer basket in a single layer, working in batches if necessary, and cook for 10 minutes. Stir, then cook for 5 minutes more. Transfer the pecans to a parchment paper–lined baking sheet and allow them to cool completely before serving.

Per Serving: Calories: 225; Fat: 24g; Protein: 3g; Total Carbs: 10g; Fiber: 3g; Net Carbs: 1g; Macros: Fat: 96%; Protein: 4%; Carbs: 0%

Down Home Biscuits

PREP TIME: 15 minutes | COOK TIME: 12 to 15 minutes | TEMPERATURE: 325°F

10 ounces (2¼ cups plus 2 tablespoons) almond flour

1½ tablespoons baking powder

1 teaspoon garlic powder

1 teaspoon sea salt

½ teaspoon freshly ground black pepper

¼ teaspoon xanthan gum

3 tablespoons unsalted butter, melted, divided

1 large egg, beaten

¾ cup heavy (whipping) cream

¾ cup shredded Cheddar cheese (optional)

In a large bowl, whisk the almond flour, baking powder, garlic powder, salt, pepper, and xanthan gum. In a small bowl, whisk 1 tablespoon of the melted butter, the egg, and the heavy cream. Add the wet mixture to the dry mixture and stir, just until the dough comes together. Stir in the Cheddar cheese (if using). Place the dough on a sheet of parchment paper and press it out evenly to a ½-inch thickness. Using a 2½-inch round cookie cutter, cut the dough into biscuits. Ball up the dough scraps, press it out again, and continue cutting biscuits until all the dough is used. Working in batches, place the biscuits in either silicone muffin cups or in a 7-inch cake pan that fits in the basket of your air fryer. Brush the tops and sides of the biscuits with the remaining 2 tablespoons of butter. Set your air fryer to 325°F. Place the muffin cups or cake pan into the basket. Cook for 12 minutes, and check for doneness. Cook for up to 3 minutes more, until golden brown.

Per Serving: Calories: 227; Fat: 19g; Protein: 7g; Total Carbs: 7g; Fiber: 3g; Net Carbs: 4g; Macros: Fat: 75%; Protein: 12%; Carbs: 13%

Veggie Frittata

SERVES 2 | PREP TIME: 7 minutes | COOK TIME: 21 to 23 minutes | TEMPERATURE: 350°F

Avocado oil spray

¼ cup diced red onion

¼ cup diced red bell pepper

¼ cup finely chopped broccoli

4 large eggs

3 ounces shredded Cheddar cheese, divided

½ teaspoon dried thyme

Sea salt

Freshly ground black pepper

Spray a 7-inch pan well with oil. Put the onion, pepper, and broccoli in the pan, place the pan in the air fryer, and set to 350°F. Cook for 5 minutes. While the vegetables cook, beat the eggs in a medium bowl. Stir in half of the cheese, and season with the thyme, salt, and pepper. Add the eggs to the pan and top with the remaining cheese. Set the air fryer to 350°F. Cook for 16 to 18 minutes, until cooked through.

Per Serving: Calories: 325; Fat: 23g; Protein: 22g; Total Carbs: 6g; Fiber: 1g; Net Carbs: 5g; Macros: Fat: 64%; Protein: 27%; Carbs: 9%

Bacon and Spinach Egg Muffins

SERVES 6 | PREP TIME: 7 minutes | COOK TIME: 12 to 14 minutes | TEMPERATURE: 300°F

6 large eggs

¼ cup heavy (whipping) cream

½ teaspoon sea salt

¼ teaspoon freshly ground black pepper

¼ teaspoon cayenne pepper (optional)

¾ cup frozen chopped spinach, thawed and drained

4 strips cooked bacon, crumbled

2 ounces shredded Cheddar cheese

In a large bowl, whisk the eggs, heavy cream, salt, black pepper, and cayenne pepper (if using). Divide the spinach and bacon among 6 silicone muffin cups. Place the muffin cups in your air fryer basket. Divide the egg mixture among the muffin cups. Top with the cheese. Set the air fryer to 300°F. Cook for 12 to 14 minutes, until the eggs are set and cooked through.

Per Serving: Calories: 180; Fat: 14g; Protein: 11g; Total Carbs: 2g; Fiber: 1g; Net Carbs: 1g; Macros: Fat: 70%; Protein: 24%; Carbs: 6%

Pumpkin-Pie Breakfast Bars

MAKES 8 BARS | PREP TIME: 15 minutes | COOK TIME: 3 hours on low

For the crust

5 tablespoons butter, softened, divided

¾ cup unsweetened shredded coconut

½ cup almond flour

¼ cup granulated erythritol

For the filling

1 (28-ounce) can pumpkin purée

1 cup heavy (whipping) cream

4 large eggs

1 ounce protein powder

1 teaspoon pure vanilla extract

4 drops liquid stevia

1 teaspoon ground cinnamon

½ teaspoon ground ginger

¼ teaspoon ground nutmeg

Pinch ground cloves

Pinch salt

Lightly grease the bottom of the insert of the slow cooker with 1 tablespoon of the butter. In a small bowl, stir the coconut, almond flour, erythritol, and remaining butter until the mixture forms into coarse crumbs. Press the crumbs into the bottom of the insert evenly to form a crust. In a medium bowl, stir the pumpkin, heavy cream, eggs, protein powder, vanilla, stevia, cinnamon, ginger, nutmeg, cloves, and salt until well blended. Spread the filling evenly over the crust. Cover and cook on low for 3 hours. Uncover and let cool for 30 minutes. Then place the insert in the refrigerator until completely chilled, about 2 hours.

Per serving: Calories: 227; Fat: 19g; Protein: 10g; Total Carbs: 8g; Fiber: 4g; Net Carbs: 4g; **Macros:** Fat: 70%; Protein: 16%; Carbs: 14%

Smoky Sausage Patties

SERVES 8 | PREP TIME: 10 minutes, plus 30 minutes to chill | COOK TIME: 9 minutes | TEMPERATURE: 400°F

1 pound ground pork	½ teaspoon fennel seeds
1 tablespoon coconut aminos	½ teaspoon dried thyme
2 teaspoons liquid smoke	½ teaspoon freshly ground
1 teaspoon dried sage	black pepper
1 teaspoon sea salt	¼ teaspoon cayenne pepper

In a large bowl, combine the pork, coconut aminos, liquid smoke, sage, salt, fennel seeds, thyme, black pepper, and cayenne pepper. Work the meat with your hands until the seasonings are fully incorporated. Shape the mixture into 8 equal-size patties. Using your thumb, make a dent in the center of each patty. Place the patties on a plate and cover with plastic wrap. Refrigerate the patties for at least 30 minutes. Working in batches if necessary, place the patties in a single layer in the air fryer, being careful not to overcrowd them. Set the air fryer to 400°F and cook for 5 minutes. Flip and cook for about 4 minutes more.

Per Serving: Calories: 152; Fat: 12g; Protein: 10g; Total Carbs: 1g; Fiber: 0g; Net Carbs: 1g; **Macros:** Fat: 71%; Protein: 26%; Carbs: 3%

Fried Chicken Breasts

SERVES 4 | PREP TIME: 10 minutes, plus 2 hours to brine | COOK TIME: 12 to 14 minutes | TEMPERATURE: 400°F

1 pound boneless, skinless	½ teaspoon sea salt
chicken breasts	½ teaspoon freshly ground
¾ cup dill pickle juice	black pepper
¾ cup almond flour	2 large eggs
¾ cup grated	Avocado oil spray
Parmesan cheese	

Place the chicken breasts in a zip-top bag or between two pieces of plastic wrap. Using a meat mallet or heavy skillet, pound the chicken to a uniform ½-inch thickness. Place the chicken in a large bowl with the pickle juice. Cover and allow to brine in the refrigerator for up to 2 hours. In a shallow dish, combine the almond flour, Parmesan cheese, salt, and pepper. In a separate, shallow bowl, beat the eggs. Drain the chicken and pat it dry with paper towels. Dip in the eggs and then in the flour mixture,

making sure to press the coating into the chicken. Spray both sides of the coated breasts with oil. Spray the air fryer basket with oil and put the chicken inside. Set the temperature to 400°F and cook for 6 to 7 minutes. Carefully flip the breasts with a spatula. Spray the breasts again with oil and continue cooking for 6 to 7 minutes more, until golden and crispy.

Per Serving: Calories: 345; Fat: 18g; Protein: 39g; Total Carbs: 8g; Fiber: 2g; Net Carbs: 6g; **Macros:** Fat: 47%; Protein: 45%; Carbs: 8%

Buffalo Chicken Wings

SERVES 4 | PREP TIME: 10 minutes | COOK TIME: 20 to 25 minutes | TEMPERATURE: 400°F

2 tablespoons baking powder	½ cup Buffalo hot sauce, such
1 teaspoon smoked paprika	as Frank's RedHot
Sea salt	¼ cup unsalted butter
Freshly ground black pepper	2 tablespoons apple
2 pounds chicken wings or	cider vinegar
chicken drumettes	1 teaspoon minced garlic
Avocado oil spray	Blue cheese or garlic ranch
⅓ cup avocado oil	dressing

In a large bowl, stir the baking powder, smoked paprika, and salt and pepper to taste. Add the chicken wings and toss to coat. Set the air fryer to 400°F. Spray the wings with oil. Place the wings in the basket in a single layer, working in batches, and cook for 20 to 25 minutes. Check with an instant-read thermometer and remove when they reach 155°F. Let rest until they reach 165°F. While the wings are cooking, whisk the avocado oil, hot sauce, butter, vinegar, and garlic in a small saucepan over medium-low heat until warm. When the wings are done cooking, toss them with the Buffalo sauce. Serve warm with the dressing.

Per Serving: Calories: 750; Fat: 64g; Protein: 34g; Total Carbs: 2g; Fiber: <1g; Net Carbs: 2g; **Macros:** Fat: 77%; Protein: 18%; Carbs: 5%

Buffalo Chicken Breakfast Muffins

SERVES 10 | PREP TIME: 7 minutes | COOK TIME: 13 to 16 minutes | TEMPERATURE: 300°F

6 ounces shredded	⅓ cup Buffalo hot sauce, such
cooked chicken	as Frank's RedHot
3 ounces blue cheese,	1 teaspoon minced garlic
crumbled	6 large eggs
2 tablespoons unsalted	Sea salt
butter, melted	Freshly ground black pepper
	Avocado oil spray

In a large bowl, stir the chicken, blue cheese, melted butter, hot sauce, and garlic. In a medium bowl or large liquid measuring cup, beat the eggs. Season with salt and pepper. Spray 10 silicone muffin cups with oil. Divide the chicken mixture among the cups, and pour the egg mixture over top. Place the cups in the air fryer and set to 300°F. Cook for 13 to 16 minutes, until the muffins are set and cooked through.

Per Serving: Calories: 120; Fat: 8g; Protein: 9g; Total Carbs: 1g; Fiber: 0g; Net Carbs: 1g; **Macros:** Fat: 60%; Protein: 30%; Carbs: 10%

Broccoli-Stuffed Chicken

SERVES 6 | PREP TIME: 10 minutes | COOK TIME: 19 to
24 minutes | TEMPERATURE: 400°F

1 tablespoon avocado oil
¼ cup chopped onion
½ cup finely chopped broccoli
4 ounces cream cheese, at
room temperature
2 ounces Cheddar cheese,
shredded
1 teaspoon garlic powder

½ teaspoon sea salt, plus additional for seasoning, divided
¼ freshly ground black
pepper, plus additional for
seasoning, divided
2 pounds boneless, skinless
chicken breasts
1 teaspoon smoked paprika

Heat a medium skillet over medium-high heat and pour in
the avocado oil. Add the onion and broccoli and cook, stirring occasionally, for 5 to 8 minutes, until the onion is tender.
Transfer to a large bowl and stir in the cream cheese, Cheddar
cheese, and garlic powder, and season to taste with salt and
pepper. Hold a sharp knife parallel to the chicken breast and
cut a long pocket into one side. Stuff the chicken pockets with
the broccoli mixture, using toothpicks to secure the pockets around the filling. In a small dish, combine the paprika,
½ teaspoon salt, and ¼ teaspoon pepper. Sprinkle this over
the outside of the chicken. Set the air fryer to 400°F. Place
the chicken in a single layer in the air fryer basket, cooking
in batches if necessary, and cook for 14 to 16 minutes, until
an instant-read thermometer reads 160°F. Place the chicken
on a plate and tent a piece of aluminum foil over the chicken.
Allow to rest for 5 to 10 minutes before serving.

Per Serving: Calories: 277; Fat: 15g; Protein: 35g; Total Carbs: 3g;
Fiber: 1g; Net Carbs: 2g; Macros: Fat: 70%; Protein: 24%; Carbs: 6%

Chicken Parmesan

SERVES 8 | PREP TIME: 25 minutes | COOK TIME: 18 to
20 minutes | TEMPERATURE: 400°F

2 pounds boneless, skinless
chicken breasts or thighs
1 cup almond flour
1 cup grated Parmesan cheese
1 teaspoon Italian seasoning
Sea salt
Freshly ground black pepper

2 large eggs
Avocado oil spray
⅓ cup sugar-free mari-
nara sauce
4 ounces fresh mozzarella
cheese, sliced or shredded

Place the chicken in a zip-top bag or between two pieces of plastic wrap. Use a meat mallet or heavy skillet to pound the chicken
to a uniform ½-inch thickness. Place the almond flour, Parmesan cheese, Italian seasoning, and salt and pepper to taste in a
large shallow bowl. In a separate shallow bowl, beat the eggs.
Dip a chicken breast in the egg, then coat it in the almond flour
mixture, making sure to press the coating onto the chicken
gently. Repeat with the remaining chicken. Set the air fryer to
400°F. Spray both sides of the chicken well with oil and place
the pieces in a single layer in the air fryer basket, working in
batches if necessary. Cook for 10 minutes. Flip the chicken with
a spatula. Spray each piece with more oil and continue cooking
for 5 minutes more. Top each chicken piece with the marinara
sauce and mozzarella. Return to the air fryer and cook for 3 to

5 minutes, until the cheese is melted and an instant-read thermometer reads 160°F. Allow the chicken to rest for 5 minutes,
then serve.

Per Serving: Calories: 306; Fat: 17g; Protein: 36g; Total Carbs: 5g;
Fiber: 2g; Net Carbs: 3g; Macros: Fat: 50%; Protein: 47%; Carbs: 3%

Lemon-Dijon Boneless Chicken

SERVES 6 | PREP TIME: 5 minutes, plus 30 minutes to 4 hours
to marinate | COOK TIME: 13 to 16 minutes |
TEMPERATURE: 400°F

½ cup sugar-free mayonnaise
1 tablespoon Dijon mustard
1 tablespoon freshly squeezed
lemon juice
1 tablespoon coconut aminos
1 teaspoon Italian seasoning

1 teaspoon sea salt
½ teaspoon freshly ground
black pepper
¼ teaspoon cayenne pepper
1½ pounds boneless, skinless
chicken breasts or thighs

In a small bowl, combine the mayonnaise, mustard, lemon juice
(if using), coconut aminos, Italian seasoning, salt, black pepper,
and cayenne pepper. Place the chicken in a shallow dish or large
zip-top plastic bag. Add the marinade, making sure all the pieces
are coated. Cover and refrigerate for at least 30 minutes or up
to 4 hours. Set the air fryer to 400°F. Arrange the chicken in a
single layer in the air fryer basket, working in batches if necessary. Cook for 7 minutes. Flip the chicken and continue cooking
for 6 to 9 minutes more, until an instant-read thermometer
reads 160°F.

Per Serving: Calories: 236; Fat: 17g; Protein: 23g; Total Carbs: 1g; Fiber:
<1g; Net Carbs: 1g; Macros: Fat: 65%; Protein: 35%; Carbs: 0%

Spiced Chicken

SERVES 8 | PREP TIME: 15 minutes | COOK TIME: 4 to 5 hours

½ cup (1 stick) butter
½ medium onion,
finely chopped
2-inch piece fresh ginger,
peeled and finely chopped
6 garlic cloves, minced
2 teaspoons salt
1 tablespoon garam masala
1 teaspoon ground turmeric
½ to 1 teaspoon red
pepper flakes

1 (14-ounce) can full-fat
coconut milk
2 tablespoons
no-sugar-added
tomato paste
2 pounds boneless, skinless
chicken breasts, cut into
1-inch pieces
¼ cup chopped fresh cilantro,
basil, or mint, for serving

In a large skillet or saucepan, melt the butter over medium heat.
Sauté the onion and ginger for 5 minutes, until softened. Add
the garlic, salt, garam masala, turmeric, and red pepper flakes
and sauté for another 2 minutes, until fragrant. Add the coconut
milk and tomato paste and whisk to combine. Bring the mixture to a simmer and remove from the heat. Place the chicken
pieces in the pot of a slow cooker. Pour the sauce mixture over
the chicken, cover, and cook on low for 4 to 5 hours, or until the
chicken is very tender. Serve the chicken and sauce mixture
garnished with chopped herbs.

Per Serving: Calories: 326; Fat: 23g; Protein: 26g; Total Carbs: 5g;
Fiber: 1g; Net Carbs: 4g; Macros: Fat: 63%; Protein: 32%; Carbs: 5%

Nashville Hot Chicken

SERVES 8 | PREP TIME: 20 minutes, plus 15 minutes to set | COOK TIME: 24 to 28 minutes | TEMPERATURE: 400°F, then 350°F

3 pounds bone-in, skin-on chicken pieces, breasts halved crosswise

1 tablespoon sea salt

1 tablespoon freshly ground black pepper

1½ cups almond flour

1½ cups grated Parmesan cheese

1 tablespoon baking powder

2 teaspoons garlic powder, divided

½ cup heavy (whipping) cream

2 large eggs, beaten

1 tablespoon vinegar-based hot sauce

Avocado oil spray

½ cup (1 stick) unsalted butter

½ cup avocado oil

1 tablespoon cayenne pepper (more or less to taste)

2 tablespoons brown sugar substitute

Sprinkle the chicken with the salt and pepper. In a large shallow bowl, whisk the almond flour, Parmesan cheese, baking powder, and 1 teaspoon of the garlic powder. In a separate bowl, whisk the heavy cream, eggs, and hot sauce. Dip the chicken pieces in the egg, then coat each with the almond flour mixture, pressing the mixture into the chicken to adhere. Allow to sit for 15 minutes to let the breading set. Set the air fryer to 400°F. Place the chicken in a single layer in the air fryer basket, being careful not to overcrowd the pieces, working in batches if necessary. Spray the chicken with oil and cook for 13 minutes. Carefully flip the chicken and spray it with more oil. Reduce the air fryer temperature to 350°F. Cook for another 11 to 15 minutes, until an instant-read thermometer reads 160°F. While the chicken cooks, heat the butter, avocado oil, cayenne pepper, brown sugar substitute, and remaining 1 teaspoon of garlic powder in a saucepan over medium-low heat. Cook until the butter is melted and the sugar substitute has dissolved. Remove the chicken from the air fryer. Use tongs to dip the chicken in the sauce. Place the coated chicken on a rack over a baking sheet, and allow it to rest for 5 minutes before serving.

Per Serving: Calories: 677; Fat: 50g; Protein: 52g; Total Carbs: 10g; Fiber: 3g; Net Carbs: 4g; Macros: Fat: 66%; Protein: 31%; Carbs: 3%

Spice-Rubbed Turkey Breast

SERVES 10 | PREP TIME: 5 minutes | COOK TIME: 45 to 55 minutes | TEMPERATURE: 350°F

1 tablespoon sea salt

1 teaspoon paprika

1 teaspoon onion powder

1 teaspoon garlic powder

½ teaspoon freshly ground black pepper

4 pounds bone-in, skin-on turkey breast

2 tablespoons unsalted butter, melted

In a small bowl, combine the salt, paprika, onion powder, garlic powder, and pepper. Sprinkle the seasonings all over the turkey. Brush the turkey with some of the melted butter. Set the air fryer to 350°F. Place the turkey in the air fryer basket, skin-side down, and cook for 25 minutes. Flip the turkey and brush it with the remaining butter. Continue cooking for another 20 to 30 minutes, until an instant-read thermometer reads 160°F.

Remove the turkey breast from the air fryer. Tent a piece of aluminum foil over the turkey, and allow it to rest for about 5 minutes before serving.

Per Serving: Calories: 278; Fat: 14g; Protein: 34g; Total Carbs: <1g; Fiber: <1g; Net Carbs: <1g; Macros: Fat: 45%; Protein: 49%; Carbs: 6%

Buffalo Chicken Tenders

SERVES 4 | PREP TIME: 15 minutes | COOK TIME: 7 to 10 minutes | TEMPERATURE: 400°F

½ cup almond flour

½ cup finely grated Parmesan cheese

1 teaspoon smoked paprika

¼ teaspoon cayenne pepper

½ teaspoon sea salt, plus additional for seasoning, divided

Freshly ground black pepper

2 large eggs

1 pound chicken tenders

Avocado oil spray

⅓ cup hot sauce, such as Frank's RedHot

2 tablespoons unsalted butter

2 tablespoons white vinegar

1 garlic clove, minced

Blue cheese dressing and crumbles for serving

In a shallow bowl, combine the almond flour, Parmesan cheese, smoked paprika, and cayenne pepper and season with salt and pepper to taste. In a separate shallow bowl, beat the eggs. One at a time, dip the chicken tenders in the eggs, then coat them with the almond flour mixture, making sure to press the coating into the chicken gently. Set the air fryer to 400°F. Place the chicken tenders in a single layer in the air fryer basket and spray them with oil. Cook for 4 minutes. Flip the tenders and spray them with more oil. Cook for 3 to 6 minutes more or until an instant-read thermometer reads 165°F. While the chicken is cooking, combine the hot sauce, butter, vinegar, garlic, and ½ teaspoon of salt in a small saucepan over medium-low heat. Heat until the butter is melted, whisking to combine. Toss the chicken tenders with the sauce. Serve warm with blue cheese dressing and blue cheese crumbles.

Per Serving: Calories: 337; Fat: 20g; Protein: 37g; Total Carbs: 4g; Fiber: 2g; Net Carbs: 2g; Macros: Fat: 53%; Protein: 44%; Carbs: 3%

Barbecue Turkey Meatballs

SERVES 4 | PREP TIME: 20 minutes | COOK TIME: 9 to 12 minutes | TEMPERATURE: 400°F

1 pound ground turkey

½ teaspoon sea salt, plus additional to season the ground turkey

Freshly ground black pepper

1 large egg, beaten

1 teaspoon gelatin

½ cup almond meal

½ tablespoon chili powder

2½ teaspoons smoked paprika, divided

1 teaspoon onion powder

2 teaspoons garlic powder, divided

Avocado oil spray

¾ cup sugar-free ketchup

1 tablespoon yellow mustard

1 tablespoon apple cider vinegar

2 tablespoons brown sugar substitute

1 teaspoon liquid smoke

Place the ground turkey in a large bowl and season with salt and pepper. Place the beaten egg in a bowl and sprinkle with the gelatin. Allow to sit for 5 minutes, then whisk to combine. Pour the gelatin mixture over the ground turkey and add the almond meal, chili powder, 1 teaspoon of smoked paprika, onion powder, and 1 teaspoon of garlic powder. Mix gently with your hands until combined. Form the mixture into 1½-inch balls. Set the air fryer to 400°F. Spray the meatballs with oil and place in the air fryer basket in a single layer. Cook for 5 minutes. Flip the meatballs and spray them with more oil. Cook for 4 to 7 minutes more, until an instant-read thermometer reads 165°F. While the meatballs cook, place the ketchup, mustard, apple cider vinegar, and brown sugar substitute in a small saucepan over medium heat. Bring to a simmer and cook for 5 minutes. Reduce the heat to low and add the remaining 1½ teaspoons of smoked paprika, liquid smoke, remaining 1 teaspoon of garlic powder, and ½ teaspoon of salt. Cook for 5 minutes more, stirring occasionally, until thickened. Toss the meatballs with the sauce and serve warm.

Per Serving: Calories: 412; Fat: 24g; Protein: 38g; Total Carbs: 15g; Fiber: 3g; Net Carbs: 6g; **Macros:** Fat: 52%; Protein: 37%; Carbs: 11%

Chicken Kiev

SERVES 8 | PREP TIME: 25 minutes, plus 4 hours to chill | COOK TIME: 14 to 18 minutes | TEMPERATURE: 350°F

½ cup (1 stick) unsalted butter, at room temperature
1 teaspoon minced garlic
2 tablespoons chopped fresh parsley
½ teaspoon freshly ground black pepper
2 pounds boneless, skinless chicken breasts
Sea salt
¾ cup almond flour
¾ cup grated Parmesan cheese
⅛ teaspoon cayenne pepper
2 large eggs
Avocado oil spray

In a medium bowl, combine the butter, garlic, parsley, and black pepper. Form the mixture into a log and wrap it tightly with parchment paper or plastic wrap. Refrigerate for at least 2 hours, until firm. Place the chicken breasts in a zip-top bag or between two pieces of plastic wrap. Pound the chicken with a meat mallet or heavy skillet to an even ¼-inch thickness. Place a pat of butter in the center of each chicken breast and wrap the chicken tightly around the butter from the long side, tucking in the short sides as you go. Secure with toothpicks. Season the outside of the chicken with salt. Wrap the stuffed chicken tightly with plastic wrap and refrigerate at least 2 hours or overnight. In a shallow bowl, combine the almond flour, Parmesan cheese, and cayenne pepper. In another shallow bowl, beat the eggs. Dip each piece of chicken in the eggs, then coat it in the almond flour mixture, using your fingers to press the breading gently into the chicken. Set the air fryer to 350°F. Spray the chicken with oil and place it in a single layer in the air fryer basket, working in batches if necessary. Cook for 8 minutes. Flip the chicken, then spray it again with oil. Cook for 6 to 10 minutes more, until an instant-read thermometer reads 165°F.

Per Serving: Calories: 333; Fat: 23g; Protein: 31g; Total Carbs: 3g; Fiber: 1g; Net Carbs: 2g; **Macros:** Fat: 62%; Protein: 37%; Carbs: 1%

Maple-Glazed Salmon with a Kick

SERVES 4 | PREP TIME: 5 minutes | COOK TIME: 23 minutes | TEMPERATURE: 300°F, then 400°F

½ cup maple syrup substitute, such as ChocZero sugar-free maple syrup
1 tablespoon grated fresh ginger
2 tablespoons coconut aminos
2 tablespoons freshly squeezed lemon juice
1 teaspoon minced garlic
Sea salt
Freshly ground black pepper
1 pound (1½-inch-thick) salmon fillets
Avocado oil spray

In a small dish that fits inside your air fryer, combine the maple syrup substitute with the ginger, coconut aminos, lemon juice, and garlic. Season with salt and pepper. Set the air fryer to 300°F. Place the dish in the basket and cook for 15 minutes, stirring every 5 minutes. Divide the glaze between 2 bowls and allow it to cool slightly. Brush the salmon with the glaze from one bowl, and spray both sides of the fillets with oil. Place the fillets in a single layer in the air fryer basket, skin-side up. Set the air fryer to 400°F and cook for 7 minutes. Flip and cook for 1 minute longer or until an instant-read thermometer reads about 125°F for medium-rare. Let rest for 5 minutes, then serve with the reserved sauce from the second bowl.

Per Serving: Calories: 215; Fat: 4g; Protein: 23g; Total Carbs: 33g; Fiber: 28g; Net Carbs: 5g; **Macros:** Fat: 17%; Protein: 43%; Carbs: 40%

Fish Fillets with Lemon-Dill Sauce

SERVES 4 | PREP TIME: 5 minutes | COOK TIME: 7 minutes | TEMPERATURE: 400°F, then 325°F

1 pound snapper, grouper, or salmon fillets
Sea salt
Freshly ground black pepper
1 tablespoon avocado oil
¼ cup sour cream
¼ cup sugar-free mayonnaise
2 tablespoons fresh dill, chopped, plus more for garnish
1 tablespoon freshly squeezed lemon juice
½ teaspoon grated lemon zest

Pat the fish dry with paper towels and season well with salt and pepper. Brush with the avocado oil. Set the air fryer to 400°F. Place the fillets in the air fryer basket and cook for 1 minute. Lower the air fryer temperature to 325°F and continue cooking for 5 minutes. Flip the fish and cook for 1 minute more or until an instant-read thermometer reads 145°F. (If using salmon, cook it to 125°F for medium-rare.) While the fish is cooking, make the sauce by combining the sour cream, mayonnaise, dill, lemon juice, and lemon zest in a medium bowl. Season with salt and pepper and stir until combined. Refrigerate until ready to serve. Serve the fish with the sauce, garnished with the remaining dill.

Per Serving: Calories: 304; Fat: 19g; Protein: 30g; Total Carbs: 2g; Fiber: 0g; Net Carbs: 2g; **Macros:** Fat: 56%; Protein: 39%; Carbs: 5%

Shrimp Caesar Salad

SERVES 4 | PREP TIME: 10 minutes, plus 15 minutes to marinate | COOK TIME: 4 to 6 minutes | TEMPERATURE: 400°F

12 ounces fresh large shrimp, peeled and deveined

1 tablespoon plus 1 teaspoon freshly squeezed lemon juice, divided

¼ cup olive oil or avocado oil, divided

2 garlic cloves, minced, divided

¼ teaspoon sea salt, plus additional to season the marinade

¼ teaspoon freshly ground black pepper, plus additional to season the marinade

⅓ cup sugar-free mayonnaise

2 tablespoons freshly grated Parmesan cheese

1 teaspoon Dijon mustard

1 tinned anchovy, mashed

12 ounces romaine hearts, torn

Place the shrimp in a large bowl. Add 1 tablespoon of lemon juice, 1 tablespoon of olive oil, and 1 minced garlic clove. Season with salt and pepper. Toss well and refrigerate for 15 minutes. While the shrimp marinates, make the dressing: In a blender, combine the mayonnaise, Parmesan cheese, Dijon mustard, the remaining 1 teaspoon of lemon juice, the anchovy, the remaining minced garlic clove, ¼ teaspoon of salt, and ¼ teaspoon of pepper. Process until smooth. With the blender running, slowly stream in the remaining 3 tablespoons of oil. Transfer the mixture to a jar; seal and refrigerate until ready to serve. Remove the shrimp from its marinade and place it in the air fryer basket in a single layer. Set the air fryer to 400°F and cook for 2 minutes. Flip the shrimp and cook for 2 to 4 minutes more, until the flesh turns opaque. Place the romaine in a large bowl and toss with the desired amount of dressing. Top with the shrimp and serve immediately.

Per Serving: Calories: 329; Fat: 30g; Protein: 16g; Total Carbs: 4g; Fiber: 2g; Net Carbs: 2g; **Macros:** Fat: 82%; Protein: 18%; Carbs: 0%

Crab Cakes

SERVES 4 | PREP TIME: 10 minutes, plus 1 hour to chill | COOK TIME: 14 minutes | TEMPERATURE: 400°F

Avocado oil spray cup red onion, diced

¼ cup red bell pepper, diced

8 ounces lump crabmeat, picked over for shells

3 tablespoons almond flour

1 large egg, beaten

1 tablespoon sugar-free mayonnaise

2 teaspoons Dijon mustard

⅛ teaspoon cayenne pepper

Sea salt

Freshly ground black pepper

Tartar sauce, for serving

Lemon wedges, for serving

Spray an air fryer–friendly baking pan with oil. Put the onion and red bell pepper in the pan and give them a quick spray with oil. Place the pan in the air fryer basket. Set the air fryer to 400°F and cook the vegetables for 7 minutes, until tender. Transfer the vegetables to a large bowl. Add the crabmeat, almond flour, egg, mayonnaise, mustard, and cayenne pepper and season with salt and pepper. Stir until the mixture is well combined. Form the mixture into four 1-inch-thick cakes. Cover

with plastic wrap and refrigerate for 1 hour. Place the crab cakes in a single layer in the air fryer basket and spray them with oil. Cook for 4 minutes. Flip the crab cakes and spray with more oil. Cook for 3 minutes more, until the internal temperature of the crab cakes reaches 155°F. Serve with tartar sauce and a squeeze of fresh lemon juice.

Per Serving: Calories: 121; Fat: 8g; Protein: 11g; Total Carbs: 3g; Fiber: 1g; Net Carbs: 2g; **Macros:** Fat: 60%; Protein: 36%; Carbs: 4%

Scallops with Lemon-Butter Sauce

SERVES 4 | PREP TIME: 5 minutes, plus 15 minutes to chill | COOK TIME: 15 minutes | TEMPERATURE: 350°F

1 pound large sea scallops

Sea salt

Freshly ground black pepper

Avocado oil spray

¼ cup unsalted butter

1 tablespoon freshly squeezed lemon juice

1 teaspoon minced garlic

¼ teaspoon red pepper flakes

Pat the scallops dry with a paper towel. Season the scallops with salt and pepper, then place them on a plate and refrigerate for 15 minutes. Spray the air fryer basket with oil, and arrange the scallops in a single layer. Spray the top of the scallops with oil. Set the air fryer to 350°F and cook for 6 minutes. Flip the scallops and cook for 6 minutes more, until an instant-read thermometer reads 145°F. While the scallops cook, place the butter, lemon juice, garlic, and red pepper flakes in a small ramekin. When the scallops have finished cooking, remove them from the air fryer. Place the ramekin in the air fryer and cook until the butter melts, about 3 minutes. Stir. Toss the scallops with the warm butter and serve.

Per Serving: Calories: 203; Fat: 12g; Protein: 19g; Total Carbs: 3g; Fiber: 0g; Net Carbs: 3g; **Macros:** Fat: 53%; Protein: 37%; Carbs: 10%

Marinated Swordfish Skewers

SERVES 4 | PREP TIME: 10 minutes, plus 30 minutes to marinate | COOK TIME: 6 to 8 minutes | TEMPERATURE: 400°F

1 pound filleted swordfish

¼ cup avocado oil

2 tablespoons freshly squeezed lemon juice

1 tablespoon minced fresh parsley

2 teaspoons Dijon mustard

Sea salt

Freshly ground black pepper

3 ounces cherry tomatoes

Cut the fish into 1½-inch chunks, picking out any remaining bones. In a large bowl, whisk the oil, lemon juice, parsley, and Dijon mustard. Season to taste with salt and pepper. Add the fish and toss to coat the pieces. Cover and marinate the fish chunks in the refrigerator for 30 minutes. Remove the fish from the marinade. Thread the fish and cherry tomatoes on 4 skewers, alternating as you go. Set the air fryer to 400°F. Place the skewers in the air fryer basket and cook for 3 minutes. Flip the skewers and cook for 3 to 5 minutes longer, until the fish is cooked through and an instant-read thermometer reads 140°F.

Per Serving: Calories: 315; Fat: 20g; Protein: 29g; Total Carbs: 2g; Fiber: <1g; Net Carbs: 2g; **Macros:** Fat: 57%; Protein: 37%; Carbs: 6%

Coconut Shrimp

SERVES 4 | PREP TIME: 15 minutes | COOK TIME: 17 minutes | TEMPERATURE: 400°F

¾ cup unsweetened shredded coconut

¾ cup coconut flour

1 teaspoon garlic powder

¼ teaspoon cayenne pepper

Sea salt

Freshly ground black pepper

2 large eggs

1 pound fresh extra-large or jumbo shrimp, peeled and deveined

Avocado oil spray

In a medium bowl, combine the shredded coconut, coconut flour, garlic powder, and cayenne pepper. Season to taste with salt and pepper. In a small bowl, beat the eggs. Pat the shrimp dry with paper towels. Dip each shrimp in the eggs and then the coconut mixture. Gently press the coating to the shrimp to help it adhere. Set the air fryer to 400°F. Spray the shrimp with oil and place them in a single layer in the air fryer basket, working in batches if necessary. Cook the shrimp for 9 minutes, then flip and spray them with more oil. Cook for 8 minutes more, until the center of the shrimp is opaque and cooked through.

Per Serving: Calories: 362; Fat: 17g; Protein: 35g; Total Carbs: 20g; Fiber: 11g; Net Carbs: 9g; Macros: Fat: 42%; Protein: 39%; Carbs: 19%

Crispy Fish Sticks

SERVES 4 | PREP TIME: 10 minutes, plus 30 minutes to freeze | COOK TIME: 9 minutes | TEMPERATURE: 400°F

1 pound cod fillets

1½ cups almond flour

2 teaspoons Old Bay seasoning

½ teaspoon paprika

Sea salt

Freshly ground black pepper

¼ cup sugar-free mayonnaise

1 large egg, beaten

Avocado oil spray

Tartar sauce for serving

Cut the fish into ¾-inch-wide strips. In a shallow bowl, stir the almond flour, Old Bay seasoning, paprika, and salt and pepper to taste. In another shallow bowl, whisk the mayonnaise and egg. Dip the cod strips in the egg mixture, then the almond flour, gently pressing with your fingers to help adhere the coating. Place the coated fish on a parchment paper–lined baking sheet and freeze for 30 minutes. Spray the air fryer basket with oil. Set the air fryer to 400°F. Place the fish in the basket in a single layer, and spray each piece with oil. Cook for 5 minutes. Flip and spray with more oil. Cook for 4 minutes more, until the internal temperature reaches 140°F. Serve with the tartar sauce.

Per Serving: Calories: 439; Fat: 33g; Protein: 31g; Total Carbs: 9g; Fiber: 5g; Net Carbs: 4g; Macros: Fat: 68%; Protein: 28%; Carbs: 4%

Sweet and Spicy Salmon

SERVES 4 | PREP TIME: 5 minutes | COOK TIME: 10 to 12 minutes | TEMPERATURE: 400°F

½ cup sugar-free mayonnaise

2 tablespoons brown sugar substitute, such as Sukrin Gold

2 teaspoons Dijon mustard

1 canned chipotle chile in adobo sauce, diced

1 teaspoon adobo sauce (from the canned chipotle)

16 ounces salmon fillets

Salt

Freshly ground black pepper

In a small food processor, combine the mayonnaise, brown sugar substitute, Dijon mustard, chipotle pepper, and adobo sauce. Process for 1 minute until everything is combined and the brown sugar substitute is no longer granular. Season the salmon with salt and pepper. Spread half of the sauce over the fish, and reserve the remainder of the sauce for serving. Set the air fryer to 400°F. Place the salmon in the air fryer basket. Cook for 5 minutes. Flip the salmon and cook for 5 to 7 minutes more, until an instant-read thermometer reads 125°F (for medium-rare). Serve warm with the remaining sauce.

Per Serving: Calories: 326; Fat: 25g; Protein: 23g; Total Carbs: 7g; Fiber: 0g; Net Carbs: 1g; Macros: Fat: 69%; Protein: 28%; Carbs: 3%

Garlic Shrimp

SERVES 4 | PREP TIME: 5 minutes | COOK TIME: 8 to 10 minutes | TEMPERATURE: 350°F

1 pound fresh large shrimp, peeled and deveined

1 tablespoon avocado oil

2 teaspoons minced garlic, divided

½ teaspoon red pepper flakes

Sea salt

Freshly ground black pepper

2 tablespoons unsalted butter, melted

2 tablespoons chopped fresh parsley

Place the shrimp in a large bowl and toss with the avocado oil, 1 teaspoon of minced garlic, and red pepper flakes. Season with salt and pepper. Set the air fryer to 350°F. Arrange the shrimp in a single layer in the air fryer basket, working in batches if necessary. Cook for 6 minutes. Flip the shrimp and cook for 2 to 4 minutes more, until the internal temperature of the shrimp reaches 120°F. (The time it takes to cook will depend on the size of the shrimp.) While the shrimp are cooking, melt the butter in a small saucepan over medium heat and stir in the remaining 1 teaspoon of garlic. Transfer the cooked shrimp to a large bowl, add the garlic butter, and toss well. Top with the parsley and serve warm.

Per Serving: Calories: 220; Fat: 11g; Protein: 28g; Total Carbs: 1g; Fiber: <1g; Net Carbs: 1g; Macros: Fat: 45%; Protein: 51%; Carbs: 4%

Bacon Cheeseburger Meatloaf

SERVES 6 | PREP TIME: 20 minutes | COOK TIME: 40 to 43 minutes | TEMPERATURE: 400°F

¼ cup beef broth

2 tablespoons heavy (whipping) cream

2½ teaspoons unflavored gelatin

Avocado oil spray

¼ cup chopped onion

4 ounces (½ cup) keto-friendly tomato sauce

⅓ cup sugar-free mayonnaise

2 tablespoons keto-friendly ketchup

1 large egg, beaten

1 pound ground beef

Sea salt

Freshly ground black pepper

4 slices Cheddar cheese

8 ounces sliced bacon, cooked and crumbled

1 small tomato, sliced

Combine the broth and heavy cream in a small bowl. Sprinkle the gelatin evenly over the top. Set aside. Spray a small skillet with oil and place it over medium-high heat. Once the oil is hot, add the onion and cook for 5 minutes or until soft. Reduce the heat to medium-low, then stir the gelatin mixture and add it to the skillet, along with the tomato sauce.

Cook, stirring occasionally, until the mixture is reduced by half, about 10 minutes. Meanwhile, stir the mayonnaise and ketchup in a small bowl. In a large bowl, combine the onion mixture with the egg and ground beef. Season with salt and pepper. Mix well to combine. Place the meatloaf mixture in a small loaf pan that fits inside your air fryer. Place the pan in the air fryer basket. Set the air fryer to 400°F and cook for 20 minutes. Top the meatloaf with the mayonnaise sauce, cheese, crumbled bacon, and tomato slices. Cook for 5 to 8 minutes more, until the cheese is melted and an instant-read thermometer reads 160°F.

Per Serving: Calories: 489; Fat: 41g; Protein: 25g; Total Carbs: 3g; Fiber: 1g; Net Carbs: 2g; Macros: Fat: 75%; Protein: 20%; Carbs: 5%

Garlic-Marinated Flank Steak

SERVES 6 | PREP TIME: 5 minutes, plus 2 hours to marinate | COOK TIME: 8 to 10 minutes (for medium-rare) | TEMPERATURE: 400°F

½ cup avocado oil

¼ cup coconut aminos

1 shallot, minced

1 tablespoon minced garlic

2 tablespoons chopped fresh oregano, or 2 teaspoons dried

1½ teaspoons sea salt

1 teaspoon freshly ground black pepper

¼ teaspoon red pepper flakes

2 pounds flank steak

In a blender, combine the avocado oil, coconut aminos, shallot, garlic, oregano, salt, black pepper, and red pepper flakes. Process until smooth. Place the steak in a zip-top plastic bag or shallow dish with the marinade. Seal the bag or cover the dish and marinate in the refrigerator for at least 2 hours or overnight. Remove the steak from the bag and discard the marinade. Set the air fryer to 400°F. Place the steak in the air fryer basket (if needed, cut into sections and work in batches). Cook for 4 to 6 minutes, flip the steak, and cook for another 4 minutes or until the internal temperature reaches 120°F in the thickest part for medium-rare (or as desired).

Per Serving: Calories: 304; Fat: 23g; Protein: 16g; Total Carbs: 4g; Fiber: <1g; Net Carbs: 4g; Macros: Fat: 68%; Protein: 21%; Carbs: 11%

Greek Beef Kebabs with Tzatziki

SERVES 6 | PREP TIME: 15 minutes, plus 4 hours to marinate | COOK TIME: 8 to 10 minutes | TEMPERATURE: 400°F

1 pound boneless sirloin steak, cut into 2-inch chunks

¼ cup avocado oil

2 teaspoons minced garlic

2 teaspoons dried oregano

Sea salt

Freshly ground black pepper

1 small red onion, cut into wedges

½ cup cherry tomatoes

Tzatziki sauce

4 ounces feta cheese, crumbled

Place the steak in a shallow dish. In a blender, combine the avocado oil, garlic, oregano, and salt and pepper to taste. Blend until smooth, then pour over the steak. Cover the dish with plastic wrap and allow to marinate in the refrigerator for at least 4 hours or overnight. Thread the steak, onion, and cherry tomatoes onto 6 skewers, alternating as you go. (If using wooden skewers, first

soak them in water for 30 minutes). Set the air fryer to 400°F. Place the skewers in the basket and cook for 5 minutes. Flip and cook for 3 to 5 minutes more. Transfer the kebabs to serving plates. Drizzle with tzatziki sauce and sprinkle with the crumbled feta cheese.

Per Serving: Calories: 307; Fat: 25g; Protein: 18g; Total Carbs: 3g; Fiber: 1g; Net Carbs: 2g; Macros: Fat: 73%; Protein: 23%; Carbs: 4%

Short Ribs with Chimichurri

SERVES 4 | PREP TIME: 15 minutes, plus 45 minutes to rest | COOK TIME: 13 minutes | TEMPERATURE: 400°F

1 pound boneless short ribs

1½ teaspoons sea salt, divided

½ teaspoon freshly ground black pepper, divided

½ cup fresh parsley leaves

½ cup fresh cilantro leaves

1 teaspoon minced garlic

1 tablespoon freshly squeezed lemon juice

½ teaspoon ground cumin

¼ teaspoon red pepper flakes

2 tablespoons extra-virgin olive oil

Avocado oil spray

Pat the short ribs dry with paper towels. Sprinkle the ribs all over with 1 teaspoon salt and ¼ teaspoon black pepper. Let sit at room temperature for 45 minutes. Meanwhile, place the parsley, cilantro, garlic, lemon juice, cumin, red pepper flakes, the remaining ½ teaspoon salt, and the remaining ¼ teaspoon black pepper in a blender or food processor. With the blender running, slowly drizzle in the olive oil. Blend for about 1 minute, until the mixture is smooth and well combined. Set the air fryer to 400°F. Spray both sides of the ribs with oil. Place in the basket and cook for 8 minutes. Flip and cook for another 5 minutes, until an instant-read thermometer reads 125°F for medium-rare (or to your desired doneness). Allow the meat to rest for 5 to 10 minutes, then slice. Serve warm with the chimichurri sauce.

Per Serving: Calories: 329; Fat: 24g; Protein: 21g; Total Carbs: 7g; Fiber: 1g; Net Carbs: 6g; Macros: Fat: 66%; Protein: 26%; Carbs: 8%

Grilled Rib Eye Steaks with Horseradish Cream

SERVES 8 | PREP TIME: 5 minutes, plus 55 minutes to rest | COOK TIME: 10 minutes | TEMPERATURE: 400°F

2 pounds rib eye steaks

Sea salt

Freshly ground black pepper

Unsalted butter, for serving

1 cup sour cream

⅓ cup heavy (whipping) cream

¼ cup prepared horseradish

1 teaspoon Dijon mustard

1 teaspoon apple cider vinegar

¼ teaspoon Swerve Confectioners sweetener

Pat the steaks dry. Season with salt and pepper and let sit at room temperature for about 45 minutes. Place the grill pan in the air fryer and set the air fryer to 400°F. Let preheat for 5 minutes. Working in batches, place the steaks in a single layer on the grill pan and cook for 5 minutes. Flip the steaks and cook for 5 minutes more, until an instant-read thermometer reads 120°F (or to your desired doneness). Transfer the steaks to a plate and top each with a pat of butter. Tent with foil and let rest for 10 minutes. Combine the sour cream, heavy cream, horseradish, Dijon mustard, vinegar, and Swerve in a bowl. Stir until smooth. Serve the steaks with the horseradish cream.

Per Serving: Calories: 322; Fat: 22g; Protein: 23g; Total Carbs: 6g; Fiber: <1g; Net Carbs: 6g; **Macros:** Fat: 61%; Protein: 29%; Carbs: 10%

Goat Cheese–Stuffed Flank Steak

SERVES 6 | PREP TIME: 10 minutes | COOK TIME: 14 minutes | TEMPERATURE: 400°F

1 pound flank steak
1 tablespoon avocado oil
½ teaspoon sea salt
½ teaspoon garlic powder

¼ teaspoon freshly ground black pepper
2 ounces goat cheese, crumbled
1 cup baby spinach, chopped

Place the steak in a large zip-top bag or between two pieces of plastic wrap. Using a meat mallet or heavy-bottomed skillet, pound the steak to an even ¼-inch thickness. Brush both sides of the steak with the avocado oil. Mix the salt, garlic powder, and pepper in a small dish. Sprinkle this mixture over both sides of the steak. Sprinkle the goat cheese over top, and top that with the spinach. Starting at one of the long sides, roll the steak up tightly. Tie the rolled steak with kitchen string at 3-inch intervals. Set the air fryer to 400°F. Place the steak roll-up in the air fryer basket. Cook for 7 minutes. Flip the steak and cook for an additional 7 minutes, until an instant-read thermometer reads 120°F for medium-rare (adjust the cooking time for your desired doneness).

Per Serving: Calories: 165; Fat: 9g; Protein: 18g; Total Carbs: 1g; Fiber: 1g; Net Carbs: 0g; **Macros:** Fat: 49%; Protein: 44%; Carbs: 7%

Garlic Steak

SERVES 6 | PREP TIME: 5 minutes, plus 1 hour to marinate | COOK TIME: 10 minutes | TEMPERATURE: 400°F

½ cup olive oil
2 tablespoons minced garlic
Sea salt
Freshly ground black pepper

1½ pounds New York strip or top sirloin steak
Unsalted butter, for serving

In a bowl or blender, combine the olive oil, garlic, and salt and pepper to taste. Place the steak in a shallow bowl or zip-top bag. Pour the marinade over the meat, seal, and marinate in the refrigerator for at least 1 hour and up to 24 hours. Place a grill pan or basket in the air fryer, set it to 400°F, and let preheat for 5 minutes. Place the steak on the grill pan in a single layer, working in batches if necessary, and cook for 5 minutes. Flip the steak and cook for another 5 minutes, until an instant-read thermometer reads 120°F for medium-rare (or cook to your desired doneness). Transfer the steak to a plate, and let rest for 10 minutes before serving.

Per Serving: Calories: 386; Fat: 32g; Protein: 25g; Total Carbs: 1g; Fiber: 0g; Net Carbs: 0g; **Macros:** Fat: 74%; Protein: 26%; Carbs: 0%

Sausage-Stuffed Peppers

SERVES 6 | PREP TIME: 15 minutes | COOK TIME: 28 to 30 minutes | TEMPERATURE: 350°F

Avocado oil spray
8 ounces Italian sausage, casings removed

½ cup chopped mushrooms
¼ cup diced onion
1 teaspoon Italian seasoning

Sea salt
Freshly ground black pepper
1 cup keto-friendly marinara sauce

3 bell peppers, halved and seeded
3 ounces provolone cheese, shredded

Spray a large skillet with oil and place it over medium-high heat. Add the sausage and cook for 5 minutes, breaking up the meat with a wooden spoon. Add the mushrooms, onion, and Italian seasoning, and season with salt and pepper. Cook for 5 minutes more. Stir in the marinara sauce and cook until heated through. Scoop the sausage filling into the bell pepper halves. Set the air fryer to 350°F. Arrange the peppers in a single layer in the air fryer basket, working in batches if necessary. Cook for 15 minutes. Top the stuffed peppers with the cheese and cook for 3 to 5 minutes more, until the cheese is melted and the peppers are tender.

Per Serving: Calories: 186; Fat: 12g; Protein: 11g; Total Carbs: 8g; Fiber: 2g; Net Carbs: 6g; **Macros:** Fat: 58%; Protein: 24%; Carbs: 18%

Pork Kebabs

SERVES 4 | PREP TIME: 15 minutes, plus 2 hours to marinate | COOK TIME: 6 to 8 minutes | TEMPERATURE: 375°F

¼ cup coconut aminos
¼ cup sugar-free ketchup
2 tablespoons freshly squeezed lime juice
2 tablespoons brown sugar substitute, such as Swerve or Sukrin Gold
1 teaspoon minced garlic
Sea salt
Freshly ground black pepper

1 cup stevia-sweetened ginger ale, such as Zevia brand (optional)
1 pound pork tenderloin, cut into 1½-inch cubes
1 red bell pepper, cut into 1½-inch pieces
1 small red onion, cut into 1½-inch pieces

In a small bowl, whisk the coconut aminos, ketchup, lime juice, brown sugar substitute, garlic, and salt and pepper to taste. Whisk in the ginger ale (if using). Place the pork in a shallow dish and pour the marinade over top. Cover the dish with plastic wrap and let the pork marinate in the refrigerator for 2 to 4 hours. Thread the marinated pork cubes, red bell pepper, and onion on skewers, alternating as you go. Set the air fryer to 375°F. Place the kebabs in the air fryer basket in a single layer and cook for 6 to 8 minutes, until an instant-read thermometer reads 145°F.

Per Serving: Calories: 271; Fat: 9g; Protein: 34g; Total Carbs: 14g; Fiber: 1g; Net Carbs: 7g; **Macros:** Fat: 30%; Protein: 50%; Carbs: 20%

Cream Cheese Sausage Balls

SERVES 12 | PREP TIME: 10 minutes | COOK TIME: 10 minutes | TEMPERATURE: 350°F

1¾ cups almond flour
1 tablespoon baking powder
½ teaspoon sea salt
¼ teaspoon freshly ground black pepper
¼ teaspoon cayenne pepper

1 pound fresh pork sausage, casings removed, crumbled
8 ounces Cheddar cheese, shredded
8 ounces cream cheese, at room temperature, cut into chunks

In a large mixing bowl, combine the almond flour, baking powder, salt, black pepper, and cayenne pepper. Add the sausage, Cheddar cheese, and cream cheese. Stir to combine, and then, using clean hands, mix until all of the ingredients are well incorporated. Form the mixture into 1½-inch balls. Set the air fryer to 350°F. Arrange the sausage balls in a single layer in the air fryer basket, working in batches if necessary. Cook for 5 minutes. Flip the sausage balls and cook for 5 minutes more.

Per Serving: Calories: 386; Fat: 27g; Protein: 16g; Total Carbs: 5g; Fiber: 2g; Net Carbs: 3g; **Macros:** Fat: 63%; Protein: 17%; Carbs: 20%

Parmesan-Breaded Boneless Pork Chops

SERVES 4 | PREP TIME: 15 minutes | COOK TIME: 9 to 14 minutes | TEMPERATURE: 400°F

2 large eggs
½ cup finely grated
  Parmesan cheese
½ cup almond flour or finely
  crushed pork rinds
1 teaspoon paprika
½ teaspoon dried oregano

½ teaspoon garlic powder
Salt
Freshly ground black pepper
1¼ pounds (1-inch-thick)
  boneless pork chops
Avocado oil spray

Beat the eggs in a shallow bowl. In a separate bowl, combine the Parmesan cheese, almond flour, paprika, oregano, garlic powder, and salt and pepper to taste. Dip the pork chops into the eggs, then coat them with the Parmesan mixture, gently pressing the coating onto the meat. Spray the breaded pork chops with oil. Set the air fryer to 400°F. Place the pork chops in the air fryer basket in a single layer, working in batches if necessary. Cook for 6 minutes. Flip the chops and spray them with more oil. Cook for another 3 to 8 minutes, until an instant-read thermometer reads 145°F. Allow the pork chops to rest for at least 5 minutes, then serve.

Per Serving: Calories: 351; Fat: 20g; Protein: 38g; Total Carbs: 4g; Fiber: 2g; Net Carbs: 2g; **Macros:** Fat: 51%; Protein: 43%; Carbs: 6%

Sweet-and-Sour Pork Chops

SERVES 4 | PREP TIME: 10 minutes | COOK TIME: 6 hours on low

3 tablespoons extra-virgin
  olive oil, divided
1 pound boneless pork chops
½ cup granulated erythritol
¼ cup chicken broth
¼ cup tomato paste

2 tablespoons coconut aminos
2 tablespoons red chili paste
2 teaspoons minced garlic
¼ teaspoon salt
¼ teaspoon freshly ground
  black pepper

Lightly grease the insert of the slow cooker with 1 tablespoon of the olive oil. In a large skillet over medium-high heat, heat the remaining 2 tablespoons of the olive oil. Add the pork chops, brown for about 5 minutes, and transfer to the insert. In a medium bowl, stir the erythritol, broth, tomato paste, coconut aminos, chili paste, garlic, salt, and pepper. Add the sauce to the chops. Cover and cook on low for 6 hours. Serve warm.

Per serving: Calories: 297; Fat: 20g; Protein: 24g; Total Carbs: 8g; Fiber: 2g; Net Carbs: 6g; **Macros:** Fat: 63%; Protein: 32%; Carbs: 5%

Herb-Braised Pork Chops

SERVES 6 | PREP TIME: 15 minutes | COOK TIME: 7 to 8 hours on low

¼ cup extra-virgin olive
  oil, divided
1½ pounds pork loin chops
Salt, for seasoning
Freshly ground black pepper,
  for seasoning
1 cup chicken broth

½ sweet onion, chopped
2 teaspoons minced garlic
1 teaspoon dried thyme
1 teaspoon dried oregano
1 cup heavy (whipping) cream
1 tablespoon chopped fresh
  basil, for garnish

Lightly grease the insert of the slow cooker with 1 tablespoon of the olive oil. In a large skillet over medium-high heat, heat the remaining 3 tablespoons of the olive oil. Lightly season the pork with salt and pepper. Add the pork to the skillet and brown for about 5 minutes. Transfer the chops to the insert. In a medium bowl, stir the broth, onion, garlic, thyme, and oregano. Add the broth mixture to the chops. Cover and cook on low for 7 to 8 hours. Stir in the heavy cream. Serve topped with the basil.

Per serving: Calories: 522; Fat: 45g; Protein: 27g; Total Carbs: 2g; Fiber: 0g; Net Carbs: 2g; **Macros:** Fat: 76%; Protein: 21%; Carbs: 3%

Slow Cooker Pulled Pork

SERVES 6 TO 8 | PREP TIME: 10 minutes | COOK TIME: 6-7 hours

½ cup extra-virgin olive
  oil, divided
2 pounds boneless pork loin,
  untrimmed and cut into
  4 to 6 large chunks
6 garlic cloves, crushed with
  the back of a knife

2 teaspoons ground cumin
1½ teaspoons salt
1 teaspoon smoked paprika
1 teaspoon red pepper flakes
¼ cup red wine or apple
  cider vinegar

In a slow cooker, heat 2 tablespoons of olive oil on high heat. Place the pork pieces in a single layer in the heated oil. Add the garlic, cumin, salt, paprika, and red pepper flakes and stir to coat the meat. Brown the pork on all sides, and reduce the heat to low. Add the vinegar, cover, and cook on low for 6 hours, or until the pork is very tender. Using a slotted spoon, transfer the pork to a large bowl and shred with two forks. Return the pork to the slow cooker and toss to combine with the cooking liquid.

Per Serving: Calories: 426; Fat: 31g; Protein: 33g; Total Carbs: 2g; Fiber: <1g; Net Carbs: 2g; **Macros:** Fat: 65%; Protein: 31%; Carbs: 4%

Pancetta-and-Brie–Stuffed Pork Tenderloin

SERVES 4 | PREP TIME: 20 minutes | COOK TIME: 8 hours on low

1 tablespoon extra-virgin
  olive oil
2 (½-pound) pork tenderloins
4 ounces pancetta, cooked
  crispy and chopped

4 ounces triple-cream Brie
1 teaspoon minced garlic
1 teaspoon chopped fresh basil
⅛ teaspoon freshly ground
  black pepper

Lightly grease the insert of the slow cooker with the olive oil. Place the pork on a cutting board and make a lengthwise cut, holding the knife parallel to the board, through the center of the meat without cutting right through. Open the meat up like a book and cover it with plastic wrap. Pound the meat with a mallet or rolling pin until each piece is about ½ inch thick. Lay the butterflied pork on a clean work surface. In a small bowl, stir the pancetta, Brie, garlic, basil, and pepper. Divide the cheese mixture between the tenderloins and spread it evenly over the meat leaving about 1-inch around the edges. Roll the tenderloin up and secure with toothpicks. Place the pork in the insert, cover, and cook on low for 8 hours. Remove the toothpicks and serve.

Per Serving: Calories: 423; Fat: 32g; Protein: 34g; Total Carbs: 1g; Fiber: 0g; Net Carbs: 1g; **Macros:** Fat: 68%; Protein: 30%; Carbs: 2%

Dijon Pork Chops

SERVES 4 | PREP TIME: 10 minutes | COOK TIME: 8 hours on low

1 tablespoon extra-virgin olive oil	1 teaspoon maple extract
1 cup chicken broth	4 (4-ounce) boneless pork chops
1 sweet onion, chopped	1 cup heavy (whipping) cream
¼ cup Dijon mustard	1 teaspoon chopped fresh thyme, for garnish
1 teaspoon minced garlic	

Lightly grease the insert of the slow cooker with the olive oil. Add the broth, onion, Dijon mustard, garlic, and maple extract to the insert, and stir to combine. Add the pork chops. Cover and cook on low for 8 hours. Stir in the heavy cream. Serve topped with the thyme.

Per Serving: Calories: 490; Fat: 42g; Protein: 22g; Total Carbs: 6g; Fiber: 1g; Net Carbs: 5g; **Macros:** Fat: 76%; Protein: 19%; Carbs: 5%

Cranberry Pork Roast

SERVES 6 | PREP TIME: 15 minutes | COOK TIME: 7 to 8 hours on low

3 tablespoons extra-virgin olive oil, divided	½ cup cranberries
2 tablespoons butter	½ cup chicken broth
2 pounds pork shoulder roast	½ cup granulated erythritol
1 teaspoon ground cinnamon	2 tablespoons Dijon mustard
¼ teaspoon allspice	Juice and zest of ½ orange
¼ teaspoon salt	1 scallion, white and green parts, chopped, for garnish
⅛ teaspoon freshly ground black pepper	

Lightly grease the insert of the slow cooker with 1 tablespoon of the olive oil. In a large skillet over medium-high heat, heat the remaining 2 tablespoons of the olive oil and the butter. Lightly season the pork with cinnamon, allspice, salt, and pepper. Add the pork to the skillet and brown on all sides for about 10 minutes. Transfer to the insert. In a small bowl, stir the cranberries, broth, erythritol, mustard, and orange juice and zest, and add the mixture to the pork. Cover and cook on low for 7 to 8 hours. Serve topped with the scallion.

Per Serving: Calories: 492; Fat: 40g; Protein: 26g; Total Carbs: 4g; Fiber: 1g; Net Carbs: 3g; **Macros:** Fat: 73%; Protein: 21%; Carbs: 6%

Pork-and-Sauerkraut Casserole

SERVES 6 | PREP TIME: 15 minutes | COOK TIME: 9 to 10 hours on low

3 tablespoons extra-virgin olive oil, divided	1 (28-ounce) jar sauerkraut, drained
2 tablespoons butter	1 cup chicken broth
2 pounds pork shoulder roast	½ sweet onion, thinly sliced
	¼ cup granulated erythritol

Lightly grease the insert of the slow cooker with 1 tablespoon of the olive oil. In a large skillet over medium-high heat, heat the remaining 2 tablespoons of the olive oil and the butter. Add the pork to the skillet and brown on all sides for about 10 minutes. Transfer to the insert and add the sauerkraut, broth, onion, and erythritol. Cover and cook on low for 9 to 10 hours. Serve warm.

Per Serving: Calories: 516; Fat: 42g; Protein: 28g; Total Carbs: 7g; Fiber: 4g; Net Carbs: 3g; **Macros:** Fat: 73%; Protein: 22%; Carbs: 5%

Carnitas

SERVES 8 | PREP TIME: 15 minutes | COOK TIME: 9 to 10 hours on low

3 tablespoons extra-virgin olive oil, divided	1 teaspoon ground coriander
2 pounds pork shoulder, cut into 2-inch cubes	1 teaspoon ground cumin
2 cups diced tomatoes	½ teaspoon salt
2 cups chicken broth	1 avocado, peeled, pitted, and diced, for garnish
½ sweet onion, chopped	1 cup sour cream, for garnish
2 chipotle peppers, chopped	2 tablespoons chopped cilan-tro, for garnish
Juice of 1 lime	

Lightly grease the insert of the slow cooker with 1 tablespoon of the olive oil. In a large skillet over medium-high heat, heat the remaining 2 tablespoons of the olive oil. Add the pork and brown on all sides for about 10 minutes. Transfer to the insert and add the tomatoes, broth, onion, peppers, lime juice, corian-der, cumin, and salt. Cover and cook on low for 9 to 10 hours. Shred the cooked pork with a fork and stir the meat into the sauce. Serve topped with the avocado, sour cream, and cilantro.

Per Serving: Calories: 508; Fat: 41g; Protein: 29g; Total Carbs: 7g; Fiber: 3g; Net Carbs: 4g; **Macros:** Fat: 73%; Protein: 22%; Carbs: 5%

Asian Pork Spare Ribs

SERVES 4 | PREP TIME: 10 minutes | COOK TIME: 9 to 10 hours on low

1 tablespoon extra-virgin olive oil	3 tablespoons coconut aminos
2 pounds pork spare ribs	3 tablespoons sesame oil
1 tablespoon Chinese five-spice powder	2 tablespoons apple cider vinegar
2 teaspoons garlic powder	1 tablespoon granulated erythritol
½ cup chicken broth	

Lightly grease the insert of the slow cooker with the olive oil. Season the ribs with the five-spice powder and garlic powder, and place upright on their ends in the insert. Add the broth, coconut aminos, sesame oil, apple cider vinegar, and erythritol to the bottom of the insert, stirring to blend. Cover and cook on low for 9 to 10 hours. Serve warm.

Per Serving: Calories: 518; Fat: 37g; Protein: 36g; Total Carbs: 4g; Fiber: 0g; Net Carbs: 4g; **Macros:** Fat: 65%; Protein: 32%; Carbs: 3%

Bacon-Wrapped Pork Loin

SERVES 8 | PREP TIME: 15 minutes | COOK TIME: 9 to 10 hours on low

3 tablespoons extra-virgin olive oil, divided
2 pounds pork shoulder roast
1 teaspoon garlic powder
1 teaspoon onion powder

8 bacon strips, uncooked
¼ cup chicken broth
2 teaspoons chopped thyme
1 teaspoon chopped oregano

Lightly grease the insert of the slow cooker with 1 tablespoon of the olive oil. Rub the pork all over with the garlic powder and onion powder. In a large skillet over medium-high heat, heat the remaining 2 tablespoons of the olive oil. Add the pork to the skillet and brown on all sides for about 10 minutes. Let stand about 10 minutes to cool. Wrap the pork with the bacon slices, place in the insert, and add the broth, thyme, and oregano. Cover and cook on low for 9 to 10 hours. Serve warm.

Per serving: Calories: 493; Fat: 40g; Protein: 31g; Total Carbs: 1g; Fiber: 0g; Net Carbs: 1g; **Macros:** Fat: 73%; Protein: 26%; Carbs: 1%

Lemon Pork

SERVES 6 | PREP TIME: 15 minutes | COOK TIME: 7 to 8 hours on low

3 tablespoons extra-virgin olive oil, divided
1 tablespoon butter
2 pounds pork loin roast
½ teaspoon salt

¼ teaspoon freshly ground black pepper
¼ cup chicken broth
Juice and zest of 1 lemon
1 tablespoon minced garlic
½ cup heavy (whipping) cream

Lightly grease the insert of the slow cooker with 1 tablespoon of the olive oil. In a large skillet over medium-high heat, heat the remaining 2 tablespoons of the olive oil and the butter. Lightly season the pork with salt and pepper. Add the pork to the skillet and brown the roast on all sides for about 10 minutes. Transfer it to the insert. In a small bowl, stir the broth, lemon juice and zest, and garlic. Add the broth mixture to the roast. Cover, and cook on low for 7 to 8 hours. Stir in the heavy cream and serve.

Per serving: Calories: 448; Fat: 31g; Protein: 39g; Total Carbs: 1g; Fiber: 0g; Net Carbs: 1g; **Macros:** Fat: 65%; Protein: 34%; Carbs: 1%

Smoky Pork Tenderloin

SERVES 6 | PREP TIME: 5 minutes | COOK TIME: 19 to 22 minutes | TEMPERATURE: 400°F

1½ pounds pork tenderloin
1 tablespoon avocado oil
1 teaspoon chili powder
1 teaspoon smoked paprika

1 teaspoon garlic powder
1 teaspoon sea salt
1 teaspoon freshly ground black pepper

Pierce the tenderloin all over with a fork and rub the oil all over the meat. In a small dish, stir the chili powder, smoked paprika,

garlic powder, salt, and pepper. Rub the spice mixture all over the tenderloin. Set the air fryer to 400°F. Place the pork in the air fryer basket and cook for 10 minutes. Flip the tenderloin and cook for 9 to 12 minutes more, until an instant-read thermometer reads at least 145°F. Allow the tenderloin to rest for 5 minutes, then slice and serve.

Per Serving: Calories: 255; Fat: 12g; Protein: 34g; Total Carbs: 1g; Fiber: <1g; Net Carbs: 1g; **Macros:** Fat: 42%; Protein: 53%; Carbs: 5%

Pork Taco Bowls

SERVES 4 | PREP TIME: 15 minutes, plus 30 minutes to marinate | COOK TIME: 13 to 16 minutes | TEMPERATURE: 400°F

2 tablespoons avocado oil
2 tablespoons freshly squeezed lime juice
1 pound boneless pork shoulder
2 tablespoons taco seasoning
½ small head cabbage, cored and thinly sliced

Sea salt
Freshly ground black pepper
1 cup shredded Cheddar cheese
¼ cup diced red onion
¼ cup diced tomatoes
1 avocado, sliced
1 lime, cut into wedges

In a small dish, whisk the avocado oil and lime juice. Pierce the pork all over with a fork and spread half of the oil mixture over it. Sprinkle with the taco seasoning and allow to sit at room temperature for 30 minutes. Place the cabbage in a large bowl and toss with the remaining oil mixture. Season with salt and pepper. Set the air fryer to 400°F. Place the pork in the air fryer basket and cook for 13 to 16 minutes, until an instant-read thermometer reads 145°F. Allow the pork to rest for 10 minutes, then chop or shred the meat. Place the cabbage in serving bowls. Top each serving with some pork, Cheddar cheese, red onion, tomatoes, and avocado. Serve with lime wedges.

Per Serving: Calories: 521; Fat: 41g; Protein: 25g; Total Carbs: 17g; Fiber: 7g; Net Carbs: 10g; **Macros:** Fat: 71%; Protein: 19%; Carbs: 10% 146

Tomato and Bacon Zoodles

SERVES 2 | PREP TIME: 10 minutes | COOK TIME: 15 to 22 minutes | TEMPERATURE: 400°F

8 ounces sliced bacon
½ cup grape tomatoes
1 large zucchini, spiralized
½ cup ricotta cheese
¼ cup heavy (whipping) cream

⅓ cup finely grated Parmesan cheese, plus more for serving
Sea salt
Freshly ground black pepper

Set the air fryer to 400°F. Arrange the bacon strips in a single layer in the air fryer basket—some overlapping is okay because the bacon will shrink, but cook in batches if needed. Cook for 8 minutes. Flip the bacon strips and cook for 2 to 5 minutes more, until the bacon is crisp. Remove the bacon from the air fryer. Put the tomatoes in the air fryer basket and cook for 3 to 5 minutes, until they are just starting to burst. Remove the tomatoes from the air fryer. Put the zucchini noodles in the air fryer and cook for 2 to 4 minutes, to the desired doneness. Meanwhile, combine the ricotta, heavy cream, and Parmesan in a saucepan over medium-low heat. Cook, stirring often, until warm and combined. Crumble the bacon. Place the zucchini, bacon, and tomatoes in a bowl. Toss with the ricotta sauce. Season with salt and pepper, and sprinkle with additional Parmesan.

Per Serving: Calories: 535; Fat: 40g; Protein: 35g; Total Carbs: 11g; Fiber: 2g; Net Carbs: 9g; **Macros:** Fat: 67%; Protein: 26%; Carbs: 7%

Chocolate Chip–Pecan Biscotti

SERVES 10 | PREP TIME: 15 minutes | COOK TIME: 20 to 22 minutes | TEMPERATURE: 325°F, Then 300°F

1¼ cups almond flour	1 large egg, beaten
¾ teaspoon baking powder	1 teaspoon pure vanilla extract
½ teaspoon xanthan gum	⅓ cup chopped pecans
¼ teaspoon sea salt	¼ cup stevia-sweetened chocolate chips
3 tablespoons unsalted butter, at room temperature	
⅓ cup Swerve Confectioners sweetener	

In a large bowl, combine the almond flour, baking powder, xanthan gum, and salt. Line a 7-inch cake pan that fits inside your air fryer with parchment paper. In the bowl of a stand mixer, beat the butter and Swerve. Add the beaten egg and vanilla, and beat for about 3 minutes. Add the almond flour mixture to the butter-and-egg mixture; beat until just combined. Stir in the pecans and chocolate chips. Transfer the dough to the prepared pan, and press it into the bottom. Set the air fryer to 325°F and cook for 12 minutes. Remove from the air fryer and let cool for 15 minutes. Using a sharp knife, cut the cookie into thin strips, then return the strips to the cake pan with the bottom sides facing up. Set the air fryer to 300°F. Cook for 8 to 10 minutes. Remove from the air fryer and let cool completely on a wire rack.

Per Serving: Calories: 148; Fat: 14g; Protein: 4g; Total Carbs: 11g; Fiber: 2g; Net Carbs: 3g; **Macros:** Fat: 85%; Protein: 11%; Carbs: 4%

Pecan Squares

SERVES 8 | PREP TIME: 20 minutes | COOK TIME: 22 minutes | TEMPERATURE: 325°F

1 cup almond flour	¼ cup unsalted butter, at room temperature
1½ tablespoons Swerve Confectioners sweetener	½ cup brown sugar substitute
5 tablespoons cold unsalted butter, cut into cubes	¼ cup maple syrup substitute
3 teaspoons pure vanilla extract, divided	1 tablespoon heavy (whipping) cream
	1¼ cups chopped pecans

Line a 7-inch pan that is at least 2-inches deep with parchment paper. Stir the almond flour and Swerve in the bowl of a stand mixer. Add the cold butter and 1 teaspoon of vanilla, and beat until the mixture comes together, 3 to 4 minutes. Press the crust into the prepared pan. Place the pan in the air fryer basket and set the air fryer to 325°F. Cook for 8 minutes. Remove the basket from the air fryer and allow the crust to cool. While the crust cooks, combine the ¼ cup of butter, brown sugar substitute, and maple syrup substitute in a saucepan over medium heat. Cook until the butter is melted and the mixture is thick and bubbly, about 5 minutes. Stir in the heavy cream, remaining

2 teaspoons of vanilla, and chopped pecans. Pour the mixture on top of the crust. Place the basket back in the air fryer and cook for 14 minutes or until set. Remove the pan from the air fryer and let cool completely. Carefully remove the pastry from the pan and cut it into squares.

Per Serving: Calories: 350; Fat: 34g; Protein: 5g; Total Carbs: 28g; Fiber: 10g; Net Carbs: 3g; **Macros:** Fat: 87%; Protein: 6%; Carbs: 7%

Air-Fried Vanilla and Chocolate Layer Cake

SERVES 8 | PREP TIME: 15 minutes | COOK TIME: 1 hour

For the cake layers

Nonstick cooking spray	10 large eggs, divided
1 cup coconut flour, divided	¼ cup coconut milk, divided
¼ cup vanilla protein powder	24 drops vanilla-flavored liquid stevia, divided
1 cup melted butter-flavored coconut oil, divided	2 tablespoons unsweetened cocoa powder
1 cup erythritol, divided	
1 teaspoon baking soda, divided	

For the frosting

½ cup melted butter-flavored coconut oil	12 to 24 drops vanilla-flavored liquid stevia
¼ cup unsweetened cocoa powder	2 tablespoons sugar-free coconut yogurt (optional but recommended)

Spray a small round cake pan (small enough to fit in an air fryer) with nonstick spray. In a blender, combine ½ cup of coconut flour, the vanilla protein powder, ½ cup of coconut oil, ½ cup of erythritol, ½ teaspoon of baking soda, 5 eggs, 2 tablespoons of coconut milk, and 12 drops of liquid stevia and purée until smooth. Pour the vanilla cake batter into the prepared pan, place in the air fryer and air-fry at 400°F for 12 to 15 minutes, until a spatula doesn't stick to the sides. Remove the vanilla layer from the air fryer. Invert it onto a plate, then return it to the cake pan and put back in the air fryer to cook on the other side. Reduce the temperature to 370°F and bake for another 15 minutes, or until a toothpick inserted in the center comes out clean. Remove from the air fryer and let cool for 20 to 30 minutes. Using the remaining cake ingredients, repeat to make the chocolate layer, but use the chocolate protein powder instead of vanilla and add the cocoa powder. Let cool for 20 to 30 minutes when done baking. In a mixing bowl, combine the oil with the cocoa powder, liquid stevia, and coconut yogurt (if using), then mix until it forms a frosting-like consistency. Stack the cake layers and use a butter knife to spread the frosting all over the cake.

Per Serving: Calories: 620; Fat: 52g; Protein: 16g; Total Carbs: 22g; Fiber: 12g; Net Carbs: 10g; **Macros:** Fat: 75%; Protein: 11%; Carbs: 14%

Slow Cooker Breakfast Sausage

SERVES 8 | PREP TIME: 10 minutes | COOK TIME: 3 hours on low

1 tablespoon extra-virgin olive oil	1 sweet onion, chopped
2 pounds ground pork	½ cup almond flour
2 large eggs	2 teaspoons minced garlic
	2 teaspoons dried oregano

1 teaspoon dried thyme
1 teaspoon fennel seeds
1 teaspoon freshly ground black pepper
½ teaspoon salt

Lightly grease the insert of the slow cooker with the olive oil. In a large bowl, stir the pork, eggs, onion, almond flour, garlic, oregano, thyme, fennel seeds, pepper, and salt until well mixed. Transfer the meat mixture to the slow cooker's insert and shape it into a loaf, leaving about ½ inch between the sides and meat. Cover, and if your slow cooker has a temperature probe, insert it. Cook on low until it reaches an internal temperature of 150°F, about 3 hours. Slice in any way you prefer and serve.

Per serving: Calories: 341; Fat: 27g; Protein: 21g; Total Carbs: 1g; Fiber: 0g; Net Carbs: 1g; **Macros:** Fat: 73%; Protein: 25%; Carbs: 2%

Slow Cooker Huevos Rancheros

SERVES 8 | PREP TIME: 10 minutes | COOK TIME: 3 hours on low

1 tablespoon extra-virgin olive oil
10 large eggs
1 cup heavy (whipping) cream
1 cup shredded Monterey Jack cheese, divided
1 cup prepared or home-made salsa
1 scallion, white and green parts, chopped
1 jalapeño pepper, chopped
½ teaspoon chili powder
½ teaspoon salt
1 avocado, chopped, for garnish
1 tablespoon chopped cilantro, for garnish

Lightly grease the insert of the slow cooker with the olive oil. In a large bowl, whisk the eggs, heavy cream, ½ cup of the cheese, salsa, scallion, jalapeño, chili powder, and salt. Pour the mixture into the insert and sprinkle the top with the remaining ½ cup of cheese. Cover and cook until the eggs are firm, about 3 hours on low. Let the eggs cool slightly, then cut into wedges and serve garnished with avocado and cilantro.

Per serving: Calories: 302; Fat: 26g; Protein: 13g; Total Carbs: 5g; Fiber: 2g; Net Carbs: 3g; **Macros:** Fat: 76%; Protein: 17%; Carbs: 7%

Slow Cooker Mediterranean Eggs

SERVES 4 | PREP TIME: 10 minutes | COOK TIME: 5 to 6 hours on low

1 tablespoon extra-virgin olive oil
12 large eggs
½ cup coconut milk
½ teaspoon dried oregano
½ teaspoon freshly ground black pepper
¼ teaspoon salt
2 cups chopped spinach
1 tomato, chopped
¼ cup chopped sweet onion
1 teaspoon minced garlic
½ cup crumbled goat cheese

Lightly grease the insert of the slow cooker with the olive oil. In a large bowl, whisk the eggs, coconut milk, oregano, pepper, and salt, until well blended. Add the spinach, tomato, onion, and garlic, and stir to combine. Pour the egg mixture into the insert and top with the crumbled goat cheese. Cover and cook on low 5 to 6 hours, until it is set like a quiche. Serve warm.

Per serving: Calories: 349; Fat: 27g; Protein: 23g; Total Carbs: 5g; Fiber: 1g; Net Carbs: 4g; **Macros:** Fat: 67%; Protein: 25%; Carbs: 8%

Greek Frittata with Olives, Artichoke Hearts & Feta

SERVES 6 | PREP: 10 minutes | COOK: 6 hours on low or 3 hours on high

1 tablespoon unsalted butter, ghee, or extra-virgin olive oil
½ (14-ounce) can artichoke hearts, drained and diced
½ (12-ounce) jar roasted red bell peppers, drained and diced
½ cup pitted Kalamata olives, drained and halved
4 scallions (both white and green parts), sliced
12 large eggs
2 tablespoons heavy (whipping) cream
1 tablespoon minced fresh oregano or 1 teaspoon dried oregano
½ teaspoon kosher salt
¼ teaspoon freshly ground black pepper
8 ounces crumbled feta cheese

Generously coat the inside of the slow cooker insert with the butter. Layer the artichoke hearts in the bottom of the cooker. Next, layer the roasted bell peppers, then the olives, and finally the scallions. In a large bowl, beat the eggs, then whisk in the heavy cream, oregano, salt, and pepper. Pour the egg mixture over the layered vegetables. Sprinkle the feta cheese over the top. Cover and cook for 6 hours on low or 3 hours on high. Serve hot, warm, or at room temperature.

Per Serving: Calories: 310; Fat: 25g; Protein: 17g; Total Carbs: 9g; Fiber: 4g; Net Carbs: 5g; Cholesterol: 471mg; **Macros:** Fat: 70%; Protein: 20%; Carbs: 10%

Slow Cooker Layered Egg Casserole

SERVES 12 | PREP TIME: 10 minutes | COOK TIME: 4 hours on low

1 tablespoon extra-virgin olive oil
1 pound breakfast sausage
1 zucchini, chopped
1 red bell pepper, finely chopped
½ sweet onion, chopped
12 ounces shredded Cheddar cheese
12 large eggs
1 cup heavy (whipping) cream
½ teaspoon salt
½ teaspoon freshly ground black pepper

Lightly grease the insert of the slow cooker with the olive oil. Arrange half of the sausage in the bottom of the insert. Top with half of the zucchini, pepper, and onion. Top the vegetables with half of the cheese. Repeat, creating another layer. In a medium bowl, whisk the eggs, heavy cream, salt, and pepper. Pour the egg mixture over the casserole. Cover and cook on low for 4 hours. Serve warm.

Per serving: Calories: 338; Fat: 29g; Protein: 18g; Total Carbs: 2g; Fiber: 0g; Net Carbs: 2g; **Macros:** Fat: 77%; Protein: 21%; Carbs: 2%

Slow Cooker Spanakopita Frittata

SERVES 8 | PREP TIME: 10 minutes | 5 to 6 hours on low

1 tablespoon extra-virgin olive oil
12 large eggs
1 cup heavy (whipping) cream
2 teaspoons minced garlic
2 cups chopped spinach
½ cup feta cheese
Cherry tomatoes, halved, for garnish (optional)
Yogurt, for garnish (optional)
Parsley, for garnish (optional)

Lightly grease the insert of the slow cooker with the olive oil. In a medium bowl, whisk the eggs, heavy cream, garlic, spinach, and feta. Pour the mixture into the slow cooker. Cover and cook on low 5 to 6 hours. Serve topped with the tomatoes, a dollop of yogurt, and parsley, if desired.

Per serving: Calories: 247; Fat: 22g; Protein: 11g; Total Carbs: 2g; Fiber: 0g; Net Carbs: 2g; **Macros:** Fat: 79%; Protein: 18%; Carbs: 3%

Crustless Wild Mushroom–Kale Quiche

SERVES 8 | PREP TIME: 10 minutes | COOK TIME: 5 to 6 hours on low

1 tablespoon extra-virgin olive oil	¼ teaspoon freshly ground black pepper
12 large eggs	⅛ teaspoon salt
1 cup heavy (whipping) cream	2 cups coarsely chopped wild mushrooms (shiitake, portabella, oyster, enoki)
1 tablespoon chopped fresh thyme	
1 tablespoon chopped fresh chives	1 cup chopped kale
	1 cup shredded Swiss cheese

Lightly grease the insert of the slow cooker with the olive oil. In a medium bowl, whisk the eggs, heavy cream, thyme, chives, pepper, and salt. Stir in the mushrooms and kale. Pour the mixture into the slow cooker and top with the cheese. Cover and cook on low 5 to 6 hours. Serve warm.

Per serving: Calories: 289; Fat: 24g; Protein: 15g; Total Carbs: 5g; Fiber: 1g; Net Carbs: 4g; **Macros:** Fat: 73%; Protein: 20%; Carbs: 7%

Bacon-and-Eggs Breakfast Casserole

SERVES 8 | PREP TIME: 15 minutes | COOK TIME: 5 to 6 hours on low

1 tablespoon bacon fat or extra-virgin olive oil	½ sweet onion, chopped
12 large eggs	2 teaspoons minced garlic
1 cup coconut milk	¼ teaspoon freshly ground black pepper
1 pound bacon, chopped and cooked crisp	⅛ teaspoon salt
	Pinch red pepper flakes

Lightly grease the insert of the slow cooker with the bacon fat or olive oil. In a medium bowl, whisk together the eggs, coconut milk, bacon, onion, garlic, pepper, salt, and red pepper flakes. Pour the mixture into the slow cooker. Cover and cook on low for 5 to 6 hours. Serve warm.

Per serving: Calories: 526; Fat: 43g; Protein: 32g; Total Carbs: 3g; Fiber: 0g; Net Carbs: 3g; **Macros:** Fat: 73%; Protein: 24%; Carbs: 3%

Vegetable Omelet

SERVES 8 | PREP TIME: 15 minutes | COOK TIME: 4 to 5 hours on low

1 tablespoon extra-virgin olive oil	½ cup chopped cauliflower
10 large eggs	½ cup chopped broccoli
½ cup heavy (whipping) cream	1 red bell pepper, chopped
1 teaspoon minced garlic	1 scallion, white and green parts, chopped
¼ teaspoon salt	4 ounces goat cheese, crumbled
⅛ teaspoon freshly ground black pepper	2 tablespoons chopped parsley, for garnish

Lightly grease the insert of the slow cooker with the olive oil. In a medium bowl, whisk the eggs, heavy cream, garlic, salt, and pepper. Stir in the cauliflower, broccoli, red bell pepper, and scallion. Pour the mixture into the slow cooker. Sprinkle the top with goat cheese. Cover and cook on low for 4 to 5 hours. Serve topped with the parsley.

Per serving: Calories: 200; Fat: 16g; Protein: 11g; Total Carbs: 2g; Fiber: 1g; Net Carbs: 1g; **Macros:** Fat: 73%; Protein: 22%; Carbs: 5%

Sausage-Stuffed Peppers

SERVES 4 | PREP TIME: 15 minutes | COOK TIME: 4 to 5 hours on low

1 tablespoon extra-virgin olive oil	½ cup coconut milk
4 bell peppers, tops cut off and seeds removed	1 scallion, white and green parts, chopped
1 cup breakfast sausage, crumbled	½ teaspoon freshly ground black pepper
6 large eggs	1 cup shredded Cheddar cheese

Line a slow cooker insert with foil and grease the foil with the olive oil. Place the four peppers in the slow cooker and evenly fill them with the sausage crumbles. In a medium bowl, whisk together the eggs, coconut milk, scallion, and pepper. Pour the egg mixture into the four peppers. Next, sprinkle the cheese over them. Cook on low for 4 to 5 hours, until the eggs are set. Serve warm.

Per serving: Calories: 450; Fat: 36g; Protein: 25g; Total Carbs: 8g; Fiber: 3g; Net Carbs: 5g; **Macros:** Fat: 71%; Protein: 22%; Carbs: 7%

Dill-Asparagus Bake

SERVES 8 | PREP TIME: 10 minutes | COOK TIME: 4 to 5 hours on low

1 tablespoon extra-virgin olive oil	2 teaspoons chopped fresh dill
10 large eggs	2 cups chopped asparagus spears
¾ cup coconut milk	1 cup chopped cooked bacon
½ teaspoon salt	
¼ teaspoon freshly ground black pepper	

Lightly grease the insert of the slow cooker with the olive oil. In a medium bowl, whisk together the eggs, coconut milk, salt, pepper, and dill. Stir in the asparagus and bacon. Pour the mixture into the slow cooker. Cover and cook on low for 4 to 5 hours. Serve warm.

Per serving: Calories: 225; Fat: 18g; Protein: 14g; Total Carbs: 3g; Fiber: 1g; Net Carbs: 2g; **Macros:** Fat: 70%; Protein: 24%; Carbs: 6%

Slow Cooker Grain-Free Zucchini Bread

SERVES 12 | PREP: 15 minutes | COOK: 6 hours on low or 3 hours on high

⅓ cup unsalted butter, melted and cooled slightly, plus more for coating the pan	1½ teaspoons baking powder
	½ teaspoon baking soda
1 cup almond flour	½ teaspoon xanthan gum (optional)
⅓ cup coconut flour	1½ teaspoons pure vanilla extract
2 teaspoons ground cinnamon	

½ teaspoon baking soda
½ teaspoon fine sea salt
3 large eggs
1 cup erythritol
1 teaspoon stevia powder
2 cups shredded zucchini
½ cup chopped walnuts
    or pecans

Generously coat a loaf pan with butter. In a medium bowl, stir the almond flour, coconut flour, cinnamon, baking powder, baking soda, sea salt, and xanthan gum (if using). In a large bowl, beat the eggs, then whisk in the melted butter, vanilla, erythritol, and stevia. Stir the dry ingredients into the egg mixture. Gently fold in the zucchini and walnuts. Transfer the batter to the prepared loaf pan and spread it into an even layer with a rubber spatula or the back of a spoon. Wad four pieces of aluminum foil into balls and put them on the bottom of the slow cooker insert. Place the filled loaf pan on top of the foil balls. Cover and cook for 6 hours on low or 3 hours on high. Remove the pan from the slow cooker and invert the loaf onto a cooling rack. Let cool completely. Wrap in foil or plastic wrap and refrigerate. Slice and serve chilled.

Per Serving: Calories: 213; Fat: 20g; Protein: 6g; Total Carbs: 6g; Fiber: 3g; Net Carbs: 3g; Macros: Fat: 80%; Protein: 10%; Carbs: 10%

Cheddar Cheese Soup

SERVES 6 | PREP TIME: 15 minutes | COOK TIME: 6 hours on low

1 tablespoon butter
5 cups chicken broth
1 cup coconut milk
2 celery stalks, chopped
1 carrot, chopped
½ sweet onion, chopped
Pinch cayenne pepper
8 ounces cream cheese, cubed
2 cups shredded Cheddar cheese
Salt, for seasoning
Freshly ground black pepper, for seasoning
1 tablespoon chopped fresh thyme, for garnish

Lightly grease the insert of the slow cooker with the butter. Place the broth, coconut milk, celery, carrot, onion, and cayenne pepper in the insert. Cover and cook on low for 6 hours. Stir in the cream cheese and Cheddar, then season with salt and pepper. Serve topped with the thyme.

Per Serving: Calories: 406; Fat: 36g; Protein: 15g; Total Carbs: 7g; Fiber: 1g; Net Carbs: 6g; Macros: Fat: 79%; Protein: 15%; Carbs: 6%

Sausage-Sauerkraut Soup

SERVES 6 | PREP TIME: 15 minutes | COOK TIME: 6 hours on low

1 tablespoon extra-virgin olive oil
6 cups beef broth
1 pound organic sausage, cooked and sliced
2 cups sauerkraut
2 celery stalks, chopped
1 sweet onion, chopped
2 teaspoons minced garlic
2 tablespoons butter
1 tablespoon hot mustard
½ teaspoon caraway seeds
½ cup sour cream
2 tablespoons chopped fresh parsley, for garnish

Lightly grease the insert of the slow cooker with the olive oil. Place the broth, sausage, sauerkraut, celery, onion, garlic, butter, mustard, and caraway seeds in the insert. Cover and cook on

low for 6 hours. Stir in the sour cream. Serve topped with the parsley.

Per Serving: Calories: 332; Fat: 28g; Protein: 15g; Total Carbs: 6g; Fiber: 2g; Net Carbs: 4g; Macros: Fat: 75%; Protein: 18%; Carbs: 7%

Slow Cooker Grain-Free Pumpkin Loaf

SERVES 12 | PREP: 15 minutes | COOK: 6 hours on low or 3 hours on high

½ cup (1 stick) unsalted butter, melted and cooled slightly, plus more for coating the pan
12 large eggs
1 cup pumpkin purée
1½ teaspoons pure vanilla extract
1 cup erythritol
2 teaspoons ground cinnamon
1 teaspoon stevia powder
1 teaspoon fine sea salt
1 cup coconut flour
1 teaspoon baking powder

Generously coat a loaf pan with butter. In a large bowl, beat the eggs, then whisk in the pumpkin, melted butter, vanilla, erythritol, cinnamon, stevia powder, and sea salt until combined. Add the coconut flour and baking powder and beat until smooth. Transfer the batter to the prepared loaf pan and spread it into an even layer with a rubber spatula or the back of a spoon. Wad four pieces of aluminum foil into balls and put them on the bottom of the slow cooker insert. Place the filled loaf pan on top of the foil balls. Cover and cook for 6 hours on low or 3 hours on high. Remove the pan from the slow cooker and invert the loaf onto a cooling rack. Let cool completely. Wrap in foil or plastic wrap and refrigerate. Slice and serve chilled.

Per Serving: Calories: 207; Fat: 18g; Protein: 7g; Total Carbs: 6g; Fiber: 2g; Net Carbs: 4g; Macros: Fat: 76%; Protein: 14%; Carbs: 10%

Spiced-Pumpkin Chicken Soup

SERVES 6 | PREP TIME: 15 minutes | COOK TIME: 6 hours on low

1 tablespoon extra-virgin olive oil
4 cups chicken broth
2 cups coconut milk
1 pound pumpkin, diced
½ sweet onion, chopped
1 tablespoon grated fresh ginger
2 teaspoons minced garlic
½ teaspoon ground cinnamon
¼ teaspoon ground nutmeg
¼ teaspoon freshly ground black pepper
¼ teaspoon salt
Pinch ground allspice
1 cup heavy (whipping) cream
2 cups chopped cooked chicken

Lightly grease the insert of the slow cooker with the olive oil. Place the broth, coconut milk, pumpkin, onion, ginger, garlic, cinnamon, nutmeg, pepper, salt, and allspice in the insert. Cover and cook on low for 6 hours. Using an immersion blender or a regular blender, purée the soup. If you removed the soup from the insert to purée, add it back to the pot, and stir in the cream and chicken. Keep heating the soup on low for 15 minutes to heat the chicken through.

Per serving: Calories: 389; Fat: 32g; Protein: 16g; Total Carbs: 10g; Fiber: 5g; Net Carbs: 5g; Macros: Fat: 73%; Protein: 16%; Carbs: 11%

Cheesy Bacon-Cauliflower Soup

SERVES 6 | PREP TIME: 15 minutes | COOK TIME: 6 hours on low

1 tablespoon extra-virgin olive oil	2 cups chopped cauliflower
4 cups chicken broth	1 sweet onion, chopped
2 cups coconut milk	3 teaspoons minced garlic
2 cups chopped cooked chicken	½ cup cream cheese, cubed
1 cup chopped cooked bacon	2 cups shredded Cheddar cheese

Lightly grease the insert of the slow cooker with the olive oil. Place the broth, coconut milk, chicken, bacon, cauliflower, onion, and garlic in the insert. Cover and cook on low for 6 hours. Stir in the cream cheese and Cheddar and serve.

Per Serving: Calories: 540; Fat: 44g; Protein: 35g; Total Carbs: 7g; Fiber: 1g; Net Carbs: 6g; Macros: Fat: 70%; Protein: 25%; Carbs: 5%

Turkey-Potpie Soup

SERVES 8 | PREP TIME: 20 minutes | COOK TIME: 7 to 8 hours on low

1 tablespoon extra-virgin olive oil	2 teaspoons chopped fresh thyme
4 cups chicken broth	1 cup cream cheese, diced
½ pound skinless turkey breast, cut into ½-inch chunks	2 cups heavy (whipping) cream
2 celery stalks, chopped	1 cup green beans, cut into 1-inch pieces
1 carrot, diced	Salt, for seasoning
1 sweet onion, chopped	Freshly ground black pepper, for seasoning
2 teaspoons minced garlic	

Lightly grease the insert of the slow cooker with the olive oil. Place the broth, turkey, celery, carrot, onion, garlic, and thyme in the insert. Cover and cook on low for 7 to 8 hours. Stir in the cream cheese, heavy cream, and green beans. Season with salt and pepper and serve.

Per serving: Calories: 415; Fat: 35g; Protein: 20g; Total Carbs: 7g; Fiber: 2g; Net Carbs: 5g; Macros: Fat: 74%; Protein: 19%; Carbs: 7%

Chicken-Nacho Soup

SERVES 8 | PREP TIME: 15 minutes | COOK TIME: 6 hours on low

3 tablespoons extra-virgin olive oil, divided	2 cups coconut milk
1 pound ground chicken	1 tomato, diced
1 sweet onion, diced	1 jalapeño pepper, chopped
1 red bell pepper, chopped	2 cups shredded Cheddar cheese
2 teaspoons minced garlic	½ cup sour cream, for garnish
2 tablespoons taco seasoning	1 scallion, white and green parts, chopped, for garnish
4 cups chicken broth	

Lightly grease the insert of the slow cooker with 1 tablespoon of the olive oil. In a large skillet over medium-high heat, heat the remaining 2 tablespoons of the olive oil. Add the chicken and sauté until it is cooked through, about 6 minutes. Add the onion, red bell pepper, garlic, and taco seasoning, and sauté for

an additional 3 minutes. Transfer the chicken mixture to the insert, and stir in the broth, coconut milk, tomato, and jalapeño pepper. Cover and cook on low for 6 hours. Stir in the cheese. Serve topped with the sour cream and scallion.

Per serving: Calories: 434; Fat: 35g; Protein: 22g; Total Carbs: 9g; Fiber: 2g; Net Carbs: 7g; Macros: Fat: 73%; Protein: 20%; Carbs: 7%

Faux Lasagna Soup

SERVES 6 | PREP TIME: 20 minutes | COOK TIME: 6 hours on low

3 tablespoons extra-virgin olive oil, divided	1 (28-ounce) can diced tomatoes, undrained
1 pound ground beef	1 zucchini, diced
½ sweet onion, chopped	1½ tablespoons dried basil
2 teaspoons minced garlic	2 teaspoons dried oregano
4 cups beef broth	4 ounces cream cheese
	1 cup shredded mozzarella

Lightly grease the insert of the slow cooker with 1 tablespoon of the olive oil. In a large skillet over medium-high heat, heat the remaining 2 tablespoons of the olive oil. Add the ground beef and sauté until it is cooked through, about 6 minutes. Add the onion and garlic and sauté for an additional 3 minutes. Transfer the meat mixture to the insert. Stir in the broth, tomatoes, zucchini, basil, and oregano. Cover and cook on low for 6 hours. Stir in the cream cheese and mozzarella and serve.

Per serving: Calories: 472; Fat: 36g; Protein: 30g; Total Carbs: 9g; Fiber: 3g; Net Carbs: 6g; Macros: Fat: 67%; Protein: 25%; Carbs: 8%

Chicken-Bacon Soup

SERVES 8 | PREP TIME: 15 minutes | COOK TIME: 8 hours on low

1 tablespoon extra-virgin olive oil	2 teaspoons minced garlic
6 cups chicken broth	1½ cups heavy (whipping) cream
3 cups cooked chicken, chopped	1 cup cream cheese
1 sweet onion, chopped	1 cup cooked chopped bacon
2 celery stalks, chopped	1 tablespoon chopped fresh parsley, for garnish
1 carrot, diced	

Lightly grease the insert of the slow cooker with the olive oil. Add the broth, chicken, onion, celery, carrot, and garlic. Cover and cook on low for 8 hours. Stir in the heavy cream, cream cheese, and bacon. Serve topped with the parsley.

Per serving: Calories: 488; Fat: 37g; Protein: 27g; Total Carbs: 11g; Fiber: 1g; Net Carbs: 10g; Macros: Fat: 69%; Protein: 22%; Carbs: 9%

Curried Broccoli, Cheddar & Toasted Almond Soup

SERVES 6 | PREP: 10 minutes | COOK: 6 hours on low or 3 hours on high

2 tablespoons unsalted butter, cubed	2 garlic cloves, minced
8 ounces broccoli stems, peeled and chopped	½ cup sliced toasted almonds, divided
½ onion, diced	6 cups vegetable broth or chicken broth

1 tablespoon curry powder
Kosher salt
Freshly ground white pepper
¾ cup heavy (whipping) cream

1½ cups shredded white Cheddar cheese
½ cup sour cream

In the slow cooker insert, combine the butter, broccoli, onion, garlic, ¼ cup of almonds, broth, and curry powder. Season with salt and pepper. Cover and cook for 6 hours on low or 3 hours on high. Stir in the heavy cream, then stir in the Cheddar cheese by the handful until thoroughly melted and incorporated. Use an immersion or countertop blender to purée the soup until smooth, working in batches if necessary. Serve hot, garnished with the sour cream and the remaining ¼ cup of almonds.

Per Serving: Calories: 455; Fat: 37g; Protein: 17g; Total Carbs: 15g; Fiber: 2g; Net Carbs: 13g; Macros: Fat: 71%; Protein: 15%; Carbs: 14%

Chicken Chowder with Bacon

SERVES 6 | PREP: 15 minutes | COOK: 8 hours on low

12 ounces bacon
¼ cup (½ stick) unsalted butter or ghee, at room temperature, divided
12 ounces boneless, skinless chicken breast, diced
6 ounces cremini mushrooms, sliced
2 celery stalks, diced
1 leek (white and pale green parts), halved lengthwise and thinly sliced crosswise

1 onion, thinly sliced
1 shallot, finely chopped
4 garlic cloves, minced
1 tablespoon minced fresh thyme
1 teaspoon kosher salt
1 teaspoon freshly ground black pepper
2 cups chicken broth
1 cup heavy (whipping) cream
8 ounces cream cheese, at room temperature

In a large skillet, cook the bacon over medium heat until crisp. Transfer to a paper towel–lined plate to drain. Crumble into small pieces and set aside. Spread 2 tablespoons of butter over the bottom of the slow cooker insert. Add the chicken, cooked bacon, mushrooms, celery, leek, onion, shallot, garlic, thyme, salt, and pepper. In a medium bowl, whisk the chicken broth, heavy cream, cream cheese, and remaining 2 tablespoons of butter until well combined and smooth. Pour the mixture over the ingredients in the slow cooker and stir to mix. Cover and cook for 8 hours on low. Serve hot.

Per Serving: Calories: 573; Fat: 45g; Protein: 31g; Total Carbs: 12g; Fiber: 1g; Net Carbs: 11g; Macros: Fat: 70%; Protein: 22%; Carbs: 8%

Mulligatawny Soup with Cauliflower Rice

SERVES 6 | PREP: 10 minutes | COOK: 6 hours on low

6 cups chicken broth
2 cups canned coconut milk
¾ cup coconut cream
3 tablespoons curry powder
2 tablespoons erythritol

1 teaspoon kosher salt
8 ounces boneless, skinless chicken thighs, diced
1 cup riced cauliflower
3 cups baby spinach

In the slow cooker, combine the chicken broth, coconut milk, coconut cream, curry powder, erythritol, salt, chicken, and cauliflower. Cover and cook for 6 hours on low. Just before serving, stir in the spinach until it is wilted. Serve hot.

Per Serving: Calories: 388; Fat: 31g; Protein: 17g; Total Carbs: 14g; Fiber: 2g; Net Carbs: 12g; Macros: Fat: 70%; Protein: 17%; Carbs: 13%

Homemade Sausage Soup

SERVES 6 | PREP TIME: 15 minutes | COOK TIME: 6 hours on low

3 tablespoons olive oil, divided
1½ pounds sausage, without casing
6 cups chicken broth
2 celery stalks, chopped
1 carrot, diced

1 leek, thoroughly cleaned and chopped
2 teaspoons minced garlic
2 cups chopped kale
1 tablespoon chopped fresh parsley, for garnish

Lightly grease the insert of the slow cooker with 1 tablespoon of the olive oil. In a large skillet over medium-high heat, heat the remaining 2 tablespoons of the olive oil. Add the sausage and sauté until it is cooked through, about 7 minutes. Transfer the sausage to the insert, and stir in the broth, celery, carrot, leek, and garlic. Cover and cook on low for 6 hours. Stir in the kale. Serve topped with the parsley.

Per Serving: Calories: 383; Fat: 31g; Protein: 21g; Total Carbs: 5g; Fiber: 1g; Net Carbs: 4g; Macros: Fat: 73%; Protein: 22%; Carbs: 5%

Cheeseburger Soup

SERVES 8 | PREP TIME: 15 minutes | COOK TIME: 6 hours on low

3 tablespoons olive oil, divided
1 pound ground beef
1 sweet onion, chopped
2 teaspoons minced garlic
6 cups beef broth
1 (28-ounce) can diced tomatoes
2 celery stalks, chopped

1 carrot, chopped
1 cup heavy (whipping) cream
2 cups shredded Cheddar cheese
½ teaspoon freshly ground black pepper
1 scallion, white and green parts, chopped, for garnish

Lightly grease the insert of the slow cooker with 1 tablespoon of the olive oil. In a large skillet over medium-high heat, heat the remaining 2 tablespoons of the olive oil. Add the ground beef and sauté until it is cooked through, about 6 minutes. Add the onion and garlic and sauté for an additional 3 minutes. Transfer the beef mixture to the insert, and stir in the broth, tomatoes, celery, and carrot. Cover and cook on low for 6 hours. Stir in the heavy cream, cheese, and pepper. Serve hot, topped with the scallion.

Per Serving: Calories: 413; Fat: 32g; Protein: 26g; Total Carbs: 8g; Fiber: 2g; Net Carbs: 6g; Macros: Fat: 68%; Protein: 25%; Carbs: 7%

Jambalaya Soup

SERVES 8 | PREP TIME: 15 minutes | COOK TIME: 6 to 7 hours on low

1 tablespoon extra-virgin olive oil
6 cups chicken broth
1 (28-ounce) can diced tomatoes
1 pound spicy organic sausage, sliced

1 cup chopped cooked chicken
1 red bell pepper, chopped
½ sweet onion, chopped
1 jalapeño pepper, chopped
2 teaspoons minced garlic

3 tablespoons Cajun
 seasoning
½ pound medium shrimp,
 peeled, deveined,
 and chopped

½ cup sour cream, for garnish
1 avocado, diced, for garnish
2 tablespoons chopped cilantro, for garnish

Lightly grease the insert of the slow cooker with the olive oil. Add the broth, tomatoes, sausage, chicken, red bell pepper, onion, jalapeño pepper, garlic, and Cajun seasoning. Cover and cook on low for 6 to 7 hours. Stir in the shrimp and leave on low for 30 minutes, or until the shrimp are cooked through. Serve topped with the sour cream, avocado, and cilantro.

Per serving: Calories: 400; Fat: 31g; Protein: 24g; Total Carbs: 9g; Fiber: 4g; Net Carbs: 5g; **Macros:** Fat: 68%; Protein: 23%; Carbs: 9%

Creamy Chicken Stew

SERVES 6 | PREP TIME: 20 minutes | COOK TIME: 6 hours on low

3 tablespoons extra-virgin
 olive oil, divided
1 pound boneless chicken
 thighs, diced into
 1½-inch pieces
½ sweet onion, chopped
2 teaspoons minced garlic
2 cups chicken broth

2 celery stalks, diced
1 carrot, diced
1 teaspoon dried thyme
1 cup shredded kale
1 cup coconut cream
Salt, for seasoning
Freshly ground black pepper,
 for seasoning

Lightly grease the insert of the slow cooker with 1 tablespoon of the olive oil. In a large skillet over medium-high heat, heat the remaining 2 tablespoons of the olive oil. Add the chicken and sauté until it is just cooked through, about 7 minutes. Add the onion and garlic and sauté for an additional 3 minutes. Transfer the chicken mixture to the insert, and stir in the broth, celery, carrot, and thyme. Cover and cook on low for 6 hours. Stir in the kale and coconut cream. Season with salt and pepper, and serve warm.

Per serving: Calories: 276; Fat: 22g; Protein: 17g; Total Carbs: 6g; Fiber: 2g; Net Carbs: 4g; **Macros:** Fat: 68%; Protein: 23%; Carbs: 9%

Simple Chicken-Vegetable Soup

SERVES 6 | PREP TIME: 15 minutes | COOK TIME: 7 to 8 hours on low

1 tablespoon extra-virgin
 olive oil
4 cups chicken broth
2 cups coconut milk
2 cups diced chicken breast
½ sweet onion, chopped
2 celery stalks, chopped

1 carrot, diced
½ cup chopped cauliflower
2 teaspoons minced garlic
1 teaspoon chopped thyme
1 teaspoon chopped oregano
¼ teaspoon freshly ground
 black pepper

Lightly grease the insert of the slow cooker with the olive oil. Add the broth, coconut milk, chicken, onion, celery, carrot, cauliflower, garlic, thyme, oregano, and pepper. Cover and cook on low for 7 to 8 hours. Serve warm.

Per serving: Calories: 299; Fat: 25g; Protein: 14g; Total Carbs: 8g; Fiber: 3g; Net Carbs: 5g; **Macros:** Fat: 72%; Protein: 18%; Carbs: 10%

Beef Stew

SERVES 6 | PREP TIME: 15 minutes | COOK TIME: 8 hours on low

3 tablespoons extra-virgin
 olive oil, divided
1 (2-pound) beef chuck roast,
 cut into 1-inch chunks
½ teaspoon salt
¼ teaspoon freshly ground
 black pepper
2 cups beef broth
1 cup diced tomatoes

¼ cup apple cider vinegar
1½ cups cubed pumpkin, cut
 into 1-inch chunks
½ sweet onion, chopped
2 teaspoons minced garlic
1 teaspoon dried thyme
1 tablespoon chopped fresh
 parsley, for garnish

Lightly grease the insert of the slow cooker with 1 tablespoon of the olive oil. Lightly season the beef chucks with salt and pepper. In a large skillet over medium-high heat, heat the remaining 2 tablespoons of the olive oil. Add the beef and brown on all sides, about 7 minutes. Transfer the beef to the insert and stir in the broth, tomatoes, apple cider vinegar, pumpkin, onion, garlic, and thyme. Cover and cook on low heat for about 8 hours, until the beef is very tender. Serve topped with the parsley.

Per Serving: Calories: 461; Fat: 34g; Protein: 32g; Total Carbs: 10g; Fiber: 3g; Net Carbs: 7g; **Macros:** Fat: 65%; Protein: 27%; Carbs: 8%

Curried Vegetable Stew

SERVES 6 | PREP TIME: 15 minutes | COOK TIME: 7 to 8 hours on low

1 tablespoon extra-virgin
 olive oil
4 cups coconut milk
1 cup diced pumpkin
1 cup cauliflower florets
1 red bell pepper, diced
1 zucchini, diced

1 sweet onion, chopped
2 teaspoons grated
 fresh ginger
2 teaspoons minced garlic
1 tablespoon curry powder
2 cups shredded spinach
1 avocado, diced, for garnish

Lightly grease the insert of the slow cooker with the olive oil. Add the coconut milk, pumpkin, cauliflower, bell pepper, zucchini, onion, ginger, garlic, and curry powder. Cover and cook on low for 7 to 8 hours. Stir in the spinach. Garnish each bowl with a spoonful of avocado and serve.

Per serving: Calories: 502; Fat: 44g; Protein: 7g; Total Carbs: 19g; Fiber: 10g; Net Carbs: 9g; **Macros:** Fat: 79%; Protein: 6%; Carbs: 15%

Turkey-Vegetable Stew

SERVES 6 | PREP TIME: 20 minutes | COOK TIME: 7 to 8 hours on low

3 tablespoons extra-virgin
 olive oil, divided
1 pound boneless turkey
 breast, cut into 1-inch pieces
1 leek, thoroughly cleaned
 and sliced
2 teaspoons minced garlic
2 cups chicken broth
1 cup coconut milk

2 celery stalks, chopped
2 cups diced pumpkin
1 carrot, diced
2 teaspoons chopped thyme
Salt, for seasoning
Freshly ground black pepper,
 for seasoning
1 scallion, white and green
 parts, chopped, for garnish

Lightly grease the insert of the slow cooker with 1 tablespoon of the olive oil. In a large skillet over medium-high heat, heat the remaining 2 tablespoons of the olive oil. Add the turkey and sauté until browned, about 5 minutes. Add the leek and garlic and sauté for an additional 3 minutes. Transfer the turkey mixture to the insert and stir in the broth, coconut milk, celery, pumpkin, carrot, and thyme. Cover and cook on low for 7 to 8 hours. Season with salt and pepper. Serve topped with the scallion.

Per serving: Calories: 356; Fat: 27g; Protein: 21g; Total Carbs: 11g; Fiber: 4g; Net Carbs: 7g; **Macros:** Fat: 65%; Protein: 23%; Carbs: 12%

Simple Texas Chili

SERVES 4 | PREP TIME: 20 minutes | COOK TIME: 7 to 8 hours on low

¼ cup extra-virgin olive oil
1½ pounds beef sirloin, cut into 1-inch chunks
1 sweet onion, chopped
2 green bell peppers, chopped
1 jalapeño pepper, seeded, finely chopped
2 teaspoons minced garlic
1 (28-ounce) can diced tomatoes
1 cup beef broth
3 tablespoons chili powder
½ teaspoon ground cumin
¼ teaspoon ground coriander
1 cup sour cream, for garnish
1 avocado, diced, for garnish
1 tablespoon cilantro, chopped, for garnish

Lightly grease the insert of the slow cooker with 1 tablespoon of the olive oil. In a large skillet over medium-high heat, heat the remaining 2 tablespoons of the olive oil. Add the beef and sauté until it is cooked through, about 8 minutes. Add the onion, bell peppers, jalapeño pepper, and garlic, and sauté for an additional 4 minutes. Transfer the beef mixture to the insert and stir in the tomatoes, broth, chili powder, cumin, and coriander. Cover and cook on low for 7 to 8 hours. Serve topped with the sour cream, avocado, and cilantro.

Per serving: Calories: 487; Fat: 38g; Protein: 26g; Total Carbs: 17g; Fiber: 7g; Net Carbs: 10g; **Macros:** Fat: 66%; Protein: 20%; Carbs: 14%

Simple Spaghetti Squash

SERVES 8 | PREP TIME: 15 minutes | COOK TIME: 6 hours on low

1 small spaghetti squash, washed
½ cup chicken stock
¼ cup butter
Salt, for seasoning
Freshly ground black pepper, for seasoning

Place the squash and chicken stock in the insert of the slow cooker. The squash should not touch the sides of the insert. Cook on low for 6 hours. Let the squash cool for 10 minutes and cut in half. Scrape out the squash strands into a bowl with a fork. When finished, add the butter and toss to combine. Season with salt and pepper and serve.

Per Serving: Calories: 98; Fat: 7g; Protein: 1g; Total Carbs: 6g; Fiber: 3g; Net Carbs: 3g; **Macros:** Fat: 69%; Protein: 26%; Carbs: 5%

Chipotle Chicken Chili

SERVES 6 | PREP TIME: 20 minutes | COOK TIME: 7 to 8 hours on low

3 tablespoons extra-virgin olive oil, divided
1 pound ground chicken
½ sweet onion, chopped
2 teaspoons minced garlic
1 (28-ounce) can diced tomatoes
1 cup chicken broth
1 cup diced pumpkin
1 green bell pepper, diced
3 tablespoons chili powder
1 teaspoon chipotle chili powder
1 cup sour cream, for garnish
1 cup shredded Cheddar cheese, for garnish

Lightly grease the insert of the slow cooker with 1 tablespoon of the olive oil. In a large skillet over medium-high heat, heat the remaining 2 tablespoons of the olive oil. Add the chicken and sauté until it is cooked through, about 6 minutes. Add the onion and garlic and sauté for an additional 3 minutes. Transfer the chicken mixture to the insert and stir in the tomatoes, broth, pumpkin, bell pepper, chili powder, and chipotle chili powder. Cover and cook on low for 7 to 8 hours. Serve topped with the sour cream and cheese.

Per serving: Calories: 390; Fat: 30g; Protein: 22g; Total Carbs: 14g; Fiber: 5g; Net Carbs: 9g; **Macros:** Fat: 65%; Protein: 21%; Carbs: 14%

Slow Keto Chili

SERVES 2 (2 CUPS PER SERVING) | PREP TIME: 10 minutes | COOK TIME: 2 hours

1 tablespoon avocado oil
¼ medium white onion, diced
¼ green bell pepper, diced
2 garlic cloves, minced
12 ounces ground beef
1 (12-ounce) can tomato sauce
1 tablespoon coconut aminos
2 cups beef broth
½ teaspoon ground cumin
½ teaspoon garlic powder
¼ teaspoon chili powder
¼ teaspoon paprika
¼ teaspoon dried oregano
¼ teaspoon cayenne pepper
¼ teaspoon freshly ground black pepper
¼ teaspoon pink Himalayan salt

In a large skillet, heat the oil over medium heat. Add the onion, bell pepper, and garlic, and sauté for 5 to 7 minutes, until soft. Add the ground beef and cook until it is browned and no longer pink. Transfer the mixture to a slow cooker. Add the tomato sauce, coconut aminos, broth, cumin, garlic powder, chili powder, paprika, oregano, cayenne, black pepper, and salt. Stir to combine everything. Cook on high for 2 hours, stirring occasionally.

Per Serving: Calories: 663; Fat: 51g; Protein: 35g; Total Carbs: 16g; Fiber: 4g; Net Carbs: 12g; **Macros:** Fat: 69%; Protein: 21%; Carbs: 10%

Vegetarian Mole Chili

SERVES 8 | PREP: 15 minutes | COOK: 8 hours on low or 4 hours on high

¼ cup coconut oil
1 pound firm tofu, diced
1 (15-ounce) can diced tomatoes, with juice
1 onion, diced
3 garlic cloves, minced
1 or 2 jalapeño peppers, seeded and minced
3 tablespoons unsweetened cocoa powder
2 tablespoons chili powder
1½ teaspoons paprika

1½ teaspoons ground cumin
1 teaspoon ground cinnamon
1 teaspoon kosher salt
½ teaspoon dried oregano
2½ cups sour cream, divided

2 cups shredded Cheddar cheese
1 avocado, peeled, pitted, and sliced

In the slow cooker, combine the coconut oil, tofu, tomatoes and their juice, onion, garlic, jalapeños, cocoa powder, chili powder, paprika, cumin, cinnamon, salt, and oregano. Cover and cook for 8 hours on low or 4 hours on high. Just before serving, stir in 1½ cups of sour cream. Serve hot, garnished with the remaining 1 cup of sour cream, Cheddar cheese, and avocado.

Per Serving: Calories: 392; Fat: 34g; Protein: 15g; Total Carbs: 9g; Fiber: 2g; Net Carbs: 7g; **Macros:** Fat: 78%; Protein: 15%; Carbs: 7%

Cheese-Stuffed Peppers

SERVES 6 | PREP: 15 minutes | COOK: 7 hours on low

3 large bell peppers (any color), halved lengthwise, seeded, and ribbed
1 cup riced cauliflower
1 cup diced tomatoes
1 onion, diced
2 garlic cloves, minced
¼ cup (½ stick) unsalted butter or ghee melted

8 ounces cream cheese, cut into small pieces
2 cups shredded Cheddar cheese, divided
2 large eggs, lightly beaten
1 teaspoon kosher salt
½ teaspoon freshly ground black pepper
1 cup vegetable broth

Place the pepper halves in the slow cooker with the open sides up. In a large bowl, mix the cauliflower, tomatoes, onion, garlic, butter, cream cheese, 1½ cups of Cheddar cheese, eggs, salt, and pepper. Spoon the cheese mixture into the peppers, dividing equally. Sprinkle the remaining ½ cup of Cheddar cheese over the top. Pour the vegetable broth around the peppers. Cover and cook for 7 hours on low. Serve hot.

Per Serving: Calories: 404; Fat: 34g; Protein: 16g; Total Carbs: 10g; Fiber: 2g; Net Carbs: 8g; **Macros:** Fat: 74%; Protein: 17%; Carbs: 9%

Deep-Dish Cauliflower Crust Pizza with Olives

SERVES 4 | PREP: 15 minutes | COOK: 6 hours on low or 3 hours on high

3 cups riced cauliflower
3 cups shredded Fontina cheese, divided
1 cup grated Parmesan cheese, divided
1 large egg, lightly beaten
1 teaspoon dried Italian seasoning

¼ teaspoon kosher salt
Coconut oil, for coating the slow cooker insert
1 cup tomato sauce
4 ounces mascarpone cheese
1 cup Kalamata olives, pitted and halved
½ teaspoon dried rosemary

In a large bowl, stir the cauliflower, 1 cup of Fontina cheese, ½ cup of Parmesan cheese, egg, Italian seasoning, and salt. Mix well. Coat the inside of the slow cooker insert with coconut oil and then press the cauliflower mixture into it in an even layer that is just slightly higher around the edges. In a medium bowl, stir the tomato sauce and mascarpone. Pour the mixture over the crust, spreading it into an even layer. Top with the remaining 2 cups of Fontina cheese and ½ cup of Parmesan cheese. Sprinkle the olives and rosemary over the top. Put the lid on the slow cooker, but prop it slightly open with a chopstick or wooden spoon. Cook for 6 hours on low or 3 hours on high. When finished, let the pizza sit in the slow cooker for 10 or 15 minutes more before serving. Serve warm.

Per Serving: Calories: 423; Fat: 33g; Protein: 25g; Total Carbs: 8g; Fiber: 2g; Net Carbs: 6g; **Macros:** Fat: 70%; Protein: 25%; Carbs: 5%

Vegan Pumpkin Curry

SERVES 4 | PREP: 15 minutes | COOK: 6 hours on low

2 tablespoons coconut oil, melted
1½ pounds extra-firm tofu, cut into 1-inch cubes
12 ounces cremini or button mushrooms, halved or quartered
½ cup diced onion
2 garlic cloves, minced
1 tablespoon grated fresh ginger

3 tablespoons curry powder
1 teaspoon ground cumin
1 teaspoon kosher salt
½ teaspoon cayenne pepper
1 (14-ounce) can coconut milk
¼ cup chopped macadamia nuts
¼ cup chopped fresh cilantro

Coat the inside of the slow cooker insert with the coconut oil. Add the tofu, mushrooms, onion, garlic, ginger, curry powder, cumin, salt, cayenne, and coconut milk. Cover and cook for 6 hours on low. Serve hot, garnished with the macadamia nuts and cilantro.

Per Serving: Calories: 350; Fat: 29g; Protein: 16g; Total Carbs: 11g; Fiber: 1g; Net Carbs: 10g; **Macros:** Fat: 70%; Protein: 20%; Carbs: 10%

Thai Green Curry with Tofu & Vegetables

SERVES 4 | PREP: 15 minutes | COOK: 7 hours on low

2 tablespoons coconut oil
½ onion, diced
1 tablespoon minced fresh ginger
2 garlic cloves, minced
1 pound firm tofu, diced
½ green bell pepper, seeded and sliced

1 (14-ounce) can coconut milk
¼ cup Thai green curry paste
1 tablespoon erythritol
1 teaspoon kosher salt
½ teaspoon turmeric
¼ cup chopped fresh cilantro, for garnish

In a medium skillet, heat the coconut oil over medium-high heat. Add the onion and sauté until softened, about 5 minutes. Stir in the ginger and garlic and then transfer the mixture to the slow cooker. Mix in the tofu, green bell pepper, coconut milk, curry paste, erythritol, salt, and turmeric. Cover and cook for 7 hours on low. Serve hot, garnished with the cilantro.

Per Serving: Calories: 380; Fat: 31g; Protein: 15g; Total Carbs: 15g; Fiber: 6g; Net Carbs: 9g; **Macros:** Fat: 70%; Protein: 15%; Carbs: 15%

Slow Cooker Eggplant Parmesan

SERVES 6 | PREP: 10 minutes | COOK: 8 hours on low or 4 hours on high

2 tablespoons coconut oil
2 cups tomato sauce
8 ounces mascarpone cheese

8 ounces eggplant, peeled and thinly sliced
3 cups shredded Fontina cheese

1 cup grated Parmesan cheese   1 cup coarsely ground
                                 almond meal

Coat the inside of the slow cooker insert with the coconut oil. In a medium bowl, stir the tomato sauce and mascarpone. Coat the bottom of the insert with ½ cup of sauce. Arrange several eggplant slices in a single layer, or slightly overlapping, over the sauce. Top with a bit of Fontina cheese, a bit of Parmesan cheese, a sprinkling of almond meal, and more sauce. Continue layering until you've used all the ingredients, ending with a layer of sauce, then cheese, and then almond meal. Cover and cook for 8 hours on low or 4 hours on high. Serve hot.

Per Serving: Calories: 536; Fat: 43g; Protein: 29g; Total Carbs: 13g; Fiber: 5g; Net Carbs: 8g; **Macros:** Fat: 70%; Protein: 9%; Carbs: 21%

Enchilada Casserole

SERVES 6 | PREP: 15 minutes | COOK: 6 hours on low or 3 hours on high

1 tablespoon coconut oil   1 teaspoon kosher salt
4 large eggs   2 (7-ounce) cans whole
2 cups sour cream   roasted green chiles,
12 ounces cream cheese, at   drained and seeded
  room temperature   1 pound frozen spin-
1½ cups grated Cheddar   ach, thawed
  cheese, divided   3 cups enchilada sauce
1 cup heavy (whipping) cream   ¼ cup chopped fresh cilantro
1 teaspoon dried oregano   4 scallions, sliced

Coat the inside of the slow cooker insert with the coconut oil. In a large bowl, beat the eggs, then whisk in the sour cream, cream cheese, 1 cup of Cheddar cheese, heavy cream, oregano, and salt. Lay several strips of green chiles in a single layer on the bottom of the slow cooker to cover it. Dollop one-third of the cheese mixture on top, distributing it evenly. Spread it out with the back of the spoon. Top with one-third of the spinach, and then 1 cup of enchilada sauce. Repeat twice more with the remaining ingredients. Sprinkle the remaining ½ cup of Cheddar cheese over the top layer. Cover and cook for 6 hours on low or 3 hours on high. Serve hot, garnished with the cilantro and scallions.

Per Serving: Calories: 865; Fat: 77g; Protein: 36g; Total Carbs: 12g; Fiber: 2g; Net Carbs: 10g; **Macros:** Fat: 79%; Protein: 16%; Carbs: 5%

Mushroom No-Meatballs in Tomato Sauce

SERVES 4 | PREP: 15 minutes | COOK: 6 hours on low or 3 hours on high

2 tablespoons coconut oil,   10 ounces mushrooms,
  plus more for coating the   roughly chopped
  slow cooker insert   2 tablespoons almond flour
½ onion, diced   1½ teaspoons dried basil
1 garlic clove, minced   1 teaspoon dried oregano
1½ cups raw walnuts   ¾ teaspoon kosher salt
                                 1½ cups tomato sauce

Coat the inside of the slow cooker insert with coconut oil. In a large skillet, heat 2 tablespoons of coconut oil over medium-high heat. Add the onion and garlic and sauté until softened, about 5 minutes. Meanwhile, in a food processor, combine the walnuts, mushrooms, almond flour, basil, oregano, and salt. Pulse

until everything is minced and well combined. Add the cooked onion and garlic and pulse again until combined. Form the nut mixture into 1½-inch balls and place them in the slow cooker. Pour the tomato sauce over the top. Cover and cook for 6 hours on low or 3 hours on high. Serve hot.

Per Serving: Calories: 367; Fat: 34g; Protein: 13g; Total Carbs: 14g; Fiber: 5g; Net Carbs: 9g; **Macros:** Fat: 74%; Protein: 13%; Carbs: 13%

Squash Boats Filled with Spinach-Artichoke Gratin

SERVES 4 | PREP: 10 minutes | COOK: 6 hours on low or 3 hours on high

1 tablespoon coconut oil   ½ cup chopped arti-
1½ cups grated Parmesan   choke hearts
  cheese, divided   2 small delicata squashes,
½ cup sour cream   halved lengthwise
¼ cup mayonnaise   and seeded
½ onion, diced   1 cup shredded Fon-
3 garlic cloves, minced   tina cheese
Kosher salt   1 tablespoon chopped fresh
Freshly ground black pepper   flat-leaf parsley
1 cup chopped baby spinach

Coat the inside of the slow cooker insert with the coconut oil. In a medium bowl, stir ¾ cup of Parmesan cheese, sour cream, mayonnaise, onion, and garlic until well combined. Season with salt and pepper. Add the spinach and artichoke hearts and stir gently to mix. Spoon the mixture into the squash halves, dividing evenly. Place the filled halves in the slow cooker in a single layer. Sprinkle the Fontina cheese and remaining ¾ cup of Parmesan over the top. Cover and cook for 6 hours on low or 3 hours on high. Serve hot, garnished with the parsley.

Per Serving: Calories: 416; Fat: 32g; Protein: 21g; Total Carbs: 13g; Fiber: 2g; Net Carbs: 11g; **Macros:** Fat: 70%; Protein: 19%; Carbs: 11%

White Chicken Chili

SERVES 6 | PREP TIME: 5 minutes | COOK TIME: 3 hours 30 minutes

2 pounds boneless, skinless   1 tablespoon cumin
  chicken breasts   1 teaspoon minced garlic
1 (4-ounce) can chopped   4½ cups chicken broth or
  green chiles   bone broth
½ small onion, chopped   12 ounces (1½ bricks)
2 jalapeño peppers, minced,   cream cheese
  with or without seeds   ⅔ cup heavy (whipping) cream
  depending on taste   1 teaspoon xanthan gum

In a slow cooker, combine the chicken, green chiles, onion, jalapeños, cumin, garlic, and broth. Cook on high for 3 hours. Using two forks, shred the chicken inside the slow cooker. Melt the cream cheese in the microwave. Add it to the slow cooker along with the heavy cream, and stir. Add the xanthan gum, and stir until well incorporated. Cover, cook for another 30 minutes on high, and serve.

Per Serving: (2 cups): Calories: 506; Fat: 33g; Protein: 45g; Total Carbs: 6.5g; Fiber: 0.5g; Net Carbs: 6g; **Macros:** Fat: 59%; Protein: 36%; Carbs: 5%

Coconut Chicken Curry

SERVES 6 | PREP TIME: 15 minutes | COOK TIME: 7 to 8 hours on low

3 tablespoons extra-virgin olive oil, divided
1½ pounds boneless chicken breasts
½ sweet onion, chopped
1 cup quartered baby bok choy
1 red bell pepper, diced
2 cups coconut milk
2 tablespoons almond butter

1 tablespoon red Thai curry paste
1 tablespoon coconut aminos
2 teaspoons grated fresh ginger
Pinch red pepper flakes
¼ cup chopped peanuts, for garnish
2 tablespoons chopped cilantro, for garnish

Lightly grease the insert of the slow cooker with 1 tablespoon of the olive oil. In a large skillet over medium-high heat, heat the remaining 2 tablespoons of the olive oil. Add the chicken and brown for about 7 minutes. Transfer the chicken to the slow cooker and add the onion, baby bok choy, and bell pepper. In a medium bowl, whisk the coconut milk, almond butter, curry paste, coconut aminos, ginger, and red pepper flakes, until well blended. Pour the sauce over the chicken and vegetables, and mix to coat. Cover and cook on low for 7 to 8 hours. Serve topped with the peanuts and cilantro.

Per Serving: Calories: 543; Fat: 42g; Protein: 35g; Total Carbs: 10g; Fiber: 5g; Net Carbs: 5g; **Macros**: Fat: 68%; Protein: 25%; Carbs: 7%

Mandarin Orange Chicken

SERVES 6 | PREP: 10 minutes | COOK: 6 hours on low

1½ pounds bone-in, skin-on chicken thighs
1 tablespoon Chinese five-spice powder
½ teaspoon kosher salt
6 bacon slices, diced
1 large orange, sliced
1 small red chile pepper, very thinly sliced, or ½ teaspoon red pepper flakes
1 garlic clove, minced
1 tablespoon minced fresh ginger

¼ cup Asian sesame paste
2 tablespoons soy sauce or tamari
1 tablespoon freshly squeezed lime juice
1 tablespoon toasted sesame oil
1 tablespoon erythritol
¼ cup (½ stick) unsalted butter, cubed
½ cup chopped macadamia nuts

Season the chicken thighs all over with the five-spice powder and salt. Set aside. In a large skillet, cook the bacon over medium-high heat until crisp and browned, about 5 minutes. Transfer the bacon to the slow cooker. To the slow cooker, add the orange slices, red chile pepper, garlic, ginger, sesame paste, soy sauce, lime juice, sesame oil, and erythritol. Stir to mix. Return the skillet to medium-high heat and add the seasoned chicken, skin-side down. Cook until browned, about 3 minutes per side. Arrange the browned chicken in the slow cooker, skin-side up. Top with the butter pieces. Cover and cook for 6 hours on low. Serve hot, garnished with the macadamia nuts.

Per Serving: Calories: 641; Fat: 56g; Protein: 27g; Total Carbs: 10g; Fiber: 3g; Net Carbs: 7g; **Macros**: Fat: 76%; Protein: 18%; Carbs: 6%

Garlicky Braised Chicken Thighs

SERVES 4 | PREP TIME: 15 minutes | COOK TIME: 7 to 8 hours on low

¼ cup extra-virgin olive oil, divided
1½ pounds boneless chicken thighs
1 teaspoon paprika
Salt
Freshly ground black pepper

1 sweet onion, chopped
4 garlic cloves, thinly sliced
½ cup chicken broth
2 tablespoons freshly squeezed lemon juice
½ cup Greek yogurt

Lightly grease the insert of the slow cooker with 1 tablespoon of the olive oil. Season the thighs with the paprika and salt and pepper to taste. In a large skillet over medium-high heat, heat the remaining olive oil. Add the chicken and brown for 5 minutes, turning once. Transfer the chicken to the insert and add the onion, garlic, broth, and lemon juice. Cover and cook on low for 7 to 8 hours. Stir in the yogurt and serve.

Per Serving: Calories: 434; Fat: 36g; Protein: 22g; Total Carbs: 5g; Fiber: 1g; Net Carbs: 4g; **Macros**: Fat: 75%; Protein: 20%; Carbs: 5%

Chicken Mole

SERVES 6 | PREP TIME: 15 minutes | COOK TIME: 7 to 8 hours on low

3 tablespoons extra-virgin olive oil or ghee, divided
2 pounds boneless chicken thighs and breasts
Salt
Freshly ground black pepper
1 sweet onion, chopped
1 tablespoon minced garlic
1 (28-ounce) can diced tomatoes

4 dried chile peppers, soaked in water for 2 hours and chopped
3 ounces dark chocolate, chopped
¼ cup natural peanut butter
1½ teaspoons ground cumin
¾ teaspoon ground cinnamon
½ teaspoon chili powder
½ cup coconut cream
2 tablespoons chopped cilantro, for garnish

Lightly grease the insert of the slow cooker with 1 tablespoon of the olive oil. In a large skillet over medium-high heat, heat the remaining 2 tablespoons of the olive oil. Lightly season the chicken with salt and pepper, add to the skillet, and brown for about 5 minutes, turning once. Add the onion and garlic and sauté for an additional 3 minutes. Transfer the chicken, onion, and garlic to the slow cooker, and stir in the tomatoes, chiles, chocolate, peanut butter, cumin, cinnamon, and chili powder. Cover and cook on low for 7 to 8 hours. Stir in the coconut cream, and serve hot, topped with the cilantro.

Per Serving: Calories: 386; Fat: 30g; Protein: 19g; Total Carbs: 11g; Fiber: 5g; Net Carbs: 6g; **Macros**: Fat: 69%; Protein: 19%; Carbs: 12%

Chicken Cacciatore

SERVES 6 | PREP TIME: 15 minutes | COOK TIME: 8 hours on low

3 tablespoons extra-virgin olive oil, divided
2 pounds boneless chicken thighs

Salt
Freshly ground black pepper
1 (14-ounce) can stewed tomatoes

2 cups chicken broth	1 tablespoon minced garlic
1 cup quartered button mushrooms	1 tablespoon dried oregano
	1 teaspoon dried basil
½ sweet onion, chopped	Pinch red pepper flakes

Lightly grease the insert of the slow cooker with 1 tablespoon of the olive oil. Lightly season the chicken thighs with salt and pepper. In a large skillet over medium-high heat, heat the remaining 2 tablespoons of the olive oil. Add the chicken thighs and brown for about 8 minutes, turning once. Transfer the chicken to the insert and add the tomatoes, broth, mushrooms, onion, garlic, oregano, basil, and red pepper flakes. Cover and cook on low for 8 hours. Serve warm.

Per Serving: Calories: 425; Fat: 32g; Protein: 27g; Total Carbs: 8g; Fiber: 1g; Net Carbs: 7g; **Macros:** Fat: 67%; Protein: 25%; Carbs: 8%

Creamy Lemon Chicken

SERVES 6 | PREP TIME: 10 minutes | COOK TIME: 7 to 8 hours on low

3 tablespoons extra-virgin olive oil	½ teaspoon salt
	⅛ teaspoon pepper, depending on taste
2 tablespoons butter	
1½ pounds boneless chicken thighs	1½ cups chicken broth
	Juice and zest of 1 lemon
½ sweet onion, diced	1 tablespoon Dijon mustard
2 teaspoons minced garlic	1 cup heavy (whipping) cream
2 teaspoons dried oregano	

Lightly grease the insert of the slow cooker with 1 tablespoon of the olive oil. In a large skillet over medium-high heat, heat the remaining 2 tablespoons of the olive oil and the butter. Add the chicken and brown for 5 minutes, turning once. Transfer the chicken to the insert and add the onion, garlic, oregano, salt, and pepper. In a small bowl, whisk the broth, lemon juice and zest, and mustard. Pour the mixture over the chicken. Cover and cook on low for 7 to 8 hours. Remove from the heat, stir in the heavy cream, and serve.

Per Serving: Calories: 400; Fat: 34g; Protein: 22g; Total Carbs: 2g; Fiber: 0g; Net Carbs: 2g; **Macros:** Fat: 76%; Protein: 22%; Carbs: 2%

Hungarian Chicken

SERVES 4 | PREP TIME: 10 minutes | COOK TIME: 7 to 8 hours on low

1 tablespoon extra-virgin olive oil	2 teaspoons minced garlic
	2 teaspoons paprika
2 pounds boneless chicken thighs	¼ teaspoon salt
	1 cup sour cream
½ cup chicken broth	1 tablespoon chopped parsley, for garnish
Juice and zest of 1 lemon	

Lightly grease the insert of the slow cooker with the olive oil. Place the chicken thighs in the insert. In a small bowl, stir the broth, lemon juice and zest, garlic, paprika, and salt. Pour the broth mixture over the chicken. Cover and cook on low for 7 to 8 hours. Turn off the heat and stir in the sour cream. Serve topped with the parsley.

Per Serving: Calories: 404; Fat: 32g; Protein: 23g; Total Carbs: 4g; Fiber: 0g; Net Carbs: 4g; **Macros:** Fat: 73%; Protein: 23%; Carbs: 4%

Bacon-Mushroom Chicken

SERVES 8 | PREP TIME: 15 minutes | COOK TIME: 7 to 8 hours on low

3 tablespoons coconut oil, divided	1 sweet onion, diced
	1 tablespoon minced garlic
¼ pound bacon, diced	½ cup chicken broth
2 pounds boneless chicken (breasts, thighs, drumsticks)	2 teaspoons chopped thyme
	1 cup coconut cream
2 cups quartered button mushrooms	

Lightly grease the insert of the slow cooker with 1 tablespoon of the coconut oil. In a large skillet over medium-high heat, heat the remaining 2 tablespoons of the coconut oil. Add the bacon and cook until it is crispy, about 5 minutes. Using a slotted spoon, transfer the bacon to a plate and set aside. Add the chicken to the skillet and brown for 5 minutes, turning once. Transfer the chicken and bacon to the insert and add the mushrooms, onion, garlic, broth, and thyme. Cover and cook on low for 7 to 8 hours. Stir in the coconut cream and serve.

Per Serving: Calories: 406; Fat: 34g; Protein: 22g; Total Carbs: 5g; Fiber: 2g; Net Carbs: 3g; **Macros:** Fat: 74%; Protein: 21%; Carbs: 5%

Roasted Chicken Dinner

SERVES 8 | PREP TIME: 15 minutes | COOK TIME: 7 to 8 hours on low

¼ cup extra-virgin olive oil, divided	1 lemon, quartered
	6 thyme sprigs
1 (3-pound) chicken	4 garlic cloves, crushed
Salt	3 bay leaves
Freshly ground black pepper	1 sweet onion, quartered

Lightly grease the insert of the slow cooker with 1 tablespoon of the olive oil. Rub the remaining olive oil all over the chicken and season with salt and pepper. Stuff the lemon quarters, thyme, garlic, and bay leaves into the cavity of the chicken. Place the onion quarters on the bottom of the slow cooker and place the chicken on top so it does not touch the bottom of the insert. Cover and cook on low for 7 to 8 hours, or until the internal temperature reaches 165°F on an instant-read thermometer. Serve warm.

Per Serving: Calories: 427; Fat: 34g; Protein: 29g; Total Carbs: 2g; Fiber: 0g; Net Carbs: 2g; **Macros:** Fat: 71%; Protein: 27%; Carbs: 2%

Herb-Infused Turkey Breast

SERVES 6 | PREP TIME: 25 minutes | COOK TIME: 7 to 8 hours on low

3 tablespoons extra-virgin olive oil, divided	2 teaspoons dried thyme
	1 teaspoon dried oregano
1½ pounds boneless turkey breasts	1 avocado, peeled, pitted, and chopped
Salt	1 tomato, diced
Freshly ground black pepper	½ jalapeño pepper, diced
1 cup coconut milk	1 tablespoon chopped cilantro
2 teaspoons minced garlic	

Lightly grease the insert of the slow cooker with 1 tablespoon of the olive oil. In a large skillet over medium-high heat, heat the remaining 2 tablespoons of the olive oil. Lightly season the turkey with salt and pepper. Add the turkey to the skillet and brown for about 7 minutes, turning once. Transfer the turkey to the insert and add the coconut milk, garlic, thyme, and oregano. Cover and cook on low for 7 to 8 hours. In a small bowl, stir the avocado, tomato, jalapeño pepper, and cilantro. Serve the turkey topped with the avocado salsa.

Per Serving: Calories: 347; Fat: 27g; Protein: 25g; Total Carbs: 5g; Fiber: 3g; Net Carbs: 2g; **Macros:** Fat: 67%; Protein: 28%; Carbs: 5%

Turkey-Pumpkin Ragout

SERVES 6 | PREP TIME: 15 minutes | COOK TIME: 8 hours on low

1 tablespoon extra-virgin olive oil	1½ cups chicken broth
1 pound boneless turkey thighs, cut into 1½-inch chunks	1½ cups coconut milk
	2 teaspoons chopped fresh thyme
3 cups cubed pumpkin, cut into 1-inch chunks	½ cup coconut cream
1 red bell pepper, diced	Salt, for seasoning
½ sweet onion, cut in half and sliced	Freshly ground black pepper, for seasoning
1 tablespoon minced garlic	12 slices cooked bacon, chopped, for garnish

Lightly grease the insert of the slow cooker with the olive oil. Add the turkey, pumpkin, red bell pepper, onion, garlic, broth, coconut milk, and thyme. Cover and cook on low for 8 hours. Stir in the coconut cream and season with salt and pepper. Serve topped with the bacon.

Per Serving: Calories: 418; Fat: 34g; Protein: 25g; Total Carbs: 6g; Fiber: 1g; Net Carbs: 5g; **Macros:** Fat: 71%; Protein: 23%; Carbs: 6%

Thyme Turkey Legs

SERVES 6 | PREP TIME: 15 minutes | COOK TIME: 7 to 8 hours on low

3 tablespoons extra-virgin olive oil, divided	2 teaspoons poultry seasoning
2 pounds boneless turkey legs	½ cup chicken broth
Salt	2 tablespoons chopped fresh parsley, for garnish
Freshly ground black pepper	
1 tablespoon dried thyme	

Lightly grease the insert of the slow cooker with 1 tablespoon of the olive oil. In a large skillet over medium-high heat, heat the remaining 2 tablespoons of the olive oil. Generously season the turkey with salt and pepper. Sprinkle with thyme and poultry seasoning. Add the turkey to the skillet and brown for about 7 minutes, turning once. Transfer the turkey to the slow cooker and add the broth. Cover and cook on low for 7 to 8 hours. Serve topped with the parsley.

Per Serving: Calories: 363; Fat: 29g; Protein: 28g; Total Carbs: 1g; Fiber: 0g; Net Carbs: 1g; **Macros:** Fat: 69%; Protein: 30%; Carbs: 1%

Easy "Roasted" Duck

SERVES 8 | PREP TIME: 15 minutes | COOK TIME: 7 to 8 hours on low

3 tablespoons extra-virgin olive oil, divided	4 garlic cloves, crushed
1 (2½-pound) whole duck, giblets removed	6 thyme sprigs, chopped
	1 cinnamon stick, broken into several pieces
Salt, for seasoning	1 sweet onion, coarsely chopped
Freshly ground black pepper, for seasoning	¼ cup chicken broth

Lightly grease the insert of the slow cooker with 1 tablespoon of the olive oil. Rub the remaining 2 tablespoons of the olive oil all over the duck and season with salt and pepper. Stuff the garlic, thyme, and cinnamon into the cavity of the duck. Place the onion on the bottom of the slow cooker and place the duck on top so it does not touch the bottom of the insert, and pour in the broth. Cover and cook on low for 7 to 8 hours, or until the internal temperature reaches 180°F on an instant-read thermometer. Serve warm.

Per Serving: Calories: 364; Fat: 28g; Protein: 29g; Total Carbs: 2g; Fiber: 1g; Net Carbs: 1g; **Macros:** Fat: 67%; Protein: 31%; Carbs: 2%

Duck Legs Braised in Olive Oil with Chive Cream

SERVES 4 TO 6 | PREP: 10 minutes, plus overnight to brine | COOK: 6 hours on low

For the sauce

1½ cups sour cream	¾ teaspoon kosher salt
3 tablespoons heavy (whipping) cream	¼ teaspoon freshly ground black pepper
¼ cup chopped fresh chives, plus additional for garnish	

For the duck

2 tablespoons kosher salt	1 teaspoon freshly ground black pepper
4 garlic cloves, minced	
4 duck legs	4 to 5 cups extra-virgin olive oil or melted coconut oil

Mash the salt and garlic to make a paste. Rub the paste all over the duck legs. Arrange the duck in a single layer in a baking dish and season with the pepper. Cover the pan loosely with aluminum foil and refrigerate overnight. Rinse the duck legs and pat them very dry with paper towels. Arrange the duck, skin-side up, in the slow cooker. Pour the olive oil over the duck to cover it completely. Cover and cook for 6 hours on low. When finished, remove the duck from the oil. Remove and discard the skin, pull the meat from the bones, and shred the meat. In a small bowl, stir all the ingredients until well combined. Refrigerate until ready to use. Serve the meat topped with the cream sauce and garnish with additional chives.

Per Serving: Calories: 710; Fat: 59g; Protein: 39g; Total Carbs: 9g; Fiber: 2g; Net Carbs: 7g; **Macros:** Fat: 75%; Protein: 22%; Carbs: 3%

Duck with Turnips in Cream

SERVES 8 | PREP: 15 minutes | COOK: 7 hours on low

2 turnips, peeled and diced	2 tablespoons unsalted butter or ghee, melted
2 celery stalks, diced	

1 (3- to 4-pound) duck, giblets removed, rinsed and patted dry
1 teaspoon kosher salt
Freshly ground black pepper
2 tablespoons coconut oil
1 lemon, quartered
1 small onion, quartered
2 fresh rosemary sprigs
4 or 5 fresh thyme sprigs
¾ cup heavy (whipping) cream

In the slow cooker, toss the turnips and celery with the butter. Generously season the duck with salt and pepper. In a large skillet, heat the coconut oil over medium-high heat. Add the duck, breast-side down, and cook until browned, about 5 minutes per side. Pierce the skin in several places with a small sharp knife or the tines of a fork. Insert the lemon quarters, onion quarters, rosemary, and thyme into the duck cavity and place the duck, breast-side up, in the slow cooker on top of the vegetables. Cover and cook for 7 hours on low. Remove the duck from the slow cooker and let it rest for about 10 minutes before carving. While the duck is resting, stir the heavy cream into the juices and vegetables in the slow cooker. Serve the duck over the vegetables and sauce.

Per Serving: Calories: 831; Fat: 83g; Protein: 20g; Total Carbs: 3g; Fiber: 0g; Net Carbs: 3g; **Macros:** Fat: 90%; Protein: 9%; Carbs: 1%

Classic Sauerbraten

SERVES 6 | PREP TIME: 15 minutes | COOK TIME: 9 to 10 hours on low

3 tablespoons extra-virgin olive oil, divided
2 pounds beef brisket
Salt, for seasoning
Freshly ground black pepper, for seasoning
1 sweet onion, cut into eighths
1 carrot, cut into chunks
2 celery stalks, cut into chunks
¾ cup beef broth
½ cup German-style mustard
¼ cup apple cider vinegar
½ teaspoon ground cloves
2 bay leaves

Lightly grease the insert of the slow cooker with 1 tablespoon of the olive oil. In a large skillet over medium-high heat, heat the remaining 2 tablespoons of the olive oil. Season the beef with salt and pepper. Add the beef to the skillet and brown on all sides for 6 minutes. Place the onion, carrot, and celery in the bottom of the insert and the beef on top of the vegetables. In a small bowl, whisk the broth, mustard, apple cider vinegar, and cloves, and add to the beef along with the bay leaves Cover and cook on low for 9 to 10 hours. Remove the bay leaves before serving.

Per serving: Calories: 507; Fat: 42g; Protein: 29g; Total Carbs: 3g; Fiber: 1g; Net Carbs: 2g; **Macros:** Fat: 75%; Protein: 23%; Carbs: 2%

Pesto Roast Beef

SERVES 8 | PREP TIME: 5 minutes | COOK TIME: 9 to 10 hours on low

1 tablespoon extra-virgin olive oil
2 pounds beef chuck roast
¾ cup prepared pesto
½ cup beef broth

Lightly grease the insert of the slow cooker with the olive oil. Slather the pesto all over the beef. Place the beef in the insert and pour in the broth. Cover and cook on low for 9 to 10 hours. Serve warm.

Per serving: Calories: 530; Fat: 43g; Protein: 32g; Total Carbs: 2g; Fiber: 0g; Net Carbs: 2g; **Macros:** Fat: 73%; Protein: 25%; Carbs: 2%

Salisbury Steak

SERVES 6 | PREP TIME: 20 minutes | COOK TIME: 6 hours on low

3 tablespoons extra-virgin olive oil, divided
1½ pounds ground beef
½ cup almond flour
¼ cup heavy (whipping) cream
1 scallion, white and green parts, chopped
1 large egg
1 teaspoon minced garlic
2 cups sliced mushrooms
½ sweet onion, chopped
1½ cups beef broth
1 tablespoon Dijon mustard
¾ cup heavy (whipping) cream
Salt, for seasoning
Freshly ground black pepper, for seasoning
2 tablespoons chopped fresh parsley, for garnish

Lightly grease the insert of the slow cooker with 1 tablespoon of the olive oil. In a medium bowl, mix the beef, almond flour, heavy cream, scallion, egg, and garlic. Form into 6 patties about 1 inch thick. In a large skillet over medium-high heat, heat the remaining 2 tablespoons of the olive oil. Pan sear the patties on both sides, about 5 minutes, and transfer the patties to the insert. In the skillet, sauté the mushrooms and onion for 3 minutes. Whisk in the broth and mustard and transfer the sauce to the insert. Cover and cook on low for 6 hours. Remove the patties to a plate and whisk the cream into the sauce. Season the sauce with salt and pepper. Serve the patties topped with the sauce and garnished with the parsley.

Per serving: Calories: 500; Fat: 39g; Protein: 33g; Total Carbs: 5g; Fiber: 2g; Net Carbs: 3g; **Macros:** Fat: 70%; Protein: 26%; Carbs: 4%

Tomato-Braised Beef

SERVES 4 | PREP TIME: 15 minutes | COOK TIME: 7 to 8 hours on low

3 tablespoons extra-virgin olive oil, divided
1 pound beef chuck roast, cut into 1-inch cubes
Salt, for seasoning
Freshly ground black pepper, for seasoning
1 (15-ounce) can diced tomatoes
2 tablespoons tomato paste
2 teaspoons minced garlic
2 teaspoons dried basil
1 teaspoon dried oregano
½ teaspoon whole black peppercorns
1 cup shredded mozzarella cheese, for garnish
2 tablespoons chopped parsley, for garnish

Lightly grease the insert of the slow cooker with 1 tablespoon of the olive oil. In a large skillet over medium-high heat, heat the remaining 2 tablespoons of the olive oil. Season the beef with salt and pepper. Add the beef to the skillet and brown for 7 minutes. Transfer the beef to the insert. In a medium bowl, stir the tomatoes, tomato paste, garlic, basil, oregano, and peppercorns, and add the tomato mixture to the beef in the insert. Cover and cook on low for 7 to 8 hours. Serve topped with the cheese and parsley.

Per serving: Calories: 539; Fat: 43g; Protein: 30g; Total Carbs: 7g; Fiber: 2g; Net Carbs: 5g; **Macros:** Fat: 72%; Protein: 22%; Carbs: 6%

Beef and Bell Peppers

SERVES 6 | PREP TIME: 15 minutes | COOK TIME: 9 to 10 hours on low

3 tablespoons extra-virgin olive oil, divided

1 pound beef tenderloin, cut into 1-inch chunks

½ sweet onion, chopped

2 teaspoons minced garlic

1 red bell pepper, diced

1 yellow bell pepper, diced

2 cups coconut cream

1 cup beef broth

3 tablespoons coconut aminos

1 tablespoon hot sauce

1 scallion, white and green parts, chopped, for garnish

1 tablespoon sesame seeds, for garnish

Lightly grease the insert of the slow cooker with 1 tablespoon of the olive oil. In a large skillet over medium-high heat, heat the remaining 2 tablespoons of the olive oil. Add the beef and brown for 6 minutes. Transfer to the insert. In the skillet, sauté the onion and garlic for 3 minutes. Transfer the onion and garlic to the insert along with the red pepper, yellow pepper, coconut cream, broth, coconut aminos, and hot sauce. Cover and cook on low for 9 to 10 hours. Serve topped with the scallion and sesame seeds.

Per serving: Calories: 441; Fat: 34g; Protein: 25g; Total Carbs: 11g; Fiber: 4g; Net Carbs: 7g; **Macros:** Fat: 70%; Protein: 23%; Carbs: 7%

Ginger Beef

SERVES 8 | PREP TIME: 15 minutes | COOK TIME: 9 to 10 hours on low

¼ cup extra-virgin olive oil, divided

2 pounds beef boneless chuck roast

½ teaspoon salt

½ cup beef broth

¼ cup Paleo or low-carb ketchup

2 tablespoons apple cider vinegar

2 tablespoons grated fresh ginger

Lightly grease the insert of the slow cooker with 1 tablespoon of the olive oil. In a large skillet over medium-high heat, heat the remaining 3 tablespoons of the olive oil. Season the beef with salt. Add the beef to the skillet and brown for 6 minutes. Transfer the beef to the insert. In a small bowl, stir the broth, ketchup, apple cider vinegar, and ginger. Add the broth mixture to the beef. Cover and cook on low for 9 to 10 hours. Serve warm.

Per serving: Calories: 481; Fat: 39g; Protein: 29g; Total Carbs: 4g; Fiber: 0g; Net Carbs: 4g; **Macros:** Fat: 73%; Protein: 24%; Carbs: 3%

Carne Asada

SERVES 8 | PREP TIME: 15 minutes | COOK TIME: 9 to 10 hours on low

½ cup extra-virgin olive oil, divided

¼ cup lime juice

2 tablespoons apple cider vinegar

2 teaspoons minced garlic

1½ teaspoons paprika

1 teaspoon ground cumin

1 teaspoon chili powder

¼ teaspoon cayenne pepper

1 sweet onion cut into eighths

2 pounds beef rump roast

1 cup sour cream, for garnish

Lightly grease the insert of the slow cooker with 1 tablespoon of the olive oil. In a small bowl, whisk the remaining olive oil, lime juice, apple cider vinegar, garlic, paprika, cumin, chili powder, and cayenne until well blended. Place the onion in the bottom of the insert and the beef on top of the vegetable. Pour the sauce over the beef. Cover and cook on low for 9 to 10 hours. Shred the beef with a fork. Serve topped with the sour cream.

Per serving: Calories: 538; Fat: 44g; Protein: 31g; Total Carbs: 3g; Fiber: 1g; Net Carbs: 2g; **Macros:** Fat: 74%; Protein: 23%; Carbs: 3%

Beef Goulash

SERVES 6 | PREP TIME: 15 minutes | COOK TIME: 9 to 10 hours on low

1 tablespoon extra-virgin olive oil

1½ pounds beef, cut into 1-inch pieces

½ sweet onion, chopped

1 carrot, cut into ½-inch-thick slices

1 red bell pepper, diced

2 teaspoons minced garlic

1 cup beef broth

¼ cup tomato paste

1 tablespoon Hungarian paprika

1 bay leaf

1 cup sour cream

2 tablespoons chopped fresh parsley, for garnish

Lightly grease the insert of the slow cooker with the olive oil. Add the beef, onion, carrot, red bell pepper, garlic, broth, tomato paste, paprika, and bay leaf to the insert. Cover and cook on low for 9 to 10 hours. Remove the bay leaf and stir in the sour cream. Serve topped with the parsley.

Per serving: Calories: 548; Fat: 42g; Protein: 32g; Total Carbs: 8g; Fiber: 2g; Net Carbs: 6g; **Macros:** Fat: 70%; Protein: 24%; Carbs: 6%

Braised Beef Short Ribs

SERVES 8 | PREP TIME: 10 minutes | COOK TIME: 7 to 8 hours on low

1 tablespoon extra-virgin olive oil

2 pounds beef short ribs

1 sweet onion, sliced

2 cups beef broth

2 tablespoons granulated erythritol

2 tablespoons balsamic vinegar

2 teaspoons dried thyme

1 teaspoon hot sauce

Lightly grease the insert of the slow cooker with the olive oil. Place the ribs, onion, broth, erythritol, balsamic vinegar, thyme, and hot sauce in the insert. Cover and cook on low for 7 to 8 hours. Serve warm.

Per Serving: Calories: 473; Fat: 43g; Protein: 18g; Total Carbs: 2g; Fiber: 0g; Net Carbs: 2g; **Macros:** Fat: 82%; Protein: 16%; Carbs: 2%

Stuffed Meatballs

SERVES 6 | PREP TIME: 30 minutes | COOK TIME: 5 to 6 hours on low

3 tablespoons extra-virgin olive oil, divided

1½ pounds ground beef

1 large egg

¼ cup grated Parmesan cheese

2 teaspoons minced garlic

2 teaspoons dried basil

½ teaspoon salt

¼ teaspoon freshly ground black pepper

6 ounces mozzarella, cut into 16 small cubes

4 cups marinara sauce

Lightly grease the insert of the slow cooker with 1 tablespoon of the olive oil. In large bowl, combine the beef, egg, Parmesan, garlic, basil, salt, and pepper until well mixed. Shape the mixture into 16 meatballs and press a mozzarella piece into the center of each, making sure to completely enclose the cheese. In a large skillet over medium-high heat, heat the remaining 2 tablespoons of the olive oil. Add the meatballs and brown all over, about 10 minutes. Transfer the meatballs to the insert and add the marinara sauce. Cover and cook on low for 5 to 6 hours. Serve warm.

Per serving: Calories: 508; Fat: 36g; Protein: 39g; Total Carbs: 6g; Fiber: 2g; Net Carbs: 4g; **Macros:** Fat: 65%; Protein: 31%; Carbs: 4%

Balsamic Roast Beef

SERVES 8 | PREP TIME: 15 minutes | COOK TIME: 7 to 8 hours on low

3 tablespoons of extra-virgin olive oil, divided	1 tablespoon minced garlic
2 pounds boneless beef chuck roast	1 tablespoon granulated erythritol
1 cup beef broth	½ teaspoon red pepper flakes
½ cup balsamic vinegar	1 tablespoon chopped fresh thyme

Lightly grease the insert of the slow cooker with 1 tablespoon of the olive oil. In a large skillet over medium-high heat, heat the remaining 2 tablespoons of the olive oil. Add the beef and brown on all sides, about 7 minutes total. Transfer to the insert. In a small bowl, whisk the broth, balsamic vinegar, garlic, erythritol, red pepper flakes, and thyme until blended. Pour the sauce over the beef. Cover and cook on low for 7 to 8 hours. Serve warm.

Per Serving: Calories: 476; Fat: 39g; Protein: 28g; Total Carbs: 1g; Fiber: 0g; Net Carbs: 1g; **Macros:** Fat: 74%; Protein: 25%; Carbs: 1%

Slow Cooker Barbacoa Pulled Beef with Cilantro Cauliflower Rice

SERVES 6-8 | PREP TIME: 10 minutes | COOK TIME: 8 hours

For the Barbacoa

5 pounds round roast	4 garlic cloves, minced
½ cup beef broth	3 tablespoons apple cider vinegar
¼ cup lime juice, fresh squeezed	1 tablespoon salt
1 medium yellow onion, peeled and cut in half	2 teaspoons dried oregano

For the cilantro cauliflower rice

2 heads cauliflower, riced	Juice from 2 limes
¼ cup avocado oil	½ cup fresh chopped cilantro, chopped
4 garlic cloves, minced	
2 teaspoons salt	

Put all ingredients in 6-quart slow cooker. Cook on low for 8 hours or high for 4 hours. The beef is done when it easily falls apart with forks. Shred the beef with two forks before serving. In a large skillet, heat the avocado oil over medium heat. Add the garlic and cook until soft, about 3 to 5 minutes. Add the cauliflower "rice" and stir to combine. Season with salt and cook for about 5 minutes stirring

frequently until the cauliflower softens. Remove from heat and transfer to a serving bowl. Add lime juice and fresh cilantro and toss gently to combine.

Per Serving: Calories: 562; Fat: 30g; Protein: 65g; Total Carbs: 8g; Fiber: 2g; Net Carbs: 6g; **Macros:** Fat: 48%; Protein: 46%; Carbs: 6%

Corned Beef & Cabbage with Horseradish Cream

SERVES 8 TO 10 | PREP: 10 minutes | COOK: 8 hours on low

For the horseradish cream

1½ cups sour cream	1 teaspoon kosher salt
1 cup prepared horseradish	½ teaspoon freshly ground black pepper
2 tablespoons Dijon mustard	
1½ teaspoons white wine vinegar	

For the beef

1 head cabbage, cut into wedges	½ teaspoon ground allspice
1 onion, chopped	½ teaspoon ground marjoram
½ cup (1 stick) unsalted butter or ghee, melted	½ teaspoon ground thyme
1½ cups water	½ teaspoon kosher salt
½ teaspoon ground coriander	½ teaspoon freshly ground black pepper
½ teaspoon ground mustard	1 (3-pound) corned beef brisket

In a medium bowl, stir all the ingredients. Cover and chill until ready to serve. In the slow cooker, toss the cabbage wedges, onion, and butter, and then spread them out in an even layer. Add the water. In a small bowl, stir the coriander, mustard, allspice, marjoram, thyme, salt, and pepper. Rub the spice mixture all over the corned beef. Place the beef on top of the vegetables in the slow cooker. Cover and cook for 8 hours on low. Let the meat rest for 5 to 10 minutes before slicing. Serve with the vegetables and horseradish cream.

Per Serving: Calories: 681; Fat: 57g; Protein: 29g; Total Carbs: 13g; Fiber: 4g; Net Carbs: 9g; **Macros:** Fat: 75%; Protein: 19%; Carbs: 6%

Fiery Curry Beef

SERVES 6 | PREP TIME: 10 minutes | COOK TIME: 7 to 8 hours on low

1 tablespoon extra-virgin olive oil	2 tablespoons hot curry powder
1 pound beef chuck roast, cut into 2-inch pieces	1 tablespoon coconut aminos
1 sweet onion, chopped	2 teaspoons grated fresh ginger
1 red bell pepper, diced	2 teaspoons minced garlic
2 cups coconut milk	1 cup shredded baby bok choy

Lightly grease the insert of the slow cooker with the olive oil. Add the beef, onion, and bell pepper to the insert. In a medium bowl, whisk the coconut milk, curry, coconut aminos, ginger, and garlic. Pour the sauce into the insert and stir to combine. Cover and cook on low for 7 to 8 hours. Stir in the bok choy and let stand 15 minutes. Serve warm.

Per Serving: Calories: 504; Fat: 42g; Protein: 23g; Total Carbs: 10g; Fiber: 3g; Net Carbs: 7g; **Macros:** Fat: 75%; Protein: 19%; Carbs: 6%

Slow Cooker Beef-Stuffed Cabbage in Creamy Tomato Sauce

SERVES 4 | PREP: 20 minutes | COOK: 8 hours on low or 4 hours on high

1 pound (70% lean) ground beef

4 bacon slices, finely diced

1 cup shredded Gruyère cheese

1 small onion, finely diced

1 large egg, beaten

½ cup almond meal

1 teaspoon garlic powder

1 teaspoon kosher salt

¼ teaspoon freshly ground black pepper

12 whole cabbage leaves, lightly steamed in the microwave

1 (14.5-ounce) can tomato sauce

1 tablespoon red wine vinegar or apple cider vinegar

2 teaspoons soy sauce or tamari

1 teaspoon erythritol or ⅓ teaspoon stevia powder

1 teaspoon paprika

¼ teaspoon ground allspice

1½ cups sour cream

In a large bowl, mix the ground beef, bacon, Gruyère cheese, onion, egg, almond meal, garlic powder, salt, and pepper. Place a handful of the meat mixture in the center of each of the softened cabbage leaves, dividing equally. Fold two sides of the leaf over the filling, and then roll it up like a burrito. Place each roll, seam-side down, in the slow cooker (it's okay to stack the rolls if necessary). In a medium bowl, stir the tomato sauce, vinegar, soy sauce, erythritol, paprika, and allspice. Pour the sauce mixture over the rolls. Cover and cook for 8 hours on low or 4 hours on high. Turn off the slow cooker and let the cabbage rolls rest for 10 to 15 minutes. Carefully remove the cabbage rolls from the slow cooker and arrange them on a serving platter. Stir the sour cream into the sauce in the cooker, then pour it over the cabbage rolls. Serve warm.

Per Serving: Calories: 782; Fat: 60g; Protein: 45g; Total Carbs: 20g; Fiber: 6g; Net Carbs: 14g; **Macros:** Fat: 70%; Protein: 23%; Carbs: 7%

Slow Cooker Brisket

SERVES 8 | PREP TIME: 15 minutes | COOK TIME: 8 hours

1 teaspoon garlic powder

1 teaspoon Lawry's seasoned salt

1 teaspoon minced onion

½ teaspoon freshly ground black pepper

4- to 6-pound beef brisket

3 to 4 cups beef broth or bone broth

In a small bowl, mix the garlic powder, seasoned salt, minced onion, and pepper. Spread it on all sides of the meat. Place the meat into the slow cooker. If the brisket is too big, cut it to fit. Pour the broth over the meat, cover, and cook for 8 hours on low. Serve topped with its own juice.

Per Serving: Calories: 538; Fat: 36g; Protein: 50g; Total Carbs: 1g; Fiber: 0g; Net Carbs: 1g; **Macros:** Fat: 61%; Protein: 38%; Carbs: 1%

Savory Stuffed Peppers

SERVES 4 | PREP TIME: 25 minutes | COOK TIME: 6 hours on low

3 tablespoons extra-virgin olive oil, divided

1 pound ground beef

½ cup finely chopped cauliflower

1 tomato, diced

½ sweet onion, chopped

2 teaspoons minced garlic

2 teaspoons dried oregano

1 teaspoon dried basil

4 bell peppers, tops cut off and seeded

1 cup shredded Cheddar cheese

½ cup chicken broth

1 tablespoon basil, sliced into thin strips, for garnish

Lightly grease the insert of the slow cooker with 1 tablespoon of the olive oil. In a large skillet over medium-high heat, heat the remaining 2 tablespoons of the olive oil. Add the beef and sauté until it is cooked through, about 10 minutes. Add the cauliflower, tomato, onion, garlic, oregano, and basil. Sauté for an additional 5 minutes. Spoon the meat mixture into the bell peppers and top with the cheese. Place the peppers in the slow cooker and add the broth to the bottom. Cover and cook on low for 6 hours. Serve warm, topped with the basil.

Per serving: Calories: 571; Fat: 41g; Protein: 38g; Total Carbs: 12g; Fiber: 3g; Net Carbs: 9g; **Macros:** Fat: 65%; Protein: 28%; Carbs: 7%

Mediterranean Meatloaf

SERVES 8 | PREP TIME: 15 minutes | COOK TIME: 7 to 8 hours on low

3 tablespoons extra-virgin olive oil, divided

½ sweet onion, chopped

2 teaspoons minced garlic

1 pound ground beef

1 pound ground pork

½ cup almond flour

½ cup heavy (whipping) cream

2 large eggs

2 teaspoons dried oregano

1 teaspoon dried basil

¼ teaspoon salt

¼ teaspoon freshly ground black pepper

¾ cup tomato purée

1 cup goat cheese

Lightly grease the insert of the slow cooker with 1 tablespoon of the olive oil. In a medium skillet over medium-high heat, heat the remaining 2 tablespoons of the olive oil. Add the onion and garlic and sauté until the onion is softened, about 3 minutes. In a large bowl mix the onion mixture, beef, pork, almond flour, heavy cream, eggs, oregano, basil, salt, and pepper until well combined. Transfer the meat mixture to the insert and form into a loaf with about ½-inch gap on the sides. Spread the tomato purée on top of the meatloaf and sprinkle with goat cheese. Cover and cook on low for 7 to 8 hours. Serve warm.

Per serving: Calories: 410; Fat: 29g; Protein: 32g; Total Carbs: 4g; Fiber: 1g; Net Carbs: 3g; **Macros:** Fat: 65%; Protein: 32%; Carbs: 3%

Deconstructed Cabbage Rolls

SERVES 4 | PREP TIME: 15 minutes | COOK TIME: 7 to 8 hours on low

3 tablespoons extra-virgin olive oil, divided

1 pound ground beef

1 sweet onion, chopped

2 cups finely chopped cauliflower

2 teaspoons minced garlic

1 teaspoon dried thyme

¼ teaspoon salt

¼ teaspoon freshly ground black pepper

4 cups shredded cabbage

2 cups marinara sauce

½ cup cream cheese

Lightly grease the insert of the slow cooker with 1 tablespoon of the olive oil. Press the ground beef along bottom of the insert. In a medium skillet over medium-high heat, heat the remaining 2 tablespoons of the olive oil. Add the onion, cauliflower, garlic, thyme, salt, and pepper, and sauté until the onion is softened, about 3 minutes. Add the cabbage and sauté for an additional 5 minutes. Transfer the cabbage mixture to the insert, pour the marinara sauce over the cabbage, and top with the cream cheese. Cover and cook on low for 7 to 8 hours. Stir before serving.

Per serving: Calories: 547; Fat: 42g; Protein: 34g; Total Carbs: 10g; Fiber: 4g; Net Carbs: 6g; **Macros:** Fat: 70%; Protein: 25%; Carbs: 5%

Pork Chile Verde

SERVES 4 | PREP TIME: 5 minutes | COOK TIME: 8 hours

1 pound pork shoulder	1 quart chicken bone broth
1 yellow onion, halved and cut into thick slices	Sea salt
	Freshly ground black pepper
2 garlic cloves, smashed	1 small avocado, pitted, peeled, and thinly sliced
1 (16-ounce) jar fire-roasted salsa verde	½ cup full-fat sour cream

Place the pork shoulder into a medium-size slow cooker and scatter the sliced onion and garlic over it. Season generously with salt and pepper. Pour the salsa verde and chicken broth into the slow cooker, cover, and cook on low for 8 hours. Shred the pork with two forks, and season with salt and pepper. Serve with avocado and sour cream.

Per Serving: Calories: 496; Fat: 37g; Protein: 29g; Total Carbs: 11g; Fiber: 3g; Net Carbs: 8g; **Macros:** Fat: 67%; Protein: 23%; Carbs: 10%

Pork Loin with Creamy Gravy

SERVES 6 | PREP: 10 minutes | COOK: 8 hours on low

1 tablespoon kosher salt	2 onions, sliced
2 teaspoons freshly ground black pepper	¼ cup water
	2 tablespoons soy sauce or tamari
4 garlic cloves, minced	1 cup heavy (whipping) cream
1 (3-pound) bone-in pork loin roast	

In a small bowl, stir the salt, pepper, and garlic to form a paste. Rub the seasoning mixture all over the pork roast. Arrange the onions in the bottom of the slow cooker. Pour in the water and soy sauce. Place the roast on top of the onions. Cover and cook for 8 hours on low. Remove the roast from the slow cooker and let it rest for 10 minutes. While the roast is resting, transfer the remaining liquid and onions from the slow cooker to a blender. Add the heavy cream and process into a smooth sauce. Slice the pork and serve it with the gravy spooned over the top.

Per Serving: Calories: 524; Fat: 36g; Protein: 44g; Total Carbs: 6g; Fiber: 1g; Net Carbs: 5g; **Macros:** Fat: 64%; Protein: 33%; Carbs: 3%

Southeast Asian Lemongrass Pork

SERVES 6 | PREP: 10 minutes, plus overnight to marinate | COOK: 8 hours on low

¼ cup coconut oil, melted	3 tablespoons minced lemongrass (white part only)
1 tablespoon apple cider vinegar	
	3 garlic cloves, minced

2 teaspoons kosher salt	1 onion, sliced
1 teaspoon freshly ground black pepper	1 (2-inch) piece fresh ginger, peeled and cut into thin slices
2 pounds boneless pork shoulder or butt roast, top fatty layer scored in a criss-cross pattern	1 (14-ounce) can coconut milk

In a small bowl, stir the coconut oil, cider vinegar, lemongrass, garlic, salt, and pepper. Place the pork in a baking dish and rub the seasoning mixture all over it. Cover and refrigerate overnight. In the morning, remove the pork from the refrigerator 30 to 60 minutes before you plan to cook it so it can come to room temperature. You could also complete the next step and then set a delay timer to start the slow cooker 30 to 60 minutes later, if you prefer. Cover the bottom of the slow cooker with the onion and ginger slices in an even layer. Top with the marinated pork, along with any accumulated juices in the dish. Pour the coconut milk over the top. Cover and cook for 8 hours on low. Shred the meat using two forks. Serve immediately.

Per Serving: Calories: 547; Fat: 43g; Protein: 34g; Total Carbs: 6g; Fiber: 2g; Net Carbs: 4g; **Macros:** Fat: 71%; Protein: 25%; Carbs: 4%

Slow Cooker Pork Chops with Creamy Bacon-and-Artichoke Sauce

SERVES 4 | PREP TIME: 5 minutes | COOK TIME: 2 hours on high or 4 hours on low

2 tablespoons olive oil	8 slices smoked bacon, roughly chopped
4 bone-in pork chops, about 1½ inches thick	1 tablespoon onion powder
Salt	1 teaspoon garlic powder
Freshly ground black pepper	¼ cup heavy (whipping) cream
14 ounces canned artichokes, drained and halved	¼ cup grated Parmesan cheese
	½ teaspoon xanthan gum (optional)

In a large skillet, heat the oil over medium heat. Season the pork chops with salt and pepper on both sides. Working in batches, sear for 2 to 3 minutes on each side, until nicely browned. Place the pork chops in the bowl of a large slow cooker. Add the artichokes, bacon, onion powder, and garlic powder. Cover and cook on low heat for 4 to 6 hours or on high for 2 to 3 hours. Until the pork has reached an internal temperature of at least 145°F. Once cooked, transfer to a plate to rest. In the slow cooker, combine the heavy cream, Parmesan, and xanthan gum (if using), stir well, and cook for 1 minute, until thickened. Serve the pork chops with the sauce poured over top.

Per Serving: Calories: 655; Fat: 49g; Protein: 42g; Total Carbs: 11g; Fiber: 5g; Net Carbs: 6g; **Macros:** Fat: 66%; Protein: 26%; Carbs: 8%

Pork Loin with Ginger Cream Sauce

SERVES 6 | PREP: 15 minutes | COOK: 8 hours on low

For the pork

1 tablespoon erythritol	1 teaspoon ground ginger
2 teaspoons kosher salt	½ teaspoon ground cinnamon
1 teaspoon garlic powder	½ teaspoon ground cloves

½ teaspoon red pepper flakes
¼ teaspoon freshly ground
   black pepper

For the sauce
2 tablespoons unsalted butter
3 tablespoons minced
   fresh ginger
2 shallots, minced

1 (2-pound) pork
   shoulder roast
½ cup water

1 tablespoon minced garlic
⅔ cup dry white wine
1 cup heavy (whipping) cream

In a small bowl, stir the erythritol, salt, garlic powder, ginger, cinnamon, cloves, red pepper flakes, and black pepper. Rub the seasoning mixture all over the pork and place it in the slow cooker. Pour the water into the cooker around the pork. Cover and cook for 8 hours on low. Remove the pork from the slow cooker and let it rest for about 5 minutes. While the pork rests, melt the butter in a small saucepan over medium heat. Stir in the ginger, shallots, and garlic. Add the white wine and bring to a boil. Cook, stirring, until the liquid is reduced to about ¼ cup, about 5 minutes. Whisk in the heavy cream and continue to boil, stirring, until the sauce thickens, 3 to 5 minutes more. Slice the pork and serve it with the sauce spooned over the top.

Per Serving: Calories: 488; Fat: 40g; Protein: 27g; Total Carbs: 5g; Fiber: 1g; Net Carbs: 4g; **Macros:** Fat: 67%; Protein: 22%; Carbs: 11%

Mustard-Herb Pork Chops

SERVES 4 | PREP: 5 minutes | COOK: 8 hours on low or 4 hours on high

¾ cup chicken or beef broth
2 tablespoons coconut
   oil, melted
1 tablespoon Dijon mustard
2 garlic cloves, minced
1 tablespoon paprika
1 tablespoon onion powder

1 teaspoon dried oregano
1 teaspoon dried basil
1 teaspoon dried parsley
1 onion, thinly sliced
4 thick-cut boneless
   pork chops
1 cup heavy (whipping) cream

In the slow cooker, stir the broth, coconut oil, mustard, garlic, paprika, onion powder, oregano, basil, and parsley. Add the onion and pork chops and toss to coat. Cover and cook for 8 hours on low or 4 hours on high. Transfer the chops to a serving platter. Transfer the remaining juices and onion in the slow cooker to a blender, add the heavy cream, and process until smooth. Pour the sauce over the pork chops and serve hot.

Per Serving: Calories: 470; Fat: 32g; Protein: 39g; Total Carbs: 7g; Fiber: 2g; Net Carbs: 5g; **Macros:** Fat: 62%; Protein: 33%; Carbs: 5%

Slow Cooker Pulled Pork with Cabbage Slaw

SERVES 8 | PREP TIME: 30 minutes | COOK TIME: 8½ hours

For the slaw
¾ cup shredded cabbage
¼ cup shredded carrot
⅛ cup sliced scallions
3 tablespoons mayonnaise

1 teaspoon mustard
¼ teaspoon salt
¼ teaspoon freshly ground
   black pepper

For the rub
¼ cup stevia, or other sugar
   substitute
1 tablespoon paprika
2 teaspoons garlic powder

2 teaspoons onion powder
2 teaspoons mustard powder
1 teaspoon ground cumin
1 teaspoon salt

1 teaspoon freshly ground
   black pepper

½ teaspoon chili powder

For the pork
1 (4- to 5-pound) boneless
   pork shoulder roast
2½ tablespoons olive oil
¾ cup light beer

3 tablespoons apple
   cider vinegar
3 tablespoons tomato paste
8 low-carb buns or lettuce
   wraps (optional)

In a large bowl, combine the cabbage, carrots, scallions, mayonnaise, mustard, salt, and pepper. Mix thoroughly. Refrigerate until ready to serve. In a medium bowl, mix the stevia, paprika, garlic powder, onion powder, mustard powder, cumin, salt, pepper, and chili powder. Cover the pork shoulder with the rub, massaging it thoroughly into the meat. In a large skillet over medium-high heat, heat the olive oil for 1 minute. Add the pork to the skillet, browning on all sides for about 3 minutes per side. Once browned, remove the pork from the skillet and set aside. Pour the beer into the skillet and scrape the bottom of the pan to loosen any browned bits. Remove the skillet from the heat and pour the drippings into a large slow cooker. To the slow cooker, add the apple cider vinegar and tomato paste. Whisk to combine with the pork drippings. Place the pork in the slow cooker and spoon some of the liquid over it. Cover. Cook on low for 8 hours until the internal temperature is between 180°F and 200°F. Remove the pork from the slow cooker and place it in a large bowl to cool. In a large skillet over high heat, add the remaining liquid from the slow cooker and bring to a boil. Lower the heat to medium-low and reduce the liquid by at least half over the next 10 minutes. Using two forks, shred the cooled pork until you have bite-size chunks. Pour the reduced liquid over the meat. Mix until it is coated evenly. Serve the shredded pork with the slaw on its own, or on a low-carb bun or a lettuce wrap (if using).

Per Serving: Calories: 750; Fat: 58.8g; Protein: 44.4g; Total Carbs: 7.3g; Fiber: 1.8g; Net Carbs: 5.5g; **Macros:** Fat: 72%; Protein: 24%; Carbs: 4%

Slow Cooker Pork Carnitas

SERVES 4 | PREP TIME: 5 minutes | COOK TIME: 8 to 10 hours on low

1 tablespoon extra-virgin
   olive oil
1 (1½-pound) boneless pork
   shoulder
2 teaspoons dried oregano
1 teaspoon ground cumin
⅛ teaspoon ground cloves

Zest and juice of 1 orange
Sea salt
Freshly ground black pepper
1 red onion, halved and sliced
4 garlic cloves,
   roughly chopped
1 cinnamon stick

Coat the interior of the slow cooker with the olive oil. Season the pork with the oregano, cumin, cloves, orange zest, salt, and pepper. Place the pork in the slow cooker. Scatter the onion slices, garlic, and cinnamon stick around the pork. Sprinkle with the orange juice. Cook on low for 8 to 10 hours, or until the meat is tender. Shred with two forks before serving.

Per Serving: Calories: 599; Fat: 44g; Protein: 41g; Total Carbs: 7g; Fiber: 1g; Net Carbs: 6g; **Macros:** Fat: 68%; Protein: 27%; Carbs: 5%

Slow Cooker Ranch Favorite Texas-Style Pulled Pork

SERVES 8 | PREP TIME: 15 minutes | COOK TIME: 8 hours

1 tablespoon paprika
1 tablespoon monk fruit/ erythritol blend sweetener
2½ teaspoons kosher salt, divided
1 teaspoon freshly ground black pepper
2 teaspoons garlic powder
1 teaspoon chili powder
1 teaspoon onion powder
½ teaspoon cayenne pepper
½ teaspoon dry mustard

1 (5-pound) bone-in pork butt
2 tablespoons yellow mustard
½ cup diced onion
½ cup sugar-free barbecue sauce
1¼ tablespoons apple cider vinegar
1 tablespoon gluten-free Worcestershire sauce
Diced purple onion, for garnish
Chopped fresh cilantro, for garnish

In a small bowl, stir the paprika, sweetener, 2 teaspoons of salt, the black pepper, garlic powder, chili powder, onion powder, cayenne, and dry mustard. Pat the pork butt dry with paper towels and trim excess fat. Rub the entire outside of the pork butt with yellow mustard and generously season the pork butt with the spice mix. Rub the seasoning into the roast. Reserve any remaining seasoning. Add the onion to the slow cooker and place the pork butt on top of the onion. Cover the slow cooker and cook on low heat for 8 hours. Remove the pork butt from the cooker. Remove the bone and shred the pork butt with two forks and set aside. Strain the juices from the slow cooker into a small saucepan and bring to a boil over high heat. Cook, uncovered, for about 10 minutes until reduced. Stir in the barbecue sauce, vinegar, Worcestershire sauce, and remaining ½ teaspoon of salt. Pour the sauce over the shredded pork and season with any remaining rub. Serve topped with purple onion and cilantro.

Per Serving: Calories: 504; Fat: 40g; Protein: 33g; Total Carbs: 3g; Fiber: 1g; Net Carbs: 2g; Macros: Fat: 71%; Protein: 26%; Carbs: 3%

Smoked Sausage with Cabbage & Onions

SERVES 6 | PREP: 5 minutes | COOK: 7 hours on low

1 tablespoon extra-virgin olive oil
1½ pounds cabbage, cut into wedges
1 onion, halved and thinly sliced
½ teaspoon kosher salt
½ teaspoon freshly ground black pepper

1 cup chicken broth
¼ cup (½ stick) unsalted butter or ghee, melted
1 tablespoon spicy brown mustard
2 pounds smoked pork sausage, such as kielbasa, cut into 3-inch lengths

Coat the inside of the slow cooker insert with the olive oil. Put the cabbage wedges and onions in the slow cooker. Sprinkle with salt and pepper and then add the chicken broth, butter, and mustard. Toss to coat the cabbage and onions. Top with the sausage pieces. Cover and cook for 7 hours on low. Serve hot.

Per Serving: Calories: 486; Fat: 38g; Protein: 22g; Total Carbs: 14g; Fiber: 4g; Net Carbs: 10g; Macros: Fat: 70%; Protein: 19%; Carbs: 11%

Slow Cooker Saucy Sausage-and-Beef Meatballs

SERVES 4 | PREP TIME: 10 minutes | COOK TIME: 15 minutes, plus 2 hours on high or 4 hours on low

1 (15-ounce) can tomato sauce
¼ cup beef, chicken, or vegetable broth
2 teaspoons minced garlic
1 teaspoon dried oregano
1 teaspoon onion powder
¼ cup grated Parmesan cheese

1 pound pork sausage
½ pound lean ground beef
½ cup pork rind crumbs
1 large egg, beaten
1 tablespoon Italian seasoning
1 tablespoon olive oil

In a slow cooker, combine the tomato sauce, broth, garlic, oregano, onion powder, and Parmesan. Stir well and set aside. In a large bowl, combine the sausage, ground beef, pork rind crumbs, egg, and Italian seasoning. Use your hands to mix well. Form the mixture into 1-inch balls; you'll get about 24 meatballs. In a large skillet, heat the oil over medium heat. Working in batches, cook the meatballs for 5 to 6 minutes, turning to brown on all sides. Drop them into the slow cooker. Cover and cook on high for 2 hours or low for 4 hours.

Per Serving: Calories: 620; Fat: 51g; Protein: 32g; Total Carbs: 9g; Fiber: 2g; Net Carbs: 7g; Macros: Fat: 73%; Protein: 21%; Carbs: 6%

Pork Belly with Brussels Sprouts & Turnips

SERVES 6 TO 8 | PREP: 10 minutes | COOK: 8 hours on low

2 tablespoons paprika
2 tablespoons onion powder
2 tablespoons garlic powder
1 tablespoon kosher salt
1 tablespoon freshly ground black pepper

2 pounds pork belly, thickly sliced
1 pound Brussels sprouts, halved
1 medium turnip, peeled and diced
4 bay leaves

In a small bowl, stir the paprika, onion powder, garlic powder, salt, and pepper. Rub the mixture all over the pork belly slices. In the bottom of the slow cooker, arrange the Brussels sprouts, turnip, and bay leaves in an even layer. Lay the pork over the vegetables. Cover and cook for 8 hours on low. Discard the bay leaves and serve hot.

Per Serving: Calories: 848; Fat: 80g; Protein: 18g; Total Carbs: 14g; Fiber: 5g; Net Carbs: 9g; Macros: Fat: 85%; Protein: 9%; Carbs: 6%

Pork & Sausage Meatballs with Mushroom Ragout

SERVES 4 | PREP: 20 minutes | COOK: 8 hours on low

For the meatballs

1½ pounds sweet Italian sausage, casings removed
8 ounces ground pork
1 cup almond meal
½ cup pine nuts
2 cups finely grated Parmesan cheese, divided

1 large egg, beaten
1 teaspoon rubbed sage
1 teaspoon dried oregano
½ teaspoon kosher salt
¼ teaspoon freshly grated nutmeg

For the sauce

¼ cup (½ stick) unsalted butter, melted

1 (14.5-ounce) can diced tomatoes, with juice

¼ cup tomato paste
½ ounce dried porcini mushrooms, crumbled
1 teaspoon dried oregano
1 teaspoon dried thyme

½ teaspoon fennel seeds
½ teaspoon kosher salt
¼ teaspoon red pepper flakes
1 cup heavy (whipping) cream

In a large bowl, thoroughly mix the sausage, ground pork, almond meal, and pine nuts. Add 1 cup of Parmesan cheese, egg, sage, oregano, salt, and nutmeg. Mix well. Form the mixture into 12 meatballs. In the slow cooker, stir the butter, tomatoes and their juice, tomato paste, mushrooms, oregano, thyme, fennel seeds, salt, and red pepper flakes. Nestle the meatballs in the sauce. Cover and cook for 8 hours on low. Just before serving, stir in the heavy cream. Serve hot, garnished with the remaining 1 cup of Parmesan cheese.

Per Serving: Calories: 951; Fat: 70g; Protein: 63g; Total Carbs: 22g; Fiber: 7g; Net Carbs: 15g; **Macros:** Fat: 68%; Protein: 25%; Carbs: 7%

Tunisian Lamb Ragout

SERVES 6 | PREP TIME: 15 minutes | COOK TIME: 8 hours on low

¼ cup extra-virgin olive oil
1½ pounds lamb shoulder, cut
  into 1-inch chunks
1 sweet onion, chopped
1 tablespoon minced garlic
4 cups pumpkin, cut into
  1-inch pieces
2 carrots, diced

1 (14.5-ounce) can diced
  tomatoes
3 cups beef broth
2 tablespoons ras el hanout
1 teaspoon hot chili powder
1 teaspoon salt
1 cup Greek yogurt

Lightly grease the slow cooker insert with 1 tablespoon olive oil. Place a large skillet over medium–high heat and add the remaining oil. Brown the lamb for 6 minutes, then add the onion and garlic. Sauté 3 minutes more, then transfer the lamb and vegetables to the insert. Add the pumpkin, carrots, tomatoes, broth, ras el hanout, chili powder, and salt to the insert and stir to combine. Cover and cook on low for 8 hours. Serve topped with yogurt.

Per Serving: Calories: 447; Fat: 35g; Protein: 22g; Total Carbs: 12g; Fiber: 3g; Net Carbs: 9g; **Macros:** Fat: 70%; Protein: 21%; Carbs: 9%

Slow Cooker All-in-One Lamb-Vegetable Dinner

SERVES 4 | PREP TIME: 10 minutes | COOK TIME: 6 hours on low

¼ cup extra-virgin olive
  oil, divided
1 pound boneless lamb chops,
  about ½-inch thick
Salt, for seasoning
Freshly ground black pepper,
  for seasoning
½ sweet onion, sliced

½ fennel bulb, cut into
  2-inch chunks
1 zucchini, cut into
  1-inch chunks
¼ cup chicken broth
2 tablespoons chopped fresh
  basil, for garnish

Lightly grease the insert of the slow cooker with 1 tablespoon of the olive oil. Season the lamb with salt and pepper. In a medium bowl, toss the onion, fennel, and zucchini with the remaining 3 tablespoons of the olive oil and then place half

of the vegetables in the insert. Place the lamb on top of the vegetables, cover with the remaining vegetables, and add the broth. Cover and cook on low for 6 hours. Serve topped with the basil.

Per Serving: Calories: 431; Fat: 37g; Protein: 21g; Total Carbs: 5g; Fiber: 2g; Net Carbs: 3g; **Macros:** Fat: 77%; Protein: 20%; Carbs: 3%

Wild Mushroom Lamb Shanks

SERVES 6 | PREP TIME: 15 minutes | COOK TIME: 7 to 8 hours on low

3 tablespoons extra-virgin
  olive oil, divided
2 pounds lamb shanks
½ pound wild mushrooms,
  sliced
1 leek, thoroughly cleaned
  and chopped
2 celery stalks, chopped
1 carrot, diced

1 tablespoon minced garlic
1 (15-ounce) can crushed
  tomatoes
½ cup beef broth
2 tablespoons apple
  cider vinegar
1 teaspoon dried rosemary
½ cup sour cream, for garnish

Lightly grease the insert of the slow cooker with 1 tablespoon of the olive oil. In a large skillet over medium-high heat, heat the remaining 2 tablespoons of the olive oil. Add the lamb; brown for 6 minutes, turning once; and transfer to the insert. In the skillet, sauté the mushrooms, leek, celery, carrot, and garlic for 5 minutes. Transfer the vegetables to the insert along with the tomatoes, broth, apple cider vinegar, and rosemary. Cover and cook on low for 7 to 8 hours. Serve topped with the sour cream.

Per serving: Calories: 475; Fat: 36g; Protein: 31g; Total Carbs: 11g; Fiber: 5g; Net Carbs: 6g; **Macros:** Fat: 70%; Protein: 25%; Carbs: 5%

Slow Cooker Braised Lamb with Fennel

SERVES 4 | PREP: 15 minutes | COOK: 8 hours on low

1½ pounds lamb stew meat,
  cut into 2-inch pieces
1 teaspoon kosher salt
½ teaspoon freshly ground
  black pepper
¼ cup (½ stick) unsalted
  butter, ghee, or coconut oil
1 onion, sliced
1 cup sliced fennel
1 (14.5-ounce) can diced tomatoes, drained

½ cup dry red wine
2 tablespoons tomato paste
2 garlic cloves, minced
2 teaspoons paprika
Pinch stevia powder
1 cinnamon stick
1 cup heavy (whipping) cream
¾ cup chopped pistachios
2 tablespoons chopped
  fresh mint

Season the lamb with the salt and pepper. In a large skillet, heat the butter over medium-high heat. Add the lamb and cook until browned on all sides, about 8 minutes. Transfer the meat to the slow cooker. Return the skillet to medium-high heat and add the onion and fennel. Sauté until softened, about 3 minutes. Stir in the tomatoes, red wine, tomato paste, garlic, paprika, stevia, and cinnamon. Bring to a boil. Transfer the sauce to the cooker. Cover and cook for 8 hours on low. Just before serving, discard the cinnamon stick and stir in the heavy cream. Serve hot, garnished with the pistachios and mint.

Per Serving: Calories: 686; Fat: 60g; Protein: 28g; Total Carbs: 13g; Fiber: 3g; Net Carbs: 10g; **Macros:** Fat: 75%; Protein: 17%; Carbs: 8%

Curried Lamb

SERVES 6 | PREP TIME: 15 minutes | COOK TIME: 7 to 8 hours on low

3 tablespoons extra-virgin olive oil, divided	½ sweet onion, sliced
1½ pounds lamb shoulder chops	¼ cup curry powder
Salt, for seasoning	1 tablespoon grated fresh ginger
Freshly ground black pepper, for seasoning	2 teaspoons minced garlic
3 cups coconut milk	1 carrot, diced
	2 tablespoons chopped cilantro, for garnish

Lightly grease the insert of the slow cooker with 1 tablespoon of the olive oil. In a large skillet over medium-high heat, heat the remaining 2 tablespoons of the olive oil. Season the lamb with salt and pepper. Add the lamb to the skillet and brown for 6 minutes, turning once. Transfer to the insert. In a medium bowl, stir the coconut milk, onion, curry, ginger, and garlic. Add the mixture to the lamb along with the carrot. Cover and cook on low for 7 to 8 hours. Serve topped with the cilantro.

Per serving: Calories: 490; Fat: 41g; Protein: 26g; Total Carbs: 10g; Fiber: 5g; Net Carbs: 5g; **Macros:** Fat: 74%; Protein: 20%; Carbs: 6%

Slow Cooker Lamb Stew with Turnips

SERVES 4 | PREP TIME: 15 minutes | COOK TIME: 3 hours on high or 6 hours on low

1 pound boneless lamb stewing meat, roughly chopped	2 teaspoons onion powder
1 pound turnips, peeled and chopped	1 teaspoon minced garlic
1 (8-ounce) package white mushrooms, sliced	Salt
1 (14-ounce) can beef broth	Freshly ground black pepper
	Chopped fresh parsley, for garnish

In a slow cooker bowl, combine the lamb, turnips, mushrooms, broth, onion powder, and garlic. Stir well. Cook on high for 3 hours or low for 6 hours. Season with salt and pepper to taste. Use a slotted spoon to transfer the lamb and vegetables to a serving dish, then spoon over some of the sauce. Garnish with parsley and serve.

Per Serving: Calories: 298; Fat: 17g; Protein: 26g; Total Carbs: 11g; Fiber: 3g; Net Carbs: 8g; **Macros:** Fat: 50%; Protein: 35%; Carbs: 15%

Rosemary Lamb Chops

SERVES 4 | PREP TIME: 15 minutes | COOK TIME: 6 hours on low

3 tablespoons extra-virgin olive oil, divided	½ cup chicken broth
1½ pounds lamb shoulder chops	1 sweet onion, sliced
Salt, for seasoning	2 teaspoons minced garlic
Freshly ground black pepper, for seasoning	2 teaspoons dried rosemary
	1 teaspoon dried thyme

Lightly grease the insert of the slow cooker with 1 tablespoon of the olive oil. In a large skillet over medium-high heat, heat the remaining 2 tablespoons of the olive oil. Season the lamb with salt and pepper. Add the lamb to the skillet and brown for 6 minutes, turning once. Transfer the lamb to the insert, and add the broth, onion, garlic, rosemary, and thyme. Cover and cook on low for 6 hours. Serve warm.

Per serving: Calories: 380; Fat: 27g; Protein: 31g; Total Carbs: 3g; Fiber: 1g; Net Carbs: 2g; **Macros:** Fat: 65%; Protein: 32%; Carbs: 3%

Tender Lamb Roast

SERVES 6 | PREP TIME: 10 minutes | COOK TIME: 7 to 8 hours on low

1 tablespoon extra-virgin olive oil	1 tablespoon cumin
2 pounds lamb shoulder roast	2 teaspoons minced garlic
Salt, for seasoning	1 teaspoon paprika
Freshly ground black pepper, for seasoning	1 teaspoon chili powder
1 (14.5-ounce) can diced tomatoes	1 cup sour cream
	2 teaspoons chopped fresh parsley, for garnish

Lightly grease the insert of the slow cooker with the olive oil. Lightly season the lamb with salt and pepper. Place the lamb in the insert and add the tomatoes, cumin, garlic, paprika, and chili powder. Cover and cook on low for 7 to 8 hours. Stir in the sour cream. Serve topped with the parsley.

Per serving: Calories: 523; Fat: 43g; Protein: 28g; Total Carbs: 6g; Fiber: 1g; Net Carbs: 5g; **Macros:** Fat: 74%; Protein: 21%; Carbs: 5%

Pumpkin-Nutmeg Pudding

SERVES 8 | PREP: 15 minutes | COOK: 6 to 7 hours on low

¼ cup melted butter, divided	1 cup almond flour
2½ cups canned pumpkin puree	½ cup granulated erythritol
2 cups coconut milk	2 ounces protein powder
4 eggs	1 teaspoon baking powder
1 tablespoon pure vanilla extract	1 teaspoon ground cinnamon
	¼ teaspoon ground nutmeg
	Pinch ground cloves

Lightly grease the insert of the slow cooker with 1 tablespoon of the butter. In a large bowl, whisk the remaining butter, pumpkin, coconut milk, eggs, and vanilla until well blended. In a small bowl, stir the almond flour, erythritol, protein powder, baking powder, cinnamon, nutmeg, and cloves. Add the dry ingredients to the wet ingredients and stir to combine. Pour the mixture into the insert. Cover and cook on low for 6 to 7 hours. Serve warm.

Per Serving: Calories: 265; Fat: 22g; Protein: 13g; Total Carbs: 8g; Fiber: 3g; Net Carbs: 5g; **Macros:** Fat: 70%; Protein: 18%; Carbs: 12%

Chocolate–Peanut Butter Fudge

SERVES 12 | PREP: 10 minutes | COOK: 2 hours on low, plus 4 hours to chill

Coconut oil, for coating the
 slow cooker insert
1½ cups heavy (whip-
 ping) cream
1 cup all-natural peanut butter
1 tablespoon unsalted
 butter, melted

1 teaspoon pure
 vanilla extract
4 ounces unsweetened
 chocolate, chopped
½ cup erythritol
1 teaspoon stevia powder

Generously coat the inside of the slow cooker insert with coconut oil. In the slow cooker, stir the heavy cream, peanut butter, butter, vanilla, chocolate, erythritol, and stevia. Cover and cook for 2 hours on low, stirring occasionally. Line a small, rimmed baking sheet with parchment or wax paper. Transfer the cooked fudge to the prepared sheet and refrigerate for at least 4 hours. Cut into squares and serve chilled.

Per Serving: Calories: 246; Fat: 23g; Protein: 7g; Total Carbs: 8g; Fiber: 3g; Net Carbs: 5g; Macros: Fat: 79%; Protein: 10%; Carbs: 11%

Chocolate Walnut Fudge

SERVES 12 | PREP: 15 minutes | COOK: 2 hours on low, plus 3 hours to cool, overnight to chill

Coconut oil, for coating the
 slow cooker insert and a
 baking dish
1 cup canned coconut milk
4 ounces unsweetened chocolate, chopped
1 cup erythritol

2 teaspoons stevia powder
¼ teaspoon fine sea salt
2 teaspoons pure
 vanilla extract
1 cup chopped
 toasted walnuts

Generously coat the inside of the slow cooker insert with coconut oil. In a large bowl, whisk the coconut milk into a uniform consistency. Add the chocolate, erythritol, stevia powder, and sea salt. Stir to mix well. Pour into the slow cooker. Cover and cook for 2 hours on low. When finished, stir in the vanilla. Let the fudge sit in the slow cooker, with the lid off, until it cools to room temperature, about 3 hours. Coat a large baking dish with coconut oil and set aside. Stir the fudge until it becomes glossy, about 10 minutes. Stir in the walnuts. Transfer the mixture to the prepared baking dish and smooth it into an even layer with a rubber spatula. Refrigerate overnight. Serve chilled, cut into small pieces.

Per Serving: Calories: 128; Fat: 13g; Protein: 3g; Total Carbs: 4g; Fiber: 2g; Net Carbs: 2g; Macros: Fat: 87%; Protein: 6%; Carbs: 7%

Cinnamon-Cocoa Almonds

SERVES 8 | PREP: 5 minutes | COOK: 2 hours on high

3 cups raw almonds
3 tablespoons coconut
 oil, melted
Kosher salt
¼ cup erythritol

1 tablespoon unsweetened
 cocoa powder
1 tablespoon ground
 cinnamon

In the slow cooker, stir the almonds and coconut oil until the nuts are well coated. Season with salt. Mix in the erythritol,

cocoa powder, and cinnamon. Cover and cook for 2 hours on high, stirring every 30 minutes. Transfer the nuts to a large, rimmed baking sheet and spread them out to cool quickly. Serve immediately or store in a covered container for up to 3 weeks.

Per Serving: Calories: 275; Fat: 23g; Protein: 8g; Total Carbs: 9g; Fiber: 5g; Net Carbs: 4g; Macros: Fat: 75%; Protein: 12%; Carbs: 13%

Chocolate Pot de Crème

SERVES 6 | PREP TIME: 10 minutes | COOK TIME: 3 hours on low

6 large egg yolks
2 cups heavy (whip-
 ping) cream
⅓ cup cocoa powder
1 tablespoon pure
 vanilla extract

½ teaspoon liquid stevia
Whipped coconut cream, for
 garnish (optional)
Shaved dark chocolate, for
 garnish (optional)

In a medium bowl, whisk the yolks, heavy cream, cocoa powder, vanilla, and stevia. Pour the mixture into a 1½-quart baking dish and place the dish in the insert of the slow cooker. Pour in enough water to reach halfway up the sides of the baking dish. Cover and cook on low for 3 hours. Remove the baking dish from the insert and cool to room temperature on a wire rack. Chill the dessert completely in the refrigerator and serve, garnished with the whipped coconut cream and shaved dark chocolate (if desired).

Per serving: Calories: 198; Fat: 18g; Protein: 5g; Total Carbs: 4g; Fiber: 1g; Net Carbs: 3g; Macros: Fat: 82%; Protein: 10%; Carbs: 8%

Spicy Chai Custard

SERVES 8 | PREP: 10 minutes | COOK: 5 hours on low, plus 1 to 2 hours to cool

4 cups canned coconut milk
4 chai tea bags
1 tablespoon coconut oil
8 large eggs, lightly beaten

1 cup erythritol or 1 teaspoon
 stevia powder
2 teaspoons stevia powder
1 teaspoon pure vanilla
 extract or vanilla bean paste

In a medium saucepan, heat the coconut milk over medium-high heat until it simmers. Remove from the heat and add the tea bags. Steep for 5 to 10 minutes. Remove and discard the tea bags. Generously coat the inside of the slow cooker insert with the coconut oil. In the insert, stir the tea-infused coconut milk, eggs, erythritol, stevia powder, and vanilla until well combined. Cover and cook for 5 hours on low. Turn off the cooker and let cool in the slow cooker for 1 to 2 hours. Serve immediately.

Per Serving: Calories: 375; Fat: 35g; Protein: 8g; Total Carbs: 7g; Fiber: 3g; Net Carbs: 4g; Macros: Fat: 84%; Protein: 9%; Carbs: 7%

Coconut Custard

SERVES 8 | PREP: 5 minutes | COOK: 5 hours on low, plus 1 to 2 hours to cool

1 tablespoon coconut oil
8 large eggs, lightly beaten
4 cups canned coconut milk

1 cup erythritol or 1 teaspoon
 stevia powder
2 teaspoons stevia powder
1 teaspoon coconut extract

Generously coat the inside of the slow cooker insert with the coconut oil. In the insert, stir the eggs, coconut milk, erythritol, stevia powder, and coconut extract until well combined. Cover and cook for 5 hours on low. Turn off the cooker and let cool in the slow cooker for 1 to 2 hours. Serve immediately.

Per Serving: Calories: 375; Fat: 35g; Protein: 8g; Total Carbs: 7g; Fiber: 3g; Net Carbs: 4g; **Macros:** Fat: 84%; Protein: 9%; Carbs: 7%

Tempting Lemon Custard

SERVES 4 | PREP TIME: 10 minutes | COOK TIME: 3 hours on low

5 large egg yolks	1 teaspoon pure
¼ cup freshly squeezed	vanilla extract
lemon juice	⅓ teaspoon liquid stevia
1 tablespoon lemon zest	2 cups heavy (whipping) cream
	1 cup whipped coconut cream

In a medium bowl, whisk the yolks, lemon juice and zest, vanilla, and liquid stevia. Whisk in the heavy cream and divide the mixture between 4 (4-ounce) ramekins. Place a rack at the bottom of the insert of the slow cooker and place the ramekins on it. Pour in enough water to reach halfway up the sides of the ramekins. Cover and cook on low for 3 hours. Remove the ramekins from the insert and cool to room temperature. Chill the ramekins completely in the refrigerator and serve topped with whipped coconut cream.

Per serving: Calories: 319; Fat: 30g; Protein: 7g; Total Carbs: 3g; Fiber: 0g; Net Carbs: 3g; **Macros:** Fat: 86%; Protein: 10%; Carbs: 4%

Vanilla Pudding

SERVES 2 | PREP TIME: 5 minutes, plus 1 hour to chill | COOK TIME: 10 minutes

1 cup cream	3 tablespoons erythritol
3 egg yolks	½ teaspoon vanilla extract

In a medium saucepan over medium-low heat, whisk together the cream, egg yolks, and erythritol. Whisk gently every 1 to 2 minutes until the mixture is bubbling and thick, about 10 minutes total. Remove from the heat and stir in the vanilla. Chill in the refrigerator for at least 1 hour before serving.

Per serving: Calories: 478; Fat: 49g; Protein: 7g; Total Carbs: 22g; Fiber: 0g; Net Carbs: 4g; **Macros:** Fat: 92%; Protein: 6%; Carbs: 2%

Pumpkin Spice Pudding

SERVES 10 | PREP: 5 minutes | COOK: 8 hours on low

3 tablespoons melted coconut	½ cup erythritol
oil, plus more for coating the	¼ cup almond flour
slow cooker insert	2 teaspoons pumpkin
2 cups canned coconut milk	pie spice
1½ cups puréed pumpkin	1 teaspoon stevia powder
4 large eggs, lightly beaten	1 teaspoon baking powder
1 tablespoon pure	
vanilla extract	

Generously coat the inside of the slow cooker insert with coconut oil. In the insert, stir 3 tablespoons of coconut oil, coconut

milk, pumpkin, eggs, vanilla, erythritol, almond flour, pumpkin pie spice, stevia powder, and baking powder until smooth. Cover and cook for 8 hours on low. Serve warm.

Per Serving: Calories: 215; Fat: 19g; Protein: 4g; Total Carbs: 7g; Fiber: 3g; Net Carbs: 4g; **Macros:** Fat: 79%; Protein: 8%; Carbs: 13%

Pumpkin-Ginger Pudding

SERVES 8 | PREP TIME: 5 minutes | COOK TIME: 3 to 4 hours on low

1 tablespoon coconut oil	1 tablespoon grated
2 cups pumpkin purée	fresh ginger
1½ cups coconut milk	¾ teaspoon liquid stevia
2 eggs	Pinch ground cloves
½ cup almond flour	1 cup whipped coconut cream
1 ounce protein powder	

Lightly grease the insert of the slow cooker with coconut oil. In a large bowl, stir pumpkin, coconut milk, eggs, almond flour, protein powder, ginger, liquid stevia, and cloves. Transfer the mixture to the insert. Cover and cook on low 3 to 4 hours. Serve warm with whipped coconut cream.

Per serving: Calories: 217; Fat: 19g; Protein: 8g; Total Carbs: 7g; Fiber: 4g; Net Carbs: 3g; **Macros:** Fat: 78%; Protein: 12%; Carbs: 10%

Spicy Chai Custard

SERVES 8 | PREP: 10 minutes | COOK: 5 hours on low, plus 1 to 2 hours to cool

4 cups canned coconut milk	2 teaspoons stevia powder
4 chai tea bags	1 teaspoon pure vanilla
1 tablespoon coconut oil	extract or vanilla
8 large eggs, lightly beaten	bean paste
1 cup erythritol or 1 teaspoon	
stevia powder	

In a medium saucepan, heat the coconut milk over medium-high heat until it simmers. Remove from the heat and add the tea bags. Steep for 5 to 10 minutes. Remove and discard the tea bags. Generously coat the inside of the slow cooker insert with the coconut oil. In the insert, stir the tea-infused coconut milk, eggs, erythritol, stevia powder, and vanilla until well combined. Cover and cook for 5 hours on low. Turn off the cooker and let cool in the slow cooker for 1 to 2 hours.

Per Serving: Calories: 375; Fat: 35g; Protein: 8g; Total Carbs: 7g; Fiber: 3g; Net Carbs: 4g; **Macros:** Fat: 84%; Protein: 9%; Carbs: 7%

Chocolate & Coconut Pudding

SERVES 10 | PREP: 10 minutes | COOK: 8 hours on low

3 tablespoons melted coconut	1 teaspoon pure
oil, plus more for coating the	vanilla extract
slow cooker insert	½ cup erythritol
4 ounces unsweetened	¼ cup almond flour
chocolate, chopped	1 teaspoon stevia powder
2 cups canned coconut milk	1 teaspoon baking powder
4 large eggs, lightly beaten	
2 teaspoons coconut extract	

Generously coat the inside of the slow cooker insert with coconut oil. In a microwave-safe bowl or measuring cup, combine 3 tablespoons of coconut oil with the chocolate. Microwave for 1 minute on high. Stir, and then microwave in 30-second intervals, stirring in between, until the chocolate is melted and smooth. Transfer to the prepared insert. Stir in the coconut milk, eggs, coconut and vanilla extracts, erythritol, almond flour, stevia powder, and baking powder until smooth. Cover and cook for 8 hours on low. Serve warm.

Per Serving: Calories: 223; Fat: 19g; Protein: 5g; Total Carbs: 8g; Fiber: 3g; Net Carbs: 5g; **Macros:** Fat: 77%; Protein: 9%; Carbs: 14%

Berry-Pumpkin Compote

SERVES 10 | PREP TIME: 10 minutes | COOK TIME: 3 to 4 hours on low

1 tablespoon coconut oil
2 cups diced pumpkin
1 cup cranberries
1 cup blueberries
½ cup granulated erythritol
Juice and zest of 1 orange

½ cup coconut milk
1 teaspoon ground cinnamon
½ teaspoon ground allspice
¼ teaspoon ground nutmeg
1 cup whipped cream

Lightly grease the insert of the slow cooker with the coconut oil. Place the pumpkin, cranberries, blueberries, erythritol, orange juice and zest, coconut milk, cinnamon, allspice, and nutmeg in the insert. Cover and cook on low for 3 to 4 hours. Let the compote cool for 1 hour and serve warm with a generous scoop of whipped cream.

Per serving: Calories: 113; Fat: 9g; Protein: 4g; Total Carbs: 7g; Fiber: 3g; Net Carbs: 4g; **Macros:** Fat: 72%; Protein: 7%; Carbs: 21%

Blackberry Cobbler

SERVES 10 | PREP TIME: 15 minutes | COOK TIME: 3 to 4 hours on low

For the filling
1 tablespoon coconut oil
6 cups blackberries

½ cup granulated erythritol
1 teaspoon ground cinnamon

For the topping
2 cups ground almonds
½ cup granulated erythritol
1 tablespoon baking powder

½ teaspoon salt
1 cup heavy (whipping) cream
½ cup butter, melted

For the filling: Lightly grease the insert of a 4-quart slow cooker with the coconut oil. Add the blackberries, erythritol, and cinnamon to the insert. Mix to combine. For the topping: In a large bowl, stir the almonds, erythritol, baking powder, and salt. Add the heavy cream and butter and stir until a thick batter forms. Drop the batter by the tablespoon on top of the blackberries. Cover and cook on low for 3 to 4 hours. Serve warm.

Per serving: Calories: 281; Fat: 31g; Protein: 8g; Total Carbs: 10g; Fiber: 6g; Net Carbs: 4g; **Macros:** Fat: 75%; Protein: 11%; Carbs: 14%

Slow Cooker Sour-Cream Cheesecake

SERVES 10 | PREP TIME: 15 minutes, plus time to chill | COOK TIME: 5 to 6 hours on low

¼ cup butter, melted, divided
1 cup ground almonds

¾ cup plus 1 tablespoon granulated erythritol, divided

¼ teaspoon ground cinnamon
12 ounces cream cheese, at room temperature
2 large eggs

2 teaspoons pure vanilla extract
1 cup sour cream

Lightly grease a 7-inch springform pan with 1 tablespoon of the butter. In a small bowl, stir the almonds, 1 tablespoon of the erythritol, and cinnamon until blended. Add the remaining 3 tablespoons of the butter and stir until coarse crumbs form. Press the crust mixture into the springform pan along the bottom and about 2 inches up the sides. In a large bowl, using a handheld mixer, beat the cream cheese, eggs, vanilla, and remaining ¾ cup of the erythritol. Beat the sour cream into the cream-cheese mixture until smooth. Spoon the batter into the springform pan and smooth out the top. Place a wire rack in the insert of the slow cooker and place the springform pan on top. Cover and cook on low for 5 to 6 hours, or until the cheesecake doesn't jiggle when shaken. Cool completely before removing from the pan. Chill completely before serving.

Per Serving: Calories: 279; Fat: 25g; Protein: 8g; Total Carbs: 4g; Fiber: 1g; Net Carbs: 3g; **Macros:** Fat: 81%; Protein: 13%; Carbs: 6%

Peanut Butter Cheesecake

SERVES 10 | PREP TIME: 15 minutes, plus time to chill | COOK TIME: 5 to 6 hours on low

¼ cup butter, melted, divided
1 cup ground almonds
2 tablespoons cocoa powder
1 cup granulated erythritol, divided
12 ounces cream cheese, room temperature

½ cup natural peanut butter
2 large eggs, room temperature
1 teaspoon pure vanilla extract

Lightly grease a 7-inch springform pan with 1 tablespoon butter. In a small bowl, stir the almonds, cocoa powder, and ¼ cup erythritol until blended. Add the remaining 3 tablespoons of the butter and stir until coarse crumbs form. Press the crust mixture into the springform pan along the bottom and about 2 inches up the sides. In a large bowl, using a handheld mixer, beat the cream cheese and peanut butter until smooth. Beat in the remaining ¾ cup of the erythritol, eggs, and vanilla. Spoon the batter into the springform pan and smooth out the top. Place a wire rack in the insert of a slow cooker and place the springform pan on the wire rack. Cover and cook on low for 5 to 6 hours, or until the cheesecake doesn't jiggle when shaken. Cool completely before removing from the pan. Chill before serving.

Per Serving: Calories: 311; Fat: 28g; Protein: 11g; Total Carbs: 5g; Fiber: 2g; Net Carbs: 3g; **Macros:** Fat: 80%; Protein: 14%; Carbs: 6%

Blueberry Crisp

SERVES 8 | PREP TIME: 10 minutes | COOK TIME: 3 to 4 hours on low

5 tablespoons coconut oil, melted, divided
4 cups blueberries
¾ cup plus 2 tablespoons granulated erythritol

1 cup ground pecans
1 teaspoon baking soda
½ teaspoon ground cinnamon
2 tablespoons coconut milk
1 large egg

Lightly grease a 4-quart slow cooker with 1 tablespoon of the coconut oil. Add the blueberries and 2 tablespoons of erythritol to the insert. In a large bowl, stir the remaining ¾ cup of the erythritol, ground pecans, baking soda, and cinnamon until well mixed. Add the coconut milk, egg, and remaining coconut oil, and stir until coarse crumbs form. Top the contents in the insert with the pecan mixture. Cover and cook on low for 3 to 4 hours. Serve warm.

Per serving: Calories: 222; Fat: 19g; Protein: 9g; Total Carbs: 9g; Fiber: 4g; Net Carbs: 5g; **Macros:** Fat: 72%; Protein: 14%; Carbs: 14%

Tender Pound Cake

SERVES 8 | PREP TIME: 10 minutes | COOK TIME: 5 to 6 hours on low

1 tablespoon coconut oil
2 cups almond flour
1 cup granulated erythritol
½ teaspoon cream of tartar
Pinch salt

1 cup butter, melted
5 large eggs
2 teaspoons pure
  vanilla extract

Lightly grease an 8-by-4-inch loaf pan with the coconut oil. In a large bowl, stir the almond flour, erythritol, cream of tartar, and salt, until well mixed. In a small bowl, whisk the butter, eggs, and vanilla. Add the wet ingredients to the dry ingredients and stir to combine. Transfer the batter to the loaf pan. Place the loaf pan in the insert of the slow cooker. Cover and cook until a toothpick inserted in the center comes out clean, about 5 to 6 hours on low. Serve warm.

Per serving: Calories: 281; Fat: 29g; Protein: 5g; Total Carbs: 1g; Fiber: 0g; Net Carbs: 1g; **Macros:** Fat: 90%; Protein: 8%; Carbs: 2%

Almond Golden Cake

SERVES 8 | PREP TIME: 15 minutes |
COOK TIME: 3 hours on low

½ cup coconut oil, divided
1½ cups almond flour
½ cup coconut flour
½ cup granulated erythritol
2 teaspoons baking powder

3 large eggs
½ cup coconut milk
2 teaspoons pure
  vanilla extract
½ teaspoon almond extract

Line the insert of a 4-quart slow cooker with aluminum foil and grease the aluminum foil with 1 tablespoon of the coconut oil. In a medium bowl, mix the almond flour, coconut flour, erythritol, and baking powder. In a large bowl, whisk the remaining coconut oil, eggs, coconut milk, vanilla, and almond extract. Add the dry ingredients to the wet ingredients and stir until well blended. Transfer the batter to the insert and use a spatula to even the top. Cover and cook on low for 3 hours, or until a toothpick inserted in the center comes out clean. Remove the cake from the insert and cool completely before serving.

Per serving: Calories: 234; Fat: 22g; Protein: 6g; Total Carbs: 3g; Fiber: 1g; Net Carbs: 2g; **Macros:** Fat: 84%; Protein: 11%; Carbs: 5%

Delectable Peanut Butter Cup Cake

SERVES 8 | PREP TIME: 15 minutes | COOK TIME: 3 to 4 hours on low

2 tablespoons coconut
  oil, divided

1 cup almond flour

1 cup granulated erythritol, divided
1 teaspoon baking powder
¼ teaspoon salt
¾ cup natural peanut butter

½ cup heavy (whipping) cream
1 teaspoon pure
  vanilla extract
1 cup boiling water
¼ cup cocoa powder

Lightly grease the insert of a 4-quart slow cooker with 1 tablespoon of the coconut oil. In a large bowl, stir the almond flour, ½ cup of the erythritol, baking powder, and salt. In a medium bowl, whisk the peanut butter, heavy cream, and vanilla until smooth. Add the peanut butter mixture to the dry ingredients and stir to combine. Transfer the batter to the insert and spread it out evenly. In a small bowl, stir the remaining ½ cup of the erythritol, boiling water, and cocoa powder. Pour the chocolate mixture over the batter. Cover and cook on low for 3 to 4 hours. Let the cake stand for 30 minutes and serve warm.

Per serving: Calories: 244; Fat: 20g; Protein: 11g; Total Carbs: 6g; Fiber: 3g; Net Carbs: 3g; **Macros:** Fat: 70%; Protein: 20%; Carbs: 10%

Coconut-Raspberry Cake

SERVES 10 | PREP: 10 minutes | COOK: 3 hours, plus 3 to 4 hours to cool

½ cup melted coconut oil, plus more for coating the slow cooker insert
2 cups almond flour
1 cup unsweetened shredded coconut
1 cup erythritol or 1 teaspoon stevia powder

¼ cup unsweetened, unflavored protein powder
2 teaspoons baking soda
¼ teaspoon fine sea salt
4 large eggs, lightly beaten
¾ cup canned coconut milk
1 teaspoon coconut extract
1 cup raspberries, fresh
  or frozen

Generously coat the inside of the slow cooker insert with coconut oil. In a large bowl, stir the almond flour, coconut, erythritol, protein powder, baking soda, and sea salt. Whisk in the eggs, coconut milk, ½ cup of coconut oil, and coconut extract. Gently fold in the raspberries. Transfer the batter to the prepared slow cooker, cover, and cook for 3 hours on low. Turn off the slow cooker and let the cake cool for several hours, to room temperature. Serve at room temperature.

Per Serving: Calories: 405; Fat: 38g; Protein: 11g; Total Carbs: 10g; Fiber: 5g; Net Carbs: 5g; **Macros:** Fat: 80%; Protein: 10%; Carbs: 10%

Warm Gingerbread

SERVES 8 | PREP TIME: 10 minutes | COOK TIME: 3 hours on low

1 tablespoon coconut oil
2 cups almond flour
¾ cup granulated erythritol
2 tablespoons coconut flour
2 tablespoons ground ginger
2 teaspoons baking powder
2 teaspoons ground cinnamon
½ teaspoon ground nutmeg

¼ teaspoon ground cloves
Pinch salt
¾ cup heavy (whipping) cream
½ cup butter, melted
4 large eggs
1 teaspoon pure
  vanilla extract

Lightly grease the insert of the slow cooker with coconut oil. In a large bowl, stir the almond flour, erythritol, coconut flour, ginger, baking powder, cinnamon, nutmeg, cloves, and salt. In a medium bowl, whisk the heavy cream, butter, eggs, and vanilla. Add the wet ingredients to the dry ingredients and stir to combine. Spoon the batter into the insert. Cover and cook on low for 3 hours, or until a toothpick inserted in the center comes out clean. Serve warm.

Per serving: Calories: 259; Fat: 23g; Protein: 7g; Total Carbs: 6g; Fiber: 3g; Net Carbs: 3g; **Macros:** Fat: 80%; Protein: 11%; Carbs: 9%

Carrot Cake

SERVES 8 | PREP TIME: 15 minutes | COOK TIME: 3 hours on low

½ cup coconut oil, melted, divided	1 teaspoon baking powder
1 cup granulated erythritol	1 teaspoon ground cinnamon
2 large eggs	½ teaspoon baking soda
¼ cup almond milk	½ teaspoon ground ginger
2 teaspoons pure vanilla extract	¼ teaspoon ground nutmeg
	Pinch ground allspice
1½ cups almond flour	1 cup finely shredded carrots

Lightly grease a 7-inch springform pan with 1 tablespoon of the coconut oil. In a large bowl, using a handheld mixer, beat the remaining coconut oil, erythritol, eggs, almond milk, and vanilla until blended. In a medium bowl, stir the almond flour, baking powder, cinnamon, baking soda, ginger, nutmeg, and allspice. Add the dry ingredients to the wet ingredients and stir to combine. Stir in the carrots until uniformly mixed. Spoon the batter into the springform pan and smooth out the top. Place a wire rack in the insert of the slow cooker and place the springform pan on the wire rack. Cover and cook on low for 3 hours, or until a toothpick inserted in the center comes out clean. Cool the cake and serve.

Per serving: Calories: 199; Fat: 20g; Protein: 4g; Total Carbs: 4g; Fiber: 2g; Net Carbs: 2g; **Macros:** Fat: 90%; Protein: 5%; Carbs: 5%

Lime-Raspberry Custard Cake

SERVES 8 | PREP TIME: 15 minutes | COOK TIME: 3 hours on low

1 teaspoon coconut oil	½ cup coconut flour
6 large eggs, separated	¼ teaspoon salt
2 cups heavy (whipping) cream	Juice and zest of 2 limes
	½ cup raspberries
¾ cup granulated erythritol	

Lightly grease a 7-inch springform pan with the coconut oil. In a large bowl, using a handheld mixer, beat the egg whites until stiff peaks form, about 5 minutes. In a large bowl, whisk the yolks, heavy cream, erythritol, coconut flour, salt, and lime juice and zest. Fold the egg whites into the mixture. Transfer the batter to the springform pan and sprinkle the raspberries over the top. Place a wire rack in the insert of the slow cooker and place the springform pan on the wire rack. Cover and cook on low for 3 hours, or until a toothpick inserted in the center comes out clean. Remove the cover and allow the cake to cool to room temperature. Place the springform pan in the refrigerator for at least 2 hours, until the cake is firm. Carefully remove the sides of the springform pan. Slice and serve.

Per serving: Calories: 165; Fat: 15g; Protein: 6g; Total Carbs: 4g; Fiber: 1g; Net Carbs: 3g; **Macros:** Fat: 80%; Protein: 15%; Carbs: 5%

Slow Cooker Tangy Lemon Cake with Lemon Glaze

SERVES 8 | PREP: 10 minutes | COOK: 6 hours on low or 3 hours on high

For the glaze

½ cup boiling water	2 tablespoons freshly squeezed lemon juice
2 tablespoons unsalted butter or Ghee, melted	¼ cup erythritol

For the cake

Coconut oil, for coating the insert	½ cup (1 stick) unsalted butter or ghee melted and cooled slightly
2 cups almond flour	
½ cup erythritol	½ cup heavy (whipping) cream
2 teaspoons baking powder	Grated zest and juice of 2 lemons
3 large eggs	

In a small bowl, stir all the ingredients. Set aside. Coat the inside of the slow cooker insert with coconut oil. In a medium bowl, mix the almond flour, erythritol, and baking powder. In a large bowl, beat the eggs, then whisk in the butter, heavy cream, lemon zest, and lemon juice. Add the dry ingredients to the wet ingredients. Stir to mix well. Transfer the batter to the insert and spread evenly with a rubber spatula. Pour the glaze over the cake batter. Cover and cook for 6 hours on low or 3 hours on high. Serve warm or at room temperature.

Per Serving: Calories: 420; Fat: 40g; Protein: 11g Total Carbs: 10g; Fiber: 4g; Net Carbs: 6g; **Macros:** Fat: 82%; Protein: 9%; Carbs: 9%

Brownie Chocolate Cake

SERVES 12 | PREP TIME: 10 minutes | COOK TIME: 3 hours on low

½ cup plus 1 tablespoon unsalted butter, melted, divided	¼ teaspoon fine salt
	1 cup heavy (whipping) cream
1½ cups almond flour	3 large eggs, beaten
¾ cup cocoa powder	2 teaspoons pure vanilla extract
¾ cup granulated erythritol	1 cup whipped cream
1 teaspoon baking powder	

Generously grease the insert of the slow cooker with 1 tablespoon of the melted butter. In a large bowl, stir the almond flour, cocoa powder, erythritol, baking powder, and salt. In a medium bowl, whisk the remaining ½ cup of the melted butter, heavy cream, eggs, and vanilla until well blended. Whisk the wet ingredients into the dry ingredients and spoon the batter into the insert. Cover and cook on low for 3 hours, and then remove the insert from the slow cooker and let the cake sit for 1 hour. Serve warm with the whipped cream.

Per serving: Calories: 185; Fat: 16g; Protein: 5g; Total Carbs: 7g; Fiber: 1g; Net Carbs: 6g; **Macros:** Fat: 80%; Protein: 8%; Carbs: 12%

Slow Cooker Moist Ginger Cake with Whipped Cream

SERVES 10 | PREP: 15 minutes | COOK: 3 hours on low

For the cake

½ cup (1 stick) unsalted butter, melted, plus more for coating the slow cooker insert

2¼ cups almond flour

¾ cup erythritol

2 tablespoons coconut flour

1½ tablespoons ground ginger

1 tablespoon unsweetened cocoa powder

2 teaspoons baking powder

1½ teaspoons ground cinnamon

½ teaspoon ground cloves

¼ teaspoon fine sea salt

4 large eggs, lightly beaten

⅔ cup heavy (whipping) cream

1 teaspoon pure vanilla extract

For the whipped cream

1 cup heavy (whipping) cream

½ teaspoon stevia powder or ½ cup erythritol

1 teaspoon pure vanilla extract

Generously coat the inside of the slow cooker insert with butter. In a large bowl, mix the almond flour, erythritol, coconut flour, ginger, cocoa powder, baking powder, cinnamon, cloves, and sea salt. Add butter, eggs, heavy cream, and vanilla. Mix and transfer to the insert. Cover and cook for 3 hours on low. Serve warm with whipped cream. In a large bowl, use an electric mixer set on medium-high to beat the heavy cream, stevia, and vanilla until stiff peaks form, about 5 minutes.

Per Serving: Calories: 453; Fat: 43g; Protein: 12g; Total Carbs: 12g; Fiber: 5g; Net Carbs: 7g; **Macros:** Fat: 80%; Protein: 10%; Carbs: 10%

Vanilla Cheesecake

SERVES 8 | PREP: 15 minutes | COOK: 4 hours on low or 2 hours on high, plus time to chill

For the crust

1 cup toasted walnuts, ground to a meal

1 large egg, lightly beaten

2 tablespoons coconut oil, melted

1 teaspoon stevia powder

1 cup water

For the filling

2 large eggs

2 (8-ounce) packages cream cheese, at room temperature

¼ cup heavy (whipping) cream

2 teaspoons pure vanilla extract

½ cup erythritol

1 tablespoon coconut flour

½ teaspoon stevia powder

In a medium bowl, mix the walnut meal, egg, coconut oil, and stevia powder. Press the mixture into the bottom of a baking pan that fits into your slow cooker (make sure there is room to lift the pan out). Pour the water into the slow cooker insert. Place the pan in the cooker. In a large bowl, beat the eggs, then beat in the cream cheese, heavy cream, vanilla, erythritol, coconut flour, and stevia powder. Pour the mixture over the crust. Cover and cook for 4 hours on low or 2 hours on high. When finished, turn off the cooker and let the cheesecake sit inside until cooled to room temperature, up to 3 hours. Remove the pan from the slow cooker and refrigerate until chilled, about 2 hours more. Serve chilled.

Per Serving: Calories: 338; Fat: 33g; Protein: 7g; Total Carbs: 5g; Fiber: 1g; Net Carbs: 4g; **Macros:** Fat: 86%; Protein: 9%; Carbs: 5%

Chocolate–Macadamia Nut Cheesecake

SERVES 8 | PREP: 15 minutes | COOK: 4 hours on low or 2 hours on high, plus time to chill

For the crust

1 cup macadamia nuts, ground to a meal

1 large egg, lightly beaten

2 tablespoons coconut oil, melted

1 teaspoon stevia powder

1 cup water

For the filling

6 ounces unsweetened chocolate, chopped

2 large eggs

2 (8-ounce) packages cream cheese, at room temperature

¼ cup coconut cream

1 tablespoon coconut flour

1 teaspoon pure vanilla extract

½ cup erythritol

½ teaspoon stevia powder

¼ cup coarsely chopped macadamia nuts

In a medium bowl, stir the macadamia nut meal, egg, coconut oil, and stevia powder. Press the mixture into the bottom of a baking pan that fits into your slow cooker (make sure there is room on the sides so you can lift the pan out). Pour the water into the slow cooker insert. Place the pan in the cooker. In a microwave-safe bowl, heat the chocolate in the microwave for 1 minute on high. Stir and then microwave in 30-second intervals, stirring in between, until the chocolate is melted and smooth. Set aside. In a large bowl, beat the eggs, then beat in the cream cheese, coconut cream, coconut flour, vanilla, erythritol, and stevia powder. Stir in the chocolate until well incorporated. Pour the mixture over the crust. Cover and cook for 4 hours on low or 2 hours on high. When finished, turn off the slow cooker and let the cheesecake sit inside until cooled to room temperature, up to 3 hours. Remove the pan from the slow cooker and refrigerate until chilled, about 2 hours more. Sprinkle the macadamia nuts over the top and serve chilled.

Per Serving: Calories: 433; Fat: 44g; Protein: 8g; Total Carbs: 6g; Fiber: 2g; Net Carbs: 4g; **Macros:** Fat: 87%; Protein: 7%; Carbs: 6%

Toasted Almond Cheesecake

SERVES 8 | PREP: 15 minutes | COOK: 4 hours on low or 2 hours on high, plus time to chill

For the crust

1 cup toasted almonds, ground to a meal

1 large egg, lightly beaten

2 tablespoons coconut oil, melted

1 teaspoon stevia powder

1 cup water

For the filling

2 large eggs

2 (8-ounce) packages cream cheese, at room temperature

¾ cup almond butter

¼ cup coconut cream

1 teaspoon pure almond extract

¾ cup erythritol

1 tablespoon coconut flour

2 teaspoons stevia powder

In a medium bowl, mix the almond meal, egg, coconut oil, and stevia powder. Press the mixture into the bottom of a baking pan that fits into your slow cooker (make sure there is room to lift the pan out). Pour the water into the slow cooker insert. Place the pan in the cooker. In a large bowl, beat the eggs, then beat in the cream cheese, almond butter, coconut cream, almond extract, erythritol, coconut flour, and stevia powder. Pour the mixture over the crust. Cover and cook for 4 hours on low or 2 hours on high. When finished, turn off the slow cooker and let the cheesecake sit inside until cooled to room temperature, up to 3 hours. Remove the pan from the slow cooker and refrigerate until chilled, about 2 hours more. Serve chilled.

Per Serving: Calories: 538; Fat: 51g; Protein: 14g; Total Carbs: 12g; Fiber: 3g; Net Carbs: 9g; **Macros:** Fat: 82%; Protein: 9%; Carbs: 9%

Slow Cooker Chocolate Chip Cookies

SERVES 10 | PREP: 10 minutes | COOK: 2½ hours on low

¼ cup coconut oil, melted, plus more for coating the parchment
1 cup erythritol
1 teaspoon stevia powder
1 large egg, beaten
½ teaspoon pure vanilla extract

1½ cups almond flour
1¾ teaspoons baking powder
½ teaspoon fine sea salt
4 ounces unsweetened chocolate, chopped
½ cup chopped toasted walnuts

Line a slow cooker insert with enough parchment or wax paper to extend over the sides slightly. Coat the parchment with coconut oil. In a large bowl, stir the ¼ cup of melted coconut oil, erythritol, and stevia powder. Beat in the egg and vanilla. Add the almond flour, baking powder, and sea salt and beat until well combined. Gently fold in the chocolate and walnuts. Transfer the dough to the insert and press it into an even layer, covering the bottom of the insert. Cover and cook for 2½ hours on low. Using the parchment as a sling, lift the cookie out of the insert and transfer to a wire rack to cool. Cut into squares and serve warm or at room temperature.

Per Serving: Calories: 234; Fat: 23g; Protein: 6g; Total Carbs: 8g; Fiber: 4g; Net Carbs: 4g; **Macros:** Fat: 83%; Protein: 8%; Carbs: 9%

Chocolate Cake with Whipped Cream

SERVES 12 | PREP: 15 minutes | COOK: 3 hours on low

For the cake
Coconut oil, for coating the slow cooker insert
1½ cups almond flour
¾ cup erythritol
⅔ cup unsweetened cocoa powder
¼ cup unflavored, unsweetened protein powder
2 teaspoons baking powder

¼ teaspoon fine sea salt
4 large eggs, lightly beaten
¾ cup canned coconut milk
½ cup (1 stick) unsalted butter, melted
1 teaspoon pure vanilla extract
½ cup chopped toasted hazelnuts

For the whipped cream
1 cup heavy (whipping) cream
2 teaspoons stevia powder or ½ cup erythritol

1 teaspoon pure vanilla extract or hazelnut extract

Generously coat the inside of the slow cooker insert with coconut oil. In a medium bowl, whisk almond flour, erythritol, cocoa powder, protein powder, baking powder, and sea salt. Stir in the eggs, coconut milk, butter, and vanilla until well mixed. Gently fold in the hazelnuts. Transfer the batter to the prepared insert. Cover and cook for 3 hours on low. In a large bowl, use an electric mixer set on medium-high to beat the heavy cream, stevia, and vanilla until stiff peaks form, about 5 minutes. Turn off the slow cooker and let the cake cool for 30 minutes. Serve warm, topped with the whipped cream.

Per Serving: Calories: 323; Fat: 30g; Protein: 9g; Total Carbs: 8g; Fiber: 3g; Net Carbs: 5g; **Macros:** Fat: 80%; Protein: 10%; Carbs: 10%

Fudge Nut Brownies

MAKES 12 BROWNIES | PREP: 15 minutes | COOK: 4 hours on low

¼ cup unsalted butter, plus more for coating the slow cooker insert
4 ounces unsweetened chocolate, chopped
1½ cups almond flour
½ cup unsweetened cocoa powder
¼ cup coconut flour
2 teaspoons baking powder

¼ teaspoon fine sea salt
1 large ripe avocado, peeled, pitted, and mashed
¼ cup heavy (whipping) cream
3 large eggs, lightly beaten
¾ cup erythritol
¾ teaspoon stevia powder
¾ cup coarsely chopped walnuts

Coat the bottom and sides of the slow cooker insert with butter, then line the bottom with parchment or wax paper (trace the bottom of the insert on the parchment and then cut it out). In a small, microwave-safe bowl, combine ¼ cup of butter and the chocolate. Heat for 30-second intervals on high, stirring after each interval, until the chocolate is melted and the ingredients are fully incorporated. In a medium bowl, stir the almond flour, cocoa powder, coconut flour, baking powder, and salt. In a large bowl, mix the avocado and heavy cream until smooth. Add the eggs, erythritol, and stevia and mix to combine. Mix in the melted chocolate until incorporated. Add the dry ingredients to the wet ingredients and mix until incorporated. Stir in the walnuts. Transfer the mixture to the slow cooker and spread evenly. Cover and cook for 4 hours on low. Let cool for about 30 minutes in the slow cooker. Run a knife around the edge and then lift out of the insert. Cut into pieces and serve at room temperature.

Per Serving: (1 brownie) Calories: 229; Fat: 21g; Protein: 6g; Total Carbs: 10g; Fiber: 5g; Net Carbs: 5g; **Macros:** Fat: 78%; Protein: 9%; Carbs: 13%

SNACKS & APPS

Bacon-Pepper Fat Bombs

MAKES 12 FAT BOMBS | PREP TIME: 10 minutes, plus 1 hour to chill

2 ounces goat cheese, at room temperature

2 ounces cream cheese, at room temperature

¼ cup butter, at room temperature

8 bacon slices, cooked and chopped

Pinch freshly ground black pepper

Line a small baking sheet with parchment paper and set aside. In a medium bowl, stir the goat cheese, cream cheese, butter, bacon, and pepper until well combined. Use a tablespoon to drop mounds of the bomb mixture on the baking sheet and place the sheet in the freezer until the fat bombs are very firm but not frozen, about 1 hour.

Per Serving: (1 fat bomb) Calories: 89; Fat: 8g; Protein: 3g; Total Carbs: 0g; Fiber: 0g; Net Carbs: 0g; **Macros:** Fat: 84%; Protein: 15%; Carbs: 1%

Smoked Salmon Fat Bombs

MAKES 12 FAT BOMBS | PREP TIME: 10 minutes, plus 2 hours to chill

½ cup goat cheese, at room temperature

½ cup butter, at room temperature

2 ounces smoked salmon

2 teaspoons freshly squeezed lemon juice

Pinch freshly ground black pepper

Line a baking sheet with parchment paper and set aside. In a medium bowl, stir the goat cheese, butter, smoked salmon, lemon juice, and pepper until very well blended. Use a tablespoon to scoop the salmon mixture onto the baking sheet until you have 12 even mounds. Place the baking sheet in the refrigerator until the fat bombs are firm, 2 to 3 hours.

Per Serving: (2 fat bombs) Calories: 193; Fat: 18g; Protein: 8g; Total Carbs: 0g; Fiber: 0g; Net Carbs: 0g; **Macros:** Fat: 84%; Protein: 16%; Carbs: 0%

Bacon Chive Fat Bombs

MAKES 8 FAT BOMBS | PREP TIME: 5 minutes

8 ounces cream cheese, at room temperature

¼ cup butter, at room temperature

4 bacon slices, cooked, cooled, and crumbled

1 tablespoon minced chives

¼ teaspoon freshly ground black pepper

¼ cup grated Parmesan cheese

In a bowl, mix the cream cheese, butter, crumbled bacon, chives, and pepper. Divide the mixture into eight small balls. Roll the balls in the Parmesan cheese to coat lightly. Refrigerate until ready to serve.

Per Serving: (1 fat bomb): Calories: 190; Fat: 19g; Protein: 5g; Total Carbs: 1g; Fiber: 0g; Net Carbs: 1g; **Macros:** Fat: 90%; Protein: 9%; Carbs: 1%

Sun-Dried Tomato and Feta Fat Bombs

MAKES 8 FAT BOMBS | PREP TIME: 5 minutes

4 ounces cream cheese, at room temperature

¼ cup butter, at room temperature

2 ounces crumbled feta cheese

¼ cup minced sun-dried tomatoes

1 tablespoon minced fresh oregano

1 tablespoon minced fresh parsley

¼ teaspoon freshly ground black pepper

¼ cup almond flour

In a bowl, mix the cream cheese, butter, feta cheese, sun-dried tomatoes, oregano, parsley, and pepper. Divide the mixture into 8 small balls. Roll the balls in the almond flour to coat lightly. Refrigerate until ready to serve.

Per Serving: (1 fat bomb): Calories: 154; Fat: 15g; Protein: 4g; Total Carbs: 3g; Fiber: 1g; Net Carbs: 2g; **Macros:** Fat: 88%; Protein: 10%; Carbs: 2%

Avocado Chili Fat Bomb

MAKES 10 FAT BOMBS | PREP TIME: 25 minutes, plus 4 hours to chill

1 ripe avocado, peeled

⅓ cup cocoa butter

1 tablespoon freshly squeezed lime juice

1 teaspoon chopped fresh cilantro

1 teaspoon minced jalapeño pepper

1 teaspoon minced garlic

Place the avocado, cocoa butter, lime juice, cilantro, jalapeño, and garlic in a blender and pulse until smooth. Transfer the mixture to a bowl and place in the refrigerator until firm enough to roll into balls, about 1 hour. Roll into 10 balls and place in the freezer to firm up, about 3 hours. Serve frozen.

Per Serving: (1 fat bomb): Calories: 94; Fat: 10g; Protein: 0.4g; Total Carbs: 2g; Fiber: 1g; Net Carbs: 1g; **Macros:** Fat: 96%; Protein: 2%; Carbs: 2%

"Everything but the Bagel" Fat Bombs

MAKES 7 FAT BOMBS | PREP TIME: 10 minutes, plus 1 hour 30 minutes to chill

8 ounces cream cheese, at room temperature

2 cups shredded Cheddar cheese

1 (2.3-ounce) jar "Everything but the Bagel" seasoning

In a medium bowl or in a food processor, combine the cream cheese and Cheddar cheese until well mixed. Put the mixture in the refrigerator to harden for 1 hour. Line a baking sheet with parchment paper. Pour the seasoning onto a plate and set aside. Remove the cheese mixture from the refrigerator and roll it into 1-inch balls. Roll each ball in the seasoning mix until completely covered. Transfer the coated balls to the prepared baking sheet. Place the baking sheet in the refrigerator to chill for 30 minutes.

Per Serving: (2 balls): Calories: 246; Fat: 22g; Protein: 11g; Total Carbs: 1g; Fiber: 0g; Net Carbs: 1g; **Macros:** Fat: 80%; Protein: 19%; Carbs: 1%

Cheesy Dill Fat Bombs

SERVES 7 | PREP TIME: 10 minutes, plus 1 hour 30 minutes to chill

8 ounces cream cheese, at room temperature

2 cups shredded Cheddar cheese

6 mini dill pickles, finely chopped

2 tablespoons minced fresh dill

In a medium bowl or in a food processor, combine the cream cheese and Cheddar cheese until well mixed. Fold in the pickles and dill. Put the mixture in the refrigerator to harden for 1 hour. Line a baking sheet with parchment paper. Remove the cheese mixture from the refrigerator and roll it into 1-inch balls. Transfer the balls to the prepared baking sheet. Place the baking sheet in the refrigerator to chill for 30 minutes.

Per Serving: (2 balls): Calories: 254; Fat: 22g; Protein: 11g; Total Carbs: 3g; Fiber: 1g; Net Carbs: 2g; **Macros:** Fat: 78%; Protein: 17%; Carbs: 5%

Almond Crackers

SERVES 6 | PREP TIME: 5 minutes | COOK TIME: 10 to 12 minutes

2 cups almond flour

½ teaspoon sea salt

3 tablespoons olive oil

1 to 2 tablespoons ice water

Preheat the oven to 325°F. In a bowl, stir the almond flour and sea salt. Stir in the olive oil and just enough water to bind, starting with 1 tablespoon and adding more as needed. Stir until the dough comes together into a ball. Place the ball between two sheets of parchment paper and roll with a rolling pin until very thin, about the thickness of a nickel. Remove the top sheet of parchment paper. Slice the dough into individual squares or rectangles. Carefully slide the dough and parchment paper onto a rimmed baking sheet. Bake for 10 to 12 minutes, or until the crackers are golden brown and crisp. Allow to cool before storing in a covered container.

Per Serving: (2 crackers): Calories: 273; Fat: 25g; Protein: 8g; Total Carbs: 8g; Fiber: 4g; Net Carbs: 4g; **Macros:** Fat: 78%; Protein: 11%; Carbs: 11%

Nut Crackers

SERVES 12 | PREP TIME: 25 minutes | COOK TIME: 10 minutes

1 cup almond flour

2 tablespoons egg white protein powder

¼ cup ground walnuts

2 tablespoons extra-virgin olive oil

2 large egg whites

Preheat the oven to 350°F. Line a 9-by-13-inch baking dish with parchment, and set aside. In a medium bowl, stir the almond flour, egg white protein powder, and ground walnuts. Stir in the olive oil and egg whites to form a stiff dough. Press the dough evenly into the baking dish, and use a paring knife to cut the dough into 24 squares. Bake until the crackers are golden brown, about 10 minutes.

Per Serving: (2 crackers): Calories: 96; Fat: 8g; Protein: 4g; Total Carbs: 2g; Fiber: 1g; Net Carbs: 1g; **Macros:** Fat: 75%; Protein: 17%; Carbs: 8%

Seedy Crackers

SERVES 4 | PREP TIME: 20 minutes | COOK TIME: 15 minutes

1 cup almond flour

1 tablespoon sesame seeds

1 tablespoon flaxseed

1 tablespoon fennel seed

¼ teaspoon baking soda

¼ teaspoon salt

Freshly ground black pepper

1 large egg, at room temperature

1 tablespoon olive oil

Preheat the oven to 350°F. Line a baking sheet with parchment paper and set aside. In a large bowl, combine the almond flour, sesame seeds, flaxseed, fennel, baking soda, salt, and pepper and stir well. In a small bowl, whisk the egg until well beaten. Add the egg and olive oil to the dry ingredients and stir well to combine and form the dough into a ball. Place one layer of parchment paper on the countertop and place the dough on top. Cover with a second layer of parchment and using a rolling pin, roll the dough to ⅛-inch thickness, aiming for a rectangular shape. Cut the dough into 1- to 2-inch crackers, transfer the crackers to the prepared baking sheet, and bake for 10 to 15 minutes, until crispy and slightly golden.

Per Serving: Calories: 238; Fat: 21g; Protein: 9g; Total Carbs: 7g; Fiber: 4g; Net Carbs: 3g; **Macros:** Fat: 79%; Protein: 15%; Carbs: 6%

Crispy Parmesan Crackers

MAKES 8 CRACKERS | PREP TIME: 10 minutes | COOK TIME: 5 minutes

1 teaspoon butter

8 ounces Parmesan cheese, shredded or freshly grated

Preheat the oven to 400°F. Line a baking sheet with parchment paper and lightly grease the paper with the butter. Spoon the Parmesan cheese onto the baking sheet in mounds, spread evenly apart. Spread out the mounds with the back of a spoon until they are flat. Bake the crackers until the edges are browned and the centers are still pale, about 5 minutes. Remove the sheet from the oven, and remove the crackers with a spatula to paper towels. Lightly blot the tops with additional paper towels and let them completely cool.

Per Serving: (1 cracker): Calories: 133; Fat: 11g; Protein: 11g; Total Carbs: 1g; Fiber: 0g; Net Carbs: 1g; **Macros:** Fat: 70%; Protein: 29%; Carbs: 1%

Flaxseed Chips and Guacamole

SERVES 6 | PREP TIME: 10 minutes | COOK TIME: 1 hour

1 cup whole flaxseeds

½ cup vegetable broth

2 teaspoons garlic powder

2 teaspoons paprika

2 teaspoons onion powder

1 teaspoon onion salt

3 large avocados, halved

½ cup diced red onion

1 tablespoon freshly squeezed lime juice

½ teaspoon salt

¼ teaspoon ground cumin

Preheat the oven to 325°F. Line a baking sheet with parchment paper. In a large bowl, combine flaxseeds, broth, garlic powder, paprika, onion powder, and onion salt, and mix well. Spread into a thin, even layer on the prepared baking sheet and bake for 55 to 60 minutes. While the chips are baking, mash the avocado in a medium bowl. Mix in the red onion, lime juice, salt, and cumin. Cover the bowl and place it in the refrigerator until you are ready to eat. Remove the flaxseed chips from the oven and allow them to cool; then break them apart into chip-size pieces. Serve with the guacamole.

Per Serving: Calories: 328; Fat: 24g; Protein: 8g; Total Carbs: 20g; Fiber: 15g; Net Carbs: 5g; **Macros:** Fat: 66%; Protein: 10%; Carbs: 24%

Spicy Cheddar Wafers

MAKES 30 WAFERS | PREP TIME: 10 minutes, plus 2 hours to chill | COOK TIME: 25 minutes

1 cup almond flour	5 tablespoons butter, at room
2 tablespoons coconut flour	temperature
¼ teaspoon kosher salt	1 ounce cream cheese, at room
¼ teaspoon cayenne pepper	temperature
¼ teaspoon garlic powder	4 ounces Cheddar cheese,
¼ teaspoon onion powder	shredded
	¼ cup finely chopped pecans

In a small bowl, stir the almond and coconut flours, salt, cayenne, garlic powder, and onion powder. Set aside. In a large bowl and using an electric hand mixer, cream the butter and cream cheese. Add the Cheddar cheese, and mix until well combined. Add the almond flour mixture and mix to combine. Stir in the chopped pecans. Place the dough on plastic wrap or parchment paper and form it into a roll about 2½ inches thick. Wrap the dough tightly and refrigerate until firm, at least 2 hours. Preheat the oven to 300°F. Line a baking sheet with parchment paper. Slice the chilled dough into ¼-inch-thick slices and place them on the prepared baking sheet. Bake for 20 to 25 minutes, or until lightly golden brown. Cool the crackers completely on the pan before removing.

Per Serving: (3 wafers): Calories: 184; Fat: 16g; Protein: 6g; Total Carbs: 4g; Fiber: 2g; Net Carbs: 2g; **Macros:** Fat: 78%; Protein: 13%; Carbs: 9%

Triple Cheese Chips

SERVES 4 | PREP TIME: 10 minutes | COOK TIME: 7 minutes

Olive oil spray	¼ cup finely shredded
½ cup finely shredded Parmesan cheese	jalapeño Cheddar cheese
	Pinch cayenne pepper
½ cup finely shredded Cheddar cheese	

Preheat the oven to 425°F. Lightly spray a baking sheet with oil and line with parchment paper. In a medium bowl, toss the Parmesan, Cheddars, and cayenne pepper until well mixed. Drop the cheese mixture onto the baking sheet, about 1½ tablespoons per chip. Spread out the cheese with the back of a spoon, leaving a minimum of 1 inch between the edges. Bake until melted and bubbly, but do not brown, 5 to 7 minutes. Remove the chips from the baking sheet and cool on a baking rack.

Per Serving: Calories: 138; Fat: 11g; Protein: 10g; Total Carbs: 1g; Fiber: 0g; Net Carbs: 1g; **Macros:** Fat: 72%; Protein: 29%; Carbs: 1%

Parmesan Zucchini Chips

SERVES 2 | PREP TIME: 20 minutes | COOK TIME: 20 minutes

Nonstick cooking spray	1 cup grated Parmesan cheese
2 medium zucchini, cut into	1 teaspoon garlic powder
¼-inch coins	½ cup low-sugar marinara sauce
½ teaspoon salt	

Preheat the oven to 425°F. Spray a baking sheet with cooking spray. Put the zucchini slices in a medium bowl and sprinkle with the salt. Set aside for 15 minutes. In a separate bowl, combine the Parmesan cheese and garlic powder. Blot the zucchini with a paper towel and place on the prepared baking sheet. Sprinkle each zucchini coin with a generous amount of the cheese mixture. Bake for 15 to 20 minutes, or until the cheese topping is bubbling. Serve with the marinara sauce for dipping.

Per Serving: Calories: 249; Fat: 13g; Protein: 21g; Total Carbs: 12g; Fiber: 3g; Net Carbs: 9g; **Macros:** Fat: 47%; Protein: 34%; Carbs: 19%

Crispy Kale Chips

SERVES 2 | PREP TIME: 5 minutes | COOK TIME: 25 minutes

2 cups kale, cleaned, leaves trimmed from stalk	½ teaspoon freshly ground black pepper
1 tablespoon olive oil	½ teaspoon onion powder
½ teaspoon salt	½ teaspoon garlic powder

Preheat the oven to 300°F. In a large bowl, add kale leaves and the olive oil. Toss to coat the leaves evenly with the oil. Add the salt, pepper, onion powder, and garlic powder to the bowl. Toss again to coat the leaves evenly. On a parchment-lined baking sheet, spread the kale into an even layer. Place the sheet in the preheated oven. Bake for 10 minutes, rotate the baking sheet, then bake for an additional 15 minutes. Remove the baking sheet from the oven. Cool the kale on the tray for 3 minutes before serving.

Per Serving: Calories: 99; Fat: 7g; Total Carbs: 8.3g; Net Carbs: 7.2g; Fiber: 1.2g; Protein: 2.2g; **Macros:** Fat: 64%; Protein: 4%; Carbs: 32%

Margarita Pizza Chips

SERVES 8 | PREP TIME: 10 minutes | COOK TIME: 10 minutes

16 slices deli salami	Pinch pepper
2 medium tomatoes, cut into	8 ounces fresh mozzarella, cut
¼-inch-thick slices	into 16 pieces
Pinch salt	16 fresh basil leaves

Preheat the oven to 375°F. Line a rimmed baking sheet with parchment paper. Line a plate with paper towels. Lay the salami on the parchment paper and bake for 9 minutes, until the salami browns on the edges and begins to shrink. While the salami bakes, season the tomatoes with salt and pepper and set aside. Transfer the salami it to the prepared plate to drain excess oil for a couple of minutes. Turn the oven to broil. Place the crisp salami on the prepared baking sheet. Top each slice with a slice of tomato, a basil leaf, and a mozzarella slice. Return the baking sheet to the oven and broil for 60 to 90 seconds, until the cheese begins to bubble. Allow the bites to cool for 2 to 3 minutes, then transfer to a dish and serve.

Per Serving: Calories: 155; Fat: 12g; Protein: 9g; Total Carbs: 1g; Fiber: <1g; Net Carbs: 1g; **Macros:** Fat: 72%; Protein: 25%; Carbs: 3%

Garlic Pepperoni Chips

SERVES 4 | PREP TIME: 5 minutes | COOK TIME: 10 minutes | TOTAL TIME: 15 minutes

6 ounces pepperoni slices	½ teaspoon garlic powder

Preheat the oven to 425°F. On a parchment-lined baking sheet, lay out the pepperoni slices about ½ inch apart. Sprinkle the slices with the garlic powder. Place the sheet in the preheated oven. Bake for 7 to 8 minutes. Remove the tray and flip each slice. Bake for another 2 to 3 minutes, or until the pepperoni slices are golden brown and crispy.

Per Serving: (1½ ounces pepperoni): Calories: 200; Fat: 17g; Protein: 8.6g; Total Carbs: 0.2g; Fiber: 0g; Net Carbs: 0.2g; **Macros:** Fat: 81%; Protein: 18%; Carbs: 1%

Savory Party Mix

SERVES 12 | PREP TIME: 5 minutes | COOK TIME: 20 minutes

½ cup pecans
½ cup cashews
½ cup pistachios
½ cup peanuts
½ cup almonds
½ cup pumpkin seeds

½ cup sunflower seeds
2 teaspoons onion powder
1 teaspoon garlic powder
½ teaspoon salt
2 tablespoons olive oil

Preheat the oven to 350°F. Line a baking sheet with parchment paper. In a large bowl, combine the pecans, cashews, pistachios, peanuts, almonds, pumpkin seeds, and sunflower seeds. Stir in the onion powder, garlic powder, and salt. Pour in the oil. Toss well to thoroughly coat the nuts and seeds with the oil. Spread the mixture in a single layer on the prepared baking sheet and bake for 10 minutes. Stir well and place back in the oven to bake for 10 additional minutes. Remove from the oven and allow to cool completely before serving.

Per Serving: (⅓ cup): Calories: 214; Fat: 18g; Protein: 6g; Total Carbs: 7g; Fiber: 2g; Net Carbs: 5g; **Macros:** Fat: 76%; Protein: 11%; Carbs: 13%

Dips Herby Yogurt Dip

SERVES 6 | PREP TIME: 10 minutes

1 cup plain Greek yogurt
¼ cup extra-virgin olive oil
¼ cup chopped fresh parsley
1 tablespoon freshly squeezed lemon juice
1 tablespoon chopped fresh dill or 1 teaspoon dried dill

1 tablespoon chopped fresh oregano or 1 teaspoon dried oregano
1 teaspoon garlic powder
1 teaspoon salt
½ teaspoon freshly ground black pepper
Assorted raw vegetables, for serving

In a medium bowl, combine the yogurt, olive oil, parsley, lemon juice, dill, oregano, garlic powder, salt, and pepper and whisk well until smooth and creamy. Serve with raw vegetables or atop grilled meats or fish.

Per Serving: (¼ cup): Calories: 118; Fat: 11g; Protein: 4g; Total Carbs: 2g; Fiber: <1g; Net Carbs: 2g; **Macros:** Fat: 84%; Protein: 14%; Carbs: 2%

Bacon Guacamole

SERVES 4 | PREP TIME: 5 minutes | COOK TIME: 10 minutes

4 bacon slices
2 avocados, peeled, pitted, and diced
½ cup chopped yellow onion

⅓ cup chopped tomato
2 teaspoons minced garlic
1 jalapeño pepper, minced
1 serrano pepper, minced

1 tablespoon chopped fresh cilantro
1 teaspoon freshly squeezed lime juice

¼ teaspoon cayenne pepper
¼ teaspoon salt
⅛ teaspoon freshly ground black pepper

Heat a large skillet over medium-high heat. Add the bacon. Cook for 3 minutes. Flip and cook for another 2 to 3 minutes. Transfer the cooked bacon to paper towels to cool. Once cooled, chop the bacon and set aside. In a large bowl, combine the avocados, onion, and tomato. Add the garlic, jalapeño pepper, and serrano pepper. Gently fold the ingredients together. Before the ingredients are fully incorporated, add the cilantro, chopped bacon, lime juice, cayenne pepper, salt, and black pepper to the bowl. Mix all ingredients. Serve immediately.

Per Serving: Calories: 259; Fat: 23g; Protein: 5g; Total Carbs: 12g; Fiber: 8g; Net Carbs: 4g; **Macros:** Fat: 75%; Protein: 8%; Carbs: 17%

Coconut Tzatziki

SERVES 4 | PREP TIME: 10 minutes, plus overnight to chill

1 cup grated cucumber, with the liquid squeezed out
½ cup plain Greek yogurt
½ cup coconut milk
1 teaspoon minced garlic

2 tablespoons freshly squeezed lemon juice
2 tablespoons coconut oil, melted
1 teaspoon chopped fresh dill
Pinch sea salt

In a medium bowl, stir the cucumber, yogurt, coconut milk, garlic, lemon juice, coconut oil, dill, and salt. Refrigerate overnight in a sealed container. Serve.

Per Serving: Calories: 149; Fat: 12g; Protein: 4g; Total Carbs: 4g; Fiber: 1g; Net Carbs: 3g; **Macros:** Fat: 78%; Protein: 11%; Carbs: 11%

Tzatziki Dip with Vegetables

SERVES 4 | PREP TIME: 5 minutes | COOK TIME: 0 minutes

5 ounces plain Greek yogurt
¼ cup mayonnaise
½ cup diced, peeled cucumbers
1 teaspoon minced fresh dill
1 teaspoon minced fresh garlic

Sea salt
Freshly ground black pepper
4 celery stalks, halved and sliced into 3-inch pieces
2 carrots, halved and sliced into 3-inch pieces

In a small bowl, mix the yogurt, mayonnaise, cucumbers, dill, and garlic. Season to taste with salt and pepper. Serve alongside the vegetables.

Per Serving: (¼ cup dip and 6 to 8 vegetable pieces) Calories: 162; Fat: 14g; Protein: 3g; Total Carbs: 9g; Fiber: 2g; Net Carbs: 7g; **Macros:** Fat: 78%; Protein: 7%; Carbs: 15%

Lemon-Turmeric Aioli

MAKES 1 CUP | PREP TIME: 5 minutes

1 cup mayonnaise
Juice and zest of 1 lemon
2 garlic cloves, very finely minced
1 teaspoon monk fruit extract (optional)

¼ to ½ teaspoon ground cayenne pepper or red pepper flakes (optional)
½ to 1 teaspoon ground turmeric

In a small bowl, combine the mayo, lemon juice and zest, garlic, monk fruit extract (if using), turmeric, and cayenne (if using) and whisk well until smooth and creamy.

Per Serving: (2 tablespoons): Calories: 254; Fat: 28g; Protein: 1g; Total Carbs: 1g; Fiber: <1g; Net Carbs: 1g; **Macros:** Fat: 99%; Carbs: <1%; Protein: <1%

Guacamole

SERVES 4 | PREP TIME: 5 minutes

2 large avocados, pitted and peeled
2 tablespoons extra-virgin olive oil
¼ teaspoon sea salt

Juice of 1 lime
1 jalapeño pepper, ribs and seeds removed, minced
1 garlic clove, minced
1 small shallot, minced

Mash the avocado, olive oil, salt, and lime juice in a bowl, or use a mortar and pestle. Fold in the pepper, garlic, and shallot. Serve immediately.

Per Serving: (about ⅓ cup): Calories: 212; Fat: 20g; Protein: 2g; Total Carbs: 10g; Fiber: 6g; Net Carbs: 4g; **Macros:** Fat: 84%; Protein: 2%; Carbs: 14%

Olive and Artichoke Tapenade

SERVES 8 | PREP TIME: 10 minutes, plus 1 hour to marinate

1 cup pitted finely chopped Kalamata olives
1 cup finely chopped artichoke hearts
¼ cup extra-virgin olive oil or avocado oil

2 teaspoons dried rosemary, oregano, parsley, basil, or thyme
1 garlic clove, finely minced
½ to 1 teaspoon red pepper flakes

In a medium bowl, combine the olives, artichoke hearts, olive oil, rosemary, garlic, and red pepper flakes and stir to combine. Marinate in the refrigerator, covered, for at least 1 hour before serving to allow flavors to blend.

Per Serving: (¼ cup): Calories: 94; Fat: 9g; Protein: 1g; Total Carbs: 3g; Fiber: 3g; Net Carbs: 0g; **Macros:** Fat: 86%; Protein: 4%; Carbs: 10%

Baba Ghanoush

SERVES 8 | PREP TIME: 15 minutes | COOK TIME: 45 minutes

1 medium eggplant (1 to 1½ pounds)
¼ cup tahini
2 tablespoons freshly squeezed lemon juice
2 tablespoons olive oil, plus more for drizzling

1 teaspoon garlic powder
½ teaspoon salt
6 sliced Kalamata olives, for garnish
Chopped parsley, for garnish

Preheat the oven to 350°F. Place aluminum foil on the middle rack, place the eggplant on the aluminum foil, and bake for 45 to 60 minutes, or until the eggplant is fork-tender and the skin very wrinkly. Remove from the oven and cut the eggplant lengthwise. Scoop out the insides, discarding the skins, drain the liquid, and place the insides in a food processor or blender. Add the tahini, lemon juice, olive oil, garlic powder, and salt to the food processor, and blend into a paste for 2 minutes. Transfer to a serving bowl or plate, and garnish with the olives, parsley, and a drizzle of olive oil.

Per Serving: (2 tablespoons): Calories: 86; Fat: 6.5g; Protein: 2g; Total Carbs: 6.5g; Fiber: 2.5g; Net Carbs: 4g; **Macros:** Fat: 63%; Protein: 9%; Carbs: 28%

Cauliflower Hummus

SERVES 12 | PREP TIME: 15 minutes

3 cups chopped cooked cauliflower
¼ cup freshly squeezed lemon juice
¼ cup extra-virgin olive oil

2 tablespoons tahini paste
2 tablespoons egg white protein powder
1 teaspoon minced garlic
½ teaspoon sea salt

In a food processor, pulse the cauliflower, lemon juice, olive oil, tahini, egg white protein powder, garlic, and salt until the hummus is smooth.

Per Serving: (¼ cup): Calories: 72; Fat: 6g; Protein: 2g; Total Carbs: 2g; Fiber: 1g; Net Carbs: 1g; **Macros:** Fat: 78%; Protein: 11%; Carbs: 11%

Zucchini Hummus

SERVES 4 | PREP TIME: 5 minutes

1 medium zucchini, peeled and diced
1 garlic clove
2 tablespoons lemon juice

¼ cup tahini
3 tablespoons extra-virgin olive oil
½ teaspoon sea salt

In a blender, purée the zucchini, garlic, lemon juice, tahini, olive oil, and sea salt until very smooth.

Per Serving: Calories: 190; Fat: 18g; Protein: 3g; Total Carbs: 6g; Fiber: 2g; Net Carbs: 4g; **Macros:** Fat: 85%; Protein: 6%; Carbs: 9%

French Onion Dip

SERVES 4 | PREP TIME: 5 minutes | COOK TIME: 45 minutes

2 tablespoons butter
1½ cups chopped yellow onion
¾ teaspoon salt, divided
1 cup sour cream
½ cup mayonnaise

1 teaspoon minced garlic
1 teaspoon Worcestershire sauce
½ teaspoon freshly ground black pepper

In a large skillet over medium-high heat, melt the butter. Add the onions and ¼ teaspoon of salt. Cook for 1 to 2 minutes. Reduce the heat to medium-low. Allow the onions to caramelize for 35 to 40 minutes, stirring occasionally. Remove the onions from the heat. Allow them to cool while preparing the remaining ingredients. In a medium bowl, mix the sour cream, mayonnaise, garlic, Worcestershire sauce, pepper, and remaining ½ teaspoon of salt. Add the cooled onions to the mixture. Stir to combine. Before serving, cover and refrigerate the dip for 1 hour to allow the flavors to meld, or overnight for the best-tasting results.

Per Serving: Calories: 207; Fat: 18.4g; Protein: 1.7g; Total Carbs: 9.4g; Fiber: 1g; Net Carbs: 8.4g; **Macros:** Fat: 79%; Protein: 17%; Carbs: 4%

Pimento Cheese

SERVES 4 TO 6 | PREP TIME: 5 minutes

4 ounces cream cheese, at room temperature

¼ cup mayonnaise

2 tablespoons pimentos, drained and chopped

½ teaspoon salt

¼ to ½ teaspoon ground cayenne pepper or red pepper flakes

1 cup freshly shredded Cheddar cheese

In a medium bowl, combine the cream cheese, mayonnaise, pimentos, salt, and cayenne pepper and whisk until well combined and smooth and creamy. Stir in the cheese and mix until well incorporated. Serve chilled.

Per Serving: (2 tablespoons): Calories: 340; Fat: 33g; Protein: 9g; Total Carbs: 3g; Fiber: <1g; Net Carbs: 3g; Macros: Fat: 87%; Protein: 11%; Carbs: 2%

Roasted Red Pepper Dip

SERVES 6 | PREP TIME: 20 minutes | COOK TIME: 6 minutes

3 red bell peppers, halved and seeded

2 tablespoons melted coconut oil

1 cup cream cheese

2 tablespoons hemp hearts

2 tablespoons chopped fresh parsley

2 tablespoons chopped fresh basil

2 tablespoons freshly squeezed lemon juice

Pinch red pepper flakes

Sea salt

Freshly ground black pepper

Preheat the oven to broil. Place the bell peppers on a baking tray and massage to coat with the coconut oil. Broil them skin-side up until the peppers are tender and the skin is charred, about 6 minutes. Let the peppers cool for 10 minutes and scrape off the skin. Place the peppers, cream cheese, hemp hearts, parsley, basil, lemon juice, and red pepper flakes in a food processor or blender and pulse until smooth and creamy. Season with salt and pepper.

Per Serving: Calories: 208; Fat: 20g; Protein: 5g; Total Carbs: 6g; Fiber: 2g; Net Carbs: 4g; Macros: Fat: 87%; Protein: 10%; Carbs: 3%

Spinach-Artichoke Dip

SERVES 8 | PREP TIME: 5 minutes | COOK TIME: 25 minutes

2 tablespoons butter

2 tablespoons minced garlic

1¼ cups spinach, chopped

1¾ cups artichoke hearts, chopped

8 ounces cream cheese

1 cup Parmesan cheese, divided

½ cup shredded mozzarella cheese

½ cup shredded Gruyère cheese

3 tablespoons sour cream

1 tablespoon mayonnaise

½ teaspoon salt

½ teaspoon freshly ground black pepper

½ teaspoon paprika

Preheat the oven to 375°F. In a large skillet over medium-high heat, melt the butter. Add the garlic. Cook for 1 minute. Add the chopped spinach and cook for 1 to 2 minutes more. Add the artichokes and cook for an additional minute. Transfer the spinach and artichoke mixture to a large bowl. Reduce the heat under the skillet to medium-low. Add the cream cheese to the pan. Melt until creamy. Add ½ cup of Parmesan cheese, the mozzarella cheese, and the Gruyère cheese. Stir until the cheeses melt, about 2 minutes. Pour the melted cheeses over the spinach and artichoke mixture. Stir to combine. Add the sour cream, mayonnaise, salt, pepper, and paprika. Stir to incorporate. Transfer the spinach and artichoke mixture to a 9-inch-square pan. Sprinkle with the remaining ½ cup of Parmesan cheese. Bake for 20 to 25 minutes, or until the top is browned and bubbling. Cool the dip for 5 minutes before serving.

Per Serving: Calories: 259; Fat: 20.3g; Protein: 12.5g; Total Carbs: 9.4g; Fiber: 3.6g; Net Carbs: 5.8g; Macros: Fat: 68%; Protein: 19%; Carbs: 13%

Queso Dip

SERVES 6 | PREP TIME: 5 minutes | COOK TIME: 10 minutes

½ cup coconut milk

½ jalapeño pepper, seeded and diced

1 teaspoon minced garlic

½ teaspoon onion powder

2 ounces goat cheese

6 ounces Cheddar cheese, shredded

¼ teaspoon cayenne pepper

Place a medium pot over medium heat and add the coconut milk, jalapeño, garlic, and onion powder. Bring the liquid to a simmer and then whisk in the goat cheese until smooth. Add the Cheddar cheese and cayenne and whisk until the dip is thick, 30 seconds to 1 minute.

Per Serving: Calories: 213; Fat: 19g; Protein: 10g; Total Carbs: 2g; Fiber: 0g; Net Carbs: 2g; Macros: Fat: 79%; Protein: 19%; Carbs: 2%

Queso Blanco Dip

SERVES 8 | PREP TIME: 5 minutes | COOK TIME: 10 minutes

½ cup heavy (whipping) cream

3 ounces cream cheese

1 cup shredded Monterey Jack cheese

1 cup shredded queso blanco or other white Cheddar cheese

1 (4.5-ounce) can diced green chiles, drained

½ teaspoon freshly ground black pepper

½ teaspoon ground cumin

In a small saucepan over medium heat, melt the heavy cream and cream cheese, whisking until totally melted. Stir in the Monterey Jack cheese and queso blanco and the green chiles. Remove from the heat and add the pepper and cumin. Stir well and serve.

Per Serving: (2 tablespoons): Calories: 202; Fat: 18g; Protein: 8g; Total Carbs: 2g; Fiber: 0g; Net Carbs: 2g; Macros: Fat: 80%; Protein: 16%; Carbs: 4%

Buffalo Chicken Dip

SERVES 8 | PREP TIME: 10 minutes | COOK TIME: 40 minutes

½ cup butter

1 teaspoon minced garlic

4 boneless chicken thighs

¼ cup sour cream

¼ teaspoon salt

¼ teaspoon freshly ground black pepper

¼ teaspoon cayenne pepper

¼ teaspoon paprika

8 ounces (1 package) cream cheese, at room temperature

½ cup hot sauce, additional as needed

½ cup ranch dressing

1 cup shredded mozza-
rella cheese

½ cup shredded
Cheddar cheese

Preheat the oven to 450°F. Heat a large skillet with a cover over medium-high heat. Add the butter and melt. Add the garlic and chicken to the skillet. Cook for 3 minutes. Reduce the heat to medium. Turn the chicken so it cooks on all sides, cooking for 12 to 15 minutes total. It should reach 165°F. When cooked, remove the chicken to a large bowl. Set aside to cool. Shred the cooled chicken into bite-size pieces. Add the sour cream, salt, black pepper, cayenne pepper, and paprika to the shredded chicken. Mix well. In a 9-inch-square pan, spread the cream cheese over the bottom and up the sides, coating evenly. Pour the chicken mixture over the cream cheese layer. Drizzle the hot sauce and ranch dressing over the chicken mixture, distributing evenly. Top with the mozzarella and Cheddar cheeses. Using a butter knife, swirl the ingredients together in the pan. Place the pan in the preheated oven. Bake for 15 minutes, or until the top layer is browned and bubbling. Remove the pan from the oven. Cool the dip for 5 minutes before serving.

Per Serving: Calories: 358; Fat: 31.4g; Protein: 21.2g; Total Carbs: 3g; Fiber: 0.2g; Net Carbs: 2.8g; **Macros:** Fat: 74%; Protein: 22%; Carbs: 4%

Taco Layer Dip

SERVES 6 | PREP TIME: 20 minutes | COOK TIME: 20 minutes

1 tablespoon olive oil

½ pound ground beef

1 tablespoon chili powder

2 teaspoons ground cumin

1 teaspoon paprika

½ teaspoon garlic powder

1 red bell pepper, chopped

½ red onion, chopped

½ cup chopped black olives

1 cup shredded Ched-
dar cheese

1 cup sour cream

1 tablespoon chopped fresh
cilantro

Preheat the oven to 400°F. Heat the olive oil in a large skillet and brown the ground beef until cooked through, about 10 minutes. Stir in the chili powder, cumin, paprika, and garlic powder. Spread the ground beef in a 9-by-13-inch casserole dish and top with bell pepper, red onion, black olives, and Cheddar cheese. Bake in the oven until the cheese is bubbly and melted, about 10 minutes. Top with sour cream and cilantro and serve.

Per Serving: Calories: 319; Fat: 26g; Protein: 13g; Total Carbs: 8g; Fiber: 1g; Net Carbs: 7g; **Macros:** Fat: 73%; Protein: 16%; Carbs: 11%

Crab and Artichoke Dip

SERVES 6 | PREP TIME: 10 minutes | COOK TIME: 25 minutes

2 tablespoons extra-virgin
olive oil

½ small onion, diced

½ cup chopped arti-
choke hearts

1 cup frozen spinach, thawed
and drained

2 garlic cloves, minced

8 ounces cream cheese, at
room temperature

4 ounces crab meat

1 teaspoon smoked paprika

1 teaspoon salt or Old Bay
seasoning

½ to 1 teaspoon red
pepper flakes

¼ cup mayonnaise

¼ cup freshly shredded
Parmesan cheese

Preheat the oven to 375°F. In a medium skillet, heat the olive oil over medium heat. Sauté the onion for 6 minutes, until tender. Add the artichokes and spinach and sauté for another 4 to 5 minutes, or until the vegetables are tender and any water has evaporated. Add the cream cheese and garlic and, stirring constantly, cook for 3 to 4 minutes, until the cheese is melted and creamy. Reduce the heat to low and stir in the crab meat, paprika, salt, and red pepper flakes. Remove from the heat and stir in the mayonnaise until creamy and well combined. Transfer the mixture to an 8-by-8-inch glass baking dish, spreading it out evenly. Top with the Parmesan and bake for 8 to 10 minutes, until the cheese is melted and lightly browned. Serve warm with raw vegetables such as cucumber rounds, celery, or red peppers.

Per Serving: (⅓ cup): Calories: 308; Fat: 29g; Protein: 8g; Total Carbs: 6g; Fiber: 1g; Net Carbs: 5g; **Macros:** Fat: 85%; Protein: 10%; Carbs: 5%

Smoked Salmon and Cucumber Bites

SERVES 2 | PREP TIME: 10 minutes

½ English cucumber, cut into
8 to 12 slices

4 ounces cold smoked
salmon or lox

½ cup sour cream

5 sprigs fresh dill,
roughly chopped

Freshly ground black pepper

Top each cucumber slice with a small piece of the salmon and a generous spoonful of sour cream. Garnish with a pinch of fresh dill over the sour cream. Season with pepper.

Per Serving: Calories: 179; Fat: 13g; Protein: 12g; Total Carbs: 4g; Fiber: 1g; Net Carbs: 3g; **Macros:** Fat: 65%; Protein: 27%; Carbs: 8%

Black Forest Ham, Cheese, and Chive Roll-Ups

SERVES 2 | PREP TIME: 10 minutes

6 slices Black forest ham
(about 5 ounces total)

3 ounces cream cheese, at
room temperature

1 tablespoon chopped
fresh chives

¼ cup shredded Monterey
Jack cheese

½ teaspoon garlic powder

½ teaspoon onion powder

⅛ teaspoon salt

⅛ teaspoon freshly ground
black pepper

On a cutting board, lay out the six ham slices. Spread ½ ounce of cream cheese on each ham slice, covering evenly. Distribute the chives evenly over each piece of ham. Top evenly with the Monterey Jack cheese. Sprinkle each piece with the garlic powder, onion powder, salt, and pepper. Roll up each slice and enjoy. If desired, slice each roll crosswise into 1-inch pieces, and serve.

Per Serving: (3 roll-ups): Calories: 345; Fat: 27g; Protein: 21g; Total Carbs: 6g; Fiber: 1g; Net Carbs: 5g; **Macros:** Fat: 68%; Protein: 25%; Carbs: 7%

Cheesy Shrimp Spread

MAKES 1½ CUPS | PREP TIME: 10 minutes

6 ounces cream cheese,
softened

¼ cup mayonnaise

6 ounces cooked
shrimp, chopped

1 tablespoon freshly squeezed
  lemon juice
1 tablespoon chopped scallion
1 teaspoon chopped fresh dill

Pinch red pepper flakes
Sea salt
Freshly ground black pepper

In a food processor, pulse the cream cheese, Mayonnaise, shrimp, lemon juice, scallion, dill, and red pepper flakes until the spread is thick and well blended. Season the spread with salt and pepper. Refrigerate in a sealed container for up to 4 days.

Per Serving: (3 tablespoons): Calories: 130; Fat: 10g; Protein: 7g; Total Carbs: 3g; Fiber: 0g; Net Carbs: 3g; **Macros:** Fat: 69%; Protein: 22%; Carbs: 9%

Avocado and Smoked Salmon Stack with Dill Caper Sauce

SERVES 1 | PREP TIME: 5 minutes

2 ounces smoked salmon
½ avocado, sliced
¼ cup cucumber, diced
2 tablespoon plain unsweetened coconut yogurt

2 tablespoons chopped
  fresh dill
1 teaspoon chopped capers
¼ teaspoon caper juice
¼ teaspoon freshly squeezed
  lemon juice

Layer the salmon, avocado, and cucumber on a plate. In a small bowl, mix the coconut yogurt, dill, capers, caper juice, and lemon juice until well combined. Top the salmon stack with the Dill Caper sauce and serve.

Per Serving: Calories: 411; Fat: 35g; Protein: 14g; Total Carbs: 10g; Fiber: 6g; Net Carbs: 4g; **Macros:** Fat: 77%; Protein: 13%; Carbs: 10%

Salmon Salad Sushi Bites

SERVES 4 TO 6 | PREP TIME: 20 minutes

2 large cucumbers, peeled
8 ounces canned or fresh
  red salmon, bones and
  skin removed
¼ cup mayonnaise
1 tablespoon sesame oil

2 teaspoons miso paste
1 teaspoon sriracha or other
  hot sauce
1 nori seaweed sheet, crumbled
½ medium ripe avocado,
  thinly sliced

Slice the cucumber into 1-inch segments and using a spoon, scrape the seeds out of the center of each segment and stand up on a plate. In a medium bowl, combine the salmon, mayonnaise, sesame oil, miso, sriracha, and nori and mix until creamy. Spoon the salmon mixture into the center of each cucumber segment and top with a slice of avocado. Serve chilled.

Per Serving: (2 pieces): Calories: 289; Fat: 24g; Protein: 13g; Total Carbs: 8g; Fiber: 3g; Net Carbs: 5g; **Macros:** Fat: 75%; Protein: 18%; Carbs: 7%

BLTA Wraps

SERVES 4 | PREP TIME: 5 minutes

16 slices cooked bacon
1 avocado, pitted, peeled,
  and diced
12 cherry tomatoes, halved

2 tablespoons mayonnaise
Salt
Freshly ground black pepper
8 large iceberg lettuce leaves

Roughly chop the bacon and transfer it to a large bowl. Add the avocado, tomatoes, and mayonnaise. Season with salt and

pepper and stir well to combine. Arrange the lettuce on four plates and divide the bacon mixture among the leaves. Serve immediately.

Per Serving: Calories: 329; Fat: 27g; Protein: 14g; Total Carbs: 9g; Fiber: 5g; Net Carbs: 4g; **Macros:** Fat: 72%; Protein: 18%; Carbs: 10%

Party Deli Pinwheels

SERVES 2 | PREP TIME: 10 minutes, plus 5 to 10 minutes to chill

1 low-carb tortilla
3 tablespoons cream cheese,
  at room temperature
2 ounces (2 or 3 slices) oven
  roasted turkey

2 ounces (2 or 3 slices) fresh
  smoked uncured ham
2 slices provolone cheese
2 slices Cheddar cheese

Lay the tortilla on a plate and spread with the cream cheese. Layer the meats and cheeses around the tortilla until it's covered. Roll the tortilla up and refrigerate for 5 to 10 minutes or longer. Cut the roll into 8 slices and serve on a plate or platter.

Per Serving: (4 pinwheels) Calories: 484; Fat: 32g; Protein: 31g; Total Carbs: 18g; Fiber: 9g; Net Carbs: 9g; **Macros:** Fat: 60%; Protein: 26%; Carbs: 14%

Turkey Spinach Roll-Ups

SERVES 1 | PREP TIME: 5 minutes

4 slices (2 ounces) deli
  turkey breast
¼ cup cream cheese

¼ cup thinly sliced
  fresh spinach
2 tablespoons thinly sliced
  fresh basil (optional)

Lay one slice of the turkey on a cutting board. Top with 1 tablespoon of the cream cheese, a quarter of the spinach, and ½ tablespoon of the basil (if using). Roll the meat around the filling into a tight cylinder. Repeat with the remaining turkey, cream cheese, spinach, and basil.

Per Serving: Calories: 260; Fat: 21g; Protein: 14g; Total Carbs: 5g; Fiber: 0g; Net Carbs: 5g; **Macros:** Fat: 73%; Protein: 22%; Carbs: 5%

Smoked Salmon and Goat Cheese Pinwheels

SERVES 4 | PREP TIME: 15 minutes

4 ounces goat cheese
¼ cup extra-virgin olive
  oil, divided
1 tablespoon finely
  chopped capers
1 tablespoon minced
  red onion

1 teaspoon dried dill
¼ to ½ teaspoon red
  pepper flakes
6 ounces smoked wild-caught
  salmon (not cut nova bits),
  thinly sliced into 2 rough
  rectangles

In a small bowl, mix the goat cheese, 2 tablespoons of olive oil, capers, onion, dill, and red pepper flakes. Lay out the slices of smoked salmon on a large plate or serving dish. Top each slice with the goat cheese mixture and spread to evenly coat. Starting at the narrow end, roll the salmon to form a log. Slice each log into 1-inch segments and arrange on the platter. Drizzle the pinwheels with the remaining 2 tablespoons of olive oil and serve chilled.

Per Serving: Calories: 274; Fat: 24g; Protein: 14g; Total Carbs: 1g; Fiber: <1g; Net Carbs: 1g; **Macros:** Fat: 79%; Protein: 20%; Carbs: 1%

Dilled Tuna Salad Sandwich

SERVES 4 | PREP TIME: 10 minutes

4 keto sandwich rounds

2 (4-ounce) cans tuna, packed in olive oil

2 tablespoons avocado oil mayonnaise with 1 to 2 teaspoons freshly squeezed lemon juice and/or zest

1 very ripe avocado, peeled, pitted, and mashed

1 tablespoon chopped fresh capers (optional)

1 teaspoon chopped fresh dill or ½ teaspoon dried dill

Cut each round of keto sandwich rounds or bread in half and set aside. In a medium bowl, place the tuna and the oil from cans. Add the aioli, avocado, capers (if using), and dill and blend well with a fork. Toast sandwich rounds and fill each with one-quarter of the tuna salad, about ⅓ cup.

Per Serving: (1 sandwich): Calories: 436; Fat: 36g; Protein: 23g; Total Carbs: 5g; Fiber: 3g; Net Carbs: 2g; **Macros:** Fat: 74%; Protein: 21%; Carbs: 5%

Tuna Salad Wrap

SERVES 2 | PREP TIME: 5 minutes

2 (5-ounce) cans tuna packed in olive oil, drained

3 tablespoons mayonnaise

1 tablespoon chopped red onion

2 teaspoons dill relish

¼ teaspoon pink Himalayan sea salt

¼ teaspoon freshly ground black pepper

Pinch of dried or fresh dill

2 low-carb tortillas

2 romaine lettuce leaves

¼ cup grated Cheddar cheese

In a medium bowl, combine the tuna, mayonnaise, onion, relish, salt, pepper, and dill. Place a lettuce leaf on each tortilla, then split the tuna mixture evenly between the wraps, spreading it evenly over the lettuce. Sprinkle the Cheddar on top of each, then fold the tortillas and serve.

Per Serving: Calories: 549; Fat: 33g; Protein: 42g; Total Carbs: 21g; Fiber: 16g; Net Carbs: 5g; **Macros:** Fat: 54%; Protein: 31%; Carbs: 15%

Prosciutto-Wrapped Mozzarella

SERVES 4 | PREP TIME: 10 minutes

8 slices (4 ounces) prosciutto

16 small bocconcini

1 teaspoon minced rosemary

Freshly ground black pepper

Slice the prosciutto in half lengthwise. Wrap one slice of prosciutto around each of the bocconcini and secure with a toothpick. Set the balls on a serving platter and sprinkle with the rosemary and pepper.

Per Serving: (4 balls): Calories: 170; Fat: 14g; Protein: 13g; Total Carbs: 1g; Fiber: 0g; Net Carbs: 1g; **Macros:** Fat: 72%; Protein: 26%; Carbs: 2%

Macadamia Nut Cream Cheese Log

SERVES 8 | PREP TIME: 10 minutes, plus 30 minutes to chill

1 (8-ounce) brick cream cheese, cold

1 cup finely chopped macadamia nuts

Place the cream cheese on a piece of parchment paper or wax paper. Roll the paper around the cream cheese, then roll the wrapped cream cheese with the palm of your hands lengthwise on the cream cheese, using the paper to help you roll the cream cheese into an 8-inch log. Open the paper and sprinkle the macadamia nuts all over the top and sides of the cream cheese until the log is entirely covered in nuts. Chill in the refrigerator for 30 minutes before serving. Serve on a small plate, cut into 8 even slices.

Per Serving: Calories: 285; Fat: 29g; Protein: 4g; Total Carbs: 4g; Fiber: 1g; Net Carbs: 3g; **Macros:** Fat: 90%; Protein: 5%; Carbs: 5%

Mediterranean Cucumber Bites

SERVES 4 | PREP TIME: 10 minutes

8 ounces cream cheese, at room temperature

2 tablespoons chopped flat-leaf parsley

⅓ cup diced black olives

1 bell pepper, diced

2 cucumbers, halved lengthwise and seeded

2 tablespoons sliced scallions

In a small bowl, mix the cream cheese, parsley, olives, and bell pepper. Fill each cucumber cavity with the cream cheese mixture. Sprinkle with the scallions, slice into 1-inch pieces, and serve.

Per Serving: (½ cucumber) Calories: 253; Fat: 21g; Protein: 6g; Total Carbs: 10g; Fiber: 2g; Net Carbs: 8g; **Macros:** Fat: 75%; Protein: 9%; Carbs: 16%

Caprese Skewers

SERVES 1 | PREP TIME: 5 minutes

12 small mozzarella balls, about 1 ounce

12 grape tomatoes

12 small basil leaves

Alternating between the ingredients, thread six mozzarella balls, six tomatoes, and six basil leaves onto a bamboo skewer. Repeat with the remaining ingredients on a second skewer. Refrigerate until ready to serve.

Per Serving: Calories: 97; Fat: 5g; Protein: 5g; Total Carbs: 6g; Fiber: 0g; Net Carbs: 6g; **Macros:** Fat: 46%; Protein: 21%; Carbs: 21%

Turmeric Cauliflower "Pickles"

SERVES 6 | PREP TIME: 10 minutes | COOK TIME: 5 minutes, plus 3 days to ferment

1 cauliflower head, cut into florets

⅔ cup white vinegar

⅓ cup water

½ cup powdered monk fruit sweetener

1 tablespoon sea salt

1 teaspoon ground coriander

1 teaspoon turmeric powder

1 bay leaf

1 teaspoon peppercorns

Place the cauliflower florets in large mason jars. In a medium saucepan over medium heat, combine the vinegar, water, monk fruit sweetener, salt, coriander, turmeric, bay leaf, and peppercorns. Bring the brine to a low simmer for 5 minutes. Remove the pan from the heat and allow it to cool. Once the brine has cooled, pour it over the cauliflower in the jars. Be sure to fill the jars all the way to the top to ensure that the cauliflower is completely covered. Close the jars to make them as airtight as possible. Store the jars in the refrigerator for 3 days to ferment before eating.

Per Serving: Calories: 26; Fat: <1g; Protein: 2g; Total Carbs: 5g; Fiber: 3g; Net Carbs: 2g; **Macros:** Fat: 2%; Protein: 27%; Carbs: 71%

Anti-Inflammatory Power Bites

MAKES ABOUT 1 DOZEN | PREP TIME: 20 minutes

1 cup unsweetened almond butter	¼ cup unsweetened coconut flakes
½ cup ground flaxseed	¼ cup roasted pumpkin seeds
¼ cup almond or coconut flour	¼ cup chia seeds
¼ cup unsweetened cocoa powder	1 teaspoon ground cinnamon
	1 to 2 teaspoons monk fruit extract (optional)

In a large bowl, combine the almond butter, flaxseed, almond flour, cocoa powder, coconut flakes, pumpkin seeds, chia seeds, cinnamon, and sweetener (if using). Using your hands, mix everything and shape the mixture into 12 (1-inch) balls. Place them in a single layer on a baking sheet or large container. Cover and refrigerate at least 1 hour before serving.

Per Serving: (1 bite): Calories: 214; Fat: 18g; Protein: 8g; Total Carbs: 9g; Fiber: 6g; Net Carbs: 3g; **Macros:** Fat: 76%; Protein: 15%; Carbs: 9%

Marinated Antipasto Veggies

SERVES 8 | PREP TIME: 10 minutes, plus 24 hours to marinate

1 (14-ounce) can artichoke hearts, drained and quartered	4 small garlic cloves, peeled and crushed with the back of a knife
1 cup halved small button mushrooms	1 tablespoon roughly chopped fresh rosemary leaves
8 small snack-sized sweet peppers, seeded and halved or 2 medium bell peppers, cut into 1-inch-thick strips	1 tablespoon chopped fresh oregano or 1 teaspoon dried oregano
¾ cup extra-virgin olive oil	1 to 2 teaspoons red pepper flakes
	1 teaspoon salt

In a medium bowl, combine the artichoke hearts, mushrooms, peppers, olive oil, garlic, rosemary, oregano, red pepper flakes, and salt. Toss to combine well. Store the mixture in an airtight (preferably glass) container in the refrigerator and marinate for at least 24 hours before serving.

Per Serving: Calories: 218; Fat: 22g; Protein: 1g; Total Carbs: 5g; Fiber: 2g; Net Carbs: 3g; **Macros:** Fat: 91%; Protein: 2%; Carbs: 7%

Grilled Avocados

SERVES 8 | PREP TIME: 5 minutes | COOK TIME: 5 minutes

4 avocados, cut in half lengthwise, pitted	¼ cup olive oil
	1 teaspoon salt

Preheat the grill to medium-high heat. Brush or drizzle the olive oil on the cut side of each avocado, and season with the salt. Lay cut-side down, grill 5 minutes, and serve.

Per Serving: (½ avocado): Calories: 173; Fat: 17g; Protein: 1g; Total Carbs: 5.5g; Fiber: 4.5g; Net Carbs: 1g; **Macros:** Fat: 85%; Protein: 2%; Carbs: 13%

Roasted Brussels Sprouts with Tahini-Yogurt Sauce

SERVES 4 | PREP TIME: 10 minutes | COOK TIME: 35 minutes

1 pound Brussels sprouts, trimmed and halved lengthwise	½ teaspoon garlic powder
	¼ teaspoon freshly ground black pepper
6 tablespoons extra-virgin olive oil, divided	¼ cup plain Greek yogurt
1 teaspoon salt, divided	¼ cup tahini
	Zest and juice of 1 lemon

Preheat the oven to 425°F. Line a baking sheet with aluminum foil or parchment paper and set aside. Place the Brussels sprouts in a large bowl. Drizzle with ¼ cup olive oil, ½ teaspoon salt, the garlic powder, and pepper and toss well to coat. Place the Brussels sprouts in a single layer on the baking sheet, reserving the bowl, and roast for 20 minutes, tossing halfway through, until browned and crispy. Remove from the oven and return to the reserved bowl. In a small bowl, whisk the yogurt, tahini, lemon zest and juice, remaining 2 tablespoons olive oil, and remaining ½ teaspoon salt. Drizzle over the roasted sprouts and toss to coat. Serve warm.

Per Serving: Calories: 358; Fat: 30g; Protein: 7g; Total Carbs: 15g; Fiber: 6g; Net Carbs: 9g; **Macros:** Fat: 75%; Protein: 8%; Carbs: 17%

Avocado Deviled Eggs

SERVES 4 | PREP TIME: 20 minutes

6 hard-boiled eggs	1 teaspoon minced fresh cilantro
½ ripe avocado	1 teaspoon minced jalapeño pepper
1 tablespoon freshly squeezed lime juice	Sea salt

Peel the hard-boiled eggs and carefully cut them in half lengthwise. Remove the yolks and set them aside in a small bowl. Mash the egg yolks, avocado, lime juice, cilantro, and jalapeño until well combined and creamy. Season with salt. Spoon the yolk mixture into the center of the egg whites, distributing evenly, and serve.

Per Serving: Calories: 155; Fat: 11g; Protein: 10g; Total Carbs: 3g; Fiber: 2g; Net Carbs: 1g; **Macros:** Fat: 64%; Protein: 26%; Carbs: 10%

Bacon-Cheese Deviled Eggs

MAKES 12 | PREP TIME: 15 minutes

6 hard-boiled eggs, peeled

¼ cup mayonnaise

¼ avocado, chopped

¼ cup finely shredded
   Swiss cheese

½ teaspoon Dijon mustard

Freshly ground black pepper

6 bacon slices, cooked
   and chopped

Halve each of the eggs lengthwise. Carefully remove the yolk and place the yolks in a medium bowl. Place the whites, hollow-side up, on a plate. Mash the yolks with a fork and add the mayonnaise, avocado, cheese, and Dijon mustard. Stir until well mixed. Season the yolk mixture with the black pepper. Spoon the yolk mixture back into the egg white hollows and top each egg half with the chopped bacon. Store the eggs in an airtight container in the refrigerator for up to 1 day.

Per Serving: (1 deviled egg): Calories: 85; Fat: 7g; Protein: 6g; Total Carbs: 2g; Fiber: 0g; Net Carbs: 2g; **Macros:** Fat: 70%; Protein: 25%; Carbs: 5%

Bacon Deviled Eggs

SERVES 4 | PREP TIME: 5 minutes | COOK TIME: 15 minutes

6 large eggs

3 to 4 bacon slices (½ cup
   when chopped, depending
   on thickness)

1½ tablespoons mayonnaise

1 tablespoon mustard

½ teaspoon paprika, divided

⅛ teaspoon salt

⅛ teaspoon freshly ground
   black pepper

Bring a large pot half filled with water to a boil. Gently place the eggs in the water, being careful not to crack the shells. Cook for 10 minutes. Remove the pot from the water. Set aside to cool. While the eggs cook, heat a large skillet over medium-high heat. Add the bacon to the skillet. Cook for 3 minutes. Flip and cook for 2 to 3 minutes more, or until crisp. Transfer the bacon to paper towels to drain. Once the eggs cool, peel them, and cut them in half lengthwise. Scoop the yolks into a medium bowl. Add the mayonnaise, mustard, ¼ teaspoon paprika, salt, and pepper. Stir to combine. Chop the bacon into small pieces. Divide into two equal amounts (about ¼ cup each). Add ¼ cup of bacon to the yolks. Mix well to combine. Place the egg whites cut-side up on a plate. Spoon an equal amount of the yolk mixture into each. Use the remaining ¼ cup of bacon and ¼ teaspoon of paprika to garnish the eggs, and serve.

Per Serving: (3 stuffed egg halves): Calories: 283; Fat: 21g; Protein: 20g; Total Carbs: 3g; Fiber: 1g; Net Carbs: 2g; **Macros:** Fat: 67%; Protein: 28%; Carbs: 5%

Green Chile Deviled Eggs

SERVES 12 | PREP TIME: 10 minutes | COOK TIME: 10 minutes

6 hard-boiled eggs, peeled
   and halved lengthwise

3 ounces cream cheese, at
   room temperature

2½ tablespoons mayonnaise

2½ tablespoons canned mild
   green chilies

¼ teaspoon kosher salt

½ teaspoon Worcester-
   shire sauce

⅛ teaspoon garlic powder

3 or 4 drops hot sauce

2 crispy cooked bacon
   slices, chopped

Using a small spoon, scoop the egg yolks into a small bowl. Using a fork, break up the yolks, mashing them. Add the cream cheese and mayonnaise and continue to mash until smooth. Stir in the green chilies, salt, Worcestershire sauce, garlic powder, and hot sauce. Spoon or pipe the egg yolk mixture into the egg whites. Top each with crispy bacon.

Per Serving: (2 halves): Calories: 172; Fat: 16g; Protein: 6g; Total Carbs: 1g; Fiber: 0g; Net Carbs: 1g; **Macros:** Fat: 84%; Protein: 14%; Carbs: 2%

Southern Fried Deviled Eggs

MAKES 16 | PREP TIME: 15 minutes | COOK TIME: 20 minutes

4 to 5 cups avocado oil for
   frying (or enough to fill your
   pan about 2 inches deep)

8 hard-boiled eggs, plus
   2 large eggs

1 cup finely crushed pork skins

¼ cup mayonnaise

¼ cup sour cream

2 teaspoons Dijon mustard

1 teaspoon salt

½ teaspoon freshly ground
   black pepper

Paprika, for garnish

Pour the oil into a deep, medium heavy-bottomed pan, and place on the stove over medium heat. Cut the boiled eggs in half lengthwise. Scoop out the yolks, place the yolks in a small bowl, and set the yolks and egg white boats aside. Pour the crushed pork skins into a shallow bowl. In another shallow bowl, whisk the two uncooked eggs. Take an egg white boat, dip both sides in the pork skins, then submerge it in the whisked eggs and then back in the pork skins. Place on a plate, and repeat with the remaining egg white boats. Using a slotted spoon, gently lower 2 or 3 of the boats into the oil. Cook for about 3 minutes, flipping halfway through, until golden brown. Transfer onto another plate lined with paper towels. Working in batches, repeat with the remaining boats. With a fork, mash the egg yolks. Add the mayonnaise, sour cream, Dijon mustard, salt, and pepper, and mix well. Using a piping bag, resealable bag with the corner cut off, or spoon, fill each boat with yolk mixture, and garnish with paprika.

Per Serving: (2 deviled eggs): Calories: 257; Fat: 22g; Protein: 12g; Total Carbs: 1g; Fiber: 0g; Net Carbs: 1g; **Macros:** Fat: 79%; Protein: 19%; Carbs: 2%

Antipasto Skewers

SERVES 12 | PREP TIME: 10 minutes

12 Kalamata olives

12 slices thick-cut salami

12 pimento-stuffed
   green olives

12 marinated baby
   mozzarella balls

12 slices thick-cut
   summer sausage

12 grape tomatoes

On a 7-inch wooden or bamboo knotted skewer, thread the ingredients in this order: Kalamata olive, salami (end to end), green olive, mozzarella ball, summer sausage (end to end), grape tomato. Repeat with the remaining skewers. Plate and serve.

Per Serving: (1 skewer): Calories: 255; Fat: 22g; Protein: 11g; Total Carbs: 2.5g; Fiber: 0.5g; Net Carbs: 2g; **Macros:** Fat: 78%; Protein: 17%; Carbs: 5%

Rosemary Roasted Almonds

SERVES 4 | PREP TIME: 5 minutes | COOK TIME: 15 minutes

1½ cups almonds
1 tablespoon olive oil
1 tablespoon chopped fresh
  rosemary

½ teaspoon salt
½ teaspoon freshly ground
  black pepper
¼ teaspoon ground ginger

Preheat the oven to 325°F. In a medium bowl, combine the almonds and olive oil. Mix until the almonds are evenly coated. Add the rosemary, salt, pepper, and ginger to the almonds. Stir to combine. On a baking sheet covered with aluminum foil, spread the almonds into an even layer. Place the sheet in the preheated oven. Bake for 15 minutes, or until toasted.

Per Serving: (½ cup): Calories: 240; Fat: 21.5g; Protein: 7.6g; Total Carbs: 8.4g; Fiber: 4.9g; Net Carbs: 3.5g; **Macros:** Fat: 76%; Protein: 12%; Carbs: 12%

Smoked Almonds

SERVES 10 | PREP TIME: 5 minutes | COOK TIME: 45 minutes

1 pound raw almonds
2 tablespoons butter, melted
2 tablespoons liquid smoke

2 tablespoons Worcester-
  shire sauce
1 tablespoon salt

Preheat the oven to 200°F. Line a baking dish with aluminum foil. Put the almonds in a large mixing bowl and set aside. In a small bowl, mix the butter, liquid smoke, and Worcestershire sauce. Pour the mixture over the almonds and stir. Sprinkle in the salt and mix again. Spread the almonds evenly on the prepared baking dish and place in the oven. Cook for 45 minutes, stirring well every 10 minutes. Once cooked, transfer the nuts to paper towels to drain.

Per Serving: (about 27 almonds) Calories: 305; Fat: 25g; Protein: 10g; Total Carbs: 10g; Fiber: 6g; Net Carbs: 4g; **Macros:** Fat: 74%; Protein: 13%; Carbs: 13%

Spicy Barbecue Pecans

SERVES 8 | PREP TIME: 15 minutes | COOK TIME: 20 minutes

2½ tablespoons butter, melted
1 tablespoon gluten-free
  Worcestershire sauce
1 tablespoon tamari, or
  gluten-free soy sauce
1 teaspoon kosher salt

½ teaspoon chili powder
½ teaspoon garlic powder
¼ teaspoon cayenne pepper
¼ teaspoon dry mustard
2 cups pecan halves

Preheat the oven to 325°F. Line a baking sheet with parchment paper. Set aside. In a medium bowl, stir the melted butter, Worcestershire sauce, tamari, salt, chili powder, garlic powder, cayenne, and mustard. Add the pecans and toss to coat well. Pour the coated pecans on the baking sheet and spread into a single layer. Bake for 18 to 20 minutes, stirring once halfway through the cooking time. Keep a close eye on them to ensure they don't burn. Spread the pecan halves on paper towels to cool completely before packing in an airtight container for storage.

Per Serving: (¼ cup): Calories: 270; Fat: 26g; Protein: 4g; Total Carbs: 5g; Fiber: 4g; Net Carbs: 1g; **Macros:** Fat: 87%; Protein: 6%; Carbs: 7%

Texas Trash

SERVES 10 TO 12 | PREP TIME: 15 minutes | COOK TIME: 1 hour, 15 minutes

1½ (5-ounce) bags pork rinds,
  broken into bite-size pieces
½ cup raw almonds
½ cup raw pecans
½ cup raw Brazil nuts
6 tablespoons melted butter
2 tablespoons Worcester-
  shire sauce
2 teaspoons hot sauce or
  sriracha

½ teaspoon onion powder
½ teaspoon garlic powder
½ teaspoon paprika
½ teaspoon kosher salt
¼ teaspoon celery salt
1½ cups Cheddar cheese
  crisps, purchased or
  homemade

Preheat the oven to 250°F. Line a baking sheet with parchment paper. In a large bowl, mix the pork rinds, almonds, pecans, and Brazil nuts. In a small bowl, whisk the melted butter, Worcestershire sauce, hot sauce, onion powder, garlic powder, paprika, salt, and celery salt. Pour the butter mixture over the pork rinds and nuts, and toss to coat. Pour everything onto the baking sheet and spread it evenly. Bake for 1 hour to 1 hour and 15 minutes, stirring every 15 minutes. The pork rinds should be crispy, not soggy. Remove from the oven, add the cheese crisps, and gently toss to incorporate them into the warm mixture. Transfer the Texas trash onto paper towels to cool.

Per Serving: (⅓ cup): Calories: 388; Fat: 32g; Protein: 21g; Total Carbs: 4g; Fiber: 2g; Net Carbs: 2g; **Macros:** Fat: 74%; Protein: 22%; Carbs: 4%

Marinated Artichokes

MAKES 2 CUPS | PREP TIME: 10 minutes, plus 24 hours to marinate

2 (13¾-ounce) cans artichoke
  hearts, drained and
  quartered
¾ cup extra-virgin olive oil
4 small garlic cloves, crushed
  with the back of a knife
1 tablespoon fresh rose-
  mary leaves

2 teaspoons chopped fresh
  oregano or 1 teaspoon
  dried oregano
1 teaspoon red pepper flakes
  (optional)
1 teaspoon salt

In a medium bowl, combine the artichoke hearts, olive oil, garlic, rosemary, oregano, red pepper flakes (if using), and salt. Refrigerate in an airtight container and marinate for at least 24 hours before using. Refrigerate for up to 2 weeks.

Per Serving (¼ cup): Calories: 275; Fat: 27g; Protein: 4g; Total Carbs: 11g; Fiber: 4g; Net Carbs: 7g; **Macros:** Fat: 88%; Protein: 5%; Carbs: 7%

Fennel and Orange Marinated Olives

SERVES 12 | PREP TIME: 10 minutes | COOK TIME: 2 hours

1 cup almonds, prefera-
  bly Marcona
¾ cup extra-virgin olive oil
1 orange, peeled and very
  thinly sliced
½ fennel bulb, thinly sliced

1 small red onion, thinly sliced
1 sprig fresh rosemary
Pinch red pepper flakes
2 tablespoons red
  wine vinegar

Preheat the oven to 300°F. In a shallow baking dish, toss all of the ingredients. Cover with foil and bake for 1½ hours. Remove the foil and continue baking for another 20 to 30 minutes. Allow the mixture to cool to room temperature before serving.

Per Serving: (about ⅓ cup): Calories: 243; Fat: 24g; Protein: 3g; Total Carbs: 7g; Fiber: 3g; Net Carbs: 4g; **Macros:** Fat: 85%; Protein: 5%; Carbs: 10%

Baked Olives and Feta

SERVES 6 | PREP TIME: 5 minutes | COOK TIME: 30 minutes

Nonstick cooking spray
1 (6-ounce) can black olives, drained
1 (6-ounce) jar green olives, drained
14 ounces feta cheese, crumbled
2 tablespoons minced fresh rosemary
2 tablespoons minced fresh thyme
2 tablespoons olive oil

Preheat the oven to 350°F. Spray an 8-inch-square baking dish with cooking spray. Pour the olives into the prepared dish. Stir in the feta cheese, rosemary, and thyme. Drizzle the olive oil on top and mix well until the olives and cheese are well coated. Bake for 22 to 25 minutes. Turn the oven to low broil and broil for an additional 2 to 4 minutes, or until the olives are browned. Remove from the oven and serve warm.

Per Serving: Calories: 284; Fat: 24g; Protein: 10g; Total Carbs: 7g; Fiber: 2g; Net Carbs: 5g; **Macros:** Fat: 76%; Protein: 14%; Carbs: 10%

Baked Feta Blocks

SERVES 8 | PREP TIME: 5 minutes | COOK TIME: 20 minutes

2 (8-ounce) blocks of feta cheese
1 pint grape or cherry tomatoes
6 ounces Kalamata olives
2 tablespoons roughly chopped fresh oregano
1 lemon, cut into wedges
2 tablespoons extra-virgin olive oil
Sea salt
Freshly ground black pepper
Handful fresh basil leaves, for garnish

Preheat the oven to 300°F. Place the feta blocks side by side in a rectangular baking dish. Top with the tomatoes, olives, oregano, and lemon wedges. Drizzle with the olive oil and season with salt and pepper. Bake for 20 minutes, or until the cheese is warmed through and the tomatoes are soft. Squeeze the baked lemon wedges over the dish and top with the fresh basil leaves before serving.

Per Serving: Calories: 207; Fat: 18g; Protein: 8g; Total Carbs: 5g; Fiber: 0g; Net Carbs: 5g; **Macros:** Fat: 78%; Protein: 15%; Carbs: 7%

Goat Cheese Nuggets

MAKES 16 NUGGETS | PREP TIME: 20 minutes, plus chilling time

8 ounces goat cheese
3 oil-packed sun-dried tomatoes
1 teaspoon coconut oil
½ cup walnuts, coarsely ground
Pinch red pepper flakes

In a blender, blend the goat cheese, sun-dried tomatoes, coconut oil, and red pepper flakes until well combined. Transfer the cheese mixture to a small bowl, and refrigerate until it is firm enough to roll into balls. Roll the goat cheese mixture into 16 small balls, and roll the balls in the ground walnuts until they are completely coated.

Per Serving: (1 nugget): Calories: 96; Fat: 8g; Protein: 5g; Total Carbs: 1g; Fiber: 0g; Net Carbs: 1g; **Macros:** Fat: 75%; Protein: 21%; Carbs: 4%

Almond Fried Goat Cheese

SERVES 6 | PREP TIME: 20 minutes, plus time to chill | COOK TIME: 10 minutes

1 (16-ounce) goat cheese log
1½ cups almond meal, divided
2 eggs, beaten
1 tablespoon chopped fresh parsley
¼ teaspoon sea salt
¼ teaspoon freshly ground black pepper
½ cup avocado oil

Place the goat cheese log in the freezer for 30 minutes to firm it up. Add ½ cup of almond meal to a small bowl. Add the eggs to a second bowl. Place the remaining almond meal, parsley, salt, and pepper in a third bowl, stirring to combine. Slice the goat cheese into ½-inch-thick slices using dental floss or fishing line. Carefully dredge the goat cheese in the almond meal, then the eggs, and finally the almond-parsley mixture until entirely breaded. Heat the oil in a large skillet over medium-high heat. Fry the breaded cheese until golden brown, turning once, about 10 minutes in total.

Per Serving: Calories: 569; Fat: 52g; Protein: 22g; Total Carbs: 4g; Fiber: 2g; Net Carbs: 2g; **Macros:** Fat: 82%; Protein: 15%; Carbs: 3%

Feta Cheese Kebabs

SERVES 4 | PREP TIME: 25 minutes | COOK TIME: 6 minutes

8 ounces feta cheese, cut into 12 chunks
1 large carrot, cut into 8 ribbons and blanched until tender crisp
1 zucchini, cut into 12 slices
½ red onion, cut into 8 wedges
2 tablespoons extra-virgin olive oil
Sea salt
Freshly ground black pepper
1 tablespoon black sesame seeds

Preheat the oven to broil. Line a baking sheet with aluminum foil, and set the oven rack about 4 inches from the heat. Thread the feta, carrot (doubled over), zucchini, and onion onto 4 metal skewers or onto wood skewers that have been soaked in water for 30 minutes. Brush the kebabs generously with olive oil on all sides, and place them on the baking sheet. Season the kebabs with salt and pepper. Broil the kebabs until the vegetables and cheese are lightly browned, turning to brown all sides, for about 6 minutes in total. Sprinkle with the sesame seeds, and serve immediately.

Per Serving: (1 kebab): Calories: 243; Fat: 20g; Protein: 10g; Total Carbs: 7g; Fiber: 2g; Net Carbs: 5g; **Macros:** Fat: 73%; Protein: 16%; Carbs: 11%

Loaded Feta

MAKES 1½ CUPS | PREP TIME: 5 minutes

⅓ cup extra-virgin olive oil
2 teaspoons dried rosemary
1 teaspoon dried oregano
1 teaspoon dried thyme

1 to 2 teaspoons red pepper
 flakes, to taste
½ teaspoon salt
8 ounces feta cheese, cut into
 ½-inch cubes

In a medium bowl or large glass jar, whisk the olive oil, rosemary, oregano, thyme, red pepper flakes, and salt. Add the feta and toss to coat, being sure not to crumble the feta. Store, covered, in the refrigerator for up to 4 days. Let sit at room temperature for at least 30 minutes before serving to allow the oil to return to liquid.

Per Serving: (⅓ cup): Calories: 311; Fat: 30g; Protein: 8g; Total Carbs: 3g; Fiber: 1g; Net Carbs: 2g; **Macros:** Fat: 87%; Protein: 10%; Carbs: 3%

Buffalo Roasted Cauliflower

SERVES 3 | PREP TIME: 5 minutes | COOK TIME: 20 minutes

2 cups cauliflower florets
1 tablespoon olive oil
1 teaspoon garlic powder
1 teaspoon onion powder
¼ teaspoon salt
⅛ teaspoon freshly ground
 black pepper

¼ cup butter
⅓ cup hot sauce
1 tablespoon white vinegar
¼ teaspoon Worcester-
 shire sauce

For the bleu cheese sauce

2 tablespoons bleu cheese
 dressing

2 tablespoons sour cream
⅛ cup crumbled bleu cheese

Preheat the oven to 425°F. In a large bowl, combine the cauliflower florets, olive oil, garlic powder, onion powder, salt, and pepper. Mix well to season evenly. On a parchment-lined baking sheet, spread the cauliflower into an even layer. Bake for 20 minutes, or until the edges of the cauliflower pieces begin to brown. In a large skillet over medium-high heat, add the butter and melt. Add the hot sauce, vinegar, and Worcestershire sauce. Whisk over medium-high heat until the mixture is bubbling. Remove the skillet from the heat. In a small bowl, whisk the bleu cheese dressing and sour cream. Fold in the crumbled bleu cheese. Cover and refrigerate until ready to serve. In a large bowl, toss the cooked cauliflower with the buffalo sauce to coat. Allow the cauliflower to cool for 1 to 2 minutes before serving with the bleu cheese sauce.

Per Serving: Calories: 340; Fat: 33g; Protein: 7g; Total Carbs: 7g; Fiber: 2g; Net Carbs: 5g; **Macros:** Fat: 85%; Protein: 8%; Carbs: 7%

Jalapeño Poppers

SERVES 1 | PREP TIME: 10 minutes | COOK TIME: 15 minutes | TOTAL TIME: 25 minutes

6 jalapeño peppers
½ teaspoon minced garlic
2 tablespoons cream cheese,
 at room temperature
¼ teaspoon salt

⅛ teaspoon freshly ground
 black pepper
4 ounces Monterey Jack
 cheese, cubed
1 teaspoon olive oil

Preheat the oven to 450°F. Wash the jalapeños and cut off the tops. Using a small knife, cut the jalapeños top to bottom without cutting through to the other side. Gently open the peppers and remove the seeds and veins. Set the peppers aside. To a small bowl, add the minced garlic, cream cheese, salt, and pepper. Mix well to combine. Stuff the jalapeños with the Monterey Jack cheese so they are full but will still close. With a small spoon or knife, spread an equal amount of cream cheese inside each jalapeño, over the Monterey Jack, to help bind the pepper together. Close the peppers and place them on a baking sheet. Drizzle the jalapeños with olive oil and place the baking sheet in the preheated oven. Bake for 15 minutes, or until browned.

Per Serving: (6 cheese-stuffed jalapeños): Calories: 254; Fat: 21.5g; Protein: 9.8g; Total Carbs: 7.8g; Fiber: 3.6g; Net Carbs: 4.2g; **Macros:** Fat: 73%; Protein: 15%; Carbs: 12%

Cheesy Pork Rind Nachos

SERVES 1 | PREP TIME: 10 minutes | COOK TIME: 5 minutes

1½ ounces pork rinds
⅓ cup shredded Mexican
 cheese blend
⅛ cup diced tomato

1 garlic clove, minced
¼ teaspoon cumin
⅛ cup sour cream
Fresh cilantro for garnish

Arrange the pork rinds on a large microwaveable plate, being careful not to overlap them. Sprinkle the cheese evenly over all the pork rinds, covering each one to the edges. Top with the tomatoes and garlic. Season with the cumin. Place the plate in a microwave. Cook on high for 1 minute, 15 seconds. Check to see if the cheese has melted. If needed, cook for another 15 to 30 seconds, checking frequently. Make sure not to overcook, or the pork rinds will become soggy. Remove the plate from the microwave. Garnish the nachos with sour cream and cilantro. Serve.

Per Serving: Calories: 461; Fat: 33.4g; Protein: 36.7g; Total Carbs: 4.5g; Fiber: 0g; Net Carbs: 4.5g; **Macros:** Fat: 64%; Protein: 32%; Carbs: 15%

Jalapeño Firecrackers

SERVES 8 | PREP TIME: 20 minutes | COOK TIME: 20 minutes

8 (3- to 4-inch) jalapeños
 halved lengthwise
 and seeded
6 ounces cream cheese

¼ cup sugar-free apricot
 preserves
⅛ teaspoon red pepper flakes
16 pieces bacon, room
 temperature

Set the grill to low heat, and make a flat-bottom boat with aluminum foil large enough to hold 16 jalapeño halves, or use a grill mat. In a small bowl, mash the cream cheese, apricot preserves, and red pepper flakes until well incorporated. Using a butter knife, fill each of the jalapeño halves with the cream cheese mixture. Starting at the stem end of the jalapeño, lay a piece of bacon lengthwise across the cream cheese down toward the pointed end, and then wrap bacon around the jalapeño all the way back to the stem end so the entire jalapeño is covered lengthwise. This keeps the cream cheese from bubbling out. Repeat with remaining peppers and bacon slices. Place the jalapeños cream cheese–side down on the foil boat or mat, cook for 10 minutes, flip, and cook for an additional 10 minutes.

Per Serving: (2 jalapeño halves): Calories: 163; Fat: 13g; Protein: 7g; Total Carbs: 5g; Fiber: 1.5g; Net Carbs: 3.5g; **Macros:** Fat: 73%; Protein: 17%; Carbs: 10%

Spicy Jalapeño Chips and Ranch

SERVES 8 | PREP TIME: 5 minutes | COOK TIME: 20 minutes

5 medium jalapeños, very thinly sliced, with or without seeds depending on taste
1 tablespoon olive oil
½ teaspoon garlic powder
½ teaspoon minced onion

1 (7-ounce) package Havarti cheese slices
½ packet ranch dressing mix
½ cup sour cream
½ cup mayonnaise
1 tablespoon jalapeño juice, from a jar, or more or less

Preheat the oven to 450°F, line a baking sheet with parchment paper, and place a paper towel on a plate. Place the sliced jalapeños in a resealable bag with the olive oil. Seal, and massage and turn the bag to coat the slices. Spread the jalapeño slices on baking sheet, and then season with the garlic powder and minced onion. Roast for 10 to 15 minutes, until crisp. Remove from the oven, and transfer onto the paper towel. Place a new parchment paper on the baking sheet, and reduce the oven temperature to 400°F. Cut the cheese slices into quarters, and place on the lined baking sheet with a little space between them. Place a jalapeño slice in the middle of each piece of cheese. Bake for 5 to 7 minutes, or until the edges are brown. Remove from the oven, allow to cool for a few minutes, and then transfer to a plate or bowl. In a small bowl, stir the ranch dressing mix, sour cream, mayonnaise, and jalapeño juice. Serve with the jalapeño cheese chips.

Per Serving: (5 chips with dip): Calories: 251; Fat: 23g; Protein: 6g; Total Carbs: 3.5g; Fiber: 0g; Net Carbs: 3.5g; **Macros:** Fat: 84%; Protein: 10%; Carbs: 6%

Sriracha Artichoke Bites

SERVES 12 | PREP TIME: 15 minutes | COOK TIME: 35 minutes

For the scoops
Oil or nonstick cooking spray, for greasing
1½ cups grated mozzarella cheese

2 ounces (¼ cup) cream cheese
½ cup almond flour
2 tablespoons flaxseed meal
¼ teaspoon salt

For the artichoke dip
Oil or nonstick cooking spray, for greasing
1 (14-ounce) can water-packed artichoke hearts, rinsed, drained, and chopped
½ cup sour cream
½ cup mayonnaise

1 tablespoon sriracha sauce
1 teaspoon garlic powder
¼ teaspoon salt
½ cup grated Parmesan cheese
2 scallions, chopped, for garnish

Preheat the oven to 350°F, and grease the back sides of two mini muffin tins. In a microwave-safe bowl, melt the mozzarella cheese and cream cheese in 20-second increments until the mozzarella is melted and smooth. Remove from the microwave, and mix in the almond flour, flaxseed, and salt, and work into a ball of dough (it will be greasy). Spread a sheet of parchment paper on the counter. Split the dough in two, and place one on the parchment paper and one aside. Place another sheet of parchment paper over the top of the dough on the parchment paper, and with a rolling pin, roll the dough out very thin, 1/16 to 1/8 inch thick. Repeat this step with the remaining half of the dough. Cut circles of dough using a 2¼-inch round cookie cutter or something similar. Set the muffin pans upside down, and place a circle of dough flat on top of each of the mounds. Repeat until all the tops are covered. Bake for 10 to 15 minutes, turning the pans about halfway through, until completely golden brown. The dough will melt into a scoop. Remove from the oven, let cool 1 minute, and then gently pop them off and allow them to cool. Store in an airtight container until ready to fill. Preheat the oven to 350°F, and grease a small baking dish. In a medium bowl, stir the artichoke hearts, sour cream, mayonnaise, sriracha, garlic powder, and salt. Pour the mixture into the prepared baking dish, cover loosely with aluminum foil, and bake for 20 minutes. Remove from the oven. When cool enough to handle, spoon the mixture into the scoops. Sprinkle with the Parmesan, garnish with the scallions, and serve.

Per Serving: (2 artichoke bites): Calories: 216; Fat: 18g; Protein: 7g; Total Carbs: 6.5g; Fiber: 1.5g; Net Carbs: 5g; **Macros:** Fat: 75%; Protein: 13%; Carbs: 12%

Maple Bacon-Wrapped Brussels Sprouts

SERVES 20 | PREP TIME: 10 minutes | COOK TIME: 30 minutes

20 Brussels sprouts
¾ cup sugar-free maple-flavored syrup, divided
20 bacon slices, cut in half
2 cups mayonnaise

2 teaspoons sriracha sauce
2 teaspoons Dijon mustard
1 teaspoon salt
1 teaspoon freshly ground black pepper

Preheat the oven to 400°F, and line a baking sheet with parchment paper. Trim the ends off the Brussels sprouts, remove any wilted leaves, and halve the sprouts lengthwise. Drizzle ¼ cup of syrup on the bacon slices. Roll each Brussels sprout half with a piece of bacon, syrup-side out. Secure with a toothpick, and set them down on the parchment paper, leaving a little room between each sprout. Bake for 30 minutes, or until the bacon is crispy and the Brussels sprouts are fork-tender, rotating the pan halfway through. In a small bowl, mix the mayonnaise, ½ cup syrup, sriracha, Dijon mustard, salt, and pepper. Serve the Brussels sprouts with the dip.

Per Serving: (2 sprouts with dip): Calories: 217; Fat: 21g; Protein: 5g; Total Carbs: 3.5g; Fiber: 0.5g; Net Carbs: 1.5g; **Macros:** Fat: 87%; Protein: 10%; Carbs: 3%

Sausage and Spinach–Stuffed Mushrooms

SERVES 15 | PREP TIME: 15 minutes | COOK TIME: 35 minutes

15 whole button mushrooms, or cremini mushrooms, cleaned and stemmed (reserve the stems)
3 tablespoons butter
2 tablespoons finely chopped onion

2 garlic cloves, minced
¼ teaspoon kosher salt
1 cup fresh spinach, chopped
8 ounces spicy pork sausage
1 tablespoon gluten-free Worcestershire sauce

1 tablespoon chopped
   fresh parsley
⅓ cup shredded Parme-
   san cheese, plus more
   for garnish

½ cup shredded
   Fontina cheese

Preheat the oven to 400°F. Line a baking sheet with parchment. Set aside. Finely chop the reserved mushroom stems and set aside. In a sauté pan or skillet over medium to medium-high heat, melt the butter. Add the onion, garlic, mushroom stems, and salt. Cook for 7 to 10 minutes, or until the onion is translucent and soft, and the liquid from the mushroom stems is almost gone. Stir in the spinach and cook for about 2 minutes, just until the spinach wilts. Remove from the heat to cool. In a medium bowl, stir the sausage, Worcestershire sauce, parsley, and cooled spinach mixture. Add the Parmesan and Fontina cheeses and mix until thoroughly combined. Stuff each mushroom cap with about 1 tablespoon of filling, depending on their size. The filling should be heaping. Arrange the stuffed mushrooms on the baking sheet. Sprinkle with a little Parmesan cheese. Bake for 20 to 25 minutes, or until cooked through and browned.

Per Serving: Calories: 100; Fat: 8g; Protein: 5g; Total Carbs: 2g; Fiber: 0g; Net Carbs: 2g; **Macros:** Fat: 72%; Protein: 20%; Carbs: 8%

Pigs in a Blanket

SERVES 9 | PREP TIME: 10 minutes, plus 15 minutes to sit | COOK TIME: 25 minutes

2 cups grated mozza-
   rella cheese
2½ ounces (5 tablespoons)
   cream cheese
½ cup coconut flour

1 large egg
½ teaspoon garlic salt
6 smoked sausages, cut
   into thirds (check the
   carb count)

Preheat the oven to 350°F, and line a baking sheet with parchment paper. In a large microwave-safe bowl, combine the mozzarella and cream cheese, and melt in 20-second increments until the mozzarella is melted and smooth. Remove from the microwave, and mix. Add the flour, egg, and garlic salt, mixing well with your hands. Using your hands, form into a ball of dough. Allow to sit for about 15 minutes. Divide the dough into 18 sections. With damp hands, roll a dough section into a ball, place the ball in the palm of your hand, and flatten it out. Place a sausage on the dough, and wrap the dough around the sausage completely. Place on the lined baking sheet, and repeat with the remaining dough and sausage. Bake for 20 to 25 minutes, or until golden brown, rotating the pan halfway through. Serve warm.

Per Serving: (2 pigs): Calories: 187; Fat: 14g; Protein: 10g; Total Carbs: 5g; Fiber: 2.5g; Net Carbs: 2.5g; **Macros:** Fat: 68%; Protein: 21%; Carbs: 11%

Tofu Fries

SERVES 2 | PREP TIME: 15 minutes | COOK TIME: 15 minutes | TOTAL TIME: 30 minutes

Oil for frying
1 package (12 ounces)
   extra-firm tofu, sliced into
   ¼-inch slices

1 tablespoon salt
2 teaspoons freshly ground
   black pepper
1 teaspoon ground cumin

1 teaspoon dried parsley
1 teaspoon garlic powder
½ teaspoon onion powder
¼ teaspoon paprika

¼ teaspoon cayenne pepper
Sugar-free ketchup
   for serving

In a large pot, heat about 4 inches of oil to 350°F. Dry each tofu slice thoroughly between paper towels or a dishcloth. In a medium bowl, mix the salt, black pepper, cumin, parsley, garlic powder, onion powder, paprika, and cayenne pepper. Dredge the tofu fries in the spice mixture and set aside. Working in batches, add a few fries at a time to the oil so they do not stick together. Cook each batch for about 4 minutes, or until golden brown. Remove from the oil with a slotted spoon. Set aside on paper towels to drain. Repeat the process with the remaining tofu strips, working in batches as needed. Serve with sugar-free ketchup.

Per Serving: (6 ounces tofu fries): Calories: 197; Fat: 14.3g; Protein: 14.7g; Total Carbs: 6.5g; Fiber: 2.5g; Net Carbs: 4g; **Macros:** Fat: 59%; Protein: 28%; Carbs: 13%

Avocado "Fries"

SERVES 6 | PREP TIME: 10 minutes | COOK TIME: 15 minutes

1 or 2 medium semi-firm avo-
   cado(s), peeled, pitted, and
   cut lengthwise into 1-inch-
   thick sticks
1 cup almond flour

1 tablespoon ground flaxseed
1 teaspoon ground paprika
¼ teaspoon cayenne pepper
1 cup unsweetened hemp milk
1 teaspoon sea salt

Preheat the oven to 420°F. Line a baking sheet with parchment paper. If you don't have parchment paper, use aluminum foil or a greased pan. In a mixing bowl, whisk the almond flour, flaxseed, paprika, and cayenne. Pour the hemp milk into a separate bowl and set aside. Dip the avocado sticks in the hemp milk, then immediately roll them in the dry mixture until well coated. Place the coated avocado sticks on the prepared baking sheet. Bake for 7 minutes on one side, then flip the fries and bake for another 5 minutes until golden brown and crisp. Remove the fries from the oven and sprinkle with the salt.

Per Serving: Calories: 170; Fat: 16g; Protein: 7g; Total Carbs: 5g; Fiber: 3g; Net Carbs: 2g; **Macros:** Fat: 75%; Protein: 15%; Carbs: 10%

Jicama Nachos

SERVES 6 | PREP TIME: 10 minutes | COOK TIME: 5 minutes

1 lime, halved
½ medium jicama, peeled and
   thinly sliced
1 cup jarred cashew queso
1 small Roma tomato,
   finely diced

¼ cup finely diced
   yellow onion
1 jalapeño pepper, seeded and
   finely diced
¼ cup sliced olives
2 tablespoons coarsely
   chopped fresh cilantro

In a medium bowl, squeeze the lime halves directly over the jicama and set the jicama aside. In a small saucepan, heat the cashew queso until it is warm and a little steam is rising from the surface. If the cheese becomes too thick, stir in a little water to thin it out. Arrange the jicama "nacho chips" on a plate and pour the queso on top. Top with the tomato, onion, and jalapeño. Finish by sprinkling the nachos with the olives and cilantro.

Per Serving: Calories: 79; Fat: 4g; Protein: 3g; Total Carbs: 11g; Fiber: 5gm; Net Carbs: 6g; **Macros:** Fat: 39%; Protein: 13%; Carbs: 48%

Cheesy Cauliflower Breadsticks

SERVES 6 | PREP TIME: 25 minutes | COOK TIME: 35 minutes

1 head cauliflower, riced
4 large egg whites
½ cup grated Cheddar cheese, divided
½ cup grated Parmesan cheese, divided
1 teaspoon dried oregano
¼ teaspoon salt

Preheat the oven to 450°F. Line a baking sheet with parchment paper. Place the cauliflower to a microwave-safe bowl and cook in the microwave for 7 minutes. Remove and allow to cool for 5 minutes. Pour the cooked cauliflower into a cheesecloth or clean kitchen towel and squeeze to remove as much moisture as possible. The drier the cauliflower, the better the result. In a medium mixing bowl, combine the cauliflower, egg whites, ¼ cup of the Cheddar cheese, ¼ cup of Parmesan cheese, oregano, and salt. Mix until a dough forms. Place the dough on top of the parchment paper on the baking sheet. Use a rolling pin to roll it out into a rectangle or circle about ¼ inch thick. Cook the cauliflower crust for 16 to 18 minutes or until light golden brown. Remove the baking sheet from the oven and top the crust with the remaining ¼ cup of Cheddar and ¼ cup of Parmesan cheese. Bake for an additional 5 minutes. Turn the oven to low broil and broil for 3 minutes, or until the cheese is bubbling. Remove from the oven, cut into 12 breadsticks, and serve warm.

Per Serving: (2 breadsticks) Calories: 93; Fat: 5g; Protein: 9g; Total Carbs: 3g; Fiber: 1g; Net Carbs: 2g; **Macros:** Fat: 48%; Protein: 39%; Carbs: 13%

Soft-Baked Pretzels with Spicy Mustard Dip

MAKES 10 PRETZELS | PREP TIME: 20 minutes, plus rising time | COOK TIME: 25 to 30 minutes, plus cooling time

For the spicy mustard dip

¼ cup mayonnaise
¼ cup prepared yellow mustard
1½ teaspoons prepared horseradish
1 teaspoon Tabasco sauce
½ teaspoon sea salt
½ teaspoon onion powder
¼ teaspoon red pepper flakes
¼ teaspoon freshly ground black pepper
¼ teaspoon garlic powder

For the pretzels

1 tablespoon yeast
1 teaspoon sugar
3 tablespoons warm water
2 cups shredded part-skim mozzarella cheese, melted
2 tablespoons cream cheese, at room temperature
¾ cup coconut flour
2 teaspoons baking powder
¼ teaspoon xanthan gum
2 large eggs, at room temperature
1 large egg white, at room temperature
Coarse sea salt

In a medium bowl, combine the mayonnaise, mustard, prepared horseradish, Tabasco, salt, onion powder, red pepper flakes, pepper, and garlic powder. Cover, and refrigerate for at least 30 minutes to allow the flavors to develop. Refrigerate the mustard sauce for up to 5 days. Put the yeast and sugar in a small bowl. Add the warm water, and stir. Cover the bowl with a kitchen towel, and leave to rest for 10 minutes. The yeast has properly proofed when it expands and bubbles. While the yeast is proofing, line a large baking sheet with parchment paper. Put the mozzarella cheese in a large microwave-safe bowl. Microwave in 30-second increments, making sure to stir each time, until fully melted. Add the cream cheese to the melted mozzarella, and mix until combined. Using a rubber spatula, stir in the coconut flour, baking powder, and xanthan gum. Add the whole eggs and proofed yeast, and combine well. Once the dough comes together, lightly knead the dough with wet hands. Divide the dough into 10 equal balls, being sure to keep your hands wet so the dough doesn't stick. Roll each ball between your hands to form a pretzel stick about ¾-inch thick. Place the pretzels on the prepared baking sheet. Smooth any cracks on the surface or sides of the pretzels with your hands. In a small bowl, use a whisk to beat the egg white until foamy, and brush onto the pretzels with a pastry brush. Allow the pretzels to rest and slightly rise in a warm, draft-free place for 30 minutes. While the pretzels are rising, preheat the oven to 375°F. Sprinkle the pretzels with coarse sea salt. Bake for 25 to 30 minutes, or until the pretzels are golden brown. Allow to cool for 2 to 3 minutes in the pan, then transfer to a wire rack to cool fully.

Per Serving: Calories: 169; Fat: 11g; Protein: 10g; Total Carbs: 8g; Fiber: 4g; Net Carbs: 4g; **Macros:** Fat: 59%; Protein: 24%; Carbs: 17%

Garlic Breadsticks

MAKES 8 | PREP TIME: 15 minutes, plus 30 minutes to rest | COOK TIME: 15 minutes

1 cup almond flour
2 tablespoons coconut flour
2 teaspoons baking powder
1 teaspoon garlic powder
¼ teaspoon salt
2½ cups grated mozzarella cheese
½ cup grated Cheddar cheese
2 ounces (¼ cup) cream cheese
2 large eggs
2 tablespoons garlic salt

Preheat the oven to 400°F, and line a baking sheet with parchment paper. In a small bowl, stir the almond flour, coconut flour, baking powder, garlic powder, and salt. Set aside. In a medium microwave-safe bowl, combine the mozzarella, Cheddar, and cream cheese. Heat in 30-second increments until the mixture is melted and smooth. Remove the cheese from the microwave, and stir to blend. Add half the flour mixture, and mix. Add the eggs and remaining flour mixture, and mix until incorporated. Let the dough rest for 30 minutes to make it easier to work with. Spread a piece of parchment paper on the counter. With damp hands, make a ball out of the dough, and split it in half. Place half the ball on the parchment paper on the counter, and split it into 4 equal parts. Using your palms, roll each part into a 6- to 8-inch breadstick. Place the 4 breadsticks on the baking sheet. Repeat with the remaining dough to make 8 breadsticks total. Sprinkle the garlic salt over the breadsticks. Bake for 13 to 15 minutes, or until golden brown, turning halfway through. Remove from the oven, and serve.

Per Serving: (1 breadstick): Calories: 254; Fat: 20g; Protein: 14g; Total Carbs: 4g; Fiber: 2g; Net Carbs: 2g; **Macros:** Fat: 74%; Protein: 22%; Carbs: 4%

Classic Mozzarella Sticks

SERVES 4 | PREP TIME: 10 minutes | COOK TIME: 15 minutes | TOTAL TIME: 1½ hours

2 ounces powdered Parmesan cheese

1 teaspoon Italian seasoning

1 large egg

5 mozzarella cheese sticks

Oil for frying

Pizza sauce or ranch dressing, for serving

In a large bowl, combine the powdered Parmesan cheese and Italian seasoning. In another bowl, whisk the egg for 1 minute. On a cutting board, slice each mozzarella stick crosswise into thirds for 15 pieces total. Dip one piece of the mozzarella into the egg and then roll it in the seasoned Parmesan cheese. Re-dip the piece of cheese in the egg, and then again in the Parmesan cheese. Roll the cheese-covered mozzarella piece between your hands so the coating adheres. Repeat with remaining mozzarella pieces. Freeze the cheese sticks for at least 1 hour. When ready to cook, preheat 1 inch of oil in a large pan to 350°F. Place 2 to 3 cheese sticks in the pan at a time, being careful not to overcrowd. Cook for 4 to 6 minutes, turning halfway through. Transfer to paper towels to drain. Repeat with the remaining pieces.

Per Serving: (about 4 pieces): Calories: 275; Fat: 22g; Protein: 21g; Total Carbs: 2g; Fiber: 0g; Net Carbs: 2g; Macros: Fat: 68%; Protein: 29%; Carbs: 3%

Bacon-Wrapped Mozzarella Sticks

SERVES 2 | PREP TIME: 10 minutes | COOK TIME: 5 minutes | TOTAL TIME: 15 minutes

Oil for frying

2 mozzarella string cheese pieces

4 bacon slices

In a large saucepan, heat 2 inches of oil to 350°F. Cut each string cheese stick in half widthwise. Wrap each half of string cheese in one slice of bacon. Secure with a toothpick. Keep the ends of the cheese stick exposed for better cooking. Once the oil is hot, drop the bacon-wrapped cheese pieces into the oil. Cook for 2 to 3 minutes, or until the bacon is thoroughly browned. Transfer to paper towels to drain. Serve alone or with sugar-free marinara sauce.

Per Serving: (2 bacon-wrapped cheese sticks): Calories: 381; Fat: 29.3g; Protein: 27.5g; Total Carbs: 1.7g; Fiber: 0g; Net Carbs: 1.7g; Macros: Fat: 69%; Protein: 29%; Carbs: 2%

Prosciutto and Cream Cheese Stuffed Mushrooms

SERVES 4 | PREP TIME: 5 minutes | COOK TIME: 20 minutes | TOTAL TIME: 27 minutes

¾ cup cream cheese, at room temperature

¼ cup sour cream

4 slices prosciutto, chopped

1 teaspoon chopped fresh parsley

¼ teaspoon salt

⅛ teaspoon freshly ground black pepper

16 small button mushrooms, stemmed, gills removed

1 tablespoon olive oil

Preheat the oven to 400°F. In a large bowl, mix the cream cheese and sour cream. Add the prosciutto, parsley, salt, and pepper. Stir to combine. Spoon equal amounts of the cream cheese and prosciutto mixture into the mushrooms. On a parchment-lined baking sheet, arrange the mushrooms, cream cheese-side up. Drizzle with the olive oil. Bake for 20 minutes, or until slightly browned. Remove the baking sheet from the oven. Cool for 1 to 2 minutes before serving.

Per Serving: (4 stuffed mushrooms): Calories: 279; Fat: 25g; Protein: 12g; Total Carbs: 3g; Fiber: 1g; Net Carbs: 2g; Macros: Fat: 79%; Protein: 17%; Carbs: 4%

Brown Sugar Bacon Smokies

SERVES 10 | PREP TIME: 15 minutes | COOK TIME: 45 minutes

¾ cup brown erythritol blend

1 pound bacon, cut into thirds

1 (14-ounce) package smoked cocktail franks

Preheat the oven to 400°F, and line a baking sheet with parchment paper. Pour the brown sweetener into a shallow bowl. Wrap a piece of bacon around a smokie, roll in the sweetener, secure the bacon with a toothpick, and lay on the baking sheet. Repeat with the remaining bacon and smokies. Bake for 30 to 35 minutes, until the bacon is crisp.

Per Serving: (4 smokies): Calories: 240; Fat: 16g; Protein: 10g; Total Carbs: 14g; Fiber: 0g; Net Carbs: 0g; Macros: Fat: 60%; Protein: 17%; Carbs: 23%

Cheesy Baked Meatballs

SERVES 12 | PREP TIME: 20 minutes | COOK TIME: 40 minutes

¼ cup olive oil, plus more for greasing

2 garlic cloves, minced

1 (10-ounce) can diced tomatoes with green chiles, like Ro-tel

1 (8-ounce) can tomato sauce

1 teaspoon salt, divided

¼ teaspoon freshly ground black pepper, divided

1½ pounds ground beef

½ cup crushed pork skins

¼ cup grated Parmesan cheese

1 large egg

½ teaspoon garlic powder

½ cup grated mozzarella cheese

½ cup grated Parmesan cheese

Preheat the oven to 375°F, and lightly grease a 9-by-13-inch baking dish. In a medium pot over medium-low heat, heat the olive oil. Add the garlic, and sauté for 1 or 2 minutes. Reduce heat to low, and add the diced tomatoes, tomato sauce, ½ teaspoon salt, and ⅛ teaspoon pepper. Cook, stirring occasionally, while you make the meatballs. In a large bowl, combine the ground beef, pork skins, Parmesan, egg, garlic powder, and remaining ½ teaspoon salt and ⅛ teaspoon pepper. Mix well, scoop, and roll into 24 balls about 1½ inches in diameter, and place side by side in the prepared baking dish. Bake for 20 minutes, remove from the oven, cover with the sauce, and top with the grated mozzarella. Bake for another 20 minutes, covering lightly with aluminum foil if the cheese begins to get too brown. Garnish with the Parmesan, and serve.

Per Serving: (2 meatballs): Calories: 220; Fat: 15g; Protein: 16g; Total Carbs: 3.5g; Fiber: 0.5g; Net Carbs: 3g; Macros: Fat: 63%; Protein: 30%; Carbs: 7%

Hot Dog Rolls

SERVES 4 | PREP TIME: 10 minutes | COOK TIME: 15 minutes | TOTAL TIME: 30 minutes

1½ cups shredded mozza-
　rella cheese
2 tablespoons cream cheese,
　at room temperature
¾ cup almond flour

1 large egg
1 teaspoon minced garlic
1 teaspoon Italian seasoning
4 hot dogs

Preheat the oven to 425°F. In a large microwaveable bowl, combine the mozzarella cheese and cream cheese. Microwave on high for 1 minute. Remove, stir, and microwave again for 30 seconds more. The mixture will be very hot. Add the almond flour, egg, garlic, and Italian seasoning to the cheese mixture. Stir to incorporate fully. With wet hands, divide the dough into four equal pieces. Shape one piece of dough around each hot dog, encasing the hot dog completely. Place the dough-wrapped hot dogs onto a parchment-lined baking sheet. Use a fork to poke holes into each piece of dough so it doesn't bubble up during cooking. Put the baking sheet into the preheated oven. Bake for 7 to 8 minutes. Remove the tray from the oven. Check for bubbles (prick with a fork, if formed). Turn the dogs over. Return to the oven for another 6 to 7 minutes. Remove the sheet from the oven. Cool the hot dog rolls for 3 to 5 minutes before serving.

Per Serving: (1 hot dog roll): Calories: 435; Fat: 34.7g; Protein: 18.6g; Total Carbs: 7.6g; Fiber: 2.3g; Net Carbs: 5.3g; Macros: Fat: 74%; Protein: 18%; Carbs: 8%

Empanadas

SERVES 10 | PREP TIME: 10 minutes | COOK TIME: 22 minutes

For the filling

½ pound 80 percent lean
　ground beef
½ teaspoon kosher salt
½ teaspoon ground cinnamon
¼ teaspoon ground cumin
¼ teaspoon chili powder
¼ teaspoon freshly ground
　black pepper

2 ounces canned diced toma-
　toes with green chiles
1 tablespoon minced onion
1 tablespoon minced garlic
½ cup shredded Cheddar
　cheese

For the dough

1¾ cups mozzarella cheese
¾ cup almond flour
2 tablespoons cream cheese

1 large egg
1 teaspoon kosher salt

Preheat the oven to 350°F. Line a baking sheet with parchment paper. In a large skillet, heat the beef over medium-high heat. Cook the beef until browned and fully cooked, about 10 minutes. Drain the grease. Add the salt, cinnamon, cumin, chili powder, pepper, tomatoes and green chiles, onion, and garlic to the skillet and stir until combined with the beef. In a medium microwave-safe bowl, mix the mozzarella cheese and almond flour. Add the cream cheese and microwave on high for 1 minute. Stir the mixture, then microwave again on high for 30 seconds. Remove from the microwave and mix in the egg and salt until combined. Roll out the dough into a rectangle between 2 pieces of parchment paper (about ¼-inch thick). Using a large circle cutter or the edge of a drinking glass, cut 10 (4-inch diameter)

circles out of the dough and place them on the baking sheet. (You may need to roll the dough scraps to get more circles.) Place a spoonful of filling and about 2½ teaspoons of Cheddar cheese on top of each circle of dough. Fold the dough over to enclose the filling and pinch the edges closed, forming a half-circle. Use a fork to crimp the edges and to ensure the meat won't leak out. Bake for 10 to 12 minutes or until the dough begins to brown. Serve.

Per Serving: Calories: 201; Fat: 16g; Protein: 12g; Total Carbs: 3g; Fiber: 1g; Net Carbs: 2g; Macros: Fat: 70%; Protein: 25%; Carbs: 5%

Beef Taquitos

SERVES 4 | PREP TIME: 15 minutes | COOK TIME: 30 minutes

1 tablespoon olive oil
½ red onion, spiralized
1 garlic clove, minced
2 teaspoons tomato paste
8 ounces ground beef
Salt

Freshly ground black pepper
1 tablespoon taco seasoning
1 large zucchini, spiralized
6 ounces shredded cheese
　of choice
¼ cup sour cream, for serving

Preheat the oven to 350°F. Line a baking sheet with parchment paper. In a large skillet over medium-high heat, heat the olive oil. Add the red onion and sauté for 2 to 3 minutes. Stir in the garlic and cook for 1 to 2 minutes more. Add the tomato paste and ground beef to the pan, stirring well to combine. Season with salt and pepper and stir in the taco seasoning. Cook for 7 to 8 minutes, or until the meat has cooked through and is completely browned. Add the zucchini, cook for 1 to 2 minutes, and remove from the heat. While the beef cooks, separate the shredded cheese into 4 equal piles on the prepared baking sheet. The cheese will spread a bit when baking so do two at a time if you don't have a large baking sheet. Bake for 8 to 10 minutes, or until the edges begin to brown. Let cool slightly for just a couple of minutes—you want them to still be a little warm so they'll be pliable. To assemble the taquitos, spoon about 2 heaping tablespoons of the beef and zucchini mixture onto the taco shells. Carefully roll them and set aside. Let the rolls rest for a few minutes before serving. Serve with a side of sour cream for dipping.

Per Serving: (1 taquito): Calories: 390; Fat: 31g; Protein: 22g; Total Carbs: 7g; Fiber: 2g; Net Carbs: 5g; Macros: Fat: 70%; Protein: 23%; Carbs: 7%

Cheesy Chicken Taquitos

PREP TIME: 15 minutes | COOK TIME: 45 minutes | TAQUITOS: 12

12 large (deli-sliced) slices
　Cheddar cheese
3 ounces (6 tablespoons)
　cream cheese
¼ cup tomato salsa
1 tablespoon fresh lime juice
1 teaspoon chili powder
1 teaspoon garlic salt

½ teaspoon freshly ground
　black pepper
2 cups cooked shred-
　ded chicken
¾ cup sour cream
1 or 2 scallions, chopped,
　for garnish

Preheat the oven to 375°F, and line two baking sheets with parchment paper. Lay 6 pieces of Cheddar cheese on each baking sheet an equal distance apart. In a medium skillet over medium heat, mix the cream cheese, salsa, lime juice, chili powder, garlic salt, and pepper. Add the shredded chicken, and mix until heated through. Set aside. Place the baking sheets in the oven for 6 to 10 minutes, or until the edges are brown and the cheese is bubbly. Remove the sheets from the oven and allow to cool for a couple of minutes. When cool enough to handle, peel the cheese off the parchment paper and place on a clean piece of parchment paper. Spoon 1/12 of the chicken mixture onto each piece of cheese and wrap tightly. Place the taquitos on a serving dish, top each with 1 tablespoon of sour cream, and sprinkle with scallions to garnish.

Per Serving: (1 taquito): Calories: 177; Fat: 13g; Protein: 12g; Total Carbs: 2g; Fiber: 0g; Net Carbs: 2g; **Macros:** Fat: 68%; Protein: 27%; Carbs: 5%

Thai Chicken Skewers with Peanut Sauce

SERVES 4 | PREP TIME: 10 minutes | COOK TIME: 12 to 15 minutes

1 pound boneless, skinless chicken thighs	2 tablespoons low-sodium soy sauce
1 tablespoon toasted sesame oil	Juice of 1 lime
Sea salt	1 teaspoon minced ginger
Freshly ground black pepper	1 teaspoon minced garlic
1/3 cup natural peanut butter	Pinch red pepper flakes

Preheat the oven to 400°F. Slice the chicken lengthwise into 2-inch-long pieces. Thread the chicken pieces onto four bamboo skewers. Brush the skewered chicken with the sesame oil and season with salt and pepper. Bake for 12 to 15 minutes, or until the chicken is cooked through to an internal temperature of 165°F. Meanwhile, combine the peanut butter, soy sauce, lime juice, ginger, garlic, and red pepper flakes in a small jar. Cover tightly with a lid and shake vigorously. Thin with 2 to 3 tablespoons of water until the sauce reaches the desired consistency. Serve each skewer with 2 tablespoons of the peanut sauce on the side.

Per Serving: (1 skewer) Calories: 316; Fat: 20g; Protein: 31g; Total Carbs: 5g; Fiber: 1g; Net Carbs: 4g; **Macros:** Fat: 57%; Protein: 39%; Carbs: 4%

Sriracha Wings

SERVES 5 | PREP TIME: 10 minutes | COOK TIME: 1 hour

1 (2½-pound) package chicken wings (20 to 22 wings), patted dry	½ cup sriracha sauce
1 tablespoon garlic powder	1 teaspoon sesame oil
1 tablespoon baking powder	1 teaspoon soy sauce
½ teaspoon salt	1 teaspoon brown erythritol blend
¼ teaspoon freshly ground black pepper	2 tablespoons sesame seeds, for garnish

Preheat the oven to 425°F, and line a baking sheet with parchment paper. Spread the chicken wings on the lined baking sheet. In a small bowl, stir the garlic powder, baking powder, salt, and pepper. Sprinkle half the mixture evenly on top of the chicken wings, flip them over, and sprinkle with the other half of the mixture. Bake for 25 minutes, flip the wings over, and cook for 25 minutes more. In a medium bowl, whisk the sriracha, sesame

oil, soy sauce, and brown sweetener. Dip the wings in the mixture to coat evenly, and place back on the baking sheet. Bake for another 10 minutes and remove from the oven. Garnish with sesame seeds and serve.

Per Serving: (4 wings): Calories: 299; Fat: 21g; Protein: 26g; Total Carbs: 6.5g; Fiber: 0.5g; Net Carbs: 5g; **Macros:** Fat: 59%; Protein: 32%; Carbs: 9%

Bacon-Wrapped Jalapeño Chicken

SERVES 6 | PREP TIME: 20 minutes | COOK TIME: 45 minutes

2 tablespoons seasoned salt	1 pound boneless skinless chicken tenderloins (10 to 12 tenderloins), patted dry
2 tablespoons garlic powder	
2 tablespoons freshly ground black pepper	10 to 12 slices uncooked bacon
	3 jalapeños, seeded and cut lengthwise into 4 slices

Preheat the oven to 375°F. Line a rimmed baking sheet with parchment paper and set aside. In a small bowl, mix the seasoned salt, garlic powder, and pepper. Lay a tenderloin in the seasonings, then remove it. Lay a slice of jalapeño across the tenderloin, and wrap both the chicken and the jalapeño with a slice of bacon. Place the wrapped tenderloin on the prepared baking sheet. Repeat with the remaining tenderloins. Bake for 45 minutes.

Per Serving: (2 tenderloins) Calories: 303; Fat: 22g; Protein: 23g; Total Carbs: 2g; Fiber: 0g; Net Carbs: 2g; **Macros:** Fat: 66%; Protein: 31%; Carbs: 3%

Latkes with Sour Cream

SERVES 12 | PREP TIME: 15 minutes | COOK TIME: 45 minutes

1 (2-pound) head cauliflower, stems trimmed and florets coarsely chopped	½ cup grated Cheddar cheese
	2 large eggs
2 tablespoons olive oil	3 tablespoons coconut flour
½ teaspoon freshly ground black pepper	2 tablespoons mayonnaise
½ teaspoon garlic powder	2 tablespoons olive oil, for frying
½ teaspoon salt	1 cup sour cream
½ cup grated mozzarella cheese	2 scallions, chopped, for garnish

Preheat the oven to 450°F, and line a baking sheet with parchment paper. Place the cauliflower in a gallon resealable bag, add the olive oil, seal, and massage and turn the bag to coat. Empty the cauliflower onto the baking sheet, and spread in a single layer. Season the cauliflower with the pepper, garlic powder, and salt. Roast for 30 minutes. Remove from the oven, and when cool enough to handle, coarsely chop and place in a medium bowl. Add the mozzarella, Cheddar, eggs, flour, and mayonnaise, and mix well. In a medium nonstick skillet over medium heat, heat the olive oil. Using a large spoon, scoop the mixture, drop it in the pan, and pat down into a patty. Working in batches and being careful not to crowd the pan, cook for 2 to 3 minutes, or until golden brown on one side. Flip, and cook 2 more minutes on the other side. Remove from the skillet, and transfer to a paper towel–lined plate. Top warm latkes with a spoonful of sour cream and garnish with the scallions.

Per Serving: (1 latke with sour cream): Calories: 156; Fat: 13g; Protein: 5g; Total Carbs: 4.5g; Fiber: 1.5g; Net Carbs: 3g; **Macros:** Fat: 75%; Protein: 13%; Carbs: 12%

Goat Cheese and Basil Pizza

MAKES 1 (14-INCH) PIZZA (8 SLICES) | PREP TIME: 15 minutes | COOK TIME: 30 to 40 minutes, plus 15 minutes to cool

For the sauce

2 tablespoons extra-virgin olive oil

2 garlic cloves, crushed

1 (14-ounce) can crushed tomatoes

1 teaspoon Italian seasoning

1 teaspoon dried basil

1 teaspoon dried oregano

1 teaspoon sea salt

¼ teaspoon red pepper flakes

For the crust

Extra-virgin olive oil, for greasing the pan

3 cups shredded mozzarella cheese

¼ cup cream cheese

2 large eggs, at room temperature

1¼ cups almond flour, sifted

¼ cup coconut flour

For the toppings

1 cup crumbled goat cheese

½ cup fresh basil, chiffonade

2 teaspoons minced fresh rosemary

Heat the olive oil in a medium saucepan over medium-high heat. Sauté the garlic until translucent. Add the crushed tomatoes, Italian seasoning, basil, oregano, salt, and red pepper flakes. Lower the heat to a simmer, and cook the sauce until it has reduced and thickened, for about 15 minutes. Preheat the oven to 375°F. Lightly grease a 14-inch pizza pan with olive oil. Put the mozzarella cheese in a medium microwave-safe bowl. Microwave in 30-second increments, making sure to stir each time, until fully melted. Add the cream cheese to the melted mozzarella, and combine well. Allow the mixture to cool slightly and then stir in the eggs, almond flour, and coconut flour. Using wet hands, press the dough into the pizza pan, and stretch to cover it. Pierce the surface of the pizza crust all over with a fork. Bake for 10 minutes, then check for any large bubbles that may have formed, and poke with a fork to deflate them. Continue baking for another 5 to 10 minutes, or until golden brown on top. Take the pan out of the oven, and allow to cool for at least 15 minutes. To make the toppings and finish the pizza: Spread the sauce evenly over the crust, and sprinkle the goat cheese on top. Add the basil and rosemary. Bake for another 15 to 20 minutes, or until the cheese is melted.

Per Serving: Calories: 356; Fat: 27g; Protein: 22g; Total Carbs: 10g; Fiber: 4g; Net Carbs: 6g; **Macros:** Fat: 68%; Protein: 25%; Carbs: 7%

Pesto Cauliflower Sheet-Pan "Pizza"

SERVES 4 | PREP TIME: 10 minutes | COOK TIME: 35 minutes

1 head cauliflower, trimmed

¼ cup extra-virgin olive oil

1 teaspoon salt

½ teaspoon freshly ground black pepper

1 teaspoon garlic powder

¼ cup pesto

1 cup shredded whole-milk mozzarella or Italian cheese blend

½ cup crumbled feta cheese

Preheat the oven to 425°F. Remove the stem and bottom leaves from a head of cauliflower and carefully break into large florets—the larger, the better. Thinly slice each floret from top to stem to about ¼-inch thickness. Line a large rimmed baking sheet with aluminum foil and drizzle with the olive. Lay the cauliflower out in a single layer on the oiled sheet. Sprinkle with salt, pepper, and garlic powder. Place in the oven and roast until softened, 15 to 20 minutes. Remove from the oven and spread the pesto evenly over top of the cauliflower. Sprinkle with the shredded cheese and feta, return to the oven, and roast for 10 more minutes, or until the cheese is melted and the cauliflower is soft. Turn the broiler to low and broil until browned and bubbly on top, 3 to 5 minutes. Remove from the oven, allow to cool slightly, and cut into large squares to serve.

Per Serving: Calories: 346; Fat: 30g; Protein: 12g; Total Carbs: 7g; Fiber: 2g; Net Carbs: 5g; **Macros:** Fat: 78%; Protein: 14%; Carbs: 8%

Pepperoni Supreme Pizza

MAKES 1 (14-INCH) PIZZA (8 SLICES) | PREP TIME: 15 minutes | COOK TIME: 30 to 40 minutes

For the sauce

2 tablespoons extra-virgin olive oil

2 garlic cloves, crushed

1 (14-ounce) can crushed tomatoes

1 teaspoon Italian seasoning

1 teaspoon dried basil

1 teaspoon dried oregano

1 teaspoon sea salt

¼ teaspoon red pepper flakes

For the crust

Extra-virgin olive oil, for greasing the pan

3 cups shredded mozzarella cheese

2 tablespoons cream cheese

2 large eggs, at room temperature

1¼ cups almond flour, measured and sifted

¼ cup coconut flour

For the toppings

1 cup shredded mozzarella cheese

¼ cup sliced pepperoni

¼ cup chopped onions

¼ cup chopped green bell pepper

¼ cup sliced mushrooms

¼ cup sliced black olives

¼ cup grated Parmesan cheese

Heat the olive oil in a medium saucepan over medium-high heat. Sauté the garlic until translucent. Add the crushed tomatoes, Italian seasoning, basil, oregano, salt, and red pepper flakes. Lower the heat to a simmer, and cook the sauce until it has reduced and thickened, for about 15 minutes. Preheat the oven to 375°F. Lightly grease a 14-inch pizza pan with olive oil. Put the mozzarella cheese in a medium microwave-safe bowl. Microwave in 30-second increments, making sure to stir each time, until fully melted. Add the cream cheese to the melted mozzarella, and combine well. Allow the mixture to cool slightly and then stir in the eggs, almond flour, and coconut flour. Using wet hands, press the dough into the pizza pan, and stretch to cover it. Pierce the surface of the pizza crust all over with a fork. Bake for 10 minutes, then check for any large bubbles that may have formed, and poke with a fork to deflate them. Continue baking for another 5 to 10 minutes, or until golden brown on top. Take the pan out of the oven, and allow to cool for at least 15 minutes. Spread the sauce evenly over the crust, and sprinkle the mozzarella cheese on top. Add the pepperoni, onions, bell pepper, mushrooms, olives, and Parmesan cheese, and bake for another 15 to 20 minutes, or until all the toppings are cooked and the cheese is slightly browned around the edges. Serve hot.

Per Serving: Calories: 384; Fat: 28g; Protein: 25g; Total Carbs: 12g; Fiber: 4g; Net Carbs: 8g; **Macros:** Fat: 66%; Protein: 26%; Carbs: 8%

Meat Crust Pizza

SERVES 8 | PREP TIME: 5 minutes | COOK TIME: 28 minutes

2 pounds Italian sausage, casings removed

4 ounces low-carb pizza sauce

1 cup shredded mozzarella cheese

3 ounces crumbled goat cheese

1 red bell pepper, seeded and diced

Preheat the oven to 350°F. Line a baking sheet with foil and form the sausage into a 14-inch circle (about ½-inch thick) in the middle of the baking sheet. Bake the sausage until cooked through, about 18 minutes. Remove from the oven and drain any excess grease. Then spread the pizza sauce on the meat crust, leaving a ½-inch border around the edges. Sprinkle the mozzarella and goat cheeses on the sauce and top with the bell pepper. Cook until the cheese is melted, about 10 minutes. Cut the pizza into slices and serve.

Per Serving: Calories: 472; Fat: 41g; Protein: 22g; Total Carbs: 3g; Fiber: 1g; Net Carbs: 2g; **Macros:** Fat: 78%; Protein: 19%; Carbs: 3%

Bacon and Egg Pizza

MAKES 1 (14-INCH) PIZZA (8 SLICES) | PREP TIME: 15 minutes | COOK TIME: 30 to 40 minutes

For the crust

Extra-virgin olive oil, for greasing the pan

3 cups shredded mozzarella cheese

¼ cup cream cheese

2 large eggs, at room temperature

1¼ cups almond flour, measured and sifted

¼ cup coconut flour

For the toppings

1 tablespoon extra-virgin olive oil

1 cup shredded mozzarella cheese

5 slices cooked bacon, crumbled

4 large eggs, at room temperature

2 tablespoons grated Parmesan cheese

2 tablespoons minced chives

Preheat the oven to 375°F. Lightly grease a 14-inch pizza pan with olive oil. Put the mozzarella cheese in a medium microwave-safe bowl. Microwave in 30-second increments, making sure to stir each time, until fully melted. Add the cream cheese to the melted mozzarella, and combine well. Allow the mixture to cool slightly and then stir in the eggs, almond flour, and coconut flour. Using

wet hands, press the dough into the pizza pan, and stretch to cover it. Pierce the surface of the pizza crust all over with a fork. Bake for 10 minutes, then check for any large bubbles that may have formed, and poke with a fork to deflate them. Continue baking for another 5 to 10 minutes, or until golden brown on top. Take the pan out of the oven, and allow to cool for at least 15 minutes. Spread the olive oil evenly over the crust. Sprinkle on the mozzarella cheese, then the bacon. Carefully crack the eggs on the top, spacing them evenly. Sprinkle on the Parmesan cheese. Bake for 15 to 20 minutes, or until the eggs are cooked. Garnish with the chives, then cut and serve hot.

Per Serving: Calories: 401; Fat: 29g; Protein: 28g; Total Carbs: 9g; Fiber: 3g; Net Carbs: 6g; **Macros:** Fat: 65%; Protein: 28%; Carbs: 7%

SWEETS & TREATS

Chocolate Sea Salt Almonds

SERVES 8 | PREP TIME: 10 minutes, plus 30 minutes to chill

4 ounces low-carb chocolate, chopped

1 tablespoon coconut oil

1 cup dry-roasted almonds

Sea salt

Line a rimmed baking sheet with parchment paper. In a small saucepan over medium-low heat, melt the chocolate and coconut oil together while stirring constantly. Remove from the heat and pour into a small bowl. Add the almonds to the chocolate and stir. Using a teaspoon, remove a cluster of almonds and place it on the baking sheet. Immediately sprinkle with a bit of sea salt. Repeat with the remaining nuts. Place the baking sheet in the refrigerator for 30 minutes or until set.

Per Serving: (1 cluster): Calories: 187; Fat: 15g; Protein: 6g; Total Carbs: 7g; Fiber: 4g; Net Carbs: 3g; **Macros:** Fat: 72%; Protein: 13%; Carbs: 15%

Salted Caramels

MAKES 24 | PREP TIME: 3 to 5 minutes | COOK TIME: 10 to 15 minutes, plus 2 hours to chill

1 cup allulose

¼ teaspoon sea salt

¼ cup heavy (whipping) cream

½ teaspoon vanilla extract

Line a baking pan with wax paper and set aside. In a small saucepan, brown the butter over medium heat for about 3 minutes, stirring often. Add the allulose and stir until well combined. Simmer for about 7 minutes, until melted, then stir in the salt. Once it starts to bubble, add the heavy cream and vanilla and stir constantly, making sure it doesn't boil over. Once combined, reduce the heat and allow to gently simmer for about 3 minutes, until reduced slightly. Remove the caramel sauce from the heat and pour it evenly into the prepared baking pan. Refrigerate for a couple of hours or overnight, until cool and hardened. Cut the caramel into 24 pieces and serve.

Per Serving: (1 piece): Calories: 6; Fat: 1g; Protein: 0g; Total Carbs: 0g; Fiber: 0g; Net Carbs: 0g; **Macros:** Fat: 97%; Protein: 1%; Carbs: 2%

Salted Caramel Cashew Brittle

SERVES 6 | **PREP TIME:** 10 minutes | **COOK TIME:** 5 minutes, plus 1 hour to chill

½ cup butter
¼ cup brown erythritol, granulated

4 ounces raw unsalted cashews
¼ cup natural cashew butter
Coarse sea salt

Line a rimmed baking sheet with parchment paper. In a small saucepan over low heat, stir the butter until it melts. Add the erythritol, cashews, and cashew butter. Mix until thoroughly combined and melted. Pour the mixture onto the prepared baking sheet. Sprinkle salt on top. Refrigerate the baking sheet to harden for about 1 hour. Remove the brittle from the sheet and break it into about 12 pieces.

Per Serving: (2 pieces): Calories: 321; Fat: 29g; Protein: 5g; Total Carbs: 10g; Fiber: 1g; Net Carbs: 9g; **Macros:** Fat: 81%; Protein: 7%; Carbs: 12%

White Chocolate Bark

SERVES 12 | **PREP TIME:** 15 minutes (plus 2 hours of freezing time)

Nonstick cooking spray
6 ounces coconut butter
1 ounce coconut oil
¼ cup protein powder
¼ cup powdered erythritol

2 tablespoons unsweetened coconut milk
2 teaspoons vanilla extract
2 tablespoons sugar-free chocolate chips

Coat a 9-inch square baking dish with nonstick spray. In a blender, combine the coconut butter, coconut oil, protein powder, erythritol, coconut milk, and vanilla. Blend until completely smooth. Pour the mixture into the prepared baking dish. Sprinkle with the chocolate chips and freeze for at least 2 hours before cutting or breaking into pieces and digging in.

Per Serving (1 ounce): Calories: 176; Fat: 16g; Protein: 3g; Total Carbs: 5g; Fiber: 3g; Net Carbs: 2g; **Macros:** Fat: 82%; Protein: 11%; Carbs: 7%

Almond Chocolate Bark

MAKES 15 PIECES | **PREP TIME:** 5 to 10 minutes, plus 20 minutes to chill

¾ cup coconut oil
¼ cup confectioners' erythritol–monk fruit blend; less sweet: 3 tablespoons

3 tablespoons dark cocoa powder
½ cup slivered almonds
¾ teaspoon almond extract

Line a baking sheet with parchment paper and set aside. In the microwave-safe bowl, melt the coconut oil in the microwave in 10-second intervals. In the medium bowl, whisk the melted coconut oil, sweetener, and cocoa powder until combined. Stir in the slivered almonds and almond extract. Pour the mixture into the prepared baking sheet and spread evenly. Put it in the freezer for about 20 minutes, or until the chocolate bark is solid. Once the chocolate bark is solid, break apart into 15 roughly even pieces to serve. Freeze the chocolate bark in an airtight container.

Per Serving: (1 piece): Calories: 117; Fat: 13g; Protein: 1g; Total Carbs: 1g; Fiber: 1g; Net Carbs: 0g; **Macros:** Fat: 94%; Protein: 3%; Carbs: 3%

Dairy-Free Chocolate Truffles

MAKES 16 | **PREP TIME:** 10 minutes | **COOK TIME:** 5 minutes, plus 40 minutes to chill

¼ cup coconut milk
5 ounces sugar-free dark chocolate, finely chopped

1 tablespoon solid coconut oil, at room temperature
¼ cup unsweetened cocoa powder, for coating

Line the baking sheet with parchment paper. In the small saucepan, heat the coconut milk over medium heat for about 3 minutes, until hot. Stir in the chocolate and let sit in the coconut milk for 5 minutes, then whisk carefully until all of the chocolate is melted and the texture is smooth and glossy. Add the coconut oil and whisk until combined. Refrigerate until firm and set, about 30 minutes. Using a small cookie scoop or spoon, scoop out the truffles, and shape into 1-inch balls. Move quickly, and only lightly touch the chocolate or it will melt in your hands. Roll the truffles in the cocoa powder and place on the baking sheet. Refrigerate for 10 minutes to set before serving.

Per Serving: (1 truffle): Calories: 74; Fat: 6g; Protein: 2g; Total Carbs: 3g; Fiber: 2g; Net Carbs: 1g; **Macros:** Fat: 77%; Protein: 8%; Carbs: 15%

Candied Bacon Fudge

MAKES 24 BARS | **PREP TIME:** 10 minutes | **COOK TIME:** 40 minutes, plus 30 minutes to chill

½ cup granulated erythritol–monk fruit blend
6 bacon slices
½ cup (1 stick) unsalted butter, at room temperature
4 ounces unsweetened baking chocolate, coarsely chopped

1 cup confectioners' erythritol–monk fruit blend; less sweet: ½ cup
8 ounces cream cheese, at room temperature
¼ cup dark cocoa powder
1 teaspoon vanilla extract
1 cup chopped pistachios

Preheat the oven to 350°F. Line a baking sheet with aluminum foil. Line a baking pan with parchment paper and set aside. Put the sweetener in a small shallow bowl, and dip the bacon slices to evenly coat both sides. Place the coated bacon on the baking sheet and bake for 30 to 40 minutes, or until fully cooked. Once cooled, break the bacon into smaller pieces and set aside. In the small microwave-safe bowl, melt the butter and baking chocolate in the microwave in 30-second intervals, then set aside. In the medium bowl, using an electric mixer on medium high, mix the confectioners' sweetener, cream cheese, dark cocoa powder, and vanilla until well combined, scraping the bowl once or twice, as needed. Add the melted chocolate mixture and combine until fully incorporated. Fold in three-quarters of the candied bacon and the chopped pistachios. Spread the batter into the prepared baking pan. Sprinkle the remaining candied bacon on top of the fudge. Freeze for about 30 minutes or until the fudge firms. Cut the fudge into 24 squares and serve.

Per Serving: (1 piece): Calories: 141; Fat: 13g; Protein: 3g; Total Carbs: 4g; Fiber: 2g; Net Carbs: 2g; **Macros:** Fat: 81%; Protein: 9%; Carbs: 10%

Pralines

MAKES 18 CLUSTERS | PREP TIME: 5 minutes |
COOK TIME: 15 minutes, plus 20 minutes to cool

¼ cup (½ stick) unsalted
   butter, at room temperature
¼ cup granulated erythritol–
   monk fruit blend

1½ cups pecan halves
½ teaspoon salt
2 tablespoons heavy (whipping) cream

Line the baking sheet with parchment paper. In the skillet, melt the butter over medium-high heat. Using the silicone spatula, stir in the sweetener until it is dissolved in the butter. Stir in the pecan halves and salt. Once the pecans are completely covered in the glaze, add the heavy cream and quickly stir. When the heavy cream bubbles and evaporates, remove from the heat immediately. Quickly spoon clusters of 4 to 5 pecan halves onto the baking sheet and allow to fully cool and set, 15 to 20 minutes, before enjoying.

Per Serving: (1 cluster): Calories: 85; Fat: 9g; Protein: 1g; Total Carbs: 1g; Fiber: 1g; Net Carbs: 0g; Macros: Fat: 91%; Protein: 3%; Carbs: 6%

Chocolate Peppermint Fudge

MAKES 24 BARS | PREP TIME: 10 minutes |
COOK TIME: 5 minutes, plus 30 minutes to chill

½ cup (1 stick) unsalted butter,
   at room temperature
4 ounces unsweetened baking
   chocolate, coarsely chopped
1 cup confectioners' erythritol–monk fruit blend; less
   sweet: ½ cup

8 ounces cream cheese, at
   room temperature
¼ cup dark cocoa powder
1 teaspoon vanilla extract
1½ teaspoons pepper-
   mint extract

Line the baking sheet with parchment paper. In the microwave-safe bowl, melt the butter and baking chocolate in the microwave in 30-second intervals, then set aside. In the large mixing bowl, using an electric mixer on medium high, mix the confectioners' sweetener, cream cheese, cocoa powder, vanilla, and peppermint extract until well combined, scraping the bowl once or twice, as needed. Add the melted chocolate mixture and mix until fully incorporated. Evenly spread the batter into the prepared baking pan. Freeze for about 30 minutes, or until the fudge firms. Cut the fudge into 24 squares and serve.

Per Serving: (1 piece): Calories: 99; Fat: 10g; Protein: 1g; Total Carbs: 2g; Fiber: 1g; Net Carbs: 1g; Macros: Fat: 87%; Protein: 6%; Carbs: 7%

Cinnamon-Dusted Almonds

MAKES 2½ CUPS | PREP TIME: 5 minutes |
COOK TIME: 45 minutes, plus 20 minutes to cool

2½ cups whole raw almonds
2 tablespoons unsalted
   butter, melted
1 large egg white
½ teaspoon vanilla extract

¼ cup brown or golden erythritol–monk fruit blend; less
   sweet: 2 tablespoons
1 teaspoon ground cinnamon
¼ teaspoon sea salt

Preheat the oven to 275°F. Line the baking sheet with parchment paper and set aside. In a large bowl, toss the almonds in the melted butter. In another large bowl, using an electric mixer on medium high, lightly beat the egg white for about 1 minute, until frothy. Add the vanilla to the egg white and mix until just combined. Add the almonds and stir until well coated. In the small bowl, combine the sweetener, cinnamon, and salt and sprinkle over the nut mixture. Toss to coat and spread evenly on the baking sheet. Bake for 45 minutes, stirring occasionally, until golden. Allow to cool fully, 15 to 20 minutes, before eating.

Per Serving: (¼ cup): Calories: 384; Fat: 34g; Protein: 13g; Total Carbs: 13g; Fiber: 8g; Net Carbs: 5g; Macros: Fat: 74%; Protein: 12%; Carbs: 14%

Cinnamon-Glazed Pecans

SERVES 10 | PREP TIME: 5 minutes | COOK TIME: 25 to
30 minutes

½ cup (1 stick) butter
2½ cups pecan halves
1 teaspoon vanilla extract

2 teaspoons cinnamon
1 cup sugar-free granu-
   lated sugar

Line a baking sheet with parchment paper and set aside. In a skillet over medium heat, melt the butter. Add the pecans, vanilla, and cinnamon, and cook, stirring occasionally, for 2 minutes. Reduce the heat to low and cook, stirring occasionally, for another 10 minutes. Add the sweetener and cook for another 10 to 15 minutes, until the pecans take on a glazed look. Spread on the baking sheet and let cool.

Per Serving: (¼ cup) Calories: 289; Fat: 29g; Protein: 3g; Total Carbs: 4g; Fiber: 3g; Net Carbs: 1g; Macros: Fat: 90%; Protein: 4%; Carbs: 6%

Coconut Truffles

MAKES 12 TRUFFLES | PREP TIME: 10 minutes, plus 15 minutes
to chill

½ cup stevia, or other sugar
   substitute
2 teaspoons coconut extract

½ cup unsweetened shred-
   ded coconut

In a medium bowl, mix the cream cheese, stevia, and coconut extract. Scoop into balls, 1 to 2 tablespoons in size. It should yield about 12. Roll the balls in the coconut flakes. Chill the truffles for 15 minutes before serving.

Per Serving: (1 truffle): Calories: 98; Fat: 9g; Protein: 2g; Total Carbs: 2g; Fiber: 1g; Net Carbs: 1g; Macros: Fat: 84%; Protein: 8%; Carbs: 8%

Chocolate-Covered Bacon

SERVES 4 | PREP TIME: 15 minutes, plus 1 hour to chill | COOK
TIME: 20 minutes

8 bacon slices
1½ tablespoons coconut oil
3 tablespoons unsweetened
   chocolate chips or pieces

1 teaspoon stevia, or other
   sugar substitute

Preheat the oven to 425°F. Skewer each bacon slice accordion-style on wooden skewers. Place on a baking sheet. Bake for 15 minutes, until crisp. Remove the bacon from the oven and cool completely. In a medium saucepan over low heat, melt the coconut oil and chocolate. Whisk in the stevia. Transfer the bacon to a sheet of parchment paper. With a pastry brush, coat one side of each bacon slice with the chocolate. Flip. Coat the other side of each piece with the remaining chocolate. Refrigerate for 1 hour before serving.

Per Serving: (2 slices): Calories: 165; Fat: 13g; Protein: 9g; Total Carbs: 3g; Fiber: 1g; Net Carbs: 2g; **Macros:** Fat: 71%; Protein: 22%; Carbs: 7%

Chocolate-Coconut Treats

MAKES 16 TREATS | **PREP TIME:** 10 minutes, plus 30 minutes to chill | **COOK TIME:** 3 minutes

⅓ cup coconut oil

¼ cup unsweetened cocoa powder

4 drops liquid stevia

Pinch sea salt

¼ cup shredded unsweetened coconut

Line a 6-inch-square baking dish with parchment paper and set aside. In a small saucepan over low heat, stir the coconut oil, cocoa, stevia, and salt for about 3 minutes. Stir in the coconut and press the mixture into the baking dish. Refrigerate until the mixture is hard, about 30 minutes.

Per Serving: (1 treat): Calories: 43; Fat: 5g; Protein: 1g; Total Carbs: 1g; Fiber: 0g; Net Carbs: 1g; **Macros:** Fat: 88%; Protein: 6%; Carbs: 6%

Chocolate Peanut Butter Cups

SERVES 6 | **PREP TIME:** 20 minutes

Nonstick cooking spray

¼ cup coconut oil, divided

½ cup creamy natural peanut butter, divided

2 tablespoons unsweetened cocoa powder

8 or 10 drops liquid stevia, divided

¼ teaspoon vanilla extract

Spray the cups of a 12-cup mini muffin pan with cooking spray. In a small bowl, whisk 2 tablespoons of the coconut oil, ¼ cup of the peanut butter, cocoa powder, and 4 or 5 drops of the stevia until well combined. Fill the bottom of each muffin cup with about 2 teaspoons of the mixture. Place in the freezer to set for about 8 minutes. While the chocolate layer is freezing, in a small bowl, combine the remaining ingredients and mix well. Remove the muffin tin from the freezer and top each chocolate layer with 2 teaspoons of peanut butter mixture. Place the muffin tin back in the freezer and freeze for a further 8 minutes. Use a butter knife to remove the cups from the tin and place them in a resealable plastic freezer bag. Store in the freezer.

Per Serving: (3 cups): Calories: 224; Fat: 20g; Protein: 5g; Total Carbs: 5g; Fiber: 2g; Net Carbs: 3g; **Macros:** Fat: 82%; Protein: 9%; Carbs: 9%

Cookie Dough Balls

SERVES 2 | **PREP TIME:** 10 minutes (plus 1 hour freezing time)

2 scoops protein powder

2 tablespoons coconut flour

2 teaspoons erythritol

1 tablespoon coconut oil

1½ teaspoons vanilla extract

¼ cup water or unsweetened nondairy milk of choice

2 teaspoons sugar-free chocolate chips (optional)

2 teaspoons freeze-dried strawberries (optional)

2 teaspoons nuts of your choice (optional)

2 teaspoons cocoa powder (optional)

In a large bowl, mix the protein powder, coconut flour, erythritol, coconut oil, vanilla, water, and, if using, the chocolate chips, strawberries, nuts, and cocoa powder until well combined. Roll the batter into 10 to 12 balls and put them on a plate. The dough balls can be enjoyed at room temperature, or you can freeze them for 1 hour before serving.

Per Serving: Calories: 191; Fat: 11g; Protein: 12g; Total Carbs: 11g; Fiber: 6g; Net Carbs: 5g; **Macros:** Fat: 52%; Protein: 25%; Carbs: 23%

Almond Butter Fudge

MAKES 36 PIECES | **PREP TIME:** 10 minutes, plus 2 hours to chill

1 cup coconut oil, at room temperature

1 cup almond butter

¼ cup heavy (whipping) cream

10 drops liquid stevia

Pinch sea salt

Line a 6-inch-square baking dish with parchment paper and set aside. In a medium bowl, whisk the coconut oil, almond butter, heavy cream, stevia, and salt until very smooth. Spoon the mixture into the baking dish and smooth the top with a spatula. Refrigerate until the fudge is firm, about 2 hours. Cut into 36 pieces and store the fudge in an airtight container in the freezer.

Per Serving: (2 pieces): Calories: 204; Fat: 22g; Protein: 3g; Total Carbs: 3g; Fiber: 1g; Net Carbs: 2g; **Macros:** Fat: 90%; Protein: 5%; Carbs: 5%

Chocolate Fudge

SERVES 12 | **PREP TIME:** 5 minutes, plus 30 minutes to freeze

1 cup coconut oil

¼ cup cacao powder

½ teaspoon stevia or 4 drops liquid stevia extract

1 teaspoon vanilla extract

¼ cup almond butter

¼ teaspoon pink Himalayan salt

Line a 5-inch square dish with parchment paper overhanging the sides. In a small saucepan, melt the coconut oil over low heat. Add the cacao and stevia, and stir until completely smooth. Remove from the heat, and stir in the vanilla. Pour the mixture into the prepared dish. Swirl the almond butter over the top, and sprinkle with the salt. Freeze for 30 minutes or until solid and firm. Using the parchment paper as handles, carefully transfer the fudge to a cutting board. Cut the fudge into squares, and store them in a sealed container in the freezer.

Per Serving: Calories: 235; Fat: 23g; Protein: 2g; Total Carbs: 5g; Fiber: 2g; Net Carbs: 3g; **Macros:** Fat: 88%; Protein: 4%; Carbs: 8%

Grilled Cantaloupe

SERVES 4 | **PREP TIME:** 15 minutes | **COOK TIME:** 10 minutes

1 small cantaloupe, cut into 1-inch-thick slices, seeded, with the rind intact

2 tablespoons melted coconut oil

½ teaspoon ground cinnamon

Pinch ground cloves

Pinch sea salt

½ cup heavy (whipping) cream

Preheat the grill to medium and clean the grates. Or preheat a grill pan on the stovetop. Brush the cut edges of the melon with coconut oil. Sprinkle the slices with cinnamon, cloves, and salt. Grill the melon slices until they are tender and very lightly charred, turning once, about 10 minutes total. Transfer the melon to a plate and set aside. Whip the cream until fluffy and thick, about 5 minutes. Serve the grilled cantaloupe with whipped cream.

Per Serving: Calories: 201; Fat: 18g; Protein: 2g; Total Carbs: 10g; Fiber: 1g; Net Carbs: 9g; **Macros:** Fat: 80%; Protein: 4%; Carbs: 16%

Grilled Sweet Peaches

SERVES 6 | PREP TIME: 40 minutes | COOK TIME: 15 minutes

2 tablespoons coconut oil	½ teaspoon ground cinnamon
2 teaspoons honey	3 peaches, cut in half and
1 teaspoon gluten-free	pits removed
vanilla extract	½ teaspoon salt

Combine the coconut oil, honey, vanilla, and cinnamon in a small bowl. Heat your grill or grill pan to medium high heat. Grill your peaches for 7 to 8 minutes on each side. Top each peach half with 1 teaspoon of the coconut and sprinkle with salt.

Per Serving: Calories: 75; Fat: 5g; Protein: 1g; Total Carbs: 9g; Fiber: 1g; Net Carbs: 8g; **Macros:** Fat: 54%; Protein: 3%; Carbs: 43%

Chocolate-Covered Strawberries

MAKES 15 | PREP TIME: 10 minutes | COOK TIME: 5 minutes, plus 15 minutes to chill

5 ounces sugar-free dark	15 medium whole strawberries,
chocolate chips	fresh or frozen
1 tablespoon vegetable short-	
ening or lard	

Line the baking sheet with parchment paper and set aside. In the microwave-safe bowl, combine the chocolate and shortening. Melt in the microwave in 30-second intervals, stirring in between. Dip the strawberries into the melted chocolate mixture and place them on the prepared baking sheet. Freeze the strawberries for 10 to 15 minutes to set before serving.

Per Serving: (3 strawberries): Calories: 217; Fat: 18g; Protein: 4g; Total Carbs: 11g; Fiber: 5g; Net Carbs: 6g; **Macros:** Fat: 73%; Protein: 8%; Carbs: 19%

Mint Chocolate Fat Bombs

MAKES 6 FAT BOMBS | PREP TIME: 10 minutes, plus time to chill

⅔ cup coconut oil, melted	¼ teaspoon peppermint
1 tablespoon erythritol,	extract
granulated	2 tablespoons unsweetened
	cocoa powder

In a small bowl, mix the coconut oil, erythritol, and peppermint extract. Use a silicone mold or an ice cube tray and fill six of the cups only halfway with the mixture. Note: You will have mixture left in the bowl. Place the mold in the refrigerator for 5 minutes. Stir the cocoa powder into the remaining mixture. Pour a cocoa layer on top of each peppermint layer and place the mold back in the refrigerator until set. Use a butter knife to remove the bombs

from the mold (they should just pop right out) and place them in a resealable freezer bag. Store in the refrigerator or freezer.

Per Serving: (1 fat bomb) Calories: 229; Fat: 25g; Protein: 0g; Total Carbs: 1g; Fiber: 1g; 2g; Net Carbs: 0g; **Macros:** Fat: 98%; Protein: 0%; Carbs: 2%

Salted Macadamia Fat Bomb

SERVES 8 | PREP TIME: 10 minutes plus 1 hour to chill

½ cup no-sugar-added maca-	1 to 2 teaspoons monk fruit
damia nut butter	extract (optional)
½ cup coconut oil	1½ teaspoons salt, divided
¼ cup coconut flour	¼ cup finely chopped maca-
	damia nuts

In a mixing bowl, combine the macadamia nut butter, coconut oil, coconut flour, monk fruit extract (if using), and ½ teaspoon of salt and stir well with a spatula to combine. Using your hands, form the mixture into 8 (1-inch) diameter balls. In a small bowl, combine the nuts and remaining 1 teaspoon of salt. Roll balls in the nuts and refrigerate at least 1 hour to harden before serving.

Per Serving: (1 fat bomb): Calories: 254; Fat: 26g; Protein: 1g; Total Carbs: 7g; Fiber: 4g; Net Carbs: 3g; **Macros:** Fat: 92%; Protein: 2%; Carbs: 6%

Roasted Strawberries with Whipped Cream

SERVES 6 | PREP TIME: 10, plus 30 minutes to chill | COOK TIME: 10 minutes

1 cup coconut cream, refriger-	3 cups strawberries, stems
ated overnight	removed and halved
2 teaspoons raw honey	2 teaspoons gluten-free
	vanilla extract

In a medium bowl, use an electric mixer to beat the coconut cream and honey for 5 to 10 minutes or until fluffy. Refrigerate the whipped cream for 30 minutes to allow it to firm. Preheat the oven to 375°F. Line a baking sheet with parchment paper. In another medium bowl, toss the strawberries and vanilla together. Spread the strawberries in a single layer on the baking sheet and bake for 10 minutes. Top the roasted strawberries with the chilled whipped cream.

Per Serving: Calories: 166; Fat: 12g; Protein: 2g; Total Carbs: 11g; Fiber: 3g; Net Carbs: 8g; **Macros:** Fat: 71%; Protein: 4%; Carbs: 25%

Lime-Coconut Fat Bomb

SERVES 8 | PREP TIME: 10 minutes plus 1 hour to chill

½ cup coconut oil	Juice and zest of 1 lime
½ cup coconut flour	1 to 2 teaspoons monk fruit
½ cup unsweetened flaked	extract (optional)
coconut, divided	½ teaspoon salt

In a mixing bowl, combine the coconut oil, coconut flour, ¼ cup of coconut, lime juice and zest, monk fruit extract (if using), and salt and stir well with a spatula to combine. Using your hands, form the mixture into 8 (1-inch) diameter balls. Place the remaining ¼ cup of coconut in a shallow dish and roll the balls in the coconut. Refrigerate for at least 1 hour to harden before serving.

Per Serving: (1 fat bomb): Calories: 186; Fat: 18g; Protein: 1g; Total Carbs: 6g; Fiber: 3g; Net Carbs: 3g; **Macros:** Fat: 87%; Protein: 2%; Carbs: 11%

Coconut Lemon Fat Bombs

MAKES 16 FAT BOMBS | PREP TIME: 15 minutes, plus 1 hour to freeze

2 ounces cream cheese	2 tablespoons freshly
¼ cup butter	squeezed lemon juice
¼ cup coconut oil	1 teaspoon lemon extract
¼ cup heavy (whipping) cream	1 teaspoon stevia, or other sugar substitute

In a medium microwaveable bowl, combine the cream cheese, butter, and coconut oil. Microwave on high in short 10-second intervals until the mixture begins to melt. Once melted, add the heavy cream. Whisk thoroughly to combine. Mix in the lemon juice, lemon extract, and stevia. Pour the mixture evenly into an ice cube tray. Freeze for at least 1 hour to solidify, preferably overnight. Enjoy within 2 hours.

Per Serving: (1 fat bomb): Calories: 81; Fat: 9g; Protein: 0g; Total Carbs: 0g; Fiber: 0g; Net Carbs: 0g; **Macros:** Fat: 100%; Protein: 0%; Carbs: 0%

Chocolate Peanut Butter Fat Bombs

MAKES 16 FAT BOMBS | PREP TIME: 15 minutes, plus 1 hour to freeze

¼ cup butter	2 tablespoons unsweetened
¼ cup coconut oil	cocoa powder
¼ cup heavy (whipping) cream	1 teaspoon pure
2 tablespoons powdered	vanilla extract
peanut butter, like PB2	1 teaspoon stevia, or other sugar substitute

To a medium microwaveable bowl, add the butter and coconut oil. Microwave on high in short 10-second intervals until the mixture begins to melt. Once melted, add the heavy cream. Whisk thoroughly to combine. Mix in the powdered peanut butter, cocoa powder, vanilla, and stevia. Pour the mixture evenly into an ice cube tray. Freeze for at least 1 hour to solidify, preferably overnight. Enjoy within 2 hours.

Per Serving: (1 fat bomb): Calories: 73; Fat: 8g; Protein: 1g; Total Carbs: 1g; Fiber: 1g; Net Carbs: 0g; **Macros:** Fat: 90%; Protein: 5%; Carbs: 5%

Nut Butter Cup Fat Bomb

SERVES 8 | PREP TIME: 5 minutes, plus 12 hours to freeze

½ cup crunchy almond butter (no-sugar-added)	1 teaspoon vanilla extract
½ cup extra-virgin olive oil	1 teaspoon ground cinnamon (optional)
¼ cup ground flaxseed	1 to 2 teaspoons sugar-free
2 tablespoons unsweetened cocoa powder	sweetener of choice (optional)

In a large bowl, combine the almond butter, olive oil, flaxseed, cocoa powder, vanilla, cinnamon (if using), and sweetener (if

using) and stir well to combine. Pour into 8 mini muffin liners and freeze until solid, at least 12 hours. Store in the freezer for 1 month.

Per Serving (1 fat bomb): Calories: 240; Fat: 24g; Protein: 3g; Total Carbs: 5g; Fiber: 2g; Net Carbs: 3g; **Macros:** Fat: 88%; Protein: 5%; Carbs: 7%

Peanut Butter Cookie Dough Fat Bombs

SERVES 8 | PREP TIME: 5 minutes

½ cup natural peanut butter	6 to 7 drops liquid stevia
¼ cup coconut oil, melted	Pinch sea salt
¼ cup butter, at room temperature	

In a small mixing bowl, mix the peanut butter, oil, butter, stevia, and sea salt together. Scoop 1 tablespoon of the mixture into a mini muffin paper, repeating until all the dough is used. Refrigerate the bombs in a covered container to firm up for at least 30 minutes.

Per Serving: Calories: 215; Fat: 21g; Protein: 4g; Total Carbs: 3g; Fiber: 1g; Net Carbs: 2g; **Macros:** Fat: 88%; Protein: 7%; Carbs: 5%

Marzipan Fat Bomb

SERVES 8 | PREP TIME: 5 minutes

1½ cup almond flour	2 teaspoons almond extract
½ to 1 cup powdered sugar-free sweetener of choice	½ cup extra-virgin olive oil or avocado oil

Add the almond flour and sweetener to a food processor and run until the mixture is very finely ground. Add the almond extract and pulse until combined. With the processor running, stream in the olive oil until the mixture starts to form a large ball. Using your hands, form the marzipan into eight (1-inch) diameter balls, pressing to hold the mixture together.

Per Serving (1 fat bomb): Calories: 157; Fat: 17g; Protein: 2g; Total Carbs: 0g; Fiber: 0g; Net Carbs: 0g; **Macros:** Fat: 94%; Protein: 4%; Carbs: 2%

Pumpkin Spice Fat Bombs

MAKES 16 FAT BOMBS | PREP TIME: 10 minutes, plus 1 hour chilling time

½ cup butter, at room temperature	3 tablespoons chopped almonds
½ cup cream cheese, at room temperature	4 drops liquid stevia
⅓ cup pure pumpkin purée	½ teaspoon ground cinnamon
	¼ teaspoon ground nutmeg

Line an 8-inch-square baking pan with parchment paper and set aside. In a small bowl, whisk the butter and cream cheese until very smooth. Add the pumpkin purée and whisk until blended. Stir in the almonds, stevia, cinnamon, and nutmeg. Spread the pumpkin mixture evenly into the pan. Freeze for about 1 hour.

Per Serving: (1 fat bomb) Calories: 87; Fat: 9g; Protein: 1g; Total Carbs: 1g; Fiber: 0g; Net Carbs: 1g; **Macros:** Fat: 90%; Protein: 5%; Carbs: 5%

Creamy Banana Fat Bombs

MAKES 12 FAT BOMBS | PREP TIME: 10 minutes, plus 1 hour chilling time

1¼ cups cream cheese, at room temperature

¾ cup heavy (whipping) cream

1 tablespoon pure banana extract

6 drops liquid stevia

Line a baking sheet with parchment paper and set aside. In a medium bowl, beat the cream cheese, heavy cream, banana extract, and stevia until smooth and very thick, about 5 minutes. Gently spoon the mixture onto the baking sheet in mounds, leaving some space between each mound. Refrigerate until firm, about 1 hour.

Per serving: Calories: 134; Fat: 12g; Protein: 3g; Total Carbs: 1g; Fiber: 0g; Net Carbs: 1g; **Macros:** Fat: 88%; Protein: 9%; Carbs: 3%

Lime Almond Fat Bomb

MAKES 16 | PREP TIME: 20 minutes, plus time to chill | COOK TIME: 2 minutes

½ cup coconut oil

2 tablespoons cocoa butter

Juice and zest of 1 lime

½ teaspoon vanilla extract

½ cup coconut flour

½ cup almond flour

1 teaspoon Swerve

½ cup almond meal

In a small saucepan over medium heat, stir the coconut oil, cocoa butter, lime juice, lime zest, and vanilla until the mixture is smooth and melted, about 2 minutes. Remove from the heat and set aside. In a medium bowl, stir the coconut flour, almond flour, and Swerve until well combined. Add in the coconut oil mixture and stir until well blended. Until firm enough to form into balls, about 1 hour. Roll the fat bombs into balls and roll them in the almond meal to coat. Freeze the balls in a sealed container until very firm, about 3 hours. Serve frozen.

Per Serving: Calories: 130; Fat: 12g; Protein: 2g; Total Carbs: 4g; Fiber: 2g; Net Carbs: 2g; **Macros:** Fat: 83%; Protein: 6%; Carbs: 11%

Blueberry Fat Bombs

MAKES 12 FAT BOMBS | PREP TIME: 10 minutes, plus 3 hours chilling time

½ cup coconut oil, at room temperature

½ cup cream cheese, at room temperature

½ cup blueberries, mashed with a fork

6 drops liquid stevia

Pinch ground nutmeg

Line a mini muffin tin with paper liners and set aside. In a medium bowl, stir the coconut oil and cream cheese until well blended. Stir in the blueberries, stevia, and nutmeg until combined. Divide the blueberry mixture into the muffin cups and freeze until set, about 3 hours. Freeze the fat bombs in an airtight container until you wish to eat them.

Per serving: Calories: 115; Fat: 12g; Protein: 1g; Total Carbs: 1g; Fiber: 0g; Net Carbs: 1g; **Macros:** Fat: 94%; Protein: 3%; Carbs: 3%

Spiced-Chocolate Fat Bombs

MAKES 12 FAT BOMBS | PREP TIME: 10 minutes, plus 15 minutes chilling time | COOK TIME: 4 minutes

¾ cup coconut oil

¼ cup cocoa powder

¼ cup almond butter

⅛ teaspoon chili powder

3 drops liquid stevia

Line a mini muffin tin with paper liners and set aside. Put a small saucepan over low heat and add the coconut oil, cocoa powder, almond butter, chili powder, and stevia. Heat until the coconut oil is melted, then whisk to blend. Spoon the mixture into the muffin cups and refrigerate until the bombs are firm, about 15 minutes.

Per Serving: (1 fat bomb) Calories: 117; Fat: 12g; Protein: 2g; Total Carbs: 2g; Fiber: 0g; Net Carbs: 2g; **Macros:** Fat: 92%; Protein: 4%; Carbs: 4%

Key Lime Pie Fat Bombs

MAKES 16 FAT BOMBS | PREP TIME: 5 minutes, plus 15 minutes to chill

8 ounces cream cheese

2 teaspoons lime zest

2 tablespoons lime juice

¼ teaspoon liquid stevia

½ cup shredded unsweetened coconut, finely ground

½ cup macadamia nuts, finely ground

¼ teaspoon sea salt

In a medium bowl, mix the cream cheese, lime zest, lime juice, and liquid stevia. In a shallow dish, mix the coconut, macadamia nuts, and sea salt. Divide the cream cheese mixture into 16 small balls, about 1 tablespoon each. Roll the balls in the coconut mixture. Refrigerate the balls in a covered container for at least 15 minutes before serving.

Per Serving: (1 fat bomb): Calories: 98; Fat: 10g; Protein: 2g; Total Carbs: 3g; Fiber: 1g; Net Carbs: 2g; **Macros:** Fat: 96%; Protein: 2%; Carbs: 2%

Salted Caramel Fudge Fat Bombs

SERVES 32 | PREP TIME: 15 minutes | COOK TIME: 8 minutes | CHILL TIME: 1 hour

4 ounces unsweetened chocolate, roughly chopped

½ cup (1 stick) butter

½ cup allulose blend sweetener

½ cup heavy (whipping) cream

Sea salt

Line an 8- or 9-inch loaf pan with plastic wrap. Set aside. Place the chocolate in a medium heat-resistant bowl. In a medium saucepan over medium heat, combine the butter and sweetener. Melt the butter and bring the mixture to a boil. Cook for 3 to 5 minutes, or until golden, stirring often. Add the cream and cook for 2 to 3 minutes more. Stir in a pinch of salt. Set aside to cool for 5 to 7 minutes. Pour the warm butter mixture over the chopped chocolate. Let sit for 1 minute. Stir until smooth and the chocolate is completely melted. Pour the fudge into the prepared loaf pan and spread it evenly. Sprinkle the top of the fudge with salt. Refrigerate for 45 minutes to 1 hour, or until firm. This fudge can be served at room temperature once it's been completely chilled.

Per Serving: (1 fat bomb): Calories: 62; Fat: 6g; Protein: 1g; Total Carbs: 1g; Fiber: 1g; Net Carbs: 0g; **Macros:** Fat: 88%; Protein: 6%; Carbs: 6%

Butter Pecan Cheesecake Truffle Fat Bombs

SERVES 24 | PREP TIME: 10 minutes |
COOK TIME: 5 minutes | CHILL TIME: 20 minutes

3 tablespoons butter
¼ cup finely chopped pecans
8 ounces cream cheese, at room temperature

3 tablespoons powdered monk fruit/erythritol blend sweetener (confectioners' sugar style)
1 teaspoon vanilla extract

In a small skillet over medium-low heat, melt the butter. Add the pecans and sauté for 3 to 4 minutes, until the pecans are toasted and the butter is golden. Set aside the pan to cool. In a medium bowl, using an electric hand mixer, beat the cream cheese, sweetener, and vanilla until smooth. Stir in the pecans and browned butter. Cover and refrigerate the mixture for 15 to 20 minutes, or until firm enough to roll. Drop by the ½ tablespoon onto parchment paper and roll each portion into a ball.

Per Serving: (1 fat bomb): Calories: 62; Fat: 6g; Protein: 1g; Total Carbs: 1g; Fiber: 0g; Net Carbs: 1g; **Macros:** Fat: 88%; Protein: 6%; Carbs: 6%

Cowboy Cookie Dough Fat Bombs

SERVES 12 | PREP TIME: 10 minutes |
COOK TIME: 5 minutes | CHILL TIME: 20 minutes

3 tablespoons butter
⅓ cup almond flour
1 teaspoon coconut flour
1 tablespoon plus 1 teaspoon monk fruit/erythritol blend sweetener
1 ounce cream cheese, at room temperature
½ teaspoon vanilla extract

⅛ teaspoon ground cinnamon
Pinch kosher salt
3 tablespoons sugar-free semisweet chocolate chips, roughly chopped
2 tablespoons finely chopped pecans
1 tablespoon desiccated unsweetened coconut

In a small skillet over medium-low heat, melt the butter and cook it for 4 to 6 minutes, stirring often, until it starts to foam. The solids in the butter should be the color of caramel and the aroma should be nutty. Cook for 1 minute more and remove the skillet from the heat. Set aside to cool. In a medium bowl, stir the cooled browned butter, almond and coconut flours, sweetener, cream cheese, vanilla, cinnamon, and salt to combine. Stir in the chocolate chips, pecans, and coconut. Refrigerate the dough for 15 to 20 minutes, or until firm. Drop the dough by the ½ tablespoon onto a piece of parchment paper and roll each portion into a ball.

Per Serving: Calories: 53; Fat: 5g; Protein: 1g; Total Carbs: 1g; Fiber: 1g; Net Carbs: 0g; **Macros:** Fat: 86%; Protein: 7%; Carbs: 7%

Cookie Dough Fat Bombs

MAKES 18 | PREP TIME: 5 minutes | CHILL TIME: 1 hour 15 minutes

8 ounces cream cheese, at room temperature

½ cup (1 stick) unsalted butter, at room temperature

¾ cup almond flour
½ cup granulated erythritol–monk fruit blend; less sweet: ¼ cup

1 teaspoon vanilla extract
¼ teaspoon sea salt
¼ cup chocolate chips

Line the baking sheet with parchment paper and set aside. In the medium bowl, using an electric mixer on high, blend the cream cheese and butter, scraping the bowl once or twice, as needed. Add the almond flour, sweetener, vanilla, and salt and mix until fully incorporated. Fold in the chocolate chips. Refrigerate the mixture for 1 hour until firm (like ice cream). Using a small cookie scoop or spoon, scoop the fat bombs into 1 tablespoon-size mounds and place onto the baking sheet. Refrigerate for about 15 minutes to allow the fat bombs to firm before serving.

Per Serving: (1 piece): Calories: 124; Fat: 12g; Protein: 2g; Total Carbs: 2g; Fiber: 1g; Net Carbs: 1g; **Macros:** Fat: 88%; Protein: 6%; Carbs: 6%

Cheesecake Fat Bombs

MAKES 30 | PREP TIME: 10 minutes | CHILL TIME: 1 hour

8 ounces cream cheese, at room temperature
½ cup (1 stick) unsalted butter, at room temperature

3 tablespoons confectioners' erythritol–monk fruit blend
3 tablespoons coconut oil
½ teaspoon vanilla extract

In the large mixing bowl, using an electric mixer on high, beat the cream cheese and butter for 2 to 3 minutes, until light and fluffy, stopping and scraping the bowl once or twice, as needed. Add the confectioners' sweetener, coconut oil, and vanilla and mix until well combined. Scoop the mixture into a pastry bag and pipe into the molds or cupcake liners. Freeze the molds for 1 hour to firm. Pop out the fat bombs to serve.

Per Serving: (1 piece): Calories: 65; Fat: 7g; Protein: 0g; Total Carbs: 0g; Fiber: 0g; Net Carbs: 0g; **Macros:** Fat: 95%; Protein: 3%; Carbs: 2

Cinnamon Roll Fat Bomb

MAKES 16 | PREP TIME: 15 minutes, plus 45 minutes to chill

¼ cup butter, at room temperature
2 ounces cream cheese, at room temperature
¼ cup brown sugar replacement
½ cup almond flour
1 teaspoon ground cinnamon

1 tablespoon creamy almond butter
1 tablespoon coconut oil, melted
½ tablespoon powdered erythritol
1 teaspoon ground cinnamon
½ teaspoon vanilla extract

In a large bowl, beat the butter and cream cheese. Add the brown sugar replacement and beat until well combined. Add the flour and cinnamon and beat until thoroughly blended. Cover and refrigerate for 15 to 20 minutes, until the dough solidifies. Line a baking sheet with parchment paper. Using a tablespoon, scoop the mixture out of the bowl and use your hands to roll it into balls. Place the balls on the baking sheet. Refrigerate the balls for 1 hour or freeze for 15 minutes, until solid to the touch. While the cinnamon rolls are hardening, make the icing. In a small bowl, whisk the almond butter, coconut oil, erythritol, cinnamon, and vanilla. Drizzle the icing mixture evenly over the cold cinnamon balls. Refrigerate or freeze again until the frosting sets. Let sit at room temperature for 5 minutes before serving.

Per Serving: (1 bomb): Calories: 72; Fat: 7g; Protein: 1g; Total Carbs: 5g; Fiber: 1g; Net Carbs: 1g; **Macros:** Fat: 88%; Protein: 6%; Carbs: 6%

Strawberry Cheesecake Fat Bombs

MAKES 12 FAT BOMBS | PREP TIME: 10 minutes, plus 4 hours to freeze | COOK TIME: 12 minutes

Nonstick cooking spray	2 tablespoons powdered
⅓ cup frozen strawberries	erythritol
4½ tablespoons cream cheese	½ teaspoon vanilla extract
4½ tablespoons butter	

Spray the cups of a 12-cup mini muffin tin with cooking spray. In a small saucepan over low heat, bring the strawberries to a simmer and cook for 10 minutes while stirring, until all the excess liquid has evaporated, leaving just the strawberries. Set aside. In the bowl of a stand mixer, combine the cream cheese, butter, erythritol, and vanilla, and mix on low for 3 to 4 minutes or until fluffy. Pour in the strawberries and mix for another 1 to 2 minutes. Using a 2-inch cookie scoop, scoop the mixture into the mini muffin cups. Freeze to set for 4 hours. Use a butter knife to remove the bombs from the tin (they should just pop right out) and place the bombs in a resealable freezer bag. Store in the freezer.

Per Serving: (1 fat bomb): Calories: 58; Fat: 6g; Protein: 0g; Total Carbs: 1g; Fiber: 0g; Net Carbs: 1g; **Macros:** Fat: 93%; Protein: 0%; Carbs: 7%

Cinnamon Coconut Fat Bomb

MAKES 12 | PREP TIME: 10 minutes, plus time to chill

½ cup cocoa butter	2 tablespoons almond butter
½ cup coconut oil	2 tablespoons Swerve
½ cup finely shredded	¾ teaspoon ground cinnamon
unsweetened coconut	

Place the cocoa butter, coconut oil, coconut, almond butter, Swerve, and cinnamon in a blender and pulse until very well combined. Spoon the mixture into an ice cube tray, pressing it in firmly. Freeze the fat bombs until very firm, 2 to 3 hours. Pop the fat bombs out of the tray and place them in a container. Serve frozen.

Per Serving: Calories: 198; Fat: 22g; Protein: 1g; Total Carbs: 2g; Fiber: 1g; Net Carbs: 1g; **Macros:** Fat: 98%; Protein: 1%; Carbs: 1%

Chocolate Almond Fat Bombs

MAKES 12 | PREP TIME: 5 minutes | COOK TIME: 5 minutes

¾ cup coconut oil	½ teaspoon vanilla extract
6 tablespoons cocoa powder	24 whole raw almonds
2 tablespoons powdered	Coarse sea salt
erythritol	

Place 12 candy molds or miniature muffin tin liners on a large baking sheet. In a small saucepan over medium heat, melt the coconut oil. Add the cocoa powder, erythritol, and vanilla, and whisk well to combine. Spoon the mixture into the candy molds.

Drop 2 almonds into each mold. Refrigerate until the chocolate is set. Remove the bombs from the molds and press a pinch of coarse sea salt onto the top of each chocolate.

Per Serving: Calories: 138; Fat: 15g; Protein: 1g; Total Carbs: 2g; Fiber: 1g; Net Carbs: 1g; **Macros:** Fat: 95%; Protein: 2%; Carbs: 3%

Creamy Tiramisu Fat Bomb

MAKES 12 | PREP TIME: 15 minutes, plus time to chill

½ cup cream cheese	1 tablespoon Swerve
½ cup mascarpone cheese	½ teaspoon liquid
¼ cup cocoa butter	coffee extract
¼ cup almond flour	½ cup almond meal
1 tablespoon cacao powder	

Place the cream cheese, mascarpone, cocoa butter, almond flour, cacao powder, Swerve, and coffee extract in a blender and pulse until very well mixed and smooth. Scoop the mixture into balls, 2 tablespoons each, and place them on a baking sheet. Freeze the balls until firm, about 1 hour. Roll the balls in the almond meal and place them in a container and cover. Serve frozen. Freeze for up to 1 month in a sealed container.

Per Serving: Calories: 156; Fat: 15g; Protein: 2g; Total Carbs: 2g; Fiber: 1g; Net Carbs: 1g; **Macros:** Fat: 87%; Protein: 5%; Carbs: 8%

Chai Tea Cookies

MAKES 1 DOZEN | PREP TIME: 10 minutes | COOK TIME: 20 minutes

½ cup (1 stick) butter, at room	½ teaspoon baking powder
temperature	½ teaspoon ground cinnamon
⅓ cup granulated sugar-free	½ teaspoon ground
sweetener	cardamom
1 large egg	½ teaspoon ground ginger
½ teaspoon vanilla extract	½ teaspoon salt
1 cup almond flour	¼ teaspoon freshly ground
1 cup coconut flour	black pepper
½ teaspoon xanthan gum	

Preheat the oven to 350°F. Line a baking sheet with parchment paper and set aside. In a large bowl, using an electric mixer on medium, cream the butter and sweetener until smooth. Add the egg and vanilla and beat well. Add in the almond and coconut flours, xanthan gum, baking powder, cinnamon, cardamom, ginger, salt, and pepper, and stir until well incorporated. Using a spoon, place 1-inch mounds of the dough, onto the baking sheet about 1-inch apart. Bake the cookies for 15 to 18 minutes, until set and lightly golden. Refrigerate at least 1 hour before serving.

Per Serving: (1 cookie): Calories: 170; Fat: 14g; Protein: 4g; Total Carbs: 13g; Fiber: 5g; Net Carbs: 8g; **Macros:** Fat: 74%; Protein: 9; Carbs: 17%

Peanut Butter–Chocolate Chip Cookies

MAKES 16 COOKIES | PREP TIME: 10 minutes | COOK TIME: 10 to 15 minutes, plus 15 minutes to cool

1 cup sugar-free natural	8 tablespoons (1 stick)
peanut butter	unsalted butter, softened
1 cup granulated erythritol–	1 large egg, at room
monk fruit blend	temperature

1 cup almond flour, measured and sifted

1 teaspoon baking powder

½ teaspoon sea salt

½ cup sugar-free chocolate chips

Sea salt flakes (optional)

Preheat the oven to 350°F. Line a baking sheet with parchment paper. In a large bowl, using an electric mixer, beat the peanut butter, erythritol–monk fruit blend, butter, and egg until well combined. Add the almond flour, baking powder, and salt. Beat the mixture until fully incorporated. Fold in the chocolate chips. Using a tablespoon or small cookie scoop, evenly space spoonfuls of the cookie dough on the baking sheet. Lightly flatten the cookies with the back of the spoon, then use the tines of a fork to make a crisscross design. Sprinkle with sea salt flakes (if using). Bake for 10 to 12 minutes, or until lightly browned around the edges. Allow to cool on the baking sheet for at least 15 minutes before eating and storing, as these cookies can be fragile.

Per Serving: Calories: 225; Fat: 20g; Protein: 6g; Total Carbs: 9g; Fiber: 2g; Net Carbs: 7g; **Macros:** Fat: 80%; Protein: 11%; Carbs: 9%

Lemon Cookies

MAKES 24 COOKIES | PREP TIME: 10 minutes, plus 30 minutes to chill | COOK TIME: 15 minutes, plus cooling time

For the cookies

¾ cup coconut flour

1½ teaspoons baking powder

¼ teaspoon sea salt

¾ cup granulated erythritol–monk fruit blend

½ cup (1 stick) unsalted butter, at room temperature

4 ounces (about ½ cup) cream cheese, at room temperature

1 tablespoon grated lemon zest

1 teaspoon liquid lemon extract

4 large eggs, at room temperature

1 tablespoon heavy whipping cream

For the lemon icing

½ cup confectioners' erythritol–monk fruit blend

2 tablespoons freshly squeezed lemon juice

¼ teaspoon liquid lemon extract

1 to 2 tablespoons heavy (whipping) cream

Preheat the oven to 350°F. Line a baking sheet with parchment paper. In a medium bowl, mix the coconut flour, baking powder, and salt. In a large bowl, using an electric mixer on medium speed, cream the sweetener, butter, cream cheese, lemon zest, and lemon extract. Add the eggs one at a time, beating well after each addition. Add the heavy whipping cream, and mix until fully incorporated. Add the dry ingredients to the wet, and mix well until the dough is formed. Refrigerate the dough for 30 minutes before baking. Using a tablespoon or a small cookie scoop, measure out the cookie dough. Roll each scoop of cookie dough into a small ball. Lay the balls out evenly on the baking sheet. Lightly flatten the balls with your palms. Bake for 15 minutes, or until lightly browned around the edges. Allow to cool completely on a wire rack before icing. To make the lemon icing and finish the cookies In a medium bowl, combine the confectioners' erythritol–monk fruit blend with the lemon juice and lemon extract. Add 1 tablespoon heavy whipping cream to thin the icing, and add another tablespoon if necessary. Drizzle over tops of the fully

cooled cookies, and allow the icing to set for about 15 minutes before eating.

Per Serving: Calories: 82; Fat: 7g; Protein: 2g; Total Carbs: 3g; Fiber: 2g; Net Carbs: 1g; **Macros:** Fat: 77%; Protein: 10%; Carbs: 13%

Chocolate Chunk Cookies

MAKES 16 COOKIES | PREP TIME: 10 minutes | COOK TIME: 10 to 15 minutes, plus cooling time

¾ cup (1½ sticks) unsalted butter, at room temperature

½ cup golden or brown granulated erythritol–monk fruit blend

½ cup granulated erythritol–monk fruit blend

1 tablespoon sugar-free maple syrup

½ teaspoon pure vanilla extract

2 large eggs, at room temperature

1 tablespoon unflavored gelatin powder

2 cups almond flour, measured and sifted

¼ cup coconut flour

2 teaspoons baking powder

¼ teaspoon salt

½ cup roughly chopped sugar-free chocolate bar

Preheat the oven to 350°F. Line a baking sheet with parchment paper. In a large bowl, using an electric mixer on medium speed, beat the butter, sweetener, maple syrup, and vanilla until light and fluffy. Add the eggs one at a time, mixing well after each addition. Sprinkle in the gelatin powder, and combine well. Mix in the almond flour, coconut flour, baking powder, and salt. Fold in the chocolate chunks. Drop the dough onto the baking sheet by heaping tablespoons spaced about 2 inches apart. Flatten the cookies slightly with your palm. Bake for 12 to 15 minutes, or until golden. Allow to cool completely on a wire rack before eating or storing.

Per Serving: Calories: 211; Fat: 19g; Protein: 5g; Total Carbs: 9g; Fiber: 3g; Net Carbs: 6g; **Macros:** Fat: 81%; Protein: 9%; Carbs: 10%

Double Chocolate Peppermint Cookies

MAKES 16 COOKIES | PREP TIME: 15 minutes | COOK TIME: 15 to 20 minutes, plus cooling time

For the cookies

2 ounces (2 squares) unsweetened baking chocolate

8 ounces (about 1 cup) cream cheese, at room temperature

1 cup granulated erythritol–monk fruit blend

½ cup (1 stick) unsalted butter, at room temperature

1 teaspoon liquid peppermint extract

4 large eggs, at room temperature

1 cup coconut flour

¼ cup unsweetened cocoa powder

2 teaspoons baking powder

1 teaspoon instant espresso coffee

¼ teaspoon sea salt

For the icing and topping

¼ cup (½ stick) unsalted butter

2 ounces (2 squares) unsweetened baking chocolate

½ cup confectioners' erythritol–monk fruit blend

1 teaspoon coconut oil

1 teaspoon instant espresso coffee

Pinch sea salt

5 sugar-free peppermint candies, crushed

Preheat the oven to 350°F. Line a baking sheet with parchment paper. Put the baking chocolate in a microwave-safe bowl. Microwave in 10-second increments, until fully melted. In a large bowl, using an electric mixer on high speed, combine the cream cheese, sweetener, butter, and peppermint extract. Add the eggs one at a time, making sure they are fully incorporated into the batter. Add the chocolate, and beat the dough until it's very well mixed. Mix in the coconut flour, unsweetened cocoa powder, baking powder, instant espresso coffee, and salt. Using a tablespoon or small cookie scoop, evenly space spoonfuls of the cookie dough on the prepared baking sheet. Slightly flatten the cookies using your palms. Bake for 15 to 20 minutes, being careful not to overbake. Place the cookies on a wire rack to cool completely before icing. Put the butter and baking chocolate in a microwave-safe bowl. Microwave in 10-second increments, until fully melted. Add the confectioners' sweetener and stir. Mix in the coconut oil, instant espresso coffee, and salt. Once the cookies have cooled completely, spread about 1 teaspoon of icing on each cookie. Sprinkle with the peppermint candies. Make sure to add the candies before the icing sets so that they stick to the cookies. Allow to set for at least 5 minutes before eating.

Per Serving: Calories: 220; Fat: 20g; Protein: 5g; Total Carbs: 10g; Fiber: 5g; Net Carbs: 5g; **Macros:** Fat: 82%; Protein: 9%; Carbs: 9%

Chocolate Sandwich Cookies

SERVES 7 | PREP TIME: 20 minutes | COOK TIME: 15 minutes

For the cookies

¼ cup coconut flour
¼ cup unsweetened cocoa powder
¼ cup water
2 tablespoons tapioca flour
2 tablespoons xanthan gum
¼ cup coconut butter

1 tablespoon unsweetened coconut milk
1 large egg
1 teaspoon vanilla extract
2 tablespoons xylitol-sweetened honey
1 tablespoon erythritol

For the cream filling

3 tablespoons coconut butter, melted
1 tablespoon protein powder
2 tablespoons water

½ teaspoon vanilla extract
1 tablespoon xylitol-sweetened honey

Preheat the oven to 350°F. Line a baking sheet with parchment paper. In a mixing bowl, combine the coconut flour, cocoa powder, water, tapioca flour, xanthan gum, coconut butter, coconut milk, egg, vanilla extract, honey, and erythritol and mix well. Transfer the cookie dough to the prepared baking sheet and use a rolling pin to roll it out ⅛-inch thick. Bake in the oven for about 15 minutes, or until soft but no longer sticky. While the cookies are baking, in a medium bowl, whisk the coconut butter, protein powder, water, vanilla extract, and honey until smooth. Let the baked cookie dough cool for at 5 minutes, then use a round cookie cutter to cut out 12 or 14 cookies. Let the cookies cool for 15 to 20 minutes. Spread the cream filling on half of the cookies, then sandwich them with the remaining cookies and serve.

Per Serving: (1 sandwich cookie): Calories: 368; Fat: 24g; Protein: 10g; Total Carbs: 28g; Fiber: 12g; Net Carbs: 16g; **Macros:** Fat: 60%; Protein: 12%; Carbs: 28%

Sugar Cookie Balls

MAKES 24 | PREP TIME: 15 minutes, plus 1 hour to chill | COOK TIME: 10 minutes

1 cup (2 sticks) butter
1 cup granulated erythritol blend, divided
5 large eggs
3 ounces (6 tablespoons) cream cheese, room temperature

1 teaspoon vanilla extract
1¾ cups coconut flour
2 teaspoons baking powder
⅛ teaspoon salt

In a large bowl, cream the butter, ¾ cup of sweetener, eggs, cream cheese, and vanilla. In a small bowl, sift the flour, baking powder, and salt. Slowly add the flour mixture to the creamed mixture, and mix until incorporated. Cover with plastic wrap, and refrigerate for at least 1 hour so they don't spread while baking. Preheat the oven to 350°F, and line a baking sheet with parchment paper. Using a cookie scoop, scoop the dough onto the baking sheet, 1 inch apart. Sprinkle the cookies with the remaining ¼ cup of sweetener. Bake for 12 minutes, being sure not to overbake. Allow to cool on the baking sheet before removing.

Per Serving: (2 cookie balls): Calories: 130; Fat: 11g; Protein: 3g; Total Carbs: 13g; Fiber: 3.5g; Net Carbs: 1.5g; **Macros:** Fat: 76%; Protein: 9%; Carbs: 5%

Chocolate Chip Brownies

MAKES 16 BROWNIES | PREP TIME: 10 minutes | COOK TIME: 20 to 25 minutes, plus 30 minutes to cool

10 tablespoons unsalted butter, plus more to grease the pan
1¼ cups granulated erythritol–monk fruit blend
¾ cup dark unsweetened cocoa powder
1 ounce (1 square) unsweetened baking chocolate, roughly chopped
1 teaspoon instant coffee (optional)

¼ teaspoon sea salt
3 large eggs, at room temperature
2 teaspoons pure vanilla extract
¾ cup almond flour, measured and sifted
1 teaspoon baking powder
½ cup sugar-free chocolate chips

Preheat the oven to 325°F. Lightly grease the 8-inch-square baking pan with butter. In a medium saucepan, bring 1 cup water to a boil over medium-high heat. Set a glass mixing bowl over the saucepan, making sure the bowl doesn't touch the water. Add the butter, sweetener, cocoa powder, baking chocolate, instant coffee (if using), and salt to the bowl. Whisk occasionally until fully melted and combined. Allow the mixture to cool slightly, and pour it into a large bowl. Add the eggs one at a time to the chocolate mixture. Add the vanilla, and mix well. Add the almond flour and baking powder, and gently stir with a rubber spatula until just combined. Fold in the chocolate chips. Pour the brownie mixture into the prepared pan, and bake for 20 to 25 minutes. Allow the brownies to cool for at least 30 minutes in the pan before slicing.

Per Serving: Calories: 160; Fat: 14g; Protein: 3g; Total Carbs: 9g; Fiber: 3g; Net Carbs: 6g; **Macros:** Fat: 79%; Protein: 8%; Carbs: 13%

Peanut Butter Cookies

MAKES 30 COOKIES | PREP TIME: 10 minutes | COOK TIME: 30 minutes

¾ cup butter, at room temperature

1 cup plus 2 tablespoons Swerve or another non-caloric sweetener

1 cup natural peanut butter

2 large egg

1 teaspoon vanilla extract

2 cups almond flour

2 tablespoons coconut flour

1 teaspoon sea salt

1 teaspoon baking soda

Preheat the oven to 350°F. Line a baking sheet with parchment paper. In a large bowl, beat the butter and Swerve until light and fluffy, about 1 minute. Add the peanut butter, eggs, and vanilla extract, and beat until fully emulsified, another minute. Stir in the almond flour, coconut flour, sea salt, and baking soda. Using one-third of the mixture, form 10 equal-size cookies on the baking sheet. Flatten each cookie with the back of a fork that has been dipped in Swerve. Bake for 10 minutes, or until barely golden brown around the edges. Transfer to a cooling rack and repeat with the remaining cookie dough, making 20 cookies total.

Per Serving: (1 cookie): Calories: 146; Fat: 13g; Protein: 4g; Total Carbs: 4g; Fiber: 2g; Net Carbs: 2g; Macros: Fat: 80%; Protein: 10%; Carbs: 10%

Avocado Brownies

SERVES 12 TO 14 | PREP TIME: 5 to 10 minutes | COOK TIME: 25 minutes

Nonstick cooking spray or 1 tablespoon coconut oil

1 avocado, halved, pitted, and peeled

2 tablespoons vanilla protein powder

2 tablespoons chocolate protein powder

¼ cup unsweetened cocoa powder

¼ cup erythritol

1 large egg

1½ teaspoons vanilla extract

3 tablespoons unsweetened coconut milk

Powdered erythritol, for serving

Preheat the oven to 350°F. Coat a 9-inch-square baking dish with nonstick spray. In a blender, puree the avocado, protein powders, cocoa, erythritol, egg, vanilla extract, and coconut milk and until smooth. Pour the batter into the baking dish and bake for 20 to 25 minutes, or until a toothpick inserted in the center comes out clean. Let the brownies cool for at least 10 minutes, cut into squares, and serve with a sprinkle of powdered erythritol.

Per Serving: Calories: 61; Fat: 5g; Protein: 2g; Total Carbs: 2g; Fiber: 2g; Net Carbs: 1g; Macros: Fat: 74%; Protein: 13%; Carbs: 13%

No-Bake Coconut Cookies

MAKES 12 COOKIES | PREP TIME: 10 minutes, plus 30 minutes to chill | COOK TIME: 5 minutes

2 tablespoons butter

⅔ cup crunchy natural peanut butter

5 or 6 drops liquid stevia

1½ tablespoons unsweetened cocoa powder

1 cup finely shredded unsweetened coconut flakes

Line a baking sheet with parchment paper. In a medium saucepan over medium heat, melt the butter. Add the peanut butter and cocoa powder, and stir well. Remove from the heat and add

the stevia. Stir in the coconut flakes and mix until all the ingredients are well combined. Scoop the dough in small spoonfuls onto the prepared baking sheet. Place the baking sheet in the refrigerator for 30 minutes to set.

Per Serving: (1 cookie): Calories: 153; Fat: 13g; Protein: 4g; Total Carbs: 5g; Fiber: 2g; Net Carbs: 3g; Macros: Fat: 76%; Protein: 11%; Carbs: 13%

Lemon Snowball Cookies

MAKES 12 COOKIES | PREP TIME: 5 minutes | COOK TIME: 20 minutes

½ cup coconut flour

2 tablespoons collagen peptides powder

¼ teaspoon baking soda

¼ cup coconut oil, melted

¼ cup granular erythritol

Dash of salt

½ tablespoon beef gelatin powder

3 tablespoons water, divided

2 tablespoons lemon juice

2 teaspoons lemon zest

½ teaspoon gluten-free vanilla extract

6 tablespoons confectioner erythritol

Preheat the oven to 325°F. Line a baking sheet with parchment paper. In a medium bowl, mix the coconut flour, collagen, baking soda, coconut oil, erythritol, and salt. In a small bowl, prepare the gelatin by vigorously whisking in 1 tablespoon of room-temperature water, followed immediately by 2 tablespoons of just under boiling hot water. Immediately pour the gelatin mixture into the dough mixture, followed by the lemon juice, zest, and vanilla extract. Roll the dough into 1½-inch balls, then gently roll them in 3 tablespoons of confectioner erythritol. Place the balls on the baking sheet. Bake the cookies for about 18 minutes or until they start to turn golden. Let the cookies cool slightly, then roll them again in the remaining 3 tablespoons of confectioner erythritol.

Per Serving: Calories: 83; Fat: 6g; Protein: 2g; Total Carbs: 6g; Fiber: 4g; Net Carbs: 2g; Macros: Fat: 62%; Protein: 10%; Carbs: 28%

Coconut Cookies

MAKES 6 COOKIES | PREP TIME: 5 minutes, plus 10 minutes to freeze

2 tablespoons butter

⅔ cup almond butter

1 tablespoon cacao powder (optional)

1 teaspoon stevia or 8 drops liquid stevia extract

1 cup unsweetened shredded coconut

Line a baking sheet with parchment paper. In a small saucepan, melt the butter over medium heat. Pour the melted butter into a medium bowl, stir in the almond butter, and mix until smooth. Mix in the cocoa powder (if using). Add the stevia and coconut, and mix thoroughly. Drop 2-inch spoonfuls of the mixture onto the baking sheet. Freeze for at least 10 minutes or until they are completely solidified. Transfer the cookies to a sealed container, and store in the refrigerator.

Per Serving: (1 cookie): Calories: 315; Fat: 31g; Protein: 5g; Total Carbs: 10g; Fiber: 4g; Net Carbs: 6g; Macros: Fat: 82%; Protein: 6%; Carbs: 12%

Nutty Shortbread Cookies

MAKES 18 COOKIES | PREP TIME: 10 minutes, plus 30 minutes to chill | COOK TIME: 10 minutes

½ cup butter, at room temperature, plus additional for greasing the baking sheet

½ cup granulated sweetener

1 teaspoon alcohol-free pure vanilla extract

1½ cups almond flour

½ cup ground hazelnuts

Pinch sea salt

In a medium bowl, cream the butter, sweetener, and vanilla until well blended. Stir in the almond flour, ground hazelnuts, and salt until a firm dough is formed. Roll the dough into a 2-inch cylinder and wrap it in plastic wrap. Place the dough in the refrigerator for at least 30 minutes until firm. Preheat the oven to 350°F. Line a baking sheet with parchment paper and lightly grease the paper with butter. Unwrap the chilled cylinder, slice the dough into 18 cookies, and place the cookies on the baking sheet. Bake the cookies until firm and lightly browned, about 10 minutes. Allow the cookies to cool on the baking sheet for 5 minutes and then transfer them to a wire rack to cool completely.

Per Serving: (1 cookie): Calories: 105; Fat: 10g; Protein: 3g; Total Carbs: 2g; Fiber: 1g; Net Carbs: 1g; Macros: Fat: 85%; Protein: 9%; Carbs: 6%

Almond Cookies

MAKES 18 COOKIES | PREP TIME: 5 minutes | COOK TIME: 15 minutes

2 cups almond flour

¾ cup confectioners' erythritol blend

½ teaspoon baking powder

¼ teaspoon salt

¼ teaspoon xanthan gum

2 tablespoons cold butter, cubed or grated

2 tablespoons buttermilk

2 tablespoons cream cheese, room temperature

½ teaspoon almond extract

18 almonds

Preheat the oven to 325°F, and line a baking sheet with parchment paper. In a medium bowl, sift the almond flour, confectioners' sweetener, baking powder, salt, and xanthan gum. Add the butter, buttermilk, cream cheese, and almond extract, and using your hands or a stand mixer on low, mix to incorporate. Scoop the dough using a cookie scoop, and roll into a ball in the palm of your hand. Place on the baking sheet, and press down just a bit to make a cookie about 2 inches in diameter. Repeat with remaining dough. You don't need to leave much space between them; they don't spread. Press an almond into the center of each cookie. Bake for 15 to 17 minutes, or until the edges are golden brown. They will seem undercooked, but don't overbake. Allow to cool completely before removing from the baking sheet. They will harden as they cool.

Per Serving: (1 cookie): Calories: 116; Fat: 8g; Protein: 3g; Total Carbs: 8g; Fiber: 2g; Net Carbs: 6g; Macros: Fat: 82%; Protein: 13%; Carbs: 5%

Chocolate Chip Cookies

MAKES 16 COOKIES | PREP TIME: 10 minutes | COOK TIME: 20 minutes

2 cups almond flour

½ cup Swerve or another non-caloric sweetener

1 teaspoon baking powder

½ teaspoon sea salt

3 tablespoons butter

2 tablespoons milk

1 tablespoon vanilla extract

½ cup dark chocolate chips, at least 60 percent cacao

½ cup roughly chopped pecans

Preheat the oven to 350°F. Line a baking sheet with parchment paper. In a medium bowl, mix the almond flour, Swerve, baking powder, and sea salt. Add the butter, milk, and vanilla, and stir to mix. Fold in the chocolate chips and pecans. Using half of the mixture, form 8 equal-size cookies on the baking sheet. Flatten each gently with the palm of your hand. Bake for 10 minutes, or until barely golden brown around the edges. Transfer to a cooling rack and repeat with the remaining cookie dough, making another 8 cookies.

Per Serving: (1 cookie): Calories: 144; Fat: 13g; Protein: 4g; Total Carbs: 6g; Fiber: 2g; Net Carbs: 4g; Macros: Fat: 75%; Protein: 10%; Carbs: 15%

Pecan Sandies

MAKES 24 COOKIES | PREP TIME: 10 minutes, plus 45 minutes to chill | COOK TIME: 35 to 40 minutes, plus cooling time

2½ cups almond flour, measured and sifted

¾ cup granulated erythritol–monk fruit blend

½ cup finely chopped pecans (optional)

1 teaspoon baking powder

½ teaspoon sea salt

1 cup (2 sticks) unsalted butter, very cold

1½ teaspoons pure vanilla extract

Preheat the oven to 300°F. In a medium bowl, whisk the almond flour, sweetener, chopped pecans (if using), baking powder, and salt. Take the butter out of the refrigerator, and cut it into about 30 small slices. Use your fingers to rub the pieces of butter and vanilla into the flour mixture, for about 5 minutes, or until the dough comes together. Press the dough into a 10-inch-square baking pan. Refrigerate for at least 45 minutes. Use the tines of a fork to poke holes in the top of the pecan sandies. Bake for 35 to 40 minutes, or until the edges are light golden brown. Allow the shortbread to cool in the pan completely before slicing.

Per Serving: Calories: 153; Fat: 15g; Protein: 3g; Total Carbs: 3g; Fiber: 2g; Net Carbs: 1g; Macros: Fat: 88%; Protein: 8%; Carbs: 4%

Chocolate Chip Cookie Dough Balls

MAKES 18 TO 20 | PREP TIME: 10 minutes, plus 15 minutes to chill

½ cup unsalted butter, at room temperature

⅓ cup Swerve sweetener

½ teaspoon vanilla extract

¼ teaspoon salt

2 cups almond flour

½ cup dark chocolate chips

In the bowl of a stand mixer, combine the butter, Swerve, vanilla, and salt. Beat until the mixture is light and fluffy. Add the almond flour and continue to mix on low until a dough forms. Fold in the chocolate chips until just barely combined. Refrigerate the dough for about 15 minutes to set. Line a baking sheet with parchment paper. Using a 2-inch cookie scoop, scoop balls of dough onto the prepared baking sheet and chill. Refrigerate in a sealed container until ready to eat.

Per Serving: (1 ball): Calories: 122; Fat: 10g; Protein: 2g; Total Carbs: 6g; Fiber: 1g; Net Carbs: 5g; **Macros:** Fat: 74%; Protein: 6%; Carbs: 20%

Pistachio Cookies

SERVES 8 | PREP TIME: 10 minutes | COOK TIME: 20 minutes, plus 30 minutes to cool

For the cookies

1 cup coconut flour

1½ teaspoons baking powder

¼ teaspoon salt

1 cup granulated erythritol–monk fruit blend; less sweet: ¾ cup

½ cup (1 stick) unsalted butter, at room temperature

4 ounces cream cheese, at room temperature

1 teaspoon vanilla extract

4 large eggs, at room temperature

¼ cup finely chopped pistachios, plus more for garnish

For the vanilla icing

½ cup confectioners' erythritol–monk fruit blend

3 tablespoons heavy (whipping) cream

1 teaspoon vanilla extract

Preheat the oven to 350°F. Line the baking sheet with parchment paper and set aside. In the medium bowl, stir the coconut flour, baking powder, and salt and set aside. In the large bowl, using an electric mixer on medium, beat the sweetener, butter, cream cheese, and vanilla until fully combined, scraping the bowl once or twice, as needed. Add the eggs, one at a time, mixing well after each addition. Add the dry ingredients to the wet mixture, stirring until fully combined. Stir in the pistachios and refrigerate the dough for at least 30 minutes. Using a cookie scoop or spoon, drop the dough in tablespoon-size cookies onto the baking sheet, evenly spaced, leaving about 1 inch between the cookies. Flatten each ball slightly. Bake for 15 to 18 minutes, or until lightly browned around the edges. Cool on the rack for 30 minutes. In the small bowl, combine the confectioners' sweetener, heavy cream, and vanilla. Using a fork, drizzle the icing on top of the cooled cookies and top with chopped pistachios before serving.

Per Serving: (3 cookies): Calories: 272; Fat: 27g; Protein: 5g; Total Carbs: 4g; Fiber: 1g; Net Carbs: 3g; **Macros:** Fat: 86%; Protein: 8%; Carbs: 6%

Pumpkin Cookies

SERVES 8 | PREP TIME: 10 minutes, plus 1 hour to chill | COOK TIME: 25 minutes, plus 30 minutes to cool

For the cookies

¾ cup coconut flour

1½ teaspoons baking powder

1 teaspoon ground cinnamon

½ teaspoon ground ginger

¼ teaspoon ground nutmeg

¼ teaspoon salt

¾ cup granulated erythritol–monk fruit blend; less sweet: ½ cup

½ (1 stick) unsalted butter, at room temperature

4 ounces cream cheese, room temperature

½ teaspoon vanilla extract

4 large eggs, at room temperature

½ cup canned pumpkin puree

For the icing

½ cup confectioners' erythritol–monk fruit blend

4 to 5 tablespoons heavy (whipping) cream, divided

Preheat the oven to 350°F. Line the baking sheet with parchment paper and set aside. In the medium bowl, combine the coconut flour, baking powder, cinnamon, ginger, nutmeg, and salt and set aside. In the large bowl, using an electric mixer on high, beat the sweetener, butter, cream cheese, and vanilla until fully combined, scraping the bowl once or twice, as needed. Add the eggs, one at a time, mixing well after each addition, then stir in the pumpkin puree. Add the dry ingredients to the wet mixture and mix on low until combined. Chill the cookie dough for 45 minutes to 1 hour. Using a cookie scoop or spoon, drop the dough in tablespoon-size cookies onto the baking sheet, evenly spaced, and leaving about 1 inch between the cookies. Flatten each ball slightly. Bake for 20 to 25 minutes, or until lightly browned around the edges. Remove the cookies from the oven and let them cool on the rack for 30 minutes. While the cookies bake, in a small bowl, combine the confectioners' sweetener with 2 tablespoons of heavy cream, adding 1 tablespoon more at a time, if needed. The icing should be runny enough to easily drizzle. Using a pastry bag or fork, drizzle the cookies with the icing. Let the icing set on the cookies for about 10 minutes before eating.

Per Serving: (2 cookies): Calories: 246; Fat: 24g; Protein: 5g; Total Carbs: 4g; Fiber: 1g; Net Carbs: 3g; **Macros:** Fat: 86%; Protein: 8%; Carbs: 6%

Salted Peanut Butter Cookies

SERVES 8 | PREP TIME: 10 minutes | COOK TIME: 40 minutes

1 cup all-natural peanut butter (no added sugar)

1 cup granulated erythritol–monk fruit blend; less sweet: ½ cup

½ cup (1 stick) unsalted butter, at room temperature

1 large egg, at room temperature

1 cup almond flour

1 teaspoon baking powder

½ teaspoon sea salt

Preheat the oven to 350°F. Line the baking sheet with parchment paper. In the large bowl, using an electric mixer on medium high, combine the peanut butter, sweetener, butter, and egg and mix until combined, scraping the bowl once or twice, as needed. Add the almond flour and baking powder. Mix on low until fully incorporated. Using a small cookie scoop or spoon, place tablespoon-size cookies on the baking sheet and flatten them with the tines of a fork to make a crisscross design. Sprinkle the tops with the salt. Bake for 10 to 12 minutes, until lightly browned around the edges. Allow the cookies to cool completely before eating.

Per Serving: (3 cookies): Calories: 360; Fat: 32g; Protein: 11g; Total Carbs: 3g; Fiber: 2g; Net Carbs: 1g; **Macros:** Fat: 82%; Protein: 14%; Carbs: 4%

Easy Peasy Peanut Butter Cookies

15 COOKIES | PREP TIME: 15 minutes | COOK TIME: 7 to 12 minutes

½ cup coconut flour	2 tablespoons butter, at room
¼ cup sugar-free sweetener	temperature
½ teaspoon baking soda	2 large eggs
¼ cup (low-carb or handmade) peanut butter	1 teaspoon vanilla extract

Preheat the oven to 350°F. Line a baking sheet with parchment paper and set aside. In a large bowl, mix the flour, sweetener, and baking soda. Add the peanut butter, butter, eggs, and vanilla, and mix well to incorporate. Drop by even spoonfuls onto the baking sheet to make 15 cookies. Using the back of a fork, press the cookies down a little and make decorative criss-cross marks. Cook for 7 to 8 minutes for soft cookies or 10 to 12 minutes for crispy cookies.

Per Serving: (1 cookie) Calories: 70; Fat: 5g; Protein: 3g; Total Carbs: 3g; Fiber: 2g; Net Carbs: 1g; Macros: Fat: 66%; Protein: 17%; Carbs: 17%

Lemon-Poppyseed Cookies

SERVES 4 | PREP TIME: 5 minutes | COOK TIME: 10 minutes

Nonstick cooking spray	3 tablespoons fresh grated
1 cup almond butter	lemon zest
¾ cup monk fruit sweetener	Juice of 1 lemon
¼ cup chia seeds	1 tablespoon poppy seeds

Preheat the oven to 350°F. Grease a baking sheet with cooking spray and set aside. In a large bowl, combine the almond butter with the sweetener, chia seeds, lemon zest, lemon juice, and poppy seeds. Mix well, kneading the mixture with your hands. Roll pieces of the dough into cookie-size balls and place them on the baking sheet, spacing them evenly, as they do spread. Bake the cookies for 8 minutes, until golden. Transfer the cookies to a cooling rack.

Per Serving: Calories: 460; Fat: 39g; Protein: 13g; Total Carbs: 21g; Fiber: 12g; Net Carbs: 9g; Macros: Fat: 72%; Protein: 17%; Carbs: 21%

Iced Gingerbread Cookies

SERVES 24 | PREP TIME: 15 minutes, plus 30 minutes to chill | COOK TIME: 15 minutes, plus 20 minutes to cool

2 cups brown or golden erythritol–monk fruit blend; less sweet: 1¼ cups	½ teaspoon ground nutmeg
	¼ teaspoon ground cloves
3 large eggs	3 cups almond flour
¼ cup (½ stick) unsalted butter, at room temperature	1 tablespoon psyllium husk powder
1 tablespoon molasses or 1 teaspoon molasses extract (optional)	1½ teaspoons baking powder
	¼ teaspoon salt
	¼ cup confectioners' erythritol–monk fruit blend
1 teaspoon vanilla extract	1 tablespoon heavy (whipping) cream
4 teaspoons ground cinnamon	
3 tablespoons ground ginger	

Preheat the oven to 325°F. Line the baking sheet with parchment paper and set aside. In the large bowl, using an electric mixer on high, beat the sweetener, eggs, butter, molasses (if using), and vanilla until fully incorporated, scraping the bowl once or twice, as needed. Add the cinnamon, ginger, nutmeg, and cloves to the mixture and stir to combine. Add the almond flour, psyllium powder, baking powder, and salt and beat on medium high until well incorporated. Place the dough between two sheets of parchment paper and flatten with a rolling pin. Refrigerate the dough for 30 minutes. Using a small cookie cutter or small-mouthed glass jar, cut the dough into cookies and place them about 1 inch apart, evenly spaced, on the prepared baking sheet. Bake for 12 to 15 minutes, until golden brown. Allow them to cool completely on the cooling rack, 15 to 20 minutes. In the small bowl, combine the sweetener with the heavy cream 1 teaspoon at a time to make the icing. The icing should have a runny consistency. Drizzle the cooled cookies.

Per Serving: (1 cookie): Calories: 106; Fat: 9g; Protein: 3g; Total Carbs: 5g; Fiber: 2g; Net Carbs: 3g; Macros: Fat: 71%; Protein: 12%; Carbs: 17%

Snickerdoodle Cookies

48 COOKIES | PREP TIME: 15 minutes | COOK TIME: 13 minutes

1½ cups (3 sticks) butter, at room temperature	1 tablespoon vanilla extract
	1¼ cups coconut flour
1½ cups granulated sweetener, divided	2 teaspoons cinnamon, divided
6 large eggs plus 1 additional yolk	1 teaspoon baking soda
	1 teaspoon cream of tartar
½ cup heavy (whipping) cream	½ teaspoon salt

Preheat the oven to 325°F. Line a baking sheet with parchment paper and set aside. In a large bowl, cream the butter, 1 cup of sweetener, eggs and additional yolk, heavy cream, and vanilla. In a small bowl, mix the coconut flour, 1 teaspoon of cinnamon, baking soda, cream of tartar, and salt. Add the flour mixture to the butter mixture and mix well. In another small bowl, mix the remaining ½ cup of sweetener and the remaining 1 teaspoon of cinnamon. Using a cookie scoop, scoop the dough and roll it into a ball, then roll the ball in the sweetener and cinnamon mixture. Place the dough balls on the prepared baking sheet and pat to flatten them slightly. Bake for 13 minutes, turning the baking sheet halfway through the baking time. Let the cookies rest a few minutes before transferring to a wire rack.

Per Serving: (3 cookies) Calories: 286; Fat: 24g; Protein: 5g; Total Carbs: 13g; Fiber: 8g; Net Carbs: 5g; Macros: Fat: 75%; Protein: 7%; Carbs: 18%

Pecan Chocolate Chip Cookies

SERVES 16 | PREP TIME: 10 minutes | COOK TIME: 15 minutes, plus 20 minutes to cool

¾ cup (1½ sticks) unsalted butter, at room temperature	1 tablespoon unflavored gelatin
½ cup golden or brown erythritol–monk fruit blend	2 cups almond flour, sifted
	¼ cup coconut flour
½ cup granulated erythritol–monk fruit blend	2 teaspoons baking powder
	¼ teaspoon salt
1 tablespoon sugar-free maple syrup	4 ounces sugar-free chocolate chips
2 large eggs	1 cup chopped pecans

Preheat the oven to 350°F. Line the baking sheet with parchment paper and set aside. In the large bowl, beat the butter, sweeteners, and maple syrup until light and fluffy. Add the eggs, one at a time, mixing well after each addition. Sprinkle in the gelatin and combine well. Mix in the almond flour, coconut flour, baking powder, and salt. Fold in the chocolate chips and pecans. Drop the dough by heaping tablespoons onto the prepared baking sheet, spacing them evenly about 2 inches apart. Flatten the cookies slightly. Bake for 12 to 15 minutes, until golden. Cool on the rack for 15 to 20 minutes before serving.

Per Serving: (1 cookie): Calories: 253; Fat: 24g; Protein: 5g; Total Carbs: 6g; Fiber: 4g; Net Carbs: 2g; **Macros:** Fat: 82%; Protein: 8%; Carbs: 10%

Carrot Cake Cookies

SERVES 12 | PREP TIME: 10 minutes, plus 30 minutes to chill | COOK TIME: 15 minutes, plus 30 minutes to cool

For the cookies

½ cup (1 stick) unsalted butter, at room temperature, plus more for greasing	¾ cup granulated erythritol–monk fruit blend; less sweet: ½ cup
¾ cup coconut flour	4 ounces cream cheese, at room temperature
2 teaspoons ground cinnamon	½ teaspoon vanilla extract
1½ teaspoons baking powder	4 large eggs
½ teaspoon ground ginger	¾ cup finely shredded carrots
¼ teaspoon ground nutmeg	¼ cup finely chopped walnuts (optional)
¼ teaspoon salt	

For the cream cheese icing

1 cup confectioners' erythritol–monk fruit blend	3 to 4 tablespoons heavy (whipping) cream
¼ cup (½ stick) unsalted butter, at room temperature	1 teaspoon vanilla extract
2 ounces cream cheese, at room temperature	¼ teaspoon ground cinnamon

Preheat the oven to 350°F. Lightly grease the baking sheet with butter and set aside. In a large bowl, combine the coconut flour, cinnamon, baking powder, ginger, nutmeg, and salt and set aside. In another large bowl, using an electric mixer on medium high, beat the sweetener, butter, cream cheese, and vanilla until fully combined, scraping the bowl once or twice, as needed. Add the eggs, one at a time, mixing well after each addition. Add the dry ingredients to the wet mixture and beat until fully combined. Fold in the shredded carrots, and walnuts (if using). Refrigerate the cookie dough for 30 minutes. Using a cookie scoop or spoon, drop the dough in tablespoon-size cookies onto the baking sheet, evenly spaced and leaving about 1 inch between the cookies. Flatten each ball slightly. Bake for 15 minutes, or until lightly browned around the edges. Allow the cookies to cool on the cooling rack for 30 minutes. In the medium bowl, using an electric mixer on high, mix the confectioners' sweetener, butter, and cream cheese for 1 to 2 minutes until smooth, scraping the bowl

once or twice, as needed. Add 3 tablespoons of heavy cream, the vanilla, and cinnamon and mix well. Add the additional 1 tablespoon of cream to thin the icing, if necessary. Using a fork, drizzle the cooled cookies with icing before serving.

Per Serving: (2 cookies): Calories: 213; Fat: 21g; Protein: 3g; Total Carbs: 3g; Fiber: 1g; Net Carbs: 2g; **Macros:** Fat: 88%; Protein: 7%; Carbs: 5%

Fudgy Brownies

MAKES 16 | PREP TIME: 15 minutes | COOK TIME: 20 minutes

5 tablespoons butter, at room temperature	2 large eggs at room temperature
⅔ cup granular erythritol	1 teaspoon vanilla extract
1 cup almond flour	3 tablespoons unsweetened vanilla almond milk
⅓ cup unsweetened cocoa powder	½ cup sugar-free chocolate chips or chopped walnuts, divided
1 teaspoon baking powder	
¼ teaspoon sea salt	

Preheat the oven to 350°F. Line an 8-inch-square baking dish with parchment paper. In a large bowl, beat the butter and erythritol until the sweetener dissolves. In another large bowl, whisk the flour, cocoa powder, baking powder, and salt. Beat half of this dry mixture into the butter; then beat in 1 egg. Repeat with the remaining dry mix and the remaining egg. Beat in the vanilla, then the almond milk until just incorporated. Gently fold in half the chocolate chips. Pour the mixture into the prepared dish and top evenly with the remaining chocolate chips. Bake for 20 minutes or until a toothpick inserted in the middle of the dish comes out clean. Let the brownies cool at room temperature for at least 30 minutes before slicing and serving.

Per Serving: (1 brownie): Calories: 106; Fat: 10g; Protein: 3g; Total Carbs: 14g; Fiber: 3g; Net Carbs: 2g; **Macros:** Fat: 85%; Protein: 11%; Carbs: 4%

Coconut Macaroons

SERVES 4 | PREP TIME: 5 minutes | COOK TIME: 15 minutes

Nonstick cooking spray	2 tablespoons coconut oil
1 cup unsweetened coconut flakes	¼ teaspoon vanilla extract
½ cup coconut milk	¼ teaspoon sea salt
⅓ cup monk fruit sweetener	

Preheat the oven to 350°F. Line a baking sheet with parchment paper and grease it with cooking spray. In a high-powered blender, pulse the coconut flakes until they are meal-like. Transfer the coconut to a large bowl and add the coconut milk, sweetener, coconut oil, vanilla, and salt. Knead the mixture with your hands to create a dough. Roll pieces of the dough into bite-size balls and place them on the baking sheet. Bake for 15 minutes, checking often to avoid burning. When you see the bottom edges of the macaroons become golden, remove them from the oven. Transfer the macaroons to a cooling rack and allow them to cool for 20 minutes before serving.

Per Serving: Calories: 212; Fat: 22g; Protein: 1g; Total Carbs: 5g; Fiber: 2g; Net Carbs: 3g; **Macros:** Fat: 89%; Protein: 2%; Carbs: 9%

Coconut Lime Macaroons

MAKES 12 MACAROONS | PREP TIME: 5 minutes | COOK TIME: 10-12 minutes

1½ cups shredded unsweet-
ened coconut flakes
2 teaspoons raw honey
2 tablespoons collagen peptides powder

2 tablespoons coconut flour
¼ cup coconut butter
1 tablespoons lime juice
1½ teaspoon lime zest, plus
extra for garnish

Preheat the oven to 350°F. Line a baking sheet with parchment paper. Mix all the ingredients in a medium bowl using your hands to break apart any coconut butter clumps. Roll the mixture into 1½-inch balls and place them on the baking sheet. Bake the cookies for 10 to 12 minutes or until the outsides start to brown. Remove them from the oven and garnish each macaroon with extra lime zest.

Per Serving: Calories: 164; Fat: 15g; Protein: 3g; Total Carbs: 9g; Fiber: 5g; Net Carbs: 4g; **Macros:** Fat: 75%; Protein: 5%; Carbs: 20%

Chewy "Noatmeal" Chocolate Chip Cookies

SERVES 20 | PREP TIME: 15 minutes | COOK TIME: 18 minutes

½ cup (1 stick) butter
¼ cup creamy almond butter
⅓ cup plus 1 tablespoon
monk fruit/erythritol blend
sweetener
1 large egg
1 teaspoon vanilla extract
1¼ cups almond flour

1 tablespoon
unflavored gelatin
¾ teaspoon baking soda
¼ teaspoon kosher salt
½ cup sugar-free choco-
late chips
⅓ cup unsweetened desic-
cated coconut

Preheat the oven to 350°F. Line a baking sheet with parchment paper. In a small skillet over medium-low heat, melt the butter and cook it for about 10 minutes, stirring often, until browned and nutty. The solids in the butter should be the color of caramel. Remove from the heat and set aside to cool. In a large bowl, using an electric hand mixer, cream the browned butter, almond butter, and sweetener until light and fluffy. Add the egg and vanilla, and mix until combined. Add the almond flour, gelatin, baking soda, and salt. Mix well until thoroughly incorporated. Stir in the chocolate chips and coconut. Scoop the cookies onto the baking sheet, about 1 generous tablespoon each, and flatten slightly. Bake for 7 to 8 minutes, or until golden around the edges. Let cool on the sheet pan for at least 10 minutes before removing. Store in an airtight container.

Per Serving: (1 cookie): Calories: 99; Fat: 9g; Protein: 2g; Total Carbs: 2g; Fiber: 1g; Net Carbs: 1g; **Macros:** Fat: 84%; Protein: 8%; Carbs: 8%

Almond Butter Oatmeal Cookies

MAKES 18 TO 20 | PREP TIME: 10 minutes, plus 20 minutes to chill | COOK TIME: 10 minutes

1 cup unsweetened, unsalted
almond butter, creamy but
not liquid

¼ cup sugar-free
maple-flavored syrup

1 tablespoon brown sugar
substitute
1¼ teaspoons ground
cinnamon

½ tablespoon baking powder
¼ teaspoon sea salt
1 large egg, beaten

Line 2 baking sheets with parchment paper. In a large bowl, beat the almond butter, syrup, brown sugar substitute, cinnamon, baking powder, salt, and egg until well combined. Scoop tablespoons of dough onto the baking sheets, leaving a 1-inch between each cookie because they will spread when baking. Press down gently to form them into cookies. Preheat the oven to 350°F and refrigerate the baking sheets for 20 minutes. Bake the cookies 1 sheet at a time for about 10 minutes, until golden around the edges. Keep the second sheet refrigerated while the other bakes. Cool the cookies completely before removing them from the baking sheet to avoid crumbling.

Per Serving: (1 cookie): Calories: 93; Fat: 8g; Protein: 3g; Total Carbs: 4g; Fiber: 2g; Net Carbs: 2g; **Macros:** Fat: 77%; Protein: 13%; Carbs: 10%

Chocolate-Drizzled Pecan Shortbread

SERVES 12 | PREP TIME: 10 minutes, plus 45 minutes to chill | COOK TIME: 40 minutes

For the shortbread

2½ cups almond flour, sifted
¾ cup granulated erythritol–
monk fruit blend
½ cup finely chopped pecans
1 teaspoon baking powder

½ teaspoon sea salt
1 cup (2 sticks) unsalted
butter, chilled and
thinly sliced
1½ teaspoons vanilla extract

For the chocolate drizzle

5 ounces sugar-free dark
chocolate chips

1 teaspoon coconut oil

Preheat the oven to 300°F. In the medium bowl, whisk the almond flour, sweetener, pecans, baking powder, and salt. Add the butter and vanilla to the flour mixture. Using your fingers, rub the pieces of butter into the flour mixture, working the mixture for about 5 minutes until the dough comes together. Press the dough into the baking pan and refrigerate for at least 45 minutes. Using a fork, make a few indents with the tines on top of the shortbread. Bake for 35 to 40 minutes, or until the edges are lightly golden brown. Remove and let cool in the pan completely before slicing into 24 bars. In the small microwave-safe bowl, melt the chocolate and coconut oil together in the microwave in 30-second intervals. Using a fork or a pastry bag, drizzle the cooled bars with melted chocolate. Allow the chocolate to set before serving.

Per Serving: (2 bars): Calories: 331; Fat: 32g; Protein: 6g; Total Carbs: 8g; Fiber: 4g; Net Carbs: 4g; **Macros:** Fat: 84%; Protein: 7%; Carbs: 9%

Classic Chocolate Brownies

SERVES: 12 | Prep time: 10 minutes | COOK TIME: 30 minutes

½ cup (1 stick) butter, plus
more for greasing
1½ ounces unsweetened
Baker's Chocolate

1¼ cups powdered erythritol
7 tablespoons cocoa powder
¼ teaspoon salt
3 large eggs, beaten

2 tablespoons water   1¼ cups almond flour
1½ teaspoons vanilla extract

Preheat the oven to 350°F. Butter an 8-inch-square baking dish. Fill a medium saucepan with 2 inches of water and bring to a simmer over medium heat. Place a large glass bowl over the pot to create a double boiler. Put the butter and chocolate in the bowl and stir until melted. Add the erythritol, cocoa powder, and salt, and whisk until the sweetener is dissolved. Remove from the heat. Allow to cool for a few minutes. Whisk in the eggs a little at a time. Whisk in the water and vanilla. Gradually add the almond flour and stir to combine. Pour the batter into the baking dish and use a rubber spatula to spread it out evenly. Bake for about 30 minutes or until a toothpick inserted comes out clean. Allow to cool completely before cutting and serving.

Per Serving: Calories: 158; Fat: 15g; Protein: 4g; Total Carbs: 4g; Fiber: 2g; Net Carbs: 2g; Macros: Fat: 82%; Protein: 10%; Carbs: 8%

Fluffy Lime-Meringue Clouds

SERVES 4 | PREP TIME: 30 minutes | COOK TIME: 3 hours

For the meringues
4 large egg whites   1 teaspoon pure
½ teaspoon plus   vanilla extract
  ¼ teaspoon stevia

For the lime curd
2 large eggs   ¼ cup freshly squeezed
2 teaspoons lime zest   lime juice
                            3 tablespoons coconut oil

For the topping
1 cup heavy (whipping) cream

Preheat the oven to 200°F. Cover a baking sheet with parchment paper, and set aside. In a large bowl, beat the egg whites, ½ teaspoon stevia, and vanilla until the whites form stiff peaks, about 8 minutes. Scoop the egg whites onto the baking sheet to form 4 mounds, and make a well in the center of each mound to create a bowl. Bake the meringues until they are crisp and set, about 3 hours. While the meringues are baking, in a small saucepan over medium heat, whisk the eggs, lime zest, and ¼ teaspoon stevia until the eggs are pale and slightly thickened, about 3 minutes. Whisk in the lime juice and coconut oil until the mixture starts to bubble, about 5 minutes. Remove the saucepan from the heat. Strain the curd through a fine mesh sieve into a small bowl. Cover the curd with plastic wrap, pressing it right on the surface of the curd, and refrigerate until completely cooled. In a medium bowl, beat the cream until it forms soft peaks. Place 1 meringue on each plate, and evenly divide the lime curd among the meringues. Top the dessert with the whipped cream, and serve.

Per Serving: Calories: 260; Fat: 24g; Protein: 8g; Total Carbs: 3g; Fiber: 0g; Net Carbs: 3g; Macros: Fat: 83%; Protein: 12%; Carbs: 5%

French Meringues

MAKES 30 | PREP TIME: 20 minutes | COOK TIME: 2 hours

4 large egg whites   ¼ teaspoon sea salt
¼ teaspoon cream of tartar

½ cup granulated   ¼ cup powdered
  erythritol-monk fruit blend   erythritol-monk fruit blend
                            ½ teaspoon vanilla extract

Preheat the oven to 200°F. Line the baking sheet with parchment paper and set aside. In the large bowl, using an electric mixer on medium, beat the egg whites, cream of tartar, and salt for 1 to 2 minutes, until foamy and the egg whites begin to turn opaque. Continue to whip the egg whites, adding in the granulated and powdered sweetener about 1 teaspoon at a time and scraping the bowl once or twice. Once all the sweetener has been added, increase the mixer speed to high and whip for 5 to 7 minutes, until the meringue is glossy and very stiff. Using a rubber spatula, gently fold in the vanilla. Scoop the meringue into the pastry bag fitted with a French star tip and pipe 2-inch-diameter kisses onto the baking sheet. Alternatively, spoon the meringue onto the sheet. Bake for 2 hours, or until crisp and lightly browned. Allow to cool completely on the cooling rack before serving.

Per Serving: (3 meringues): Calories: 8; Fat: 0g; Protein: 2g; Total Carbs: 0g; Fiber: 0g; Net Carbs: 0g; Macros: Fat: 3%; Protein: 88%; Carbs: 9%

No-Bake Brownie Bites

18 BROWNIE BITES | PREP TIME: 15 minutes, plus 1 hour to chill

¼ cup coconut flour   2 tablespoons butter, at room
½ cup unsweetened baking   temperature
  cocoa powder   3 tablespoons peanut butter
½ cup sugar-free confection-   1 teaspoon vanilla extract
  ers' sugar   1 tablespoon water
6 ounces cream cheese, at   ¼ teaspoon salt
  room temperature

Line a baking sheet with parchment paper and set aside. Put all the ingredients into a large bowl and mix with your hands or a spatula. Until it has the consistency of play dough. Refrigerate for 30 minutes. Using a cookie scoop, drop a scoop of dough into your hand, roll it into a ball, and place it on the baking sheet. Repeat with the remaining dough. Freeze the balls for 30 minutes.

Per Serving: (1 brownie bite) Calories: 89; Fat: 7g; Protein: 2g; Total Carbs: 4g; Fiber: 2g; Net Carbs: 2g; Macros: Fat: 72%; Protein: 10%; Carbs: 18%

Pumpkin Cheesecake Brownies

MAKES 16 | PREP TIME: 15 minutes, plus 35 minutes to chill | COOK TIME: 25 minutes, plus 15 minutes to cool

For the brownies
¾ cup (1½ sticks) unsalted   3 large eggs, at room
  butter, at room temperature,   temperature
  plus more for greasing   1 teaspoon vanilla extract
4 ounces unsweetened baking   1 cup almond flour, sifted
  chocolate, coarsely chopped 1 teaspoon baking powder
1¼ cups granulated erythri-   ¼ teaspoon sea salt
  tol–monk fruit blend; less
  sweet: 1 cup

For the pumpkin cheesecake swirl

8 ounces cream cheese, at room temperature	1 teaspoon vanilla extract
	1 teaspoon ground cinnamon
½ cup canned pumpkin puree	½ teaspoon ground ginger
¼ cup granulated erythritol–monk fruit blend	¼ teaspoon ground nutmeg
	¼ teaspoon ground allspice
1 large egg, at room temperature	

Preheat the oven to 350°F. Line the bottom of the 8-by-8-inch baking pan with parchment paper and grease the sides of the pan with butter. In the small microwave-safe bowl, melt the chocolate and butter together in the microwave, in 30-second intervals, until fully melted. Stir well and allow to cool for 5 minutes. In a medium bowl, using an electric mixer on low, whisk the chocolate mixture and sweetener until fully combined. With the mixer on medium high, add the eggs, one at a time, until well combined, scraping the bowl once or twice, as needed. Mix in the vanilla until the batter is smooth and the sweetener has fully dissolved. Stir in the almond flour, baking powder, and salt until fully blended, being careful not to overmix. Spread two-thirds of the batter into the bottom of the baking pan and set aside. In another medium bowl, using an electric mixer on medium high, combine the cream cheese, pumpkin puree, sweetener, egg, vanilla, cinnamon, ginger, nutmeg, and allspice and mix, scraping the bowl once or twice, as needed, until well combined. Pour the cheesecake swirl on the top of the brownie batter. Then add the remainder of the brownie mix, by spoonfuls, on top of the cheesecake layer. Using a knife, gently swirl the two batters together. Bake for 20 to 25 minutes, or until the center is just set but still jiggles. Allow the brownies to fully cool on the rack, about 15 minutes. Refrigerate the cooled brownies for 30 to 35 minutes before slicing into 16 squares before serving.

Per Serving: (1 brownie): Calories: 228; Fat: 21g; Protein: 5g; Total Carbs: 5g; Fiber: 2g; Net Carbs: 3g; **Macros:** Fat: 83%; Protein: 9%; Carbs: 8%

Blondies

MAKES 24 | PREP TIME: 10 minutes | COOK TIME: 35 minutes

¼ cup (½ stick) unsalted butter, at room temperature, plus more for greasing	1 teaspoon vanilla extract
	2 large eggs
	½ cup almond flour
1 cup brown or golden erythritol–monk fruit blend; less sweet: ½ cup	2½ tablespoons coconut flour
	1 teaspoon baking powder
4 ounces cream cheese, at room temperature	¼ teaspoon xanthan gum (optional)
	⅛ teaspoon sea salt

Preheat the oven to 350°F. Grease a baking pan with butter and set aside. In the large bowl, using an electric mixer on medium high, beat the sweetener, cream cheese, butter, and vanilla until combined. Add the eggs, one at a time, mixing well after each addition, scraping the bowl once or twice, as needed. Fold in the almond flour, coconut flour, baking powder, xanthan gum (if using), and salt. Spread the batter evenly into the prepared

baking pan. Bake for 30 to 35 minutes, or until golden brown. Allow the blondies to cool completely before slicing into 24 bars and serving.

Per Serving: (1 blondie): Calories: 53; Fat: 5g; Protein: 2g; Total Carbs: 1g; Fiber: 0g; Net Carbs: 1g; **Macros:** Fat: 84%; Protein: 10%; Carbs: 6%

Blueberry Cheesecake Bars

SERVES 12 | PREP TIME: 15 minutes | COOK TIME: 40 minutes

For the blueberry compote

2 cups blueberries, fresh or frozen	2 tablespoons lemon juice
	Zest of 1 lemon
2 teaspoons powdered erythritol	

For the crust

2 cups almond flour	½ teaspoon ground cinnamon
2 teaspoons powdered erythritol	¾ cup (1½ sticks) butter, melted

For the filling

16 ounces cream cheese, at room temperature	½ cup powdered erythritol
	2 teaspoons vanilla extract
2 large eggs, at room temperature	

In a small saucepan, combine the blueberries, sweetener, lemon juice, and lemon zest and cook over medium heat for 15 minutes, stirring occasionally. While the compote cooks, preheat the oven to 350°F, and butter a 9-by-13-inch baking dish. In a large bowl, combine all the ingredients and stir well to combine. Press the mixture into the baking dish and bake for 12 minutes. Remove from the oven. In a large mixing bowl, combine all the ingredients and use a hand mixer to mix well. Pour the filling into the prebaked crust and use a spatula to spread it evenly. Spoon the blueberry compote over the top of the filling. Use a knife to swirl the compote into the filling. Bake for 35 to 40 minutes or until the cheesecake is set. When cool, refrigerate for at least 1 hour to set up before cutting and serving.

Per Serving: Calories: 324; Fat: 31g; Protein: 6g; Total Carbs: 8g; Fiber: 2g; Net Carbs: 6g; **Macros:** Fat: 83%; Protein: 7%; Carbs: 10%

Fudge Brownies

SERVES 12 | PREP TIME: 15 minutes | COOK TIME: 20 minutes

Nonstick cooking spray	¼ cup unsweetened cocoa powder
¾ cup (1½ sticks) butter	
2 ounces dark chocolate squares (80 percent or higher), broken into chunks	½ cup almond flour
	⅔ cup Swerve sweetener
	½ teaspoon baking powder
	3 large eggs, beaten

Preheat the oven to 350°F. Grease an 8-inch-square baking dish with cooking spray. In a small saucepan over low heat, melt the butter and dark chocolate while stirring. When melted, add the cocoa powder and stir until combined. Set aside. In a small bowl, combine the almond flour, Swerve, and baking powder. In a separate bowl, pour in the eggs and then slowly mix in the dark chocolate mixture for about 1 minute to make sure everything is well combined. Pour the flour mixture into the chocolate mixture and stir until a batter forms. Spread the batter into the prepared baking dish and cook for 18 to 20 minutes, or until a toothpick inserted into the center comes out clean. Remove from the oven and allow to cool before cutting into 12 squares.

Per Serving: (1 brownie): Calories: 163; Fat: 15g; Protein: 3g; Total Carbs: 4g; Fiber: 1g; Net Carbs: 3g; **Macros:** Fat: 83%; Protein: 7%; Carbs: 10%

No-Bake Coconut Chocolate Squares

MAKES 24 SQUARES | PREP TIME: 10 minutes, plus 45 minutes to chill

1½ cups coconut oil, at room temperature, divided
1 cup shredded unsweetened coconut
¼ teaspoon liquid stevia, divided
½ cup unsweetened cocoa powder
½ teaspoon vanilla extract
⅛ teaspoon sea salt

Line an 8-inch-square baking dish with parchment paper. In a bowl, mix 1 cup of the coconut oil, coconut, and ⅛ teaspoon of liquid stevia. Spread the mixture in the baking dish and smooth it down with a spatula. Place it in the freezer for 15 minutes to set. Melt the remaining ½ cup of coconut oil in a glass measuring cup. Whisk in the cocoa powder, vanilla extract, sea salt, and remaining ⅛ teaspoon of stevia. Pour the chocolate mixture over the chilled coconut layer. Refrigerate and allow to set for 30 minutes. Slice into 24 squares.

Per Serving: (1 square): Calories: 144; Fat: 16g; Protein: 1g; Total Carbs: 2g; Fiber: 1g; Net Carbs: 1g; **Macros:** Fat: 98%; Protein: 1%; Carbs: 1%

Raspberry Cheesecake Squares

MAKES 12 SQUARES | PREP TIME: 10 minutes | COOK TIME: 25 to 30 minutes

½ cup coconut oil, melted
½ cup cream cheese, at room temperature
6 large eggs
3 tablespoons granulated sweetener
1 teaspoon alcohol-free pure vanilla extract
½ teaspoon baking powder
¾ cup raspberries

Preheat the oven to 350°F. Line an 8-inch-square baking dish with parchment paper and set aside. In a large bowl, beat the coconut oil and cream cheese until smooth. Beat in the eggs, scraping down the sides of the bowl at least once. Beat in the sweetener, vanilla, and baking powder until smooth. Spoon the batter into the baking dish and use a spatula to smooth out the top. Scatter the raspberries on top. Bake until the center is firm, about 25 to 30 minutes. Allow the cheesecake to cool completely before cutting into 12 squares.

Per Serving: (1 square): Calories: 176; Fat: 18g; Protein: 6g; Total Carbs: 3g; Fiber: 1g; Net Carbs: 2g; **Macros:** Fat: 85%; Protein: 11%; Carbs: 4%

Peanut Butter Cake Bars

SERVES 12 | PREP TIME: 10 minutes | COOK TIME: 45 minutes, plus 20 minutes to cool

¾ cup (1½ sticks) unsalted butter, at room temperature, plus more for greasing
2 cups granulated erythritol–monk fruit blend; less sweet: 1½ cups
8 ounces cream cheese, at room temperature
1 teaspoon vanilla extract
2¼ cups all-natural peanut butter (no added sugar), divided
½ cup sour cream
5 large eggs, at room temperature
2 cups almond flour
1 cup whey protein or an additional 1 cup almond flour
2 teaspoons baking powder
¼ teaspoon salt

Preheat the oven to 350°F. Grease a baking sheet with butter and set aside. In the large bowl, using an electric mixer on medium high, cream the sweetener, cream cheese, butter, and vanilla for 2 to 3 minutes, stopping and scraping the bowl once or twice, as needed, until light and fluffy. Add half the peanut butter and sour cream. Add the eggs, one at a time, until fully incorporated. Stir in the almond flour, whey protein, baking powder, and salt. Spread evenly into the prepared pan. Bake for 40 to 45 minutes, or until a toothpick inserted into the center comes out clean. Cool on the rack for 20 minutes. While the bars are cooling, in a microwave-safe bowl, melt the remaining peanut butter in the microwave in 20-second intervals. Drizzle on top of the bars and allow to set for 10 minutes before slicing into 24 bars to serve.

Per Serving: (2 bars): Calories: 638; Fat: 53g; Protein: 26g; Total Carbs: 8g; Fiber: 3g; Net Carbs: 5g; **Macros:** Fat: 75%; Protein: 16%; Carbs: 9%

Snickerdoodle Bars

SERVES 24 | PREP TIME: 10 minutes | COOK TIME: 30 to 40 minutes, plus cooling time

½ cup (1 stick) unsalted butter, at room temperature, plus more to grease the pan
2 cups granulated erythritol–monk fruit blend, plus 3 tablespoons
8 ounces (about 1 cup) cream cheese, at room temperature
2 teaspoons pure vanilla extract
5 large eggs, at room temperature
1 cup almond flour, measured and sifted
⅓ cup coconut flour
½ teaspoon baking soda
½ teaspoon cream of tartar
½ teaspoon xanthan gum (optional)
¼ teaspoon sea salt
2 teaspoons ground cinnamon

Preheat the oven to 350°F. Grease a 10-inch-square baking pan with butter. In a large bowl, using an electric mixer on medium speed, beat 2 cups sweetener, cream cheese, butter, and vanilla. Add the eggs one at a time, mixing well after each addition. Fold in the almond flour, coconut flour, baking soda, cream of tartar, xanthan gum (if using) and salt. Pour the batter into the prepared pan, and spread evenly. In a small bowl, combine the remaining 3 tablespoons of sweetener and the cinnamon. Sprinkle the mixture on top of the batter. Bake for 30 to 35 minutes, or until golden brown. Allow to cool completely in the pan on a wire rack before slicing into bars.

Per Serving: Calories: 116; Fat: 11g; Protein: 3g; Total Carbs: 3g; Fiber: 1g; Net Carbs: 2g; **Macros:** Fat: 85%; Protein: 10%; Carbs: 5%

Bourbon Pecan Pie Bars

SERVES 12 | PREP TIME: 15 minutes | COOK TIME: 35 minutes

Nonstick cooking spray	2 large eggs, beaten
1 cup almond flour	⅔ cup allulose blend
3 tablespoons coconut flour	sweetener
2 tablespoons monk fruit/	¼ cup heavy (whipping) cream
erythritol blend sweetener	2 tablespoons bourbon
¼ teaspoon ground cinnamon	1 teaspoon vanilla extract
Kosher salt	1½ cups chopped pecans
½ cup (1 stick) butter, melted, divided	

Preheat the oven to 350°F. Lightly coat an 8-inch-square baking pan with cooking spray. In a medium bowl, stir the almond and coconut flours, sweetener, cinnamon, and a pinch of salt; mix well. Stir in ¼ cup of melted butter and press the mixture firmly into the bottom of the prepared pan. Bake the crust for 8 to 10 minutes until it is golden brown around the edges. In another medium bowl, whisk the eggs, sweetener, heavy cream, remaining ¼ cup of melted butter, the bourbon, vanilla, and ¼ teaspoon salt until blended well. Sprinkle the pecans evenly over the crust. Pour the egg mixture over the pecans. Bake for 20 to 25 minutes, or until set. Cool completely in the pan before cutting into 12 bars. Refrigerate in a sealed container for up to 1 week.

Per Serving: Calories: 258; Fat: 24g; Protein: 4g; Total Carbs: 6g; Fiber: 4g; Net Carbs: 2g; **Macros:** Fat: 84%; Protein: 6%; Carbs: 10%

Lemon Cheesecake Bars

SERVES 8 | PREP TIME: 10 minutes, plus 2 hours to chill | COOK TIME: 10 minutes

½ cup butter, melted	8 ounces (1 package)
½ cup almond flour	cream cheese
1 cup boiling water	2 tablespoons freshly
⅓ cup sugar-free lemon gelatin mix	squeezed lemon juice

Preheat the oven to 350°F. In a medium bowl, mix the melted butter and the almond flour. Transfer the mixture to an 8-inch-square baking pan. Press the mixture firmly into the bottom. Bake for 10 minutes. Remove from the oven. Set aside to cool. In a large bowl, combine the boiling water and gelatin. Stir for about 2 minutes to dissolve. Add the cream cheese and lemon juice. Mix well to combine. Pour the cream cheese mixture over the cooled crust. Refrigerate for at least 2 hours until set, preferably overnight. Cut into 8 bars and serve.

Per Serving: (1 bar): Calories: 268; Fat: 25g; Protein: 7g; Total Carbs: 2g; Fiber: 1g; Net Carbs: 1g; **Macros:** Fat: 86%; Protein: 11%; Carbs: 3%

Pecan Pie Bars

SERVES 8 | PREP TIME: 15 minutes | COOK TIME: 40 minutes

2 cups coarsely chopped pecans	3 large eggs
¾ cup coconut flour	⅓ cup sugar-free maple-flavored syrup
¼ cup ground pecans	⅓ cup heavy (whipping) cream
6 tablespoons melted butter	¼ cup (½ stick) melted butter
⅛ teaspoon salt	2 teaspoons vanilla extract
2 tablespoons granulated erythritol blend, plus ⅔ cup, divided	½ teaspoon salt

Preheat the oven to 350°F. Line a baking sheet and an 8-inch square baking dish with parchment paper. Spread the coarsely chopped pecans evenly on the baking sheet. Bake for 7 to 10 minutes, shaking the tray halfway through. Remove from the oven, and allow to cool. In a small bowl, combine the flour, ground pecans, melted butter, salt, and 2 tablespoons of sweetener. Mix into a dough, and press evenly into the bottom of the baking dish. Bake for 10 to 12 minutes, until golden brown. Reduce the oven temperature to 325°F. In a medium bowl, mix together the remaining ⅔ cup of sweetener, eggs, syrup, heavy cream, butter, vanilla, salt, and chopped pecans. Pour the mixture over the crust in the baking dish. Bake for 30 to 35 minutes, until golden brown on top. Remove from the oven, cool, slice into 18 bars, and serve.

Per Serving: (1 bar): Calories: 197; Fat: 19g; Protein: 3g; Total Carbs: 13.5g; Fiber: 3g; Net Carbs: 1.5g; **Macros:** Fat: 87%; Protein: 6%; Carbs: 3%

Coconut Cinnamon Bars

SERVES 8 | PREP TIME: 5 minutes | COOK TIME: 2 hours

1 (7 ounce) bag unsweetened shredded coconut	¼ cup collagen peptides powder
6 tablespoons granular erythritol	2 teaspoons ground cinnamon
½ cup water	½ cup confectioner erythritol (like Swerve brand)
1 teaspoon gluten-free vanilla extract	2⅓ tablespoons teaspoon coconut milk

Preheat the oven to 350°F. On a baking sheet, spread the coconut flakes, and bake for 3 to 5 minutes or until the coconut barely starts to turn golden. In a medium saucepan, mix the erythritol and water over medium heat, and let it thicken and bubble for 5 minutes. Add the vanilla extract, collagen peptides, and cinnamon, and stir. Turn off the heat. Stir in the toasted coconut flakes. Line a 9-by-13-inch casserole dish with parchment paper. Press the coconut mixture into the dish firmly. Allow the coconut mixture to cool and set for 2 hours. Once cooled and firm, cut the mixture into 8 bars, and place them on a wire rack. In a small bowl, stir confectioner erythritol and coconut milk, and drizzle or pipe your icing onto each bar. Allow icing to set before serving.

Per Serving: Calories: 293; Fat: 30g; Protein: 6g; Total Carbs: 8g; Fiber: 4g; Net Carbs: 4g; **Macros:** Fat: 84%; Protein: 7%; Carbs: 9%

Cinnamon Popovers with Coconut Streusel

SERVES 12 | PREP TIME: 5 minutes | COOK TIME: 15 minutes

For the popover

¼ cup coconut oil

3 teaspoon ground cinnamon, divided

6 large eggs

½ cup coconut milk

¼ cup almond flour

3 tablespoons granular erythritol

For the topping

3 tablespoons coconut oil

3 tablespoons granular erythritol

3 tablespoons almond flour

2 teaspoons ground cinnamon

¼ cup unsweetened shredded coconut

Preheat the oven to 400°F. In a saucepan, melt the coconut oil and 1 teaspoon of ground cinnamon over medium heat. In a 12-well muffin tin, evenly pour the melted coconut oil mixture in each well. Place the muffin tin in the oven and heat for 3 minutes or until the oil sizzles. Mix the eggs, coconut milk, almond flour, the remaining 2 teaspoons of ground cinnamon, and 3 tablespoons of erythritol together in a medium bowl. Evenly pour the egg mixture into each well. Immediately place the muffin tin back in the oven, and let it cook for 10 minutes or until the popovers have significantly risen and are golden brown. While the popovers are baking, make the topping by mixing the coconut oil, erythritol, almond flour, cinnamon, and shredded coconut in a small bowl. Remove the muffin tin from the oven and top each popover evenly with the crumb mixture. Place the popovers back in the oven for an additional 3 to 5 minutes until the shredded coconut is golden brown.

Per Serving: Calories: 143; Fat: 14g; Protein: 4g; Total Carbs: 1g; Fiber: 0g; Net Carbs: 1g; **Macros:** Fat: 86%; Protein: 10%; Carbs: 4%

Ultra-Soft Pumpkin Chocolate Bars

SERVES 15 | PREP TIME: 5 minutes | COOK TIME: 30 minutes

½ cup ghee, melted

1 large egg

¾ cup pumpkin puree

½ cup packed granular erythritol

1 tablespoon vanilla extract

2 teaspoons ground cinnamon

1 teaspoon pumpkin pie spice

1¼ cups almond flour

1 cup 85% dark chocolate chips or sugar-free chocolate chips

Preheat the oven to 350°F. Line an 8-by-11-inch baking dish with parchment paper. In a large bowl, mix the ghee and egg, followed by the pumpkin puree and erythritol. Add the vanilla extract, cinnamon, pumpkin pie spice, and the almond flour. Mix well until the flour is fully incorporated. Fold in the chocolate chips. Pour the batter into the baking dish and bake for 30 to 35 minutes or until a wooden pick inserted in the middle comes out clean. Allow it to cool before slicing it into bars.

Per Serving: Calories: 150; Fat: 12g; Protein: 2g; Total Carbs: 9g; Fiber: 2g; Net Carbs: 7g; **Macros:** Fat: 71%; Protein: 6%; Carbs: 23%

Pistachio-Raspberry Chocolate Bark

SERVES 4 | PREP TIME: 5 minutes

Nonstick cooking spray

6 ounces unsweetened dark chocolate

⅓ cup monk fruit sweetener

1 tablespoon coconut oil

¼ cup pistachios, crushed

¼ cup freeze-dried raspberries

Sea salt

Line a baking sheet with parchment and grease it with nonstick spray. Using a double boiler or a bowl set over a pan of simmering water (the bowl shouldn't touch the water), slowly melt the chocolate. Once the chocolate has melted, stir in the sweetener and coconut oil and cook on low for one minute until the ingredients are mixed. Pour the chocolate mixture onto the prepared baking sheet. Tap the sheet on the countertop to spread the chocolate out evenly and remove bubbles. Before the chocolate hardens, generously sprinkle it with the pistachios, raspberries, and sea salt. Refrigerate for 2 hours to let the chocolate firm up. Break the chocolate into rough chunks.

Per Serving: Calories: 308; Fat: 20g; Protein: 4g; Total Carbs: 28g; Fiber: 1g; Net Carbs: 27g; **Macros:** Fat: 58%; Protein: 5%; Carbs: 37%

Blackberry "Cheesecake" Bites

SERVES 4 | PREP TIME: 5 minutes, plus overnight to soak and 1 hour 30 minutes to set

1½ cups almonds, soaked overnight

1 cup blackberries

⅓ cup coconut oil, melted

¼ cup coconut cream

⅓ cup monk fruit sweetener

¼ cup freshly squeezed lemon juice

Prepare a muffin tin by lining the cups with cupcake liners. Set aside. In a high-powered blender, combine the soaked almonds, blackberries, melted coconut oil, coconut cream, sweetener, and lemon juice. Blend on high until the mixture is whipped and fluffy. Divide the mixture equally among the muffin cups. Place the muffin tin in the freezer for 90 minutes to allow the cheesecake bites to set.

Per Serving: Calories: 514; Fat: 48g; Protein: 12g; Total Carbs: 18g; Fiber: 9g; Net Carbs: 9g; **Macros:** Fat: 78%; Protein: 9%; Carbs: 13%

Salted Caramel Cupcakes

MAKES 12 | PREP TIME: 20 minutes |
COOK TIME: 40 minutes, plus 20 minutes to cool

For the cupcakes

1¼ cups almond flour, sifted

1 teaspoon baking powder

¼ teaspoon salt, plus more for topping

¼ cup (½ stick) unsalted butter, at room temperature

¾ cup granulated erythritol–monk fruit blend

3½ ounces cream cheese, at room temperature

1 teaspoon vanilla extract

4 large eggs, at room temperature

For the caramel sauce

2 tablespoons unsalted butter, at room temperature

1 cup allulose

¼ cup heavy (whipping) cream

For the buttercream

¾ cup (1½ sticks) unsalted butter, at room temperature

2 to 3 tablespoons heavy (whipping) cream

1 teaspoon vanilla extract

¼ teaspoon sea salt

1½ cups confectioners' erythritol–monk fruit blend

Preheat the oven to 350°F. Line the muffin pan with cupcake liners. In the medium bowl, combine the almond flour, baking powder, and salt. Set aside. In the large bowl, using an electric mixer on medium high, cream the butter and sweetener, scraping the bowl once or twice, as needed, until the mixture is light and fluffy and well incorporated. Add the cream cheese and vanilla and mix well. Add the eggs, one at a time, making sure to mix well after each addition. Add the dry ingredients to the wet ingredients and mix well, until the batter is fully combined. Fill the prepared muffin cups with the batter. Bake for 20 to 25 minutes, until golden brown and a toothpick inserted into a cupcake comes out clean. Cool on a cooling rack for 15 to 20 minutes. While the cupcakes bake, in the saucepan, brown the butter over medium heat, stirring constantly. Once the butter begins to foam and bubble, after 2 to 4 minutes, you should begin to see browned bits on the bottom of the pan. At this point, remove from the heat immediately and continue to stir until the butter turns to a golden amber color. Add the allulose and return to the stove to cook over low heat. Once the sauce thickens, stir in the heavy cream, remove from the heat, and set aside. In the large bowl, using an electric mixer on medium-high, mix the butter, heavy cream, vanilla, and salt until well mixed, scraping the bowl once or twice, as needed. Add the confectioners' sweetener 1 tablespoon at a time, beating well after each addition until fully incorporated. Once the cupcakes have completely cooled, frost with the buttercream, drizzle on the caramel sauce, and top with salt to serve.

Per Serving: Calories: 290; Fat: 29g; Protein: 5g; Total Carbs: 3g; Fiber: 1g; Net Carbs: 2g; Macros: Fat: 90%; Protein: 7%; Carbs: 3%

Coconut-Orange Cupcakes

SERVES 6 | PREP TIME: 15 minutes | COOK TIME: 20 minutes

¼ cup powdered sugar-free sweetener	½ cup coconut flour
1 large egg	½ cup almond flour
½ cup coconut oil, melted	½ teaspoon baking powder
1 teaspoon vanilla extract	½ teaspoon salt
	Zest and juice of 1 orange

Preheat the oven to 350°F and place liners into 6 cups of a muffin tin. In a large bowl, whisk the sweetener and egg. Add the coconut oil and vanilla and whisk until well combined. In a medium bowl, whisk the coconut flour, almond flour, baking powder, and salt. Add the dry ingredients, orange juice, and zest to the wet ingredients and stir until just combined. Divide the batter evenly among the prepared muffin tin and bake for 15 to 18 minutes, until a toothpick inserted in the center of the cupcake comes out clean. Remove the cupcakes from the oven and cool for 5 minutes in the tin before transferring to a wire rack to cool completely.

Per Serving: (1 cupcake): Calories: 277; Fat: 25g; Protein: 4g; Total Carbs: 19g; Fiber: 4g; Net Carbs: 15g; Macros: Fat: 81%; Protein: 6%; Carbs: 13%

Orange-Olive Oil Cupcakes

MAKES 6 CUPCAKES | PREP TIME: 15 minutes | COOK TIME: 20 minutes

1 large egg	Zest of 1 orange
2 tablespoons powdered sugar-free sweetener (such as stevia or monk fruit extract)	1 cup almond flour
	¾ teaspoon baking powder
	⅛ teaspoon salt
½ cup extra-virgin olive oil	1 tablespoon freshly squeezed orange juice
1 teaspoon almond extract	

Preheat the oven to 350°F. Place muffin liners into 6 cups of a muffin tin. In a large bowl, whisk the egg and powdered sweetener. whisk in the olive oil, almond extract, and orange zest. In a small bowl, whisk the almond flour, baking powder, and salt. Add the dry ingredients to the wet with the orange juice and stir until just combined. Divide the batter evenly between the muffin cups and bake until a toothpick inserted in the center of the cupcake comes out clean, 15 to 18 minutes. Remove from the oven and cool for 5 minutes in the tin before cooling completely on a wire rack.

Per Serving: Calories: 211; Fat: 22g; Protein: 3g; Total Carbs: 2g; Fiber: 0g; Net Carbs: 2g; Macros: Fat: 91%; Protein: 5%; Carbs: 4%

Almond Cake

SERVES 12 | PREP TIME: 15 minutes | COOK TIME: 1 hour

Butter, for greasing	¼ teaspoon sea salt
2½ cups almond flour	3 large eggs
½ cup egg white protein powder	½ cup almond milk
	½ cup plain Greek yogurt
2 teaspoons baking powder	1 teaspoon pure vanilla extract
1 teaspoon baking soda	
1 teaspoon stevia	1 teaspoon almond extract

Preheat the oven to 300°F. Lightly grease a 9-by-4-inch loaf pan with butter, and set aside. In a large bowl, stir the almond flour, egg white protein powder, baking powder, baking soda, stevia, and salt. In a medium bowl, whisk the eggs, almond milk, yogurt, vanilla, and almond extract. Add the wet ingredients to the dry ingredients, and stir to blend well. Spoon the batter into the loaf pan, and smooth the top with a spatula. Bake until the loaf is golden and firm, about 1 hour. Cool the cake for 10 minutes in the pan, and then flip it out to cool completely on a wire rack. Serve.

Per Serving: (1 slice): Calories: 198; Fat: 16g; Protein: 5g; Total Carbs: 6g; Fiber: 3g; Net Carbs: 3g; Macros: Fat: 77%; Protein: 10%; Carbs: 13%

Tiramisu

SERVES 8 | PREP TIME: 20 minutes | COOK TIME: 45 minutes, plus 8 hours to chill

For the cake

¼ cup (½ stick) unsalted butter, at room temperature	1 teaspoon vanilla extract
¾ cup granulated erythritol–monk fruit blend	4 large eggs, at room temperature
4 ounces cream cheese, at room temperature	1¼ cups almond flour, sifted
	1 teaspoon baking powder
	½ teaspoon sea salt

For the custard

4 large egg yolks, at room temperature	¼ teaspoon sea salt
	4 ounces mascarpone cheese
½ cup granulated erythritol–monk fruit blend	1 cup heavy (whipping) cream

For the topping

¼ cup espresso or strong coffee	¼ cup unsweetened cocoa powder
2 tablespoons dark rum or ½ teaspoon rum extract	

Preheat the oven to 350°F. Line a baking sheet with parchment paper and set aside. In the large bowl, using an electric mixer on high, beat the butter and sweetener for 2 to 3 minutes, scraping the bowl once or twice, as needed, until light and fluffy and well incorporated. Add the cream cheese and vanilla and mix well. Add the eggs, one at a time, mixing well after each addition. Add the almond flour, baking powder, and salt and mix well until combined. Spread the batter evenly onto the prepared baking sheet. Bake for 25 to 30 minutes, until golden brown on top. Allow to cool fully, 15 to 20 minutes, before cutting into 1-by-3-inch slices to mimic ladyfingers. While the cake bakes, in the medium glass bowl, using an electric mixer on medium high, beat the egg yolks, sweetener and salt, scraping the bowl once or twice, as needed, until thick and lemon colored. Fill a medium saucepan with 3 inches of water and bring to a boil over high heat, then reduce the heat to a simmer. Put the glass bowl with the egg mixture over the simmering water, stirring constantly for 9 to 10 minutes, or until the mixture reaches a custard-like texture. Remove from the heat and stir in the mascarpone cheese. In the medium bowl, using an electric mixer on high, beat the heavy cream for 3 to 5 minutes, scraping the bowl once or twice, as needed, until stiff peaks form. Gently fold the mascarpone mixture into the whipped cream. Set aside. In the small bowl, combine the espresso and rum and set aside. Using a sifter, sprinkle a layer of cocoa powder onto the bottom of the loaf pan. Place a layer of the cake "fingers" in the pan. Coat the layer with the coffee-rum mixture using a pastry brush. Follow by spreading one-quarter of the custard over the top. Repeat the layers of cake, coffee, and custard ending with the custard. Top with a generous coating of cocoa powder. Cover and refrigerate for at least 8 hours or overnight before serving.

Per Serving: Calories: 415; Fat: 39g; Protein: 11g; Total Carbs: 7g; Fiber: 3g; Net Carbs: 4g; **Macros:** Fat: 84%; Protein: 10%; Carbs: 6%

Strawberry Cheesecake

SERVES 12 | PREP TIME: 10 minutes, plus 9 hours 20 minutes to chill | COOK TIME: 55 minutes

1½ cups almond flour

6 tablespoons melted butter

2 tablespoons sugar-free maple syrup

1 tablespoon brown sugar substitute

1 teaspoon ground cinnamon

¾ cup erythritol

1 cup sliced ripe strawberries

2 (8-ounce) packages cream cheese, at room temperature

1 cup sour cream, at room temperature

¾ teaspoon vanilla extract

¾ teaspoon strawberry extract

½ tablespoon lemon juice

2 large eggs, at room temperature

In a large bowl, combine the almond flour, butter, syrup, brown sugar substitute, and cinnamon then pour into a 9-inch springform pie pan. Pack it down evenly on the bottom and sides of the pan. Refrigerate for at least 20 minutes until firm to the touch. Preheat the oven to 350°F. Pulse the erythritol in a blender or food processor until powdered. Set aside. Puree the strawberries in a blender. Set aside. In a large bowl, gently beat the cream cheese and sour cream. Add the erythritol, vanilla, strawberry extract, and lemon juice. Beat in one egg at a time until fully incorporated. Pour the cheesecake mixture into the chilled pie crust. Drizzle with the pureed strawberries. Use a butter knife to swirl the puree into the cheesecake. Place the cheesecake in a large roasting pan and carefully pour hot water into the pan to reach about halfway up the side of the cheesecake dish. Lay a piece of aluminum foil loosely on top of the roasting pan. Bake for 45 to 55 minutes, until the edges are set, but the center still jiggles. Turn off the oven and crack open the oven door. Leave the cheesecake for 30 minutes. Remove the cheesecake from the water bath. Let sit at room temperature for 1 hour. Cover the cooled cheesecake with plastic wrap and refrigerate for 8 hours or overnight before serving.

Per Serving: (1 slice): Calories: 322; Fat: 31g; Protein: 7g; Total Carbs: 21g; Fiber: 2g; Net Carbs: 6g; **Macros:** Fat: 82%; Protein: 8%; Carbs: 10%

No-Bake Chocolate Raspberry Cheesecake

SERVES 14 | PREP TIME: 15 minutes | COOK TIME: 10 minutes, plus 4 hours to chill

For the crust

¼ cup (½ stick) unsalted butter

2 ounces unsweetened baking chocolate

2 cups almond flour, sifted

¼ cup granulated erythritol–monk fruit blend; less sweet: 3 tablespoons

¼ teaspoon sea salt

For the cheesecake

¼ cup (½ stick) unsalted butter

2 ounces unsweetened baking chocolate, coarsely chopped

3 cups granulated erythritol–monk fruit blend; less sweet: 2 cups

20 ounces cream cheese, at room temperature

2 cups sour cream

¼ cup unsweetened cocoa powder

For the topping

1 tablespoon coconut oil

2 tablespoons sugar-free dark chocolate chips

1 cup chopped raspberries

In a small microwave-safe bowl, melt the butter and baking chocolate together in the microwave in 30-second intervals. Add the almond flour, sweetener, and salt to the melted chocolate and combine well. Press the mixture into the pie dish and put in the refrigerator to cool until ready to fill. In another small microwave-safe bowl, melt the butter and baking chocolate together in the microwave, in 30-second intervals, and set aside. In the large bowl, using an electric mixer on medium high, beat the sweetener, cream cheese, sour cream, and cocoa powder until well combined, scraping the bowl once or twice, as needed. Gradually fold in the chocolate and butter mixture until fully combined. Scrape the cheesecake batter into the crust and spread evenly. In a third small microwave-safe bowl, melt the coconut oil and chocolate baking chips together in the microwave in 30-second intervals to make the chocolate sauce. Top the cheesecake with the raspberries and drizzle with the chocolate sauce. Cover and refrigerate for at least 4 hours or overnight to set. Cut into 14 slices and serve.

Per Serving: Calories: 414; Fat: 40g; Protein: 8g; Total Carbs: 10g; Fiber: 4g; Net Carbs: 6g; **Macros:** Fat: 84%; Protein: 7%; Carbs: 9%

Quick Pressure Cooker Cheesecake

SERVES 12 | PREP TIME: 5 minutes | COOK TIME: 30 minutes, plus 3 hours chill time

16 ounces cream cheese, at room temperature	2 large eggs, at room temperature
¼ cup sour cream	2 teaspoons lemon juice
⅔ cup powdered erythritol	2 teaspoons vanilla extract

In a large bowl, combine the cream cheese, sour cream, and erythritol. Use a hand mixer to beat them until combined. Add the eggs, one at a time, mixing after each addition. Add the lemon juice and vanilla, and mix. Do not overbeat. Butter the inside of a springform pan that fits inside your multicooker. Cover the outside of the pan with aluminum foil to prevent water entering. Pour the cheesecake mixture into the pan. Place the trivet in the bottom of the multicooker and add 1 inch of water. Lower the springform pan onto the trivet. Use the manual setting on high pressure and cook for 20 minutes. Allow a 10-minute natural release, then manually release any remaining pressure. Allow the cake to cool in the multicooker for about 10 minutes, then transfer to a rack for another 10 minutes. Chill for at least 3 hours and preferably overnight for the creamiest texture.

Per Serving: Calories: 153; Fat: 15g; Protein: 3g; Total Carbs: 2g; Fiber: 0g; Net Carbs: 2g; **Macros:** Fat: 86%; Protein: 10%; Carbs: 4%

Pumpkin-Ricotta Cheesecake

SERVES 10 TO 12 | PREP TIME: 25 minutes, plus 6 hours to set | COOK TIME: 45 minutes

1 cup almond flour	½ to ¾ cup sugar-free sweetener
½ cup butter, melted	4 large eggs
1 (14 ½-ounce) can pumpkin purée	2 teaspoons vanilla extract
8 ounces cream cheese, at room temperature	2 teaspoons pumpkin pie spice
½ cup whole-milk ricotta cheese	Whipped cream, for garnish (optional)

Preheat the oven to 350°F. Line the bottom of a 9-inch springform pan with parchment paper. In a small bowl, combine the almond flour and melted butter with a fork until well combined. Press the mixture into the bottom of the prepared pan. In a large bowl, beat the pumpkin purée, cream cheese, ricotta, and sweetener using an electric mixer on medium. Add the eggs, one at a time, beating after each addition. Stir in the vanilla and pumpkin pie spice until just combined. Pour the mixture over the crust and bake until set, 40 to 45 minutes. Allow to cool to room temperature. Refrigerate for at least

6 hours before serving. Serve chilled, garnishing with whipped cream, if desired.

Per Serving: Calories: 242; Fat: 22g; Protein: 7g; Total Carbs: 5g; Fiber: 1g; Net Carbs: 4g; **Macros:** Fat: 81%; Protein: 11%; Carbs: 8%

Italian Cream Cheesecake

SERVES 12 | PREP TIME: 15 minutes | COOK TIME: 2 hours, plus 8 hours to chill

For the crust

Nonstick cooking spray	3 tablespoons monk fruit/erythritol blend sweetener
1½ cups almond flour	¼ teaspoon rum extract
6 tablespoons butter, melted	Pinch kosher salt

For the cheesecake

3 (8-ounce) packages cream cheese, at room temperature	¾ cup sour cream, at room temperature
½ cup monk fruit/erythritol blend sweetener	½ cup canned coconut milk
	2 teaspoons vanilla extract
4 large eggs, at room temperature	1½ teaspoon coconut extract
	½ cup toasted pecans, finely chopped

Preheat the oven to 350°F. Lightly coat a 9-inch springform pan with cooking spray and line it with parchment paper. Set aside. In a medium bowl, stir the almond flour, melted butter, sweetener, rum extract, and salt until crumbly. Firmly press the crust mixture evenly into the bottom and 1 inch up the sides of the prepared pan. Bake for 10 to 12 minutes on the center rack, or until golden brown around the edges. Set the pan aside to cool completely. Wrap the outside of a springform pan tightly in two layers of foil to prevent water from leaking in during baking. Lower the oven temperature to 325°F. Place a roaster pan on the center oven rack and fill it with about 1 inch of hot water. In a large bowl and using an electric hand mixer, beat the cream cheese at medium speed until creamy. Add the sweetener and mix well to combine. One at a time, add the eggs, beating just until incorporated after each addition. Gently stir in the sour cream, coconut milk, vanilla, and coconut extract to combine. Stir in the toasted pecans. Pour the batter onto the prepared crust. Place the springform pan carefully into the center of the water bath. Bake for 60 to 70 minutes. The outer edges of the cheesecake will be set but the center of the cheesecake will be slightly jiggly and not completely set. Turn off the oven, leaving the door closed, and let the cheesecake sit in the oven for an additional 25 minutes. Remove the springform pan from the water bath and the foil, and let cool for 15 to 20 minutes on a wire rack. Run a butter knife around the edge of the pan to release the cheesecake and cool completely. Cover the cheesecake and chill for at least 8 hours, or overnight. Carefully remove the sides of the springform pan and transfer the cheesecake to a serving platter.

Per Serving: Calories: 416; Fat: 40g; Protein: 9g; Total Carbs: 5g; Fiber: 1g; Net Carbs: 4g; **Macros:** Fat: 87%; Protein: 9%; Carbs: 4%

Butter Rum Pound Cake

SERVES 15 | PREP TIME: 15 minutes | COOK TIME: 1 hour, 10 minutes

For the pound cake

Nonstick cooking spray

7 tablespoons butter

1 cup almond flour

¾ cup coconut flour

⅔ cup monk fruit/erythritol blend sweetener

2 teaspoons baking powder

1 teaspoon baking soda

½ teaspoon kosher salt

8 large eggs

¼ cup plus 2 tablespoons sour cream

¼ cup dark rum

1 teaspoon vanilla extract

Fresh whipped cream, for serving

For the glaze

¼ cup butter

¼ cup allulose blend sweetener

3 tablespoons dark rum

2 tablespoons water

Preheat the oven to 350°F. Spray a 10-cup Bundt pan. In a small skillet over medium-low heat, melt the butter and cook it for about 10 minutes, stirring often, until browned and nutty. The solids in the butter should be the color of caramel. Remove from the heat and set aside to cool. In a medium bowl, stir the almond and coconut flours, sweetener, baking powder, baking soda, and salt. In a large bowl and using an electric hand mixer, whip the eggs for about 2 minutes until light and foamy. Add the flour mixture and mix on medium speed until combined, stopping to scrape down the sides. Add the sour cream, rum, vanilla, and cooled browned butter to the batter (reserve the skillet for the glaze) and mix again until well combined. Spoon the batter evenly into the prepared pan and smooth the top. Bake for 35 to 40 minutes or until a toothpick inserted into the center comes out clean. If needed, loosely cover with aluminum foil halfway through the baking time to prevent over-browning. While the cake bakes, in the skillet used to brown the butter, combine the butter, sweetener, rum, and water. Place the skillet over medium heat and bring the mixture to a boil. Cook for 2 to 3 minutes. Pour the glaze evenly over the warm cake. Cool the cake in the pan. Turn the cake out onto a cake stand or plate of choice. Serve with a dollop of whipped cream.

Per Serving: Calories: 179; Fat: 15g; Protein: 5g; Total Carbs: 6g; Fiber: 3g; Net Carbs: 3g; Macros: Fat: 75%; Protein: 11%; Carbs: 13%

Hazelnut-Chocolate Snack Cakes

SERVES 24 | PREP TIME: 10 minutes | COOK TIME: 30 to 35 minutes, plus cooling time

2 cups granulated erythritol–monk fruit blend

8 ounces (about 1 cup) cream cheese, at room temperature

½ cup (1 stick) unsalted butter, at room temperature, plus more to grease the pan

1 teaspoon liquid hazelnut extract

5 large eggs, at room temperature

1 cup hazelnut flour

⅓ cup coconut flour

¼ cup unsweetened cocoa powder

1½ teaspoons baking powder

¼ teaspoon sea salt

1 cup chopped hazelnuts

½ cup sugar-free chocolate chips

½ cup roughly chopped unsweetened baking chocolate

Preheat the oven to 350°F. Grease a 9-by-13-inch baking pan with butter. In a large bowl, using an electric mixer, beat the sweetener cream cheese, butter, and hazelnut extract. Add the eggs one at a time, and mix well after each addition to make sure the eggs are well incorporated into the batter. Fold in the hazelnut flour, coconut flour, unsweetened cocoa powder, baking powder, and salt. Using a spatula, stir in the hazelnuts, chocolate chips, and unsweetened baking chocolate. Pour the batter into the prepared pan, and bake for 30 to 35 minutes, or until golden brown. Allow the cake to cool completely in the pan, then cut into 24 individual snack cakes.

Per Serving: Calories: 187; Fat: 17g; Protein: 4g; Total Carbs: 8g; Fiber: 3g; Net Carbs: 5g; Macros: Fat: 82%; Protein: 9%; Carbs: 9%

Cream Cheese Pound Cake

SERVES 12 | PREP TIME: 10 minutes | COOK TIME: 40 to 45 minutes

4 ounces butter, at room temperature

8 ounces cream cheese, at room temperature

1¼ cups Swerve or another non-caloric sweetener

6 large eggs

1 tablespoon vanilla extract

2 cups almond flour

⅓ cup coconut flour

1 tablespoon aluminum-free double-acting baking powder

½ teaspoon sea salt

Preheat the oven to 350°F. Line a 9-by-13-inch baking pan with parchment paper. Beat the butter, cream cheese, and Swerve with a hand mixer until smooth and creamy, about 1 minute. Add the eggs and vanilla extract, and beat until thoroughly emulsified. Stir in the almond flour, coconut flour, baking powder, and sea salt. Mix until just combined. Pour into the prepared pan. Bake for 40 to 45 minutes, or until a toothpick inserted into the center comes out clean.

Per Serving: Calories: 288; Fat: 26g; Protein: 9g; Total Carbs: 7g; Fiber: 3g; Net Carbs: 4g; Macros: Fat: 81%; Protein: 13%; Carbs: 6%

Pumpkin Pound Cake

MAKES 12 SLICES | PREP TIME: 10 minutes | COOK TIME: 45 to 50 minutes, plus 35 minutes to cool

For the pound cake

1½ cups almond flour, measured and sifted

1½ tablespoons ground cinnamon

1½ teaspoons ground ginger

1½ teaspoons pumpkin pie spice

1½ teaspoons baking powder

½ teaspoon ground nutmeg

¼ teaspoon ground allspice

⅛ teaspoon ground cloves

¼ teaspoon sea salt

¾ cup granulated erythritol–monk fruit blend

½ cup (1 stick) unsalted butter, at room temperature

¼ cup brown or golden granulated erythritol–monk fruit blend

4 ounces (about ½ cup) cream cheese, at room temperature

1 teaspoon pure vanilla extract

½ cup canned pumpkin purée

3 large eggs, at room temperature

For the icing

½ cup confectioners' erythritol–monk fruit blend

3 to 4 tablespoons heavy (whipping) cream plus more as needed

½ teaspoon pure vanilla extract

Preheat the oven to 350°F. Line a 9-by-5-inch loaf pan with parchment paper. In a medium bowl, combine the almond flour, cinnamon, ginger, pumpkin pie spice, baking powder, nutmeg, allspice, cloves, and salt. In a large bowl, using an electric mixer, cream the sweetener, butter, and brown sweetener until the mixture is light and fluffy and well incorporated. Add the cream cheese and vanilla, and mix well. Add the pumpkin purée, and mix until just incorporated. Alternate adding the eggs one at a time with the dry ingredients, and mix thoroughly after each addition. Scrape down the sides of the bowl periodically. Pour the batter into the prepared pan. Bake for 45 to 50 minutes, or until golden brown on top and a toothpick inserted into the center comes out clean. Allow to cool on a wire rack for 10 minutes before removing the cake from the pan. Then allow to cool for another 25 minutes on a wire rack until fully cooled before icing. In a small bowl, put the confectioners' sweetener, and whisk in the heavy cream and vanilla, making sure to fully incorporate the mixture. Add more heavy cream if the icing is too thick; it should be runny enough to drizzle. Once the pound cake has fully cooled, drizzle on the icing, and serve.

Per Serving: Calories: 221; Fat: 21g; Protein: 6g; Total Carbs: 6g; Fiber: 3g; Net Carbs: 3g; **Macros:** Fat: 86%; Protein: 11%; Carbs: 3%

Raspberry-Lemon Pound Cake

MAKES 10 SLICES | PREP TIME: 10 minutes | COOK TIME: 35 to 40 minutes, plus 30 to 35 minutes to cool

For the pound cake

Coconut oil, for greasing the pan

1¼ cups almond flour, measured and sifted

1¼ teaspoons baking powder

¼ teaspoon sea salt

4 ounces (about ½ cup) cream cheese, at room temperature

½ cup granulated erythritol–monk fruit blend

¼ cup (½ stick) unsalted butter, at room temperature

2 teaspoons grated lemon zest

1 teaspoon liquid lemon extract

4 large eggs, at room temperature

1 cup fresh or frozen whole raspberries

For the vanilla glaze

½ cup confectioners' erythritol–monk fruit blend

2 to 3 tablespoons heavy (whipping) cream

½ teaspoon pure vanilla extract

Preheat the oven to 350°F. Lightly grease a 9-by-5-inch loaf pan with coconut oil. In a medium bowl, combine the almond flour, baking powder, and salt. In a large bowl, using an electric mixer on medium speed, cream the cream cheese, sweetener, butter, lemon zest, and lemon extract until light and fluffy. Scrape down the sides of the bowl with a spatula. Add the eggs

one at a time, and mix on medium speed after each addition until the eggs are blended. Scrape down the sides of the bowl each time. Add the dry ingredients to the wet batter, beating on low speed until well incorporated. Reserving 2 tablespoons, gently fold the raspberries into the batter with a rubber spatula. Spread the mixture in the prepared loaf pan, and top with the reserved raspberries, pressing them into the batter. Bake the loaf for 35 to 40 minutes, or until the top springs back to the touch and a toothpick inserted into the center comes out clean. Allow the pound cake to cool in the pan for about 15 minutes. Then allow to cool on a wire rack for another 15 to 20 minutes before icing. Combine the confectioners' sweetener, 2 tablespoons heavy cream, and vanilla. Add another tablespoon of heavy cream if the glaze is too thick. Drizzle over the pound cake once it's cooled.

Per Serving: Calories: 206; Fat: 19g; Protein: 7g; Total Carbs: 5g; Fiber: 2g; Net Carbs: 3g; **Macros:** Fat: 83%; Protein: 14%; Carbs: 3%

Poppy Seed Pound Cake

SERVES 12 | PREP TIME: 10 minutes | COOK TIME: 40 minutes

¼ cup (½ stick) unsalted butter, at room temperature, plus more for greasing

1¼ cups almond flour, sifted

1 teaspoon baking powder

¼ teaspoon salt

¾ cup granulated erythritol–monk fruit blend; less sweet: ½ cup

3½ ounces cream cheese, at room temperature

1 teaspoon lemon extract

4 large eggs, at room temperature

1½ tablespoons poppy seeds

Preheat the oven to 350°F. Grease a 9-by-5-inch loaf pan with butter, line with parchment paper, and set aside. In the medium bowl, combine the almond flour, baking powder, and salt. Set aside. In the large bowl, using an electric mixer on medium high, cream the butter and sweetener for 1 to 2 minutes, until light and fluffy. Add the cream cheese and lemon extract and mix well. Add the eggs, one at a time, making sure to mix well after each addition. Add the dry ingredients to the wet ingredients and mix well. Stir in the poppy seeds and mix well. Pour the batter into the prepared loaf pan. Bake for 30 to 40 minutes, until golden brown and a toothpick inserted into the center comes out clean. Let cool for 10 to 15 minutes, then cut into 12 slices and serve.

Per Serving: Calories: 149; Fat: 14g; Protein: 5g; Total Carbs: 3g; Fiber: 2g; Net Carbs: 1g; **Macros:** Fat: 79%; Protein: 13%; Carbs: 8%

Lemon Curd Layer Cake

MAKES 12 SLICES | PREP TIME: 15 minutes | COOK TIME: 35 to 40 minutes, plus 40 minutes to cool

For the lemon curd

5 tablespoons unsalted butter

8 large egg yolks, at room temperature

1 cup granulated erythritol–monk fruit blend

1 cup freshly squeezed lemon juice

1 tablespoon grated lemon zest

½ teaspoon lemon extract

¼ teaspoon sea salt

For the cake

¼ cup (½ stick) unsalted butter, softened, plus more to grease the pans

4 ounces (about ½ cup) cream cheese, softened

1 cup granulated erythritol–monk fruit blend

4 large eggs, at room temperature

1¼ cups almond flour, measured and sifted

1 teaspoon baking powder

1 teaspoon grated lemon zest

¼ teaspoon sea salt

3 tablespoons freshly squeezed lemon juice

1 teaspoon lemon extract

Fill a saucepan two-thirds full with simmering water, then set a heat-proof bowl above it and melt the butter. Add the egg yolks one at a time, whisking quickly to incorporate each one. While continuing to whisk, add the sweetener, lemon juice, lemon zest, lemon extract, and salt. Mix until all the ingredients are combined and the lemon curd thickens, 5 to 7 minutes. Refrigerate the bowl of lemon curd with plastic wrap on the surface of the curd. Preheat the oven 350°F. Grease 2 (9-inch) cake pans with butter. In a large bowl, using an electric mixer on high speed cream the butter and cream cheese until light and fluffy. While mixing, add the sweetener. Add the eggs one at a time, mixing well after each addition. Stir in the almond flour, baking powder, lemon zest, and salt, and mix well. Add the lemon juice and lemon extract, and beat until the batter is fully mixed. Pour the batter evenly into the 2 cake pans, and bake for 35 to 40 minutes, or until a toothpick inserted into the center comes out clean. Allow the cakes to cool in their pans for 10 minutes, then remove them from their pans. Cool the cakes on a wire rack for another 30 minutes until fully cooled. Put one of the cakes on a cake stand or flat plate, and spread half the lemon curd on top. Carefully place the second cake on top, and spread the rest of the lemon curd on top.

Per Serving: Calories: 242; Fat: 22g; Protein: 7g; Total Carbs: 6g; Fiber: 1g; Net Carbs: 5g; **Macros:** Fat: 82%; Protein: 12%; Carbs: 6%

Chocolate Marble Pound Cake

SERVES 18 | PREP TIME: 10 minutes, plus 1 hour to cool | COOK TIME: 30 minutes

Oil or nonstick cooking spray

¾ cup (1½ sticks) softened butter

1½ cups granulated erythritol blend, divided

10 large eggs

4 ounces (½ brick) cream cheese, room temperature

½ cup water

1 tablespoon vanilla extract

1 (13.66-ounce) can coconut cream

2 cups coconut flour

2 teaspoons baking powder

½ teaspoon salt

¾ cup unsweetened cocoa powder

Preheat the oven to 325°F. Lightly grease a 9-by-13-inch baking dish. Using a stand or hand mixer, cream the butter, 1 cup of sweetener, eggs, cream cheese, water, and vanilla for about 2 minutes. Add the coconut cream, and mix on low until incorporated. In a small bowl, sift the flour, baking powder, and salt, and mix. Add the flour mixture to the wet mixture, and mix on low for about 30 seconds, scraping down the sides with spatula, until incorporated. Pour all but 2 or 3 cups of batter into the prepared pan. Into the remaining batter, add the remaining

½ cup of sweetener and cocoa powder, and stir together well. It should be thicker than the batter, but if it's too thick to mix, add a little more batter from the pan. Drop the chocolate mixture by equal spoonfuls across the batter in the pan, and use a knife to zigzag through the chocolate, to marble the batter. Bake for 25 to 30 minutes, testing for doneness with a knife. If the knife comes out clean, it's done. Remove from the oven and allow to completely cool before serving, at least 1 hour.

Per Serving: Calories: 239; Fat: 20g; Protein: 6g; Total Carbs: 26g; Fiber: 6.5g; Net Carbs: 3.5g; **Macros:** Fat: 75%; Protein: 10%; Carbs: 6%

90-Second Lava Cake

SERVES 1 | PREP TIME: 5 minutes | COOK TIME: 1 to 2 minutes

1 ounce unsweetened dark chocolate (100 percent cocoa), roughly chopped

1 tablespoon butter

1 tablespoon heavy (whipping) cream

¼ teaspoon vanilla extract

2 tablespoons unsweetened cocoa powder

1 to 2 teaspoons monk fruit extract or sugar-free sweetener

¼ teaspoon ground cinnamon

⅛ teaspoon salt

Unsweetened whipped cream, for serving (optional)

In a microwave-safe mug or tall ramekin, combine the chocolate, butter, cream, and vanilla and microwave for 20 to 30 seconds. Remove and whisk to blend well. Whisk in the cocoa powder, sweetener, cinnamon, and salt until smooth. Microwave on high for 60 to 90 seconds, until set on top. Serve warm, directly out of the mug or invert the ramekin onto a plate and top with whipped cream (if using).

Per Serving: Calories: 352; Fat: 34g; Protein: 7g; Total Carbs: 15g; Fiber: 4g; Net Carbs: 11g; **Macros:** Fat: 87%; Protein: 8%; Carbs: 5%

Strawberry Shortcakes

MAKES 12 SHORTCAKES | PREP TIME: 15 minutes, plus marinating time | COOK TIME: 25 to 30 minutes, plus 30 minutes to cool

For the shortcakes

¼ cup (½ stick) unsalted butter, at room temperature, plus more to grease the pan

¾ cup coconut flour

1 teaspoon baking powder

¼ teaspoon sea salt

¾ cup granulated erythritol–monk fruit blend

4 ounces (about ½ cup) cream cheese, at room temperature

1 teaspoon pure vanilla extract

4 large eggs, at room temperature

¼ cup sour cream

For the strawberry topping

1 pint fresh strawberries, sliced

2 tablespoons granulated erythritol–monk fruit blend

½ teaspoon freshly squeezed lemon juice

⅛ teaspoon sea salt

For the whipped cream

1 cup heavy (whipping) cream, divided

1 tablespoon cream cheese, at room temperature

2 tablespoons granulated erythritol–monk fruit blend	1 teaspoon pure vanilla extract

Preheat the oven to 350°F. Generously grease a 12-cup muffin pan with butter. In a medium bowl, combine the coconut flour, baking powder, and salt. In a large bowl, using an electric mixer, beat the sweetener, cream cheese, butter, and vanilla until light and fluffy. Add the eggs one at a time, mixing after each addition. Make sure to scrape down the bowl several times. Slowly add the dry ingredients to the wet ingredients while mixing on low speed. When fully combined, gently fold in the sour cream, do not overmix. Evenly pour the batter into the muffin pan, overfilling each cup just slightly. Bake for 25 to 30 minutes, or until lightly browned on top and a toothpick inserted into the center comes out clean. Allow the shortcakes to cool in the pan for about 10 minutes before removing them. Place them on a wire rack to cool fully, for about 20 minutes. In a large bowl, combine the sliced strawberries, sweetener, lemon juice, and salt. Allow the strawberries to sit at room temperature to macerate for 15 to 30 minutes. This will cause the berries to produce their own sauce. Chill a large glass or metal bowl in the refrigerator. Using an electric mixer on high speed, beat about ¼ cup of heavy cream with the cream cheese until well combined. Add the remaining ¾ cup of heavy cream, the sweetener, and vanilla. Beat on high speed with the electric mixer until soft peaks form and hold their shape. Cut each shortcake in half. Place the bottom half of the shortcake on a plate, and spoon on 1 tablespoon of the strawberry topping and 1 tablespoon of the whipped cream. Top with the other half of the shortcake, another tablespoon of whipped cream, and another tablespoon of the strawberry topping.

Per Serving: Calories: 216; Fat: 18g; Protein: 5g; Total Carbs: 9g; Fiber: 4g; Net Carbs: 5g; **Macros:** Fat: 75%; Protein: 9%; Carbs: 16%

Butter Cake with Cream Cheese Buttercream

MAKES 16 SLICES | PREP TIME: 20 minutes, plus 1 hour to chill | COOK TIME: 35 minutes

For the cake

1¼ cups (2½ sticks) butter, room temperature or softened, plus more for greasing	1 teaspoon vanilla extract
	4 cups almond flour
6 large eggs	1 cup confectioners' erythritol blend
¾ cup buttermilk	
⅔ cup water	3 teaspoons baking powder

For the icing

16 ounces (2 bricks) cream cheese, room temperature	1⅓ cups confectioners' erythritol blend
1 cup butter, room temperature	2 tablespoons water
	½ teaspoon vanilla extract

Preheat the oven to 325°F, and lightly grease two (8-inch) round cake pans. Line the bottoms with two circles of parchment paper. In a large bowl, use a stand or hand mixer to cream the butter until fluffy. Add the eggs, buttermilk, water, and vanilla, and mix. In a medium bowl, sift the almond flour, sweetener, and baking powder. Slowly add the dry mixture to the wet mixture, and mix for 2 minutes on slow to medium speed. Pour the batter into the pans and bake for 35 to 40 minutes, rotating

the pans halfway through. The cake will seem jiggly, but if the knife comes out clean, it's done. Allow the cakes to cool completely in the pans. Once cool, run a knife along the edge of each pan. Wrap the cooled cakes in plastic wrap, and refrigerate for 30 minutes or longer. With a stand or hand mixer, combine the cream cheese and butter, and beat until fluffy. Add the sweetener, water, and vanilla, and beat on high for 1 minute. Transfer the cake to a flat plate or cake board. Using an icing spatula or knife, spread a ¼-inch layer of icing evenly across the top of the top with the second layer of cake and spread a very thin layer of icing over the top and sides. Refrigerate for 30 minutes, and then spread another coating of icing over the cake. Slice into 16 slices and serve.

Per Serving: (1 slice): Calories: 502; Fat: 50g; Protein: 10g; Total Carbs: 24g; Fiber: 3g; Net Carbs: 3.5g; **Macros:** Fat: 90%; Protein: 8%; Carbs: 3%

Chocolate Mug Cake

SERVES 1 | PREP TIME: 8½ minutes | COOK TIME: 1½ minutes

Cooking spray	1 tablespoon heavy (whipping) cream
2 tablespoons cocoa powder	
2 tablespoons stevia, or other sugar substitute	½ teaspoon pure vanilla extract
Pinch salt	1 large egg, beaten
	¼ teaspoon baking powder

Spray the inside of a microwaveable mug with cooking spray. In a medium bowl, mix the cocoa powder, stevia, and salt. Add the heavy cream, vanilla, and the beaten egg. Mix to combine. Add the baking powder and mix again until there are no air bubbles. Transfer the batter to the prepared mug. Microwave on high for 1 minute, 20 seconds. Remove the cake from the microwave. Allow it to settle for 1 minute before inverting onto a plate to serve.

Per Serving: Calories: 146; Fat: 11g; Protein: 8g; Total Carbs: 8g; Fiber: 3; Net Carbs: 5g; **Macros:** Fat: 62%; Protein: 19%; Carbs: 19%

Summer Squash Mock Apple Crumble

SERVES 8 | PREP TIME: 10 minutes | COOK TIME: 1 hour, 5 minutes

For the filling

½ cup (1 stick) butter	½ teaspoon ground ginger
⅓ cup powdered erythritol	6 cups yellow summer squash, cut into ½-inch pieces
¼ cup lemon juice	
1½ teaspoons ground cinnamon	2 teaspoons vanilla extract
	Zest of 1 lemon
1 teaspoon ground nutmeg	

For the crumble

1¼ cups almond flour	½ teaspoon ground nutmeg
⅓ cup walnuts, chopped	5 tablespoons plus 1 teaspoon butter, melted
⅓ cup golden erythritol	
1 teaspoon ground cinnamon	

In a large saucepan over medium heat, melt the butter and add the erythritol, lemon juice, cinnamon, nutmeg, and ginger. Whisk to combine well and melt the sweetener. Add the squash. Simmer on medium-low heat for 35 minutes, stirring occasionally. Remove the pot from the heat and stir in the vanilla and lemon zest. Set aside. Preheat the oven to 350°F. Butter a 9-inch-square baking dish. In a large bowl, combine the almond flour, walnuts, erythritol, cinnamon, and nutmeg. Pour in the melted butter and stir well. Pour the squash mixture into the buttered baking dish. Evenly spread the crumb topping over the squash. Gently press down to lightly pack the crumb topping. Bake for 30 minutes or until the top is lightly golden brown. Allow to cool before serving.

Per Serving: Calories: 286; Fat: 28g; Protein: 4g; Total Carbs: 7g; Fiber: 3g; Net Carbs: 4g; **Macros:** Fat: 86%; Protein: 5%; Carbs: 9%

Jicama "Apple" Pie Filling

SERVES 4 | PREP TIME: 35 minutes | COOK TIME: 1 hour

1 tablespoon coconut oil
1½ cups cubed jicama
½ tablespoon ground cinnamon
½ teaspoon ground nutmeg
¼ teaspoon allspice
2 tablespoons erythritol

1½ teaspoons apple extract flavoring
½ cup sugar-free maple syrup, divided
1 cup, plus 2 tablespoons water, divided

In a large saucepan over medium-high heat, melt the coconut oil. Add the jicama and cook, stirring occasionally, for 10 minutes. Add the cinnamon, nutmeg, allspice, erythritol, apple extract, ¼ cup of syrup, and ½ cup plus 1 tablespoon of water. Stir until completely combined. Bring the mixture to a gentle boil; then reduce the heat to medium-low and simmer for 25 minutes, stirring occasionally. The mixture will thicken and become sticky, but the jicama will still be crisp. Stir in the remaining ¼ cup of syrup and ½ cup plus 1 tablespoon of water. Continue to simmer, stirring occasionally, for 20 minutes longer or until the jicama is fork-tender. Remove from the heat and let sit for 20 minutes. The sauce will be the texture of a thick but pourable caramel, and the jicama will be tender but still have a crunch.

Per Serving: (¼ recipe): Calories: 65; Fat: 4g; Protein: 0g; Total Carbs: 15g; Fiber: 7g; Net Carbs: 2g; **Macros:** Fat: 49%; Protein: <1%; Carbs: 51%

Strawberry Cream Pie

SERVES 8 | PREP TIME: 20 minutes | COOK TIME: 36 minutes, plus 5 hours to chill

For the crust

Nonstick cooking spray
4½ tablespoons butter
1½ cups almond flour

2 tablespoons monk fruit/ erythritol blend sweetener
Pinch kosher salt

For the filling

¼ cup water, divided
1½ teaspoons gelatin
1½ cups sliced fresh strawberries
3 tablespoons monk fruit/ erythritol blend sweetener
1 teaspoon balsamic vinegar
8 ounces cream cheese, at room temperature
¼ cup sour cream

3 tablespoons powdered monk fruit/erythritol blend sweetener
1 teaspoon vanilla extract
1 cup heavy (whipping) cream, whipped, plus more for garnish
Whole fresh strawberries, for garnish

Preheat the oven to 350°F. Lightly coat a 9-inch pie plate with cooking spray. Set aside. In a small skillet over medium-low heat, melt the butter and cook it for about 10 minutes, stirring often, until browned and nutty. The solids in the butter should be the color of caramel. Remove from heat and set aside to cool slightly. In a medium bowl, stir the almond flour, sweetener, salt, and browned butter to combine. Press the mixture firmly into the bottom and up the sides of the pie plate. Bake for 12 to 14 minutes, or until the edges are golden. Set aside to cool. Place 2 tablespoons of water in a small bowl and sprinkle the gelatin on top. Let sit for 5 minutes. In a medium saucepan over medium heat, combine the strawberries, remaining 2 tablespoons of water, 3 tablespoons of the sweetener, and vinegar. Bring to a boil, using a masher to break up the strawberries. Turn the heat to medium-low and simmer the strawberries for 10 to 12 minutes, or until thick. Remove from heat and stir in the gelatin mixture until fully dissolved. Set aside to cool to room temperature. In a medium bowl and using an electric hand mixer, beat the cream cheese, sour cream, sweetener, and vanilla until smooth. Stir in the strawberry mixture until well combined. Gently fold in the whipped cream. Spoon the filling into the prepared crust, cover with plastic wrap, and refrigerate for 3 to 5 hours. Garnish as desired with whipped cream and strawberries.

Per Serving: Calories: 371; Fat: 35g; Protein: 7g; Total Carbs: 7g; Fiber: 2g; Net Carbs: 5g; **Macros:** Fat: 85%; Protein: 8%

Apple Pie Bites

MAKES 12 BITES | PREP TIME: 15 minutes | COOK TIME: 25 minutes

For the crust

Oil or nonstick cooking spray, for greasing
¾ cup grated mozzarella cheese

1 ounce (2 tablespoons) cream cheese
3 tablespoons coconut flour
1 tablespoon granulated erythritol blend

For the filling

1 small jicama, peeled and chopped into ¼-inch cubes (about 2 cups)
3 tablespoons butter
2 tablespoons water

3 tablespoons brown erythritol blend
1 teaspoon cinnamon
1 teaspoon apple pie spice
½ teaspoon vanilla extract

Preheat the oven to 300°F, and grease a mini muffin pan. In a small microwave-safe bowl, slowly melt the mozzarella cheese and cream cheese in 20-second increments until the mozzarella is smooth. Remove from the microwave, and stir. Add the flour and sweetener to the cheese mixture, using your hands to work into a dough, and divide into 12 sections. Roll a section into a ball, mash it flat in the palm of your hand, and push into a hole in the muffin pan so that it fills the bottom and sides to make a shell. Repeat with remaining dough. Bake for 8 to 10 minutes, or until golden brown, and then remove from the oven and set aside to cool. In a small saucepan over medium heat, add the chopped jicama, butter, water, sweetener, cinnamon, apple pie spice, and vanilla. Cook for 8 to 10 minutes, stirring often, until the jicama softens. Remove the shells from the pan. Using a small spoon, fill each shell with the jicama filling, and serve.

Per Serving: (1 bite): Calories: 83; Fat: 7g; Protein: 2g; Total Carbs: 8g; Fiber: 2.5g; Net Carbs: 1.5g; **Macros:** Fat: 76%; Protein: 10%; Carbs: 7%

Keto-Friendly Key Lime Pie

SERVES 6 | PREP TIME: 10 minutes, plus 4 hours to chill | COOK TIME: 15 minutes

Nonstick cooking spray

2 tablespoons coconut oil, melted

1 cup almond flour

3 tablespoons coconut flour, divided

1 large egg

⅛ teaspoon salt

2 (14-ounce) cans coconut cream

⅓ cup freshly squeezed lime juice

Zest of 2 limes

2 cups heavy (whipping) cream, whipped with 2 teaspoons erythritol

Preheat the oven to 350°F. Spray a 9-inch pie plate with cooking spray. In the bowl of a food processor or a high-speed blender, combine the coconut oil, the almond flour, 1 tablespoon of the coconut flour, egg, and salt. Pulse until crumbly. Pour the mixture into the pie plate and use a fork to press the crust down evenly. Bake for about 12 minutes, then set aside to cool for 10 minutes. While the crust is cooling, in a medium bowl, use a hand mixer to mix the remaining coconut flour, the coconut cream, lime juice, and lime zest for 1 to 2 minutes. Pour the filling into the cooled crust and cover with plastic wrap. Refrigerate for at least 4 hours to set. Remove, slice, and serve topped with the whipped cream.

Per Serving: (1 slice); Calories: 814; Fat: 83g; Protein: 10g; Total Carbs: 17g; Fiber: 6g; Net Carbs: 11g; **Macros:** Fat: 87%; Protein: 4%; Carbs: 9%

"Buttermilk" Custard Pie Bars

SERVES 12 | PREP TIME: 20 minutes | COOK TIME: 45 minutes | CHILL TIME: 3 hours

For the crust

Nonstick cooking spray

1½ cups almond flour

2 tablespoons monk fruit/ erythritol blend sweetener

⅛ teaspoon ground nutmeg

Pinch kosher salt

¼ cup butter, melted

For the filling

1½ cups heavy (whipping) cream

1½ teaspoon white vinegar

6 large eggs

⅓ cup allulose blend sweetener

¼ cup coconut flour

¼ cup sour cream

¼ cup butter, melted

2 teaspoons vanilla extract

¼ teaspoon ground nutmeg

Pinch kosher salt

Preheat the oven to 350°F. Coat a 9-inch-square pan with cooking spray and line it with parchment paper. Set aside. In a medium bowl, stir the almond flour, sweetener, nutmeg, salt, and melted butter until incorporated and crumbly. Pour the crust mixture into the prepared pan and evenly press into the bottom. Bake for 8 to 10 minutes until golden brown around the edges. Set aside. Lower the oven temperature to 325°F. In a small bowl, whisk the heavy cream and vinegar. Let sit for 5 minutes. In a large bowl, whisk the eggs, sweetener, coconut

flour, sour cream, melted butter, vanilla, nutmeg, salt, and heavy cream mixture. Pour the filling over the crust. Bake for 30 to 35 minutes, or until set. If needed, place a piece of aluminum foil over the top of the bars to prevent over-browning. Let the bars cool at room temperature. Refrigerate for at least 3 hours before cutting. To serve, lift the bars from the pan using the parchment paper and place on a cutting board. Cut into 12 bars.

Per Serving: Calories: 282; Fat: 26g; Protein: 6g; Total Carbs: 6g; Fiber: 3g; Net Carbs: 3g; **Macros:** Fat: 83%; Protein: 9%; Carbs: 8%

Blackberry Cobbler

SERVES 9 | PREP TIME: 15 minutes | COOK TIME: 30 minutes

Nonstick cooking spray

1½ cups almond flour

¼ cup plus 2 tablespoons coconut flour

½ cup plus 1 tablespoon monk fruit/erythritol blend sweetener, divided

1 tablespoon baking powder

½ teaspoon kosher salt

3 large eggs, beaten

¾ cup unsweetened almond milk

2 tablespoons sour cream

1 teaspoon vanilla extract

½ cup (1 stick) butter, melted

1 cup fresh blackberries

¼ teaspoon ground cinnamon

Fresh whipped cream, for serving

Preheat the oven to 350°F. Coat a 9-inch square pan with cooking spray. Set aside. In a medium bowl, stir the almond and coconut flours, ½ cup of sweetener, the baking powder, and salt. Whisk in the eggs, almond milk, sour cream, and vanilla. Continue whisking until the batter is smooth. Stir in the melted butter until fully incorporated. Pour the batter into the prepared pan. Evenly sprinkle the blackberries over the batter and push them down slightly. In a small bowl, stir the remaining 1 tablespoon of sweetener and the cinnamon. Evenly sprinkle the cinnamon mixture over the top of the cobbler. Bake for 25 to 30 minutes, or until the top is golden brown. Let cool for 30 minutes before serving with fresh whipped cream.

Per Serving: Calories: 243; Fat: 19g; Protein: 6g; Total Carbs: 12g; Fiber: 6g; Net Carbs: 6g; **Macros:** Fat: 70%; Protein: 10%; Carbs: 20%

Fluffy Peanut Butter Pie

SERVES 8 | PREP TIME: 15 minutes | COOK TIME: 12 minutes | CHILL TIME: 3 hours

1½ cups almond flour

3 tablespoons monk fruit/ erythritol blend sweetener

2 tablespoons cocoa powder

¼ cup butter, melted

8 ounces cream cheese, at room temperature

½ cup creamy peanut butter

⅓ cup powdered monk fruit/ erythritol blend (confectioners' sugar style)

1 cup plus 2 tablespoons heavy (whipping) cream, divided

1 teaspoon vanilla extract

Pinch kosher salt

Fresh whipped cream, for serving (optional)

Sugar-free chocolate shavings, for garnish (optional)

Preheat the oven to 350°F. In a medium bowl, stir the almond flour, sweetener, cocoa powder, and melted butter to combine.

Press the mixture firmly into the bottom and up the sides of a 9-inch pie plate. Bake for 10 to 12 minutes. Set aside to cool. In a large bowl and using an electric hand mixer, combine the cream cheese, peanut butter, sweetener, 2 tablespoons of heavy cream, the vanilla, and salt. Beat at medium speed until smooth. In a medium bowl, beat the remaining 1 cup of heavy cream at medium speed until firm peaks form. Gently fold the whipped cream into the cream cheese mixture. Spoon the filling into the prepared crust. Chill for at least 3 hours before serving. Garnish with whipped cream (if using) and chocolate shavings (if using).

Per Serving: Calories: 450; Fat: 42g; Protein: 10g; Total Carbs: 8g; Fiber: 3g; Net Carbs: 5g; **Macros:** Fat: 84%; Protein: 9%; Carbs: 7%

Fresh Berry Tart

SERVES 6 | PREP TIME: 20 minutes, plus time to chill

½ cup chopped pecans
½ cup almond flour
¼ cup coconut oil

¼ teaspoon ground cinnamon
4 cups sliced strawberries

Place the pecans, almond flour, coconut oil, and cinnamon in a blender and pulse until the mixture holds together and is well mixed. Press the nut mixture into an 8-inch pie plate and chill until firm. Fill the crust with fresh berries and serve immediately.

Per Serving: Calories: 234; Fat: 21g; Protein: 4g; Total Carbs: 11g; Fiber: 5g; Net Carbs: 6g; **Macros:** Fat: 76%; Protein: 6%; Carbs: 18%; Fat: 81%; Protein: 7%; Carbs: 13%

Lemon Curd Tartlets

SERVES 5 | PREP TIME: 15 minutes | COOK TIME: 35 minutes, plus 35 minutes to cool | CHILL TIME: 20 minutes

To make the curd

¼ cup (½ stick) unsalted butter, at room temperature
7 large egg yolks
¾ cup granulated erythritol–monk fruit blend

1 tablespoon grated lemon zest
¾ cup freshly squeezed lemon juice (about 3 large lemons)
½ teaspoon lemon extract
¼ teaspoon sea salt

For the crust

¼ cup (½ stick) unsalted butter, melted, plus more for greasing
1½ cups almond flour, sifted

¼ cup granulated erythritol–monk fruit blend
2 tablespoons freshly squeezed lemon juice
¼ teaspoon sea salt

For the mousse

6 tablespoons cold water
2 teaspoons unflavored gelatin
16 ounces cream cheese
1 cup sour cream

1 cup granulated erythritol–monk fruit blend
½ teaspoon lemon extract
½ teaspoon grated lemon zest
¼ teaspoon sea salt
1 cup heavy (whipping) cream

In the small saucepan, bring 1 inch of water to a boil over medium-high heat. Set the glass mixing bowl over the saucepan (without touching the water). Add the butter to the bowl. Once melted, add the egg yolks, one at a time, whisking quickly. Add

the sweetener, lemon zest, lemon juice, lemon extract, and salt. Whisk constantly while cooking for 7 to 10 minutes, until the mixture thickens. Remove from the heat and allow the curd to fully cool at room temperature, about 15 minutes. Preheat the oven to 350°F. Grease the tart pans with butter. In a small bowl, combine the almond flour, sweetener, lemon juice, and salt. Add the melted butter and combine well. Spread the mixture evenly among the tart pans and press into their bottoms and sides. Bake for 10 to 15 minutes, until lightly browned, and cool for 15 to 20 minutes. In another small bowl, mix the cold water and gelatin and set aside. In the large bowl, using an electric mixer on high, beat the cream cheese, sour cream, sweetener, softened gelatin, lemon extract, lemon zest, and salt until fully combined. Slowly add the heavy cream. Refrigerate until all parts are chilled, about 20 minutes. Assemble the tarts by spreading the mousse mixture in the tart shells and topping with the curd. Refrigerate the assembled tarts for 15 minutes. To unmold, put one tart pan on an upturned small glass on the counter and gently slide the ring from the bottom of the tart pan down the glass. Lift the tart off and carefully slide it off the bottom of the pan and onto a serving plate. Repeat with the remaining tart pans and serve.

Per Serving: Calories: 980; Fat: 97g; Protein: 18g; Total Carbs: 16g; Fiber: 4g; Net Carbs: 12g; **Macros:** Fat: 86%; Protein: 8%; Carbs: 6%

Chocolate Mousse Pie Cups

SERVES 6 | PREP TIME: 10 minutes, plus 1 hour 30 minutes to set

¾ cup coconut flour
2 flax "eggs"
½ cup coconut oil
4 avocados, peeled, pitted, and chopped

¼ cup cacao powder
3 tablespoons monk fruit sweetener
Sea salt

Fill the cups of a muffin tin with cupcake liners. In a large mixing bowl, combine the coconut flour, flax "eggs," and coconut oil. Mix thoroughly until you have a workable dough. Scoop the dough a tablespoon at a time into the bottom of the cupcake liners, pressing it firmly to create a crust. Place the muffin tin in the refrigerator for 1 hour to allow the crusts to firm up while you create the pie filling. In a large mixing bowl, combine the avocados, cacao powder, and monk fruit sweetener. Whip with a hand mixer on high until the mixture is well blended and airy. Remove the muffin tin from refrigerator and divide the chocolate mousse mixture equally onto the prepared pie crusts. Place the tin back in the refrigerator to set for 20 to 30 minutes before serving.

Per Serving: Calories: 439; Fat: 39g; Protein: 6g; Total Carbs: 24g; Fiber: 16g; Net Carbs: 8g

Pumpkin Pie

SERVES 8 | PREP TIME: 20 minutes | COOK TIME: 1 hour, plus 1 hour to cool in the oven

For the dough

¾ cup coconut flour
¼ cup ground pecans
2 tablespoons granulated erythritol blend

⅛ teaspoon salt
6 tablespoons melted butter

For the filling

3 large eggs

1 (15-ounce) can 100 percent pure pumpkin, unsweetened

1 cup confectioners' erythritol blend

1 cup heavy (whipping) cream

1 teaspoon pumpkin pie spice

¼ teaspoon freshly ground black pepper

1 teaspoon vanilla extract

For the sugar-free whipped cream

1 cup heavy (whipping) cream

1 tablespoon confectioners' erythritol blend

½ teaspoon vanilla extract

Preheat the oven to 350°F. Stir the flour, ground pecans, sweetener, salt, and butter. Mash the mixture evenly into a pie pan, pressing up the sides. Bake for 10 to 12 minutes, until golden brown. If the edges get too brown, cover with aluminum foil. In a medium bowl, whisk the eggs and then add the pumpkin, sweetener, cream, pumpkin pie spice, pepper, and vanilla, mixing until incorporated. Pour into the pie pan, cover the outer edges of the crust with foil, and bake for 50 minutes. After baking, turn off the oven, prop open the oven door, and allow the pie to cool in the oven for about an hour. In a medium bowl, combine the cream, sweetener, and vanilla, and beat on high for 1½ minutes, or until peaks form. Refrigerate the pie and cream until time to serve. Slice pie into 8 slices, top each one with a dollop of cream, and serve.

Per Serving: Calories: 391; Fat: 36g; Protein: 6g; Total Carbs: 31.5g; Fiber: 6g; Net Carbs: 6.5g; Macros: Fat: 83%; Protein: 6%; Carbs: 7%

Pumpkin Pie

SERVES 8 | PREP TIME: 20 minutes | COOK TIME: 1 hour, plus 1 hour to cool in the oven

For the dough

¾ cup coconut flour

¼ cup ground pecans

2 tablespoons granulated erythritol blend

⅛ teaspoon salt

6 tablespoons melted butter

For the filling

3 large eggs

1 (15-ounce) can 100 percent pure pumpkin, unsweetened

1 cup confectioners' erythritol blend

1 cup heavy (whipping) cream

1 teaspoon pumpkin pie spice

¼ teaspoon freshly ground black pepper

1 teaspoon vanilla extract

For the sugar-free whipped cream

1 cup heavy (whipping) cream

1 tablespoon confectioners' erythritol blend

½ teaspoon vanilla extract

Preheat the oven to 350°F. Stir the flour, ground pecans, sweetener, salt, and butter. Mash the mixture evenly into a pie pan, pressing up the sides. Bake for 10 to 12 minutes, until golden brown. If the edges get too brown, cover with aluminum foil. In a medium bowl, whisk the eggs and then add the pumpkin, sweetener, cream, pumpkin pie spice, pepper, and vanilla, mixing until incorporated. Pour into the pie pan, cover the outer edges of the crust with foil, and bake for 50 minutes. After baking, turn off the oven, prop open the oven door, and allow the pie to cool

in the oven for about an hour. In a medium bowl, combine the cream, sweetener, and vanilla, and beat on high for 1½ minutes, or until peaks form. Refrigerate the pie and cream until time to serve. Slice pie into 8 slices, top each one with a dollop of cream, and serve.

Per Serving: Calories: 391; Fat: 36g; Protein: 6g; Total Carbs: 31.5g; Fiber: 6g; Net Carbs: 6.5g; Macros: Fat: 83%; Protein: 6%; Carbs: 7%

Raspberry Cream Cheese Tart Bars

SERVES 20 | PREP TIME: 10 minutes, plus 1 hour to chill | COOK TIME: 10 minutes

For the cookie crust

2 cups almond flour

¾ cup confectioners' erythritol blend, sifted

½ teaspoon salt

½ teaspoon baking powder

½ cup (1 stick) cold butter, grated or cubed

For the filling

16 ounces (2 bricks) cream cheese, room temperature, cubed

½ cup (1 stick) butter, room temperature, cubed

¼ cup confectioners' erythritol blend, sifted

1 teaspoon vanilla extract

5 tablespoons sugar-free raspberry jam

20 raspberries, for decoration

Preheat the oven to 350°F, and line a 9-by-13-inch pan with parchment paper so it sticks out over the top on at least two sides. Stir the almond flour, confectioners' sweetener, salt, and baking powder. Add the butter, and with your fingers, work the ingredients together until completely incorporated. Transfer the dough into the pan, and distribute evenly, until completely covers the bottom of the pan. Bake for 10 to 14 minutes, or until golden brown on top, rotating the pan halfway through. In a large bowl, combine the cream cheese, butter, confectioners' sweetener, and vanilla. Using a mixer, whip on high for 2 minutes until completely smooth. Place the jam in a microwave-safe dish, and microwave for about 20 seconds. Pour the jam into the cream cheese mixture, and fold together just until it has a marbled look. When the crust has cooled, spoon the cream cheese mixture on top, and spread evenly. Cover and refrigerate for at least an hour. Remove from the refrigerator, and use the overhanging parchment paper to lift the tart out of the pan and onto the counter. Cut the tart into 20 bars, top each one with a raspberry, and place on a tray to serve.

Per Serving: (1 bar): Calories: 220; Fat: 22g; Protein: 4g; Total Carbs: 10.5g; Fiber: 2g; Net Carbs: 2.5g; Macros: Fat: 90%; Protein: 7%; Carbs: 5%

Cinnamon Pecan "Apple" Crisp

SERVES 12 | PREP TIME: 20 minutes | COOK TIME: 1 hour 20 minutes, plus 20 minutes to cool

For the filling

2 tablespoons unsalted butter, chilled and sliced, plus more for greasing

4 chayote squash

¾ cup granulated erythritol–monk fruit blend; less sweet: ½ cup

½ cup freshly squeezed lemon juice

| 2 tablespoons ground cinnamon | ½ teaspoon cream of tartar |
| ½ teaspoon ground ginger | ¼ teaspoon ground nutmeg |

For the topping

1½ cups almond flour, sifted	¼ cup (½ stick) unsalted butter, chilled and sliced
½ cup coconut flour	½ cup pecan halves
3 tablespoons granulated erythritol–monk fruit blend	2 tablespoons ground cinnamon
1 teaspoon baking powder	2 large eggs, at room temperature
¼ teaspoon sea salt	

To make the filling: Preheat the oven to 350°F. Grease baking pan with butter and set aside. In the medium saucepan, cover the chayote squash with water and boil for 25 to 30 minutes. They should be firm but cooked through. Allow the squash to cool, 15 to 20 minutes, then peel and cut into ¼-inch-thick slices. In a medium bowl, combine the squash, sweetener, lemon juice, cinnamon, ginger, cream of tartar, and nutmeg. Combine well. Add the filling to the prepared pan and dot with the sliced butter. In another medium bowl, combine the almond flour, coconut flour, sweetener, baking powder, and salt. Add the butter and mix until crumbly and resembling coarse cornmeal. Stir in the pecans and cinnamon. Add the eggs and combine well, but do not overmix. Spoon the topping over the filling in the baking pan, being sure to break up larger pieces, and distribute evenly. Bake for 35 to 40 minutes, until hot and bubbling. Cut into 12 pieces and serve warm or cold.

Per Serving: Calories: 206; Fat: 18g; Protein: 6g; Total Carbs: 10g; Fiber: 5g; Net Carbs: 5g; **Macros:** Fat: 74%; Protein: 9%; Carbs: 17%

Mixed Berry Crisp

SERVES 12 | PREP TIME: 20 minutes | COOK TIME: 40 minutes

For the topping

½ cup (1 stick) unsalted butter, chilled and sliced, plus more for greasing	½ cup granulated erythritol–monk fruit blend; less sweet: ¼ cup
2 cups almond flour	1 teaspoon baking powder
	¼ teaspoon sea salt
	1 large egg, lightly beaten

For the filling

1 cup sliced fresh or frozen strawberries	¼ cup granulated erythritol–monk fruit blend; less sweet: 3 tablespoons
½ cup fresh or frozen blueberries	¼ teaspoon xanthan gum
½ cup fresh or frozen raspberries	

Preheat the oven to 350°F. Grease a baking pan with butter and set aside. In the large bowl, combine the almond flour, sweetener, baking powder, and salt and mix well. Mix in the butter with a fork until the pieces are pea-size. Mix in the egg until well combined. Press half the topping into the baking pan. In the medium bowl, mix the berries, sweetener, and xanthan gum. Spread the fruit in the pan and cover with the remaining topping. Bake for 40 minutes,

until the top is golden brown. Serve warm or cold. Refrigerate in an airtight container for up to 5 days.

Per Serving: Calories: 176; Fat: 16g; Protein: 4g; Total Carbs: 6g; Fiber: 3g; Net Carbs: 3g; **Macros:** Fat: 78%; Protein: 9%; Carbs: 13%

Blueberry Crumble

SERVES 15 | PREP TIME: 10 minutes | COOK TIME: 40 minutes, plus 20 minutes to cool

For the topping

3½ cups almond flour	1 cup (2 sticks) unsalted butter, chilled and sliced, plus more for greasing
1 cup granulated erythritol–monk fruit blend	
1½ teaspoons baking powder	1 large egg, lightly beaten
½ teaspoon sea salt	

For the filling

| 4 cups blueberries | 3 tablespoons freshly squeezed lemon juice |
| ½ cup granulated erythritol–monk fruit blend | ½ teaspoon xanthan gum |

In the large bowl, combine the almond flour, sweetener, baking powder, and salt. Add the butter and use a fork to mix until the pieces are pea-size. Add the beaten egg and continue to mix until well combined. Set aside. Preheat the oven to 350°F. Grease a baking dish with butter and set aside. In the medium bowl, mix the blueberries, sweetener, lemon juice, and xanthan gum. Spoon the blueberry mixture into the baking sheet and cover with the topping. Bake for 40 minutes, until the top is golden brown. Allow the crumble to cool slightly, 15 to 20 minutes, then cut into 15 pieces and serve.

Per Serving: Calories: 265; Fat: 24g; Protein: 6g; Total Carbs: 11g; Fiber: 4g; Net Carbs: 7g; **Macros:** Fat: 77%; Protein: 9%; Carbs: 14%

Strawberry Rhubarb Cobbler

SERVES 15 | PREP TIME: 15 minutes | COOK TIME: 40 minutes, plus 10 minutes to cool

For the topping

1 cup (2 sticks) unsalted butter, chilled and sliced, plus more for greasing	1 cup granulated erythritol–monk fruit blend
3½ cups almond flour	1½ teaspoons baking powder
	½ teaspoon sea salt
	1 large egg, lightly beaten

For the filling

| 3 cups sliced fresh or frozen strawberries | ½ cup granulated erythritol–monk fruit blend |
| 2 cups sliced fresh or frozen rhubarb | ½ teaspoon xanthan gum |

Preheat the oven to 350°F. Grease a baking dish with butter and set aside. In the large bowl, combine the almond flour, sweetener, baking powder, and salt. Add the butter and use a fork to mix until the pieces are pea-size. Add the beaten egg and continue to mix until well combined. Divide the topping and press half of it into the bottom of the baking dish. In the medium bowl, mix the strawberries, rhubarb, sweetener, and xanthan gum. Spoon this mixture on top of the crumb base in the baking sheet, spreading it evenly. Top with the other half of the crumb mixture. Bake for 40 minutes, until the top is golden brown. Allow to cool slightly, 5 to 10 minutes, before serving.

Per Serving: Calories: 256; Fat: 24g; Protein: 6g; Total Carbs: 8g; Fiber: 4g; Net Carbs: 4g; **Macros:** Fat: 80%; Protein: 8%; Carbs: 12%

Chocolate Whoopie Pies

SERVES 9 | PREP TIME: 10 minutes | COOK TIME: 10 minutes

For the cookies

½ cup butter, room temperature

1 cup confectioners' erythritol blend

¼ cup buttermilk

2 large eggs

½ teaspoon vanilla extract

1¼ cups almond flour

¼ cup whey protein isolate, unflavored

2 teaspoons baking powder

¼ teaspoon freshly ground black pepper

⅛ teaspoon salt

For the cream

2 cup confectioner's erythritol blend

¼ cup unsweetened cocoa powder

¼ cup (½ stick) butter, room temperature

4 ounces (½ brick) cream cheese

½ teaspoon vanilla extract

8 teaspoons boiling water

Preheat the oven to 350°F, and line a baking sheet with parchment paper. In a medium bowl with a stand or hand mixer, cream the butter, and then mix in the sweetener, buttermilk, eggs, and vanilla. In a small bowl, sift the almond flour, whey protein, baking powder, pepper, and salt. Add to the wet mixture, and mix until incorporated. Using a cookie scoop, scoop the dough and place on the baking sheet to make 18 cookies. Bake for 9 to 10 minutes, and don't overbake. Remove and set aside to cool. In a small bowl, stir the confectioners' sweetener and cocoa powder, and set aside. In a medium bowl, use a stand or hand mixer to cream together the butter, cream cheese, and vanilla. Add the cocoa mixture along with the boiling water, and mix slowly at first and then on high for 1 minute, until completely incorporated. Add the cream mixture to a piping bag or gallon resealable bag with the corner cut off. Flip 9 of the cookies over, pipe the cream evenly on each one, top each one with an additional cookie, and serve. If you don't want to pipe the cream on, use a knife or spoon to put a dollop in the center and press another cookie on top.

Per Serving: (1 whoopie pie): Calories: 306; Fat: 28g; Protein: 11g; Total Carbs: 45g; Fiber: 2.5g; Net Carbs: 2.5g; **Macros:** Fat: 82%; Protein: 14%; Carbs: 3%

Maddie's Favorite Chocolate Malt

SERVES 1 | PREP TIME: 10 minutes

1⅓ cups unsweetened almond milk

½ small avocado, peeled and pitted (about 2 tablespoons)

1 tablespoon unsweetened cocoa powder

3 or 4 ice cubes

3 to 4 teaspoons powdered monk fruit/erythritol blend sweetener

1 teaspoon maca powder, preferably gelatinized

⅛ teaspoon pink Himalayan salt

In a blender, combine the almond milk, avocado, cocoa powder, sweetener, maca powder, salt, and ice. Blend on high speed for 10 to 20 seconds, or until smooth. Pour in a glass and enjoy.

Per Serving: Calories: 260; Fat: 20g; Protein: 7g; Total Carbs: 13g; Fiber: 10g; Net Carbs: 3g; **Macros:** Fat: 70%; Protein: 11%; Carbs: 19%

Chocolate Mousse

SERVES 4 | PREP TIME: 10 minutes

3 ounces dark chocolate, 85 percent cacao

4 large eggs, separated

Pinch sea salt

1 teaspoon vanilla extract

½ cup heavy (whipping) cream

1 teaspoon liquid stevia

½ cup raspberries (optional)

In a heavy-bottomed saucepan over low heat, or in a double boiler over a pot of barely simmering water, heat the chocolate for about 5 minutes until melted. Set aside to cool. In a medium bowl, combine the egg whites and salt. Beat the eggs until stiff peaks form, about 3 minutes. Set aside. In a separate bowl, beat the heavy cream and stevia until thick, about 3 minutes. Stir the egg yolks and vanilla into the cooled, melted chocolate. Add a generous spoonful of the whipped egg whites and whipped cream to the chocolate, and mix well. Transfer the chocolate mixture and the whipped cream to the bowl with the egg whites and fold gently until combined. Divide the mousse among the serving cups. Top with raspberries, if desired.

Per Serving: Calories: 288; Fat: 26g; Protein: 9g; Total Carbs: 6g; Fiber: 1g; Net Carbs: 5g; **Macros:** Fat: 81%; Protein: 12%; Carbs: 7%

Peanut Butter Mousse

SERVES 4 | PREP TIME: 10 minutes, plus 30 minutes to chill

1 cup heavy (whipping) cream

¼ cup natural peanut butter

1 teaspoon alcohol-free pure vanilla extract

4 drops liquid stevia

In a medium bowl, beat the heavy cream, peanut butter, vanilla, and stevia until firm peaks form, about 5 minutes. Spoon the mousse into 4 bowls and place in the refrigerator to chill for 30 minutes. Serve.

Per Serving: Calories: 280; Fat: 28g; Protein: 6g; Total Carbs: 4g; Fiber: 1g; Net Carbs: 3g; **Macros:** Fat: 83%; Protein: 10%; Carbs: 7%

Pecan Pie Pudding

SERVES 1 | PREP TIME: 5 minutes

¾ cup plain Greek yogurt

½ scoop low-carb vanilla protein powder

¼ cup chopped pecans

2 tablespoons sugar-free syrup

In a small bowl, mix the Greek yogurt and protein powder until smooth and creamy. Top with the chopped pecans and syrup.

Per Serving: Calories: 381; Fat: 21g; Protein: 32g; Total Carbs: 16g; Fiber: 7g; Net Carbs: 9g; **Macros:** Fat: 50%; Protein: 34%; Carbs: 16%

Bread Pudding

SERVES 6 | PREP TIME: 10 minutes | COOK TIME: 45 minutes

4 slices low-carb bread cut into ½-inch cubes

Cooking spray

¾ cup canned coconut milk

¾ cup unsweetened vanilla almond milk

¼ cup melted butter

3 large eggs

¼ cup granular erythritol

1 tablespoon brown sugar substitute

1 teaspoon vanilla extract

½ teaspoon ground cinnamon

Preheat the oven to 375°F. Spray an 8-inch-square baking dish with cooking spray. Add the cubes to the prepared dish and set aside. In a medium saucepan over medium heat, combine the coconut milk and almond milk. Raise the heat to medium high, and just as the mixture begins to bubble, reduce the heat to medium-low. Whisk the butter into the milk until thoroughly incorporated. Slowly pour the liquid on top of the bread. Gently stir to coat. In a medium bowl, beat the eggs, erythritol, and brown sugar substitute. Beat in the vanilla and cinnamon. Keep beating until the eggs look foamy and the sweetener dissolves a bit, about 1 minute. Pour the eggs over the soaked bread cubes. Bake until set, 25 to 30 minutes. It is done when it no longer jiggles. Cool slightly before serving. Refrigerate for up to 2 days. The bread will become mushy, so it is best to reheat in a frying pan.

Per Serving: (⅙ recipe): Calories: 365; Fat: 34g; Protein: 11g; Total Carbs: 16g; Fiber: 2g; Net Carbs: 4g; Macros: Fat: 84%; Protein: 12%; Carbs: 4%

Banana Pudding

MAKES 2 CUPS | PREP TIME: 25 minutes, plus 2 hours to chill | COOK TIME: 10 minutes

1 (¼-ounce) envelope unfla-vored gelatin

½ cup water

1 cup canned coconut milk or heavy (whipping) cream

½ cup granular erythritol

1 teaspoon banana extract

In a small bowl, whisk the gelatin and water until the gelatin dissolves. Set aside. Heat the coconut milk in a medium saucepan over medium-low heat. Whisk until the milk is smooth. In a blender or food processor, pulse the erythritol a few times until it becomes powdered. Whisk it into the coconut milk and continue to cook, whisking constantly, until the milk thickens and the sweetener dissolves, about 16 minutes. Remove from the heat and very slowly add the gelatin, whisking constantly. Return the pan to medium-low heat. Whisk in the banana extract until thoroughly combined. Pour the pudding mixture into a container and cover it with plastic wrap. Make sure the plastic wrap touches the surface of the pudding to prevent film from forming. Refrigerate for at least 2 hours, preferably overnight, until set. Serve.

Per Serving: (½ cup): Calories: 108; Fat: 11g; Protein: 2g; Total Carbs: 27g; Fiber: 1g; Net Carbs: 2g; Macros: Fat: 81%; Protein: 8%; Carbs: 11%

Mexican Chocolate Pudding

SERVES 4 | PREP TIME: 10 minutes, plus 30 minutes to chill

2 ripe avocados, halved and pitted

¼ cup unsweetened cocoa powder

¼ cup canned coconut milk, plus more if needed

2 teaspoons vanilla extract

2 teaspoons monk fruit extract

1 teaspoon ground cinnamon

¼ teaspoon ground cayenne pepper

¼ teaspoon salt

Using a spoon, scoop the avocado into a blender. Add the cocoa, coconut milk, vanilla, monk fruit extract, cinnamon, cayenne, and salt, and blend well until smooth and creamy. If the mixture is too thick, add additional coconut milk, 1 tablespoon at a time, until the desired consistency is reached. Cover and refrigerate at least 30 minutes before serving.

Per Serving: Calories: 159; Fat: 14g; Protein: 3g; Total Carbs: 12g; Fiber: 7g; Net Carbs: 5g; Macros: Fat: 79%; Protein: 8%; Carbs: 13%

Almond Butter and Jelly Chia Pudding

SERVES 4 | PREP TIME: 10 minutes, plus 6 hours chilling time

1 cup unsweetened almond milk

2 tablespoons unsweetened almond butter

½ cup fresh or frozen raspberries

1 teaspoon vanilla extract

1 to 2 teaspoons monk fruit extract (optional)

½ cup chia seeds

In a blender combine the almond milk, almond butter, raspberries, vanilla, and monk fruit extract (if using) and blend until smooth. Transfer the mixture to a medium bowl and add the chia seeds, whisking well to combine. Divide the mixture between ramekins. Cover and refrigerate at least 6 hours, preferably overnight. Serve cold.

Per Serving: (½ cup): Calories: 188; Fat: 12g; Protein: 6g; Total Carbs: 14g; Fiber: 12g; Net Carbs: 2g; Macros: Fat: 57%; Protein: 13%; Carbs: 30%

Rice Pudding

SERVES 3 | PREP TIME: 20 minutes, plus 2 hours to chil | COOK TIME: 20 minutes

1 (14.5-ounce) can coconut milk

1½ tablespoons erythritol

2 cups water

Pinch sea salt

1 (8-ounce) package miracle rice

1 teaspoon vanilla extract

1½ teaspoons ground cinnamon

Pour the coconut milk into a small saucepan over medium-high heat and bring to a slow boil, whisking occasionally. Once the coconut milk begins to bubble, add the erythritol and whisk until it dissolves. Reduce the heat and simmer, whisking occasionally, for 7 to 10 minutes until the mixture thickens. When it is thick enough to cling to the back of a spoon, pour it into a bowl. Refrigerate for at least 1 hour. Meanwhile, drain and rinse the miracle rice. Bring the water and salt to a boil and add the rice. Boil for 2 minutes; then drain and rinse again under cold water. Add the rice to the thickened coconut milk mixture. Stir in the vanilla and cinnamon. Refrigerate for another hour or overnight before serving.

Per Serving: (⅓ recipe): Calories: 248; Fat: 24g; Protein: 2g; Total Carbs: 17g; Fiber: 4g; Net Carbs: 7g; Macros: Fat: 87%; Protein: 3%; Carbs: 10%

Chocolate Avocado Pudding

SERVES 1 | PREP TIME: 5 minutes

1 avocado, halved

⅓ cup coconut milk

1 teaspoon vanilla extract

2 tablespoons unsweetened cocoa powder

5 or 6 drops liquid stevia

Combine all the ingredients in a high-powered blender or food processor and blend until smooth. Serve immediately.

Per Serving: Calories: 555; Fat: 47g; Protein: 7g; Total Carbs: 26g; Fiber: 17g; Net Carbs: 9g; **Macros:** Fat: 76%; Protein: 5%; Carbs: 19%

Chocolate-Chia Pudding

SERVES 4 | PREP TIME: 10 minutes, plus 6 hours to soak

1 cup canned coconut milk

1 cup unsweetened almond milk

¼ cup chia seeds

¼ cup cocoa powder

2 tablespoons egg white protein powder

½ teaspoon stevia, or more

1 teaspoon pure vanilla extract

In a large bowl, stir the coconut milk, almond milk, chia seeds, cocoa powder, egg white protein powder, stevia, and vanilla until well blended. Refrigerate for at least 6 hours to soak. Adjust the sweetness as desired, and serve.

Per Serving: Calories: 226; Fat: 18g; Protein: 6g; Total Carbs: 10g; Fiber: 6g; Net Carbs: 4g; **Macros:** Fat: 72%; Protein: 10%; Carbs: 18%

Snickerdoodle Pudding

SERVES 1 | PREP TIME: 3 minutes

¼ cup vanilla protein powder

½ avocado, pitted and peeled

¼ cup sugar-free cinnamon maple syrup

1 teaspoon vanilla extract

½ tablespoon ground cinnamon

1 tablespoon collagen

1 tablespoon coconut or almond flour (optional)

1 tablespoon erythritol (optional)

In a blender or food processor, combine the protein powder, avocado, maple syrup, vanilla, cinnamon, collagen, flour (if using), and erythritol (if using), and blend until smooth.

Per Serving: Calories: 268; Fat: 16g; Protein: 20g; Total Carbs: 7g; Fiber: 5g; Net Carbs: 6g; **Macros:** Fat: 54%; Protein: 30%; Carbs: 16%

Whipped Cream-Chocolate Pudding Parfaits

MAKES 4 PARFAITS | PREP TIME: 20 minutes

1 avocado, peeled and pitted

¼ cup cocoa powder

¼ cup egg white protein powder

¼ cup water

¾ teaspoon stevia, divided

¼ teaspoon ground cinnamon

Pinch sea salt

1½ cups heavy (whipping) cream

In a blender, blend the avocado, cocoa powder, egg white protein powder, water, ½ teaspoon of the stevia, cinnamon, and salt until the pudding is smooth and thick, adding more water as needed to adjust the texture. Set aside. In a large bowl, whisk the heavy cream and the remaining ¼ teaspoon stevia until firm peaks form, about 5 minutes. Set up 4 parfait or regular glasses. Spoon 1 tablespoon of chocolate pudding into each of the glasses, and top each with 2 tablespoons of whipped cream. Repeat the layering until all the pudding is used up, and you end with whipped cream on the top.

Per Serving: (1 parfait): Calories: 280; Fat: 24g; Protein: 7g; Total Carbs: 9g; Fiber: 5g; Net Carbs: 4g; **Macros:** Fat: 77%; Protein: 10%; Carbs: 13%

Cookies and Cream Parfait

SERVES 1 | PREP TIME: 5 minutes

½ scoop low-carb vanilla protein powder

¾ cup plain Greek yogurt

1 Oreo cookie

¼ cup sugar-free chocolate syrup (I like Walden Farms)

In a small bowl, mix the protein powder and Greek yogurt until smooth and creamy. Remove one side of the Oreo cookie. Place it in a small resealable plastic bag and crush it with the back of a spoon. Set aside. Pour the chocolate syrup over the yogurt mixture and sprinkle with the cookie crumbles.

Per Serving: (1 parfait) Calories: 281; Fat: 13g; Protein: 19g; Total Carbs: 22g; Fiber: 3g; Net Carbs: 19g; **Macros:** Fat: 42%; Protein: 27%; Carbs: 31%

Creamy Panna Cotta

SERVES 4 | PREP TIME: 20 minutes, plus 8 hours to chill

1 tablespoon butter, softened, plus more for greasing

½ (7g) gelatin package

½ cup warm water

6 ounces cream cheese, softened

½ teaspoon pure vanilla extract

¼ teaspoon stevia

Lightly grease 4 muffin cups with butter, and set aside. In a small bowl, sprinkle the gelatin over the water, and set aside. In a medium bowl, beat the cream cheese and butter until very smooth. Beat in the gelatin mixture, vanilla, and stevia until smooth. Spoon the panna cotta mixture into the muffin cups, and refrigerate for about 8 hours to set. Run a knife around the edges of the cups, and flip the muffin tray over to remove the panna cottas. Flip them over, and serve.

Per Serving: Calories: 194; Fat: 18g; Protein: 6g; Total Carbs: 2g; Fiber: 0g; Net Carbs: 2g; **Macros:** Fat: 84%; Protein: 12%; Carbs: 4%

Double Coconut Panna Cotta

SERVES 4 | PREP TIME: 20 minutes, plus 4 hours to chill | COOK TIME: 20 minutes

2¼ teaspoons unflavored powdered gelatin

¼ cup cold water

3 cups canned coconut milk

1 tablespoon Swerve

2 teaspoons vanilla extract

½ cup shredded unsweetened coconut

In a small bowl, sprinkle the gelatin into the water and let stand for 10 to 15 minutes to soften. Then stir until dissolved. In a large saucepan, heat the coconut milk, Swerve, and vanilla over medium heat until scalded but not boiling. Remove the coconut milk mixture from the heat and whisk in the gelatin. Pour the mixture into 4 serving dishes and refrigerate until set, 3 to 4 hours. Preheat the oven to 325°F. Spread the shredded coconut on a baking sheet in a thin layer and bake until toasted and golden, stirring a few times, 5 to 10 minutes. Cool the coconut completely. Serve the panna cotta topped with toasted coconut.

Per Serving: Calories: 340; Fat: 32g; Protein: 7g; Total Carbs: 9g; Fiber: 2g; Net Carbs: 7g; **Macros:** Fat: 81%; Protein: 9%; Carbs: 10%

Vanilla Panna Cotta

SERVES 3 | **PREP TIME:** 5 minutes, plus 4 hours to chill | **COOK TIME:** 10 minutes

1 (14 ounce) can coconut milk
Pinch of salt
4 teaspoons raw honey, divided
½ teaspoon gluten-free vanilla extract
1 tablespoon beef gelatin powder

In a medium sauce pan, heat the coconut milk, salt, and 3 teaspoons of honey over medium heat for 5 minutes or until the honey is dissolved. Turn off the heat and stir in the vanilla and gelatin. Grease three ramekins with coconut oil. Pour the mixture evenly into the ramekins. Refrigerate for 4 hours or until mixture has set firmly. Dip the ramekins in warm water for 10 seconds to loosen the panna cotta from the dish. Place a plate upside down on top of the ramekin, then flip it over. The panna cotta should come out onto the plate. Drizzle each panna cotta with 1 teaspoon of honey.

Per Serving: Calories: 237; Fat: 21g; Protein: 4g; Total Carbs: 8g; Fiber: 0g; Net Carbs: 8g; **Macros:** Fat: 79%; Protein: 8%; Carbs: 13%

Strawberry Panna Cotta

SERVES 4 | **PREP TIME:** 10 minutes, plus 6 hours to chill | **COOK TIME:** 10 minutes

2 tablespoons warm water
2 teaspoons gelatin powder
2 cups heavy (whipping) cream
1 cup sliced strawberries, plus more for garnish
1 to 2 tablespoons sugar-free sweetener of choice (optional)
1½ teaspoons pure vanilla extract
4 to 6 fresh mint leaves, for garnish (optional)

Pour the warm water into a small bowl. Sprinkle the gelatin over the water and stir well to dissolve. Allow the mixture to sit for 10 minutes. In a blender, combine the cream, strawberries, sweetener (if using), and vanilla. Blend until the mixture is smooth and the strawberries are puréed. Transfer the mixture to a medium saucepan and heat over medium-low heat until just below a simmer. Remove from the heat and cool for 5 minutes. Whisking constantly, add in the gelatin mixture until smooth. Divide the custard between ramekins or small glass bowls, cover and refrigerate until set, 4 to 6 hours. Serve chilled, garnishing with additional sliced strawberries or mint leaves (if using).

Per Serving: Calories: 431; Fat: 44g; Protein: 4g; Total Carbs: 7g; Fiber: 1g; Net Carbs: 6g; **Macros:** Fat: 90%; Protein: 4%; Carbs: 6%

Crustless Cannoli

SERVES 4 | **PREP TIME:** 5 minutes

2 cups whole-milk ricotta cheese
1 teaspoon liquid stevia
1 teaspoon ground cinnamon
¼ teaspoon allspice
¼ teaspoon lemon zest
⅓ cup heavy (whipping) cream
1 ounce grated dark chocolate

In a medium bowl, stir the ricotta, stevia, cinnamon, allspice, and lemon zest. In a separate bowl, beat the heavy cream until thick and fluffy. Fold the heavy cream and grated chocolate into the ricotta mixture. Divide the mixture among the serving cups.

Per Serving: Calories: 268; Fat: 23g; Protein: 12g; Total Carbs: 5g; Fiber: 0g; Net Carbs: 5g; **Macros:** Fat: 77%; Protein: 18%; Carbs: 5%

"Frosty" Chocolate Shake

SERVES 2 | **PREP TIME:** 10 minutes, plus 30 minutes to chill

1 cup heavy (whipping) cream or coconut cream
2 tablespoons unsweetened cocoa powder
1 tablespoon almond butter
1 teaspoon vanilla extract
5 or 6 drops liquid stevia

In a medium bowl or using a stand mixer, beat the cream until fluffy, 3 to 4 minutes. Add the cocoa powder, almond butter, vanilla, and stevia. Beat the mixture for an additional 2 to 3 minutes, or until the mixture has the consistency of whipped cream. Place the bowl in the freezer for 25 to 30 minutes before serving.

Per Serving: Calories: 493; Fat: 49g; Protein: 5g; Total Carbs: 8g; Fiber: 3g; Net Carbs: 5g; **Macros:** Fat: 89%; Protein: 4%; Carbs: 7%

Blueberry Cream Cheese Bites

MAKES 16 BITES | **PREP TIME:** 15 minutes, plus 1 hour to freeze

¼ cup butter
¼ cup cream cheese
¼ cup coconut oil
¼ cup heavy (whipping) cream
¼ cup blueberries, finely chopped
1 teaspoon pure vanilla extract

In a medium microwaveable bowl, combine the butter, cream cheese, and coconut oil. Microwave on high in short 10-second intervals until the mixture begins to melt. Once melted, add the heavy cream and blueberries. Transfer the mixture to a blender. Pulse to blend in the blueberries. Add the vanilla and pulse to combine. Pour the mixture evenly into an ice cube tray. Freeze for at least 1 hour to solidify, preferably overnight.

Per Serving: (1 bite): Calories: 82; Fat: 9g; Protein: 0g; Total Carbs: 1g; Fiber: 0g; Net Carbs: 1g; **Macros:** Fat: 95%; Protein: 0%; Carbs: 5%

Macadamia Lime Bites

MAKES 16 BITES | **PREP TIME:** 5 minutes, plus 30 minutes to freeze

⅓ cup coconut oil, melted, plus more for greasing
1 cup macadamia nuts, raw or dry roasted
¼ cup unsweetened coconut milk
3 tablespoons freshly squeezed lime juice
1 teaspoon lime zest
1 teaspoon vanilla extract
½ teaspoon stevia or 4 drops liquid stevia extract
1 tablespoon coconut flour

Grease an ice cube tray with coconut oil. Combine all the ingredients in a food processor, and process until well combined. The mixture should have the consistency of a thick and creamy nut butter. Transfer the mixture to the ice cube tray, and place it in the freezer for at least 30 minutes or until the cubes are solid and firm. Transfer the bites to a sealed container, and store them in the freezer.

Per Serving: (1 bite): Calories: 111; Fat: 11g; Protein: 1g; Total Carbs: 2g; Fiber: 1g; Net Carbs: 1g; **Macros:** Fat: 89%; Protein: 3%; Carbs: 8%;

Lemon-Blueberry Ice Cream

SERVES 8 | PREP TIME: 10 minutes, plus 6 hours chilling time | COOK TIME: 25 minutes

1 cup fresh or frozen blueberries (if frozen, allow to thaw)

Juice and zest of 1 lemon

1 to 2 teaspoons monk
fruit extract

2 large egg yolks

⅓ cup powdered sugar-free
sweetener

2 cups heavy
(whipping) cream

1 teaspoon vanilla extract

Freeze the bowl of an ice cream maker for at least 12 hours, or overnight. In a medium bowl, combine the blueberries, lemon juice and zest, and monk fruit extract and mash well with the back of a fork. Alternatively, blend using an immersion blender for a smoother texture. In a large bowl, whisk the sweetener and egg yolks. In a small saucepan, heat the cream over medium heat, until just below a boil. Remove from the heat and allow to cool slightly. Slowly pour the warm cream into the egg yolk mixture, whisking constantly to avoid cooking the eggs. Return the eggs and cream to the saucepan over low heat. Whisking constantly, cook for 15 to 20 minutes, until thickened. Remove from the heat and whisk in blueberry mixture and vanilla. Transfer to a glass bowl and cool to room temperature. Cover and refrigerate for at least 6 hours. Freeze the custard in an ice cream maker according to the manufacturer's directions.

Per Serving: (½ cup): Calories: 229; Fat: 23g; Protein: 3g; Total Carbs: 15g; Fiber: 1g; Net Carbs: 14g; Macros: Fat: 90%; Protein: 5%; Carbs: 5%

Olive Oil Ice Cream

SERVES 8 | PREP TIME: 5 minutes, plus freezing time | COOK TIME: 25 minutes

4 large egg yolks

⅓ cup powdered sugar-free
sweetener (such as stevia or
monk fruit extract)

2 cups half-and-half

1 teaspoon vanilla extract

⅛ teaspoon salt

¼ cup extra-virgin olive oil

Freeze the bowl of an ice cream maker for at least 12 hours or overnight. In a large bowl, whisk the egg yolks and sugar-free sweetener. In a small saucepan, heat the half-and-half over medium heat until just below a boil. Remove from the heat and allow to cool slightly. Slowly pour the warm half-and-half into the egg mixture, whisking constantly. Return the eggs and cream to the saucepan over low heat. Whisking constantly, cook over low heat until thickened, 15 to 20 minutes. Remove from the heat and stir in the vanilla extract and salt. Whisk in the olive oil and transfer to a glass bowl. Allow to cool, cover, and refrigerate for at least 6 hours. Freeze custard in an ice cream maker according to the manufacturer's directions.

Per Serving: Calories: 292; Fat: 31g; Protein: 3g; Total Carbs: 2g; Fiber: 0g; Net Carbs: 2g; Macros: Fat: 94%; Protein: 4%; Carbs: 2%

Matcha Ice Cream

SERVES 8 | PREP TIME: 5 minutes, plus 6 hours freezing time | COOK TIME: 25 minutes

1 tablespoon matcha green
tea powder

⅛ teaspoon freshly ground
black pepper

4 large egg yolks

⅓ cup powdered sugar-free
sweetener (such as stevia or
monk fruit)

2 cups half and half (or 1 cup
heavy (whipping) cream and
1 cup whole milk)

1 teaspoon vanilla extract

¼ cup olive oil

Freeze the bowl of an ice cream maker for at least 12 hours, or overnight. In a small bowl, combine matcha powder, ginger, and pepper. Set aside. In a large bowl, whisk the egg yolks and sweetener. In a small saucepan, heat the half and half over medium heat until just below a boil. Remove from heat and allow to cool slightly. Slowly pour the warm half and half into the egg yolk mixture, whisking constantly to avoid cooking the eggs. Return the eggs and cream to the saucepan over low heat. Whisking constantly, cook for 15 to 20 minutes over low, until thickened. Remove from heat and whisk in the vanilla and matcha powder mixture. Whisking, stream in the olive oil until smooth and well combined. Transfer to a glass bowl and allow to cool to room temperature. Cover and refrigerate for at least 6 hours. Freeze the custard in an ice cream maker according to the manufacturer's directions.

Per Serving: (½ cup): Calories: 170; Fat: 16g; Protein: 4g; Total Carbs: 13g; Fiber: 0g; Net Carbs: 13g; Macros: Fat: 85%; Protein: 9%; Carbs: 6%

Rich Vanilla Ice Cream

SERVES 16 | PREP TIME: 5 minutes, plus 4 hours to chill | COOK TIME: 10 minutes

2 cups heavy
(whipping) cream

2 cups whole milk

4 large egg yolks

Pinch sea salt

1 tablespoon vanilla extract

1 teaspoon liquid stevia

In a saucepan over low heat, whisk the cream, milk, egg yolks, and salt until the eggs are thoroughly incorporated. Cook, stirring often until the mixture thickens and coats the back of a spoon, about 10 minutes, being careful not to heat over 150°F. Stir in the vanilla extract and stevia, adding more stevia to taste, if desired. Pour this mixture through a strainer into a separate dish and cover with parchment paper or plastic wrap to prevent skin from forming on the surface. Refrigerate until thoroughly chilled, about 4 hours. Transfer the mixture to an ice cream maker and freeze according to the manufacturer's instructions.

Per Serving: (½ cup): Calories: 135; Fat: 13g; Protein: 2g; Total Carbs: 2g; Fiber: 0g; Net Carbs: 2g; Macros: Fat: 88%; Protein: 6%; Carbs: 6%

Raspberry Maple Soft Serve

SERVES 2 | PREP TIME: 5 minutes, plus chilling

1 cup coconut cream, refrigerated overnight

1 cup frozen raspberries

1 teaspoon pure maple syrup

Place the coconut cream, raspberries, and maple syrup in a blender. Process until smooth and creamy. Scoop into a bowl and serve immediately if you like a soft serve texture. Alternatively if you prefer a harder ice cream texture, you can place the blended mixture into a sealed container and freeze for an hour. Stir the mixture halfway to remove any hard or frozen sections.

Per Serving: Calories: 241; Fat: 21g; Protein: 3g; Total Carbs: 10g; Fiber: 4g; Net Carbs: 6g; **Macros:** Fat: 78%; Protein: 5%; Carbs: 17%

Banana Pudding Ice Cream

SERVES 8 (MAKES 1 QUART ICE CREAM) |
PREP TIME: 15 minutes | COOK TIME: 25 minutes |
CHILL TIME: 12+ hours

For the ice cream base

1¼ cups unsweetened almond milk

1¾ cups heavy (whipping) cream, divided

¼ cup plus 2 tablespoons allulose blend sweetener, divided

Pinch kosher salt

5 large egg yolks

3 ounces cream cheese, at room temperature

1 teaspoon vanilla extract

½ teaspoon natural banana extract

For the shortbread crumble

¼ cup butter, at room temperature

2 tablespoons monk fruit/erythritol blend sweetener

1 tablespoon cream cheese, at room temperature

½ cup almond flour

1½ tablespoons coconut flour

1 teaspoon vanilla extract

Make the ice cream base. In a medium saucepan over medium-low heat, stir the almond milk, ¾ cup of heavy cream, ¼ cup of sweetener, and salt. Bring to a simmer. In a small bowl and using an electric hand mixer, beat the egg yolks with the remaining 2 tablespoons of sweetener until pale, light, and fluffy. While mixing, slowly stream about half the hot milk mixture into the eggs. Pour the egg mixture into the saucepan and cook over medium-low heat for 2 to 3 minutes. Remove the pan from the heat and whisk in the cream cheese, vanilla, and banana extract. Transfer to a container and refrigerate for 2 to 3 hours until cool. Preheat the oven to 325°F. In a medium bowl and using an electric hand mixer, cream the butter, sweetener, and cream cheese until light and fluffy. Add the almond and coconut flours and vanilla. Mix well to combine. Wrap the dough in plastic wrap and refrigerate for 30 minutes to 1 hour, or until firm. Place the dough between two pieces of parchment paper and press it out to about ¼ inch thick. Transfer the dough onto the sheet pan and remove the top piece of parchment. Bake for 10 to 12 minutes until golden brown around the edges and slightly puffed. Remove the sheet pan from the oven and break up the shortbread using a fork to create a crumble. Bake for 3 to 5 minutes, or until golden. Let cool completely on the sheet pan. Pour the ice cream mixture into the freezer container of an electric ice cream maker and freeze according to the manufacturer's instructions. Once the ice cream is the consistency of soft serve, layer it into a 1-quart freezer-safe container starting with the ice cream and sprinkling some crumble between each layer. Reserve any leftover crumble for garnish. Cover and freeze for at least 8 hours, or until firm.

Per Serving: Calories: 355; Fat: 35g; Protein: 5g; Total Carbs: 5g; Fiber: 2g; Net Carbs: 3g; **Macros:** Fat: 89%; Protein: 6%; Carbs: 5%

Mexican Chocolate Pudding

SERVES 4 | PREP TIME: 10 minutes, plus 30 minutes to chill

2 ripe avocados, halved and pitted

¼ cup unsweetened cocoa powder

¼ cup canned coconut milk, plus more if needed

2 teaspoons vanilla extract

2 teaspoons monk fruit extract

1 teaspoon ground cinnamon

¼ teaspoon ground cayenne pepper

¼ teaspoon salt

Using a spoon, scoop the avocado into a blender. Add the cocoa, coconut milk, vanilla, monk fruit extract, cinnamon, cayenne, and salt, and blend well until smooth and creamy. If the mixture is too thick, add additional coconut milk, 1 tablespoon at a time, until the desired consistency is reached. Cover and refrigerate at least 30 minutes before serving.

Per Serving: Calories: 159; Fat: 14g; Protein: 3g; Total Carbs: 12g; Fiber: 7g; Net Carbs: 5g; **Macros:** Fat: 79%; Protein: 8%; Carbs: 13%

Buttercream Pudding "Fluff"

SERVES 10 | PREP TIME: 10 minutes

2½ (8-ounce) bricks cream cheese, at room temperature

½ cup (1 stick) butter

1 tablespoon cinnamon

1 teaspoon vanilla extract

1 squirt liquid stevia

½ cup chopped pecans

2 tablespoons sugar-free brown sugar

Using a hand mixer, whip the cream cheese, butter, cinnamon, vanilla, and liquid stevia. Gently fold in the chopped pecans and brown sugar until just incorporated. Pour the mixture into a casserole or baking dish, or divide into 10 small serving bowls.

Per Serving: (⅓ cup): Calories: 329; Fat: 33g; Protein: 5g; Total Carbs: 3g; Fiber: 1g; Net Carbs: 2g; **Macros:** Fat: 90%; Protein: 6%; Carbs: 4%

French Vanilla Ice Cream with Hot Fudge

SERVES 2 | PREP TIME: 10 minutes, plus 3½ to 4 hours to freeze

1¼ cups heavy (whipping) cream, divided

¼ cup unsweetened almond milk

½ cup Swerve sweetener, divided

1½ teaspoons vanilla extract, divided

2 ounces unsweetened chocolate, chopped

Place a 9-by-5-inch loaf pan in the freezer to chill for about 20 minutes. In a medium bowl, combine ¾ cup of cream, the almond milk, ¼ cup of Swerve, and ½ teaspoon of vanilla. Mix with a handheld electric mixer for 2 minutes, or until the sweetener has dissolved. Pour the ice-cream mixture into the chilled loaf pan. Place the pan in the freezer. Every half hour, remove the pan, scrape down the sides, and whisk the mixture for about 1 minute. While the ice cream is in the freezer, combine the remaining ½ cup of cream, remaining ¼ cup of Swerve, and the chocolate in a double boiler over medium-low heat. Stir just until the chocolate melts, and then remove the mixture from the heat. Stir in the remaining 1 teaspoon of vanilla. After 3½ to 4 hours, the ice cream will be thick enough to eat. Scrape down the sides for the last time and scoop out to serve. Pour the warm sauce over the ice cream.

Per Serving: Calories: 719; Fat: 71g; Protein: 7g; Total Carbs: 13g; Fiber: 5g; Net Carbs: 8g; **Macros:** Fat: 89%; Protein: 4%; Carbs: 7%

Strawberry Avocado Ice Cream

SERVES 6 | PREP TIME: 10 minutes, plus 6 hours to freeze

3 cups halved strawberries

1 ripe avocado, chopped

½ cup heavy (whipping) cream

½ cup plain Greek yogurt

2 teaspoons Swerve

½ teaspoon vanilla extract

¼ teaspoon ground nutmeg

Place the strawberries, avocado, cream, yogurt, Swerve, vanilla, and nutmeg in a food processor or blender and purée until smooth. If you want very smooth ice cream, pass the mixture through a fine sieve to remove the seeds. Pour the mixture into a 9-by-13-inch metal baking dish and freeze it solid, about 6 hours. Just before serving, transfer the frozen mixture to a blender or food processor and pulse until it resembles soft ice cream. Only transfer the amount you wish to serve because you can only do this process once. Serve immediately after blending.

Per Serving: Calories: 166; Fat: 13g; Protein: 2g; Total Carbs: 12g; Fiber: 4g; Net Carbs: 8g; **Macros:** Fat: 70%; Protein: 5%; Carbs: 25%

Raspberry Ice Cream

SERVES 2 | PREP TIME: 10 minutes, plus 4 to 6 hours to chill

12 raspberries

1½ cups heavy (whipping) cream

1 cup cream cheese, at room temperature

¼ cup erythritol

2 tablespoons freshly squeezed lemon juice

In a blender, combine the raspberries and cream. Blend until pureed. Transfer to a glass bowl and stir in the cream cheese, erythritol, and lemon juice. Freeze for 4 to 6 hours until frozen but scoopable.

Per serving: Calories: 1022; Fat: 105g; Protein: 12g; Total Carbs: 38g; Fiber: 1g; Net Carbs: 13g; **Macros:** Fat: 92%; Protein: 5%; Carbs: 3%

Lavender Ice Cream

SERVES 4 | PREP TIME: 5 minutes, plus 5 hours to freeze

2 (14-ounce) cans coconut cream

¾ cup monk fruit sweetener

½ cup raw cashews, soaked in water overnight

¼ cup coconut oil, melted

3 tablespoons dried lavender

1 teaspoon vanilla extract

1 teaspoon almond extract

Sea salt

Combine all the ingredients in a high-powered blender and blend on high for 5 minutes until the mixture grows in volume by about one-third and becomes fluffy. Pour the mixture into a freezer-safe pan and freeze for 2 hours. Remove the mixture from the freezer and break it into chunks. Transfer the mixture to a food processor and blend until a soft-serve consistency is achieved. Spoon the ice cream into a freezer-safe pan and place back in the freezer to set for 3 hours before serving.

Per Serving: Calories: 571; Fat: 60g; Protein: 3g; Total Carbs: 10g; Fiber: 1g; Net Carbs: 9g; **Macros:** Fat: 91%; Protein: 2%; Carbs: 7%

Chocolate Coconut Milk Ice Cream

SERVES 1 | PREP TIME: 5 minutes, plus 20 to 30 minutes to chill

½ cup coconut milk

1 tablespoon heavy (whipping) cream

1 tablespoon unsweetened cocoa powder

In a large bowl, whisk the coconut milk, heavy cream, and cocoa powder for 2 minutes, until it thickens and forms stiff peaks. Transfer the mixture to a freezer-safe container. Freeze for 20 to 30 minutes, until set to your desired consistency.

Per Serving: Calories: 340; Fat: 35g; Protein: 4g; Total Carbs: 10g; Fiber: 4g; Net Carbs: 6g; **Macros:** Fat: 85%; Protein: 4%; Carbs: 11%

Mixed Berry Sherbet

SERVES 6 | PREP TIME: 15 minutes, plus 6 hours to freeze

3 cups berries (strawberries, raspberries, blueberries, and blackberries)

2 cups canned coconut milk

6 ounces firm tofu

1 tablespoon Swerve

1 tablespoon chopped fresh thyme

Place the berries, coconut milk, tofu, Swerve, and thyme in a food processor or blender and process until smooth. Press the mixture through a fine sieve to remove the seeds. Pour the mixture into a 9-by-13-inch metal baking dish. Place the baking dish in the freezer for 3 hours. Stir the partially frozen mixture, scraping the sides, then return the container to the freezer. Scrape the sides and bottom with a fork or spoon every hour until it starts to freeze solid, about 6 hours. When you are ready to serve, use a fork to scrape until the mixture is the texture of snow.

Per Serving: Calories: 289; Fat: 23g; Protein: 6g; Total Carbs: 15g; Fiber: 4g; Net Carbs: 11g; **Macros:** Fat: 72%; Protein: 8%; Carbs: 20%

Strawberries and Cream Ice Pops

MAKES 12 | PREP TIME: 10 minutes | CHILL TIME: 4 hours

2 cups heavy (whipping) cream

8 ounces cream cheese, at room temperature

¼ cup sour cream

1 tablespoon freshly squeezed lemon juice

1½ cups sliced strawberries, divided

1 cup blueberries, divided

¾ cup granulated erythritol–monk fruit blend; less sweet: ½ cup

In a blender, combine the heavy cream, cream cheese, sour cream, and lemon juice and blend until smooth. Add 1 cup of strawberries, ½ cup of blueberries, and sweetener and blend until fully combined and smooth. Spoon the remaining berries into each popsicle mold, then pour the cream mixture into each mold. Add the popsicle sticks. Freeze for 3 to 4 hours, until frozen solid. Serve immediately after unmolding.

Per Serving: (1 pop): Calories: 225; Fat: 22g; Protein: 2g; Total Carbs: 6g; Fiber: 1g; Net Carbs: 5g; **Macros:** Fat: 87%; Protein: 4%; Carbs: 9%

Sour Cream Ice Cream

SERVES 4 | PREP TIME: 10 minutes, plus time to freeze

1 cup sour cream

1 cup unsweetened almond milk

3 tablespoons egg white protein powder

2 tablespoons freshly squeezed lemon juice

½ teaspoon stevia

½ teaspoon pure vanilla extract

In a blender, blend the sour cream, almond milk, egg white protein powder, lemon juice, stevia, and vanilla until smooth.

Transfer the mixture to an ice cream maker, and freeze according to the manufacturer's directions. Serve.

Per Serving: Calories: 149; Fat: 13g; Protein: 5g; Total Carbs: 3g; Fiber: 0g; Net Carbs: 3g; **Macros:** Fat: 79%; Protein: 13%; Carbs: 8%

Strawberry Frozen Yogurt

MAKES 3 CUPS | PREP TIME: 10 minutes, plus time to freeze

1 cup canned coconut milk
1 cup plain Greek yogurt
½ cup sliced strawberries
3 tablespoons egg white protein powder
2 tablespoons coconut oil
½ teaspoon stevia

In a blender, pulse the coconut milk, yogurt, strawberries, egg white protein powder, coconut oil, and stevia until the mixture is well blended and the strawberries are chopped. Transfer the mixture to an ice cream maker, and freeze according to the manufacturer's directions. Serve.

Per Serving: (¾ cup): Calories: 140; Fat: 12g; Protein: 4g; Total Carbs: 4g; Fiber: 1g; Net Carbs: 3g; **Macros:** Fat: 76%; Protein: 12%; Carbs: 12%

Chocolate-Dipped Peanut Butter Ice Pops

MAKES 12 | PREP TIME: 10 minutes | COOK TIME: 5 minutes, plus 4 hours to chill

8 ounces cream cheese, at room temperature
1 cup all-natural peanut butter (no added sugar or salt)
¼ cup confectioners' erythritol–monk fruit blend; less sweet: 2 tablespoons
1 teaspoon vanilla extract
¼ teaspoon sea salt
2 cups heavy (whipping) cream
4 ounces sugar-free chocolate chips
2 tablespoons coconut oil

In the large bowl, using an electric mixer on medium high, beat the cream cheese, peanut butter, confectioners' sweetener, vanilla, and salt. Add the heavy cream and combine until well incorporated. Pour the mixture into the popsicle molds and add the popsicle sticks. Freeze for 3 to 4 hours, until frozen solid. In the microwave-safe bowl, melt the chocolate baking chips and coconut oil in the microwave in 30-second intervals. Cool for 5 to 10 minutes. Line a baking sheet with parchment paper. Dip the unmolded pops halfway into the melted chocolate, then place them on the prepared sheet and return them to the freezer for about 20 minutes.

Per Serving: (1 pop): Calories: 405; Fat: 37g; Protein: 9g; Total Carbs: 9g; Fiber: 3g; Net Carbs: 6g; **Macros:** Fat: 82%; Protein: 9%; Carbs: 9%

Sangria Granita

SERVES 8 | PREP TIME: 5 minutes, plus 2 hours to freeze | COOK TIME: 5 minutes

1 bottle fruity red wine, such as Tempranillo or Rioja
3 ounces brandy
1 cinnamon stick
Zest and juice of 1 orange
1 teaspoon liquid stevia

In a medium saucepan, mix the wine, brandy, cinnamon stick, and orange zest and juice. Bring to a gentle simmer for 2 minutes, then allow the mixture to steep for 10 minutes. Stir in the liquid stevia. Pour the mixture through a sieve into a

shallow glass baking dish and transfer it to the freezer. Freeze until solid, about 2 hours. Using the tines of a fork, rake through the frozen sangria to produce fine crystals. Divide the granita among the chilled serving glasses.

Per Serving: Calories: 102; Fat: 0g; Protein: 0g; Total Carbs: 3g; Fiber: 0g; Net Carbs: 3g; **Macros:** Fat: 0%; Protein: 0%; Carbs: 12%

Blueberry Mint Ice Pops

MAKES 12 POPS | PREP TIME: 20 minutes, plus time to freeze

2 cups blueberries
1 English cucumber, cut into chunks
1 cup heavy (whipping) cream
2 teaspoons Swerve
¼ cup fresh mint
Pinch ground nutmeg

Place the blueberries, cucumber, cream, Swerve, mint, and nutmeg in a blender and pulse until the mixture is very smooth. Pour the mixture into ice pop molds and freeze until firm. Serve.

Per Serving: (1 pop); Calories: 87; Fat: 7g; Protein: 1g; Total Carbs: 5g; Fiber: 1g; Net Carbs: 4g; **Macros:** Fat: 72%; Protein: 5%; Carbs: 23%

Fudge Ice Pops

MAKES 4 POPS | PREP TIME: 15 minutes, plus 3 hours to freeze | COOK TIME: 1 minute

1 ounce unsweetened chocolate
1 tablespoon coconut oil
½ avocado
½ cup unsweetened almond milk
2 tablespoons egg white protein powder
1 tablespoon cocoa powder
½ teaspoon stevia
½ teaspoon pure vanilla extract

In a small, microwave-safe bowl, microwave the chocolate and coconut oil on low power, watching carefully, until the chocolate is melted, about 1 minute. Stir, and set aside. In a blender, purée the avocado, almond milk, egg white protein powder, cocoa, stevia, and vanilla until the mixture is smooth. Pour the coconut oil mixture into the blender, and blend until well incorporated. Evenly divide the chocolate mixture among 4 ice pop molds. Place the molds in the freezer and freeze, about 3 hours. Serve.

Per Serving: (1 pop): Calories: 144; Fat: 12g; Protein: 4g; Total Carbs: 5g; Fiber: 3g; Net Carbs: 2g; **Macros:** Fat: 75%; Protein: 14%; Carbs: 11%

Vanilla-Almond Ice Pops

MAKES 8 POPS | PREP TIME: 10 minutes, plus 4 hours to freeze | COOK TIME: 5 minutes

2 cups almond milk
1 cup heavy (whipping) cream
1 vanilla bean, halved lengthwise
1 cup shredded unsweetened coconut

Place a medium saucepan over medium heat and add the almond milk, heavy cream, and vanilla bean. Bring the liquid to a simmer and reduce the heat to low. Continue to simmer for 5 minutes. Remove the saucepan from the heat and let the liquid cool. Take the vanilla bean out of the liquid and use a knife to scrape the seeds out of the bean into the liquid. Stir in the coconut and divide the liquid between the ice pop molds. Freeze until solid, about 4 hours, and enjoy.

Per Serving: (1 pop) Calories: 166; Fat: 15g; Protein: 3g; Total Carbs: 4g; Fiber: 2g; Net Carbs: 2g; **Macros:** Fat: 81%; Protein: 9%; Carbs: 10%

Orange Cream Ice Pops

MAKES 8 POPS | PREP TIME: 5 minutes, plus 3 hours to freeze

2 cups unsweetened almond milk
¾ cup cream cheese, softened
3 tablespoons egg white protein powder
2 teaspoons orange extract
2 teaspoons pure vanilla extract
½ teaspoon stevia
Pinch sea salt

In a blender, blend the almond milk, cream cheese, egg white protein powder, orange extract, vanilla, stevia, and sea salt until the mixture is very smooth. Pour the mixture into 8 ice pop molds, freeze for at least 3 hours, and serve.

Per Serving: (1 pop): Calories: 92; Fat: 8g; Protein: 4g; Total Carbs: 1g; Fiber: 0g; Net Carbs: 1g; **Macros:** Fat: 78%; Protein: 17%; Carbs: 5%

Churros and Chocolate Sauce

SERVES 9 | PREP TIME: 20 minutes | **COOK TIME:** 10 minutes

For the churros

8 cups peanut oil, for frying
½ cup almond flour
½ cup whey protein isolate, unflavored
¼ cup coconut flour
½ teaspoon psyllium husk powder
2 tablespoons granulated erythritol blend
3 large eggs
2 tablespoons olive oil
1 teaspoon vanilla extract
1 cup monk fruit granulated erythritol blend
1 teaspoon cinnamon

For the chocolate sauce

½ cup heavy (whipping) cream
½ cup unsweetened almond milk
½ cup confectioners' erythritol blend
½ cup unsweetened cocoa powder
1 teaspoon vanilla extract
½ teaspoon cinnamon

Place a large, heavy pot on the stove over medium heat. Pour enough peanut oil in the pot to fill at least ³⁄₄ inch to 1 inch deep. In a large bowl, combine the almond flour, whey protein, coconut flour, psyllium husk powder, and sweetener. Stir well with a spoon, mashing up any lumps. Add the eggs, olive oil, and vanilla, and mix well. Spoon the dough into a piping bag or gallon resealable bag with the corner cut off to make a ¹⁄₂-inch hole. In a shallow bowl, mix the sweetener and cinnamon. When the oil is hot enough to fry, pipe 3 lines of dough into the oil 4 to 5 inches long. Using a slotted spoon, flip the churros back and forth in the oil for 2 to 4 minutes, or until golden brown. Carefully lift each one out of the oil and place in the rolling sugar. Spoon the sugar across the top of each churro, and then move them to a plate. Repeat cooking and coating with the remaining batter. Heat a small saucepan over medium heat. Combine the heavy cream, almond milk, confectioners' sweetener, cocoa powder, vanilla, and

cinnamon in the pan, and whisk or stir until it comes to a boil. Reduce heat to a simmer and continue to stir for 5 more minutes. Remove from heat, and continue stirring a few minutes more while the sauce thickens. Pour the sauce in a dish for dipping, and serve with the churros.

Per Serving: (2 churros and 2 tablespoons chocolate sauce): Calories: 308; Fat: 25g; Protein: 16g; Total Carbs: 38g; Fiber: 4g; Net Carbs: 3g; **Macros:** Fat: 73%; Protein: 21%; Carbs: 6%

Crème Brûlée

SERVES 6 TO 8 | PREP TIME: 20 minutes, plus 2½ hours chilling and cooling | **COOK TIME:** 40 minutes

4 cups coconut cream
¾ cup granular erythritol
6 large egg yolks
2 teaspoons gluten-free vanilla extract

Preheat the oven to 325°F. In a medium saucepan, bring the coconut cream to a boil, remove it from the heat, and stir in the vanilla extract. Cover the pan and let it sit for 15 minutes. In a medium bowl, whisk 6 tablespoons erythritol and the egg yolks. Slowly add the cream mixture to the yolk mixture, stirring continually. Pour the custard mixture into 6 to 8 ramekins. Place the ramekins in a large roasting pan. Pour hot water into the pan so that the water comes halfway up the sides of the ramekins. Bake for 40 to 45 minutes or until the custard is set but still jiggly. Transfer the ramekins to the refrigerator for 2 hours. Remove the ramekins from the refrigerator and allow them to come to room temperature, about 30 minutes. Sprinkle the remaining erythritol evenly over the tops of each custard. Use a torch to melt the erythritol on top. Wait until the top shell hardens, then serve. If you don't have a kitchen torch, you can also broil the custards for 3 to 5 minutes or until the tops start to brown.

Per Serving: Calories: 436; Fat: 45g; Protein: 6g; Total Carbs: 8g; Fiber: 3g; Net Carbs: 5g; **Macros:** Fat: 87%; Protein: 5%; Carbs: 8%

Sweet Egg Salad

SERVES 4 | PREP TIME: 5 minutes | **COOK TIME:** 10 minutes

6 large eggs
1 scoop vanilla protein powder
1½ tablespoons powdered erythritol
1 teaspoon vanilla extract
1 tablespoon unsweetened coconut milk (optional)
½ cup sugar-free chocolate chips
Sugar-free syrup and melted butter-flavored coconut oil, for serving (optional)

Fill a large bowl with ice and water. Place the eggs in a large saucepan filled with water and bring to a boil. Cook for 10 to 12 minutes. Using a slotted spoon, carefully transfer the eggs to the ice bath to cool for 3 minutes, peel the eggs, and put them in a large bowl. Add the protein powder, erythritol, vanilla extract, and coconut milk (if using) to the bowl and mash everything together. Add the chocolate chips and mix again. Serve the egg salad drizzled, if you'd like, with syrup or the melted coconut oil.

Per Serving: Calories: 154; Fat: 10g; Protein: 11g; Total Carbs: 5g; Fiber: 2g; Net Carbs: 3g; **Macros:** Fat: 58%; Protein: 29%; Carbs: 13%

DRINKS

Buttered Coffee

SERVES 1 | PREP TIME: 15 minutes

1½ cups hot coffee
2 tablespoons unsalted butter

1½ tablespoons MCT oil, or
  coconut oil
Sugar-free sweetener

In a blender, add the coffee, butter, and oil. Blend until frothy, about 1 minute. Flavor with a sweetener of your choice and enjoy.

Per Serving: Calories: 383; Fat: 44g; Protein: 1g; Total Carbs: 0g; Fiber: 0g; Net Carbs: 0g; **Macros:** Fat: 99%; Protein: 1%; Carbs: 0%

Pumpkin Spice Latte

SERVES 1 TO 2 | PREP TIME: 5 minutes |
COOK TIME: 5 minutes

1 cup brewed coffee
½ cup unsweetened flax milk
1 scoop vanilla protein powder
½ cup canned pumpkin purée
  (not pumpkin pie filling)
1 tablespoon coconut oil
1 tablespoon erythritol

½ teaspoon pumpkin pie
  spice, plus more for serving
  (optional)
1 tablespoon collagen powder
  (optional)
Cinnamon sticks, for garnish
  (optional)

In a medium saucepan over medium heat, combine the coffee, flax milk, vanilla protein powder, pumpkin purée, coconut oil, erythritol, and pumpkin pie spice, and collagen powder (if using) and warm for about 5 minutes. Pour or spoon the latte into mugs and dust a little extra pumpkin pie spice over the top and/or garnish with cinnamon sticks (if using).

Per Serving: Calories: 254; Fat: 18g; Protein: 11g; Total Carbs: 12g; Fiber: 5g; Net Carbs: 7g; **Macros:** Fat: 64%; Protein: 18%; Carbs: 18%

Bulletproof Coffee

SERVES 1 | PREP TIME: 1 minute

8 ounces brewed hot coffee
1 tablespoon butter

1 tablespoon coconut oil

Combine all the ingredients in a large mug. Place an immersion blender all the way into the cup. Pulse a few times until the brew is thick and frothy. Enjoy immediately.

Per Serving: Calories: 219; Fat: 25g; Protein: 0g; Total Carbs: 0g; Fiber: 0g; Net Carbs: 0g; **Macros:** Fat: 100%; Protein: 0%; Carbs: 0%

Matcha Coffee

SERVES 2 | PREP TIME: 5 minutes

1 (14-ounce) can full-fat
  coconut milk
1 cup brewed black
  coffee, chilled
1 tablespoon almond butter

2 teaspoons matcha powder,
  plus more for sprinkling
1 cup ice cubes
5 to 6 drops liquid stevia or
  monk fruit

In a high-powered blender, combine the coconut milk, coffee, almond butter, matcha powder, ice, and stevia, and blend on high speed for 60 seconds. Divide the drink between two glasses and sprinkle each with a bit more matcha powder.

Per Serving: (1 drink): Calories: 508; Fat: 48g; Protein: 7g; Total Carbs: 12g; Fiber: 5g; Net Carbs: 7g; **Macros:** Fat: 85%; Protein: 6%; Carbs: 9%

Earl Grey Rose Latte

SERVES 1 | PREP TIME: 5 minutes | COOK TIME: 5 minutes

½ cup filtered water, boiling
1 Earl Grey tea bag (make sure
  the only ingredients are
  black tea and bergamot oil)
1 tablespoon dried rose petals
  (optional)

1 cup full-fat coconut milk
1 tablespoon collagen
  peptide powder
1 teaspoon MCT oil
1 teaspoon raw honey
  (optional)

Pour the boiling water into a large mug or teapot. Add the tea bag and dried rose petals (if using) and allow to steep for 4 to 5 minutes. Meanwhile, heat the coconut milk in a small saucepan over medium heat until it simmers. Remove the saucepan from heat and transfer the coconut milk to a blender. Add in the collagen, MCT oil, and honey (if using). Using a mesh strainer, pour the tea into the blender. Blend for 10 to 30 seconds or until fully combined. Pour the latte mixture into a large mug and serve.

Per Serving: Calories: 661; Fat: 62g; Protein: 15g; Total Carbs: 13g; Fiber: 5g; Net Carbs: 8g; **Macros:** Fat: 83%; Protein: 9%; Carbs: 8%

Coconut Iced Coffee

SERVES 1 | PREP TIME: 5 minutes

Ice cubes
8 ounces brewed black
  coffee, chilled
5 drops monk fruit extract
1 teaspoon vanilla extract

1 teaspoon coconut extract
1 tablespoon MCT oil
  or powder
¼ cup heavy (whipping) cream
  or coconut milk

Fill a large glass ¾ full of ice. Pour the coffee over ice. Add the monk fruit, vanilla, and coconut extracts, and MCT oil and stir until combined. Pour the heavy cream on top and allow to settle. Serve cold.

Per Serving: Calories: 335; Fat: 36g; Protein: 1g; Total Carbs: 2g; Fiber: 0g; Net Carbs: 2g; **Macros:** Fat: 96%; Protein: 1%; Carbs: 3%

Green Tea Latte

SERVES 2 | PREP TIME: 5 minutes

1½ cups brewed green tea or
  brewed matcha tea

½ cup unsweetened full-fat
  coconut milk
1 tablespoon MCT oil

Place all the ingredients in a blender, and process until smooth.

Per Serving: Calories: 342; Fat: 35g; Protein: 2g; Total Carbs: 5g; Fiber: 2g; Net Carbs: 3g; **Macros:** Fat: 92%; Protein: 3%; Carbs: 5%

Fat Chai

SERVES 1 | PREP TIME: 5 minutes | COOK TIME: 5 minutes

2 sugar-free chai tea bags
8 to 12 ounces hot water
1 tablespoon coconut oil
1 tablespoon grass-fed butter

2 tablespoons heavy
  (whipping) cream
5 to 6 drops of stevia
  (optional)

Steep both tea bags in the hot water for 5 minutes. Remove the tea bags and stir in the coconut oil, butter, and cream. Stir until well blended. Stir in the stevia (if using) and serve warm.

Per Serving: (1 drink): Calories: 323; Fat: 35g; Protein: 1g; Total Carbs: 1g; Fiber: 0g; Net Carbs: 1g; **Macros:** Fat: 98%; Protein: 1%; Carbs: 1%

Hot Cocoa

SERVES 1 | PREP TIME: 2 minutes | COOK TIME: 5 minutes (for hot chocolate)

⅓ cup full-fat coconut milk

1 cup unsweetened coconut milk

2 tablespoons unsweetened cocoa powder

2 tablespoons erythritol

2 to 5 drops chocolate-flavored liquid stevia

1 tablespoon collagen powder or "creamer" (optional)

Sugar-free marshmallow-flavored syrup, for serving (optional)

In a small saucepan over medium-low heat, combine the coconut milks, cocoa powder, erythritol, liquid stevia, and collagen powder (if using). Stir all the ingredients together and warm for about 5 minutes, or to your desired temperature. Pour the cocoa into a mug and add a little marshmallow syrup if you please.

Per Serving: Calories: 298; Fat: 26g; Protein: 5g; Total Carbs: 11g; Fiber: 5g; Net Carbs: 6g; **Macros:** Fat: 79%; Protein: 6%; Carbs: 15%

Spicy Hot Chocolate

SERVES 4 | PREP TIME: 10 minutes

1 (14-ounce) can unsweetened coconut cream

1½ cups sugar-free vanilla almond milk

¼ cup unsweetened cocoa powder

3 tablespoons brown erythritol blend

1 teaspoon ground cinnamon, plus more for sprinkling on top

1 teaspoon vanilla extract

⅛ teaspoon nutmeg

⅛ teaspoon cayenne pepper

In a small saucepan over low heat, combine the coconut cream, almond milk, cocoa powder, brown sweetener, cinnamon, vanilla, nutmeg, and cayenne pepper. Whisk occasionally until heated through. Pour into glasses, and top with a sprinkle of cinnamon.

Per Serving: Calories: 216; Fat: 21g; Protein: 1g; Total Carbs: 15g; Fiber: 3g; Net Carbs: 12g; **Macros:** Fat: 88%; Protein: 2%; Carbs: 6%

Hot Almond Chocolate

SERVES 1 | PREP TIME: 5 minutes

2 tablespoons unsweetened cocoa powder

1 cup milk, divided

2½ teaspoons liquid stevia

½ cup heavy cream

½ teaspoon almond extract

In a small saucepan over medium-low heat, whisk together the cocoa, ½ cup of milk, and the stevia until dissolved. Increase the heat to medium, add the remaining ½ cup of milk and the cream and whisk occasionally until hot, about 5 minutes. Stir in the almond extract and serve.

Per serving: Calories: 585; Fat: 52g; Protein: 13g; Total Carbs: 22g; Fiber: 4g; Net Carbs: 18g

Bloody Mary

SERVES 6 | PREP TIME: 5 minutes

For the Bloody Mary

1 (32-ounce) bottle V8 Juice, original or spicy

5 teaspoons Worcester-shire sauce

1 tablespoon prepared horseradish

¼ teaspoon freshly ground black pepper

1 teaspoon garlic salt

1 teaspoon celery salt

2 teaspoons sriracha sauce

Ice

12 ounces vodka

For the glass rim

1 tablespoon celery salt

1 tablespoon kosher salt

1 lime, cut into wedges

For garnish

6 celery stalks, ends cut off, leaves remaining

6 slices crispy bacon

12 blue cheese–stuffed olives, or your favorite

In a large pitcher, mix the V8 Juice, Worcestershire sauce, horseradish, pepper, garlic salt, celery salt, and sriracha. Refrigerate until ready to serve. In a shallow plate, mix the celery salt and kosher salt. Use one wedge of lime to rub the rims of eight (10-ounce) glasses, and then dip them into the salt mixture. Carefully fill each glass with ice, trying not to disturb the salt on the rim, and pour 2 ounces of vodka into each glass. Pour the tomato mixture over each glass, and garnish with a stalk of celery and piece of bacon. Skewer two olives on a bamboo skewer and place across the top, garnish the edge of the glass with a lime wedge or just add to the glass, and serve.

Per Serving: Calories: 256; Fat: 8g; Protein: 5g; Total Carbs: 9g; Fiber: 2g; Net Carbs: 7g; **Macros:** Fat: 26%; Protein: 8%; Carbs: 12%

Virgin (or Not) Eggnog

SERVES 4 | PREP TIME: 5 minutes

2 cups light coconut milk

1 cup full-fat coconut milk

1 scoop vanilla protein powder

1 egg or 1 tablespoon chia seeds

8 tablespoons sugar-free maple or pancake syrup

1 teaspoon nutmeg, plus more for serving (optional)

½ teaspoon ground ginger

½ teaspoon allspice

Ground cinnamon

Rum (optional)

Sugar-free whipped cream (optional)

In a blender, combine the coconut milks, protein powder (or collagen), egg (or chia seeds), syrup, nutmeg, ginger, allspice, and cinnamon to taste and blend until smooth. Pour into a glass and, if you're feeling naughty, add some rum and a bit of whipped cream on top.

Per Serving: Calories: 347; Fat: 31g; Protein: 7g; Total Carbs: 40g; Fiber: 30g; Net Carbs: 10g; **Macros:** Fat: 80%; Protein: 8%; Carbs: 12%

Chocolate Martini

SERVES 4 | PREP TIME: 10 minutes

4 teaspoons chocolate sauce

8 ounces vodka

1 cup half-and-half

Ice

Drizzle 1 teaspoon of chocolate sauce around the edges of four chilled martini glasses. In a shaker or mason jar with a lid, add the rest of the chocolate sauce, vodka, half-and-half, and ice cubes, and shake for at least 30 seconds. Pour into the glasses, straining out the ice cubes, and serve.

Per Serving: Calories: 268; Fat: 12g; Protein: 3g; Total Carbs: 14g; Fiber: 2g; Net Carbs: 12g; Macros: Fat: 40%; Protein: 4%; Carbs: 7%

Moscow Mule

SERVES 4 | PREP TIME: 5 minutes

Ice

8 ounces vodka

¼ cup freshly squeezed lime juice (about 2 limes), reserving a slice to quarter, for garnish

16 ounces sugar-free ginger beer

Mint leaves, for garnish

Add crushed ice or cubes to four copper cups or cocktail glasses. In a shaker or mason jar, add the vodka and lime juice, along with a few ice cubes, and shake. Pour over ice in glasses. Pour 4 ounces of ginger beer in each glass and stir. Add a lime quarter to each glass, garnish with mint, and serve.

Per Serving: Calories: 168; Fat: 0g; Protein: 0g; Total Carbs: 1g; Fiber: 0g; Net Carbs: 1g; Macros: Fat: 0%; Protein: 0%; Carbs: 2%

Virgin (or Not) Mojito

SERVES 1 | PREP TIME: 5 minutes

10 fresh mint leaves

¼ cup freshly squeezed lime juice

½ cup club soda

2 tablespoons erythritol, plus more for serving (optional)

Ice

1½ ounces light rum (optional)

1 lime wedge (optional)

On a cutting board, crush the mint leaves with the back of a spoon. Put the mint in a large glass and pour in the lime juice and club soda. Add the erythritol, then use the spoon you crushed the mint with to mix the contents of the glass together. Add ice, then pour in the rum and stir.

Per Serving: Calories: 35; Fat: 0g; Protein: 1g; Total Carbs: 8g; Fiber: 2g; Net Carbs: 6g; Macros: Fat: 0%; Protein: 9%; Carbs: 91%

Blueberry Mojito

SERVES 4 | PREP TIME: 10 minutes

½ cup granulated erythritol blend, plus more for the rims

2 limes, half of one cut into 8 lime wheel slices for garnish

Ice

¾ cup fresh blueberries, divided

3 tablespoons fresh lime juice

4 large mint leaves torn in pieces, and extra leaves for garnish

8 ounces white rum

1 (1-liter) bottle club soda

Place a little sweetener on a shallow plate. Rub the rim of four (10-ounce) chilled glass tumblers with lime and dip the rims into the sweetener. Add ice cubes, being careful not to disturb the sugar rim. In a shaker or mason jar with a lid, add ½ cup of blueberries, sweetener, lime juice, and mint leaves. Muddle using the back of a wooden spoon or a muddler. Add the rum and some ice to the jar and shake for at least 45 seconds.

Pour over the ice in the glasses, fill with club soda, and stir. Drop a lime wheel in the glass and one on the rim for garnish, drop the remaining blueberries equally into each glass, and serve.

Per Serving: Calories: 148; Fat: 0g; Protein: 0g; Total Carbs: 29g; Fiber: 1; Net Carbs: 28g; Macros: Fat: 0%; Protein: 0%; Carbs: 12%

Hot Buttered Rum

SERVES 4 | PREP TIME: 5 minutes | COOK TIME: 5 minutes

½ cup butter

¾ cup brown erythritol blend

¼ cup sugar-free maple-flavored syrup

½ teaspoon pumpkin pie spice

Pinch salt

2 cups water

8 ounces spiced rum

4 cinnamon sticks, for garnish

In a medium saucepan over medium heat, add the butter, sweetener, syrup, pumpkin pie spice, salt, and water, and stir until completely melted and incorporated, 3 to 4 minutes. Remove from the heat, add the rum, pour evenly into four mugs, garnish each with a cinnamon stick, stir, and serve.

Per Serving: Calories: 341; Fat: 23g; Protein: 0g; Total Carbs: 38g; Fiber: 0g; Net Carbs: 0g; Macros: Fat: 61%; Protein: 0%; Carbs: 0%

Spicy Margarita

SERVES 4 | PREP TIME: 10 minutes

¼ cup kosher salt, for garnish

½ cup freshly squeezed lime juice, plus 4 small slices for garnish

Ice

8 ounces tequila

¼ cup freshly squeezed orange juice

12 drops liquid stevia, plus more if needed

1 jalapeño, thinly sliced, with or without seeds depending on taste

Place the salt on a shallow plate. Use one of the limes to rub the rims of four glasses. Dip the glasses in the salt, and then carefully add some ice to each glass. Combine the tequila, lime juice, orange juice, stevia, and jalapeño slices and a few ice cubes in a shaker or Mason jar and shake vigorously. Taste, add a few more drops of stevia if needed, and then pour evenly into the glasses. Garnish each glass edge with a lime slice and serve.

Per Serving: Calories: 143; Fat: 0g; Protein: 0g; Total Carbs: 4g; Fiber: 0g; Net Carbs: 4g; Macros: Fat: 0%; Protein: 0%; Carbs: 11%

Lime Margarita

SERVES 1 | PREP TIME: 5 minutes

2 tablespoons coarse sea salt

Lime wedge

Ice cubes

2 ounces 100% agave tequila

6 ounces sparkling water or club soda

1 tablespoon freshly squeezed lime juice

Stevia

Spread the salt out in an even layer on a small plate. Rub a lime wedge around the rim of a glass, and dip it into the plate of salt to create a salt rim. Fill the glass with ice cubes. Pour the tequila, sparkling water, lime juice, and stevia to taste into a cocktail shaker. Shake well, pour into the glass, and enjoy.

Per Serving: Calories: 145; Fat: 0g; Protein: 0g; Total Carbs: 1g; Fiber: 0g; Net Carbs: 1g

Raspberry Mimosa

SERVES 4 | PREP TIME: 10 minutes | COOK TIME: 5 minutes

6 ounces raspberries (roughly 28 raspberries), divided
2 tablespoons granulated erythritol blend
¼ cup water
1 bottle brut or dry champagne
Mint leaves, for garnish

In a small saucepan over medium heat, add 20 raspberries, sweetener, and water. Stir until the berries break down, 3 to 4 minutes. Remove from the heat, pour into a blender, and pulse 6 to 8 times. Pour the mixture into a strainer to remove all the seeds. Use the back of a spoon to push the mixture through the strainer. Add a few tablespoons of the raspberry mixture to a champagne glass, pour 6 ounces of champagne on top, and stir. Drop two of the remaining raspberries into each glass, add mint for garnish, and serve.

Per Serving: Calories: 178; Fat: 0g; Protein: 1g; Total Carbs: 16g; Fiber: 3g; Net Carbs: 7g; **Macros:** Fat: 0%; Protein: 2%; Carbs: 16%

Sangria

SERVES 6 | PREP TIME: 15 minutes, plus 2 hours to chill

1 bottle Pinot Noir, preferably Spanish
¼ cup freshly squeezed orange juice, plus 2 slices cut in quarters, for garnish
⅓ cup sliced strawberries
⅓ cup blueberries
1 small lemon, thinly sliced
1 or 2 tablespoons sugar-free maple-flavored syrup
½ cup brandy

In a pitcher, mix the wine, orange juice, strawberries, blueberries, lemon slices, syrup, and brandy. Refrigerate for 2 to 8 hours, stirring occasionally. Pour in a glass over a small amount of ice, garnish the side of the glass with an orange quarter, and serve.

Per Serving: Calories: 160; Fat: 0g; Protein: 0g; Total Carbs: 7g; Fiber: 1; Net Carbs: 6; **Macros:** Fat: 0%; Protein: 0%; Carbs: 14%

Michelada

SERVES 1 | PREP TIME: 5 minutes

Kosher salt, for garnish
Tajín Clasico seasoning, for garnish
Lime wedge
2 dashes Tabasco sauce or any hot sauce
Pinch freshly ground black pepper
12 ounces Corona Premier beer or low-carb beer of choice, chilled

On a small plate, mix the salt with the Tajín seasoning in a 1:1 ratio. Moisten the rim of a beer mug with the lime and dip the rim into the mixture. Fill the mug with ice and squeeze the lime juice into the glass. Add the hot sauce and black pepper, then slowly pour in the beer. Mix gently and serve with the lime wedge used for squeezing.

Per Serving: Calories: 110; Fat: 0g; Protein: 0g; Total Carbs: 2g; Fiber: 0g

Frosé Slushie

SERVES 5 | PREP TIME: 5 minutes

4 cups ice
12 ounces rosé wine, chilled
½ cup frozen strawberries

Add the ice, rosé, and strawberries to a blender. Blend until smooth and serve in wine glasses.

Per Serving: Calories: 64; Fat: 0g; Protein: 0g; Total Carbs: 5g; Fiber: 0g

Vesper Martini

SERVES 1 | PREP TIME: 5 minutes

2 ounces gin
⅓ ounce sauvignon blanc or dry white wine of choice
¼ ounce vodka
Lemon twist, for garnish

Fill a shaker with ice and add the gin, wine, and vodka. Shake vigorously and strain into a glass. Twist the lemon over the drink, wipe the rim with the lemon, and drop it into the glass.

Per Serving: Calories: 153; Fat: 0g; Protein: 0g; Total Carbs: 0g; Fiber: 0g

Negroni

SERVES 1 | PREP TIME: 3 minutes

2 ounces gin
½ ounce unsweetened pomegranate juice
½ ounce dry vermouth
3 ounces club soda, chilled
Orange twist, for garnish

Fill a glass with ice. Fill a shaker with ice and add the gin, pomegranate juice, and vermouth. Shake well and strain into the glass. Top with club soda and garnish with an orange twist.

Per Serving: Calories: 161; Fat: 0g; Protein: 0g; Total Carbs: 4g; Fiber: 0g

Tequila Sunrise

SERVES 1 | PREP TIME: 5 minutes

1½ ounces silver tequila
6 ounces orange-flavored sparkling water
1 teaspoon unsweetened pomegranate juice
2 ounces club soda, chilled (optional)

Fill a glass with ice. Pour in the tequila and sparkling water and stir well. Float the pomegranate juice on top, allowing it to sink into the drink to create a "sunrise" effect. Top with club soda (if using) and serve.

Per Serving: Calories: 100; Fat: 0g; Protein: 0g; Total Carbs: 1g; Fiber: 0g

Old-Fashioned

SERVES 1 | PREP TIME: 5 minutes

½ very thin orange slice
1 teaspoon crystallized allulose or sweetener of choice
1 teaspoon water
3 dashes Angostura bitters
2½ ounces bourbon
Orange twist, for garnish

Place the orange slice, allulose, water, and bitters in the bottom of a glass and muddle. Fill the glass with ice, pour in the bourbon, and stir. Swipe the rim with the orange peel, twist to release the oils over the drink, and garnish.

Per Serving: Calories: 161; Fat: 0g; Protein: 0g; Total Carbs: 0g; Fiber: 0g

Manhattan

SERVES 1 | PREP TIME: 5 minutes

2 ounces rye whiskey
¾ ounce dry vermouth or dry white wine
3 dashes Angostura bitters
Lemon twist, for garnish

Fill a mixing glass with ice and add the whiskey, vermouth, and bitters and stir well. Strain into a glass and twist the lemon over the drink, wipe the rim with the lemon, and drop it into the glass.

Per Serving: Calories: 163; Fat: 0g; Protein: 0g; Total Carbs: 3g; Fiber: 0g

Gelatin Shooters

MAKES 20 SHOOTERS | PREP TIME: 20 minutes, plus 4 hours to chill

2 cups water

2 mint sprigs (optional)

1 (0.3-ounce) package sugar-free strawberry gelatin mix (or flavor of choice)

½ cup water or hard seltzer, chilled

½ cup vodka or booze of choice, chilled

Heat the water and mint (if using) in a small saucepan until boiling. Remove the mint sprigs and measure 1 cup of the water into a medium bowl. Whisk in the gelatin for 2 minutes. Allow the gelatin mixture to cool for 5 minutes. Whisk in the chilled water, then the chilled vodka. Place 20 (2-ounce) disposable party cups on a rimmed baking sheet, then fill each with the gelatin mixture. Refrigerate for a minimum of 4 hours to set, and refrigerate until ready to serve, or up to 1 week tightly covered.

Per Serving: (1 shooter): Calories: 13; Fat: 0g; Total Carbs: 0g; Fiber: 0g;

STAPLES

Avocado-Herb Compound Butter

MAKES 2 CUPS | PREP TIME: 25 minutes, plus 4 hours chilling time

¼ cup butter, at room temperature

1 avocado, peeled, pitted, and quartered

Juice of ½ lemon

2 teaspoons chopped cilantro

1 teaspoon chopped fresh basil

1 teaspoon minced garlic

Sea salt

Freshly ground black pepper

Place the butter, avocado, lemon juice, cilantro, basil, and garlic in a food processor and process until smooth. Season the butter with salt and pepper. Transfer the mixture to a sheet of parchment paper and shape it into a log. Place the parchment butter log in the refrigerator until it is firm, about 4 hours. Slice and serve with fish or chicken. Store unused butter wrapped tightly for up to 1 week.

Per Serving: (1 tablespoon): Calories: 22; Fat: 2g; Protein: 0g; Total Carbs: 1g; Fiber: 0g; Net Carbs: 1g; **Macros:** Fat: 86%; Protein: 3%; Carbs: 11%

Cinnamon Butter

SERVES 16 | TOTAL TIME: 1 hour, 15 minutes

1 cup butter, at room temperature

10 drops liquid stevia, or other liquid sugar substitute

1 teaspoon pure vanilla extract

1 teaspoon ground cinnamon

¼ teaspoon salt

In a medium bowl, mix the butter, stevia, vanilla, cinnamon, and salt. Spoon the butter onto a sheet of wax paper. Roll it into a long log in the center of the paper, leaving about 2 inches of paper on each side. Roll the paper around the butter and twist the ends. Chill for at least 1 one hour before using. Refrigerate for up to 2 weeks.

Per Serving: (1 tablespoon): Calories: 103; Fat: 12g; Protein: 0g; Total Carbs: 0g; Fiber: 0g; Net Carbs: 0g; **Macros:** Fat: 100%; Protein: 0%; Carbs: 0%

Horseradish Compound Butter

MAKES 24 (½-INCH) DISKS | PREP TIME: 7 minutes

1 cup butter, softened

½ cup coconut oil

1 teaspoon prepared horseradish

1 garlic clove

1 tablespoon fresh chopped basil

1 tablespoon fresh chopped oregano

½ teaspoon freshly ground black pepper

¼ teaspoon sea salt

In a blender, pulse the butter, coconut oil, horseradish, garlic, basil, oregano, pepper, and salt until well blended. Scoop the butter mixture onto a double layer of plastic wrap (about 12 inches long) lengthwise. Fold the plastic wrap over the butter mixture, creating a long tube. Twist the ends to create a tight cylinder of butter about 1 inch in diameter. Refrigerate or freeze the butter cylinder until it is very firm. Cut off a slice of butter to top vegetables, fish, or steak. Store the butter for up to 1 month.

Per Serving: (½-inch disk): Calories: 108; Fat: 12g; Protein: 0g; Total Carbs: 0g; Fiber: 0g; Net Carbs: 0g; **Macros:** Fat: 100%; Protein: 0%; Carbs: 0%

Ghee

MAKES 2 CUPS | PREP TIME: 2 minutes | COOK TIME: 6 hours on low

1 pound unsalted butter, diced

Place the butter in the insert of the slow cooker. Cook on low with the lid set slightly open for 6 hours. Pour the melted butter through a fine-mesh cheesecloth into a bowl. Cool the ghee for 30 minutes and pour into a jar. Refrigerate for up to 2 weeks.

Per Serving: (1 tablespoon): Calories: 100; Fat: 11g; Protein: 0g; Total Carbs: 0g; Fiber: 0g; Net Carbs: 0g; **Macros:** Fat: 100%; Protein: 0%; Carbs: 0%

Strawberry Butter

MAKES 3 CUPS | PREP TIME: 25 minutes

2 cups shredded unsweetened coconut

1 tablespoon coconut oil

¾ cup fresh strawberries

½ tablespoon freshly squeezed lemon juice

1 teaspoon alcohol-free pure vanilla extract

Put the coconut in a food processor and purée it until it is buttery and smooth, about 15 minutes. Add the coconut oil, strawberries, lemon juice, and vanilla to the coconut butter and process until very smooth, scraping down the sides of the bowl. Pass the butter through a fine sieve to remove the strawberry seeds, using the back of a spoon to press the butter through. Store the strawberry butter in an airtight container in the refrigerator for up to 2 weeks. Serve chicken or fish with a spoon of this butter on top.

Per Serving: (1 tablespoon): Calories: 23; Fat: 2g; Protein: 0g; Total Carbs: 1g; Fiber: 0g; Net Carbs: 1g; **Macros:** Fat: 80%; Protein: 5%; Carbs: 15%

Beef Bone Broth

YIELDS 2 QUARTS | PREP TIME: 4 minutes |
COOK TIME: 4 hours 40 minutes

1 pound beef bones	1 teaspoon sea salt
1 tablespoon apple cider vinegar	4 quarts water

Preheat the oven to 400°F. Spread the beef bones on a rimmed baking sheet. Roast uncovered for 40 minutes, or until browned. Transfer the bones to a large pot. Pour the oil from the roasting pan and use a fat separator to discard the fat. Transfer the remaining bits, to the pot. Add the vinegar, salt, and water to the pot and bring to a gentle simmer. Cook partially covered for 4 hours, skimming fat off the surface as it rises. Allow the stock to cool completely before refrigerating in a covered container for up to 1 week or freeze for up to 3 months.

Per Serving: Calories: 45; Fat: 1g; Protein: 9g; Total Carbs: 0g; Fiber: 0g; Net Carbs: 0g; **Macros:** Fat: 20%; Protein: 80%; Carbs: 0%

Rich Beef Stock

MAKES 8 TO 10 CUPS | PREP TIME: 15 minutes |
COOK TIME: 12½ hours, plus 30 minutes cooling time

2 to 3 pounds beef bones (beef marrow, knuckle bones, ribs, and any other bones)	1 carrot, washed and chopped into 2-inch pieces
8 black peppercorns	1 celery stalk, chopped into big chunks
5 thyme sprigs	½ onion, peeled and quartered
3 garlic cloves, peeled and crushed	1 gallon water
2 bay leaves	1 teaspoon extra-virgin olive oil

Preheat the oven to 350°F. Place the beef bones in a deep baking pan and roast them in the oven for about 30 minutes. Transfer the bones to a large stockpot and add the peppercorns, thyme, garlic, bay leaves, carrot, celery, and onion. Add the water, covering the bones completely bring to a boil over high heat, then reduce the heat to low so that the stock gently simmers. Check the stock every hour, for the first 3 hours, and skim off any foam from on the top. Simmer for 12 hours in total and then remove the pot from the heat. Cool the stock for about 30 minutes. Remove any large bones with tongs and strain the stock through a fine-mesh sieve. Discard the leftover vegetables and bones. Pour the stock into containers with tight-fitting lids and cool completely before refrigerating it for up to 5 days or freezing for up to 2 months.

Per Serving: (1 cup): Calories: 65; Fat: 5g; Protein: 4g; Total Carbs: 1g; Fiber: 0g; Net Carbs: 1g; **Macros:** Fat: 70%; Protein: 25%; Carbs: 5%

Chicken Bone Broth

YIELDS 2 QUARTS | PREP TIME: 5 minutes |
COOK TIME: 4 hours

1 pound chicken bones, preferably roasted	1 teaspoon sea salt
1 tablespoon apple cider vinegar	4 quarts cold water

Place the chicken bones, vinegar, and salt in a large pot. Cover with the water and bring to a simmer over medium heat. Reduce the heat to medium-low and simmer for 4 hours, or until reduced to about 2 quarts. Allow the stock to cool completely before refrigerating in a covered container for up to 1 week or freezing for up to 3 months.

Per Serving: (1 cup): Calories: 45; Fat: 1g; Protein: 9g; Total Carbs: 0g; Fiber: 0g; Net Carbs: 0g; **Macros:** Fat: 20%; Protein: 80%; Carbs: 0%

Herbed Chicken Stock

MAKES 8 CUPS | PREP TIME: 15 minutes | COOK TIME: 12 hours, plus 30 minutes cooling time

2 chicken carcasses	1 carrot, washed and chopped roughly
6 black peppercorns	1 sweet onion, peeled and quartered
4 thyme sprigs	
3 bay leaves	
2 celery stalks, cut into quarters	1 gallon cold water (enough to cover the carcasses and vegetables)

Place the chicken carcasses in a large stockpot with the peppercorns, thyme, bay leaves, celery, carrot, and onion. Add the water, covering them completely, and bring it to a boil over high heat. Reduce the heat to low and gently simmer, stirring every few hours, for 12 hours. Remove the pot from the heat and let the stock cool for 30 minutes. Remove any large bones with tongs and then strain the stock through a fine-mesh sieve. Discard the solid bits. Pour the stock into containers with tight-fitting lids and cool completely. Refrigerate for up to 5 days, or freeze for up to 3 months.

Per Serving: (1 cup): Calories: 73; Fat: 5g; Protein: 5g; Total Carbs: 2g; Fiber: 0g; Net Carbs: 2g; **Macros:** Fat: 62%; Protein: 27%; Carbs: 11%

Herbed Vegetable Broth

MAKES 8 CUPS | PREP TIME: 15 minutes | COOK TIME: 8 hours on low

1 tablespoon extra-virgin olive oil	½ cup chopped parsley
4 garlic cloves, crushed	4 thyme sprigs
2 celery stalks with greens, roughly chopped	2 bay leaves
1 sweet onion, quartered	½ teaspoon black peppercorns
1 carrot, roughly chopped	½ teaspoon salt
	8 cups water

Lightly grease the insert of the slow cooker with the olive oil. Place the garlic, celery, onion, carrot, parsley, thyme, bay leaves, peppercorns, and salt in the insert. Add the water. Cover and cook on low for about 8 hours. Strain the broth through a fine-mesh cheesecloth and throw away the solids. Refrigerate the broth in sealed containers for up to 5 days or freeze for up to 1 month.

Per Serving: (1 cup): Calories: 27; Fat: 2g; Protein: 0g; Total Carbs: 2g; Fiber: 0g; Net Carbs: 2g; Cholesterol: 0mg; **Macros:** Fat: 65%; Protein: 0%; Carbs: 35%

Fish Stock

MAKES 6 CUPS | PREP TIME: 10 minutes | COOK TIME: 1 hour

Head and bones of 3 to 4 pounds of fish or heads and peels of 2 to 3 pounds shrimp
1 unpeeled small onion, quartered
2 celery stalks, cut into 4 to 6 pieces
2 garlic cloves, smashed
2 bay leaves
2 teaspoons salt
10 black peppercorns
6 cups water
1 cup dry white wine (optional)

In a large stockpot, place the fish parts, onion, celery, garlic, bay leaves, salt, and peppercorns. Add the water and white wine (if using) and bring to a boil. Cover, reduce the heat to low, and simmer for about 45 minutes. Using a slotted spoon or a fine-mesh strainer, strain the stock, discarding all solid pieces. Refrigerate for up to 3 days or freeze for up to 3 months.

Per Serving (1 cup): Calories: 40; Fat: 2g; Carbs: 0g

Italian Seasoning

SERVES 12 (1 TABLESPOON PER SERVING) | PREP TIME: 5 minutes

2 tablespoons dried basil
2 tablespoons dried oregano
2 tablespoons dried rosemary
2 tablespoons garlic powder
2 tablespoons dried thyme
2 teaspoons red pepper flakes

Combine all the spices. Store in a sealed container at room temperature for up to 6 months.

Per Serving: Calories: 11; Fat: 0g; Protein: 0g; Total Carbs: 2g; Fiber: 1g; Net Carbs: 1g; **Macros:** Fat: 6%; Protein: 11%; Carbs: 83%

Ranch Seasoning

SERVES 10 (1 TABLESPOON PER SERVING) | PREP TIME: 5 minutes

6 tablespoons dried dill
1 tablespoon pink Himalayan salt
1 tablespoon freshly ground black pepper
1 tablespoon onion powder
1 tablespoon garlic powder

Combine all the spices. Store in a sealed container at room temperature for up to 6 months.

Per Serving: Calories: 12; Fat: 0g; Protein: 1g; Total Carbs: 3g; Fiber: 1g; Net Carbs: 2g; **Macros:** Fat: 0%; Protein: 25%; Carbs: 75%

Taco Seasoning

SERVES 8 (1 TABLESPOON PER SERVING) | PREP TIME: 5 minutes

¼ cup ground cumin
1 tablespoon garlic powder
1 tablespoon chili powder
1 tablespoon onion powder
2 teaspoons dried oregano
2 teaspoons paprika

Combine all the spices. Store in a sealed container at room temperature for up to 6 months.

Per Serving: Calories: 29; Fat: 1g; Protein: 1g; Total Carbs: 4g; Fiber: 1g; Net Carbs: 3g; **Macros:** Fat: 31%; Protein: 14%; Carbs: 55%

Buttermilk Ranch Dressing

MAKES 1½ CUPS | PREP TIME: 10 minutes

½ cup heavy (whipping) cream
1 teaspoon apple cider vinegar
½ cup mayonnaise
¼ cup sour cream
1 tablespoon freshly squeezed lemon juice
2 tablespoons chopped fresh parsley
2 tablespoons chopped fresh chives
½ teaspoon minced garlic
¼ teaspoon ground cayenne pepper
Sea salt
Freshly ground black pepper

In a small bowl, stir the heavy cream and vinegar, and set aside for 10 minutes. In a medium bowl, whisk the mayonnaise, sour cream, lemon juice, parsley, chives, garlic, cayenne pepper, and the reserved cream mixture until blended. Season with salt and pepper. Refrigerate the dressing for up to 1 week.

Per Serving: (2 tablespoons): Calories: 74; Fat: 6g; Protein: 2g; Total Carbs: 3g; Fiber: 0g; Net Carbs: 3g; **Macros:** Fat: 73%; Protein: 11%; Carbs: 16%

Lemon-Garlic Dressing

MAKES 1 CUP | PREP TIME: 10 minutes

½ cup sour cream
¼ cup extra-virgin olive oil
1 tablespoon Dijon mustard
¼ cup freshly squeezed lemon juice
2 teaspoons minced garlic
2 teaspoons chopped fresh basil
2 teaspoons chopped fresh parsley
2 teaspoons chopped fresh thyme
Sea salt
Freshly ground black pepper

In a medium bowl, whisk the sour cream, olive oil, Dijon mustard, lemon juice, garlic, basil, parsley, and thyme until well blended. Season the dressing with salt and pepper. Refrigerate the dressing in a sealed container for up to 1 week.

Per Serving: (2 tablespoons): Calories: 98; Fat: 10g; Protein: 1g; Total Carbs: 1g; Fiber: 0g; Net Carbs: 1g

Green Basil Dressing

MAKES 1 CUP | PREP TIME: 10 minutes

1 avocado, peeled and pitted
¼ cup sour cream
¼ cup extra-virgin olive oil
¼ cup chopped fresh basil
1 tablespoon freshly squeezed lime juice
1 teaspoon minced garlic
Sea salt
Freshly ground black pepper

Place the avocado, sour cream, olive oil, basil, lime juice, and garlic in a food processor and pulse until smooth. Season the dressing with salt and pepper. Refrigerate the dressing in an airtight container for 1 to 2 weeks.

Per Serving: (1 tablespoon): Calories: 173; Fat: 17g; Protein: 5g; Total Carbs: 1g; Fiber: 0g; Net Carbs: 1g; **Macros:** Fat: 86%; Protein: 11%; Carbs: 3%

Creamy Grapefruit-Tarragon Dressing

SERVES 4 TO 6 | PREP TIME: 5 minutes

½ cup avocado oil mayonnaise
2 tablespoons Dijon mustard
1 teaspoon dried tarragon or
   1 tablespoon chopped fresh
   tarragon
Zest and juice of ½ grapefruit
   (about 2 tablespoons juice)

½ teaspoon salt
¼ teaspoon freshly ground
   black pepper
1 to 2 tablespoons water
   (optional)

In a large mason jar or glass measuring cup, shake the mayonnaise, Dijon, tarragon, grapefruit zest and juice, salt, and pepper until smooth and creamy. If a thinner dressing is preferred, thin out with water.

Per Serving: (2 tablespoons): Calories: 86; Fat: 7g; Protein: 1g; Total Carbs: 6g; Fiber: 0g; Net Carbs: 6g; **Macros:** Fat: 69%; Protein: 2%; Carbs: 29%

Harissa Oil

MAKES 1 CUP | PREP TIME: 15 minutes, plus 30 minutes to steep | COOK TIME: 5 minutes

4 to 6 medium-hot dried chiles
   (ancho or guajillo work well)
2 to 4 hot dried chiles de
   árbol (optional; these are
   very hot)
2 tablespoons coriander seeds
1 tablespoon cumin seeds

1 teaspoon caraway seeds
4 large garlic cloves, chopped
2 tablespoons tomato paste
2 teaspoons smoked paprika
1 teaspoon salt
1 cup extra-virgin olive
   oil, divided

Remove the stems and tops from the dried chiles and discard any loose seeds. Place the chiles in a medium bowl and cover with boiling water. Allow to steep 30 minutes or until softened. Remove from the water, drain off any excess liquid, and roughly chop, discarding any seeds and membranes. In a large dry skillet, toast the coriander, cumin, and caraway seeds over medium-high heat until very fragrant. Transfer to the bowl of a food processor or blender. Add the chopped chiles, garlic, tomato paste, paprika, and salt and pulse until a thick paste forms. With the food processor or blender running, stream in ¾ cup olive oil until well combined. Transfer to large glass jar and stir in the remaining ¼ cup olive oil. Refrigerate in an airtight container for up to 3 weeks.

Per Serving: (2 tablespoons): Calories: 266; Fat: 26g; Protein: 2g; Total Carbs: 6g; Fiber: 1g; Net Carbs: 5g; **Macros:** Fat: 88%; Protein: 3%; Carbs: 9%

Chimichurri

SERVES 8 (2 TABLESPOONS PER SERVING) | PREP TIME: 5 minutes | COOK TIME: 5 minutes

1 cup fresh cilantro
2 cups fresh parsley
¼ cup red wine vinegar
3 garlic cloves, halved
½ teaspoon ground cumin

½ teaspoon red pepper flakes
¼ teaspoon pink Himalayan salt
¼ cup extra-virgin olive oil

Place the cilantro, parsley, vinegar, garlic, cumin, red pepper flakes, and salt in a blender or food processor. Blend until the

ingredients start to break down, about 20 seconds. Slowly pour in the oil, and continue to blend until the oil is fully incorporated.

Per Serving: Calories: 66; Fat: 6g; Protein: 1g; Total Carbs: 2g; Fiber: 1g; Net Carbs: 1g; **Macros:** Fat: 82%; Protein: 6%; Carbs: 12%

Traditional Caesar Dressing

MAKES 1½ CUPS | PREP TIME: 10 minutes, plus 10 minutes cooling time | COOK TIME: 5 minutes

2 teaspoons minced garlic
4 large egg yolks
¼ cup wine vinegar
½ teaspoon dry mustard
Dash Worcestershire sauce

1 cup extra-virgin olive oil
¼ cup freshly squeezed
   lemon juice
Sea salt
Freshly ground black pepper

In a small saucepan, add the garlic, egg yolks, vinegar, mustard, and Worcestershire sauce and whisk over low heat. Until it thickens and is bubbly, about 5 minutes. Remove the saucepan from the heat and let it stand for about 10 minutes to cool. Transfer the mixture to a large bowl and whisk in the olive oil in a thin stream. Whisk in the lemon juice and season the dressing with salt and pepper. Refrigerate the dressing in an airtight container for up to 3 days.

Per Serving: (2 tablespoons): Calories: 180; Fat: 20g; Protein: 1g; Total Carbs: 1g; Fiber: 0g; Net Carbs: 1g; **Macros:** Fat: 96%; Protein: 2%; Carbs: 2%

Ranch Dressing

SERVES 16 | PREP TIME: 10 minutes | COOK TIME: 1 hour

1 cup mayonnaise
1 cup sour cream
¼ cup buttermilk
1 tablespoon onion powder
1 tablespoon dried parsley

2 teaspoons garlic powder
½ teaspoon salt
½ teaspoon dried dill
½ teaspoon mustard powder
¼ teaspoon celery salt

In a large bowl, mix the mayonnaise, sour cream, buttermilk, onion powder, parsley, garlic powder, salt, dill, mustard powder, and celery salt. Whisk well to incorporate. Refrigerate for 1 hour before serving. Refrigerate in an airtight container for up to 2 weeks.

Per Serving: (1 tablespoon): Calories: 93; Fat: 8g; Protein: 1g; Total Carbs: 5g; Fiber: 0g; Net Carbs: 5g; **Macros:** Fat: 75%; Protein: 4%; Carbs: 21%

Mustard Shallot Vinaigrette

SERVES 8 | TOTAL TIME: 10 minutes

½ cup olive oil
½ cup apple cider vinegar
3 tablespoons Dijon mustard
1 shallot, minced

½ teaspoon salt
¼ teaspoon freshly ground
   black pepper

In a blender or food processor, add the olive oil, cider vinegar, mustard, shallot, salt, and pepper. Pulse for about 1 minute, until combined. Refrigerate in an airtight container for up to 2 weeks.

Per Serving: (1 tablespoon): Calories: 117; Fat: 13g; Protein: 0g; Total Carbs: 1g; Fiber: 0g; Net Carbs: 1g; **Macros:** Fat: 97%; Protein: 0%; Carbs: 3%

Herbed Balsamic Dressing

MAKES 1 CUP | PREP TIME: 4 minutes

1 cup extra-virgin olive oil
¼ cup balsamic vinegar
2 tablespoons chopped
  fresh oregano

1 teaspoon chopped fresh basil
1 teaspoon minced garlic
Sea salt
Freshly ground black pepper

Whisk the olive oil and vinegar in a small bowl until emulsified, about 3 minutes. Whisk in the oregano, basil, and garlic until well combined, about 1 minute. Season the dressing with salt and pepper. Refrigerate the dressing to an airtight container, for up to 1 week.

Per Serving: (1 tablespoon): Calories: 83; Fat: 9g; Protein: 0g; Total Carbs: 0g; Fiber: 0g; Net Carbs: 0g; **Macros**: Fat: 100%; Protein: 0%; Carbs: 0%

Garlic-Rosemary Infused Olive Oil

MAKES 1 CUP | PREP TIME: 5 minutes | COOK TIME: 45 minutes

1 cup extra-virgin olive oil
4 large garlic cloves, smashed

4 (4- to 5-inch) sprigs
  rosemary

In a medium skillet, heat the olive oil, garlic, and rosemary sprigs over low heat. Cook until fragrant and garlic is very tender, 30 to 45 minutes, stirring occasionally. Don't let the oil get too hot or the garlic will burn and become bitter. Remove from the heat and allow to cool slightly. Remove the garlic and rosemary with a slotted spoon and pour the oil into a glass container. Allow to cool completely before covering. Store covered at room temperature for up to 3 months.

Per Serving: (2 tablespoons): Calories: 241; Fat: 27g; Protein: 0g; Total Carbs: 1g; Fiber: 0g; Net Carbs: 1g; **Macros**: Fat: 99%; Protein: 0%; Carbs: 1%

Ginger-Lime Dressing

SERVES 8 | PREP TIME: 5 minutes

1 cup extra-virgin olive oil
Juice of 3 limes
2 inches fresh ginger, peeled
1 teaspoon ground cumin

⅓ teaspoon ground
  cardamom
1 drop liquid stevia
Sea salt

Blend the oil, lime juice, ginger, cumin, cardamom, stevia, and salt in a high-powered blender. Refrigerate the dressing in a covered container for up to 1 week.

Per Serving: Calories: 245; Fat: 27g; Protein: 0g; Total Carbs: 0g; Fiber: 0g; Net Carbs: 0g; **Macros**: Fat: 100%; Protein: 0%; Carbs: 0%

Garlic Herb Marinade

MAKES 1 CUP | PREP TIME: 15 minutes

½ cup olive oil
Juice and zest of ½ lemon
Juice and zest of ½ lime
1½ teaspoons minced garlic
2 teaspoons chopped
  fresh basil

2 teaspoons chopped
  fresh thyme
1 teaspoon chopped
  fresh oregano
¼ teaspoon sea salt

Whisk together the olive oil, lemon and lime juices and zests, garlic, basil, thyme, oregano, and salt in a medium bowl until well combined. Refrigerate the marinade in a sealed container for up to 1 week.

Per Serving: (2 tablespoons): Calories: 122; Fat: 14g; Protein: 0g; Total Carbs: 1g; Fiber: 0g; Net Carbs: 1g; **Macros**: Fat: 97%; Protein: 0%; Carbs: 3%

Lemon-Tahini Dressing

SERVES 8 TO 10 | PREP TIME: 5 minutes

½ cup tahini
¼ cup freshly squeezed lemon
  juice (about 2 to 3 lemons)
¼ cup extra-virgin olive oil

1 garlic clove, finely minced or
  ½ teaspoon garlic powder
2 teaspoons salt

In a glass mason jar with a lid, combine the tahini, lemon juice, olive oil, garlic, and salt. Cover and shake well until combined and creamy. Refrigerate for up to 2 weeks.

Per Serving: (2 tablespoons): Calories: 121; Fat: 12g; Protein: 2g; Total Carbs: 3g; Fiber: 1g; Net Carbs: 2g; **Macros**: Fat: 84%; Protein: 6%; Carbs: 10%

Lemon Poppy Seed Dressing

MAKES 1¾ CUPS | PREP TIME: 5 minutes

1 cup extra-virgin olive oil
½ cup freshly squeezed
  lemon juice
2 tablespoons apple
  cider vinegar

2 tablespoons Swerve
1 tablespoon poppy seeds
Sea salt

Place the olive oil, lemon juice, vinegar, Swerve, and poppy seeds in a medium bowl and whisk to combine well. Season with salt. Refrigerate the dressing in an airtight container for up to 2 weeks.

Per Serving: (2 tablespoons): Calories: 142; Fat: 16g; Protein: 0g; Total Carbs: 1g; Fiber: 0g; Net Carbs: 1g; **Macros**: Fat: 100%; Protein: 0%; Carbs: 0%

Bagna Cauda

SERVES 8 TO 10 | PREP TIME: 5 minutes |
COOK TIME: 20 minutes

½ cup extra-virgin olive oil
¼ cup (½ stick) butter
8 anchovy fillets, very
  finely chopped

4 large garlic cloves,
  finely minced
½ teaspoon salt
½ teaspoon freshly ground
  black pepper

In a small saucepan, heat the olive oil and butter over medium-low heat until the butter is melted. Add the anchovies and garlic and stir to combine. Add the salt and pepper and reduce the heat to low. Cook, occasionally stirring, until the anchovies are very soft and the mixture is very fragrant, about 20 minutes. Serve warm, drizzled over steamed vegetables, as a dipping sauce for raw veggies or cooked artichokes, or use as a salad dressing.

Per Serving: (2 tablespoons): Calories: 181; Fat: 20g; Protein: 1g; Total Carbs: 1g; Fiber: 0g; Net Carbs: 1g; **Macros:** Fat: 96%; Protein: 3%; Carbs: 1%

Pesto

SERVES 8 | PREP TIME: 5 minutes | COOK TIME: 0 minutes

2 cups fresh basil leaves
¼ teaspoon sea salt
1 garlic clove
½ cup extra-virgin olive oil
¼ cup ground pine nuts
¼ cup grated Parmesan cheese

In a blender, blend the basil, salt, garlic, and olive oil until mostly smooth. Stir in the pine nuts and Parmesan cheese. Serve immediately or Refrigerate in a covered container for up to two days.

Per Serving: (2 tablespoons): Calories: 158; Fat: 17g; Protein: 2g; Total Carbs: 1g; Fiber: 1g; Net Carbs: 0g; **Macros:** Fat: 97%; Protein: 2%; Carbs: 1%

Hollandaise

MAKES 2 CUPS | PREP TIME: 20 minutes |
COOK TIME: 10 minutes, plus 15 minutes cooling time

1½ cups unsalted butter
4 large egg yolks
2 teaspoons cold water
Juice of 1 small lemon, about 4 teaspoons
Pinch sea salt

Place a medium saucepan over low heat and melt the butter. Remove from the heat and let the melted butter stand for 5 minutes. Skim the foam off the top of the butter. Very slowly pour the clarified butter (it should be a clear yellow color) into a container, leaving the milky solids. Let the clarified butter cool in the container for 15 minutes. Put a medium saucepan with about 3 inches of water in it over medium heat until the water simmers gently. In a large bowl, whisk the egg yolks and 2 teaspoons of cold water until they are foamy and light, about 3 minutes. Add 3 or 4 drops of the lemon juice and whisk for about 1 minute. Place the bowl onto the mouth of the saucepan, making sure the bottom of the bowl does not touch the simmering water. Whisk the yolks until they thicken a little, about 1 to 2 minutes, then remove the bowl. Add all the clarified butter in a thin stream to the yolk mixture, whisking continuously, until the sauce is thick and smooth. Whisk in the remaining lemon juice and the salt. Use immediately.

Per Serving: (1 tablespoon): Calories: 173; Fat: 17g; Protein: 5g; Total Carbs: 1g; Fiber: 0g; Net Carbs: 1g; **Macros:** Fat: 86%; Protein: 11%; Carbs: 3%

Herb-Kale Pesto

MAKES 1½ CUPS | PREP TIME: 15 minutes

1 cup chopped kale
1 cup fresh basil leaves
3 garlic cloves
2 teaspoons nutritional yeast
¼ cup extra-virgin olive oil

Place the kale, basil, garlic, and yeast in a food processor and pulse until the mixture is finely chopped, about 3 minutes. With the food processor running, drizzle the olive oil into the pesto until a thick paste forms. Add a little water if the pesto is too thick. Refrigerate the pesto in an airtight container for up to 1 week.

Per Serving: (2 tablespoons): Calories: 44; Fat: 4g; Protein: 1g; Total Carbs: 1g; Fiber: 0g; Net Carbs: 1g; **Macros:** Fat: 82%; Protein: 9%; Carbs: 9%

Spinach Hemp Pesto

MAKES 2 CUPS | PREP TIME: 15 minutes

1 cup spinach
1 cup fresh basil
½ cup fresh oregano
¼ cup hemp hearts
2 tablespoons freshly squeezed lemon juice
2 garlic cloves
½ cup extra-virgin olive oil
Sea salt
Freshly ground black pepper

Place the spinach, basil, oregano, hemp hearts, lemon juice, and garlic in a blender and pulse until the mixture is very finely chopped. Drizzle in the olive oil in a thin stream while the blender is running, until the pesto is the desired texture. Season with salt and pepper. Refrigerate the pesto in a sealed container for up to 2 weeks.

Per Serving: (2 tablespoons): Calories: 78; Fat: 8g; Protein: 1g; Total Carbs: 1g; Fiber: 1g; Net Carbs: 0g; **Macros:** Fat: 92%; Protein: 5%; Carbs: 3%

Creamy Mayonnaise

MAKES 4 CUPS | PREP TIME: 10 minutes

2 large eggs
2 tablespoons Dijon mustard
1½ cups extra-virgin olive oil
¼ cup freshly squeezed lemon juice
Sea salt
Freshly ground black pepper

Place the eggs and mustard in the processor bowl and blend until very smooth. While the processor is running, slowly add the oil in a thin stream until the mayonnaise is thick and completely emulsified. Add the lemon juice and process until smooth. Season with salt and pepper.

Per Serving: (2 tablespoons): Calories: 61; Fat: 7g; Protein: 0g; Total Carbs: 0g; Fiber: 0g; Net Carbs: 0g; **Macros:** Fat: 97%; Protein: 2%; Carbs: 1%

Zesty Orange Aioli

SERVES 8 TO 10 | PREP TIME: 5 minutes, plus 1 hour to rest

2 large egg yolks
2 garlic cloves, finely minced
Zest and juice of 1 orange
1 ½ teaspoons salt
1 teaspoon red pepper flakes
1 cup extra-virgin olive oil

In a blender or large bowl, if using an immersion blender, combine the egg yolks, garlic, orange zest and juice, salt, and red pepper flakes and pulse until well combined and pasty. With the blender running, stream in the olive oil until just combined. Let sit at room temperature at least 1 hour before serving. Store in the refrigerator.

Per Serving: (2 tablespoons): Calories: 203, Fat: 23g; Protein: 1g; Total Carbs: 0g; Fiber: 0g; Net Carbs: 0g; **Macros:** Fat: 98%; Protein: 1%; Carbs: 1%

Chimichurri Sauce

SERVES 12 | PREP TIME: 10 minutes

1 cup extra-virgin olive oil	1 tablespoon dried oregano
½ cup fresh parsley	1 garlic clove
⅓ cup fresh cilantro	1 shallot
¼ cup fresh mint	Juice of 1 lemon

Put all the ingredients into a high-powered blender and pulse until well combined and a bit chunky. Refrigerate the chimichurri in a covered container for up to 1 week.

Per Serving: Calories: 164; Fat: 18g; Protein: 0g; Total Carbs: 1g; Fiber: 0g; Net Carbs: 1g; **Macros:** Fat: 98%; Protein: 0%; Carbs: 2%

Thai-Style Peanut Sauce

SERVES 6 | PREP TIME: 5 minutes

½ cup natural peanut butter	1 teaspoon sesame oil
1 tablespoon miso paste	⅓ cup freshly squeezed
1 shallot, peeled	lime juice
3 tablespoons peeled and finely chopped fresh ginger	2 tablespoons monk fruit sweetener

Blend the peanut butter, miso, shallot, ginger, sesame oil, lime juice, and sweetener in a high-powered blender. Refrigerate the sauce to an airtight container until ready to use.

Per Serving: Calories: 181; Fat: 15g; Protein: 7g; Total Carbs: 9g; Fiber: 2g; Net Carbs: 7g; **Macros:** Fat: 68%; Protein: 14%; Carbs: 18%

Bleu Cheese Sauce

SERVES 8 | PREP TIME: 10 minutes | COOK TIME: 1 hour | TOTAL TIME: 1¼ hours

1 tablespoon butter	¼ cup unsweetened
1 tablespoon almond flour	almond milk
½ cup chicken broth	4 ounces bleu cheese
½ cup heavy (whipping) cream	

In a large saucepan over medium-high heat, melt the butter. Add the almond flour and reduce the heat to low. Whisk for 2 to 3 minutes, and add the chicken broth, heavy cream, and almond milk. Whisk to combine. Increase the heat to medium and whisk in the bleu cheese until it melts and the sauce is creamy. Pour the sauce into a bowl and chill in the refrigerator for at least 1 hour. Refrigerate in an airtight container for up to 1 week.

Per Serving: (1 tablespoon): Calories: 98; Fat: 9g; Protein: 4g; Total Carbs: 1g; Fiber: 0g; Net Carbs: 1g; **Macros:** Fat: 80%; Protein: 16%; Carbs: 4%

Barbecue Sauce

SERVES 10 | PREP TIME: 10 minutes | COOK TIME: 30 minutes

1 tablespoon butter	1 tablespoon Worcester-
½ cup finely chopped onion	shire sauce
1½ tablespoons minced garlic	3 tablespoons mustard
1¼ cups sugar-free cola	1 teaspoon cayenne pepper
¾ cup tomato paste	1 teaspoon liquid smoke
½ cup water	½ teaspoon paprika
¼ cup sugar-free ketchup	½ teaspoon freshly ground black pepper

In a large saucepan over medium-high heat, melt the butter. Add the onion. Cook until translucent, about 4 minutes. Add the garlic and cook for 1 minute. Add the cola, tomato paste, water, ketchup, Worcestershire sauce, mustard, cayenne, liquid smoke, paprika, and pepper. Whisk well to combine. Bring the sauce to a simmer. Cook for 25 minutes, stirring occasionally, until thickened.

Per Serving: (1 tablespoon): Calories: 47; Fat: 2g; Protein: 2g; Total Carbs: 7g; Fiber: 1g; Net Carbs: 5g; **Macros:** Fat: 33%; Protein: 15%; Carbs: 52%

Garlicky Alfredo Sauce

SERVES 8 | PREP TIME: 15 minutes | COOK TIME: 12 minutes

¼ cup butter	1½ cups freshly grated
2 tablespoons minced sweet onion	Asiago cheese
2 teaspoons minced garlic	1 teaspoon chopped fresh basil
2 large egg yolks	Sea salt
1 cup heavy (whipping) cream	Freshly ground black pepper

In a large saucepan over medium heat, melt the butter. Sauté the onion and garlic until softened, about 3 minutes. Whisk in the egg yolks and cream. Bring the sauce to a boil, and reduce the heat to low, and simmer until it thickens, about 5 minutes. Whisk in the cheese and basil, and simmer for 2 minutes. Season the sauce with salt and pepper, and serve over chicken or vegetables.

Per Serving: (½ cup): Calories: 186; Fat: 18g; Protein: 6g; Total Carbs: 1g; Fiber: 0g; Net Carbs: 0g; **Macros:** Fat: 85%; Protein: 13%; Carbs: 2%

Sugar-Free Ketchup

SERVES 16 | TOTAL TIME: 1¼ hours

1½ cups tomato paste	½ teaspoon salt
¼ cup water	½ teaspoon cinnamon
¼ cup apple cider vinegar	¼ teaspoon garlic powder
2 tablespoons Worcester- shire sauce	⅛ teaspoon freshly ground black pepper
1 tablespoon mustard	⅛ teaspoon ground cloves

In a large bowl, combine the tomato paste, water, cider vinegar, Worcestershire sauce, mustard, salt, cinnamon, garlic powder, pepper, and cloves. Whisk thoroughly to combine. Transfer to an airtight container. Chill for 1 hour to allow the flavors to incorporate.

Per Serving: (1 tablespoon): Calories: 24; Fat: 0g; Protein: 1g; Total Carbs: 5g; Fiber: 1g; Net Carbs: 4; **Macros:** Fat: 0%; Protein: 20%; Carbs: 80%

Alfredo Sauce

SERVES 6 | PREP TIME: 5 minutes | COOK TIME: 10 minutes

2 tablespoons butter	⅛ teaspoon paprika
2 tablespoons almond flour	½ cup unsweetened
⅛ teaspoon freshly ground black pepper	almond milk
¼ teaspoon salt	½ cup heavy (whipping) cream
	3 tablespoons sour cream

In a large saucepan over low heat, melt the butter. Add the almond flour, pepper, salt, and paprika. Whisk until smooth.

Slowly add the almond milk, stirring constantly to avoid forming lumps. Add the heavy cream and sour cream. Continue to whisk. Cook on low for 8 to 10 minutes, or until thickened. Refrigerate in an airtight container for up to 1 week.

Per Serving: (1 tablespoon): Calories: 99; Fat: 10g; Protein: 1g; Total Carbs: 1g; Fiber: 0g; Net Carbs: 1g; **Macros:** Fat: 92%; Protein: 4%; Carbs: 4%

Classic Bolognese Sauce

SERVES 10 | PREP TIME: 15 minutes | COOK TIME: 7 to 8 hours on low

3 tablespoons extra-virgin olive oil, divided
1 pound ground pork
½ pound ground beef
½ pound bacon, chopped
1 sweet onion, chopped
1 tablespoon minced garlic

2 celery stalks, chopped
1 carrot, chopped
2 (28-ounce) cans diced tomatoes
½ cup coconut milk
¼ cup apple cider vinegar

Lightly grease the insert of the slow cooker with 1 tablespoon of the olive oil. In a large skillet over medium-high heat, heat the remaining 2 tablespoons of the olive oil. Add the pork, beef, and bacon, and sauté until cooked through, about 7 minutes. Stir in the onion and garlic and sauté for an additional 2 minutes. Transfer the meat mixture to the insert and add the celery, carrot, tomatoes, coconut milk, and apple cider vinegar. Cover and cook on low for 7 to 8 hours. Serve, or cool completely, and refrigerate in a sealed container for up to 4 days or freeze for 1 month.

Per Serving: Calories: 333; Fat: 23g; Protein: 25g; Total Carbs: 9g; Fiber: 3g; Net Carbs: 6g; **Macros:** Fat: 62%; Protein: 30%; Carbs; 8%

Hot Crab Sauce

MAKES 4 CUPS | PREP TIME: 10 minutes | COOK TIME: 5 to 6 hours on low

8 ounces cream cheese
8 ounces goat cheese
1 cup sour cream
½ cup grated Asiago cheese
1 sweet onion, finely chopped

1 tablespoon granulated erythritol
2 teaspoons minced garlic
12 ounces crabmeat, flaked
1 scallion, white and green parts, chopped

In a large bowl, stir the cream cheese, goat cheese, sour cream, Asiago cheese, onion, erythritol, garlic, crabmeat, and scallion until well mixed. Transfer the mixture to an 8-by-4-inch loaf pan and place the pan in the insert of the slow cooker. Cover and cook on low for 5 to 6 hours. Serve warm.

Per Serving: (½ cup): Calories: 361; Fat: 28g; Protein: 17g; Total Carbs: 10g; Fiber: 2g; Net Carbs: 8g; **Macros:** Fat: 70%; Protein: 20%; Carbs: 10%

Mustard Cream Sauce

SERVES 6 | PREP TIME: 5 minutes | COOK TIME: 10 minutes

1 tablespoon butter
1 tablespoon minced onion
1 teaspoon minced garlic
½ cup heavy (whipping) cream
½ cup sour cream

1 tablespoon mustard
¼ teaspoon salt
⅛ teaspoon freshly ground black pepper

In a large saucepan over low heat, melt the butter. Add the onion and garlic. Cook for 5 minutes, until tender. Add the heavy cream and sour cream. Whisk until the consistency begins to thin. Whisk in the mustard, salt, and pepper. Remove from the heat. Allow the sauce to cool. Refrigerate in an airtight container for up to 1 week.

Per Serving: (1 tablespoon): Calories: 103; Fat: 10g; Protein: 1g; Total Carbs: 2g; Fiber: 0g; Net Carbs: 2g; **Macros:** Fat: 88%; Protein: 4%; Carbs: 8%

Enchilada Sauce

MAKES 4 CUPS | PREP TIME: 10 minutes | COOK TIME: 7 to 8 hours on low

¼ cup extra-virgin olive oil, divided
2 cups puréed tomatoes
1 cup water
1 sweet onion, chopped

2 jalapeño peppers, chopped
2 teaspoons minced garlic
2 tablespoons chili powder
1 teaspoon ground coriander

Lightly grease the insert of the slow cooker with 1 tablespoon of the olive oil. Place the remaining 3 tablespoons of the olive oil, tomatoes, water, onion, jalapeño peppers, garlic, chili powder, and coriander in the insert. Cover and cook on low 7 to 8 hours. Serve over poultry or meat. Refrigerate the cooled sauce in a sealed container for up to 1 week.

Per Serving: (½ cup): Calories: 92; Fat: 8g; Protein: 2g; Total Carbs: 4g; Fiber: 2g; Net Carbs: 2g; **Macros:** Fat: 78%; Protein: 7%; Carbs: 15%

Pico de Gallo

MAKES 2 CUPS | PREP TIME: 10 minutes, plus 20 minutes to marinate

¾ cup diced white onion
¾ cup seeded and diced Roma tomatoes (about 4)
½ cup chopped fresh cilantro

3 tablespoons freshly squeezed lime juice
1 tablespoon minced jalapeño pepper
1 teaspoon salt

In a small bowl, combine all the ingredients. Allow the flavors to develop for 15 to 20 minutes before serving.

Per serving: Calories: 8; Fat: 0g; Protein: <1g; Total Carbs: 2g; Fiber: 1g; Net Carbs: 1g; **Macros:** Fat: 0%; Protein: <1%; Carbs: 99%

Teriyaki Sauce

SERVES 8 | PREP TIME: 10 minutes | COOK TIME: 15 minutes

⅓ cup olive oil
1 teaspoon minced garlic
1 tablespoon minced fresh ginger
1 cup tamari soy sauce
2 tablespoons Worcestershire sauce

2 tablespoons white vinegar
20 drops liquid stevia, or other liquid sugar substitute
½ teaspoon freshly ground black pepper
¼ teaspoon orange extract

In a large saucepan over medium-high heat, heat the olive oil for about 1 minute. Add the garlic and ginger. Cook for 1 minute, until fragrant. Add the tamari, Worcestershire sauce, vinegar, stevia, pepper, and orange extract. Whisk to combine. Bring to a boil, reduce the heat to low, and simmer for 15 minutes, until reduced by about half. Refrigerate in an airtight container or use immediately.

Per Serving: (1 tablespoon); Calories: 110; Fat: 8g; Protein: 4g; Total Carbs: 4g; Fiber: 0g; Net Carbs: 4g; **Macros:** Fat: 70%; Protein: 15%; Carbs: 15%

Pasta Sauce
SERVES 8 | PREP TIME: 5 minutes | COOK TIME: 10 minutes

3 cups diced tomatoes
¼ cup olive oil
2 tablespoons minced garlic
1 tablespoon chopped
   fresh basil

1 teaspoon onion powder
1 teaspoon red pepper flakes
½ teaspoon salt
¼ teaspoon freshly ground
   black pepper

In a blender or food processor, pulse the tomatoes once or twice so the tomatoes still have texture. In a large saucepan over medium heat, heat the olive oil. Add the garlic. Cook for 1 minute, until fragrant. Add the tomatoes, basil, onion powder, red pepper flakes, salt, and pepper. Whisk to combine. Bring the mixture to a simmer. Cook for 10 minutes. Remove from the heat and allow to cool. Refrigerate in an airtight container for up to 3 weeks.

Per Serving: (1 tablespoon): Calories: 69; Fat: 7g; Protein: 1g; Total Carbs: 3g; Fiber: 1g; Net Carbs: 2g; **Macros:** Fat: 80%; Protein: 5%; Carbs: 15%

Pizza Sauce
SERVES 16 | TOTAL TIME: 15 minutes

2 cups diced tomatoes
¼ cup olive oil
¼ cup chopped onion
2 tablespoons minced garlic
1 cup tomato paste
2 teaspoons onion powder

1 teaspoon red pepper flakes
½ teaspoon salt
¼ teaspoon freshly ground
   black pepper
3 tablespoons chopped
   fresh basil

In a blender or food processor, pulse the tomatoes once or twice so the tomatoes still have texture. In a large saucepan over medium heat, heat the olive oil for about 1 minute. Add the onion and garlic. Cook for 2 minutes, until tender. Add the tomatoes, tomato paste, onion powder, red pepper flakes, salt, and pepper to the saucepan. Stir to combine. Bring to a simmer. Cook for 10 minutes. Remove from the heat and allow to cool. Add the basil. Stir to incorporate. Refrigerate in an airtight container for up to 3 weeks.

Per Serving: (1 tablespoon): Calories: 46; Fat: 3g; Protein: 1g; Total Carbs: 4g; Fiber: 1g; Net Carbs: 3g; **Macros:** Fat: 57%; Protein: 9%; Carbs: 34%

Pesto Sauce
SERVES 14 | TOTAL TIME: 15 minutes

4 cups fresh basil, chopped
½ cup olive oil
⅓ cup pine nuts
2 garlic cloves, minced

¼ cup freshly grated Parmesan cheese
¼ cup freshly grated
   pecorino cheese
1 teaspoon salt

In a blender or food processor, add the basil, olive oil, pine nuts, and garlic. Pulse in short bursts while slowly adding the

Parmesan and pecorino cheeses. Add the salt. Blend until smooth. Refrigerate in an airtight container for up to 3 days.

Per Serving: (1 tablespoon): Calories: 106; Fat: 11g; Protein: 3g; Total Carbs: 1g; Fiber: 0g; Net Carbs: 1g; **Macros:** Fat: 86%; Protein: 10%; Carbs: 4%

Herbed Marinara Sauce
SERVES 4 | PREP TIME: 10 minutes

1 (14-ounce) can unsweetened
   whole tomatoes
2 tablespoons extra-virgin
   olive oil
2 tablespoons grated Parmesan cheese
1 tablespoon balsamic vinegar
1 teaspoon chopped
   fresh basil

1 teaspoon chopped
   fresh oregano
1 teaspoon chopped
   fresh parsley
Pinch red pepper flakes
Pinch sea salt
Pinch freshly ground
   black pepper

In a food processor, pulse the tomatoes, olive oil, Parmesan cheese, vinegar, basil, oregano, parsley, red pepper flakes, sea salt, and pepper until the sauce is smooth. Refrigerate the sauce in a sealed container for up to 5 days.

Per Serving: (½ cup): Calories: 96; Fat: 8g; Protein: 2g; Total Carbs: 4g; Fiber: 2g; Net Carbs: 2g; **Macros:** Fat: 75%; Protein: 8%; Carbs: 17%

Indonesian Peanut Sauce
MAKES 2 CUPS | PREP TIME: 5 minutes

1 cup natural peanut butter
¼ cup toasted sesame oil
¼ cup freshly squeezed
   lemon juice
2 tablespoons tahini

1 tablespoon soy sauce
½ teaspoon red pepper flakes
¼ teaspoon stevia
Water, for thinning

In a blender, blend the peanut butter, sesame oil, lemon juice, tahini, soy sauce, red pepper flakes, and stevia until very smooth. Thin the sauce with water if you want. Refrigerate the sauce in a sealed container for up to 1 week.

Per Serving: (2 tablespoons): Calories: 147; Fat: 13g; Protein: 6g; Total Carbs: 4g; Fiber: 1g; Net Carbs: 3g; **Macros:** Fat: 75%; Protein: 15%; Carbs: 10%

Herb Pesto
MAKES 2 CUPS | PREP TIME: 15 minutes

1 cup fresh basil
½ cup fresh oregano
½ cup fresh mint
¼ cup freshly squeezed
   lemon juice

½ cup walnuts
1 garlic clove
1 cup extra-virgin olive oil

In a blender, pulse the basil, oregano, mint, lemon juice, walnuts, and garlic until the mixture is very finely chopped. Drizzle in all of the olive oil in a thin stream while the blender is running. Scrape down the sides of the blender, and pulse until the pesto is uniform. Refrigerate the pesto in a sealed container up to 2 weeks.

Per Serving: (1 tablespoon): Calories: 72; Fat: 8g; Protein: 1g; Total Carbs: 1g; Fiber: 1g; Net Carbs: 0g; **Macros:** Fat: 90%; Protein: 5%; Carbs: 5%

Bacon Chutney

MAKES 1½ CUPS | PREP TIME: 10 minutes |
COOK TIME: 27 minutes

1 tablespoon coconut oil
½ pound bacon, chopped
1 sweet onion, diced
1 (14-ounce) can diced
   unsweetened tomatoes

½ teaspoon stevia
2 tablespoons apple
   cider vinegar

In a large saucepan over medium heat, heat the coconut oil. Cook the bacon until it is cooked through and crispy, about 4 minutes. Using a slotted spoon, remove the bacon to a bowl, and set aside. Sauté the onion until softened, about 3 minutes. Add the tomatoes, reserved bacon, stevia, and vinegar to the saucepan. Bring the mixture to a boil, reduce the heat to low, and simmer until the chutney is thick, about 20 minutes. Spoon the chutney into a container, and let it cool before refrigerating it, covered, for up to 1 week.

Per Serving: (1 tablespoon): Calories: 62; Fat: 5g; Protein: 4g; Total Carbs: 1g; Fiber: 0g; Net Carbs: 0g; **Macros:** Fat: 69%; Protein: 25%; Carbs: 6%

Bacon Jam

MAKES 3 CUPS | PREP TIME: 10 minutes | COOK TIME: 3 to
4 hours on high

3 tablespoons bacon fat,
   melted and divided
1 pound cooked bacon,
   chopped into ½-inch pieces
1 sweet onion, diced

½ cup apple cider vinegar
¼ cup granulated erythritol
1 tablespoon minced garlic
1 cup brewed decaffein-
   ated coffee

Lightly grease the insert of the slow cooker with 1 tablespoon of the bacon fat. Add the remaining 2 tablespoons of the bacon fat, bacon, onion, apple cider vinegar, erythritol, garlic, and coffee to the insert. Stir to combine. Cook uncovered for 3 to 4 hours on high, until the liquid has thickened and reduced. Cool completely. Refrigerate the bacon jam in a sealed container for up to 3 weeks.

Per Serving: (¼ cup): Calories: 52; Fat: 5g; Protein: 1g; Total Carbs: 1g; Fiber: 0g; Net Carbs: 1g; **Macros:** Fat: 85%; Protein: 5%; Carbs: 10%

Cinnamon-Caramel Sauce

MAKES 1 CUP | PREP TIME: 2 minutes |
COOK TIME: 10 minutes

½ cup butter
½ cup heavy (whipping) cream

1 teaspoon stevia
¼ teaspoon ground cinnamon

In a large saucepan over low heat, cook the butter until it becomes light brown and nutty smelling, about 4 minutes. Whisk in the cream, stevia, and cinnamon. Bring the mixture to a simmer, stirring constantly. Continue simmering until the sauce is thickened, about 2 minutes. Remove the saucepan from the heat, and continue to stir for at least 5 minutes, so that the sauce does not separate. Refrigerate the sauce in a sealed container for up to 4 days.

Per Serving: (2 tablespoons): Calories: 130; Fat: 14g; Protein: 1g; Total Carbs: 0g; Fiber: 0g; Net Carbs: 0g; **Macros:** Fat: 97%; Protein: 3%; Carbs: 0%

Pastry Cream

SERVES 6 | PREP TIME: 10 minutes, plus 2 hours to chill |
COOK TIME: 20 minutes

6 large egg yolks
3 cups unsweetened
   almond milk
½ teaspoon stevia

1 tablespoon arrow-
   root powder
1 teaspoon pure
   vanilla extract
1 tablespoon butter

In a medium bowl, beat the egg yolks and almond milk until well blended. Whisk the stevia and arrowroot together in a large saucepan, and gradually whisk in the milk mixture. Over medium-low heat, cook, stirring constantly, until the mixture comes to a boil and thickens, about 20 minutes. Remove the saucepan from the heat, and stir in the vanilla and butter. Transfer the pastry cream to a medium bowl, and press a piece of plastic wrap on the surface to prevent a skin from forming. Refrigerate the pastry cream until completely chilled, at least 2 hours.

Per Serving: (¾ cup): Calories: 89; Fat: 8g; Protein: 4g; Total Carbs: 1g; Fiber: 1g; Net Carbs: 0g; **Macros:** Fat: 78%; Protein: 17%; Carbs: 5%

Cheesy-Crust Pizza

SERVES 4 | PREP TIME: 10 minutes | COOK TIME: 20 to
25 minutes

1½ cups shredded mozzarella
   cheese, divided
½ cup Cheddar cheese
1 large egg
½ teaspoon garlic powder

¼ teaspoon salt
⅛ teaspoon freshly ground
   black pepper
¼ cup sugar-free pizza sauce
20 pepperoni slices

Preheat the oven to 450°F. In a large bowl, mix 1 cup of mozzarella cheese, Cheddar cheese, egg, garlic powder, salt, and pepper. Spread the cheese dough evenly on a parchment-lined 16-inch pizza pan. The crust should be thin, but without any holes. Bake the crust for 15 to 20 minutes, or until browned. Check the oven after 10 minutes to make sure it's not burning. Remove the crust from the oven. Turn the oven to broil. With paper towels, blot any excess grease from the crust. Spread the sauce over the crust. Top with the remaining ½ cup of mozzarella cheese and the pepperoni. Return the pan to the oven. Broil for 3 to 4 minutes, or until the cheese is melted and bubbling. Remove the pan from the oven. Cool the pizza for 3 to 5 minutes before slicing and serving.

Per Serving: (¼ of 16-inch pizza): Calories: 351; Fat: 27g; Protein: 24g; Total Carbs: 4g; Fiber: 0g; Net Carbs: 4g; **Macros:** Fat: 68%; Protein: 27%; Carbs: 5%

Margherita Pizza

SERVES 1 | PREP TIME: 10 minutes | COOK TIME: 5 minutes

1 tablespoon psyllium
   husk powder
¼ teaspoon salt
½ teaspoon dried oregano
2 large eggs
1 tablespoon avocado oil
3 tablespoons low-sugar marinara sauce

2 tablespoons grated Parmesan cheese
½ cup sliced mozza-
   rella cheese
1 tablespoon chopped
   fresh basil

Line a baking sheet with aluminum foil. Turn the oven to low broil. Combine the psyllium husk powder, salt, oregano, and eggs in a blender. Blend for 30 seconds. Set aside. In a medium skillet over high heat, warm the avocado oil. Pour the crust mixture into the pan, spreading it out into a circle. Cook until the edges are browned, then flip the crust and cook for an additional minute. Transfer the crust to the prepared baking sheet. Spread the marinara sauce over the top and cover with the Parmesan and mozzarella cheeses. Broil until the cheese is melted and bubbling. Top with the basil and enjoy.

Per Serving: Calories: 545; Fat: 41g; Protein: 32g; Total Carbs: 12g; Fiber: 8g; Net Carbs: 4g; **Macros:** Fat: 68%; Protein: 23%; Carbs: 9%

Barbecue Onion and Goat Cheese Flatbread

SERVES 2 | PREP TIME: 20 minutes | COOK TIME: 10 to 15 minutes

2 tablespoons coconut flour
1/8 teaspoon baking powder
4 large egg whites
1/4 teaspoon onion powder
1/4 teaspoon garlic powder
1/4 cup coconut milk

2 tablespoons sugar-free barbecue sauce
3/4 cup goat cheese, crumbled
1/2 cup sliced yellow onion
1/2 teaspoon minced garlic
1/8 teaspoon freshly ground black pepper

In a medium bowl, whisk the coconut flour, baking powder, egg whites, onion powder, garlic powder, and coconut milk until smooth. Heat a large skillet over medium-high heat. Pour the coconut batter into the skillet and tilt the skillet so the batter coats the entire pan. Cook for 2 minutes, or until the edges brown. Flip. Cook for 1 to 2 minutes more. Remove the flatbread from the skillet to a baking sheet. Preheat the oven to 425°F. Top the cooked flatbread evenly with the barbecue sauce, goat cheese, onion, garlic, and pepper. Bake for 5 to 7 minutes, or until the cheese melts. Remove it from the oven. Cool the flatbread for 2 minutes before slicing and serving.

Per Serving: (1/2 flatbread pizza): Calories: 565; Fat: 39g; Protein: 36g; Total Carbs: 17g; Fiber: 4g; Net Carbs: 13g; **Macros:** Fat: 62%; Protein: 26%; Carbs: 12%

Cauliflower Tortillas

SERVES 6 | PREP TIME: 10 minutes | COOK TIME: 20 minutes

3/4 head fresh cauliflower
2 large eggs
1/2 teaspoon salt

1/4 teaspoon freshly ground black pepper

Preheat the oven to 375°F. To the bowl of a food processor, add the cauliflower and pulse into very fine pieces. In a large microwave-safe bowl, microwave the prepared cauliflower on high, about 5 minutes. Stir the cauliflower and microwave for 2 minutes more. Stir it again. Using a dish towel or cheesecloth, drain all the excess water from the cauliflower. Return the cauliflower to the bowl. Add the eggs, salt, and pepper. Mix well to combine. On a parchment-lined baking sheet, use your hands to spread the mixture into 6 or 7 small circles, flattening them gently. Bake for 10 minutes. Remove the sheet from the oven. Carefully remove the cauliflower tortillas from the parchment and flip them. Bake for 6 to 7 minutes more. Crisp, as needed, in a lightly oiled skillet before serving.

Per Serving: (1 tortilla): Calories: 38; Fat: 2g; Protein: 3g; Total Carbs: 4g; Fiber: 2g; Net Carbs: 2g; **Macros:** Fat: 39%; Protein: 29%; Carbs: 32%

Versatile Sandwich Round

SERVES 1 | PREP TIME: 5 minutes | COOK TIME: 90 seconds

3 tablespoons almond flour
1 tablespoon extra-virgin olive oil
1 large egg

1/2 teaspoon dried rosemary, oregano, basil, thyme, or garlic powder (optional)
1/4 teaspoon baking powder
1/8 teaspoon salt

In a microwave-safe ramekin, combine the almond flour, olive oil, egg, rosemary (if using), baking powder, and salt. Mix well with a fork. Microwave for 90 seconds on high. Slide a knife around the edges of ramekin and flip to remove the bread.

Per Serving: Calories: 232; Fat: 22g; Protein: 8g; Total Carbs: 1g; Fiber: 0g; Net Carbs: 0g; **Macros:** Fat: 84%; Protein: 14%; Carbs: 2%

Almond Butter Bread

SERVES 12 | PREP TIME: 15 minutes | COOK TIME: 30 to 40 minutes

1/2 cup unflavored, unsweetened whey protein powder
1/8 teaspoon salt
2 teaspoons baking powder

1/2 cup unsweetened almond butter
4 large eggs
1 tablespoon butter for loaf pan

Heat the oven to 300°F. In a small bowl, whisk the whey, salt, and baking powder. In a large bowl, use an electric mixer to whip the almond butter until creamy. Add one egg at a time, beating well after each addition. Beat the batter until fluffy. Fold the whey mixture into the almond batter. Mix gently until smooth. Grease the inside of a loaf pan with butter. Transfer the mixture to the loaf pan and bake for 30 to 40 minutes, or until the center is set. Remove from the oven. Cool the loaf for 5 to 10 minutes. Run a knife along the inside edges of the pan to loosen the loaf, and remove it. Place the loaf on a cooling rack to cool completely, about 5 minutes more. Slice the bread, as needed, and refrigerate covered in plastic wrap.

Per Serving: (1 slice): Calories: 102; Fat: 8g; Protein: 7g; Total Carbs: 3g; Fiber: 0g; Net Carbs: 3g; **Macros:** Fat: 64%; Protein: 25%; Carbs: 11%

Coconut Almond Flour Bread

SERVES 12 | PREP TIME: 15 minutes | COOK TIME: 1 hour

10 tablespoons butter, melted, plus 1 tablespoon for the loaf pan
1 tablespoon honey
1 1/2 tablespoons apple cider vinegar

8 large eggs
3/4 cup almond flour
3/4 teaspoon baking soda
3/4 teaspoon salt
2/3 cup coconut flour

Preheat the oven to 300°F. In a small bowl, mix the butter, honey, and cider vinegar. In a medium bowl, whisk the eggs, almond flour, butter mixture, baking soda, and salt. Mix thoroughly with a hand mixer. Slowly sift the coconut flour into the bowl. Mix well to combine. Grease the inside of a loaf pan with butter. Transfer the mixture to the loaf pan, and bake for

50 to 60 minutes, until the center is set. Remove the pan from the oven. Allow it to cool for at least 15 minutes. Run a knife along the inside edges of the pan to loosen the loaf, and remove it. Place the bread on a cooling rack to cool completely, about 5 minutes more. Slice the bread into 12 slices, and refrigerate covered in plastic wrap.

Per Serving: (1 slice): Calories: 213; Fat: 17g; Protein: 5g; Total Carbs: 7g; Fiber: 3g; Net Carbs: 4g; **Macros:** Fat: 76%; Protein: 10%; Carbs: 14%

Cheesy Taco Shells

SERVES 1 | PREP TIME: 5 minutes | COOK TIME: 5 minutes

½ cup shredded Mexican cheese blend, divided

¼ teaspoon garlic salt

On a wax paper plate, arrange ¼ cup of cheese so it covers the entire plate to the edges and sprinkle with garlic salt. Microwave on high for 1½ minutes, or until the cheese has melted and is brown around the edges and golden in the middle. Remove the plate from the microwave. With a knife, gently remove the melted cheese disk from the plate. Drape it evenly over the edge of a cutting board placed on its side. Allow it to set for 3 to 5 minutes before moving. Repeat with the remaining ¼ cup of cheese. Fill the taco shells with desired ingredients and enjoy.

Per Serving: (2 shells): Calories: 246; Fat: 20g; Protein: 14g; Total Carbs: 3g; Fiber: 0g; Net Carbs: 3g; **Macros:** Fat: 73%; Protein: 23%; Carbs: 4%

Cloud Bread

SERVES 4 | PREP TIME: 10 minutes | COOK TIME: 25 to 30 minutes

3 large eggs, separated
¼ teaspoon cream of tartar
Sea salt

3 tablespoons cream cheese
1 to 2 drops liquid stevia

Preheat the oven to 300°F. Line a rimmed baking sheet with parchment paper. In a large mixing bowl, whip the egg whites, cream of tartar, and salt until stiff peaks form. In a separate bowl, beat the egg yolks, cream cheese, and stevia until smooth. Fold some of the egg white mixture into the egg yolk mixture, and then add the remaining egg white mixture. Spoon the mixture into 8 mounds on the baking sheet spreading each one out to 3 inches wide. Bake for 25 to 30 minutes or until the breads are dry and beginning to brown.

Per Serving: (2 pieces): Calories: 82; Fat: 6g; Protein: 6g; Total Carbs: 0g; Fiber: 0g; Net Carbs: 0g; **Macros:** Fat: 70%; Protein: 30%; Carbs: 0%

Coconut Pie Crust

MAKES 1 PIE CRUST | PREP TIME: 10 minutes | COOK TIME: 10 minutes

½ cup butter, melted, plus more for greasing
3 large eggs

1 cup coconut flour
¼ teaspoon stevia
¼ teaspoon sea salt

Preheat the oven to 400°F. Lightly grease a 10-inch pie pan with butter. In a medium bowl, beat the butter and eggs until blended. Stir in the coconut flousr, stevia, and salt with a fork so that the dough holds together. Gather the dough into a ball, and press it into the pie plate. Prick the entire surface with a fork. Bake the crust until light brown, about 10 minutes. Cool and fill.

Per Serving: (⅛ of the crust): Calories: 204; Fat: 16g; Protein: 6g; Total Carbs: 9g; Fiber: 6g; Net Carbs: 3g; **Macros:** Fat: 71%; Protein: 12%; Carbs: 17%

INDEX

A

Aioli
  Crab Cakes with Garlic Aioli, 116
  Grilled Burgers with Basil Aioli, 174
  Lemon-Turmeric Aioli, 236–237
  Prosciutto-Wrapped Asparagus
    and Lemon Aioli, 116
  Zesty Orange Aioli, 306
Almond
  Almond and Vanilla Pancakes, 7
  Almond Butter and Cacao Nib
    Smoothie, 5
  Almond Butter and Jelly Chia Pudding, 289
  Almond Butter Bread, 311
  Almond Butter Fudge, 257
  Almond Butter Oatmeal Cookies, 270
  Almond Butter Pancakes, 7
  Almond Cake, 276
  Almond Chocolate Bark, 255
  Almond Coconut Hot Cereal, 34
  Almond Cookies, 266
  Almond Crackers, 234
  Almond Fried Goat Cheese, 245
  Almond Golden Cake, 229
  Almond Kale Smoothie, 2
  Almond Meal–Crusted Chicken Fingers, 127
  Chia Almond "Oatmeal," 34
  Chicken Kebabs with Spicy
    Almond Sauce, 130
  Chocolate Almond Fat Bombs, 262
  Chocolate Sea Salt Almonds, 254
  Cinnamon-Cocoa Almonds, 226
  Cinnamon-Dusted Almonds, 256
  Coconut Almond Flour Bread, 311–312
  Curried Broccoli, Cheddar & Toasted
    Almond Soup, 208–209
  Hot Almond Chocolate, 298
  Lime Almond Fat Bomb, 260
  Marzipan Fat Bomb, 259
  Meatballs in Creamy Almond Sauce, 184
  Nut Butter Cup Fat Bomb, 259
  Nutty Chocolate Protein Shake, 4
  Rosemary Roasted Almonds, 244
  Smoked Almonds, 244
  Toasted Almond Cheesecake, 231–232
  Vanilla-Almond Ice Pops, 295–296
Anchovies
  Bagna Cauda, 305–306
  Rib Eye Steak with Anchovy
    Compound Butter, 169–170
  Tuscan Kale Salad with Anchovies, 67
Apple Cabbage Cumin Coleslaw, 75
Applesauce Yogurt Muffins, 43
Apricot Hot Cross Buns, 35
Artichokes
  Bacon-Artichoke Omelet, 16
  Crab and Artichoke Dip, 239
  Garlicky Broccoli Rabe with Artichokes, 82
  Greek Chicken and "Rice" Soup
    with Artichokes, 60
  Greek Frittata with Olives, Artichoke
    Hearts & Feta, 205
  Marinated Artichokes, 244
  Mediterranean Frittata, 18

  Mint-Marinated Artichoke Hearts, 80
  Olive and Artichoke Tapenade, 237
  Roasted Chicken, Artichoke, and
    Hearts of Palm Salad, 76
  Slow Cooker Pork Chops with Creamy
    Bacon-and-Artichoke Sauce, 221
  Spinach-Artichoke Dip, 238
  Squash Boats Filled with Spinach-
    Artichoke Gratin, 213
  Sriracha Artichoke Bites, 247
Arugula
  Citrus Arugula Salad, 64
  Powerhouse Arugula Salad, 68
Asparagus
  Asparagus Frittata, 18
  Asparagus Gouda Frittata, 17
  Asparagus, Mushroom & Fennel Frittata, 17
  Avocado and Asparagus Salad, 66
  Bacon-Wrapped Asparagus and Eggs, 13
  Bacon-Wrapped Asparagus Bundles, 80
  Baked Mackerel with Kale and
    Asparagus, 104–105
  Balsamic Chicken with Asparagus
    and Tomatoes, 134
  Citrus Asparagus with Pistachios, 81
  Creamy Asparagus Soup, 51
  Dill-Asparagus Bake, 206
  Eggs with Goat Cheese and Asparagus, 14
  Lemon Chicken and Asparagus Stir-Fry, 140
  Lemon Salmon and Asparagus, 108
  Lemon-Thyme Asparagus, 190
  Prosciutto-Wrapped Asparagus
    and Lemon Aioli, 80
  Roasted Asparagus with Goat Cheese, 81
  Roasted Herb-Crusted Salmon with
    Asparagus and Tomatoes, 110
  Roasted Pork Belly and Asparagus, 159
  Sautéed Asparagus with Walnuts, 81
  Teriyaki Salmon with Spicy Mayo
    and Asparagus, 106
Avocados
  Avocado and Asparagus Salad, 66
  Avocado and Eggs with Shredded
    Chicken, 13–14
  Avocado and Smoked Salmon Stack
    with Caper Sauce, 240
  Avocado Blueberry Smoothie, 4
  Avocado Brownies, 265
  Avocado Caprese Lettuce Wraps, 73
  Avocado Chicken Burger, 143–144
  Avocado Chili Fat Bomb, 233
  Avocado Coconut Smoothie, 6
  Avocado Deviled Eggs, 242
  Avocado Egg Salad, 69
  Avocado "Fries," 248
  Avocado Gazpacho, 56
  Avocado-Herb Compound Butter, 301
  Avocado-Lime Smoothie, 2–3
  Avocado-Lime Soup, 57
  Avocado-Matcha Smoothie, 1
  Avocado Pesto Zoodles, 94
  Avocado Toast, 14
  Avocado Turkey "Toast," 150
  Bacon Guacamole, 236
  BLTA Wraps, 240

  California Chicken Bake with Guacamole, 148
  Caprese Stuffed Avocados, 72
  Chicken, Avocado, and Egg Salad, 69
  Chicken Salad–Stuffed Avocados, 73
  Chicken Thigh Chili with Avocado, 136
  Chilled Avocado-Cilantro Soup, 55
  Chocolate Avocado Pudding, 289–290
  Chopped Chicken-Avocado
    Lettuce Wraps, 129
  Cold Cucumber and Avocado Soup, 56
  Crab Salad–Stuffed Avocado, 72
  Cucumber, Tomato, and Avocado Salad, 74
  Egg Baked in Avocado, 14
  Flaxseed Chips and Guacamole, 234–235
  Green Coconut Avocado Smoothie, 2
  Grilled Avocados, 242
  Grilled Shrimp with Avocado Salad, 123
  Guacamole, 237
  Guacamole Salad, 73
  Kale, Avocado & Tahini Salad, 64
  Portabella Mushroom Burger
    with Avocado, 90–91
  Salmon Cakes with Avocado, 111
  Shaved Brussels Sprouts Salad
    with Avocado Dressing, 67
  Shrimp & Avocado Salad, 79
  Smoked Salmon Avocado Sushi Roll, 107
  Southwest Meatloaf with Lime
    Guacamole, 176
  Spinach Avocado Salad, 64
  Strawberry Avocado Ice Cream, 294
  Tuna-Stuffed Avocado, 72–73
  Turkey-Stuffed Avocados, 73
  Turmeric and Avocado Egg Salad, 69

B

Baba Ghanoush, 237
Bacon. See also Pancetta
  Bacon and Berry Harvest Salad, 65–66
  Bacon-and-Egg Breakfast Casserole, 206
  Bacon and Egg Cheeseburgers, 174
  Bacon and Egg Pizza, 254
  Bacon and Spinach Egg Muffins, 192
  Bacon-Artichoke Omelet, 16
  Bacon Barbecued Chicken, 134–135
  Bacon Broccoli Crustless Quiche Cups, 26
  Bacon Cheddar Chive Scones, 41
  Bacon Cheeseburger Meatloaf, 198–199
  Bacon-Cheese Deviled Eggs, 243
  Bacon Chive Fat Bombs, 233
  Bacon Chutney, 310
  Bacon Deviled Eggs, 243
  Bacon, Egg, and Cheese Cups, 19
  Bacon Eggs Benedict Cups, 20
  Bacon Guacamole, 236
  Bacon Jam, 310
  Bacon-Mushroom Chicken, 215
  Bacon-Pepper Fat Bombs, 232–233
  Bacon Ranch Cheesy Chicken Breasts, 133
  Bacon-Wrapped Asparagus and Eggs, 13
  Bacon-Wrapped Asparagus Bundles, 80
  Bacon-Wrapped Beef Tenderloin, 170
  Bacon-Wrapped Cajun Turkey Tenderloins
    with Roasted Brussels Sprouts, 152

Bacon (*continued*)
Bacon-Wrapped Chicken, 135
Bacon-Wrapped Egg Cups, 19–20
Bacon-Wrapped Jalapeño Chicken, 129, 252
Bacon-Wrapped Jalapeño Poppers, 191
Bacon-Wrapped Mozzarella Sticks, 250
Bacon-Wrapped Pork Loin, 203
Bacon-Wrapped Pork Tenderloin, 157
Bacon-Wrapped Scallops and
    Broccolini, 118–119
Bacon-Wrapped Shrimp, 121
Beef Burgers with Bacon, 174
BLTA Wraps, 240
BLT Salad, 78
Breakfast "Sandwich," 13
Broccoli Bacon Egg Muffin Cups, 20
Broccoli Salad with Bacon, 73–74
Brussels Sprouts with Bacon, 83
Candied Bacon Fudge, 255
Cheesy Bacon-Cauliflower Soup, 208
Chicken Bacon Burgers, 144
Chicken-Bacon Soup, 208
Chicken Chowder with Bacon, 209
Chocolate-Covered Bacon, 256–257
Classic Bacon and Eggs, 13
Creamy Broccoli, Bacon, and Cheese Soup, 52
Crustless Quiche Lorraine, 24–25
Deviled Egg Salad with Bacon, 69–70
Double Bacon Cheeseburger, 175
Eggs Benedict on Grilled Portabella
    Mushroom Caps, 24
Eggs Benedict with Bacon, 23–24
Eggs Benedict with Five-Minute
    Hollandaise, 24
Essential Cobb Salad with
    Crumbled Bacon, 77
Golden Rosti, 93
Kale with Bacon, 89
Lobster BLT Salad, 71
Maple Bacon-Wrapped Brussels Sprouts, 247
Mushroom and Bacon Frittata, 17–18
Sea Scallops with Bacon Cream Sauce, 118
Slow Cooker Pork Chops with Creamy
    Bacon-and-Artichoke Sauce, 221
Spinach and Bacon Stuffed
    Chicken Thighs, 139
Spinach Salad with Bacon and
    Soft-Boiled Eggs, 78–79
Spinach Salad with Warm Bacon Dressing, 65
Tomato and Bacon Zoodles, 203–204
Turkey Bacon Ranch Casserole, 151
Bacon, Canadian
Easy Eggs Benedict, 24
Bagels
Bagels with Smoked Salmon, 27
Chorizo Bagels, 37
Everything Bagels, 36–37
Bagna Cauda, 305–306
Baklava Hot Porridge, 34
Balsamic vinegar
Balsamic Chicken with Asparagus
    and Tomatoes, 134
Balsamic Roast Beef, 219
Balsamic Teriyaki Halibut, 103
Balsamic-Thyme Pork Tenderloin, 156
Caprese Balsamic Chicken, 132
Grilled Balsamic Cabbage, 83
Herbed Balsamic Dressing, 305
Rosemary Balsamic Pork Medallions, 156
Bamboo shoots
Curried Chicken with Bamboo Shoots, 133
Shrimp, Bamboo Shoot, and
    Broccoli Stir-Fry, 124–125
Bananas
Banana Bread Blender Pancakes, 8–9
Banana Nut Muffins, 44–45
Banana Pudding, 289

Banana Pudding Ice Cream, 293
Chocolate Chip Banana Bread, 50
Chocolate, Peanut Butter, and
    Banana Shake, 4–5
Creamy Banana Fat Bombs, 260
Barbecue Sauce, 307
Barbecue Onion and Goat
    Cheese Flatbread, 311
Barbecue Turkey Meatballs, 195–196
BBQ Baby Back Ribs, 158
BBQ Chicken Skewers, 129
BBQ Chicken Wraps, 129
Spicy Barbecue Pecans, 244
Bars. *See* Cookies and bars
Basil
Avocado Caprese Lettuce Wraps, 73
Basil Butter Grilled Shrimp, 122–123
Basil Chicken Zucchini "Pasta," 133
Caprese Skewers, 241
Caprese Stuffed Avocados, 72
Caprese-Stuffed Chicken Breasts, 132
Goat Cheese and Basil Pizza, 253
Goat Cheese Caprese Salad, 75
Green Basil Dressing, 303
Grilled Burgers with Basil Aioli, 174
Halibut in Tomato Basil Sauce, 103
Herb Pesto, 309
Margarita Pizza Chips, 235
Margherita Pizza, 310–311
Pesto, 306
Pesto Sauce, 309
Roasted Red Pepper Soup with
    Basil and Goat Cheese, 52
Tomato Basil Chicken Zoodle Bowls, 136
Tomato Basil Soup, 53
Beef
Bacon and Egg Cheeseburgers, 174
Bacon Cheeseburger Meatloaf, 198–199
Bacon-Wrapped Beef Tenderloin, 170
Baked Cheesy Meatballs, 185
Balsamic Roast Beef, 219
Beef and Bell Peppers, 218
Beef and Broccoli Stir-Fry, 164
Beef Bone Broth, 302
Beef Bourguignon Stew, 171
Beef Burgers with Bacon, 174
Beef Fajitas, 164–165
Beef Goulash, 218
Beef Pho, 62
Beef Pot Roast, 171–172
Beef-Sausage Stew, 62
Beef Stew, 171, 210
Beef Stroganoff, 165
Beef Stroganoff Meatballs over Zoodles, 185
Beef-Stuffed Red Peppers, 180
Beef Taco Lasagna, 180
Beef Tacos, 183–184
Beef Taco Stew, 171
Beef Taquitos, 251
Beefy Stuffed Cornbread Casserole, 177
Braised Beef Short Ribs, 172–173, 218
Brisket Nachos, 173
Broccoli and Beef Casserole, 178
Brussels Sprouts & Ground Beef
    Scrambled Eggs, 22
Butter-Basted Rib Eye Steaks, 169
Carne Asada, 218
Cast-Iron Blackened Rib Eye with
    Parmesan Roasted Radishes, 169
Cheeseburger Casserole, 177
Cheeseburger Meatloaf, 176
Cheeseburger Soup, 209
Cheese-Stuffed Italian Meatballs, 185–186
Cheesy Baked Meatballs, 250
Cheesy Beef and Spinach Casserole, 177
Cheesy Triple Meat Baked "Spaghetti," 179

Chicken-Fried Steak Fingers
    with Gravy, 165–166
Chili con Carne, 181
Chipotle Coffee-Crusted
    Bone-In Rib Eye, 169
Cilantro Lime Taco Bowls, 183
Classic Beef Chili, 181
Classic Bolognese Sauce, 308
Classic Meatloaf, 175
Classic Prime Rib au Jus, 170
Classic Sauerbraten, 217
Classic Steak Salad, 77
Corned Beef & Cabbage with
    Horseradish Cream, 219
Corned Beef Breakfast Hash, 23
Cottage Pie, 178
Deconstructed Cabbage Rolls, 220–221
Double Bacon Cheeseburger, 175
Empanadas, 251
Essential New York Strip Steak, 167
Faux Lasagna Soup, 208
Fiery Curry Beef, 219
Five-Alarm Beef Chili, 181
Flank Steak with Kale Chimichurri, 166
Flank Steak with Orange-Herb
    Pistou, 166–167
Garlic Braised Short Ribs, 173
Garlic-Marinated Flank Steak, 199
Garlic Steak, 200
Garlic Steak Bites, 166
Garlic Studded Prime Rib with
    Thyme au Jus, 170
Ginger Beef, 218
Goat Cheese–Stuffed Flank Steak, 200
Greek Beef Kebabs with Tzatziki, 199
Grilled Burgers with Basil Aioli, 174
Grilled Hanger Steak with
    Cilantro Crema, 167–168
Grilled Rib Eye Steaks with
    Horseradish Cream, 199–200
Grilled Sirloin Steak, Roasted Red Pepper,
    and Mozzarella Lettuce Boats, 168
Grilled Sirloin Steak with Herbed Butter, 168
Grilled Steak Salad with
    Cucumber and Mint, 77
Ground Beef Cauli-Fried Rice, 182
Ground Beef Taco Salad, 183
Ground Beef Taco Salad with
    Peppers and Ranch, 78
Herbed Meatloaf, 176–177
Italian Beef Burgers, 175
Italian Meatballs, 185
Italian Wedding Soup, 61–62
Loaded Burgers, 174
Meatballs in Creamy Almond Sauce, 184
Meatballs with Spaghetti Squash, 184–185
Meatza, 182–183
Mediterranean Meatloaf, 220
Mini Burger Sliders, 175–176
Moroccan Stuffed Peppers, 180
Moussaka, 179
Mozzarella-Stuffed Burgers, 175
Oven Burgers, 176
Pan-Seared Hangar Steak with Easy
    Herb Cream Sauce, 167
Pesto Roast Beef, 217
Philly Cheesesteak Stuffed Peppers, 180
Pot Roast with Turnips and Radishes, 172
Pressure Cooker Pork-and-
    Beef Meatloaf, 190
Pressure Cooker Pot Roast with
    Sour-Cream Gravy, 190
Pressure Cooker Sloppy Joes, 190
Quick and Easy Dirty Rice Skillet, 182
Quick Fiesta Taco Salad, 78
Rib Eye Steaks with Garlic-Thyme Butter, 169

Rib Eye Steak with Anchovy
    Compound Butter, 169–170
Rich Beef Stock, 302
Rosemary Roasted Beef Tenderloin, 170–171
Salisbury Steak, 182, 217
Savory Stuffed Peppers, 220
Sheet Pan Sirloin Steak with
    Eggplant and Zucchini, 168
Short Ribs with Chimichurri, 199
Simple Reuben Casserole, 177
Simple Texas Chili, 211
Sirloin Steak Salad with Goat
    Cheese and Pecans, 77–78
Slow-Cooked Shredded Beef, 173
Slow Cooker Barbacoa Pulled Beef with
    Cilantro Cauliflower Rice, 219
Slow Cooker Beef-Stuffed Cabbage
    in Creamy Tomato Sauce, 220
Slow Cooker Brisket, 220
Slow Cooker Saucy Sausage-
    and-Beef Meatballs, 223
Slow Keto Chili, 211
Southern-Style Shepherd's Pie, 177–178
Southwest Meatloaf with Lime
    Guacamole, 176
Southwest-Style Fajita Bowls, 165
Soy-Ginger Veggie Noodle
    Steak Roll-Ups, 166
Spiced-Up Sunday Pot Roast and
    Sautéed Squash, 172
Steak with Drunken Broccoli Noodles, 164
Stuffed Meatballs, 218–219
Swedish Meatballs, 184
Tandoori Beef Fajitas, 167
Texas-Style Beef Chili, 181
Texas Taco Hash, 183
Tomato-Braised Beef, 217
Zoodles Bolognese, 182
Zucchini Lasagna, 179–180
Zucchini Meatloaf, 176
Beer
    Michelada, 300
Bell peppers
    Baked Sausage and Shrimp with Turnips
        and Green Peppers, 162–163
    Beef and Bell Peppers, 218
    Beef Fajitas, 164–165
    Beef-Stuffed Red Peppers, 180
    Cheese-Stuffed Peppers, 212
    Chicken Fajitas, 131
    Chicken Fajita Stuffed Bell Peppers, 133
    Chicken Salad–Stuffed Peppers, 147–148
    Creamy Stuffed Peppers, 92
    Grilled Sirloin Steak, Roasted Red Pepper,
        and Mozzarella Lettuce Boats, 168
    Ground Beef Taco Salad with
        Peppers and Ranch, 78
    Moroccan Stuffed Peppers, 180
    Pan-Fried Pork Chops with
        Peppers and Onions, 154
    Philly Cheesesteak Stuffed Peppers, 180
    Roasted Red Pepper Dip, 238
    Roasted Red Pepper Soup with
        Basil and Goat Cheese, 52
    Sausage-Stuffed Peppers, 200, 206
    Savory Stuffed Peppers, 220
    Shakshuka, 29
    Southwest-Style Fajita Bowls, 165
    Tandoori Beef Fajitas, 167
    Turkey and Cauliflower Rice–
        Stuffed Peppers, 149
    Unstuffed Bell Pepper Skillet, 152
Berries. See also specific
    Almond Butter and Jelly Chia Pudding, 289
    Bacon and Berry Harvest Salad, 65–66
    Berry Cheesecake Smoothie, 6
    Berry Green Smoothie, 1

Berry-Pumpkin Compote, 228
Coconut Berry Smoothie, 4
Coconut Yogurt Berry Parfait, 30
Fresh Berry Tart, 285
Lemon Berry Yogurt Parfait, 30
Mixed Berry Crisp, 287
Mixed Berry Scones with Lemon Icing, 42
Mixed Berry Sherbet, 294
PB&J Overnight Hemp, 31
Sweet 'n' Savory Toast with
    Burrata and Berries, 12
Triple Berry Smoothie, 3
Very Berry Waffles, 11
Biscuits
    Biscuits and Sausage Gravy, 28
    Biscuits with Sausage Gravy, 34–35
    Buttermilk Biscuits, 35
    Cheddar-Chive Biscuits, 35
    Down Home Biscuits, 192
    Easy Cheese Biscuits, 36
    Egg & Cheese Biscuit Casserole, 15–16
Bison
    Bison Burgers in Lettuce Wraps, 186
    Ground Bison Chile Rellenos with
        Ranchero Sauce, 186
Blackberries
    Blackberry "Cheesecake" Bites, 275
    Blackberry Cobbler, 228, 284
    Blackberry, Prosciutto, and Goat
        Cheese Flatbread, 40
Blueberries
    Avocado Blueberry Smoothie, 4
    Blueberry Cheesecake Bars, 272
    Blueberry Cream Cheese Bites, 291
    Blueberry Crisp, 228–229
    Blueberry Crumble, 287
    Blueberry Fat Bombs, 260
    Blueberry Mint Ice Pops, 295
    Blueberry Mojito, 299
    Blueberry Smoothie with
        Lemon and Ginger, 3
    Keto Blueberry Pancakes, 9
    Lemon-Blueberry Ice Cream, 292
    Lemony Chicken Salad with
        Blueberries and Fennel, 72
    Quick and Easy Blueberry Waffles, 11–12
    Spinach-Blueberry Smoothie, 3
    Toast-less Blueberry French Toast, 12–13
Bok choy
    Pesto Flounder with Bok Choy, 102
    Roasted Cod with Garlic Butter
        and Bok Choy, 101
Bourbon
    Bourbon Pecan Pie Bars, 274
    Crispy Bourbon Pork Belly, 159
    Old-Fashioned, 300
Bowls
    Breakfast Bowl with Cauliflower Hash, 26–27
    Breakfast Burrito Bowl, 29
    Carne Asada Chicken Bowls, 135
    Cilantro Lime Taco Bowls, 183
    Egg Roll in a Bowl, 163
    Go Get 'Em Green Smoothie Bowl, 30–31
    Green Goddess Buddha Bowl, 84
    Lemongrass Pork Noodle Bowls, 155
    Pork Taco Bowls, 203
    Pumpkin Pie Yogurt Bowl, 31
    Sausage Egg Roll in a Bowl, 27
    Southwest-Style Fajita Bowls, 165
    Spaghetti Squash Chicken Bowls, 136
    Tomato Basil Chicken Zoodle Bowls, 136
    Turkey Egg Roll in a Bowl, 150–151
Breads. See also Biscuits; Buns;
        Muffins; Scones
    Almond Butter Bread, 311
    Basic Sandwich Bread, 38
    in Bread Pudding, 288–289

Buttery Coconut Bread, 50
Cheesy Cauliflower Breadsticks, 249
Chocolate Chip Banana Bread, 50
Cinnamon Swirl Bread, 49–50
Classic Zucchini Bread, 37
Cloud Bread, 312
Coconut Almond Flour Bread, 311–312
Garlic Breadsticks, 249
Garlic Cloud Bread, 38–39
Herb and Olive Focaccia, 40
Iced Cranberry-Gingerbread Loaf, 49
Jalapeño Cheese Bread, 39
Nut-Free Pumpkin Bread, 50
Nut-Free Sunflower Bread, 50–51
Onion Cheddar Bread, 37–38
Onion-Garlic Pita Bread, 38
Pizza Pull-Apart Bread, 38
Pumpkin Spice Loaf with Maple Icing, 49
Savory Naan, 39–40
Slow Cooker Grain-Free Pumpkin Loaf, 207
Slow Cooker Grain-Free Zucchini
    Bread, 206–207
Slow Cooker Zucchini-Carrot Bread, 37
Soft-Baked Pretzels with Spicy
    Mustard Dip, 249
Sour Cream Corn Bread, 41
Southern Sweet Corn Bread, 41
Tex-Mex Green Chile Corn Bread, 41
Versatile Sandwich Round, 311
Broccoli
    Bacon Broccoli Crustless Quiche Cups, 26
    Beef and Broccoli Stir-Fry, 164
    Broccoli and Beef Casserole, 178
    Broccoli and Cheese Quiche Cups, 20
    Broccoli Bacon Egg Muffin Cups, 20
    Broccoli Cheddar Soup, 52
    Broccoli Quiche, 25
    Broccoli Salad with Bacon, 73–74
    Broccoli Stir-Fry, 82
    Broccoli-Stuffed Chicken, 194
    Chicken Tenderloin Packets with Broccoli,
        Radishes, and Parmesan, 135
    Creamed Broccoli, 81
    Creamy Broccoli, Bacon, and Cheese Soup, 52
    Creamy Broccoli Casserole, 81
    Creamy Broccoli Salad, 74
    Curried Broccoli, Cheddar & Toasted
        Almond Soup, 208–209
    Ham-Broccoli-Cauliflower Casserole, 161
    Mustard-Crusted Cod with
        Roasted Broccoli, 101
    Paprika Chicken with Broccoli, 128
    Ranch Broccoli Slaw, 76
    Roasted Broccoli, 81
    Seared Tuna with Steamed Turnips,
        Broccoli, and Green Beans, 114
    Sesame-Roasted Broccoli, 82
    Shrimp, Bamboo Shoot, and
        Broccoli Stir-Fry, 124–125
    Spicy Roasted Broccoli, 191
    Steak with Drunken Broccoli Noodles, 164
Broccolini, Bacon-Wrapped
        Scallops and, 118–119
Broccoli Rabe with Artichokes, Garlicky, 82
Broths and stocks
    Beef Bone Broth, 302
    Chicken Bone Broth, 302
    Fish Stock, 303
    Herbed Chicken Stock, 302
    Herbed Vegetable Broth, 302–303
    Rich Beef Stock, 302
Brownies
    Avocado Brownies, 265
    Chocolate Chip Brownies, 264
    Classic Chocolate Brownies, 270–271
    Fudge Brownies, 272–273
    Fudge Nut Brownies, 232

Brownies (*continued*)
Fudgy Brownies, 269
No-Bake Brownie Bites, 271
Pumpkin Cheesecake Brownies, 271–272
Brown Sugar Bacon Smokies, 250
Brussels sprouts
Bacon-Wrapped Cajun Turkey Tenderloins
with Roasted Brussels Sprouts, 152
Brussels Sprout Ground Pork Hash, 163
Brussels Sprouts & Ground Beef
Scrambled Eggs, 22
Brussels Sprouts Casserole, 82
Brussels Sprouts with Bacon, 83
Brussels Sprouts with Hazelnuts, 83
Crispy Brussels Sprouts, 82
Harissa Chicken and Brussels Sprouts
with Yogurt Sauce, 139
Maple Bacon-Wrapped Brussels Sprouts, 247
Pork Belly with Brussels Sprouts
& Turnips, 223
Roasted Brussels Sprouts &
Poached Eggs, 82–83
Roasted Brussels Sprouts with
Tahini-Yogurt Sauce, 242
Shaved Brussels Sprouts Salad
with Avocado Dressing, 67
Buffalo sauce
Buffalo Chicken Breakfast Muffins, 193
Buffalo Chicken Dip, 238–239
Buffalo Chicken Salad, 70–71
Buffalo Chicken Tenders, 195
Buffalo Chicken Wings, 127, 193
Buffalo Roasted Cauliflower, 246
Buns
Apricot Hot Cross Buns, 35
Sesame Burger Buns, 36
Burgers
Avocado Chicken Burger, 143–144
Bacon and Egg Cheeseburgers, 174
Beef Burgers with Bacon, 174
Bison Burgers in Lettuce Wraps, 186
Chicken Bacon Burgers, 144
Coconut Ginger Salmon Burgers, 110–111
Double Bacon Cheeseburger, 175
Grilled Burgers with Basil Aioli, 174
Italian Beef Burgers, 175
Lettuce-Wrapped Chicken Burger, 144
Loaded Burgers, 174
Mini Burger Sliders, 175–176
Mozzarella-Stuffed Burgers, 175
Oven Burgers, 176
Portabella Breakfast "Burger," 27–28
Portabella Mushroom Burger
with Avocado, 90–91
Turkey Burgers, 150
Turkey Thyme Burgers, 150
Butter
Avocado-Herb Compound Butter, 301
Basil Butter Grilled Shrimp, 122–123
Brown Butter–Lime Tilapia, 112
Butter-Basted Rib Eye Steaks, 169
Butter Cake with Cream Cheese
Buttercream, 282
Buttered Coffee, 297
Buttered Coffee Shake, 6
Butter Pecan Cheesecake
Truffle Fat Bombs, 261
Butter Rum Pound Cake, 279
Buttery Boiled Eggs, 13
Buttery Coconut Bread, 50
Cinnamon Butter, 301
Ghee, 301
Grilled Sirloin Steak with Herbed Butter, 168
Horseradish Compound Butter, 301
Hot Buttered Rum, 299
Lemon Butter Chicken, 140
Pan-Seared Butter Scallops, 118

Rib Eye Steaks with Garlic-Thyme Butter, 169
Rib Eye Steak with Anchovy
Compound Butter, 169–170
Roasted Cod with Garlic Butter
and Bok Choy, 101
Salmon in Lime Caper Brown
Butter Sauce, 108
Scallops with Lemon-Butter Sauce, 197
Strawberry Butter, 301–302
Swordfish in Tarragon-Citrus Butter, 112
Buttermilk
Buttermilk Biscuits, 35
"Buttermilk" Custard Pie Bars, 284
Buttermilk Ranch Dressing, 303

C

Cabbage and coleslaw. *See also* Sauerkraut
Apple Cabbage Cumin Coleslaw, 75
Asian Cabbage Stir-Fry, 83–84
Cabbage Sausage Hash Browns, 23
Cheesy Sausage and Cabbage Hash, 28
Cold Front Kielbasa and Cabbage Skillet, 161
Corned Beef & Cabbage with
Horseradish Cream, 219
Crisp and Creamy Southern Coleslaw, 75
Deconstructed Cabbage Rolls, 220–221
Egg Roll in a Bowl, 163
Grilled Balsamic Cabbage, 83
Hearty Lamb Cabbage Soup, 62–63
Pork with Sesame Slaw, 162
Roasted Cabbage "Steaks," 83
Sausage Egg Roll in a Bowl, 27
Sesame Ginger Slaw, 75
Slow Cooker Beef-Stuffed Cabbage
in Creamy Tomato Sauce, 220
Slow Cooker Pulled Pork with
Cabbage Slaw, 222
Smoked Sausage with Cabbage & Onions, 223
Spicy Sausage and Cabbage
Casserole, 160–161
Sweet-Braised Red Cabbage, 83
Turkey and Kale Coleslaw, 76
Turkey Egg Roll in a Bowl, 150–151
Cacao nibs
Almond Butter and Cacao Nib
Smoothie, 5
Cacao Crunch Cereal, 32–33
Cakes and cupcakes. *See also* Cheesecakes
Air-Fried Vanilla and Chocolate
Layer Cake, 204
Almond Cake, 276
Almond Golden Cake, 229
Brownie Chocolate Cake, 230
Butter Cake with Cream Cheese
Buttercream, 282
Butter Rum Pound Cake, 279
Carrot Cake, 230
Chocolate Cake with Whipped
Cream, 232
Chocolate Marble Pound Cake, 281
Chocolate Mug Cake, 282
Cinnamon "Apple" Pecan Coffee Cake, 47–48
Cinnamon Coffee Cake, 48
Coconut-Orange Cupcakes, 276
Coconut-Raspberry Cake, 229
Cream Cheese Pound Cake, 279
Delectable Peanut Butter Cup Cake, 229
Hazelnut-Chocolate Snack Cakes, 279
Lemonade Snack Cake, 48
Lemon Curd Layer Cake, 280–281
Lime-Raspberry Custard Cake, 230
90-Second Lava Cake, 281
Old-Fashioned Lemon-Lime Teacakes, 48
Orange-Olive Oil Cupcakes, 276
Peanut Butter Cake Bars, 273
Poppy Seed Pound Cake, 280

Pumpkin Pound Cake, 279–280
Raspberry-Lemon Pound Cake, 280
Salted Caramel Cupcakes, 275–276
Slow Cooker Moist Ginger Cake
with Whipped Cream, 231
Slow Cooker Tangy Lemon Cake
with Lemon Glaze, 230
Strawberry Shortcakes, 281–282
Tender Pound Cake, 229
Tiramisu, 276–277
Vanilla Cheesecake, 231
Warm Gingerbread, 229–230
Capers
Avocado and Smoked Salmon Stack
with Caper Sauce, 240
Salmon in Lime Caper Brown
Butter Sauce, 108
Caramel
Cinnamon-Caramel Sauce, 310
Salted Caramel Cashew Brittle, 255
Salted Caramel Cupcakes, 275–276
Salted Caramel Fudge Fat Bombs, 260–261
Salted Caramels, 254
Carbohydrates, v
Carrots
Carrot Cake, 230
Carrot Cake Cookies, 269
Carrot-Pumpkin Pudding, 92
Glazed Dairy-Free Carrot Cake Muffins, 44
Slow Cooker Zucchini-Carrot Bread, 37
Cashews
Kale and Cashew Stir-Fry, 89
Lemon-Cashew Smoothie, 2
Salted Caramel Cashew Brittle, 255
Casseroles
Bacon-and-Egg Breakfast Casserole, 206
Baked Omelet with Pancetta
and Swiss Cheese, 17
Beefy Stuffed Cornbread Casserole, 177
Broccoli and Beef Casserole, 178
Brussels Sprouts Casserole, 82
California Chicken Bake with Guacamole, 148
Cauliflower-Pecan Casserole, 85
Cayenne Pepper Vegetable Bake, 97
Cheeseburger Casserole, 177
Cheesy Beef and Spinach Casserole, 177
Cheesy Chicken and Rice Skillet
Casserole, 146–147
Cheesy "Hash Brown" Casserole, 28
Cheesy Spinach Bake, 93
Chicken Cordon Bleu Casserole, 137
Creamy Broccoli Casserole, 81
Creamy Chicken and Spinach Bake, 132
Creamy Shrimp and Grits Casserole, 119–120
Creamy Spaghetti Squash Bake, 94
Denver Omelet Breakfast Bake, 16
Egg & Cheese Biscuit Casserole, 15–16
Enchilada Casserole, 213
Green Bean Casserole, 88–89
Green-Chile Chicken Enchilada
Casserole, 145–146
Ham-Broccoli-Cauliflower Casserole, 161
Jalapeño Popper Chicken Casserole, 147
Mexican Egg Casserole, 15
Potluck Chicken Spaghetti
Squash Casserole, 146
Rich Sausage and Spaghetti
Squash Casserole, 162
Sausage Verde Casserole, 26
Simple Reuben Casserole, 177
Slow Cooker Layered Egg Casserole, 205
Spicy Sausage and Cabbage
Casserole, 160–161
Tofu Green Bean Casserole, 88
Tuna Casserole, 114–115
Turkey Bacon Ranch Casserole, 151
Turkey Florentine Bake, 151

Catfish
  Easy Oven-Fried Catfish, 100
  Pecan-Crusted Catfish, 100
Cauliflower
  Breaded Pork Chops with Creamy
    Mashed Cauliflower, 153
  Breakfast Bowl with Cauliflower Hash, 26–27
  Buffalo Roasted Cauliflower, 246
  Cajun Shrimp and Cauliflower Rice, 122
  Cauliflower-Cheddar Soup, 51–52
  Cauliflower Hummus, 237
  Cauliflower Mac and Cheese, 86
  Cauliflower N'Oatmeal, 33
  Cauliflower-Pecan Casserole, 85
  Cauliflower Pizza, 86
  Cauliflower Rice, 84
  Cauliflower Smoothie, 2
  Cauliflower Tortillas, 311
  Cheesy Bacon-Cauliflower Soup, 208
  Cheesy Cauliflower Breadsticks, 249
  Cheesy Cauliflower Mac 'n' Cheese, 86
  Cheesy Chicken and Rice Skillet
    Casserole, 146–147
  Cheesy Mashed Cauliflower, 85
  Chicken Taco Soup with Cauliflower Rice, 61
  Country Pork and "Rice" Soup, 62
  Crab Fried Rice, 117
  Creamed Cauliflower Soup, 51
  Cream of Cauliflower Gazpacho, 55
  Creamy Riced Cauliflower Salad, 75
  Creamy Seafood Stew with
    Cauliflower Rice, 63
  Creole Sausage and Rice, 162
  Deep-Dish Cauliflower Crust
    Pizza with Olives, 212
  Fried Ham "Rice," 161
  Garlic and Herb Baked Shrimp
    with Cauliflower Rice, 125
  Greek Chicken and "Rice" Soup
    with Artichokes, 60
  Ground Beef Cauli-Fried Rice, 182
  Ham-Broccoli-Cauliflower Casserole, 161
  Hearty Cauliflower Soup, 54–55
  Latkes with Sour Cream, 252–253
  Loaded Baked "Fauxtato" Soup, 56
  Loaded Chicken and Cauliflower Nachos, 126
  Mashed Cauliflower, 85
  Mashed Cauliflower with Yogurt, 85
  Mediterranean Cauliflower Tabbouleh, 85
  Mexican Cauliflower Rice, 84
  Moroccan Cauliflower Salad, 74
  Moroccan Salmon with Cauliflower
    Rice Pilaf, 107
  Mulligatawny Soup with Cauliflower Rice, 209
  Nutty Miso Cauliflower Rice, 84
  Pesto Cauliflower Sheet-Pan "Pizza," 253
  Pork Fried Rice, 155
  Quick and Easy Dirty Rice Skillet, 182
  Raw Tabouli, 85
  Roasted Cauliflower Lettuce Cups, 86
  Roasted Cauliflower with Parsley
    and Pine Nuts, 84
  Sausage and Cauliflower Salad, 75
  Shrimp Fried Rice, 124
  Slow Cooker Barbacoa Pulled Beef with
    Cilantro Cauliflower Rice, 219
  Thai-Inspired Peanut Roasted Cauliflower, 84
  Turkey and Cauliflower Rice–
    Stuffed Peppers, 149
  Turkey Pilaf, 151
  Turmeric Cauliflower "Pickles," 241–242
Cayenne Pepper Vegetable Bake, 97
Celeriac
  Celery Root Purée, 86–87
  Golden Rosti, 93
Cereal
  Almond Coconut Hot Cereal, 34

Baklava Hot Porridge, 34
Cacao Crunch Cereal, 32–33
Cauliflower N'Oatmeal, 33
Chia Almond "Oatmeal," 34
Chocolate Coconut "Oatmeal," 33
Cinnamon Roll "Noatmeal," 33
Granola Cereal, 32
Nutty "Oatmeal," 33–34
Pumpkin-Pecan N'Oatmeal, 33
Chaffles, 9
  Chaffle and Lox, 10
  Spaghetti Squash Chaffles, 9
Cheese. See also Cottage cheese;
    Cream cheese; Ricotta cheese
  Almond Fried Goat Cheese, 245
  Asparagus Gouda Frittata, 17
  Avocado Caprese Lettuce Wraps, 73
  Bacon and Egg Cheeseburgers, 174
  Bacon Broccoli Crustless Quiche Cups, 26
  Bacon Cheddar Chive Scones, 41
  Bacon Cheeseburger Meatloaf, 198–199
  Bacon-Cheese Deviled Eggs, 243
  Bacon, Egg, and Cheese Cups, 19
  Bacon Ranch Cheesy Chicken Breasts, 133
  Bacon-Wrapped Mozzarella Sticks, 250
  Bagels with Smoked Salmon, 27
  Baked Cheesy Meatballs, 185
  Baked Feta Blocks, 245
  Baked Olives and Feta, 245
  Baked Omelet with Pancetta
    and Swiss Cheese, 17
  Barbecue Onion and Goat
    Cheese Flatbread, 311
  Blackberry, Prosciutto, and Goat
    Cheese Flatbread, 40
  Black Forest Ham, Cheese, and
    Chive Roll-Ups, 239
  Bleu Cheese Sauce, 307
  Breakfast Burrito Bowl, 29
  Breakfast Pizza, 27
  Broccoli and Cheese Quiche Cups, 20
  Broccoli Cheddar Soup, 52
  Broccoli Quiche, 25
  Brussels Sprouts Casserole, 82
  Caprese Balsamic Chicken, 132
  Caprese Skewers, 241
  Caprese Stuffed Avocados, 72
  Caprese-Stuffed Chicken Breasts, 132
  Cast-Iron Blackened Rib Eye with
    Parmesan Roasted Radishes, 169
  Cauliflower-Cheddar Soup, 51–52
  Cauliflower Mac and Cheese, 86
  Chaffle and Lox, 10
  Chaffles, 9
  Cheddar Cheese Soup, 207
  Cheddar-Chive Biscuits, 35
  Cheeseburger Casserole, 177
  Cheeseburger Meatloaf, 176
  Cheeseburger Soup, 209
  Cheese Pork Rind Nachos, 246
  Cheese-Stuffed Italian Meatballs, 185–186
  Cheese-Stuffed Peppers, 212
  Cheese-Stuffed Pork Chops, 155
  Cheesy Bacon-Cauliflower Soup, 208
  Cheesy Baked Meatballs, 250
  Cheesy Beef and Spinach Casserole, 177
  Cheesy Cauliflower Breadsticks, 249
  Cheesy Cauliflower Mac 'n' Cheese, 86
  Cheesy Chicken and Rice Skillet
    Casserole, 146–147
  Cheesy Chicken Taquitos, 251–252
  Cheesy-Crust Pizza, 310
  Cheesy Dill Fat Bombs, 233–234
  Cheesy Garlic Rolls, 36
  Cheesy Golden Fried Haddock, 103
  Cheesy "Hash Brown" Casserole, 28
  Cheesy Mashed Cauliflower, 85

Cheesy Sausage & Egg Muffins, 20
Cheesy Sausage and Cabbage Hash, 28
Cheesy Scrambled Eggs, 21
Cheesy Shrimp Spread, 239–240
Cheesy Spinach Bake, 93
Cheesy Taco Shells, 312
Chicken and Cheese Quesadillas, 145
Chicken Brunch Pie with Cheddar
  Pecan Crust, 28–29
Chicken Cordon Bleu, 137
Chicken Cordon Bleu Casserole, 137
Chicken Parmesan, 128, 194
Chicken Quesadillas, 145
Chicken Tenderloin Packets with Broccoli,
  Radishes, and Parmesan, 135
Chiles Rellenos, 92
Classic Mozzarella Sticks, 250
Creamy Broccoli, Bacon, and Cheese Soup, 52
Creamy Broccoli Casserole, 81
Crispy Parmesan Crackers, 234
Crustless Greek Cheese Pie, 29
Crustless Quiche Lorraine, 24–25
Crustless Sausage and Green
  Chile Quiche, 25
Crustless Spanakopita, 97–98
Crustless Wild Mushroom–Kale Quiche, 206
Cucumber and Tomato Feta Salad, 74
Curried Broccoli, Cheddar & Toasted
  Almond Soup, 208–209
Denver Omelet Breakfast Bake, 16
Double Bacon Cheeseburger, 175
Easy Cheese Biscuits, 36
Egg & Cheese Biscuit Casserole, 15–16
Eggplant Lasagna, 87
Eggs with Goat Cheese and Asparagus, 14
Enchilada Casserole, 213
Fakeachini Alfredo, 94
Feta and Olive Stuffed Chicken Thighs, 140
Feta Cheese Kebabs, 245
Florentine Breakfast Sandwich, 14
Garlic Parmesan Crusted Salmon, 105
Garlic Parmesan Wings, 127
Goat Cheese and Basil Pizza, 253
Goat Cheese Caprese Salad, 75
Goat Cheese Nuggets, 245
Goat Cheese–Stuffed Flank Steak, 200
Goat Cheese Stuffed Roasted
  Peppers, 91–92
Golden Chicken Asiago, 147
Greek Frittata with Olives, Artichoke
  Hearts & Feta, 205
Greens and Parmesan Muffins, 45
Grilled Sirloin Steak, Roasted Red Pepper,
  and Mozzarella Lettuce Boats, 168
Ham and Cheese Crustless Quiche, 25
Ham and Cheese Egg Scramble, 21
Ham and Cheese Poached Egg Cups, 19
Ham and Swiss Waffles, 11
Jalapeño Cheese Bread, 39
Konjac Noodles with Spinach Hemp
  Pesto and Goat Cheese, 98
Loaded Denver Omelet, 16
Loaded Feta, 246
Margarita Pizza Chips, 235
Margherita Pizza, 310–311
Mediterranean Frittata, 18
Mexican Egg Casserole, 15
Mozzarella-Stuffed Burgers, 175
Mushrooms with Camembert, 90
Onion Cheddar Bread, 37–38
Oregano Shrimp with Tomatoes and Feta, 122
Pancetta-and-Brie–Stuffed Pork
  Tenderloin, 201–202
Parmesan Baked Tilapia, 113
Parmesan-Breaded Boneless Pork Chops, 201
Parmesan-Crusted Tilapia with
  Sautéed Spinach, 112

Cheese (continued)
Parmesan-Rosemary Radishes, 190–191
Parmesan Zucchini Chips, 235
Party Deli Pinwheels, 240
Philly Cheesesteak Stuffed Peppers, 180
Pizza Pull-Apart Bread, 38
Pork Medallions with Blue Cheese Sauce, 156
Prosciutto-Wrapped Mozzarella, 241
Queso Blanco Dip, 238
Queso Dip, 238
Roasted Asparagus with Goat
    Cheese, 81
Roasted Red Pepper Soup with
    Basil and Goat Cheese, 52
Sausage and Cheese Frittata, 19
Sausage Verde Casserole, 26
Savory Sausage Balls, 27
Simple Reuben Casserole, 177
Sirloin Steak Salad with Goat
    Cheese and Pecans, 77–78
Slow Cooker Eggplant
    Parmesan, 212–213
Slow Cooker Spanakopita Frittata, 205–206
Smoked Salmon and Goat Cheese
    Pinwheels, 240–241
Spaghetti Squash Chaffles, 9
Spanakopita Omelet, 16–17
Spicy Cheddar Wafers, 235
Spinach, Mushroom, and Cheddar Frittata, 18
Spinach Soufflé, 93
Stuffed Pork Loin with Sun-Dried
    Tomatoes and Goat Cheese, 157
Sun-Dried Tomato and Feta Fat Bombs, 233
Sweet 'n' Savory Toast with
    Burrata and Berries, 12
Triple Cheese Chips, 235
Zucchini Lasagna, 95–96, 179–180
Cheesecakes
Blackberry "Cheesecake" Bites, 275
Blueberry Cheesecake Bars, 272
Cheesecake Fat Bombs, 261
Cheesecake Smoothie, 5–6
Chocolate–Macadamia Nut Cheesecake, 231
Italian Cream Cheesecake, 278
Lemon Cheesecake Bars, 274
No-Bake Chocolate Raspberry
    Cheesecake, 277–278
Peanut Butter Cheesecake, 228
Pumpkin-Ricotta Cheesecake, 278
Quick Pressure Cooker Cheesecake, 278
Raspberry Cheesecake Squares, 273
Slow Cooker Sour-Cream Cheesecake, 228
Strawberry Cheesecake, 277
Toasted Almond Cheesecake, 231–232
Cherry-Coconut Pancakes, 6
Chia seeds
Chia Almond "Oatmeal," 34
Chia Parfait, 30
Chocolate-Chia Pudding, 290
Overnight Chia Pudding, 34
Overnight Chocolate Chia Pudding, 31
Yogurt Parfait with Chia Seeds, 30
Chicken, 126
Almond Meal–Crusted Chicken Fingers, 127
Avocado and Eggs with Shredded
    Chicken, 13–14
Avocado Chicken Burger, 143–144
Bacon Barbecued Chicken, 134–135
Bacon-Mushroom Chicken, 215
Bacon Ranch Cheesy Chicken Breasts, 133
Bacon-Wrapped Chicken, 135
Bacon-Wrapped Jalapeño Chicken, 129, 252
Baked Chicken Tenders, 138–139
Balsamic Chicken with Asparagus
    and Tomatoes, 134
Basil Chicken Zucchini "Pasta," 133
BBQ Chicken Skewers, 129

BBQ Chicken Wraps, 129
Breaded Chicken Strip Lettuce Wraps, 129
Broccoli-Stuffed Chicken, 194
Buffalo Chicken Breakfast Muffins, 193
Buffalo Chicken Dip, 238–239
Buffalo Chicken Salad, 70–71
Buffalo Chicken Tenders, 195
Buffalo Chicken Wings, 127, 193
Calabacitas Con Pollo, 146
California Chicken Bake with Guacamole, 148
Caprese Balsamic Chicken, 132
Caprese-Stuffed Chicken Breasts, 132
Carne Asada Chicken Bowls, 135
Cheesy Chicken and Rice Skillet
    Casserole, 146–147
Cheesy Chicken Taquitos, 251–252
Cheesy Triple Meat Baked "Spaghetti," 179
Chicken & Waffles, 147
Chicken Adobo, 143
Chicken and Baby Corn Chowder, 61
Chicken and Cheese Quesadillas, 145
Chicken and Dumplings, 131
Chicken, Avocado, and Egg Salad, 69
Chicken Bacon Burgers, 144
Chicken-Bacon Soup, 208
Chicken Bone Broth, 302
Chicken Breast Tenders with Riesling
    Cream Sauce, 129–130
Chicken Brunch Pie with Cheddar
    Pecan Crust, 28–29
Chicken Cacciatore, 131, 214
Chicken Caesar Salad, 77
Chicken Chowder with Bacon, 209
Chicken Cordon Bleu, 137
Chicken Cordon Bleu Casserole, 137
Chicken Cutlets with Garlic Cream Sauce, 126
Chicken Enchiladas, 131
Chicken Fajitas, 131
Chicken Fajita Stuffed Bell Peppers, 133
Chicken Kebabs with Spicy
    Almond Sauce, 130
Chicken Kiev, 196
Chicken Marsala Soup, 59
Chicken Melon Salad, 71
Chicken Milanese, 132
Chicken Mole, 214
Chicken-Nacho Soup, 208
Chicken Noodle Soup, 58
Chicken Nuggets, 139
Chicken Paprikash, 127–128
Chicken Parmesan, 128, 194
Chicken Piccata, 138
Chicken Piccata with Mushrooms, 139–140
Chicken Pot Pie, 130
Chicken Potstickers, 144–145
Chicken Quesadillas, 145
Chicken Ramen Soup, 60
Chicken Salad on Romaine Boats, 71
Chicken Salad–Stuffed Avocados, 73
Chicken Salad–Stuffed Peppers, 147–148
Chicken Shawarma, 134
Chicken Taco Soup with Cauliflower Rice, 61
Chicken Tamale Pie, 148
Chicken Tenderloin Packets with Broccoli,
    Radishes, and Parmesan, 135
Chicken Tenders, 127
Chicken Teriyaki, 136–137
Chicken Thigh Chili with Avocado, 136
Chicken Thighs with Lemon Cream Sauce, 141
Chicken Tikka Masala, 137–138
Chicken Tortilla Soup, 59
Chicken Vegetable Hash, 126
Chicken with Mushrooms,
    Port, and Cream, 137
Chipotle Chicken Chili, 211
Chopped Chicken-Avocado
    Lettuce Wraps, 129

Chorizo, Chicken, and Salsa Verde, 141
Cilantro Chili Chicken Skewers, 135
Classic Chicken Salad, 70
Coconut Chicken, 128–129
Coconut Chicken Curry, 214
Creamy Chicken and Spinach Bake, 132
Creamy Chicken Stew, 210
Creamy Lemon Chicken, 215
Crispy Chicken Paillard, 130
Crispy Chicken Thighs with Radishes
    and Mushrooms, 135
Curried Chicken Salad, 130
Curried Chicken with Bamboo Shoots, 133
Easy Chicken Soup, 58
Feta and Olive Stuffed Chicken Thighs, 140
Fiesta Lime Chicken Chowder, 59
Fried Chicken, 142–143
Fried Chicken Breasts, 193
Garlicky Braised Chicken Thighs, 214
Garlic Parmesan Wings, 127
Golden Chicken Asiago, 147
Greek Chicken and "Rice" Soup
    with Artichokes, 60
Greek Chicken Souvlaki, 140
Green-Chile Chicken Enchilada
    Casserole, 145–146
Grilled Chicken Cobb Salad, 76–77
Harissa Chicken and Brussels Sprouts
    with Yogurt Sauce, 139
Herbed Chicken Stock, 302
Herb-Infused Chicken, 141–142
Herb Roasted Whole Chicken
    with Jicama, 142
Hungarian Chicken, 215
Jalapeño-Chicken Soup, 60
Jalapeño Popper Chicken Casserole, 147
Jamaican Jerk Chicken, 142
Jambalaya Soup, 209–210
Keto Lasagna with Deli Meat
    "Noodles," 161–162
Kung Pao Chicken, 138
Lemon Butter Chicken, 140
Lemon Chicken and Asparagus Stir-Fry, 140
Lemon-Dijon Boneless Chicken, 194
Lemon-Rosemary Spatchcock
    Chicken, 133–134
Lemony Chicken Salad with
    Blueberries and Fennel, 72
Lettuce-Wrapped Chicken Burger, 144
Mandarin Orange Chicken, 214
Matzo Ball Chicken Soup, 58
Mezze Cake, 148
Moroccan Chicken and Vegetable Tagine, 134
Mulligatawny Soup with Cauliflower Rice, 209
Mustard Shallot Chicken
    Drumsticks, 142
Nashville Hot Chicken, 195
Paprika Chicken with Broccoli, 128
Peanut-Chicken Soup, 59–60
Pecan Chicken Salad, 71
Potluck Chicken Spaghetti
    Squash Casserole, 146
Roasted Chicken, Artichoke, and
    Hearts of Palm Salad, 76
Roasted Chicken Dinner, 215
Roasted Chicken Thighs and Zucchini
    with Wine Reduction, 141
Roasted Chicken with Cilantro
    Mayonnaise, 127
Roasted Herb Chicken, 143
Sesame Broiled Chicken Thighs, 140–141
Shredded Chicken, 126
Simple Chicken-Vegetable Soup, 210
Smothered Sour Cream Chicken Thighs, 145
Southern Oven-Fried Chicken, 143
Southwest-Style Chicken Soup, 60–61
Spaghetti Squash Chicken Bowls, 136

Spiced Chicken, 194
Spiced-Pumpkin Chicken Soup, 207
Spicy Creamy Chicken Soup, 60
Spicy Kung Pao Chicken, 144
Spinach and Bacon Stuffed
    Chicken Thighs, 139
Sriracha Wings, 252
Stuffed Chicken Breasts, 128
Tandoori Vegetable Chicken Skewers, 138
Thai Chicken Lettuce Cups, 137
Thai Chicken Skewers with Peanut Sauce, 252
Tomato Basil Chicken Zoodle Bowls, 136
Tom Kha Gai, 59
Tuscan Chicken, 147
White Chicken Chili, 213
White Chili, 144
Zesty Chicken Tender Salad, 76
Chiles
    Chile Relleno Scrambled Eggs, 21
    Chiles Rellenos, 92
    Crustless Sausage and Green
        Chile Quiche, 25
    Enchilada Casserole, 213
    Green-Chile Chicken Enchilada
        Casserole, 145–146
    Green Chile Deviled Eggs, 243
    Tex-Mex Green Chile Corn Bread, 41
Chilis. See Soups, stews, and chilis
Chili sauce and paste
    Cilantro Chili Chicken Skewers, 135
    Sesame-Crusted Tuna with Sweet
        Chili Vinaigrette, 114
Chimichurri, 304
    Chimichurri Sauce, 307
    Chimichurri Shrimp, 122
    Flank Steak with Kale Chimichurri, 166
    Short Ribs with Chimichurri, 199
Chips
    Crispy Kale Chips, 235
    Flaxseed Chips and Guacamole, 234–235
    Garlic Pepperoni Chips, 235–236
    Margarita Pizza Chips, 235
    Parmesan Zucchini Chips, 235
    Smoky Zucchini Chips, 191
    Spicy Cheddar Wafers, 235
    Spicy Jalapeño Chips and Ranch, 247
    Triple Cheese Chips, 235
Chives
    Bacon Cheddar Chive Scones, 41
    Bacon Chive Fat Bombs, 233
    Black Forest Ham, Cheese, and
        Chive Roll-Ups, 239
    Cheddar-Chive Biscuits, 35
    Duck Legs Braised in Olive Oil
        with Chive Cream, 216
Chocolate
    Air-Fried Vanilla and Chocolate
        Layer Cake, 204
    Almond Chocolate Bark, 255
    Avocado Brownies, 265
    Brownie Chocolate Cake, 230
    Candied Bacon Fudge, 255
    Chewy "Noatmeal" Chocolate
        Chip Cookies, 270
    Chocolate & Coconut
        Pudding, 227–228
    Chocolate Almond Fat Bombs, 262
    Chocolate Avocado Pudding, 289–290
    Chocolate Cake Donuts, 46
    Chocolate Cake with Whipped Cream, 232
    Chocolate-Chia Pudding, 290
    Chocolate Chip Banana Bread, 50
    Chocolate Chip Brownies, 264
    Chocolate Chip Cookie Dough Balls, 266–267
    Chocolate Chip Cookies, 266
    Chocolate Chip–Pecan Biscotti, 204
    Chocolate Chip Scones, 42

Chocolate, Chocolate Chip Pancakes, 8
Chocolate Chunk Cookies, 263
Chocolate Coconut Milk Ice Cream, 294
Chocolate Coconut "Oatmeal," 33
Chocolate-Coconut Treats, 257
Chocolate-Covered Bacon, 256–257
Chocolate-Covered Strawberries, 258
Chocolate-Dipped Peanut
    Butter Ice Pops, 295
Chocolate-Drizzled Pecan Shortbread, 270
Chocolate Fudge, 257
Chocolate–Macadamia Nut Cheesecake, 231
Chocolate Marble Pound Cake, 281
Chocolate Martini, 298–299
Chocolate-Mint Smoothie, 5
Chocolate Mousse, 288
Chocolate Mousse Pie Cups, 285
Chocolate Mug Cake, 282
Chocolate, Peanut Butter, and
    Banana Shake, 4–5
Chocolate Peanut Butter Cups, 257
Chocolate Peanut Butter Fat Bombs, 259
Chocolate–Peanut Butter Fudge, 226
Chocolate Peppermint Fudge, 256
Chocolate Pot de Crème, 226
Chocolate Protein Shake, 5
Chocolate Sandwich Cookies, 264
Chocolate Sea Salt Almonds, 254
Chocolate Walnut Fudge, 226
Chocolate Whoopie Pies, 288
Churros and Chocolate Sauce, 296
Cinnamon-Cocoa Almonds, 226
Classic Chocolate Brownies, 270–271
Coconut Flour–Based Chocolate
    Chip Waffles, 10
Cookie Dough Fat Bombs, 261
Cookies and Cream Parfait, 290
Cowboy Cookie Dough Fat Bombs, 261
Creamy Tiramisu Fat Bomb, 262
Crustless Cannoli, 291
Dairy-Free Chocolate Donuts, 47
Dairy-Free Chocolate Truffles, 255
Delectable Peanut Butter Cup Cake, 229
Double Chocolate Peppermint
    Cookies, 263–264
Double Chocolate Shake, 5
French Vanilla Ice Cream with Hot Fudge, 293
"Frosty" Chocolate Shake, 291
Fudge Brownies, 272–273
Fudge Nut Brownies, 232
Fudgy Brownies, 269
Hazelnut-Chocolate Snack Cakes, 279
Hot Almond Chocolate, 298
Hot Cocoa, 298
Maddie's Favorite Chocolate Malt, 288
Mexican Chocolate Pudding, 289, 293
Mint Chocolate Fat Bombs, 258
90-Second Lava Cake, 281
No-Bake Brownie Bites, 271
No-Bake Chocolate Raspberry
    Cheesecake, 277–278
No-Bake Coconut Chocolate Squares, 273
Nut Butter Cup Fat Bomb, 259
Nutty Chocolate Protein Shake, 4
Overnight Chocolate Chia Pudding, 31
Peanut Butter–Chocolate Chip
    Cookies, 262–263
Peanut Butter Cup Protein Smoothie, 4
Peanut Butter Mousse, 288
Pecan Chocolate Chip Cookies, 268–269
Pistachio-Raspberry Chocolate Bark, 275
Pumpkin Cheesecake Brownies, 271–272
Salted Caramel Fudge Fat Bombs, 260–261
Slow Cooker Chocolate Chip Cookies, 232
Spiced-Chocolate Fat Bombs, 260
Spicy Hot Chocolate, 298
Tiramisu, 276–277

Ultra-Soft Pumpkin Chocolate Bars, 275
Whipped Cream-Chocolate
    Pudding Parfaits, 290
Zucchini Chocolate Muffins, 46
Churros and Chocolate Sauce, 296
Cilantro
    Chilled Avocado-Cilantro Soup, 55
    Chimichurri, 304
    Cilantro Chili Chicken Skewers, 135
    Cilantro Lime Taco Bowls, 183
    Crab Cakes with Cilantro Crema, 115
    Grilled Hanger Steak with
        Cilantro Crema, 167–168
    Roasted Chicken with Cilantro
        Mayonnaise, 127
    Slow Cooker Barbacoa Pulled Beef with
        Cilantro Cauliflower Rice, 219
    Spice-Rubbed Roasted Pork with
        Cilantro Pesto, 157–158
Cinnamon
    Cinnamon "Apple" Pecan Coffee Cake, 47–48
    Cinnamon Butter, 301
    Cinnamon-Caramel Sauce, 310
    Cinnamon-Cocoa Almonds, 226
    Cinnamon Coconut Fat Bomb, 262
    Cinnamon Coffee Cake, 48
    Cinnamon-Dusted Almonds, 256
    Cinnamon French Toast Sticks, 12
    Cinnamon-Glazed Pecans, 256
    Cinnamon Muffins with Cream
        Cheese Frosting, 43
    Cinnamon-Nut Cottage Cheese, 31
    Cinnamon Pecan "Apple" Crisp, 286–287
    Cinnamon Popovers with
        Coconut Streusel, 275
    Cinnamon Roll Fat Bomb, 261–262
    Cinnamon Roll "Noatmeal," 33
    Cinnamon Rolls, 51
    Cinnamon Swirl Bread, 49–50
    Coconut Cinnamon Bars, 274
    Creamy Cinnamon Breakfast Pudding, 31
    Creamy Cinnamon Smoothie, 4
Citrus. See also specific
    Citrus Arugula Salad, 64
    Citrus Asparagus with Pistachios, 81
    Swordfish in Tarragon-Citrus Butter, 112
Clams
    Creamy Seafood Stew with
        Cauliflower Rice, 63
    New England Clam Chowder, 64
    Seafood Fideo, 120
    "Spaghetti" with Clams, 115
Cloud Bread, 312
Coconut
    Almond Coconut Hot Cereal, 34
    Avocado Coconut Smoothie, 6
    Buttery Coconut Bread, 50
    Cherry-Coconut Pancakes, 6
    Chocolate & Coconut
        Pudding, 227–228
    Chocolate Coconut Milk Ice Cream, 294
    Chocolate Coconut "Oatmeal," 33
    Chocolate-Coconut Treats, 257
    Cinnamon Coconut Fat Bomb, 262
    Cinnamon Popovers with
        Coconut Streusel, 275
    Coconut Almond Flour Bread, 311–312
    Coconut Berry Smoothie, 4
    Coconut Chicken, 128–129
    Coconut Chicken Curry, 214
    Coconut Cinnamon Bars, 274
    Coconut Cookies, 265
    Coconut Custard, 226
    Coconut Flaxseed Waffles, 10–11
    Coconut Flour–Based Chocolate
        Chip Waffles, 10
    Coconut Ginger Salmon Burgers, 110–111

Coconut (*continued*)
Coconut Granola, 32
Coconut Iced Coffee, 297
Coconut Lemon Fat Bombs, 259
Coconut Lime Macaroons, 270
Coconut Macaroons, 269–270
Coconut Milk Baked Haddock, 102
Coconut-Orange Cupcakes, 276
Coconut Pie Crust, 312
Coconut-Raspberry Cake, 229
Coconut Saffron Mussels, 118
Coconut Shrimp, 125, 198
Coconut Truffles, 256
Coconut Tzatziki, 236
Coconut Yogurt Berry Parfait, 30
Double Coconut Panna Cotta, 290–291
Green Coconut Avocado Smoothie, 2
Lime-Coconut Fat Bomb, 258–259
No-Bake Coconut Chocolate Squares, 273
No-Bake Coconut Cookies, 265
Ranch Wedge Salad with
    Coconut "Bacon," 64–65
Seafood Coconut Stew, 119
Shrimp Coconut Pad Thai, 122
Tropical Smoothie, 3
Turmeric Coconut Mahi-Mahi, 104
Cod
Cod Cakes, 102
Cod with Parsley Pistou, 101
Crispy Fish Sticks, 198
Crispy Fried Cod, 101
Fennel and Cod Chowder with
    Fried Mushrooms, 63
Fish Tacos, 101
Mustard-Crusted Cod with
    Roasted Broccoli, 101
Poached Cod over Brothy Veggie
    Noodles, 101–102
Roasted Cod with Garlic Butter
    and Bok Choy, 101
Coffee
Bulletproof Coffee, 297
Buttered Coffee, 297
Buttered Coffee Shake, 6
Chipotle Coffee-Crusted
    Bone-In Rib Eye, 169
Coconut Iced Coffee, 297
Coffee Smoothie, 6
Creamy Tiramisu Fat Bomb, 262
Matcha Coffee, 297
Pumpkin Spice Latte, 297
Tiramisu, 276–277
Coleslaw. *See* Cabbage and coleslaw; Salads
Cookies and bars. *See also* Brownies
Almond Butter Oatmeal Cookies, 270
Almond Cookies, 266
Blondies, 272
Blueberry Cheesecake Bars, 272
Bourbon Pecan Pie Bars, 274
"Buttermilk" Custard Pie Bars, 284
Carrot Cake Cookies, 269
Chai Tea Cookies, 262
Chewy "Noatmeal" Chocolate
    Chip Cookies, 270
Chocolate Chip Cookie Dough Balls, 266–267
Chocolate Chip Cookies, 266
Chocolate Chip–Pecan Biscotti, 204
Chocolate-Drizzled Pecan
    Shortbread, 270
Chocolate Sandwich Cookies, 264
Chocolate Whoopie Pies, 288
Coconut Cinnamon Bars, 274
Coconut Cookies, 265
Coconut Lime Macaroons, 270
Coconut Macaroons, 269–270
Double Chocolate Peppermint
    Cookies, 263–264

Easy Peasy Peanut Butter Cookies, 268
Fluffy Lime-Meringue Clouds, 271
French Meringues, 271
Iced Gingerbread Cookies, 268
Lemon Cheesecake Bars, 274
Lemon Cookies, 263
Lemon-Poppyseed Cookies, 268
Lemon Snowball Cookies, 265
No-Bake Coconut Chocolate Squares, 273
No-Bake Coconut Cookies, 265
Nutty Shortbread Cookies, 266
Peanut Butter Cake Bars, 273
Peanut Butter–Chocolate Chip
    Cookies, 262–263
Peanut Butter Cookies, 265
Pecan Chocolate Chip Cookies, 268–269
Pecan Pie Bars, 274
Pecan Sandies, 266
Pecan Squares, 204
Pistachio Cookies, 267
Pumpkin Cookies, 267
Raspberry Cream Cheese Tart Bars, 286
Salted Peanut Butter Cookies, 267
Slow Cooker Chocolate Chip Cookies, 232
Snickerdoodle Bars, 273–274
Snickerdoodle Cookies, 268
Sugar Cookie Balls, 264
Ultra-Soft Pumpkin Chocolate Bars, 275
Corn Chowder, Chicken and Baby, 61
Cottage cheese
Cinnamon-Nut Cottage Cheese, 31
Creamy Cinnamon Breakfast Pudding, 31
Greek Cottage Cheese Salad, 70
Crabmeat
Classic Crab Cakes, 115–116
Crab and Artichoke Dip, 239
Crab au Gratin, 116–117
Crab Cakes, 197
Crab Cakes with Cilantro Crema, 115
Crab Cakes with Garlic Aioli, 116
Crab Cakes with Green
    Goddess Dressing, 116
Crab Cakes with Spicy Tartar Sauce, 115
Crab Fried Rice, 197
Crab Salad Lettuce Cups, 79
Crab Salad–Stuffed Avocado, 72
Crab-Stuffed Portabella
    Mushrooms, 117
Creamy Seafood Stew with
    Cauliflower Rice, 63
Hot Crab Sauce, 308
Seafood Fideo, 120
Spicy Crab Cakes, 116
Crackers
Almond Crackers, 234
Crispy Parmesan Crackers, 234
Nut Crackers, 234
Seedy Crackers, 234
Cranberries
Cranberry Pork Roast, 202
Dairy-Free Cranberry Muffins, 43–44
Glazed Cranberry-Orange Muffins, 44
Iced Cranberry-Gingerbread Loaf, 49
Crawfish Cream Sauce, Blackened
Redfish with Spicy, 104
Cream. *See also* Whipped cream
Blackened Redfish with Spicy
    Crawfish Cream Sauce, 104
Chicken Breast Tenders with Riesling
    Cream Sauce, 129–130
Chicken with Mushrooms,
    Port, and Cream, 137
Creamed Broccoli, 81
Creamed Cauliflower Soup, 51
Creamed Mushroom and Fennel Soup, 53
Cream of Mushroom Soup, 53
Cream-Poached Trout, 113

Creamy Banana Fat Bombs, 260
Creamy Broccoli, Bacon, and Cheese Soup, 52
Creamy Lemon Chicken, 215
Creamy Seafood Stew with
    Cauliflower Rice, 63
Creamy Shrimp and Grits Casserole, 119–120
Creamy Spaghetti Squash Bake, 94
Creamy Tomato Soup, 54
Duck with Turnips in Cream, 216–217
Grilled Rib Eye Steaks with
    Horseradish Cream, 199–200
Grilled Venison Loin with Dijon
    Cream Sauce, 189
Pan-Seared Hangar Steak with Easy
    Herb Cream Sauce, 167
Pork Loin with Creamy Gravy, 221
Pork Loin with Ginger Cream Sauce, 221–222
Rainbow Trout with Cream Leek Sauce, 113
Salmon in Cream Sauce, 105
Sea Scallops with Bacon Cream Sauce, 118
Shrimp with Creamy Tomato-
    and-Spinach Sauce, 123
Slow Cooker Pork Chops with Creamy
    Bacon-and-Artichoke Sauce, 221
Spicy Creamy Chicken Soup, 60
Strawberries and Cream Ice Pops, 294
Strawberry Cream Pie, 283
Cream cheese
Bacon-Wrapped Jalapeño Poppers, 191
Berry Cheesecake Smoothie, 6
Blackberry "Cheesecake" Bites, 275
Blueberry Cheesecake Bars, 272
Blueberry Cream Cheese Bites, 291
Butter Cake with Cream Cheese
    Buttercream, 282
Butter Pecan Cheesecake
    Truffle Fat Bombs, 261
Cheesecake Fat Bombs, 261
Cheesecake Smoothie, 5–6
Chocolate–Macadamia Nut Cheesecake, 231
Cinnamon Muffins with Cream
    Cheese Frosting, 43
Cream Cheese Pancakes, 7
Cream Cheese Pound Cake, 279
Cream Cheese Pumpkin Muffins, 46
Cream Cheese Sausage Balls, 200–201
Crustless Cream Cheese and
    Spinach Quiche, 26
Garlic Cloud Bread, 38–39
Italian Cream Cheesecake, 278
Jalapeño Popper Chicken Casserole, 147
Jalapeño Poppers, 246
Lemon Cheesecake Bars, 274
Macadamia Nut Cream Cheese Log, 241
Mushroom Cream Cheese Omelet, 17
Mustard Cream Sauce, 308
No-Bake Chocolate Raspberry
    Cheesecake, 277–278
Peanut Butter Cheesecake, 228
Pimento Cheese, 238
Prosciutto and Cream Cheese
    Stuffed Mushrooms, 250
Pumpkin Cheesecake Brownies, 271–272
Pumpkin Pancakes with Maple Frosting, 8
Pumpkin-Ricotta Cheesecake, 278
Quick Pressure Cooker Cheesecake, 278
Raspberry Cheesecake Squares, 273
Raspberry Cream Cheese Tart Bars, 286
Simple Cheesy Yogurt, 30
Slow Cooker Sour-Cream Cheesecake, 228
Spiced Cream Cheese Pancakes, 7
Strawberry Cheesecake, 277
Strawberry Cheesecake Fat Bombs, 262
Toasted Almond Cheesecake, 231–232
Vanilla Cheesecake, 231
Cucumbers
Coconut Tzatziki, 236

Cold Cucumber and Avocado Soup, 56
Cool and Creamy Cucumber
    Tomato Salad, 70
Cucumber and Tomato Feta Salad, 74
Cucumber Green Smoothie, 1–2
Cucumber, Tomato, and Avocado Salad, 74
Grilled Steak Salad with
    Cucumber and Mint, 77
Mediterranean Cucumber Bites, 241
Quick Pickled Cucumbers, 87
Smoked Salmon and Cucumber Bites, 239
Smoked Salmon and Cucumber Noodles, 70
Sole with Cucumber Radish Salsa, 111–112
Spiced Cucumbers, 87
Tuna and Jicama Salad with Mint
    Cucumber Dressing, 68
Cumin Coleslaw, Apple Cabbage, 75
Cupcakes. See Cakes and cupcakes
Curry
    Coconut Chicken Curry, 214
    Curried Broccoli, Cheddar & Toasted
        Almond Soup, 208–209
    Curried Chicken Salad, 130
    Curried Chicken with Bamboo Shoots, 133
    Curried Egg Salad, 69
    Curried Lamb, 225
    Curried Salmon Fish Cakes, 110
    Curried Tuna Salad with Pepitas, 72
    Curried Vegetable Stew, 210
    Fiery Curry Beef, 219
    Halibut Curry, 100
    Sea Scallops with Curry Sauce, 118
    Thai Green Curry with Tofu
        and Vegetables, 212
    Vegan Pumpkin Curry, 212
Custards. See Puddings and custards

D

Dairy products, vi. See also specific
Desserts. See also Brownies; Cakes and
        cupcakes; Cheesecakes; Cookies and
        bars; Fat bombs; Ice cream; Ice pops;
        Pies, sweet; Puddings and custards
    Almond Chocolate Bark, 255
    Berry-Pumpkin Compote, 228
    Blackberry Cobbler, 228, 284
    Blueberry Cream Cheese Bites, 291
    Blueberry Crisp, 228–229
    Blueberry Crumble, 287
    Chocolate Chunk Cookies, 263
    Chocolate-Coconut Treats, 257
    Chocolate-Covered Bacon, 256–257
    Chocolate-Covered Strawberries, 258
    Chocolate Mousse, 288
    Chocolate Peanut Butter Cups, 257
    Chocolate Pot de Crème, 226
    Chocolate Sea Salt Almonds, 254
    Churros and Chocolate Sauce, 296
    Cinnamon-Caramel Sauce, 310
    Cinnamon-Cocoa Almonds, 226
    Cinnamon-Dusted Almonds, 256
    Cinnamon-Glazed Pecans, 256
    Cinnamon Pecan "Apple" Crisp, 286–287
    Cinnamon Popovers with
        Coconut Streusel, 275
    Coconut Truffles, 256
    Cookies and Cream Parfait, 290
    Creamy Panna Cotta, 290
    Crustless Cannoli, 291
    Dairy-Free Chocolate Truffles, 255
    Double Coconut Panna Cotta, 290–291
    Grilled Cantaloupe, 257–258
    Grilled Sweet Peaches, 258
    Macadamia Lime Bites, 291
    Mixed Berry Crisp, 287
    Mixed Berry Sherbet, 294

Pastry Cream, 310
Peanut Butter Mousse, 288
Pistachio-Raspberry Chocolate
    Bark, 275
Pralines, 256
Roasted Strawberries with
    Whipped Cream, 258
Salted Caramel Cashew Brittle, 255
Salted Caramels, 254
Sangria Granita, 295
Strawberry Frozen Yogurt, 295
Strawberry Panna Cotta, 291
Strawberry Rhubarb Cobbler, 287–288
Summer Squash Mock Apple
    Crumble, 282–283
Vanilla Panna Cotta, 291
White Chocolate Bark, 255
Dill
    Avocado and Smoked Salmon Stack
        with Caper Sauce, 240
    Cheesy Dill Fat Bombs, 233–234
    Creamy Dill and Radish "Potato" Salad, 68–69
    Dill-Asparagus Bake, 206
    Dilled Tuna Salad Sandwich, 241
    Fish Fillets with Lemon-Dill Sauce, 196
Dips and spreads
    Baba Ghanoush, 237
    Bacon Chutney, 310
    Bacon Guacamole, 236
    Bacon Jam, 310
    Bagna Cauda, 305–306
    Buffalo Chicken Dip, 238–239
    Cauliflower Hummus, 237
    Cheesy Shrimp Spread, 239–240
    Coconut Tzatziki, 236
    Crab and Artichoke Dip, 239
    Dips Herby Yogurt Dip, 236
    French Onion Dip, 237
    Guacamole, 237
    Lemon-Turmeric Aioli, 236–237
    Macadamia Nut Cream Cheese Log, 241
    Olive and Artichoke Tapenade, 237
    Pimento Cheese, 238
    Queso Blanco Dip, 238
    Queso Dip, 238
    Roasted Red Pepper Dip, 238
    Spinach-Artichoke Dip, 238
    Taco Layer Dip, 239
    Tzatziki Dip with Vegetables, 236
    Zucchini Hummus, 237
Donuts
    Baked Donut Bites with Jelly, 47
    Chocolate Cake Donuts, 46
    Dairy-Free Chocolate Donuts, 47
    Jelly Donuts, 46
    Matcha Donuts, 47
Dressings
    Buttermilk Ranch Dressing, 303
    Creamy Grapefruit-Tarragon Dressing, 304
    Ginger-Lime Dressing, 305
    Green Basil Dressing, 303
    Herbed Balsamic Dressing, 305
    Lemon-Garlic Dressing, 303
    Lemon Poppy Seed Dressing, 305
    Lemon-Tahini Dressing, 305
    Mustard Shallot Vinaigrette, 304
    Ranch Dressing, 304
    Traditional Caesar Dressing, 304
Drinks. See also Shakes; Smoothies
    Bloody Mary, 298
    Blueberry Mojito, 299
    Bulletproof Coffee, 297
    Buttered Coffee, 297
    Chocolate Martini, 298–299
    Coconut Iced Coffee, 297
    Earl Grey Rose Latte, 297
    Fat Chai, 297–298

Frosé Slushie, 300
Gelatin Shooters, 301
Green Tea Latte, 297
Hot Almond Chocolate, 298
Hot Buttered Rum, 299
Hot Cocoa, 298
Lime Margarita, 299
Manhattan, 300–301
Matcha Coffee, 297
Michelada, 300
Moscow Mule, 299
Negroni, 300
Old-Fashioned, 300
Pumpkin Spice Latte, 297
Raspberry Mimosa, 300
Sangria, 300
Spicy Hot Chocolate, 298
Spicy Margarita, 299
Tequila Sunrise, 300
Vesper martini, 300
Virgin (or Not) Eggnog, 298
Virgin (or Not) Mojito, 299
Duck
    Duck Legs Braised in Olive Oil
        with Chive Cream, 216
    Duck with Turnips in Cream, 216–217
    East "Roasted" Duck, 216
Dumplings, Chicken and, 131

E

Eggplants
    Baba Ghanoush, 237
    Eggplant Lasagna, 87
    Roasted Eggplant with Mint
        and Harissa, 87–88
    Sheet Pan Sirloin Steak with
        Eggplant and Zucchini, 168
    Slow Cooker Eggplant Parmesan, 212–213
    Spicy Pork and Eggplant Stir-Fry, 163
    Stuffed Eggplant, 88
Egg Roll in a Bowl, 163
Eggs
    Asparagus Frittata, 18
    Asparagus Gouda Frittata, 17
    Asparagus, Mushroom & Fennel Frittata, 17
    Avocado and Eggs with Shredded
        Chicken, 13–14
    Avocado Deviled Eggs, 242
    Avocado Egg Salad, 69
    Bacon-and-Egg Breakfast Casserole, 206
    Bacon and Egg Cheeseburgers, 174
    Bacon and Egg Pizza, 254
    Bacon and Spinach Egg Muffins, 192
    Bacon-Artichoke Omelet, 16
    Bacon Broccoli Crustless Quiche Cups, 26
    Bacon-Cheese Deviled Eggs, 243
    Bacon Deviled Eggs, 243
    Bacon, Egg, and Cheese Cups, 19
    Bacon Eggs Benedict Cups, 20
    Bacon-Wrapped Asparagus and Eggs, 13
    Bacon-Wrapped Egg Cups, 19–20
    Baked Eggs in Ham Cups, 19
    Baked Omelet with Pancetta
        and Swiss Cheese, 17
    Breakfast Burrito Bowl, 29
    Breakfast Pizza, 27
    Breakfast "Sandwich," 13
    Broccoli and Cheese Quiche Cups, 20
    Broccoli Bacon Egg Muffin Cups, 20
    Broccoli Quiche, 25
    Brussels Sprouts & Ground Beef
        Scrambled Eggs, 22
    Buttery Boiled Eggs, 13
    Cheesy Sausage & Egg Muffins, 20
    Cheesy Scrambled Eggs, 21
    Chicken, Avocado, and Egg Salad, 69

Eggs (*continued*)
  Chile Relleno Scrambled Eggs, 21
  Chorizo Egg Muffins, 21
  Classic Bacon and Eggs, 13
  Corned Beef Breakfast Hash, 23
  Country Garden Scramble, 23
  Creamed Spinach with Eggs, 14–15
  Crustless Cream Cheese and
      Spinach Quiche, 26
  Crustless Quiche Lorraine, 24–25
  Crustless Sausage and Green
      Chile Quiche, 25
  Crustless Wild Mushroom–Kale Quiche, 206
  Curried Egg Salad, 69
  Denver Omelet Breakfast Bake, 16
  Deviled Egg Salad with Bacon, 69–70
  Easy Eggs Benedict, 24
  Egg & Cheese Biscuit Casserole, 15–16
  Egg Baked in Avocado, 14
  Egg Breakfast Muffins, 20
  Egg Drop Soup, 55
  Eggs Benedict on Grilled Portabella
      Mushroom Caps, 24
  Eggs Benedict with Bacon, 23–24
  Eggs Benedict with Five-Minute
      Hollandaise, 24
  Eggs with Goat Cheese and Asparagus, 14
  Fluffy Lime-Meringue Clouds, 271
  French Meringues, 271
  French Toast Egg Muffins, 21
  Garlic Cloud Bread, 38–39
  Greek Frittata with Olives, Artichoke
      Hearts & Feta, 205
  Greek-Style Egg and Tomato Scramble, 22–23
  Green Chile Deviled Eggs, 243
  Ham and Cheese Crustless Quiche, 25
  Ham and Cheese Egg Scramble, 21
  Ham and Cheese Poached Egg Cups, 19
  Italian Omelet, 16
  Italian Vegetable Egg Bake, 15
  Lemon-Herb Baked Frittata, 18–19
  Loaded Denver Omelet, 16
  Loaded Miso Soup with Tofu and Egg, 53–54
  Mediterranean Frittata, 18
  Mexican Egg Casserole, 15
  Mushroom and Bacon Frittata, 17–18
  Mushroom Cream Cheese Omelet, 17
  Prosciutto Egg Cups, 19
  Roasted Brussels Sprouts &
      Poached Eggs, 82–83
  Roasted Vegetable Hash, 23
  Salmon and Egg Scramble, 22
  Sausage and Cheese Frittata, 19
  Sausage Verde Casserole, 26
  Scotch Eggs, 13
  Scrambled Eggs with Mackerel, 22
  Shakshuka, 29
  Simple Egg Salad, 69
  Simple Scrambled Eggs, 21
  Skillet-Baked Eggs with Yogurt
      and Spinach, 15
  Slow Cooker Huevos Rancheros, 205
  Slow Cooker Layered Egg Casserole, 205
  Slow Cooker Mediterranean Eggs, 205
  Slow Cooker Spanakopita Frittata, 205–206
  Southern Fried Deviled Eggs, 243
  Spanakopita Omelet, 16–17
  Spinach, Mushroom, and Cheddar Frittata, 18
  Spinach Salad with Bacon and
      Soft-Boiled Eggs, 78–79
  Spinach Soufflé, 93
  Turkey Egg Scramble, 22
  Turmeric and Avocado Egg Salad, 69
  Vegetable Omelet, 206
  Veggie Frittata, 192
Empanadas, 251
Enchiladas
  Chicken Enchiladas, 131
  Enchilada Casserole, 213
  Enchilada Sauce, 308
  Green-Chile Chicken Enchilada
      Casserole, 145–146
  Turkey Enchilada Skillet, 150
Equipment, vii
Exercise, vii

F
Fajitas
  Beef Fajitas, 164–165
  Chicken Fajitas, 131
  Chicken Fajita Stuffed Bell Peppers, 133
  Southwest-Style Fajita Bowls, 165
  Tandoori Beef Fajitas, 167
Fat bombs
  Avocado Chili Fat Bomb, 233
  Bacon Chive Fat Bombs, 233
  Bacon-Pepper Fat Bombs, 232–233
  Blueberry Fat Bombs, 260
  Butter Pecan Cheesecake
      Truffle Fat Bombs, 261
  Cheesecake Fat Bombs, 261
  Cheesy Dill Fat Bombs, 233–234
  Chocolate Almond Fat Bombs, 262
  Chocolate Peanut Butter Fat Bombs, 259
  Cinnamon Coconut Fat Bomb, 262
  Cinnamon Roll Fat Bomb, 261–262
  Coconut Lemon Fat Bombs, 259
  Cookie Dough Fat Bombs, 261
  Cowboy Cookie Dough Fat Bombs, 261
  Creamy Banana Fat Bombs, 260
  Creamy Tiramisu Fat Bomb, 260
  "Everything but the Bagel" Fat Bombs, 233
  Key Lime Pie Fat Bombs, 260
  Lime Almond Fat Bomb, 260
  Lime-Coconut Fat Bomb, 258–259
  Marzipan Fat Bomb, 259
  Mint Chocolate Fat Bombs, 258
  Nut Butter Cup Fat Bomb, 259
  Peanut Butter Cookie Dough Fat Bombs, 259
  Pumpkin Spice Fat Bombs, 259
  Salted Caramel Fudge Fat Bombs, 260–261
  Salted Macadamia Fat Bomb, 258
  Smoked Salmon Fat Bombs, 233
  Spiced-Chocolate Fat Bombs, 260
  Strawberry Cheesecake Fat Bombs, 262
  Sun-Dried Tomato and Feta Fat Bombs, 233
Fats, v, vi
Fennel
  Asparagus, Mushroom & Fennel
      Frittata, 17
  Caramelized Fennel, 88
  Creamed Mushroom and Fennel
      Soup, 53
  Fennel and Cod Chowder with
      Fried Mushrooms, 63
  Fennel and Orange Marinated
      Olives, 244–245
  Lemony Chicken Salad with
      Blueberries and Fennel, 72
  Slow Cooker Braised Lamb
      with Fennel, 224–225
  Walnut-Fennel Salad with
      Sherry Vinaigrette, 67
Fish and seafood. *See also specific*
  Chili Fish Stew, 99–100
  Fish Fillets with Lemon-Dill Sauce, 196
  Fish Stock, 303
  Fish Tacos, 101
  Ginger Scallion Steamed Fish, 105
  Nut-Crusted Baked Fish, 100
  Omega-3 Salad, 80
  Seafood Ceviche, 120
  Seafood Chowder with Lobster, 63

  Seafood Coconut Stew, 119
  Seafood Fideo, 120
  Sheet Pan Seafood Boil, 119
  Sushi, 106–107
Flatbreads
  Barbecue Onion and Goat
      Cheese Flatbread, 311
  Blackberry, Prosciutto, and Goat
      Cheese Flatbread, 40
  Rosemary Flatbread, 39
Flax Meal Tortillas, 40
Flaxseed
  Coconut Flaxseed Waffles, 10–11
  Flaxseed Chips and Guacamole, 234–235
Flounder with Bok Choy, Pesto, 102
Focaccia, Herb and Olive, 40
French Toast, 12
  Cinnamon French Toast Sticks, 12
  French Toast Egg Muffins, 21
  Toast-less Blueberry French
      Toast, 12–13
Fries
  Avocado "Fries," 248
  Tofu Fries, 248
Fruits, vi. *See also specific*
Fudge
  Almond Butter Fudge, 257
  Candied Bacon Fudge, 255
  Chocolate Fudge, 257
  Chocolate–Peanut Butter Fudge, 226
  Chocolate Peppermint Fudge, 256
  Chocolate Walnut Fudge, 226

G
Garlic
  Charred Alaskan Salmon with
      Garlic Green Beans, 106
  Cheesy Garlic Rolls, 36
  Chicken Cutlets with Garlic Cream Sauce, 126
  Crab Cakes with Garlic Aioli, 116
  Garlic and Herb Baked Shrimp
      with Cauliflower Rice, 125
  Garlic Braised Short Ribs, 173
  Garlic Breadsticks, 249
  Garlic Cloud Bread, 38–39
  Garlic Herb Marinade, 305
  Garlic Herb Marinated Tilapia, 113
  Garlicky Alfredo Sauce, 307
  Garlicky Braised Chicken Thighs, 214
  Garlicky Broccoli Rabe with Artichokes, 82
  Garlicky Green Beans, 88
  Garlicky Kale, 89
  Garlicky Shrimp with Mushrooms, 125
  Garlic-Marinated Flank Steak, 199
  Garlic Parmesan Crusted Salmon, 105
  Garlic Parmesan Wings, 127
  Garlic Pepperoni Chips, 235–236
  Garlic-Rosemary Infused Olive Oil, 305
  Garlic Shrimp, 198
  Garlic Steak, 200
  Garlic Steak Bites, 166
  Garlic Studded Prime Rib with
      Thyme au Jus, 170
  Lemon-Garlic Dressing, 303
  Lemon-Garlic Mushrooms, 191
  Onion-Garlic Pita Bread, 38
  Pan-Seared Lemon-Garlic Salmon, 109–110
  Rib Eye Steaks with Garlic-Thyme
      Butter, 169
  Roasted Cod with Garlic Butter
      and Bok Choy, 101
  Rosemary-Garlic Lamb Racks, 187
  Steamed Mussels with Garlic and Thyme, 117
Gelatin Shooters, 301
Ghee, 301
Gin

Negroni, 300
Vesper martini, 300
Ginger
    Blueberry Smoothie with
        Lemon and Ginger, 3
    Butternut Squash Soup with
        Turmeric and Ginger, 56
    Coconut Ginger Salmon Burgers, 110–111
    Ginger Beef, 218
    Ginger-Lime Dressing, 305
    Ginger Pork Meatballs, 164
    Ginger Scallion Steamed Fish, 105
    Iced Cranberry-Gingerbread Loaf, 49
    Iced Gingerbread Cookies, 268
    Pan-Seared Dijon-Ginger Salmon, 108
    Pork Loin with Ginger Cream Sauce, 221–222
    Pumpkin-Ginger Pudding, 227
    Sesame Ginger Slaw, 75
    Slow Cooker Moist Ginger Cake
        with Whipped Cream, 231
    Soy-Ginger Veggie Noodle
        Steak Roll-Ups, 166
    Warm Gingerbread, 229–230
Granola
    Coconut Granola, 32
    Granola Cereal, 32
    Keto Granola, 32
    Macadamia Nut Granola, 32
    Nut Medley Granola, 31
    Superfood Granola, 32
    Toasty Granola Bars, 33
Grapefruit-Tarragon Dressing, Creamy, 304
Gravy
    Biscuits and Sausage Gravy, 28
    Biscuits with Sausage Gravy, 34–35
    Chicken-Fried Steak Fingers
        with Gravy, 165–166
    Pork Loin with Creamy Gravy, 221
    Pressure Cooker Pot Roast with
        Sour-Cream Gravy, 190
    Smothered Pork Chops with Onion Gravy, 153
Green beans
    Buttery Green Beans, 191
    Charred Alaskan Salmon with
        Garlic Green Beans, 106
    Garlicky Green Beans, 88
    Green Bean Casserole, 88–89
    Italian Green Bean Salad, 73
    Sausage, Zucchini, and Green
        Bean Packets, 162
    Seared Tuna with Steamed Turnips,
        Broccoli, and Green Beans, 114
    Sheet Pan Salmon with Lemon
        Green Beans, 107–108
    Southern Green Beans, 88
    Tofu Green Bean Casserole, 88
    Vegan Niçoise Salad, 64
Greens. See also specific
    Braised Greens with Olives and Walnuts, 87
    Greens and Parmesan Muffins, 45
Grits
    Creamy Shrimp and Grits Casserole, 119–120
    Shrimp and "Grits," 120–121
Grocery shopping, vii
Guacamole, 237
    Bacon Guacamole, 236
    California Chicken Bake with Guacamole, 148
    Flaxseed Chips and Guacamole, 234–235
    Guacamole Salad, 73
    Southwest Meatloaf with Lime
        Guacamole, 176

H

Haddock
    Cheesy Golden Fried Haddock, 103
    Coconut Milk Baked Haddock, 102
    Crispy "Breaded" Haddock, 103
Halibut
    Baked Halibut with Herb Sauce, 102
    Baked Nutty Halibut, 103
    Balsamic Teriyaki Halibut, 103
    Halibut Curry, 100
    Halibut in Tomato Basil Sauce, 103
    Macadamia-Crusted Halibut
        with Mango Coulis, 104
Ham. See also Bacon, Canadian; Prosciutto
    Baked Eggs in Ham Cups, 19
    Black Forest Ham, Cheese, and
        Chive Roll-Ups, 239
    Chicken Cordon Bleu, 137
    Chicken Cordon Bleu Casserole, 137
    Denver Omelet Breakfast Bake, 16
    Fried Ham "Rice," 161
    Ham and Cheese Crustless Quiche, 25
    Ham and Cheese Egg Scramble, 21
    Ham and Cheese Poached Egg Cups, 19
    Ham and Swiss Waffles, 11
    Ham-Broccoli-Cauliflower Casserole, 161
    Ham-Stuffed Pork Chops, 154
    Honey Glazed Ham, 160
    Party Deli Pinwheels, 240
Harissa
    Harissa Chicken and Brussels Sprouts
        with Yogurt Sauce, 139
    Harissa Oil, 304
    Roasted Eggplant with Mint
        and Harissa, 87–88
Hazelnuts
    Brussels Sprouts with Hazelnuts, 83
    Hazelnut-Chocolate Snack Cakes, 279
Hearts of palm
    Mediterranean Spaghetti, 98
    Roasted Chicken, Artichoke, and
        Hearts of Palm Salad, 76
Hemp hearts
    Hemp Cobb Salad, 66
    Konjac Noodles with Spinach Hemp
        Pesto and Goat Cheese, 98
    PB&J Overnight Hemp, 31
    Salmon with Spinach Hemp Pesto, 108
    Spinach Hemp Pesto, 306
Herbs. See also specific
    Avocado-Herb Compound Butter, 301
    Baked Halibut with Herb Sauce, 102
    Dips Herby Yogurt Dip, 236
    Easy Herbed Tomato Bisque, 54
    Flank Steak with Orange-Herb
        Pistou, 166–167
    Garlic and Herb Baked Shrimp
        with Cauliflower Rice, 125
    Garlic Herb Marinade, 305
    Garlic Herb Marinated Tilapia, 113
    Green Herb Smoothie, 1
    Grilled Sirloin Steak with Herbed Butter, 168
    Herb and Olive Focaccia, 40
    Herb-Crusted Lamb Chops, 186–187
    Herbed Balsamic Dressing, 305
    Herbed Chicken Stock, 302
    Herbed Marinara Sauce, 309
    Herbed Meatloaf, 176–177
    Herbed Pumpkin, 92
    Herbed Ricotta–Stuffed Mushrooms, 90
    Herbed Vegetable Broth, 302–303
    Herb-Infused Chicken, 141–142
    Herb-Infused Turkey Breast, 215–216
    Herb-Kale Pesto, 306
    Herb Mustard Lamb Racks, 187
    Herb Pesto, 309
    Herb Roasted Whole Chicken
        with Jicama, 142
    Lemon-Herb Baked Frittata, 18–19
    Mustard-Herb Pork Chops, 222

Pan-Seared Hangar Steak with Easy
    Herb Cream Sauce, 167
Roasted Herb Chicken, 143
Roasted Herb-Crusted Salmon with
    Asparagus and Tomatoes, 110
Hollandaise, 306
Honey Glazed Ham, 160
Horseradish
    Corned Beef & Cabbage with
        Horseradish Cream, 219
    Grilled Rib Eye Steaks with
        Horseradish Cream, 199–200
    Horseradish Compound Butter, 301
Hummus
    Cauliflower Hummus, 237
    Zucchini Hummus, 237

I

Ice cream
    Banana Pudding Ice Cream, 293
    Chocolate Coconut Milk Ice Cream, 294
    French Vanilla Ice Cream with Hot Fudge, 293
    Lavender Ice Cream, 294
    Lemon-Blueberry Ice Cream, 292
    Matcha Ice Cream, 292
    Olive Oil Ice Cream, 292
    Raspberry Ice Cream, 294
    Raspberry Maple Soft Serve, 292–293
    Rich Vanilla Ice Cream, 292
    Sour Cream Ice Cream, 294–295
    Strawberry Avocado Ice Cream, 294
Ice pops
    Blueberry Mint Ice Pops, 295
    Chocolate-Dipped Peanut
        Butter Ice Pops, 295
    Orange Cream Ice Pops, 296
    Strawberries and Cream Ice Pops, 294
    Vanilla-Almond Ice Pops, 295–296
Ingredient staples, vi

J

Jalapeño peppers
    Bacon-Wrapped Jalapeño Chicken, 129, 252
    Bacon-Wrapped Jalapeño Poppers, 191
    Jalapeño Cheese Bread, 39
    Jalapeño-Chicken Soup, 60
    Jalapeño Firecrackers, 246–247
    Jalapeño Popper Chicken
        Casserole, 147
    Jalapeño Poppers, 246
    Spicy Jalapeño Chips and Ranch, 247
Jelly
    Baked Donut Bites with Jelly, 47
    Jelly Donuts, 46
Jicama
    Apple Pie Bites, 283–284
    Herb Roasted Whole Chicken
        with Jicama, 142
    Jicama "Apple" Pie Filling, 283
    Jicama Nachos, 248–249
    Tuna and Jicama Salad with Mint
        Cucumber Dressing, 68

K

Kale
    Almond Kale Smoothie, 2
    Baked Mackerel with Kale and
        Asparagus, 104–105
    Berry Green Smoothie, 1
    Creamy Kale Smoothie, 1
    Crispy Kale Chips, 235
    Crustless Wild Mushroom–Kale Quiche, 206
    Flank Steak with Kale Chimichurri, 166
    Garlicky Kale, 89
    Herb-Kale Pesto, 306

Kale (continued)
Italian Wedding Soup, 61–62
Kale and Cashew Stir-Fry, 89
Kale, Avocado & Tahini Salad, 64
Kale Refresher Smoothie, 1
Kale with Bacon, 89
Killer Kale Salad, 66–67
Mean Green Smoothie, 2
Pepper-Crusted Salmon with Wilted Kale, 107
Smoky Stewed Kale, 89
Spaghetti Squash & Ground Pork
Stir-Fry with Kale, 163
Turkey and Kale Coleslaw, 76
Tuscan Kale Salad with Anchovies, 67
Tuscan Kale Soup, 57
Zuppa Toscana (Sausage and Kale Soup), 62
Kebabs and skewers
Antipasto Skewers, 243
BBQ Chicken Skewers, 129
Caprese Skewers, 241
Chicken Kebabs with Spicy
Almond Sauce, 130
Cilantro Chili Chicken Skewers, 135
Feta Cheese Kebabs, 245
Greek Beef Kebabs with Tzatziki, 199
Marinated Swordfish Skewers, 197
Pork Kebabs, 200
Shrimp and Vegetable Kebabs with
Chipotle Sour Cream Sauce, 124
Tandoori Vegetable Chicken
Skewers, 138
Thai Chicken Skewers with Peanut Sauce, 252
Ketchup, Sugar-Free, 307
Ketogenic diet, iv–vii
Ketosis, v

L
Lamb
Broiled Lamb Chops with Mint Gremolata
and Pan-Fried Zucchini, 187
Curried Lamb, 225
Greek Meatball Lettuce Wraps, 189
Grilled Moroccan Spiced Lamb Chops, 187
Hearty Lamb Cabbage Soup, 62–63
Herb-Crusted Lamb Chops, 186–187
Herb Mustard Lamb Racks, 187
Lamb Chili, 188
Lamb Kofte with Yogurt Sauce, 189
Lamb Meatball Salad with
Yogurt Dressing, 188
Leg of Lamb with Sun-dried
Tomato Pest, 187–188
Rack of Lamb with Kalamata Tapenade, 186
Rosemary-Garlic Lamb Racks, 187
Rosemary Lamb Chops, 225
Savory Lamb Stew, 188–189
Simple Lamb Sausage, 188
Slow Cooker All-in-One Lamb-
Vegetable Dinner, 224
Slow Cooker Braised Lamb
with Fennel, 224–225
Slow Cooker Lamb Stew with Turnips, 225
Tender Lamb Roast, 225
Tunisian Lamb Ragout, 224
Wild Mushroom Lamb Shanks, 224
Lasagna
Beef Taco Lasagna, 180
Eggplant Lasagna, 87
Faux Lasagna Soup, 208
Keto Lasagna with Deli Meat
"Noodles," 161–162
Mixed-Vegetable Lasagna, 98
Zucchini Lasagna, 95–96, 179–180
Latkes with Sour Cream, 252–253
Lavender Ice Cream, 294
Leeks

Creamy Leek Soup, 57
Pork Chops Smothered in Caramelized
Onions & Leeks, 153
Rainbow Trout with Cream Leek
Sauce, 113
Lemongrass
Lemongrass Pork Noodle Bowls, 155
Southeast Asian Lemongrass Pork, 221
Lemons
Blueberry Smoothie with
Lemon and Ginger, 3
Chicken Thighs with Lemon Cream Sauce, 141
Coconut Lemon Fat Bombs, 259
Creamy Lemon Chicken, 215
Fish Fillets with Lemon-Dill Sauce, 196
Lemonade Snack Cake, 48
Lemon Berry Yogurt Parfait, 30
Lemon-Blueberry Ice Cream, 292
Lemon Butter Chicken, 140
Lemon-Cashew Smoothie, 2
Lemon Cheesecake Bars, 274
Lemon Chicken and Asparagus Stir-Fry, 140
Lemon Cookies, 263
Lemon Curd Layer Cake, 280–281
Lemon Curd Tartlets, 285
Lemon-Garlic Dressing, 303
Lemon-Garlic Mushrooms, 191
Lemon-Herb Baked Frittata, 18–19
Lemon–Olive Oil Breakfast Cakes, 7–8
Lemon-Poppyseed Cookies, 268
Lemon Poppy Seed Dressing, 305
Lemon Poppy Seed Muffins, 45
Lemon Pork, 203
Lemon-Rosemary Spatchcock
Chicken, 133–134
Lemon Salmon and Asparagus, 108
Lemon Smoothie, 3
Lemon Snowball Cookies, 265
Lemon-Tahini Dressing, 305
Lemon-Thyme Asparagus, 190
Lemon-Turmeric Aioli, 236–237
Lemony Chicken Salad with
Blueberries and Fennel, 72
Mixed Berry Scones with Lemon Icing, 42
Old-Fashioned Lemon-Lime Teacakes, 48
Pan-Seared Lemon-Garlic Salmon, 109–110
Prosciutto-Wrapped Asparagus
and Lemon Aioli, 80
Raspberry-Lemon Pound Cake, 280
Rosemary-Lemon Snapper
Baked in Parchment, 111
Scallops with Lemon-Butter Sauce, 197
Sheet Pan Salmon with Lemon
Green Beans, 107–108
Slow Cooker Tangy Lemon Cake
with Lemon Glaze, 230
Tempting Lemon Custard, 227
Lettuce
Avocado Caprese Lettuce Wraps, 73
Bison Burgers in Lettuce Wraps, 186
BLTA Wraps, 240
BLT Salad, 78
Breaded Chicken Strip Lettuce
Wraps, 129
Chicken Salad on Romaine Boats, 71
Chopped Chicken-Avocado
Lettuce Wraps, 129
Crab Salad Lettuce Cups, 79
Greek Meatball Lettuce Wraps, 189
Grilled Sirloin Steak, Roasted Red Pepper,
and Mozzarella Lettuce Boats, 168
Lettuce-Wrapped Chicken Burger, 144
Lobster BLT Salad, 71
Pork Larb Lettuce Wraps, 162
Roasted Cauliflower Lettuce Cups, 86
Thai Chicken Lettuce Cups, 137
Limes

Avocado-Lime Smoothie, 2–3
Avocado-Lime Soup, 57
Brown Butter–Lime Tilapia, 112
Cilantro Lime Taco Bowls, 183
Coconut Lime Macaroons, 270
Fiesta Lime Chicken Chowder, 59
Fluffy Lime-Meringue Clouds, 271
Ginger-Lime Dressing, 305
Keto-Friendly Key Lime Pie, 284
Key Lime Pie Fat Bombs, 260
Lime Almond Fat Bomb, 260
Lime-Coconut Fat Bomb, 258–259
Lime-Raspberry Custard Cake, 230
Macadamia Lime Bites, 291
Old-Fashioned Lemon-Lime
Teacakes, 48
Salmon in Lime Caper Brown
Butter Sauce, 108
Southwest Meatloaf with Lime
Guacamole, 176
Lobster
Lobster BLT Salad, 71
Seafood Chowder with Lobster, 63

M
Macadamia nuts
Chocolate–Macadamia Nut Cheesecake, 231
Macadamia-Crusted Halibut
with Mango Coulis, 104
Macadamia Lime Bites, 291
Macadamia Nut Cream Cheese Log, 241
Macadamia Nut Granola, 32
Salted Macadamia Fat Bomb, 258
Mackerel
Baked Mackerel with Kale and
Asparagus, 104–105
Mackerel Escabeche, 104
Scrambled Eggs with Mackerel, 22
Macronutrients, v
Mahi-Mahi, Turmeric Coconut, 104
Mango Coulis, Macadamia-Crusted
Halibut with, 104
Manhattan, 300–301
Maple syrup
Maple Bacon-Wrapped Brussels Sprouts, 247
Maple-Glazed Salmon with a Kick, 196
Pumpkin Pancakes with Maple Frosting, 8
Pumpkin Spice Loaf with Maple Icing, 49
Raspberry Maple Soft Serve, 292–293
Marinade, Garlic Herb, 305
Marzipan Fat Bomb, 259
Matcha powder
Avocado-Matcha Smoothie, 1
Matcha Coffee, 297
Matcha Donuts, 47
Matcha Ice Cream, 292
Matzo Ball Chicken Soup, 58
Mayonnaise. See also Aioli
Creamy Mayonnaise, 306
Radishes with Olive Mayo, 92–93
Roasted Chicken with Cilantro
Mayonnaise, 127
Teriyaki Salmon with Spicy Mayo
and Asparagus, 106
Meal planning, vii
Meatballs
Baked Cheesy Meatballs, 185
Barbecue Turkey Meatballs, 195–196
Beef Stroganoff Meatballs over Zoodles, 185
Cheese-Stuffed Italian Meatballs, 185–186
Cheesy Baked Meatballs, 250
Ginger Pork Meatballs, 164
Greek Meatball Lettuce Wraps, 189
Italian Meatballs, 185
Lamb Meatball Salad with
Yogurt Dressing, 188

Marinara Turkey Meatballs, 149
Meatballs in Creamy Almond Sauce, 184
Meatballs with Spaghetti Squash, 184–185
Mushroom No-Meatballs in
      Tomato Sauce, 213
Pork & Sausage Meatballs with
      Mushroom Ragout, 223–224
Slow Cooker Saucy Sausage-
      and-Beef Meatballs, 223
Stuffed Meatballs, 218–219
Swedish Meatballs, 184
Meatloaf
Bacon Cheeseburger Meatloaf, 198–199
Cheeseburger Meatloaf, 176
Classic Meatloaf, 175
Herbed Meatloaf, 176–177
Mediterranean Meatloaf, 220
Pressure Cooker Pork-and-
      Beef Meatloaf, 190
Southwest Meatloaf with Lime
      Guacamole, 176
Turkey Meatloaf, 149
Turkey Meatloaf Muffins, 149
Zucchini Meatloaf, 176
Meats, vi. See also specific
Keto Lasagna with Deli Meat
      "Noodles," 161–162
Meat Waffles, 11
Melons
Chicken Melon Salad, 71
Grilled Cantaloupe, 257–258
Michelada, 300
Mint. See also Peppermint
Blueberry Mint Ice Pops, 295
Blueberry Mojito, 299
Broiled Lamb Chops with Mint Gremolata
      and Pan-Fried Zucchini, 187
Chocolate-Mint Smoothie, 5
Grilled Steak Salad with
      Cucumber and Mint, 77
Mint-Marinated Artichoke Hearts, 80
Roasted Eggplant with Mint
      and Harissa, 87–88
Sautéed Zucchini with Mint and Pine Nuts, 96
Tuna and Jicama Salad with Mint
      Cucumber Dressing, 68
Virgin (or Not) Mojito, 299
Miso
Loaded Miso Soup with Tofu and Egg, 53–54
Miso Magic, 57
Nutty Miso Cauliflower Rice, 84
Moscow Mule, 299
Moussaka, 179
Muffins
Applesauce Yogurt Muffins, 43
Bacon and Spinach Egg Muffins, 192
Banana Nut Muffins, 44–45
Broccoli Bacon Egg Muffin Cups, 20
Buffalo Chicken Breakfast Muffins, 193
Cheesy Sausage & Egg Muffins, 20
Chorizo Egg Muffins, 20
Cinnamon Muffins with Cream
      Cheese Frosting, 43
"Cornbread" Muffins, 42–43
Cottage Pie Muffins, 178–179
Cream Cheese Pumpkin Muffins, 46
Dairy-Free Churro Muffins, 43
Dairy-Free Cranberry Muffins, 43–44
Egg Breakfast Muffins, 20
French Toast Egg Muffins, 20
Glazed Cranberry-Orange Muffins, 44
Glazed Dairy-Free Carrot Cake Muffins, 44
Greens and Parmesan Muffins, 45
Lemon Poppy Seed Muffins, 45
Orange Olive Oil Poppy Seed Muffins, 45
Pancake Muffins, 44
Turkey Meatloaf Muffins, 149

Zucchini Chocolate Muffins, 46
Zucchini Muffins, 45
Mushrooms
Asparagus, Mushroom & Fennel Frittata, 17
Bacon-Mushroom Chicken, 215
Beef Stroganoff, 165
Chicken Piccata with Mushrooms, 139–140
Chicken with Mushrooms,
      Port, and Cream, 137
Crab-Stuffed Portabella Mushrooms, 117
Creamed Mushroom and Fennel Soup, 53
Cream of Mushroom Soup, 53
Crispy Chicken Thighs with Radishes
      and Mushrooms, 135
Crustless Wild Mushroom–Kale Quiche, 206
Eggs Benedict on Grilled Portabella
      Mushroom Caps, 24
Fennel and Cod Chowder with
      Fried Mushrooms, 63
Garlicky Shrimp with Mushrooms, 125
Herbed Ricotta–Stuffed Mushrooms, 90
Lemon-Garlic Mushrooms, 191
Mushroom and Bacon Frittata, 17–18
Mushroom Cream Cheese Omelet, 17
Mushroom No-Meatballs in
      Tomato Sauce, 213
Mushrooms with Camembert, 90
Pork & Sausage Meatballs with
      Mushroom Ragout, 223–224
Pork Chops with Mushroom Sauce, 154
Portabella Breakfast "Burger," 27–28
Portabella Mushroom Pizza, 90
Portabella Mushroom Burger
      with Avocado, 90–91
Prosciutto and Cream Cheese
      Stuffed Mushrooms, 250
Pumpkin Seed and Swiss Chard-Stuffed
      Portabella Mushrooms, 90
Roasted Mushrooms, 89
Sausage and Spinach–Stuffed
      Mushrooms, 247–248
Slow Cooker Mushrooms, 89
Spinach, Mushroom, and Cheddar Frittata, 18
Stuffed Cremini Mushrooms, 91
Stuffed Mushrooms, 90
Stuffed Portabella Mushrooms, 91
Wild Mushroom Lamb Shanks, 224
Wild Mushroom Stroganoff, 91
Mussels
Coconut Saffron Mussels, 118
Sheet Pan Seafood Boil, 119
Spicy Italian Sausage and Mussels, 117
Steamed Mussels with Garlic and Thyme, 117
Mustard
Dijon Pork Chops, 202
Grilled Venison Loin with Dijon
      Cream Sauce, 189
Herb Mustard Lamb Racks, 187
Lemon-Dijon Boneless Chicken, 194
Mustard Cream Sauce, 308
Mustard-Crusted Cod with
      Roasted Broccoli, 101
Mustard-Herb Pork Chops, 222
Mustard Shallot Chicken Drumsticks, 142
Mustard Shallot Vinaigrette, 304
Pan-Seared Dijon-Ginger Salmon, 108
Roasted Pork Loin with Grainy
      Mustard Sauce, 158
Salmon with Tarragon-Dijon Sauce, 109
Soft-Baked Pretzels with Spicy
      Mustard Dip, 249

N

Naan, Savory, 39–40
Nachos, 126
Brisket Nachos, 173

Cheese Pork Rind Nachos, 246
Chicken-Nacho Soup, 208
Jicama Nachos, 248–249
Negroni, 300
Noodles and zoodles
Avocado Pesto Zoodles, 94
Basil Chicken Zucchini "Pasta," 133
Beef Pho, 62
Beef Stroganoff Meatballs over Zoodles, 185
Chicken Noodle Soup, 58
Keto Lasagna with Deli Meat
      "Noodles," 161–162
Konjac Noodles with Spinach Hemp
      Pesto and Goat Cheese, 98
Lemongrass Pork Noodle Bowls, 155
Mediterranean Spaghetti, 98
Pesto Zucchini Noodles, 95
Poached Cod over Brothy Veggie
      Noodles, 101–102
Pork Pho with Shirataki Noodles, 155–156
Seafood Fideo, 120
Shrimp Coconut Pad Thai, 122
Shrimp in Creamy Pesto over Zoodles, 125
Shrimp Scampi with Zucchini Noodles, 123
Smoked Salmon and Cucumber Noodles, 70
Soy-Ginger Veggie Noodle
      Steak Roll-Ups, 166
"Spaghetti" with Clams, 115
Steak with Drunken Broccoli Noodles, 164
Thai Noodle Salad, 70
Tomato and Bacon Zoodles, 203–204
Tomato Basil Chicken Zoodle Bowls, 136
Turkey Tetrazzini, 151
Vegan Pho, 58
Vegetarian Zucchini Noodle Carbonara, 95
Zoodles Bolognese, 182
Zucchini Noodles, 94
Nutmeg Pudding, Pumpkin-, 34
Nuts. See also specific
Baked Nutty Halibut, 103
Banana Nut Muffins, 44–45
Cinnamon-Nut Cottage Cheese, 31
Israeli Salad with Nuts and Seeds, 74
Nut Crackers, 234
Nut-Crusted Baked Fish, 100
Nut Medley Granola, 31
Nut-Stuffed Pork Chops, 154
Nutty Miso Cauliflower Rice, 84
Nutty "Oatmeal," 33–34
Nutty Shortbread Cookies, 266
Savory Party Mix, 236
Texas Trash, 244

O

Oils, vi. See also Olive oil
Garlic-Rosemary Infused Olive Oil, 305
Harissa Oil, 305
Old-Fashioned, 300
Olive oil
Duck Legs Braised in Olive Oil
      with Chive Cream, 216
Garlic-Rosemary Infused Olive Oil, 305
Lemon–Olive Oil Breakfast Cakes, 7–8
Olive Oil Ice Cream, 292
Orange-Olive Oil Cupcakes, 276
Orange Olive Oil Poppy Seed Muffins, 45
Tuna Slow-Cooked in Olive Oil, 114
Olives
Baked Olives and Feta, 245
Braised Greens with Olives and Walnuts, 87
Deep-Dish Cauliflower Crust
      Pizza with Olives, 212
Fennel and Orange Marinated
      Olives, 244–245
Feta and Olive Stuffed Chicken Thighs, 140

Olives (continued)
  Greek Frittata with Olives, Artichoke
      Hearts & Feta, 205
  Herb and Olive Focaccia, 40
  Olive and Artichoke Tapenade, 237
  Rack of Lamb with Kalamata Tapenade, 186
  Radishes with Olive Mayo, 92–93
  Roasted Salmon with Black Olive Salsa, 108
Omega-3 Salad, 80
Onions
  Barbecue Onion and Goat
      Cheese Flatbread, 311
  French Onion Dip, 237
  French Onion Soup, 54
  Onion Cheddar Bread, 37–38
  Onion-Garlic Pita Bread, 38
  Pan-Fried Pork Chops with
      Peppers and Onions, 154
  Pork Chops Smothered in Caramelized
      Onions & Leeks, 153
  Roasted Onions, 91
  Smoked Sausage with Cabbage & Onions, 223
  Smothered Pork Chops with Onion Gravy, 153
  Vegetarian French Onion Soup, 54
Oranges
  Coconut-Orange Cupcakes, 276
  Fennel and Orange Marinated
      Olives, 244–245
  Flank Steak with Orange-Herb
      Pistou, 166–167
  Glazed Cranberry-Orange Muffins, 44
  Mandarin Orange Chicken, 214
  Orange Cream Ice Pops, 296
  Orange-Olive Oil Cupcakes, 276
  Orange Olive Oil Poppy Seed Muffins, 45
  Spiced Orange-Pistachio Smoothie, 3
  Zesty Orange Aioli, 306
Oregano Shrimp with Tomatoes and Feta, 122
Overnight Chia Blueberry Pudding, 34

P

Pancakes
  Almond and Vanilla Pancakes, 7
  Almond Butter Pancakes, 7
  Banana Bread Blender Pancakes, 8–9
  Cherry-Coconut Pancakes, 6
  Chocolate, Chocolate Chip Pancakes, 8
  Cream Cheese Pancakes, 7
  Keto Blueberry Pancakes, 9
  Lemon–Olive Oil Breakfast Cakes, 7–8
  Pancake Muffins, 44
  Pumpkin Pancakes with Maple Frosting, 8
  Ricotta Pancakes, 8
  Spiced Cream Cheese Pancakes, 7
  Winter Squash Pancakes, 7
Pancetta
  Baked Omelet with Pancetta
      and Swiss Cheese, 17
  Pancetta-and-Brie–Stuffed Pork
      Tenderloin, 201–202
Pantry clean out, vi
Paprika
  Chicken Paprikash, 127–128
  Hungarian Chicken, 215
  Paprika Chicken with Broccoli, 128
Parsley
  Chimichurri, 304
  Chimichurri Sauce, 307
  Chimichurri Shrimp, 122
  Cod with Parsley Pistou, 101
  Mediterranean Cauliflower Tabbouleh, 85
  Raw Tabouli, 85
  Roasted Cauliflower with Parsley
      and Pine Nuts, 84
  Short Ribs with Chimichurri, 199
Pasta Sauce, 309

Pastry Cream, 310
Peaches, Grilled Sweet, 258
Peanut butter
  Chocolate-Dipped Peanut
      Butter Ice Pops, 295
  Chocolate, Peanut Butter, and
      Banana Shake, 4–5
  Chocolate Peanut Butter Cups, 257
  Chocolate Peanut Butter Fat Bombs, 259
  Chocolate–Peanut Butter Fudge, 226
  Delectable Peanut Butter Cup Cake, 229
  Easy Peasy Peanut Butter Cookies, 268
  Fluffy Peanut Butter Pie, 284–285
  Indonesian Peanut Sauce, 309
  Nutty Chocolate Protein Shake, 4
  PB&J Overnight Hemp, 31
  Peanut Butter Cake Bars, 273
  Peanut Butter Cheesecake, 228
  Peanut Butter–Chocolate Chip
      Cookies, 262–263
  Peanut Butter Cookie Dough Fat Bombs, 259
  Peanut Butter Cookies, 265
  Peanut Butter Cup Protein Smoothie, 4
  Peanut Butter Shake, 4
  Peanut Butter Smoothie, 4
  Peanut Butter Whipped Greek Yogurt, 30
  Peanut-Chicken Soup, 59–60
  Salted Peanut Butter Cookies, 267
  Thai Chicken Skewers with Peanut Sauce, 252
  Thai-Inspired Peanut Roasted Cauliflower, 84
  Thai-Style Peanut Sauce, 307
Pea Soup, Spring, 56–57
Pecans
  Bourbon Pecan Pie Bars, 274
  Butter Pecan Cheesecake
      Truffle Fat Bombs, 261
  Cauliflower-Pecan Casserole, 85
  Chicken Brunch Pie with Cheddar
      Pecan Crust, 28–29
  Chocolate Chip–Pecan Biscotti, 204
  Chocolate-Drizzled Pecan Shortbread, 270
  Cinnamon "Apple" Pecan Coffee Cake, 47–48
  Cinnamon-Glazed Pecans, 256
  Cinnamon Pecan "Apple" Crisp, 286–287
  Pecan Chicken Salad, 71
  Pecan Chocolate Chip Cookies, 268–269
  Pecan-Crusted Catfish, 100
  Pecan-Crusted Salmon, 109
  Pecan Pie Bars, 274
  Pecan Pie Pudding, 288
  Pecan Sandies, 266
  Pecan Squares, 204
  Pralines, 256
  Sirloin Steak Salad with Goat
      Cheese and Pecans, 77–78
  Slow Cooker Pumpkin-Pecan N'Oatmeal, 33
  Spicy Barbecue Pecans, 244
  Sweet and Spicy Pecans, 192
Pepitas
  Curried Tuna Salad with Pepitas, 72
  Pumpkin Seed and Swiss Chard-Stuffed
      Portabella Mushrooms, 90
Pepper-Crusted Salmon with Wilted Kale, 107
Peppermint
  Chocolate Peppermint Fudge, 256
  Double Chocolate Peppermint
      Cookies, 263–264
  Mint Chocolate Fat Bombs, 258
Pepperoni
  Garlic Pepperoni Chips, 235–236
  Pepperoni Supreme Pizza, 253–254
  Pizza Pull-Apart Bread, 38
Peppers. See also Bell peppers;
      Chiles; Jalapeño peppers
  Goat Cheese Stuffed Roasted
      Peppers, 91–92

Ground Bison Chile Rellenos with
      Ranchero Sauce, 186
  Pimento Cheese, 238
  Spicy Serrano Gazpacho, 55
Pesto, 306
  Avocado Pesto Zoodles, 94
  Herb-Kale Pesto, 306
  Herb Pesto, 309
  Konjac Noodles with Spinach Hemp
      Pesto and Goat Cheese, 98
  Leg of Lamb with Sun-dried
      Tomato Pest, 187–188
  Pesto Cauliflower Sheet-Pan "Pizza," 253
  Pesto Flounder with Bok Choy, 102
  Pesto Roast Beef, 217
  Pesto Sauce, 309
  Pesto Sautéed Vegetables, 99
  Pesto Zucchini Noodles, 95
  Salmon with Spinach Hemp Pesto, 108
  Shrimp in Creamy Pesto over Zoodles, 125
  Spice-Rubbed Roasted Pork with
      Cilantro Pesto, 157–158
  Spinach Hemp Pesto, 306
Pico de Gallo, 308
Pies, savory. See also Quiches
  Chicken Brunch Pie with Cheddar
      Pecan Crust, 28–29
  Chicken Pot Pie, 130
  Chicken Tamale Pie, 148
  Cottage Pie, 178
  Crustless Greek Cheese Pie, 29
  Southern-Style Shepherd's Pie, 177–178
Pies, sweet
  Apple Pie Bites, 283–284
  "Buttermilk" Custard Pie Bars, 284
  Chocolate Mousse Pie Cups, 285
  Coconut Pie Crust, 312
  Fluffy Peanut Butter Pie, 284–285
  Fresh Berry Tart, 285
  Jicama "Apple" Pie Filling, 283
  Keto-Friendly Key Lime Pie, 284
  Lemon Curd Tartlets, 285
  Pumpkin Pie, 285–286, 286
  Strawberry Cream Pie, 283
Pigs in a Blanket, 248
Pimento Cheese, 238
Pine nuts
  Roasted Cauliflower with Parsley
      and Pine Nuts, 84
  Sautéed Zucchini with Mint and Pine Nuts, 96
Pistachios
  Citrus Asparagus with Pistachios, 81
  Pistachio Cookies, 267
  Pistachio Pomegranate Salad, 65
  Pistachio-Raspberry Chocolate Bark, 275
  Spiced Orange-Pistachio Smoothie, 3
Pizza. See also Flatbreads
  Bacon and Egg Pizza, 254
  Breakfast Pizza, 27
  Cauliflower Pizza, 86
  Cheesy-Crust Pizza, 310
  Deep-Dish Cauliflower Crust
      Pizza with Olives, 212
  Goat Cheese and Basil Pizza, 253
  Margarita Pizza Chips, 235
  Margherita Pizza, 310–311
  Meat Crust Pizza, 254
  Meatza, 182–183
  Pepperoni Supreme Pizza, 253–254
  Pesto Cauliflower Sheet-Pan "Pizza," 253
  Pizza Pull-Apart Bread, 38
  Pizza Sauce, 309
  Portabella Mushroom Pizza, 90
  Zucchini Mini Pizzas, 96
  Zucchini Pizza Boats, 96–97
Pomegranate Salad, Pistachio, 65
Poppy seeds

Lemon-Poppyseed Cookies, 268
Lemon Poppy Seed Dressing, 305
Lemon Poppy Seed Muffins, 45
Orange Olive Oil Poppy Seed Muffins, 45
Poppy Seed Pound Cake, 280
Pork. See also Bacon; Ham; Pancetta;
    Prosciutto; Sausage
  Asian Pork Spare Ribs, 202–203
  Bacon-Wrapped Pork Loin, 203
  Bacon-Wrapped Pork Tenderloin, 157
  Baked Cheesy Meatballs, 185
  Balsamic-Thyme Pork Tenderloin, 156
  BBQ Baby Back Ribs, 158
  Breaded Pork Chops, 152–153
  Breaded Pork Chops with Creamy
      Mashed Cauliflower, 153
  Brussels Sprout Ground Pork Hash, 163
  Carnitas, 202
  Cheese-Stuffed Pork Chops, 155
  Classic Bolognese Sauce, 308
  Cottage Pie Muffins, 178–179
  Country Pork and "Rice" Soup, 62
  Cracked Pepper Fried Pork Chops, 153–154
  Cranberry Pork Roast, 202
  Crispy Bourbon Pork Belly, 159
  Dijon Pork Chops, 202
  Dry Rub Ribs, 158
  Egg Roll in a Bowl, 163
  Ginger Pork Meatballs, 164
  Glazed Pork Tenderloin, 156
  Ham-Stuffed Pork Chops, 154
  Herb-Braised Pork Chops, 201
  Italian Wedding Soup, 61–62
  Jerk Pork Tenderloin, 157
  Lemongrass Pork Noodle Bowls, 155
  Lemon Pork, 203
  Meatballs in Creamy Almond
      Sauce, 184
  Meatballs with Spaghetti
      Squash, 184–185
  Mediterranean Meatloaf, 220
  Mustard-Herb Pork Chops, 222
  Nut-Stuffed Pork Chops, 154
  Oven-Baked Country-Style Pork Ribs, 158
  Pancetta-and-Brie–Stuffed Pork
      Tenderloin, 201–202
  Pan-Fried Pork Chops with
      Peppers and Onions, 154
  Parmesan-Breaded Boneless Pork Chops, 201
  Pork & Sausage Meatballs with
      Mushroom Ragout, 223–224
  Pork Belly with Brussels Sprouts
      & Turnips, 223
  Pork Chile Verde, 221
  Pork Chops Smothered in Caramelized
      Onions & Leeks, 153
  Pork Chops with Mushroom Sauce, 154
  Pork Fried Rice, 155
  Pork Kebabs, 200
  Pork Larb Lettuce Wraps, 162
  Pork Loin with Creamy Gravy, 221
  Pork Loin with Ginger Cream Sauce, 221–222
  Pork Medallions with Blue Cheese Sauce, 156
  Pork Pho with Shirataki Noodles, 155–156
  Pork Pumpkin Ragout, 155
  Pork Ribs, 158
  Pork Spring Rolls, 164
  Pork Taco Bowls, 203
  Pork with Sesame Slaw, 162
  Pressure Cooker Pork-and-
      Beef Meatloaf, 190
  Roasted Pork Belly and Asparagus, 159
  Roasted Pork Loin with Grainy
      Mustard Sauce, 158
  Rosemary Balsamic Pork Medallions, 156
  Slow Cooker Pork Carnitas, 222

  Slow Cooker Pork Chops with Creamy
      Bacon-and-Artichoke Sauce, 221
  Slow Cooker Pulled Pork, 201
  Slow Cooker Pulled Pork with
      Cabbage Slaw, 222
  Slow Cooker Ranch Favorite Texas-
      Style Pulled Pork, 223
  Smoky Pork Tenderloin, 203
  Smothered Pork Chops with Onion Gravy, 153
  Southeast Asian Lemongrass Pork, 221
  Spaghetti Squash & Ground Pork
      Stir-Fry with Kale, 163
  Spiced Pork Chops, 153
  Spice-Rubbed Roasted Pork with
      Cilantro Pesto, 157–158
  Spicy Pork and Eggplant Stir-Fry, 163
  Sriracha Pork Belly, 159
  Stuffed Pork Loin with Sun-Dried
      Tomatoes and Goat Cheese, 157
  Swedish Meatballs, 184
  Sweet-and-Sour Pork Chops, 201
Pork Rind Nachos, Cheese, 246
Pretzels with Spicy Mustard
    Dip, Soft-Baked, 249
Prosciutto
  Blackberry, Prosciutto, and Goat
      Cheese Flatbread, 40
  Prosciutto and Cream Cheese
      Stuffed Mushrooms, 250
  Prosciutto Egg Cups, 19
  Prosciutto-Wrapped Asparagus
      and Lemon Aioli, 80
  Prosciutto-Wrapped Mozzarella, 241
Proteins, v
Puddings and custards
  Almond Butter and Jelly Chia Pudding, 289
  Banana Pudding, 289
  Bread Pudding, 288–289
  Buttercream Pudding "Fluff," 293
  Carrot-Pumpkin Pudding, 92
  Chocolate & Coconut
      Pudding, 227–228
  Chocolate Avocado Pudding, 289–290
  Chocolate-Chia Pudding, 290
  Creamy Cinnamon Breakfast Pudding, 31
  Mexican Chocolate Pudding, 289, 293
  Overnight Chia Pudding, 34
  Overnight Chocolate Chia Pudding, 31
  Pecan Pie Pudding, 288
  Pumpkin-Ginger Pudding, 227
  Pumpkin-Nutmeg Pudding, 225
  Pumpkin Spice Pudding, 227
  Rice Pudding, 289
  Snickerdoodle Pudding, 290
  Spicy Chai Custard, 227
  Tempting Lemon Custard, 227
  Vanilla Pudding, 227
  Whipped Cream-Chocolate
      Pudding Parfaits, 290
Pumpkin
  Berry-Pumpkin Compote, 228
  Carrot-Pumpkin Pudding, 92
  Cream Cheese Pumpkin Muffins, 46
  Herbed Pumpkin, 92
  Nut-Free Pumpkin Bread, 50
  Pork Pumpkin Ragout, 155
  Pumpkin Cheesecake Brownies, 271–272
  Pumpkin Cookies, 267
  Pumpkin-Ginger Pudding, 227
  Pumpkin-Nutmeg Pudding, 34
  Pumpkin Pancakes with Maple Frosting, 8
  Pumpkin Pie, 285–286, 286
  Pumpkin-Pie Breakfast Bars, 192–193
  Pumpkin Pie Smoothie, 6
  Pumpkin Pie Yogurt Bowl, 31
  Pumpkin Pound Cake, 279–280
  Pumpkin-Ricotta Cheesecake, 278

  Pumpkin Spice Fat Bombs, 259
  Pumpkin Spice Loaf with Maple Icing, 49
  Pumpkin Spice Pudding, 227
  Slow Cooker Grain-Free Pumpkin Loaf, 207
  Slow Cooker Pumpkin-Pecan N'Oatmeal, 33
  Spiced-Pumpkin Chicken Soup, 207
  Spiced Pumpkin Soup, 52
  Turkey-Pumpkin Ragout, 216
  Ultra-Soft Pumpkin Chocolate Bars, 275
  Vegan Pumpkin Curry, 212

Q

Quiches
  Bacon Broccoli Crustless Quiche Cups, 26
  Broccoli and Cheese Quiche Cups, 20
  Broccoli Quiche, 25
  Crustless Cream Cheese and
      Spinach Quiche, 26
  Crustless Quiche Lorraine, 24–25
  Crustless Sausage and Green
      Chile Quiche, 25
  Crustless Wild Mushroom–Kale Quiche, 206
  Ham and Cheese Crustless Quiche, 25
  Tuscan "Quiche" Bites, 25–26

R

Radishes
  Cast-Iron Blackened Rib Eye with
      Parmesan Roasted Radishes, 169
  Chicken Tenderloin Packets with Broccoli,
      Radishes, and Parmesan, 135
  Classic Diner Hash Browns, 29
  Creamy Dill and Radish "Potato" Salad, 68–69
  Crispy Chicken Thighs with Radishes
      and Mushrooms, 135
  Parmesan-Rosemary Radishes, 190–191
  Pot Roast with Turnips and Radishes, 172
  Radishes with Olive Mayo, 92–93
  Red Radish "Potato" Salad, 68
  Sole with Cucumber Radish Salsa, 111–112
Ranch Dressing, 304
  Bacon Ranch Cheesy Chicken Breasts, 133
  Buttermilk Ranch Dressing, 303
  Ground Beef Taco Salad with
      Peppers and Ranch, 78
  Ranch Broccoli Slaw, 76
  Ranch Wedge Salad with
      Coconut "Bacon," 64–65
  Spicy Jalapeño Chips and Ranch, 247
  Turkey Bacon Ranch Casserole, 151
Ranch Seasoning, 303
Raspberries
  Coconut-Raspberry Cake, 229
  Lime-Raspberry Custard Cake, 230
  No-Bake Chocolate Raspberry
      Cheesecake, 277–278
  Pistachio-Raspberry Chocolate Bark, 275
  Raspberry Cheesecake Squares, 273
  Raspberry Cream Cheese Tart Bars, 286
  Raspberry Ice Cream, 294
  Raspberry-Lemon Pound Cake, 280
  Raspberry Maple Soft Serve, 292–293
  Raspberry Mimosa, 300
  Raspberry Scones, 41–42
Ratatouille, 94
Redfish with Spicy Crawfish Cream
    Sauce, Blackened, 104
Rhubarb
  Strawberry Rhubarb Cobbler, 287–288
  Strawberry Rhubarb Scones, 42
Rice Pudding, 289
Ricotta cheese
  Creamy Stuffed Peppers, 92
  Eggplant Lasagna, 87
  Herbed Ricotta–Stuffed Mushrooms, 90

Ricotta cheese (*continued*)
    Pumpkin-Ricotta Cheesecake, 278
    Ricotta Pancakes, 8
    Zucchini Lasagna, 95–96, 179–180
Rolls
    Cheesy Garlic Rolls, 36
    Cinnamon Rolls, 51
Rosemary
    Garlic-Rosemary Infused Olive Oil, 305
    Lemon-Rosemary Spatchcock
        Chicken, 133–134
    Parmesan-Rosemary Radishes, 190–191
    Rosemary Balsamic Pork Medallions, 156
    Rosemary Flatbread, 39
    Rosemary-Garlic Lamb Racks, 187
    Rosemary Lamb Chops, 225
    Rosemary-Lemon Snapper
        Baked in Parchment, 111
    Rosemary Roasted Almonds, 244
    Rosemary Roasted Beef Tenderloin, 170–171
Rum
    Blueberry Mojito, 299
    Butter Rum Pound Cake, 279
    Hot Buttered Rum, 299
    Virgin (or Not) Mojito, 299

S

Saffron Mussels, Coconut, 118
Salads
    Apple Cabbage Cumin Coleslaw, 75
    Asian Shrimp Salad, 79
    Avocado and Asparagus Salad, 66
    Avocado Egg Salad, 69
    Bacon and Berry Harvest Salad, 65–66
    BLT Salad, 78
    Broccoli Salad with Bacon, 73–74
    Buffalo Chicken Salad, 70–71
    Chef Salad, 76
    Chicken, Avocado, and Egg Salad, 69
    Chicken Caesar Salad, 77
    Chicken Melon Salad, 71
    Chicken Salad on Romaine Boats, 71
    Chopped Salad, 76
    Citrus Arugula Salad, 64
    Classic Chicken Salad, 70
    Classic Club Salad, 66
    Classic Steak Salad, 77
    Classic Tuna Salad, 71
    Cool and Creamy Cucumber
        Tomato Salad, 70
    Crab Salad Lettuce Cups, 79
    Creamy Broccoli Salad, 74
    Creamy Dill and Radish "Potato" Salad, 68–69
    Creamy Riced Cauliflower Salad, 75
    Crisp and Creamy Southern Coleslaw, 75
    Cucumber and Tomato Feta Salad, 74
    Cucumber, Tomato, and Avocado
        Salad, 74
    Curried Chicken Salad, 130
    Curried Egg Salad, 69
    Curried Tuna Salad with Pepitas, 72
    Deluxe Sub Salad, 78
    Deviled Egg Salad with Bacon, 69–70
    Essential Cobb Salad with
        Crumbled Bacon, 77
    Everyday Caesar Salad, 67
    Goat Cheese Caprese Salad, 75
    Greek Cottage Cheese Salad, 70
    Greek Salad with Shrimp, 79
    Grilled Chicken Cobb Salad, 76–77
    Grilled Shrimp with Avocado Salad, 123
    Grilled Steak Salad with
        Cucumber and Mint, 77
    Ground Beef Taco Salad, 183

    Ground Beef Taco Salad with
        Peppers and Ranch, 78
    Guacamole Salad, 73
    Hemp Cobb Salad, 66
    Israeli Salad with Nuts and Seeds, 74
    Italian Garden Salad, 66
    Italian Green Bean Salad, 73
    Japanese Hibachi House Salad, 64
    Kale, Avocado & Tahini Salad, 64
    Killer Kale Salad, 66–67
    Lamb Meatball Salad with
        Yogurt Dressing, 188
    Lemony Chicken Salad with
        Blueberries and Fennel, 72
    Lobster BLT Salad, 71
    Mayo-Less Tuna Salad, 72
    Mediterranean Cauliflower Tabbouleh, 85
    Mediterranean Salad, 66
    Moroccan Cauliflower Salad, 74
    Omega-3 Salad, 80
    Pecan Chicken Salad, 71
    Pistachio Pomegranate Salad, 65
    Powerhouse Arugula Salad, 68
    Quick Fiesta Taco Salad, 78
    Ranch Broccoli Slaw, 76
    Ranch Wedge Salad with
        Coconut "Bacon," 64–65
    Raw Tabouli, 85
    Red Radish "Potato" Salad, 68
    Roasted Cauliflower Lettuce Cups, 86
    Roasted Chicken, Artichoke, and
        Hearts of Palm Salad, 76
    Sausage and Cauliflower Salad, 75
    Sesame Ginger Slaw, 75
    Shaved Brussels Sprouts Salad
        with Avocado Dressing, 67
    Shrimp & Avocado Salad, 79
    Shrimp Caesar Salad, 197
    Shrimp Ceviche Salad, 80
    Simple Egg Salad, 69
    Sirloin Steak Salad with Goat
        Cheese and Pecans, 77–78
    Smoked Salmon and Cucumber Noodles, 70
    Smoked Trout Salad, 79
    Spinach Avocado Salad, 64
    Spinach Salad with Bacon and
        Soft-Boiled Eggs, 78–79
    Spinach Salad with Warm Bacon Dressing, 65
    Strawberry Spinach Salad, 65
    Thai Chicken Lettuce Cups, 137
    Thai Noodle Salad, 70
    Traditional Greek Salad, 67
    Tuna and Jicama Salad with Mint
        Cucumber Dressing, 68
    Tuna Niçoise Salad, 68
    Turkey and Kale Coleslaw, 76
    Turmeric and Avocado Egg Salad, 69
    Tuscan Kale Salad with Anchovies, 67
    Vegan Niçoise Salad, 64
    Walnut-Fennel Salad with
        Sherry Vinaigrette, 67
    Weeknight Greek Salad, 67–68
    Zesty Chicken Tender Salad, 76
Salmon
    Avocado and Smoked Salmon Stack
        with Caper Sauce, 240
    Bagels with Smoked Salmon, 27
    Chaffle and Lox, 10
    Charred Alaskan Salmon with
        Garlic Green Beans, 106
    Coconut Ginger Salmon Burgers, 110–111
    Curried Salmon Fish Cakes, 110
    Garlic Parmesan Crusted Salmon, 105
    Glazed Salmon, 108–109
    Grilled Salmon Foil Packets, 109
    Lemon Salmon and Asparagus, 108

    Maple-Glazed Salmon with a Kick, 196
    Moroccan Salmon with Cauliflower
        Rice Pilaf, 107
    Pan-Seared Dijon-Ginger Salmon, 108
    Pan-Seared Lemon-Garlic Salmon, 109–110
    Pecan-Crusted Salmon, 109
    Pepper-Crusted Salmon with Wilted Kale, 107
    Roasted Herb-Crusted Salmon with
        Asparagus and Tomatoes, 110
    Roasted Salmon with Black Olive Salsa, 108
    Salmon and Egg Scramble, 22
    Salmon Cakes, 110
    Salmon Cakes with Avocado, 111
    Salmon Gratin, 109
    Salmon in Cream Sauce, 105
    Salmon in Lime Caper Brown
        Butter Sauce, 108
    Salmon Oscar, 110
    Salmon Poke, 106
    Salmon Salad Sushi Bites, 240
    Salmon with Spinach Hemp Pesto, 108
    Salmon with Tarragon-Dijon Sauce, 109
    Seafood Coconut Stew, 119
    Sesame Salmon, 105–106
    Sheet Pan Salmon with Lemon
        Green Beans, 107–108
    Smoked Salmon and Cucumber Bites, 239
    Smoked Salmon and Cucumber Noodles, 70
    Smoked Salmon and Goat Cheese
        Pinwheels, 240–241
    Smoked Salmon Avocado Sushi Roll, 107
    Smoked Salmon Fat Bombs, 233
    Sweet and Spicy Salmon, 198
    Teriyaki Salmon with Spicy Mayo
        and Asparagus, 106
Salsa
    Chorizo, Chicken, and Salsa Verde, 141
    Pico de Gallo, 308
    Roasted Salmon with Black Olive Salsa, 108
    Sole with Cucumber Radish Salsa, 111–112
Sandwiches and wraps
    Avocado Caprese Lettuce Wraps, 73
    Avocado Toast, 14
    BBQ Chicken Wraps, 129
    BLTA Wraps, 240
    Breaded Chicken Strip Lettuce Wraps, 129
    Chicken and Cheese Quesadillas, 145
    Chicken Quesadillas, 145
    Chopped Chicken-Avocado
        Lettuce Wraps, 129
    Dilled Tuna Salad Sandwich, 241
    Florentine Breakfast Sandwich, 14
    Greek Meatball Lettuce Wraps, 189
    Pork Larb Lettuce Wraps, 162
    Pressure Cooker Sloppy Joes, 190
    Sweet 'n' Savory Toast with
        Burrata and Berries, 12
    Tuna Salad Wrap, 241
Sangria, 300
    Sangria Granita, 295
Sauces
    Alfredo Sauce, 307–308
    Barbecue Sauce, 307
    Bleu Cheese Sauce, 307
    Chimichurri, 304
    Chimichurri Sauce, 307
    Cinnamon-Caramel Sauce, 310
    Classic Bolognese Sauce, 308
    Enchilada Sauce, 308
    Garlicky Alfredo Sauce, 307
    Herbed Marinara Sauce, 309
    Herb-Kale Pesto, 306
    Herb Pesto, 309
    Hollandaise, 306
    Hot Crab Sauce, 308
    Indonesian Peanut Sauce, 309

Mustard Cream Sauce, 308
Pasta Sauce, 309
Pesto, 306
Pesto Sauce, 309
Pizza Sauce, 309
Spinach Hemp Pesto, 306
Teriyaki Sauce, 308–309
Thai-Style Peanut Sauce, 307
Sauerkraut
Sausage-Sauerkraut Soup, 207
Simple Reuben Casserole, 177
Sausage
Baked Sausage and Shrimp with Turnips
and Green Peppers, 162–163
Beef-Sausage Stew, 62
Biscuits and Sausage Gravy, 28
Biscuits with Sausage Gravy, 34–35
Breakfast Burrito Bowl, 29
Breakfast Pizza, 27
Breakfast Sausage, 26
Brown Sugar Bacon Smokies, 250
Cabbage Sausage Hash Browns, 23
Cheesy Sausage & Egg Muffins, 20
Cheesy Sausage and Cabbage Hash, 28
Cheesy Triple Meat Baked "Spaghetti," 179
Chorizo Bagels, 37
Chorizo, Chicken, and Salsa Verde, 141
Chorizo Egg Muffins, 21
Cold Front Kielbasa and Cabbage Skillet, 161
Cream Cheese Sausage Balls, 200–201
Creole Sausage and Rice, 162
Crustless Sausage and Green
Chile Quiche, 25
Homemade Sausage Soup, 209
Hot Dog Rolls, 251
Jambalaya Soup, 209–210
Keto Lasagna with Deli Meat
"Noodles," 161–162
Meat Crust Pizza, 254
Mezze Cake, 148
Pigs in a Blanket, 248
Pizza Pull-Apart Bread, 38
Pork & Sausage Meatballs with
Mushroom Ragout, 223–224
Rich Sausage and Spaghetti
Squash Casserole, 162
Sausage and Cauliflower Salad, 75
Sausage and Cheese Frittata, 19
Sausage and Spinach–Stuffed
Mushrooms, 247–248
Sausage Egg Roll in a Bowl, 27
Sausage-Sauerkraut Soup, 207
Sausage-Stuffed Peppers, 200, 206
Sausage Verde Casserole, 26
Sausage, Zucchini, and Green
Bean Packets, 162
Savory Sausage Balls, 27
Scotch Eggs, 13
Sheet Pan Seafood Boil, 119
Shrimp and Sausage Jambalaya, 123
Simple Lamb Sausage, 188
Slow Cooker Breakfast Sausage, 204–205
Slow Cooker Saucy Sausage-
and-Beef Meatballs, 223
Smoked Sausage with Cabbage & Onions, 223
Smoky Sausage Patties, 193
Spicy Italian Sausage and Mussels, 117
Spicy Sausage and Cabbage
Casserole, 160–161
Zuppa Toscana (Sausage and Kale Soup), 62
Scallion Steamed Fish, Ginger, 105
Scallops
Bacon-Wrapped Scallops and
Broccolini, 118–119
Pan-Fried Scallops, 118
Pan-Seared Butter Scallops, 118
Salt-and-Pepper Scallops and Calamari, 119

Scallops with Lemon-Butter Sauce, 197
Sea Scallops with Bacon Cream
Sauce, 118
Sea Scallops with Curry Sauce, 118
Scones
Bacon Cheddar Chive Scones, 41
Chocolate Chip Scones, 42
Mixed Berry Scones with Lemon Icing, 42
Raspberry Scones, 41–42
Strawberry Rhubarb Scones, 42
Scotch Eggs, 13
Sea Bass, Whole Roasted, 105
Seafood. See Fish and seafood; specific
Seasonings
Italian Seasoning, 303
Ranch Seasoning, 303
Taco Seasoning, 303
Seeds. See also specific
Anti-Inflammatory Power Bites, 242
Israeli Salad with Nuts and Seeds, 74
Savory Party Mix, 236
Seedy Crackers, 234
Sesame
Pork with Sesame Slaw, 162
Sesame Broiled Chicken Thighs, 140–141
Sesame Burger Buns, 36
Sesame-Crusted Tuna with Sweet
Chili Vinaigrette, 114
Sesame Ginger Slaw, 75
Sesame-Roasted Broccoli, 82
Sesame Salmon, 105–106
Shakes. See also Smoothies
Buttered Coffee Shake, 6
Chocolate, Peanut Butter, and
Banana Shake, 4–5
Chocolate Protein Shake, 5
Creamy Snickerdoodle Shake, 4
Double Chocolate Shake, 5
"Frosty" Chocolate Shake, 291
Maddie's Favorite Chocolate Malt, 288
Nutty Chocolate Protein Shake, 4
Peanut Butter Shake, 4
Strawberries and Cream Shake, 5
Vanilla Shake, 5
Shallots
Mustard Shallot Chicken Drumsticks, 142
Mustard Shallot Vinaigrette, 304
Shellfish. See Fish and seafood; specific
Sherry Vinaigrette, Walnut-
Fennel Salad with, 67
Shrimp
Asian Shrimp Salad, 79
Bacon-Wrapped Shrimp, 121
Baked Sausage and Shrimp with Turnips
and Green Peppers, 162–163
Bang Bang Shrimp, 124
Basil Butter Grilled Shrimp, 122–123
Cajun Shrimp and Cauliflower Rice, 122
Cheesy Shrimp Spread, 239–240
Chimichurri Shrimp, 122
Coconut Shrimp, 125, 198
Creamy Seafood Stew with
Cauliflower Rice, 63
Creamy Shrimp and Grits Casserole, 119–120
Garlic and Herb Baked Shrimp
with Cauliflower Rice, 125
Garlicky Shrimp with Mushrooms, 125
Garlic Shrimp, 198
Greek Salad with Shrimp, 79
Grilled Shrimp with Avocado Salad, 123
Jambalaya Soup, 209–210
Oregano Shrimp with Tomatoes and Feta, 122
Popcorn Shrimp, 121
Roasted Shrimp and Veggies, 122
Seafood Ceviche, 120
Seafood Chowder with Lobster, 63
Seafood Coconut Stew, 119

Seafood Fideo, 120
Sheet Pan Seafood Boil, 119
Sheet-Pan Shrimp, 121
Shrimp & Avocado Salad, 79
Shrimp and "Grits," 120–121
Shrimp and Sausage Jambalaya, 123
Shrimp and Vegetable Kebabs with
Chipotle Sour Cream Sauce, 124
Shrimp, Bamboo Shoot, and
Broccoli Stir-Fry, 124–125
Shrimp Caesar Salad, 197
Shrimp Ceviche Salad, 80
Shrimp Coconut Pad Thai, 122
Shrimp Fried Rice, 124
Shrimp in Creamy Pesto over Zoodles, 125
Shrimp Scampi with Zucchini Noodles, 123
Shrimp Veracruz, 121
Shrimp with Creamy Tomato-
and-Spinach Sauce, 123
Vietnamese Shrimp Cakes, 123–124
Skewers. See Kebabs and skewers
Smoothies. See also Shakes
Almond Butter and Cacao Nib Smoothie, 5
Almond Kale Smoothie, 2
Avocado Blueberry Smoothie, 4
Avocado Coconut Smoothie, 6
Avocado-Lime Smoothie, 2–3
Avocado-Matcha Smoothie, 1
Berry Cheesecake Smoothie, 6
Berry Green Smoothie, 1
Blueberry Smoothie with
Lemon and Ginger, 3
Cauliflower Smoothie, 2
Cheesecake Smoothie, 5–6
Chocolate-Mint Smoothie, 5
Coconut Berry Smoothie, 4
Coffee Smoothie, 6
Creamy Cinnamon Smoothie, 4
Creamy Kale Smoothie, 1
Cucumber Green Smoothie, 1–2
Go Get 'Em Green Smoothie Bowl, 30–31
Green Coconut Avocado Smoothie, 2
Green Goddess Smoothie, 2
Green Herb Smoothie, 1
Green Tea Smoothie, 2
Kale Refresher Smoothie, 1
Lemon-Cashew Smoothie, 2
Lemon Smoothie, 3
Mean Green Smoothie, 2
Peanut Butter Cup Protein Smoothie, 4
Peanut Butter Smoothie, 4
Pumpkin Pie Smoothie, 6
Spiced Orange-Pistachio Smoothie, 3
Spinach-Blueberry Smoothie, 3
Spirulina Smoothie, 1
Strawberry Spinach Smoothie, 3
Triple Berry Smoothie, 3
Tropical Smoothie, 3
Vanilla Bean Smoothie, 5
Snapper
Rosemary-Lemon Snapper
Baked in Parchment, 111
Snapper Veracruz, 111
Sole
Sole Meunière, 112
Sole with Cucumber Radish Salsa, 111–112
Soups, stews, and chilis
Avocado Gazpacho, 56
Avocado-Lime Soup, 57
Beef Bourguignon Stew, 171
Beef Pho, 62
Beef-Sausage Stew, 62
Beef Stew, 171, 210
Beef Taco Stew, 171
Broccoli Cheddar Soup, 52
Butternut Squash Soup with
Turmeric and Ginger, 56

Soups, stews, and chilis (continued)
  Cauliflower-Cheddar Soup, 51–52
  Cheddar Cheese Soup, 207
  Cheeseburger Soup, 209
  Cheesy Bacon-Cauliflower Soup, 208
  Chicken and Baby Corn Chowder, 61
  Chicken-Bacon Soup, 208
  Chicken Chowder with Bacon, 209
  Chicken Marsala Soup, 59
  Chicken-Nacho Soup, 208
  Chicken Noodle Soup, 58
  Chicken Ramen Soup, 60
  Chicken Taco Soup with Cauliflower Rice, 61
  Chicken Thigh Chili with Avocado, 136
  Chicken Tortilla Soup, 59
  Chili con Carne, 181
  Chili Fish Stew, 99–100
  Chilled Avocado-Cilantro Soup, 55
  Chipotle Chicken Chili, 211
  Classic Beef Chili, 181
  Cold Cucumber and Avocado Soup, 56
  Country Pork and "Rice" Soup, 62
  Creamed Cauliflower Soup, 51
  Creamed Mushroom and Fennel Soup, 53
  Cream of Mushroom Soup, 53
  Creamy Asparagus Soup, 51
  Creamy Broccoli, Bacon, and Cheese Soup, 52
  Creamy Chicken Stew, 210
  Creamy Leek Soup, 57
  Creamy Seafood Stew with
      Cauliflower Rice, 63
  Creamy Tomato Soup, 54
  Curried Vegetable Stew, 210
  Easy Chicken Soup, 58
  Easy Herbed Tomato Bisque, 54
  Egg Drop Soup, 55
  Faux Lasagna Soup, 208
  Fennel and Cod Chowder with
      Fried Mushrooms, 63
  Five-Alarm Beef Chili, 181
  French Onion Soup, 54
  Greek Chicken and "Rice" Soup
      with Artichokes, 60
  Hearty Cauliflower Soup, 54–55
  Hearty Lamb Cabbage Soup, 62–63
  Homemade Sausage Soup, 209
  Italian Wedding Soup, 61–62
  Jalapeño-Chicken Soup, 60
  Jambalaya Soup, 209–210
  Lamb Chili, 188
  Loaded Baked "Fauxtato" Soup, 56
  Loaded Miso Soup with Tofu and Egg, 53–54
  Matzo Ball Chicken Soup, 58
  Miso Magic, 57
  Mulligatawny Soup with Cauliflower Rice, 209
  New England Clam Chowder, 64
  North African Vegetable Stew, 98
  Peanut-Chicken Soup, 59–60
  Pork Pho with Shirataki Noodles, 155–156
  Roasted Red Pepper Soup with
      Basil and Goat Cheese, 52
  Sausage-Sauerkraut Soup, 207
  Savory Lamb Stew, 188–189
  Seafood Chowder with Lobster, 63
  Seafood Coconut Stew, 119
  Simple Chicken-Vegetable Soup, 210
  Simple Texas Chili, 211
  Slow Cooker Lamb Stew with Turnips, 225
  Slow Keto Chili, 211
  Southwest-Style Chicken Soup, 60–61
  Spiced-Pumpkin Chicken Soup, 207
  Spiced Pumpkin Soup, 52
  Spicy Creamy Chicken Soup, 60
  Spicy Serrano Gazpacho, 55
  Spring Pea Soup, 56–57
  Texas-Style Beef Chili, 181
  Tomato Basil Soup, 53

  Tom Kha Gai, 59
  Turkey-Potpie Soup, 208
  Turkey-Vegetable Stew, 210–211
  Turnip and Thyme Soup, 54
  Tuscan Kale Soup, 57
  Vegan Italian Wedding Soup, 57–58
  Vegan Pho, 58
  Vegetarian French Onion Soup, 54
  Vegetarian Mole Chili, 211–212
  Watercress-Spinach Soup, 53
  Weeknight Texas Turkey Chili, 152
  White Chicken Chili, 213
  White Chili, 144
  Zuppa Toscana (Sausage and Kale Soup), 62
Sour cream
  Beef Goulash, 218
  Crab Cakes with Cilantro Crema, 115
  Grilled Hanger Steak with
      Cilantro Crema, 167–168
  Latkes with Sour Cream, 252–253
  Pressure Cooker Pot Roast with
      Sour-Cream Gravy, 190
  Shrimp and Vegetable Kebabs with
      Chipotle Sour Cream Sauce, 124
  Slow Cooker Sour-Cream Cheesecake, 228
  Smothered Sour Cream Chicken Thighs, 145
  Sour Cream Corn Bread, 41
  Sour Cream Ice Cream, 294–295
Soy-Ginger Veggie Noodle Steak Roll-Ups, 166
Spaghetti squash
  Cheesy Triple Meat Baked "Spaghetti," 179
  Creamy Spaghetti Squash Bake, 94
  Fakeachini Alfredo, 94
  Meatballs with Spaghetti Squash, 184–185
  Mediterranean Spaghetti, 98
  Potluck Chicken Spaghetti
      Squash Casserole, 146
  Rich Sausage and Spaghetti
      Squash Casserole, 162
  Simple Spaghetti Squash, 211
  Spaghetti Squash & Ground Pork
      Stir-Fry with Kale, 163
  Spaghetti Squash Chaffles, 9
  Spaghetti Squash Chicken Bowls, 136
  Twice-Baked Spaghetti Squash, 93
Spinach
  Bacon and Spinach Egg Muffins, 192
  Cheesy Beef and Spinach Casserole, 177
  Cheesy Spinach Bake, 93
  Creamed Spinach, 93
  Creamed Spinach with Eggs, 14–15
  Creamy Chicken and Spinach Bake, 132
  Crustless Cream Cheese and
      Spinach Quiche, 26
  Crustless Spanakopita, 97–98
  Cucumber Green Smoothie, 1–2
  Go Get 'Em Green Smoothie Bowl, 30–31
  Green Coconut Avocado Smoothie, 2
  Green Goddess Buddha Bowl, 84
  Green Goddess Smoothie, 2
  Konjac Noodles with Spinach Hemp
      Pesto and Goat Cheese, 98
  Mean Green Smoothie, 2
  Mediterranean Frittata, 18
  Parmesan-Crusted Tilapia with
      Sautéed Spinach, 112
  Salmon with Spinach Hemp Pesto, 108
  Sausage and Spinach–Stuffed
      Mushrooms, 247–248
  Shrimp with Creamy Tomato-
      and-Spinach Sauce, 123
  Skillet-Baked Eggs with Yogurt
      and Spinach, 15
  Slow Cooker Spanakopita Frittata, 205–206
  Spanakopita Omelet, 16–17
  Spinach and Bacon Stuffed
      Chicken Thighs, 139

  Spinach-Artichoke Dip, 238
  Spinach Avocado Salad, 64
  Spinach-Blueberry Smoothie, 3
  Spinach Hemp Pesto, 306
  Spinach, Mushroom, and Cheddar Frittata, 18
  Spinach Salad with Bacon and
      Soft-Boiled Eggs, 78–79
  Spinach Salad with Warm Bacon Dressing, 65
  Spinach Soufflé, 93
  Squash Boats Filled with Spinach-
      Artichoke Gratin, 213
  Strawberry Spinach Salad, 65
  Strawberry Spinach Smoothie, 3
  Turkey Florentine Bake, 151
  Turkey Spinach Roll-Ups, 240
  Tuscan "Quiche" Bites, 25–26
  Vegan Italian Wedding Soup, 57–58
  Watercress-Spinach Soup, 53
Spirulina Smoothie, 1
Squash. See also Spaghetti squash; Zucchini
  Butternut Squash Soup with
      Turmeric and Ginger, 56
  Calabacitas Con Pollo, 146
  Cinnamon Pecan "Apple" Crisp, 286–287
  Golden Rosti, 93
  Sautéed Summer Squash, 93–94
  Spiced-Up Sunday Pot Roast and
      Sautéed Squash, 172
  Squash Boats Filled with Spinach-
      Artichoke Gratin, 213
  Summer Squash Mock Apple
      Crumble, 282–283
  Winter Squash Pancakes, 7
Squid
  Greek Stuffed Squid, 125–126
  Salt-and-Pepper Scallops and Calamari, 119
Sriracha
  Sriracha Artichoke Bites, 247
  Sriracha Pork Belly, 159
  Sriracha Wings, 252
Stir-fries
  Asian Cabbage Stir-Fry, 83–84
  Beef and Broccoli Stir-Fry, 164
  Broccoli Stir-Fry, 82
  Green Vegetable Stir-Fry with Tofu, 99
  Kale and Cashew Stir-Fry, 89
  Lemon Chicken and Asparagus Stir-Fry, 140
  Shrimp, Bamboo Shoot, and
      Broccoli Stir-Fry, 124–125
  Spaghetti Squash & Ground Pork
      Stir-Fry with Kale, 163
  Spicy Pork and Eggplant Stir-Fry, 163
Stocks. See Broths and stocks
Strawberries
  Chocolate-Covered Strawberries, 258
  Roasted Strawberries with
      Whipped Cream, 258
  Strawberries and Cream Ice Pops, 294
  Strawberries and Cream Shake, 5
  Strawberry Avocado Ice Cream, 294
  Strawberry Butter, 301–302
  Strawberry Cheesecake, 277
  Strawberry Cheesecake Fat Bombs, 262
  Strawberry Cream Pie, 283
  Strawberry Frozen Yogurt, 295
  Strawberry Panna Cotta, 291
  Strawberry Rhubarb Cobbler, 287–288
  Strawberry Rhubarb Scones, 42
  Strawberry Shortcakes, 281–282
  Strawberry Spinach Salad, 65
  Strawberry Spinach Smoothie, 3
Sunflower Bread, Nut-Free, 50–51
Sushi, 106–107
Swiss chard
  Mean Green Smoothie, 2
  Pumpkin Seed and Swiss Chard-Stuffed
      Portabella Mushrooms, 90

Roasted Trout with Swiss Chard, 113–114
Sautéed Swiss Chard, 87
Swordfish
    Marinated Swordfish Skewers, 197
    Swordfish in Tarragon-Citrus Butter, 112

T

Tacos
    Beef Taco Lasagna, 180
    Beef Tacos, 183–184
    Beef Taco Stew, 171
    Beef Taquitos, 251
    Cheesy Chicken Taquitos, 251–252
    Cheesy Taco Shells, 312
    Chicken Taco Soup with Cauliflower Rice, 61
    Cilantro Lime Taco Bowls, 183
    Fish Tacos, 101
    Ground Beef Taco Salad, 183
    Ground Beef Taco Salad with Peppers and Ranch, 78
    Pork Taco Bowls, 203
    Taco Layer Dip, 239
    Texas Taco Hash, 183
Tahini
    Kale, Avocado & Tahini Salad, 64
    Lemon-Tahini Dressing, 305
    Roasted Brussels Sprouts with Tahini-Yogurt Sauce, 242
Tarragon
    Creamy Grapefruit-Tarragon Dressing, 304
    Salmon with Tarragon-Dijon Sauce, 109
    Swordfish in Tarragon-Citrus Butter, 112
Tartar Sauce, Crab Cakes with Spicy, 115
Tarts. See Pies, sweet
Tea. See also Matcha powder
    Chai Tea Cookies, 262
    Earl Grey Rose Latte, 297
    Fat Chai, 297–298
    Green Tea Latte, 297
    Green Tea Smoothie, 2
    Spicy Chai Custard, 226, 227
Tequila
    Lime Margarita, 299
    Spicy Margarita, 299
    Tequila Sunrise, 300
Thyme
    Balsamic-Thyme Pork Tenderloin, 156
    Garlic Studded Prime Rib with Thyme au Jus, 170
    Lemon-Thyme Asparagus, 190
    Rib Eye Steaks with Garlic-Thyme Butter, 169
    Steamed Mussels with Garlic and Thyme, 117
    Thyme Turkey Legs, 216
    Turkey Thyme Burgers, 150
    Turnip and Thyme Soup, 54
Tilapia
    Brown Butter–Lime Tilapia, 112
    Garlic Herb Marinated Tilapia, 113
    Pan-Fried Tilapia, 112–113
    Parmesan Baked Tilapia, 113
    Parmesan-Crusted Tilapia with Sautéed Spinach, 112
Tofu
    Green Vegetable Stir-Fry with Tofu, 99
    Loaded Miso Soup with Tofu and Egg, 53–54
    Thai Green Curry with Tofu and Vegetables, 212
    Tofu and Veggie Scramble, 22
    Tofu Fries, 248
    Tofu Green Bean Casserole, 88
    Tuscan "Quiche" Bites, 25–26
    Vegetarian Mole Chili, 211–212
Tomatoes
    Avocado Caprese Lettuce Wraps, 73
    Balsamic Chicken with Asparagus and Tomatoes, 134

BLTA Wraps, 240
BLT Salad, 78
Caprese Balsamic Chicken, 132
Caprese Skewers, 241
Caprese Stuffed Avocados, 72
Caprese-Stuffed Chicken Breasts, 132
Classic Bolognese Sauce, 308
Cool and Creamy Cucumber Tomato Salad, 70
Creamy Tomato Soup, 54
Cucumber and Tomato Feta Salad, 74
Cucumber, Tomato, and Avocado Salad, 74
Easy Herbed Tomato Bisque, 54
Goat Cheese Caprese Salad, 75
Greek-Style Egg and Tomato Scramble, 22–23
Halibut in Tomato Basil Sauce, 103
Herbed Marinara Sauce, 309
Leg of Lamb with Sun-dried Tomato Pest, 187–188
Lobster BLT Salad, 71
Margarita Pizza Chips, 235
Mushroom No-Meatballs in Tomato Sauce, 213
Oregano Shrimp with Tomatoes and Feta, 122
Pasta Sauce, 309
Pico de Gallo, 308
Pizza Sauce, 309
Roasted Herb-Crusted Salmon with Asparagus and Tomatoes, 110
Shakshuka, 29
Shrimp with Creamy Tomato-and-Spinach Sauce, 123
Slow Cooker Beef-Stuffed Cabbage in Creamy Tomato Sauce, 220
Stuffed Pork Loin with Sun-Dried Tomatoes and Goat Cheese, 157
Sun-Dried Tomato and Feta Fat Bombs, 233
Tomato and Bacon Zoodles, 203–204
Tomato Basil Chicken Zoodle Bowls, 136
Tomato Basil Soup, 53
Tomato-Braised Beef, 217
Tom Kha Gai, 59
Tortillas
    Cauliflower Tortillas, 311
    Flax Meal Tortillas, 40
Trout
    Cream-Poached Trout, 113
    Rainbow Trout with Cream Leek Sauce, 113
    Roasted Trout with Swiss Chard, 113–114
    Smoked Trout Salad, 79
Tuna
    Classic Tuna Salad, 71
    Curried Tuna Salad with Pepitas, 72
    Dilled Tuna Salad Sandwich, 241
    Grandma Bev's Ahi Poke, 114
    Italian Tuna Salad, 72
    Mayo-Less Tuna Salad, 72
    Seared Tuna with Steamed Turnips, Broccoli, and Green Beans, 114
    Sesame-Crusted Tuna with Sweet Chili Vinaigrette, 114
    Tuna and Jicama Salad with Mint Cucumber Dressing, 68
    Tuna Casserole, 114–115
    Tuna Niçoise Salad, 68
    Tuna Salad Wrap, 241
    Tuna Slow-Cooked in Olive Oil, 114
    Tuna-Stuffed Avocado, 72–73
Turkey
    Avocado Turkey "Toast," 150
    Bacon-Wrapped Cajun Turkey Tenderloins with Roasted Brussels Sprouts, 152
    Barbecue Turkey Meatballs, 195–196
    Herb-Infused Turkey Breast, 215–216
    Marinara Turkey Meatballs, 149
    Party Deli Pinwheels, 240

Roast Turkey, 149
Spice-Rubbed Turkey Breast, 195
Thyme Turkey Legs, 216
Turkey and Cauliflower Rice–Stuffed Peppers, 149
Turkey and Kale Coleslaw, 76
Turkey Bacon Ranch Casserole, 151
Turkey Burgers, 150
Turkey Egg Roll in a Bowl, 150–151
Turkey Egg Scramble, 22
Turkey Enchilada Skillet, 150
Turkey Florentine Bake, 151
Turkey Meatloaf, 149
Turkey Meatloaf Muffins, 149
Turkey Pilaf, 151
Turkey-Potpie Soup, 208
Turkey-Pumpkin Ragout, 216
Turkey Rissoles, 149–150
Turkey Spinach Roll-Ups, 240
Turkey-Stuffed Avocados, 73
Turkey Tetrazzini, 151
Turkey Thyme Burgers, 150
Turkey-Vegetable Stew, 210–211
Unstuffed Bell Pepper Skillet, 152
Weeknight Texas Turkey Chili, 152
Turmeric
    Butternut Squash Soup with Turmeric and Ginger, 56
    Lemon-Turmeric Aioli, 236–237
    Turmeric and Avocado Egg Salad, 69
    Turmeric Cauliflower "Pickles," 241–242
    Turmeric Coconut Mahi-Mahi, 104
Turnips
    Baked Sausage and Shrimp with Turnips and Green Peppers, 162–163
    Duck with Turnips in Cream, 216–217
    Loaded Baked "Fauxtato" Soup, 56
    Pork Belly with Brussels Sprouts & Turnips, 223
    Pot Roast with Turnips and Radishes, 172
    Seared Tuna with Steamed Turnips, Broccoli, and Green Beans, 114
    Slow Cooker Lamb Stew with Turnips, 225
    Turnip and Thyme Soup, 54
Tzatziki
    Coconut Tzatziki, 236
    Greek Beef Kebabs with Tzatziki, 199
    Tzatziki Dip with Vegetables, 236

V

Vanilla
    Air-Fried Vanilla and Chocolate Layer Cake, 204
    Almond and Vanilla Pancakes, 7
    French Vanilla Ice Cream with Hot Fudge, 293
    Rich Vanilla Ice Cream, 292
    Vanilla-Almond Ice Pops, 295–296
    Vanilla Bean Smoothie, 5
    Vanilla Belgian Waffles, 10
    Vanilla Cheesecake, 231
    Vanilla Panna Cotta, 291
    Vanilla Pudding, 227
    Vanilla Shake, 5
Vegetables, vi. See also specific
    Cayenne Pepper Vegetable Bake, 97
    Chicken Vegetable Hash, 126
    Country Garden Scramble, 23
    Creamed Vegetables, 97
    Curried Vegetable Stew, 210
    Green Vegetable Stir-Fry with Tofu, 99
    Herbed Vegetable Broth, 302–303
    Italian Vegetable Egg Bake, 15
    Marinated Antipasto Veggies, 242
    Mexican Zucchini Hash, 97
    Mixed-Vegetable Lasagna, 98
    Moroccan Chicken and Vegetable Tagine, 134

Vegetables (continued)
Moroccan Vegetable Tagine, 98–99
North African Vegetable Stew, 98
Pesto Sautéed Vegetables, 99
Poached Cod over Brothy Veggie
Noodles, 101–102
Ratatouille, 94
Roasted Shrimp and Veggies, 122
Roasted Vegetable Hash, 23
Shrimp and Vegetable Kebabs with
Chipotle Sour Cream Sauce, 124
Simple Chicken-Vegetable Soup, 210
Slow Cooker All-in-One Lamb-
Vegetable Dinner, 224
Soy-Ginger Veggie Noodle
Steak Roll-Ups, 166
Summer Vegetable Mélange, 99
Tandoori Vegetable Chicken Skewers, 138
Thai Green Curry with Tofu
and Vegetables, 212
Tofu and Veggie Scramble, 22
Turkey-Vegetable Stew, 210–211
Tzatziki Dip with Vegetables, 236
Vegetable Omelet, 206
Vegetable Vindaloo, 99
Veggie Frittata, 192
Venison
Grilled Venison Loin with Dijon
Cream Sauce, 189
Venison Pot Roast, 189
Vodka
Bloody Mary, 298
Chocolate Martini, 298–299
Gelatin Shooters, 301
Moscow Mule, 299
Vesper martini, 300

W
Waffles. See also Chaffles
Belgian-Style Waffles, 9–10
Chicken & Waffles, 147
Coconut Flaxseed Waffles, 10–11
Coconut Flour–Based Chocolate
Chip Waffles, 10
Ham and Swiss Waffles, 11
Meat Waffles, 11
Quick and Easy Blueberry Waffles, 11–12
Vanilla Belgian Waffles, 10
Very Berry Waffles, 11
Waffles with Whipped Cream, 10
Walnuts

Braised Greens with Olives and Walnuts, 87
Chocolate Walnut Fudge, 226
Sautéed Asparagus with Walnuts, 81
Walnut-Fennel Salad with
Sherry Vinaigrette, 67
Watercress-Spinach Soup, 53
Whipped cream
Chocolate Cake with Whipped Cream, 232
Roasted Strawberries with
Whipped Cream, 258
Slow Cooker Moist Ginger Cake
with Whipped Cream, 231
Strawberry Shortcakes, 281–282
Waffles with Whipped Cream, 10
Whipped Cream-Chocolate
Pudding Parfaits, 290
Wine
Chicken Breast Tenders with Riesling
Cream Sauce, 129–130
Chicken with Mushrooms,
Port, and Cream, 137
Frosé Slushie, 300
Raspberry Mimosa, 300
Roasted Chicken Thighs and Zucchini
with Wine Reduction, 141
Sangria, 300
Sangria Granita, 295
Vesper martini, 300
Wraps. See Sandwiches and wraps

Y
Yogurt
Applesauce Yogurt Muffins, 43
Coconut Yogurt Berry Parfait, 30
Cookies and Cream Parfait, 290
Dips Herby Yogurt Dip, 236
Greek Yogurt Parfait, 30
Harissa Chicken and Brussels Sprouts
with Yogurt Sauce, 139
Lamb Kofte with Yogurt Sauce, 189
Lamb Meatball Salad with
Yogurt Dressing, 188
Lemon Berry Yogurt Parfait, 30
Mashed Cauliflower with Yogurt, 85
Peanut Butter Whipped Greek Yogurt, 30
Pumpkin Pie Yogurt Bowl, 31
Roasted Brussels Sprouts with
Tahini-Yogurt Sauce, 242
Simple Cheesy Yogurt, 30
Skillet-Baked Eggs with Yogurt
and Spinach, 15

Strawberry Frozen Yogurt, 295
Yogurt Parfait with Chia Seeds, 30

Z
Zucchini
Avocado Pesto Zoodles, 94
Basil Chicken Zucchini "Pasta," 133
Beef Stroganoff Meatballs over Zoodles, 185
Broiled Lamb Chops with Mint Gremolata
and Pan-Fried Zucchini, 187
Chicken Noodle Soup, 58
Classic Zucchini Bread, 37
Greek Stewed Zucchini, 95
Mediterranean Spiralized Zucchini, 95
Mexican Zucchini Hash, 97
Parmesan Zucchini Chips, 235
Pesto Zucchini Noodles, 95
Roasted Chicken Thighs and Zucchini
with Wine Reduction, 141
Sausage, Zucchini, and Green
Bean Packets, 162
Sautéed Crispy Zucchini, 95
Sautéed Zucchini with Mint and Pine Nuts, 96
Seafood Fideo, 120
Sheet Pan Sirloin Steak with
Eggplant and Zucchini, 168
Shrimp Coconut Pad Thai, 122
Shrimp in Creamy Pesto over Zoodles, 125
Shrimp Scampi with Zucchini
Noodles, 123
Slow Cooker Grain-Free Zucchini
Bread, 206–207
Slow Cooker Zucchini-Carrot Bread, 37
Smoky Zucchini Chips, 191
"Spaghetti" with Clams, 115
Stuffed Zucchini, 96
Tomato and Bacon Zoodles, 203–204
Tomato Basil Chicken Zoodle Bowls, 136
Turkey Tetrazzini, 151
Vegetarian Zucchini Noodle
Carbonara, 95
Zoodles Bolognese, 182
Zucchini Chocolate Muffins, 46
Zucchini Fritters, 96
Zucchini Hummus, 237
Zucchini Lasagna, 95–96, 179–180
Zucchini Meatloaf, 176
Zucchini Mini Pizzas, 96
Zucchini Muffins, 45
Zucchini Noodles, 94
Zucchini Pizza Boats, 96–97

CPSIA information can be obtained
at www.ICGtesting.com
Printed in the USA
JSHW041127091221
21120JS00006B/15

9 781638 787938